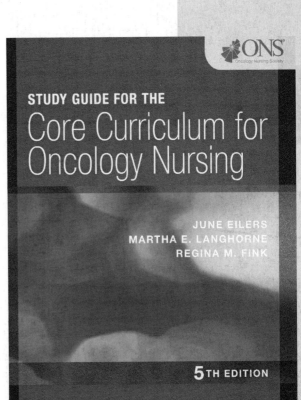
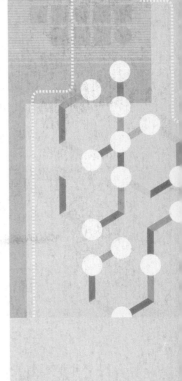

Core Curriculum for Oncology Nursing

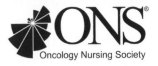
Oncology Nursing Society

Core Curriculum for Oncology Nursing

Editor:

Joanne K. Itano, RN, PhD, APRN
Associate Professor of Nursing and
Associate Vice President of Academic Affairs
University of Hawaii
Honolulu, Hawaii

Section Editors:

Jeannine M. Brant, PhD, APRN, AOCN®, FAAN
Oncology Clinical Nurse Specialist/Nurse Scientist
Billings Clinic
Billings, Montana;
Assistant Affiliate Professor
Montana State University
Bozeman, Montana

Francisco A. Conde, PhD, AOCNS®, FAAN
Advanced Practice Registered Nurse
Queens Medical Center—Oncology
Honolulu, Hawaii

Marlon G. Saria, MSN, RN, AOCNS®
Clinical Nurse Specialist
Moores Cancer Center
University of California San Diego
La Jolla, California

5TH EDITION

ELSEVIER

ELSEVIER

3251 Riverport Lane
St. Louis, Missouri 63043

CORE CURRICULUM FOR ONCOLOGY NURSING, FIFTH EDITION   ISBN: 978-1-4557-7626-9

Notices

Knowledge and best practice in this field are constantly changing. As new research and experience broaden our understanding, changes in research methods, professional practices, or medical treatment may become necessary.

Practitioners and researchers must always rely on their own experience and knowledge in evaluating and using any information, methods, compounds, or experiments described herein. In using such information or methods they should be mindful of their own safety and the safety of others, including parties for whom they have a professional responsibility.

With respect to any drug or pharmaceutical products identified, readers are advised to check the most current information provided (i) on procedures featured or (ii) by the manufacturer of each product to be administered, to verify the recommended dose or formula, the method and duration of administration, and contraindications. It is the responsibility of practitioners, relying on their own experience and knowledge of their patients, to make diagnoses, to determine dosages and the best treatment for each individual patient, and to take all appropriate safety precautions.

To the fullest extent of the law, neither the Publisher nor the authors, contributors, or editors, assume any liability for any injury and/or damage to persons or property as a matter of products liability, negligence or otherwise, or from any use or operation of any methods, products, instructions, or ideas contained in the material herein.

Previous editions copyrighted 2005, 1998, 1992, 1987 by Oncology Nursing Society.

Library of Congress Cataloging-in-Publication Data
Core curriculum for oncology nursing. – Fifth edition / volume editor, Joanne Itano ; section editors, Jeannine M. Brant, Francisco A. Conde, Marlon Garzo Saria.
   p. ; cm.
 Includes bibliographical references and index.
 ISBN 978-1-4557-7626-9 (pbk. : alk. paper)
 I. Itano, Joanne, editor. II. Brant, Jeannine M., editor. III. Conde, Francisco A., editor. IV. Saria, Marlon Garzo, editor
 [DNLM: 1. Oncology Nursing–Outlines. WY 18.2]
 RC266
 616.99'40231–dc23

                                                                    2014038270

Executive Content Strategist: Lee Henderson
Traditional Content Development Manager: Billie Sharp
Associate Content Development Specialist: Courtney Daniels
Publishing Services Manager: Pat Joiner
Project Manager: Lisa A. P. Bushey
Senior Designer: Margaret Reid

Printed in the United States of America.

Last digit is the print number: 9 8 7 6 5 4 3 2 1

Kristine Deano Abueg, RN, MSN, OCN®, CBCN
Oncology Clinical Trials Research Nurse
Kaiser Permanente, Oncology Clinical Trials
Kaiser Permanente–Roseville
Roseville, California

Roberta Bourgon, ND
Naturopathic Physician
Integrative Medicine and Hematology/Oncology
Billings Clinic
Billings, Montana

Jeannine M. Brant, PhD, APRN, AOCN®, FAAN
Oncology Clinical Nurse Specialist/Nurse Scientist
Billings Clinic
Billings, Montana;
Assistant Affiliate Professor
Montana State University
Bozeman, Montana

Christa Braun-Inglis, MS, APRN-Rx, FNP-BC, AOCNP®
Nurse Practitioner
Oncology
Kaiser Permanente
Honolulu, Hawaii

Kathleen A. Calzone, PhD, RN, APNG, FAAN
Senior Nurse Specialist, Research
National Cancer Institute
Center for Cancer Research, Genetics Branch
National Institutes of Health
Bethesda, Maryland

Dawn Camp-Sorrell, MSN, FNP, AOCN®
Oncology Nurse Practitioner
Nursing, Children's of Alabama
Birmingham, Alabama

Ellen Carr, RN, MSN, AOCN®
Nurse Case Manager
Head and Neck Oncology
Moores UCSD Cancer Center
La Jolla, California

Darlena D. Chadwick, MSN, MBA, RN
Chief Operating Officer
Hawaii Cancer Consortium
University of Hawaii Cancer Center;
Vice President of Patient Care
Oncology/Neuroscience/Endoscopy/Professional Services/
    Pathology
The Queen's Medical Center
Honolulu, Hawaii

Lani Kai Clinton, MD, PhD
Resident Physician
Pathology
John A. Burns School of Medicine
Honolulu, Hawaii

Francisco A. Conde, PhD, AOCNS®, FAAN
Advanced Practice Registered Nurse
Queens Medical Center–Oncology
Honolulu, Hawaii

Diane G. Cope, PhD, ARNP, BC, AOCNP®
Oncology Nurse Practitioner
Florida Cancer Specialists and Research Institute
Fort Myers, Florida

Stacie Corcoran, RN, MS, AOCNS®
Nurse Leader
Survivorship Program
Memorial Sloan-Kettering Cancer Center
New York, New York

Gail Wych Davidson, RN, MS, OCN®
Regional Liver Cancer Therapy Disease Management
    Coordinator
Surgical Oncology
The Arthur G. James Cancer Hospital and Richard J. Solove
    Research Institute
Columbus, Ohio

Lisa Dyk, RN, BSN, OCN®
Inpatient Cancer Care
Billings Clinic
Billings, Montana

Denice Economou, RN, MN, AOCN®
Assistant Clinical Professor
School of Nursing–UCLA
Los Angeles, California;
Senior Research Assistant/Project Director
Nursing Research and Education–City of Hope
Duarte, California

Julie Eggert, PhD, GNP-BC, AOCN®
Professional and Healthcare Genetics Doctoral Program
    Coordinator
School of Nursing, Health, Education and Human Development
Clemson University
Clemson, South Carolina;
Advanced Practice Nurse
Cancer Risk Screening Program
Upstate Oncology Associates
Bon Secours St. Francis Hospital
Greenville, South Carolina

Marie Flannery, RN, PhD, AOCN®
Assistant Professor
School of Nursing and Wilmot Cancer Center
University of Rochester
Rochester, New York

Nanette C. Fong, RN, MSN, ONP
Neuro-Oncology Nurse Practitioner
Neuro-Oncology–UCLA
Los Angeles, California

Elizabeth A. Freitas, RN, MS, OCN®, ACHPN
Adjunct Clinical Faculty
School of Nursing and Dental Hygiene
University of Hawaii at Manoa;
Clinical Nurse Specialist
Pain and Palliative Care
The Queen's Medical Center
Honolulu, Hawaii

Jacqueline J. Glover, PhD
Professor
Department of Pediatrics and the Center for Bioethics and
    Humanities
University of Colorado Anschutz Medical Campus
Aurora, Colorado

Carrie Graham, RN, MSN, ARNP
Nurse Practitioner/Teaching Associate
Department of Neurology/Division of Neuro-Oncology
University of Washington
Seattle, Washington

Stacey Danielle Green, MSN, GNP-BC, AOCNP®
Lecturer, Assistant Clinical Professor
Advanced Practice–Acute Care
Adult/Gerontology
UCLA School of Nursing;
Nurse Practitioner
Neuro-Oncology–UCLA
Los Angeles, California

Debra E. Heidrich, MSN, RN, ACHPN, AOCN®
Palliative Care Nursing Consultant
West Chester, Ohio

Dawn Hew, BSN, RN, OCN®
Registered Nurse
The Queen's Medical Center
Honolulu, Hawaii

Lori Johnson, RN, MSN, OCN®
Clinical Nurse Educator
Nursing Education, Development, and Research
UC San Diego Health System
San Diego, California

Brenda Keith, RN, MN, AOCNS®
Senior Oncology Clinical Coordinator II
BioOncology
Genentech
South San Francisco, California

HaNa Kim, PhD
Clinical Health Psychology Fellow
Behavioral Health
Tripler Army Medical Center
Honolulu, Hawaii

Angela D. Klimaszewski, MSN, RN
Technical Content Editor
Publications
Oncology Nursing Society
Pittsburgh, Pennsylvania

Sandra Kurtin, RN, MS, AOCN®, ANP
Clinical Assistant Professor of Medicine and Nursing
Hematology/Oncology
The University of Arizona Cancer Center
Tuscon, Arizona

Sally L. Maliski, PhD, RN, FAAN
Associate Dean for Academic and Student Affairs
Associate Professor
School of Nursing and David Geffen School of Medicine
Department of Urology–UCLA
Los Angeles, California

Kristen W. Maloney, MSN, RN, AOCNS®
Clinical Nurse Specialist
Oncology Nursing
The Hospital of the University of Pennsylvania
Philadelphia, Pennsylvania

Leslie V. Matthews, RN, MS, ANP, AOCNP®
Nurse Practitioner
Medical Oncology
Memorial Sloan–Kettering Cancer Center
New York, New York

Candis Morrison, PhD, CRNP
Nurse Practitioner
Division of Hematology
Johns Hopkins Bayview Medical Center
Baltimore, Maryland

Kathleen Murphy-Ende, RN, PhD, PsyD, AOCNP®
Medical Psychologist and Nurse Practitioner
Palliative-Supportive Care
Meriter Hospital
Madison, Wisconsin

Leslie Nelson, RN, MSN, AOCNS®
Nurse Manager
Phoenix Office/Ironwood
Cancer and Research Centers
Phoenix, Arizona

Paula Nelson-Marten, PhD, RN, AOCN®
Associate Professor
College of Nursing
University of Colorado
Anschutz Medical Campus
Aurora, Colorado

Patricia W. Nishimoto, BSN, MPH, DNS
Adult Oncology Clinical Nurse Specialist
Department of Medicine, Hematology/Oncology
Tripler Army Medical Center
Honolulu, Hawaii

Judy Petersen, RN, MN, AOCN®
Oncology Nurse Educator
National Cancer Institute's Cancer Information
    Service
Fred Hutchinson Cancer Research Center
Seattle, Washington

Jan Petree, RN, MS, FNP, AOCN®
Nurse Practitioner
Medical Breast Oncology, Survivorship Clinic
Women's Cancer Center
Stanford Hospital and Clinics
Stanford, California

Julie Ponto, PhD, RN, ACNS-BC, AOCNS®
Professor
Graduate Programs in Nursing
Winona State University–Rochester
Rochester, Minnesota

Krista M. Rubin, MS, FNP-BC
Nurse Practitioner
Center for Melanoma
Massachusetts General Hospital
Boston, Massachusetts

Michelle Lynne Russell, RN-C, BSN, OCN®
Clinical Nurse Case Manager
Department of Radiation Medicine and Applied
    Sciences
Rebecca and John Moores Comprehensive Cancer
    Center
University of California–San Diego
La Jolla, California

Kristi V. Schmidt, RN, MN
Clinical Oncology Specialist
Cenentech
South San Francisco, California

Terry Wilke Shapiro, RN, MSN, CRNP
Nurse Practitioner
Stem Cell Transplant Program
Division of Pediatric Hematology Oncology
Penn State University/Penn State Children's Hospital
Hershey, Pennsylvania

Brenda K. Shelton, MS, RN, CCRN, AOCN®
Associate Faculty
Acute and Chronic Adult Health
Johns Hopkins University School of Nursing;
Clinical Nurse Specialist
Oncology, Johns Hopkins Hospital
Baltimore, Maryland;
Nurse Surveyor
Joint Commission International
Oakbrook, Illinois

Mady C. Stovall, RN, MSN, ANP-BC
Neuro-Oncology Nurse Practitioner
Department of Neurosurgery
Kaiser Permanente–Northern California
Redwood City, California

Cathleen Sugarman, RN, MSN, AOCNS®
Advanced Practice Nurse
Oncology Clinical Care Line
Scripps Memorial Hospital–La Jolla
La Jolla, California

Geline Joy Tamayo, MSN, ACNS-BC, OCN®
Advanced Practice Program Director
Moores Cancer Center
UC San Diego Health System
La Jolla, California

Susan Vogt Temple, RN, MSN, AOCN®
Oncology Nurse Educator
Boehringer-Ingelheim Oncology
Boehringer-Ingelheim Pharmaceuticals, Inc.
Danbury, Connecticut

Jennifer Alisangco Tschanz, RN, MSN, FNP, AOCNP®
Nurse Practitioner
Department of Hematology Oncology
Naval Medical Center San Diego
San Diego, California

Gabriele Brunhart Tsung, RN, MSN, ANP-BC
Nurse Practitioner
Neurology–UCLA
Los Angeles, California

Kenneth Utz, PharmD, BCOP
Adjunct Clinical Professor
Skaggs School of Pharmacy
University of Montana
Missoula, Montana;
Lead Clinical Pharmacist
Pharmacy at the Billings Clinic
Billings, Montana

Carol Viele, RN, MS, OCN®
Associate Clinical Professor
Department of Physiology Nursing
University of California–San Francisco
San Francisco, California

Wendy H. Vogel, MSN, FNP, AOCNP®
Oncology Nurse Practitioner
Wellmont Cancer Institute
Kingsport, Tennessee

Kathryn Renee Waitman, DNP, FNP-C, AOCNP®
Nurse Practitioner
Oncology
Billings Clinic
Billings, Montana

Deborah Kirk Walker, DNP, CRNP, AOCN®
Assistant Professor
School of Nursing–University of Alabama at Birmingham;
Nurse Practitioner
Hematology/Oncology
Comprehensive Cancer Center at the Kirklin Clinic
University of Alabama at Birmingham
Birmingham, Alabama

Amy Walton, RN, BSN, OCN®, CMSRN
Oncology Nurse
Inpatient Cancer Care
Billings Clinic
Billings, Montana

Tracy Webb Warren, RN, BSN, OCN®
Infusion Charge Nurse, Clinical Nurse–Outpatient
The Woodlands Regional Care Center
University of Texas MD Anderson Cancer Center
Houston, Texas

Rita Wickham, PhD, RN, AOCN®
Adjunct Faculty
Adult Health Nursing
Rush College of Nursing
Chicago, Illinois;
Consultant
RSW Consulting LLC
Rapid River, Michigan

Reviewers

Karen J. Abbas, MS, RN, AOCN®
Oncology Clinical Nurse Specialist
University of Rochester Medical Center
Rochester, New York

Paula J. Anastasia, RN, MN, AOCN®
Gyn-Oncology Clinical Nurse Specialist
Cedars-Sinai Medical Center
Los Angeles, California

Tara Baney, CRNP, HS, ANP-BC, AOCN®
Nurse Practitioner
Cancer Care Partnership
Penn State–Hershey Cancer Institute
State College, Pennsylvania

Heather Belansky, MSN, RN
Clinical Trial Educator
Quintiles
Pittsburgh, Pennsylvania

Ashley Leak Bryant, PhD, RN-BC, OCN®
Assistant Professor
School of Nursing
The University of North Carolina at Chapel Hill
Chapel Hill, North Carolina

Darcy Burbage, RN, MSN, AOCN®, CBCN
Nurse Navigator
Helen F. Graham Cancer Center and Research Institute
Newark, Delaware

Kathleen D. Burns, MSN, RN, OCN®
Nurse Manager, Radiation Oncology
Hartford Hospital
Hartford, Connecticut

Susan DeCristofaro, RN, MSN, OCN®
Professional Advancement Coordinator
Boston Medical Center;
Dana Farber Cancer Institute;
Mass College of Pharmacy School of Nursing;
Boston, Massachusetts

Seth Eisenberg, RN, ASN, OCN®, BMTCN
Professional Practice Coordinator
Infusion Services
Seattle Cancer Care Alliance
Seattle, Washington

Beth Faiman, PhDc, MSN, APN-BC, AOCN®
Nurse Practitioner
Cleveland Clinic
Cleveland, Ohio

Michele E. Gaguski, MSN, RN, AOCN®,
    CHPN, APN-C
Clinical Director, Medical Oncology/Infusion Services
Atlanticare Cancer Care Institute
Egg Harbor Township, New Jersey

Catherine Glennon, RN, MHS, OCN®, NE-BC
Director of Nursing, Cancer Center
The University of Kansas Hospital
Kansas City, Kansas

Marcelle Kaplan, RN, MS, AOCN®, CBCN®
Advanced Practice Oncology Nurse Consultant and Editor
Merrick, New York

Valerie Kogut, MA, RD, LDN, CTTS
Nutrition Instructor
University of Pittsburgh School of Nursing
Pittsburgh, Pennsylvania

Denise Scott Korn, MSN, RN, OCN®
Education Specialist II
High Point Regional Health UNC Health Care
High Point, North Carolina

Joan Such Lockhart, PhD, RN, CORLN, AOCN®, CNE,
    ANEF, FAAN
Clinical Professor
Associate Dean for Academic Affairs
Duquesne University School of Nursing
Pittsburgh, Pennsylvania

Suzanne M. Mahon, RN, DNSc, AOCN®, APNG
Professor
Internal Medicine;
School of Nursing;
Saint Louis University
St. Louis, Missouri

Sandra A. Mitchell, PhD, CRNP, AOCN®
Research Scientist
Outcomes Research Branch, Applied Research Program
Division of Cancer Control and Population Sciences
National Cancer Institute
Bethesda, Maryland

Preface

On behalf of the section editors, Jeannine Brant, Francisco Conde, Marlon Saria, and myself, we are pleased to bring you the fifth edition of the *Core Curriculum for Oncology Nursing.* It has been 10 years since the previous edition, and this volume has been updated to reflect the many changes in the practice of oncology nursing since that time.

As in previous editions, the OCN® Test Blueprint is the organizing framework for the text. Sections and chapters reflect specific portions of the Test Blueprint. One of the major uses of this text is to prepare for the OCN® test. Most chapters start with an overview to provide the background knowledge necessary for the specific content area, followed by sections on assessment, problem statements and outcomes specific to the problem statements, a planning and implementation section, concluding with an evaluation statement. The easy-to-use outline format has been retained in this edition. An emphasis on QSEN competencies is designed to reduce errors in oncology nursing practice with a focus on safety and evidence-based practice. Safety-related content has been highlighted through new *Safety Alert* icons. ⚠

The content of the chapters has been updated to reflect the new discoveries in genetics, molecular biology of cancer, new drugs for new targets, changes and controversies in cancer screening, the recognition of the expanding numbers of survivors of cancer, and the important role navigators play in the continuity of care for patients and families with cancer. Some of the content has been reorganized based on the current 2013 – 2017 OCN® Test Blueprint,

and two new chapters, *Research Protocols and Clinical Trials* and *Coping Mechanisms and Skills,* have been added.

Among the recommendations of the 2013 Institute of Medicine (IOM) report, *Delivering High-Quality Cancer Care: Charting a New Course for a System in Crisis,* is the need for an adequately staffed, trained, and coordinated workforce. The report sets a goal that all individuals caring for cancer patients should have appropriate core competencies.

The Oncology Nursing Society (ONS) has been a leader in the nursing profession in establishing certification programs that formally recognize oncology nurses' specialized knowledge, skills, and expertise. To meet this IOM goal, nursing should focus on increasing the number of oncology-certified nurses and promoting the role of institutions in requiring certification. We believe this textbook will help nurses with appropriate oncology experience prepare successfully for the OCN® certification examination.

Our thanks to ONS for providing us the opportunity to revise and update this text. We want to recognize our longtime colleague, Barbara Sigler, former Director of Commercial Publications at ONS, who guided the initial process of several editions of the *Core Curriculum.* Our special thanks to Lee Henderson and Courtney Daniels of Elsevier. They have been a joy and an efficient team to work with. Finally, we thank the contributors whose expertise is what makes this book the valuable resource it is.

Aloha,
Joanne Itano

Contents

CHAPTER 1

Epidemiology, Prevention, and Health Promotion

Francisco A. Conde

OVERVIEW

I. Cancer epidemiology
   A. Definition
      1. Study of the distribution and determinants of cancer in population groups
      2. Assists in development of population-based risk profiles
   B. Global cancer statistics (International Agency for Research on Cancer and Cancer Research, 2012)
      1. Cancer is a leading cause of disease worldwide.
      2. Cancer incidence worldwide
         a. Worldwide, approximately 12.7 million people were diagnosed with cancer in 2008.
         b. The cancer rate is projected to increase by 75% to 22 million new cases in 2030 primarily because of increasing aging population, tobacco use, reproductive, dietary, and hormonal risk factors.
         c. The top five most commonly diagnosed cancers are lung (13%), breast (11%), colorectal (10%), stomach (8%), and prostate (7%).
            (1) Lung, breast, colorectal, stomach and prostate cancers make up nearly 50% of all cases diagnosed.
            (2) Lung cancer is the most common cancer in men.
            (3) Breast cancer is the most common cancer in women.
               (a) Incidence rate of breast cancer in Europe is more than double that in Africa (World Cancer Research Fund International, 2013).
               (b) In 2008, the age-standardized rate for new cases of breast cancer was 67 per 100,000 population in Europe and 28 per 100,000 in Africa.

            (4) More than 70% of prostate cancer cases are diagnosed in more developed regions of the world.
               (a) In 2008, 644,000 cases of prostate cancer were diagnosed in more developed regions of the world and 255,000 cases in less developed regions.
      3. Cancer mortality worldwide
         a. An estimated 756 million people died from the disease in 2008.
         b. The top five most common causes of death from cancer are lung (18%), stomach (10%), liver (9%), colorectum (6%), and breast (6%).
         c. About 64% of cancer-related deaths are seen in less developed regions of the world (International Agency for Research on Cancer and Cancer Research, 2011).
   C. Cancer statistics in the United States (U.S.) (American Cancer Society [ACS], 2013a)
      1. Cancer incidence in U.S.
         a. Estimated 1,660,290 new cancer cases in 2013 (ACS, 2013a).
            (1) Estimates exclude basal cell and squamous cell skin cancers and in situ carcinomas, except urinary bladder.
         b. For both sexes combined, the top five most commonly diagnosed cancers are prostate (14.4%), breast (14.1%), lung (13.7%), colorectal (8.6%), and melanoma of the skin (4.6%).
         c. Among women, the five most common cancers are breast (29%), lung (14%), colorectal (9%), uterine (6%), and thyroid (6%).
         d. Among men, the five most common cancers are prostate (28%), lung (14%), colorectal (9%), urinary bladder (6%), and melanoma of the skin (5%).

1

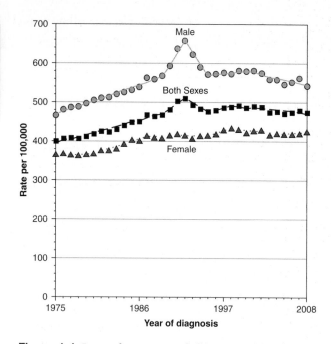

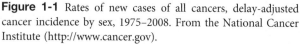

Figure 1-1 Rates of new cases of all cancers, delay-adjusted cancer incidence by sex, 1975–2008. From the National Cancer Institute (http://www.cancer.gov).

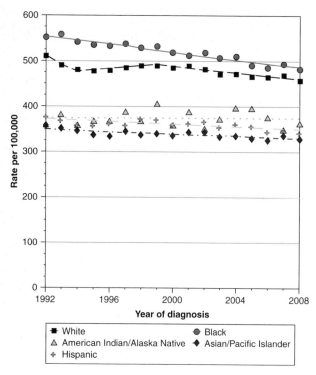

Figure 1-2 Rates of new cases of all cancers by race/ethnicity, 1992–2008. From the website of the National Cancer Institute (http://www.cancer.gov).

e. Trends in cancer incidence rates (National Cancer Institute [NCI], 2013a)
  (1) For all cancers combined, the cancer incidence rate steadily declined from 488.44 in 1998 to 473.95 per 100,000 in 2008 (Figure 1-1).
    (a) Among men, the incidence rates declined from 580.29 in 2000 to 543.09 per 100,000 in 2008.
    (b) Among women, the cancer incidence rate significantly declined from 1998 to 2005 and was stable from 2005 to 2008.
  (2) For all races, cancer incidence rates declined from 1992 to 2008 (Figure 1-2).
  (3) Cancer sites with increasing incidence trends from 1975 to 2008
    (a) Cancers with annual percentage changes of 1% or more per year include melanoma of the skin, cancer of the kidney, and thyroid, pancreas, and liver and intrahepatic bile duct cancers.
  (4) Cancer sites with decreasing incidence trends from 1975 to 2008
    (a) In addition to the four leading cancers (prostate, breast, lung, and colorectal cancer), incidence rates of other cancer sites are also decreasing, including cancers of the ovary, stomach, uterine, cervix, and larynx.
2. Cancer mortality in U.S.
  a. Estimated 580,350 deaths from cancer in 2013

  (1) One of every four deaths is caused by cancer.
  b. Cancer is the second leading cause of death in the U.S., second only to heart disease.
  c. Among women, the five leading causes of cancer-related deaths are lung (26%), breast (14%), colorectal (9%), pancreas (7%), and ovary (5%).
  d. Among men, the five leading causes of cancer-related deaths are lung (28%), prostate (10%), colorectal (9%), pancreas (6%), and liver and intrahepatic bile duct (5%).
  e. Trends in cancer mortality rates (NCI, 2013b)
    (1) For all cancers combined, cancer mortality rates steadily declined from 215.22 in 1991 to 175.86 per 100,000 in 2008 (Figure 1-3).
      (a) Among men, mortality rates declined from 278.21 in 1991 to 215.22 in 2008.
      (b) Among women, cancer incidence rates significantly declined from 175.67 in 1991 to 148.75 per 100,000 in 2008.
    (2) For all races, cancer mortality rates declined from 1992 to 2008 (Figure 1-4).
    (3) Cancer sites with increasing mortality trends from 1975 to 2008

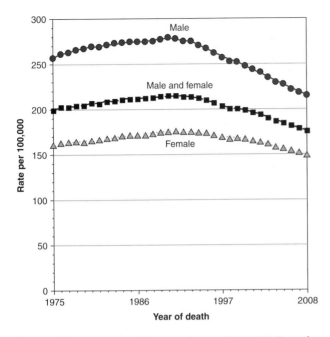

Figure 1-3 Death rates of all cancers by sex, 1975–2008. From the website of the National Cancer Institute (http://www.cancer.gov).

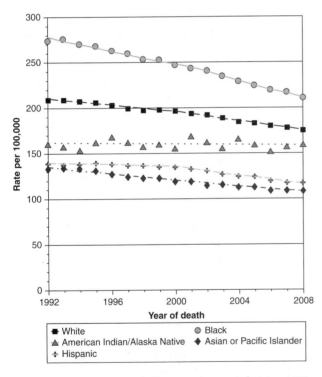

Figure 1-4 Death rates of all cancers by race/ethnicity, 1975–2008. From the website of the National Cancer Institute (http://www.cancer.gov).

(a) Include cancers of the liver and intrahepatic bile duct and pancreatic cancers.

(4) Cancer sites with decreasing incidence trends from 1997 to 2008

(a) In addition to the four leading cancers (lung, prostate, breast, and

colorectal cancer), mortality rates of other cancer sites, including cancers of the stomach and ovary, leukemia, and non-Hodgkin lymphoma, are also decreasing.

3. Cancer survival statistics in the U.S.

a. Between 2002 and 2008, the 5-year relative survival rate for all cancers was 68%, up from 49% from 1975 to 1977 (ACS, 2013a).

b. As of January 1, 2012, the NCI estimated that there were 13.7 million cancer survivors in the United States.

(1) 59% of cancer survivors are 65 years of age or older.

(2) Among all cancer survivors, 54.3% were female and 45.7% were male (Altekruse et al., 2011).

(3) 64% of cancer survivors have survived 5 years or more.

(4) Most common cancer sites in the survivor population are breast (22%), prostate (20%), colorectum (9%), and gynecologic sites (8%).

4. Cancer health disparities

a. Definition of "cancer health disparities"— adverse differences in incidence, prevalence, mortality, survivorship, and burden of cancer or related health conditions that exist among specific population groups in the U.S. (NCI, 2013c)

(1) Population groups may be characterized by age, disability, education, race/ethnicity, gender, income, poverty, lack of health insurance, geographic location, and medically underserved.

b. Statistics on race/ethnicity and cancer for 2000–2004 (NCI, 2013c)

(1) For all racial/ethnic groups combined, the age-adjusted cancer incidence rate was 470.1 per 100,000.

(a) African Americans have the highest incidence rate of cancer (504.1), followed by whites (477.5), Hispanic/Latino (356.0), Asian/Pacific Islander (314.9), and American Indian/Alaskan Native (297.6).

(2) For all racial/ethnic groups combined, the age-adjusted cancer mortality rate was 192.7 per 100,000.

(a) African Americans have the highest mortality rate of cancer (238.8), followed by whites (190.7), American Indian/Alaskan Native (160.4), Hispanic/Latino (129.1), and Asian/Pacific Islander (115.5).

(3) For breast cancer, white women have the highest incidence rate; however, the

highest mortality rate is seen among African American women.

(4) For cervical cancer, Hispanic/Latina women have the highest incidence rate; however, the highest mortality rate is seen among African American women.

(5) For prostate cancer, African American men have the highest incidence and mortality rates than other ethnic groups in the U.S.

  (a) African American men are more than twice as likely as white men to die from prostate cancer.

  (b) The lowest incidence rate is seen in American Indian/Alaska Native men.

  (c) The lowest mortality rate is seen in Asian/Pacific Islander men.

(6) For both lung and colorectal cancers, African Americans have the highest incidence and mortality rates than other ethnic groups in the U.S.

(7) Asians/Pacific Islanders have the highest incidence and mortality rates of liver and stomach cancers than other ethnic groups in the U.S.

(8) American Indians/Alaska Natives have the highest incidence and mortality rates of kidney cancer in the U.S.

c. Cancer rates in other population groups

(1) Age

  (a) The risk of developing cancer increases with age (ACS, 2013a).

  (b) Approximately 77% of all cancers are diagnosed in persons 55 years or older.

(2) Gender

  (a) Women have a 1 in 3 lifetime risk of developing cancer.

  (b) Men have a 1 in 2 lifetime risk of developing cancer.

(3) Geography—significant incidence and mortality differences exist in different locations.

  (a) Example: White women who live in Appalachia have a significantly higher risk of developing cervical cancer than other white women in the U.S. (NCI, 2013c).

  (b) Migratory data demonstrate adoption of the cancer pattern of the area to which migration occurs, suggesting lifestyle, behavioral, and environmental factors as causative or exacerbating.

(4) Socioeconomic status (SES)

  (a) Low SES is associated with increased risk of lung cancer, cervical cancer, stomach cancer, and cancer of the head and neck.

  (b) Tobacco use has increased among poorer populations.

  (c) More advanced disease at diagnosis is found among poor populations and those who live in rural areas.

  (d) High SES is associated with increased risk of breast, prostate, and colon cancers.

(5) Economic, social, and cultural factors may create barriers to accessing information and preventive services.

II. Cancer prevention

  A. Tobacco use

    1. Single largest preventable cause of disease and premature death in the U.S. (ACS, 2013b)

      a. Smoking responsible for approximately 443,000 premature deaths each year

      b. Accounts for at least 30% of all cancer deaths

      c. Increases the risk of cancers of the lung, mouth, nasal cavities, larynx, pharynx, oral cavity, esophagus, stomach, colorectum, liver, pancreas, kidney, bladder, and uterine cervix and ovary and myeloid leukemia

    2. Exposure to secondhand smoke is a risk factor for lung cancer and cardiovascular disease (U.S. Department of Health and Human Services, 2006).

      a. About 43% of nonsmokers in the U.S. have detectable levels of cotinine.

      b. About 60% of children, aged 3 to 11 years, are exposed to secondhand smoke.

    3. Smoking and gender

      a. In 2011, 21.6% of adult men and 16.5% of adult women were current smokers (ACS, 2013b).

      b. Between 2005 and 2011, smoking prevalence decreased from 20.9% to 19.0%.

        (1) Among men, smoking declined from 23.9% to 21.6%.

        (2) Among women, smoking declined from 18.1% to 16.5%.

    4. Smoking and health disparities

      a. Adults without a high school degree are three times more likely to be current smokers than those with a college degree.

      b. Among current smokers, the highest percentage is found in American Indians/Alaska Natives.

      c. Those who are uninsured are twice as likely to be current smokers than those who are insured.

      d. The state of Kentucky has the highest smoking prevalence.

5. Cigar smoking
   a. Increases the risk of cancers of the lung, oral cavity, larynx, esophagus, and probably pancreas
   b. Cigar smokers: 4 to 10 times more likely to die from laryngeal, oral, or esophageal cancers than nonsmokers
   c. Estimated 10.4% of men and 3.1% of women currently smoke cigars
   d. Cigar use highest among African Americans (9.2%), those with less than high school education (10%), and those with household income greater than $20,000 per year
6. Smokeless tobacco
   a. Chewing tobacco and snuff not safe substitutes for smoking cigarettes or cigars (ACS, 2013b)
   b. Increases the risk of oral, pancreatic, and esophageal cancers
   c. Electronic cigarettes or "e-cigarettes"
      (1) Battery-operated devices in which the inhaled vapor is produced from cartridges that contain nicotine, flavor, and other chemicals
      (2) Use may lead nonsmokers, especially children, to begin smoking
      (3) Are not currently regulated as tobacco products by the U.S. Food and Drug Administration (FDA)
7. Healthy People 2020 goals regarding tobacco use (U.S. Department of Health and Human Services, 2013)
   a. Reduce the percentage of adults who currently smoke to 12%
   b. Reduce the percentage of adults who currently use smokeless tobacco to 0.3%
   c. Reduce the percentage of adults who currently smoke cigars to 0.2%

B. Obesity
   1. Definitions (World Health Organization, 2013a)
      a. Classification of overweight and obesity by body mass index (BMI) (Table 1-1)
         (1) Overweight or pre-obese: BMI range between 25.0 and 29.9 kg/m^2
         (2) Obese: BMI of 30.0 kg/m^2 or higher
   2. Obesity, physical inactivity, and poor nutrition are major risk factors for cancer (ACS, 2013b).
      a. Second only to tobacco use
      b. Responsible for about one quarter to one third of all cancers in the U.S.
      c. Overweight and obesity contribute to 14% to 20% of all cancer-related deaths.
      d. Increase the risk of cancers of the breast (in postmenopausal women), esophagus, colorectum, gallbladder, liver, pancreas,

Table 1-1

Classification of Overweight and Obesity by Body Mass Index (BMI)

	Obesity Class	BMI (kg/m^2)
Underweight		<18.5
Normal		18.5–24.9
Overweight		25.0–29.9
Obesity	I	30.0–34.9
	II	35.0–39.9
Extreme obesity	III	≥40

Data from National Institutes of Health, National Health, Lung, and Blood Institute. (1998). *Clinical guidelines on the identification, evaluation and treatment of overweight and obesity in adults: the evidence report* (NIH Publication. No. 98-4083). Bethesda: GPO.

kidney, endometrium, cervix, ovary, and prostate; multiple myeloma; non-Hodgkin lymphoma; and myeloid leukemia
      e. Obesity and gender (ACS, 2013b)
         (1) Obesity rates for men and women are similar.
            (a) Among men, obesity rate is 35.5%.
            (b) Among women, obesity rate is 35.8%.
      f. Obesity and race/ethnicity (ACS, 2013b)
         (1) African American men (40%) have the highest rates of obesity compared with non-Hispanic white men (37%) and Hispanic men (37%).
         (2) African American women (59%) have the highest rates of obesity compared with non-Hispanic white women (32%) and Hispanic women (46%).

C. Diet
   1. Foods and beverages high in calories—may contribute to altered amounts and distribution of body fat, insulin resistance, and higher concentrations of growth factors that promote cancer growth (ACS, 2013b)
   2. Processed and red meats (ACS, 2013b; Sinha, Cross, Graubard, Leitzmann, & Schatzkin, 2009)
      a. Associated with increased risk of cancers of the colorectum, prostate, and pancreas
      b. Nitrates or other substances used to preserve processed meats involved in carcinogenesis
   3. Vegetables and fruits
      a. Only 15% of adults reported eating three or more servings of vegetables daily in 2011.
      b. Associated with decreased risk of lung, esophageal, stomach, and colorectal cancers
      c. High intake of whole-grain foods associated with decreased risk of colorectal cancer (Aune et al., 2011)

D. Alcohol consumption
   1. Risk factor for cancers of the mouth, pharynx, larynx, esophagus, liver, colorectum, pancreas, and breast

2. Has synergistic effect with tobacco
E. Ultraviolet radiation
  1. Primarily from the sun
  2. Significant risk factor for melanoma and basal and squamous cell skin cancers
      a. Basal cell carcinoma—most common skin cancer; is rarely deadly; influenced by both long-term and intermittent sun exposure
      b. Squamous cell carcinoma—often begins with small scaly lesions called *solar keratoses* or *actinic keratoses*; linked to cumulative time in the sun; both squamous and basal cell cancers typically found on the head, neck, and arms, areas of the body most frequently exposed to sunlight
      c. Melanoma
          (1) Estimated 76,690 new cancers and 9480 deaths from melanoma in 2011 (ACS, 2013a)
          (2) Incidence increasing over the past 30 years because of increased exposure to solar ultraviolet radiation and indoor tanning booths (Cust et al., 2011)
F. Viral exposures (World Health Organization, 2013b)
  1. Hepatitis B virus infection is associated with liver cancer.
  2. Human immunodeficiency virus (HIV) infection results in immunosuppression that increases the risk of Kaposi sarcoma and B-cell lymphomas.
  3. Epstein-Barr virus (EBV)
      a. Endemic in human population because more than 90% of adults worldwide are seropositive
      b. Causes infectious mononucleosis
      c. Associated with Burkitt lymphoma, nasopharyngeal cancers, undifferentiated parotid carcinoma, Hodgkin disease, B-cell lymphoma, and gastric carcinomas
  4. Human papillomavirus (HPV)
      a. Cervical cancer (Castellsagué et al., 2014; Dahlström et al., 2011)
          (1) More than 100 types of HPV
          (2) Approximately 70% of cervical cancers caused by HPV types 16 or 18
      b. Oral cancer
          (1) HPV-16 detected in a substantial proportion of squamous cell carcinomas of the soft palate, tonsils, and base of the tongue
          (2) HPV-16 detected in 60% to 70% of all HPV-associated cancers of the oral cavity and oropharynx (Chaturvedi et al., 2011; Marur, D'Souza, Westra, & Forastiere, 2010; Smith et al., 2007)
  5. Human T-cell lymphotropic virus 1 (HTLV-1)
      a. Associated with T-cell leukemias

G. Occupational exposures
  1. Occupational cancer risks
      a. Account for about 4% of cancers
      b. Introduction of effective regulation of workplace exposures in the middle years of the twentieth century believed to have reduced these risks substantially
      c. Asbestos: single most important known occupational carcinogen
          (1) Asbestos-related lung cancer and mesothelioma peaked during the middle to late 1980s because of extensive occupational exposure in shipyards during World War II.
          (2) Occupations exposed to asbestos include mining, shipyards, railroads, constructions, boiler plants, firefighting, oil refineries, and paper, textile, and steel mills (Dodson & Hammar, 2011).
          (3) Occupational exposures to asbestos fibers, environmental smoke, radon, or all of these factors have a synergistic role in elevating the risk of smoking-related lung cancer.
      d. Special population concerns
          (1) Blue collar workers—tend to have higher smoking rates that increase risks associated with occupational exposures
          (2) African Americans—discriminatory work assignments have historically resulted in placement in more hazardous jobs—steel, rubber, and chemical industries
          (3) Steel workers—increased rates of lung cancer
          (4) Rubber workers—increased rates of prostate cancer
          (5) Chemical workers—increased rates of bladder cancer
          (6) Miners—increased exposure to uranium and radon with a subsequent increase in gastric cancer and birth defects
H. Hormonal agents and antineoplastic drugs
  1. Hormone replacement therapy (HRT)
      a. Combined estrogen-progesterone HRT given to postmenopausal women increases risk of breast cancer (Manson et al., 2013)
      b. Estrogens may have a protective role in preventing colorectal cancer (Barzi, Lenz, Labonte, & Lenz, 2013).
      c. Long-term use of HRT increases risk of endometrial cancer (Trabert et al., 2013)
  2. Selective estrogen receptor modulators
      a. Include tamoxifen and raloxifene
      b. FDA-approved for use to reduce risk of breast cancer

    c. Have been shown to reduce breast cancer incidence by up to 50% among high-risk women (Fisher et al., 1998; Vogel et al., 2006)

  3. Use of oral contraceptives associated with breast cancer but may reduce the risk of cancers of ovary and uterus

  4. Daughters of women who took diethylstilbestrol (DES) during pregnancy had an increased incidence of clear cell adenocarcinoma (CCA) of the vagina, especially in their late teens and early 20s. However, after age 25, the incidence of CCA among DES-exposed daughters has decreased by over 80% (Troisi et al., 2007).

  5. Anabolic steroids may be associated with liver cancer.

  6. Certain fertility drugs (i.e., menotropins [Pergonal]) may increase the risk for ovarian cancer.

  7. Growth hormones given to children may increase the risk for leukemia.

  8. Immunosuppressive agents (for organ recipients) increase the risk of non-Hodgkin lymphoma.

  9. Prior exposure to antineoplastic agents (especially alkylating agents) and radiation therapy increases the risk of secondary cancers.

III. Health promotion

  A. American Cancer Society guidelines on nutrition and physical activity for cancer prevention (Kushi et al., 2012)

    1. Nutrition: Consume a healthy diet with emphasis on plant sources.

      a. Choose foods and beverages in amounts that help achieve and maintain a healthy weight.

        (1) Eat smaller portions of high-calorie foods.

        (2) Choose vegetables, whole fruit, and other low-calorie foods.

        (3) Limit consumption of sugar-sweetened beverages.

        (4) Avoid consuming large portion sizes.

      b. Limit consumption of processed and red meats.

        (1) Minimize consumption of processed meats.

        (2) Choose fish, poultry, or beans as an alternative to red meat.

        (3) For red meat, select lean cuts and eat smaller portions.

        (4) Prepare meat, fish, or poultry by baking, broiling, or poaching rather than frying or charbroiling.

      c. Eat at least 2½ cups of vegetables and fruits per day.

      d. Choose whole-grain instead of refined-grain products.

      e. Limit alcohol intake to no more than two drinks per day for men and one drink per day for women (ACS, 2013b).

    2. Physical activity (Kushi et al., 2012)

      a. Intensity, duration, and frequency of physical activity to reduce cancer risk unknown

      b. ACS recommendations.

        (1) Adults—at least 150 minutes of moderate-intensity activity per week or 75 minutes of vigorous-intensity activity per week.

        (2) Children—at least 60 minutes of moderate- or vigorous-intensity activity each day, with vigorous activity on at least 3 days each week.

        (3) Limiting sedentary behavior such as sitting, lying down, and watching television

  B. ACS guidelines on nutrition and physical activity for cancer survivors (Rock et al., 2012)

    1. Achieve and maintain a healthy weight.

      a. Limit consumption of high-calorie foods and beverages.

      b. Increase physical activity.

    2. Engage in regular physical activity.

      a. Return to normal daily activities as soon as possible following diagnosis.

      b. Exercise at least 150 minutes per week.

      c. Include strength training at least 2 days per week.

      d. Consume foods high in vegetables, fruits, and whole grains.

  C. Vaccination

    1. HPV vaccine for prevention of cervical cancer and other genital cancers (ACS, 2013b)

      a. Gardasil and Cervarix: two FDA-approved vaccines

        (1) Recommendations for females

          (a) Routine vaccination at 11 to 12 years of age (may start at 9 years of age) with three doses of either Gardasil or Cervarix

          (b) Vaccination at 13 to 26 years of age for those who have not been previously vaccinated or have not completed the three-dose series

        (2) Recommendations for males

          (a) Routine vaccination at 11 to 12 years of age (may start at 9 years of age) with three doses of Gardasil

          (b) Vaccination at 13 to 26 years of age for those who have not been previously vaccinated or have not completed the three-dose series

          (c) Vaccination of men through 26 years of age who have a weakened immune system or who engage in same-sex behaviors

2. Hepatitis B vaccine (Centers for Disease Control and Prevention [CDC], 2013)
   a. Recommendations for babies
      (1) First dose: at birth
      (2) Second dose: 1-2 months of age
      (3) Third dose: 6-18 months of age
   b. For children, adolescents, and adults
      (1) All unvaccinated children, adolescents, and adults at risk for hepatitis B infection should be vaccinated.

D. Measures to prevent skin cancer (ACS, 2013b)
   1. Avoid direct exposure to the sun between the hours of 10 AM and 4 PM, when ultraviolet rays are most intense.
   2. Wear hats with a brim wide enough to shade the face, ears, and neck, as well as clothing that covers as much as possible of the arms, legs, and torso.
   3. Cover exposed skin with a sunscreen lotion with a sun protection factor (SPF) of 30 or higher.
   4. Avoid indoor tanning booths and sun lamps.

E. Screening and early detection of cancer (see Chapter 2)

ASSESSMENT

I. Conduct a thorough medical history and physical examination.
   A. Obtain demographic information such as age, race/ethnicity, gender, education, employment status and place of employment, insurance coverage, and area of residence.
   B. Assess for comorbidities (e.g., hepatitis infection) and previous and current medications (e.g., hormone replacement therapy).
   C. Assess for any lifestyle risk factors such as tobacco use, alcohol consumption, exposure to ultraviolet radiation, weight, nutrition, and level of physical activity.
   D. Assess for any occupational exposures such as exposure to asbestos, benzene, and other chemicals.
   E. Assess for personal and family histories of cancer.
   F. Include any previous treatment with radiotherapy, chemotherapy, or both.
   G. Motivation for preventive behavior (health belief model)
      1. Perceived susceptibility to cancer—evidence indicates that individuals at risk often are unaware of their risks. (Ask, "How likely do you feel you are to develop cancer?")
      2. Perceived severity of cancer. (Ask, "How serious do you feel cancer is?")
      3. Perceived benefits of preventive behavior. (Ask, "Do you think you can decrease your risk for

cancer by not smoking [or the habit in question]?")
      4. Perceived barriers to preventive action. (Ask, "What problems do you think you may have lowering the fat content in your diet [or the behavior in question]?")

PROBLEM STATEMENTS AND OUTCOME IDENTIFICATION

I. Ineffective Health Maintenance (NANDA-I), related to insufficient knowledge of cancer prevention and health promotion activities
   A. Expected outcome
      1. Patient will assume responsibility for own wellness as measured by the following:
         a. Describing personal risk factors for cancer based on family history, age, exposures, and lifestyle
         b. Stating intent to adopt behavioral strategies for reducing cancer risk(s) (e.g., smoking cessation, dietary modification, weight reduction, exercise, safe sex practices)

PLANNING AND IMPLEMENTATION

I. Interventions to promote or improve health maintenance
   A. Provide education regarding health promotion activities.
      1. Tobacco cessation
         a. U.S. Public Health Service "5 A" model in treating smokers who are willing to quit (Fiore & Jaén, 2008)
            (1) Ask patient about smoking status.
            (2) Advise to quit.
            (3) Assess for willingness or readiness to quit.
               (a) Use motivational interviewing techniques such as asking, "Have you considered quitting?"
            (4) Assist in quitting.
               (a) Discuss options for quitting such as use of medications (over-the-counter and prescription) to aid smoking cessation.
               (b) Assist patient with developing a quit plan.
               (c) Offer relevant and culturally appropriate cessation materials, cessation programs, and public cessation hotlines.
            (5) Arrange a follow-up visit.
         b. For smokers who are unwilling to quit, the U.S. Public Health Service (USPHS) recommends brief motivational interventions that can help increase attempts to quit.
      2. Proper nutrition

3. Physical activity
4. Measures to limit sun exposure
   a. Educate persons of all ages about skin cancer prevention.
5. Prevention of viral exposures
   a. Offer vaccinations for hepatitis B and HPV.
   b. Discuss safe sex practices.
   c. Counsel against intravenous (IV) drug use, or educate about and facilitate access to sterile needle and syringe programs.
6. Avoidance of occupational carcinogen exposures
   a. Use protective clothing and devices, and follow safety procedures when exposure is unavoidable.
B. Refer to specialists (e.g., dietician, tobacco addiction treatment specialist), as needed.
C. Encourage participation in chemoprevention trials.

EVALUATION

The oncology nurse systematically and regularly evaluates the patient's and the family's responses to interventions to determine progress toward the achievement of expected outcomes. Relevant data are collected, and actual findings are compared with expected findings. Nursing diagnoses, outcomes, and plans of care are reviewed and revised, as necessary.

References

Altekruse, S. F., Kosary, C. L., Krapcho, M., Neyman, N., Aminou, R., Waldron, W., et al. (2011). *SEER cancer statistics review, 1975–2007*. Bethesda, MD: National Cancer Institute.

American Cancer Society. (2013a). *Cancer facts & figures, 2013*. Atlanta: Author.

American Cancer Society. (2013b). *Cancer prevention & early detection: Facts & figures, 2013*. Atlanta: Author.

Aune, D., Chan, D. S., Lau, R., Vieira, R., Greenwood, D. C., Kampman, E., et al. (2011). Dietary fibre, whole grains, and risk of colorectal cancer: Systematic review and dose-response meta-analysis of prospective studies. *British Medical Journal, 343*, 1–20. http://dx.doi.org/10.1136/bmj.d6617.

Barzi, A., Lenz, A. M., Labonte, M. J., & Lenz, H. J. (2013). Molecular pathways: Estrogen pathway in colorectal cancer. *Clinical Cancer Research, 19*(21), 5842–5848.

Castellsagué, X., Pawlita, M., Roura, E., Margall, N., Waterboer, T., Bosch, F. X., et al. (2014). Prospective seroepidemiologic study on the role of Human Papillomavirus and other infections in cervical carcinogenesis: Evidence from the EPIC cohort. *International Journal of Cancer, 135*(2), 440–452. http://dx.doi.org/10.1002/ijc.28665.

Centers for Disease Control. (2013). *Hepatitis B vaccine information statements*. http://www.cdc.gov/vaccines/hcp/vis/vis-statements/hep-b.html/. Accessed 20.11.13.

Chaturvedi, A. K., Engels, E. A., Pfeiffer, R. M., Hernandez, B. Y., Xiao, W., Kim, E., et al. (2011). Human papillomavirus and rising oropharyngeal cancer incidence in the United States. *Journal of Clinical Oncology, 29*(32), 4294–4301.

Cust, A. E., Armstrong, B. K., Goumas, C., Jenkins, M. A., Schmid, H., Hopper, J. L., et al. (2011). Sunbed use during adolescence and early adulthood is associated with increased risk of early-onset melanoma. *International Journal of Cancer, 128*(10), 2425–2435.

Dahlström, L. A., Andersson, K., Luostarinen, T., Thoresen, S., Ögmundsdottír, H., Tryggvadottír, L., et al. (2011). Prospective seroepidemiologic study of human papillomavirus and other risk factors in cervical cancer. *Cancer Epidemiology, Biomarkers & Prevention, 20*(12), 2541–2550.

Dodson, R. F., & Hammar, S. P. (Eds.). (2011). *Asbestos: Risk assessment, epidemiology, and health effects* (2nd ed.). Boca Raton, FL: CRC Press.

Fiore, M. C., & Jaén, C. R. (2008). A clinical blueprint to accelerate the elimination of tobacco use. *JAMA: The Journal of the American Medical Association, 299*(17), 2083–2085.

Fisher, B., Costantino, J. P., Wickerham, D. L., Redmond, C. K., Kavanah, M., Cronin, W. M., et al. (1998). Tamoxifen for prevention of breast cancer: Report of the National Surgical Adjuvant Breast and Bowel Project P-1 Study. *Journal of the National Cancer Institute, 90*(18), 1371–1388.

International Agency for Research on Cancer and Cancer Research (2011). *Cancer worldwide*. http://publications.cancerresearchuk.org/downloads/Product/CS_CS_WORLD.pdf/. Accessed 25.11.13.

International Agency for Research on Cancer and Cancer Research (2012). *World cancer factsheet*. http://publications.cancerresearchuk.org/downloads/product/CS_FS_WORLD_A4.pdf/. Accessed 25.11.13.

Kushi, L. H., Doyle, C., McCullough, M., Rock, C. L., Demark-Wahnefried, W., Bandera, E. V., et al. (2012). American Cancer Society guidelines on nutrition and physical activity for cancer prevention. *CA: A Cancer Journal for Clinicians, 62*(1), 30–67.

Manson, J. E., Chlebowski, R. T., Stefanick, M. L., Aragaki, A. K., Rossouw, J. E., Prentice, R. L., et al. (2013). Menopausal hormone therapy and health outcomes during the intervention and extended poststopping phases of the Women's Health Initiative randomized trials update and overview of health outcomes for WHI update and overview of health outcomes for WHI. *JAMA: The Journal of the American Medical Association, 310*(13), 1353–1368.

Marur, S., D'Souza, G., Westra, W. H., & Forastiere, A. A. (2010). HPV-associated head and neck cancer: A virus-related cancer epidemic. *The Lancet Oncology, 11*(8), 781–789.

National Cancer Institute. (2013a). *Cancer trends progress report—2011/2012 incidence update*. http://progressreport.cancer.gov/doc_detail.asp?pid=1&did=2009&chid=93&coid=920/. Accessed 20.11.13.

National Cancer Institute. (2013b). *Cancer trends progress report—2011/2012 mortality update*. http://progressreport.cancer.gov/doc_detail.asp?pid=1&did=2011&chid=106&coid=1029&mid=/. Accessed 20.11.13.

National Cancer Institute. (2013c). *Cancer health disparities*. http://www.cancer.gov/cancertopics/factsheet/disparities/cancer-health-disparities/. Accessed 20.11.13.

National Institutes of Health, National Health, Lung, and Blood Institute. (1998). *Clinical guidelines on the identification, evaluation and treatment of overweight and obesity in adults: The evidence report* (NIH Publication. No. 98-4083). Bethesda, MD: U.S. Government Printing Office.

Rock, C. L., Doyle, C., Demark-Wahnefried, W., Meyerhardt, J., Courneya, K. S., Schwartz, A. L., et al. (2012). Nutrition and physical activity guidelines for cancer survivors. *CA: A Cancer Journal for Clinicians, 62*(4), 242–274.

Sinha, R., Cross, A. J., Graubard, B. I., Leitzmann, M. F., & Schatzkin, A. (2009). Meat intake and mortality: A prospective study of over half a million people. *Archives of Internal Medicine, 169*(6), 562–571.

Smith, E. M., Ritchie, J. M., Pawlita, M., Rubenstein, L. M., Haugen, T. H., Turek, L. P., et al. (2007). Human papillomavirus seropositivity and risks of head and neck cancer. *International Journal of Cancer, 120*(4), 825–832.

Trabert, B., Wentzensen, N., Yang, H. P., Sherman, M. E., Hollenbeck, A. R., Park, Y., et al. (2013). Is estrogen plus progestin menopausal hormone therapy safe with respect to endometrial cancer risk? *International Journal of Cancer, 132*(2), 417–426.

Troisi, R., Hatch, E. E., Titus-Ernstoff, L., Hyer, M., Palmer, J. R., Robboy, S. J., et al. (2007). Cancer risk in women prenatally exposed to diethylstilbestrol. *International Journal of Cancer, 121*(2), 356–360.

U.S. Department of Health and Human Services. (2013). *Healthy people 2020.* Washington, D.C.: Office of Disease Prevention and Health Promotion. http://www.healthypeople.gov/2020/default.aspx/. Accessed 25.11.13.

U.S. Department of Health and Human Services. (2006). *The health consequences of involuntary exposure to tobacco smoke: A report of the surgeon general.* Washington, DC: U.S. Department of Health and Human Services, Centers for Disease Control and Prevention, National Center for Chronic Disease Prevention and Health Promotion, Office on Smoking and Health.

Vogel, V. G., Costantino, J. P., Wickerham, D. L., Cronin, W. M., Cecchini, R. S., Atkins, J. N., et al. (2006). Effects of tamoxifen vs. raloxifene on the risk of developing invasive breast cancer and other disease outcomes. *JAMA: The Journal of the American Medical Association, 295*(23), 2727–2741.

World Cancer Research Fund International. (2013). *Cancer facts and figures.* http://www.wcrf.org/cancer_statistics/cancer_facts/index.php/, Accessed 25.11.13.

World Health Organization. (2013a). *BMI classification.* http://apps.who.int/bmi/index.jsp?introPage=intro_3.html/. Accessed 25.11.13.

World Health Organization. (2013b). *Viral cancers.* http://www.who.int/vaccine_research/diseases/viral_cancers/en/index1.html/. Accessed 25.11.13.

CHAPTER 2

Screening and Early Detection

Candis Morrison

OVERVIEW

I. Rationale for early detection
  A. The most effective treatment for cancer is prevention (primary prevention).
  B. Early detection of cancer (secondary prevention) and effective therapy (tertiary prevention) may result in decreased morbidity and mortality.

II. Definitions
  A. Secondary prevention—measures taken to identify potential for development or existence of a disease in asymptomatic individuals
    1. Involves development of risk profiles and use of screening guidelines to both enhance screening efficacy and decrease the risks and costs of the screening test(s)
    2. Multiple organizations publish cancer screening guidelines, including the American Cancer Society (ACS), National Comprehensive Cancer Network (NCCN), and United States Preventive Services Task Force (USPSTF)
    3. Attempts to balance risks versus benefits of the screening tests by diagnosing disease early enough to favorably affect morbidity and mortality while also minimizing potential harms of the screening itself—pain and complications of procedures(s), cost, and false positives that may provoke anxiety and unnecessary procedures (Esserman & Flowers, 2011)
  B. Diagnosis—clinical problem-solving process applied to asymptomatic individuals who either screen positive or present in an already symptomatic state
  C. Incidence—number of new cases identified in a specified population in a defined period (generally 1 year)
  D. Prevalence—percentage of all individuals with disease at a given point in time in a specified population
    1. Includes new and existing cases
    2. Often expressed as a proportion of disease cases per 100,000 persons

III. Attributes of effective screening tests
  A. Validity—accuracy of screening test
    1. Ability to discriminate between those with the cancer in question and those who are cancer free
    2. Measured by sensitivity and specificity (ideally, both would be 100%), although in reality, they are inversely related (Mandel & Smith, 2011)
      a. Sensitivity—measure of the test's ability to correctly identify persons with the disease (true positives) among the population screened; 100% sensitivity = no false negatives
      b. Specificity—measure of the test's ability to correctly identify persons who do not have the disease in the group being screened (test will not be positive in anyone who does not have the cancer); 100% specificity = no false positives
  B. Predictive value
    1. Influenced by the prevalence of the disease in the population as well as the sensitivity and specificity of the test(s) used
    2. Can only be determined after evaluation of positive screens
      a. Positive predictive value—the percentage of persons who screen positive who actually have the disease
    3. Negative predictive value—the percentage of persons who screen negative who do not have the disease
  C. Ease of administration (i.e., noninvasive)
  D. Acceptability to those screened; more acceptable if:
    1. Safe (few potential complications) and relatively painless
    2. Convenient (ideal if the test can be performed during health care visits)
    3. Inexpensive (Mandel & Smith, 2011)
  E. Readily available to those who meet screening criteria

F. Evidence from randomized clinical trials (RCTs), which have demonstrated that the screening test reduces mortality, improves quality of life, or both and that potential benefits are greater than the risks associated with the testing
   1. Currently, evidence exists to recommend screening for breast, prostate, cervical, lung, and colorectal cancer screening in defined populations, although controversy exists for all cancers, with the exception of cervical cancer, in which screening is associated with the strongest evidence of screening's ability to decrease mortality.
   2. Screening for other cancers (by means other than routine history and physical examination) is not recommended because of either lack of evidence to support efficacy, evidence that its harms outweigh its benefits, or both.
IV. Screening biases that threaten validity of screening tests and programs
   A. RCTs are generally required to overcome biases prior to widespread acceptance of screening recommendations.
   B. Survival rates alone cannot be used to determine the efficacy of screening.
   C. Types of screening biases
      1. Lead time bias
         a. Screening allows cancer to be diagnosed earlier (prior to signs or symptoms), thus giving a false sense of lengthened survival; in reality, decrease in mortality not attributable to early diagnosis and treatment
         b. Most notable when short follow-up periods are used (5-year survival rates) versus overall survival statistics
      2. Length time bias
         a. Screening most often performed on asymptomatic individuals who will generally have more indolent cancers (aggressive cancers generally cause earlier symptoms promoting evaluation), which improves survival rates
         b. Favorable outcomes possibly attributable to growth properties of tumor rather than to benefits of the screening
      3. Selection bias
         a. Those choosing to undergo cancer screening, or "select in," differ from those who do not (maybe healthier, more likely to adhere to health recommendations, and/or have better access to care).
         b. Favorable outcomes may be attributable to characteristics of "select ins" rather than to screening itself (Mandel & Smith, 2011).

   4. Overdiagnosis
      a. Diagnosis of an indolent cancer in a person who, if not screened, would not have been diagnosed nor have needed treatment
      b. For very slow-growing tumors, especially in older individuals, screening may not afford a survival benefit and instead may cause unnecessary treatment, anxiety, cost, and pain (Esserman & Flowers, 2011).
V. Characteristics of the cancers that justify the risks and costs associated with screening
   A. Screening should be directed toward an important health problem (e.g., high incidence, morbidity, mortality rates).
   B. Natural history provides a window of opportunity for early detection.
   C. Effective treatment is available to alter the natural history of the disease (reduce cause-specific mortality) and is more effective if initiated during the presymptomatic stage.
   D. A suitable screening test that is safe, precise, and validated is available.
   E. Screening schedule strategy (timing and frequency) mirrors the course of the cancer; that is, designated ages to begin and end screening reflect the natural history of disease in the population at risk.
   F. The benefit of screening should outweigh the risks and be cost-effective (in relation to expenditure on medical care as a whole).
   G. There should be a plan in place for managing and monitoring the screening program, as well as accepted quality assurance standards.
   H. Potential screening participants should receive adequate information regarding risks and potential benefits of participation.
VI. Screening modalities for early detection of cancer
   A. Imaging—for example, low-dose computed tomography (LDCT) for lung cancer screening and mammography for breast cancer screening
   B. Cytologic specimens—for example, Pap smear for cervical cancer
   C. Chemical assays—for example, fecal occult blood test for colorectal cancer
   D. Biomarkers or tumor markers—for example, prostate-specific antigen (PSA) for prostate cancer
      1. Substances that may be produced by the tumor or the body's reaction to the cancer and may be detected in abnormal quantities; most often found in blood, body fluids, or tissues
      2. The markers may be used to assess response to therapy, detect recurrences earlier, determine tumor's origin, and target therapy.
      3. Although attractive for screening, because most body fluids are easily accessible and are useful adjuncts in cancer care, most currently available

biomarkers or tumor markers are neither sensitive nor specific.

4. PSA is the only marker used in cancer screening programs, and its efficacy (ability to decrease mortality) remains controversial.

E. Proteomics

1. Study of the structure, function, and patterns of expression of proteins

2. May lead to the development of new biomarkers to be used for cancer screening

3. Currently used to target therapies for several cancers; e.g., colon cancer's vulnerability to 5-fluorouracil (Espino, Belluci, Petricoin, & Liotta, 2011)

VII. Screening guidelines for specific cancers

A. Breast cancer

1. Risk prediction—based on average age of 60 years for women in the United States

a. Gail model

(1) Tools, such as the Gail Model, have been developed to help estimate a woman's personal risk and have been incorporated into screening guidelines. This model incorporates characteristics (age, age of menarche, age at first live birth, number of first-degree relatives with breast cancer, number of previous benign breast biopsies, atypical hyperplasia in a previous breast biopsy, and race) in an effort to assess 5-year and lifetime risks of developing breast cancer (Gail et al., 1989). Other tools also incorporate genetic factors.

b. Genetic testing for *BRCA1* and *BRCA2* gene mutations

(1) Responsible for approximately 20% to 25% of hereditary breast cancers (about 5% to 10% of all breast cancers in women and 4% to 40% in men) (NCCN, 2013)

(2) Not currently recommended for the general population

(3) May be offered to family members of persons with features indicating an increased likelihood of a *BRCA* mutation (ACS, 2013a; NCCN, 2013)

(a) Multiple cases of early breast cancer in family

(b) Strong family history of other cancers, such as ovarian and pancreatic cancers

(c) Ashkenazi Jewish heritage

(d) More than one primary cancer in the same person

(e) Male breast cancer

(f) Individual from a family with known positive *BRCA1* and *BRCA2* mutations

(g) Triple-negative breast cancer

(h) Early age of onset

(i) Diagnosed at age 45 years or younger

(ii) Diagnosed at age 50 years or younger with one or more close blood relative with breast cancer at age 50 years or younger

(iii) Diagnosed at age 50 years or younger with more than one close blood relative with ovarian, fallopian tube, or primary peritoneal cancer at any age

2. Impact of screening on breast cancer mortality

a. Confirmation from outcome data from RCTs that screening reduces mortality, especially among women aged 50 to 74 years (Esserman & Flowers, 2011)

b. Smaller tumors at diagnosis associated with increased chance of survival

(1) Risk for nodal metastasis 3% in tumors less than 5 millimeters (mm) versus 15% in tumors greater than 5 mm

(2) Requires less invasive surgeries and less need for aggressive treatment such as chemotherapy (Esserman & Flowers, 2011)

c. With use of adjuvant therapy such as hormone therapy and trastuzumab (Herceptin), difficult to determine the impact of breast cancer screening on survival; two thirds of survival attributed to adjuvant therapy and one third to screening (Kalanger, Zelen, Langmark, & Adami, 2010)

3. Cost of screening—$7 to $10 billion per year in the United States spent for screening and diagnostic evaluation (Esserman & Flowers, 2011)

4. Screening controversy

a. Considerable variability regarding how screening is implemented, particularly the ages at which to start screening, as well as its frequency

b. Screening impact not clear in many subpopulations—that is, young patients—because cancer is more difficult to detect and is often associated with more aggressive tumor biology (Esserman & Flowers, 2011)

c. Breast self-examination (BSE) was recommended routinely in the past but is no longer endorsed because of its mixed efficacy results for finding early-stage tumors and its association with high rates of false positives that require biopsies.

(1) A meta-analysis of two large RCTs (nearly 400,000 women) detected no significant difference in disease-related mortality at 15 years (Kosters & Gotzsche, 2008).

d. Digital mammography (uses digital receptors and computers to display images) is widely available, but RCTs have not shown digital mammography to be more effective than traditional mammography for screening to date (U.S. Preventive Services Task Force [USPSTF], 2009).

5. Screening modalities
   a. Screening mammography
      (1) Remains primary screening modality
      (2) Sensitivity and specificity highly dependent on the experience and competency of person interpreting study
      (3) Breast Imaging-Reporting and Data System (BI-RADS) developed by the American Society of Radiology to provide uniform reporting schema
         (a) Consists of seven categories of mammographic findings, each with terminology and follow-up recommendations (American College of Radiology [ACR], 2003)
            (i) Category 0: Additional imaging evaluation or comparison with prior mammogram needed
            (ii) Category 1: Negative
            (iii) Category 2: Benign (noncancerous)
            (iv) Category 3: Probably benign—follow-up in a short time frame
            (v) Category 4: Suspicious abnormality—biopsy should be considered
            (vi) Category 5: Highly suggestive of malignancy—biopsy strongly recommended
            (vii) Category 6: Known biopsy-proven malignancy
   b. Clinical breast examination (CBE) by health care provider
   c. Breast self-awareness (formerly, BSE)
6. Modalities used to evaluate any screening abnormalities, high-risk groups, or both
7. Includes ultrasonography and magnetic resonance imaging (MRI)
8. Modalities used for diagnosis

a. Biopsy of abnormalities found on screening (fine-needle aspiration, core biopsy, or excisional biopsy)

9. Breast cancer screening recommendations (Table 2-1).

B. Colorectal cancer (CRC)
   1. Screening modalities
      a. Guaiac-based fecal occult blood test (gFOBT)—remains only CRC screening method proven consistently effective in RCTs (Church & Mandel, 2011)
         (1) Must evaluate any positive test with imaging, endoscopy, or both
         (2) Three consecutive stool specimens optimal
         (3) Not procured by rectal examination (use stool cards)
         (4) May detect any source of blood, including dietary sources, so not specific for CRCs or precancerous lesions
         (5) Requires avoidance of some medications and vitamin supplements
      b. Fecal immunochemical test (FIT) or immunochemical fecal occult blood test (iFOBT)
         (1) Requires three consecutive stool samples collected by patient at home
         (2) Uses antibodies specific to human globin; therefore greater specificity than FOBT while maintaining sensitivity
         (3) Not affected by diet, medications, or both
         (4) Has superior sensitivity and specificity compared with traditional FOBT (Pox, 2011).
      c. Stool deoxyribonucleic acid (sDNA) not widely available or uniformly endorsed pending RCT results
         (1) Assesses for the presence of certain DNA mutations shed in stool that are known to be associated with cancerous and precancerous lesions; does not test for presence of blood
         (2) Not affected by diet or medications
      d. Barium enema
         (1) Relatively noninvasive method to visualize entire colon
         (2) Does not facilitate biopsy or removal of lesions, so positive findings require flexible sigmoidoscopy or colonoscopy
         (3) Less sensitive than CT
         (4) Currently only used as alternative for patients unable to undergo colonoscopy

Table 2-1

Breast Cancer Screening Recommendations

Organization	Population	Test and Schedule
ACS, 2013a	Women ages 20-39 years (yr)	CBE every 3 yr, with option of BSE monthly, or less If women choose to perform BSE, instruction regarding BSE benefits and limitations should begin for women in their 20s. Clinician should review technique periodically and emphasize the importance of immediately reporting any new findings.
	Women starting at age 40 yr and continued indefinitely	CBE annually Mammography annually (as long as woman in good health)
	High-risk women (those with a >15% to 20% lifetime risk) should initiate annual mammography at age 30 yr.	Annual mammography MRI screening may be added to annual mammography.
NCCN, 2013	Average-risk women Age 25-39 yr	CBE every 1-3 yr Breast awareness
	Ages ≥40 yr	Annual CBE, annual mammography, breast awareness
	Increased risk in women ≥ 35 yr with 5-yr risk of invasive cancer ≥1.7% per Gail Model	CBE every 6-12 mo Annual mammography Breast awareness Consider risk reduction strategies (e.g., prophylactic surgery (bilateral salpingo-oophorectomy), chemoprevention (tamoxifen, raloxifene, or exemestane), or both.
	Lobular carcinoma in situ (LCIS) (any age)	Begin CBE, mammography, and breast awareness at diagnosis.
	Women ≥ 30 yr with lifetime risk > 20% (family history)	CBE every 6-12 mo, breast awareness, annual mammography
	Women who have received thoracic (mantle) irradiation between ages 10 and 30 yr	For women < 25 yr: • CBE every 6-12 mo, beginning 8-10 yr after RT For women ≥25 yr • CBE every 6-12 mo, annual mammography, MRI recommended annually, breast awareness
	Women with known genetic predisposition (hereditary breast and ovarian cancers)	CBE every 6-12 mo, annual mammogram, and breast MRI starting at age 25 yr (or individualized by earliest age onset in family) Consider risk reduction strategies.
	Men with known genetic predisposition	Breast awareness, CBE every 6-12 mo beginning at age 35 yr. Consider baseline mammography at age 40 yr (annual mammography if abnormal results, gynecomastia or parenchymal or glandular breast density on baseline study)
USPSTF, 2009	Women 50-75 yr	Mammography every 2 yr

Insufficient evidence to support screening women older than 75 yr, use of CBE, teaching of BSE, or use of MRI or digital mammography. Moderate evidence supports screening in women age 40-49 yr. Evidence to recommend BSE or to assess additional benefits of CBE (beyond screening mammography in women > 40 yr) is insufficient.

ACS, American Cancer Society; *BSE*, breast self-examination; *CBE*, clinical breast examination; *MRI*, magnetic resonance imaging; *NCCN*, National Comprehensive Cancer Network; *RT*, radiotherapy; *USPSTF*, U.S. Preventive Services Task Force.

Data from American Cancer Society. (2013a). *Breast cancer: early detection.* http://www.cancer.ort/breastcancer/moreinformation/breastcancerearlydetection/breast-cancer-early-detection-acs-recs. Accessed 12.06.13; National Comprehensive Cancer Network. (2013). *NCCN clinical practice guidelines. Breast cancer screening. Version 1:2013. Breast cancer screening and diagnosis.* www.nccn.org/professionals/physician_gls/pdf/breast-screening.pdf Accessed 12.06.13; U.S. Preventive Services Task Force. (2009). *Screening for breast cancer.* http://www.uspreventiveservicestaskforce.org/uspstf/uspsbrca.htm. Accessed 12.06.13.

e. Flexible sigmoidoscopy
   (1) Uses 60-cm or longer scope
   (2) Allows more thorough examination of rectum and left colon
   (3) Has ability to identify 60% to 83% of polyps and cancers and thus reduce CRC mortality by 31% (Atkin et al., 2010)
f. Colonoscopy
   (1) Allows for complete examination of rectum, from left and right colon to cecum
   (2) Preferred screening method because it can both visualize most lesions and permit removal of polyps, thus preventing development of CRC
   (3) Limitations
      (a) Sensitivity of procedure dependent on the experience level of endoscopist performing the procedure
      (b) Sophistication of equipment
      (c) Effectiveness of bowel preparation by patient prior to procedure
      (d) Preparation unpleasant
      (e) Most invasive screening test (Church & Mandel, 2011)
g. CT colonography also known as virtual colonoscopy (VC)
   (1) Noninvasive method to examine colon and rectum for polyps and cancers
   (2) Requires bowel preparation
   (3) Good option for older adults and frail patients
   (4) If lesions detected, lower endoscopy needed for biopsy, which requires a second bowel preparation
   (5) Insufficient data to recommend its use as solitary screening test; multicenter RCTs currently being conducted (NCCN, 2012b)
h. Capsule endoscopy
   (1) Noninvasive procedure that uses a miniature camera and light source contained in a capsule that is swallowed by the patient
   (2) Used to detect sources of obscure gastrointestinal (GI) bleeding not explained by endoscopy
   (3) Requires bowel preparation
   (4) Has the advantage of its ability to visualize small bowel
   (5) Not deemed to have screening utility
2. Genetic testing
   a. Not used for screening general population
   b. Recommended for those with one or more of the following (National Cancer Institute [NCI], 2013):

(1) Strong family history of CRC, polyps, or both
(2) Personal history of adenoma or CRC
(3) Multiple primary cancers in patient with CRC
(4) Family history of other cancers consistent with known syndromes causing inherited risk of CRC (e.g., endometrial cancer)
(5) Early age at CRC diagnosis
3. Diagnosis
   a. Involves tissue or polyp sampling for pathologic examination
   b. CRCs believed to have begun as polyps (adenomas) that underwent additional mutations to become invasive adenocarcinoma; thus, excision of polyps can prevent cancer, as well as cure it.
   c. On the basis of observational studies, average time required for a polyp to develop into an invasive malignancy is 10 years; thus, timing of screening based on this biologic evidence (Church & Mandel, 2011)
4. Screening controversy
   a. Although colonoscopy is the preferred screening method, no direct evidence suggests that colonoscopy improves mortality.
   b. Even if the noninvasive screening test (e.g., FOBT, VC, capsule endoscopy) is positive, colonoscopy is still required for cancer diagnosis.
5. CRC screening recommendations (Table 2-2)
C. Cervical cancer
   1. Modalities for cervical cancer screening
      a. Pap smear
         (1) Principle screening tool for cervical cancer
         (2) Cellular specimen from cervix is fixed and stained on a slide for pathology review and interpretation
         (3) Morphologic changes of precancerous cells, cervical intraepithelial neoplasm (CIN) identified
         (4) Bethesda system, developed in 1988 and updated in 2001, used for reporting uniform cervical cytology results
            (a) Includes both descriptive diagnosis as well as evaluation of specimen adequacy (Solomon et al., 2002)
            (b) Used in more than 90% of laboratories in the United States
         (5) Low sensitivity of single Pap test because of both sampling error, in which cancerous cells do not get collected, and reading error; cumulative sensitivity of several tests is high
         (6) Incidence and mortality rates from cervical cancer decreased by use of Pap test (Daly & Rader, 2011).

Table 2-2

Colorectal Cancer Screening Recommendations

Organization	Population	Test and Schedule
ACS, 2013b	Age ≥ 50 years (yr) Average risk	Annual gFOBT or FIT Plus one of the following tests that can find polyps: • Flexible sigmoidoscopy every 5 yr • Double-contrast barium enema every 5 yr • CT colonography every 5 yr • Colonoscopy every 10 yr (also required if any of the above tests are positive)
NCCN, 2012b	Age ≥ 50 yr Average risk	One of the following: • FOBT, FIT, or stool test annually, with or without flexible sigmoidoscopy, every 5 yr • Flexible sigmoidoscopy alone every 5 yr • CT colonography every 5 yr • Colonoscopy every 10 yr (preferred)
USPSTF, 2008	Age 50-75 yr Average risk	One of the following: • Annual high-sensitivity FOBT • High-sensitivity FOBT every 3 yr combined with • Flexible sigmoidoscopy every 5 yr • Screening colonoscopy every 10 yr

ACS, American Cancer Society; *CT*, computed tomography; *FIT*, fecal immunochemical test; *gFOBT*, guaiac-based fecal occult blood test; *NCCN*, National Comprehensive Cancer Network; *USPSTF*, U.S. Preventive Services Task Force.

Data from American Cancer Society. (2013b). *Cancer facts and figures 2013*. Atlanta: American Cancer Society; NCCN. (2012b). *NCCN clinical practice guidelines in oncology. Colorectal cancer screening. Version V.1.2012.* http://www.nccn.org/professionals/physician_gls/pdf/colorectal_screening.pdf. Accessed 10/3/13; U.S. Preventive Services Task Force. (2008). *Screening for colorectal cancer.* http://www.uspreventiveservicestaskforce.org/uspstf08/colocancer/colors.htm. Accessed 10.03.13.

(7) Pap testing to begin at age 21 and performed every 3 to 5 years; yearly screening no longer recommended, because generally takes 10 to 20 years for cervical cancer to develop (ACS, 2013b)

b. Human papilloma virus (HPV) test

(1) HPV DNA assay is performed on liquid-based Pap specimen to identify if the oncogenic viral types are present (either as primary screening or as a "reflex test" if an abnormal Pap is reported).

(2) Positive test only indicates viral infection (which may be transient), not its oncogenic potential. Women with persistent infection with an oncogenic HPV have a much higher risk of developing cervical cancer compared with non–HPV-infected women.

2. Diagnosis

a. Colposcopy—primary method for evaluation of abnormal Pap tests

(1) Involves viewing the cervix though a long focal length dissecting microscope at magnification

(2) Acetic acid (4%) applied before viewing, which allows a directed biopsy of any grossly visible abnormalities

3. Controversy

a. Controversy exists regarding frequency, ways to implement HPV testing into routine screening practices, and the lack of applicability in developing countries (because of expense and lack of equipment and clinicians).

4. Cervical cancer screening recommendations (Table 2-3)

D. Prostate cancer (PC)

1. Screening modalities

a. Digital rectal examination (DRE)

b. Serum PSA

(1) PSA, a glycoprotein produced by prostatic epithelial cells, is the only tumor marker currently used in screening.

(2) Limited sensitivity and specificity

(a) Levels may be affected by age, presence of benign prostatic hypertrophy (BPH), inflammation, urethral or prostatic trauma, and ejaculation within recent 48 hours, as well as medications, including androgen deprivation therapy, 5-alpha-areductase inhibitors (i.e., finasteride), and ketoconazole.

(b) It is important to monitor PSA velocity and absolute quantitative PSA.

Table 2-3

Cervical Cancer Screening Recommendations

Organization	Population	Test and Schedule
ACS, 2013b, NCCN, 2012a	Between ages 21-29 yr	• Cytology (Pap test) alone every 3 yr • HPV testing is only needed after abnormal Pap results and is not recommended for routine screening in this age group.
	Ages 30-65 yr	HPV with Pap test every 5 yr (preferred) or every 3 yr with Pap alone (acceptable)
	Age > 65 yr	Women > 65 yr who have undergone regular cervical cancer testing with normal results should no longer be screened.
	Women who have had a hysterectomy should stop cervical cancer screening unless surgery was done to remove cervical cancer or precancerous lesion.	
USPSTF, 2012b	Ages 21-65 yr	Pap test every 3 yr or for women ages 30 to 65 yr who want to lengthen the screening interval, screening with a combination of Pap test and HPV testing every 5 yr

ACS, American Cancer Society; *HPV,* human papilloma virus; *NCCN,* National Comprehensive Cancer Network; *USPSTF,* U.S. Preventive Services Task Force.

Data from American Cancer Society. (2013b). *Cancer facts and figures 2013.* Atlanta: American Cancer Society; NCCN. (2012a). *NCCN clinical practice guidelines in oncology. Cervical cancer screening. Version 2.2012.* http://www.nccn.org/professionals/physician_gls/pdf/cervical_screening.pdf. Accessed 10.03.13; U.S. Preventive Services Task Force (2012b). *Screening for cervical cancer.* http://www.uspreventiveservicestaskforce.org/uspstf/uspscerv.htm. Accessed 10.03.13.

(3) Laboratory variability ranges from 20% to 25%.

(4) PSA assays are not interchangeable; therefore, the same assay should be used for longitudinal monitoring.

2. Diagnosis
   a. Ultrasound-guided prostatic biopsy is performed when PC is suspected.
      (1) Multiple areas of the prostate gland are biopsied.
      (2) Tumor histologic grade is based on the Gleason score (Gleason & Mellinger, 1974).
3. Controversy
   a. Use of PSA for prostate cancer screening is no longer unanimously recommended.
      (1) More than 70% of PCs are diagnosed with localized disease, which offers the greatest chance for cure.
      (2) PSA screening has not correlated with decreases in PC mortality and has instead prompted the use of aggressive therapies, which may cause significant side effects in many men who would never have required treatment either because of age or tumor growth pattern.
      (3) Currently, no reliable method is available to differentiate aggressive versus indolent disease prior to biopsy.
      (4) The level of PSA that should provoke biopsy is not clear, and the lower the PSA, the lower is the chance that the man has the disease (NCCN, 2012c).
      (5) Results of the European Randomized Study of Screening for Prostate Cancer demonstrated that 1055 men must be screened to identify 37 men who have PC.

Their treatment only prevents one PC death over 11 years of follow-up (Schroeder et al., 2012).

4. Prostate cancer screening recommendations (Table 2-4)

E. Lung cancer
   1. Modalities for lung cancer screening
      a. Chest x-ray (CXR)—no RCT evidence of effect on lung cancer mortality
      b. Sputum cytology with or without CXR—no RCT has demonstrated benefit of sputum cytology (NCCN, 2014).
      c. LDCT
         (1) Most sensitive test available
         (2) 20% reduction in lung cancer mortality demonstrated by National Lung Screening Trial using LDCT versus plain CXR in 53,454 high-risk participants (Aberle et al., 2011)
         (3) Screening not recommended for general population; screening to be considered for those between 55 and 80 years of age with at least a 30-pack-year smoking history and either continue to smoke or have quit less than 15 years ago (Humphrey et al., 2013; USPSTF, 2013)
   2. Controversy
      a. Tools currently available for lung cancer screening do not meet several of the criteria for screening.
      b. Screening would prevent 3.9 deaths over 6 years per 1000 persons (equates to screening 256 persons screened annually for 3 years to prevent one lung cancer death over 6 years).
      c. Cost of screened per life saved is not known, although it is likely very high, because approximately 95% false-positive results

Table 2-4

Prostate Cancer Screening Recommendations

Organization	Population	Test and Schedule
ACS, 2013b	Men with at least a 10-yr life expectancy should be given information regarding potential risks versus benefits and uncertainties associated with prostate cancer screening to allow them to make an informed consent to proceed.	
	Age 50 yr, if man chooses to proceed	PSA with or without DRE Those with PSA < 2.5 ng/mL may be retested every 2 yr. If PSA is ≥ 2.5, annual testing should be performed.
	Men at high risk who have one or more of the following: • African-American ethnicity • A father or brother diagnosed with PC before age 65	May begin screening starting at age 45 yr. Screening should include PSA with or without DRE. Frequency of testing depends on PSA level.
NCCN, 2012c	Age 40: Begin risk-benefit discussions about DRE and PSA.	For men who choose to proceed with screening, offer PSA and DRE. • If PSA < 1.0 ng/mL, repeat screening at age 45 yr. • If PSA is again < 1.0, offer next screening at age 50 yr and annually thereafter. • If PSA is ≥ 1.0 ng/mL, or patient is African American, has family history, or is taking 5-alpha-reductase inhibitors, annual DRE and PSA testing
USPTF, 2012a	USPTF recommends no screening for prostate cancer.	

ACS, American Cancer Society; *DRE,* digital rectal examination; *NCCN,* National Comprehensive Cancer Network; *ng/mL,* nanograms per milliliter; *PSA,* prostate-specific antigen; *USPSTF,* U.S. Preventive Services Task Force.

Data from American Cancer Society. (2013b). *Cancer facts and figures 2013.* Atlanta: American Cancer Society; NCCN. (2012). *NCCN guidelines. Version 2.2012. Prostate cancer early detection.* USPSTF (2012a). *Screening for prostate cancer.* http://www.nccn.org/professionals/physician_gls/pdf/prostate_detection.pdf. Accessed 12.06.13.

occurred, requiring additional tests, ongoing screening, and a relatively low absolute number of deaths prevented, 73 per 100,000 person-years (Aberle et al., 2011).
d. LDCT is expensive and not widely available.
e. Smoking prevention and cessation remain the most effective methods for decreasing lung cancer mortality rates.
3. Lung cancer screening guidelines (Table 2-5)

ASSESSMENT

I. History
  A. Demographics—age, gender, race, date and place of birth, occupation
  B. Chief complaint—brief description of reason for seeking care
  C. History of present illness: If presenting because of symptom(s), a complete symptom analysis is necessary: onset of symptom(s), location, duration, characteristics, any aggravating and relieving factors, and timing.
  D. Current medications (prescription, vitamins, herbals)
  E. Allergies (medications and environmental)
  F. Past medical history—previous state of health, previous cancer and cancer treatment, HPV vaccination, chronic illnesses, surgeries, hospitalizations
  G. Family history—medical and cancer histories in relatives

H. Social history (e.g., smoking [report in pack-years smoked and date stopped, if applicable], alcohol [quantify and date usage], illicit drug use [drug/route/dates used], sexual habits, dietary habits, sleep patterns, and exercise)
  I. Occupational history (any relevant exposures)
  J. Review of systems (Table 2-6)
II. Physical examination
  A. Even in the absence of symptoms, cancer-related physical assessment should include examination of the skin, mouth, neck, lymph nodes, breasts, cervix, pelvis, testicles, rectum, and prostate.
  B. Specific foci of physical examination are presented in Table 2-7.
III. Health counseling
  A. Teach and reinforce healthy lifestyle behaviors.
    1. Tobacco avoidance
    2. Maintaining a healthy weight
    3. Regular physical activity
    4. Eating a balanced diet that includes vegetables and fruits
    5. Limiting alcohol intake
    6. Skin protection from the sun
    7. Knowing personal family history and risks
    8. Maintaining regular checkups and cancer screening tests
  B. Teach BSE or testicular self-examination.
  C. Shared decision making regarding screening for cancers for which population-based screening is controversial

Table 2-5

Lung Cancer Screening Guidelines

Organization	Population	Test and Schedule
ACS, 2013b	Age 55-74 yr at high risk • Smoking history ≥ 30 pack-years in those who are currently smoking or quit within 15 yr	Low LDCT after a process of informed and shared decision making regarding limitations, potential benefits, potential harms associated with screening Smoking cessation remains a priority for clinical attention.
NCCN, 2014	Age 55-74 yr at high risk: • Current smokers with 30 pack-year history of smoking • History of ≥ 30 pack-years of smoking and quit within 15 years • History of ≥ 20 pack-years of smoking and one additional risk factor such as occupational exposure to arsenic, chromium, asbestos, nickel, cadmium, beryllium, silica, diesel fumes, coal smoke, soot • Residential exposure to radon • History of other cancers such as lymphoma, head and neck cancer, or other smoking-related cancers; family history of lung cancer in a first-degree relative; personal history of COPD, pulmonary fibrosis	LDCT Frequency of future screenings determined by findings.
	Moderate risk: • Age ≥ 50 yr with 20 or more pack-year history of smoking or second-hand smoke exposure, but no additional risk factors	Routine lung cancer screening not recommended
	Low risk: • Age < 50 yr and/or <20 pack-year history of smoking	Routine lung cancer screening not recommended
USPSTF, 2013	Age 55-79 yr with a 30 or more pack-year history; have smoked within the past 15 yr	Annual LDCT in persons who can undergo surgical resection if tumor is discovered because of comorbidities that shorten life expectancy

ACS, American Cancer Society; *LDCT,* low-dose computed tomography; *NCCN,* National Comprehensive Cancer Network; *USPSTF,* United States Preventative Services Task Force.

Data from American Cancer Society. (2013b). *Cancer facts and figures 2013.* Atlanta: American Cancer Society; NCCN. (2014). *NCCN clinical practice guidelines in oncology. Lung cancer screening.* Version 1.2013. http://www.nccn.org/professionals/physician_gls/pdf/lung_screening.pdf. Accessed 12.06.13; U.S. Preventive Services Task Force (2013). *Screening for lung cancer.* http://www.uspreventiveservicestaskforce.org/uspstf13/lungcan/lungcanfinalrs.htm. Accessed 12.06.13.

Table 2-6

Review of Cancer Related Symptoms

System	History Components or Symptoms: Particular Focus on Recent Change
Constitutional	Fatigue, malaise, recent weight gain or loss, previous and present level of activity Current performance status (note if changed, and when)
Skin	Changes in warts or moles; bleeding, nonhealing lesions, change in sensation History of skin cancer (record type, dates, treatment)
Head and neck	Pain, tenderness; mouth lesions; difficulty swallowing or chewing; hoarseness; discharge from eyes, ears, and nose; epistaxis.
Respiratory	Cough, pain, dyspnea, hemoptysis, shortness of breath Date and result of last imaging
Cardiac	Dyspnea, orthopnea, chest pain, edema, palpitations, dizziness
Gastrointestinal	Change in appetite, pain, reflux, nausea, vomiting, change in bowel pattern Dates and results of prior CRC screenings
Genitourinary	Change in urinary pattern, nocturia, dysuria, hematuria, change in force or caliber of stream, pain Testicular pain or masses Dates and results of prior PSA assessments

Continued

Table 2-6

Review of Cancer Related Symptoms—cont'd

System	History Components or Symptoms: Particular Focus on Recent Change
Gynecologic	Vaginal discharge, nonmenstrual or intermenstrual bleeding, bloating, enlarged abdominal girth Dates and results of prior Pap screens
Breasts	Change in appearance, skin, vascular pattern, nipple direction, inversion Mass in breast or axillae Dates and results of prior mammograms Any prior biopsies and results
Endocrine	Flushing, sweating, orthostasis, tachycardia, palpitations, polyuria, polydipsia
Hematologic/immunologic	Bruising, anemia, petechiae, purpura, bleeding disorder, anemia, fatigue, fever, infections, night sweats, chills, frequent infections, vaccines (especially HPV), enlarged lymph nodes, early satiety
Musculoskeletal	Pain and stiffness in bones and joints, limitation of movement, back pain, neck pain (history of trauma)
Neurologic	Headache, vertigo. seizures, syncope, visual disturbances Sensory, motor, memory or cognitive deficits Facial weakness, speech problems Personality change

CRC, Colorectal cancer; *HPV,* human papilloma virus; *PSA,* prostate-specific antigen.

Table 2-7

Physical Examination Foci

System	Components of Examination
Skin	Inspect (cutaneous and mucous membrane surfaces, especially sun-exposed areas such as face, chest, back, arms, legs, scalp, interdigital webs, axillae; palms of hands and soles of feet deserve particular attention). Note presence of rash, petechiae, bruising, ulcerations of color and surface, scaling, or bleeding.
Head, eyes	Inspect (shape, symmetry, nodules, masses, color of conjunctivae and sclerae, symmetry of pupils, reactivity, eye movements).
Ear, nose, and throat	Inspect (symmetry, presence of discharge, integrity of tissues—note polyps, exudate, friability, bleeding).
Oral cavity	Inspect (for color and integrity of mucous membranes, tongue, under tongue, lesions or plaques). Palpate (note masses and/or tenderness).
Neck	Inspect and palpate (entire neck for nodes—note, size, shape consistency, mobility, tenderness). Palpate thyroid (enlargement, consistency, nodules).
Chest	Inspect (symmetry, use of accessory muscles to breath.) Percuss for dullness. Auscultate (breath sounds—note presence of crackles, rhonchi, wheeze).
Breasts	Perform clinical breast examination with patient in upright and supine positions. Inspect (symmetry, dimpling, skin changes, irregular venous pattern, nipple direction, and nipple discharge). Palpate (for masses, including axillae for lymph nodes).
Abdomen	Inspect (symmetry, herniations, presence of surgical scars, abnormal vascular patterns). Auscultate (bowel sounds). Percuss (liver and spleen size). Palpate (for tenderness masses, inguinal lymph nodes.) Measure (organomegaly, masses, nodes).
Female genital	Inspect (masses, lesions, discharge or bleeding). Palpate (masses, tenderness, shape and consistency of abdominal organs, including uterus, ovaries, and colon).
Pelvic	Inspect (mucosal integrity and color of vaginal wall and cervix; presence of lesions, polyps, bleeding, or friability; discharge; constriction; nodules; masses). Perform Pap test.
Male genital	Inspect (for masses, shape of scrotum, cutaneous lesions, nodules.) Palpate (for tenderness, masses, consistency, contour, scrotal contents—testes, epididymis).
Rectal, prostate	Inspect (external lesions, hemorrhoids). Perform digital rectal examination (DRE) (note sphincter tone, masses, tenderness, constriction, bleeding). Assess and order stool test for occult blood with fecal occult blood test (FOBT) or fecal immunochemical test (FIT) (if indicated). In males, palpate prostate (note size, symmetry, consistency—firmness, tenderness, nodules).

PROBLEM STATEMENTS AND OUTCOME IDENTIFICATION

I. Readiness for Enhanced Health Management (NANDA-I)
   A. Expected outcome: Patient identifies personal risk factors for cancer.
   B. Expected outcome: Patient discusses recommendations for cancer screening and early detection.
   C. Expected outcome: Patient participates in recommended cancer screening and early detection activities.

II. Deficient Community Health (NANDA-I)
   A. Expected outcome: Individuals in the community participate in cancer screening programs.

PLANNING AND IMPLEMENTATION

I. Interventions to improve patient participation in screening programs
   A. Assess motivation and willingness of patient to learn.
   B. Identify cultural influences regarding health and health-seeking behaviors.
   C. Provide patient with personalized risk of developing cancer by use of health history and risk profiles.
   D. Assess barriers to participation in screening programs and implement strategies to overcome them—for example, transportation, child care, and cost.
   E. Provide teaching on the risk and benefits of screening based on patient's learning style (written, verbal, audiovisual presentation, or combination of these).

II. Interventions to provide education and follow-up care for clients with positive screening test results
   A. Identify resources for cancer education and information.
   B. Discuss implications of positive screening test results, and describe confirmatory evaluation.
   C. Reinforce importance of timely evaluation.
   D. Facilitate referral for further evaluation.
   E. Ensure adherence and follow-up for persons with positive screenings for cancer.
   F. Partner with the ACS and other organizations to facilitate transportation, arrange child care, and/or address other requirements to assist clients with positive screening results to receive required care.

III. Interventions to promote population-based screening programs
   A. Target high-risk groups (e.g., older adults, ethnic minority, poor) within respective community.
   B. Use media resources and community organizations (e.g., schools, churches, town hall meetings) to publicize benefits of screening and early detection.
   C. Collect data regarding outcomes of short-term measures.

   1. Number of individuals in the target population offered screening
   2. Number and proportion of those in the target population who were screened
   3. Number and proportion of the target population examined through multiple screening
   4. Number of preclinical cancers detected in persons with positive screening results leading to definitive diagnosis or follow-up
   5. Cost per cancer detected
   6. Sensitivity, specificity, positive and negative predictive values of the test(s)
   7. Costs of follow-up of false-positive results
   D. Collect data on long-term measures to use to evaluate and modify program.
   1. Stage distribution of detected cancers
   2. Case-fatality rate of screened individuals
   3. Site-specific cancer mortality rate of screened target population
   4. Total costs of screening the population
   5. Impact of early detection on quality of life (positive and negative)
   E. Routinely review screening guidelines and tests for incorporation into program.
   F. Employ skilled health care educators to ensure that the target population understands the disease and the importance of screening and early detection; the screening method being used, with the specific procedure planned, including potential risks; and plans designed for further evaluation and treatment, if deemed necessary on the basis of screening test results.

EVALUATION

The oncology nurse systematically and regularly evaluates the individual's and the population's responses to interventions to determine progress toward the achievement of expected outcomes. Relevant data are collected, actual findings are compared with expected findings (screening population's incidence of cancer, stage at diagnosis), and mortality statistics are compared with those of the nonscreened population as well as national averages. Nursing diagnoses, outcomes, and plans of care are reviewed and revised, as necessary.

References

Aberle, D. R., Adams, A. M., Berg, C. D., Black, W. G., Clapp, J. D., Fagerstrom, R. M., et al. (2011). Reduced lung-cancer mortality with low-dose computed tomographic screening. *New England Journal of Medicine*, 365, 395–409.

American Cancer Society. (2013a). *Breast cancer: Early detection.* http://www.cancer.org/cancer/breastcancer/moreinformation/ breastcancerearlydetection/breast-cancer-early-detection-toc.

American Cancer Society. (2013b). *Cancer facts and figures 2013.* Atlanta, GA: American Cancer Society.

American College of Radiology (ACR). (2003). *Breast imaging reporting and data system atlas (BI-RADS Atlas).* Reston, VA: American College of Radiology.

Atkin, W. S., Edwards, R., Kralj-Hans, I., Wooldrage, K., Hart, A. R., Northover, J. M., et al. (2010). Once-only flexible sigmoidoscopy screening in prevention of colorectal cancer: A multicenter randomized controlled trial. *The Lancet, 375*(9726), 1624–1633.

Church, T. R., & Mandel, J. S. (2011). Screening for gastrointestinal cancers. In V. T. Devita, T. S. Lawrence, S. A. Rosenberg, R. A. DePinho, & R. A. Wineburg (Eds.), *Cancer: Principles and practice of oncology.* (9th ed., pp. 596–602). Philadelphia, PA: Wolters Kluwer Health/Lippincott Williams & Wilkins.

Daly, M. B., & Rader, J. S. (2011). Screening for gynecologic cancers. In V. T. Devita, T. S. Lawrence, S. A. Rosenberg, R. A. DePinho, & R. A. Wineburg (Eds.), *Cancer: Principles and practice of oncology.* (9th ed., pp. 603–609). Philadelphia: Wolters Kluwer Health/Lippincott Williams & Wilkins.

Espino, V., Belluci, C., Petricoin, E. F., & Liotta, L. A. (2011). Early detection using proteomics. In V. T. Devita, T. S. Lawrence, S. A. Rosenberg, R. A. DePinho, & R. A. Wineburg (Eds.), *Cancer: Principles and practice of oncology* (9th ed., pp. 585–596). Philadelphia: Wolters Kluwer Health/Lippincott Williams & Wilkins.

Esserman, L. J., & Flowers, C. I. (2011). Screening for breast cancer. In V. T. Devita, T. S. Lawrence, S. A. Rosenberg, R. A. DePinho, & R. A. Wineburg (Eds.), *Cancer: Principles and practice of oncology* (9th ed., pp. 610–617). Philadelphia: Wolters Kluwer Health/Lippincott Williams & Wilkins.

Gail, M. H., Brinton, L. A., Byar, D. P., Corle, D. K., Green, S. B., Schairer, C., et al. (1989). Projecting individualized probabilities of developing breast cancer for white females who are being examined annually. *Journal of the National Cancer Institute, 81*(24), 1879–1886.

Gleason, D. F., & Mellinger, G. T. (1974). Prediction of prognosis for prostatic adenocarcinoma by combined histologic grading and clinical staging. *Journal of Urology, 111*(1), 58–64.

Humphrey, L. L., Deffebach, M., Pappas, M., Baumann, C., Artis, K., Mitchel, J. P., et al. (2013). Screening for lung cancer with low-dose computed tomography. A systematic review to update the U.S. Preventive Services Task Force recommendation. *Annals of Internal Medicine, 159*(6), 411–420.

Kalanger, M., Zelen, M., Langmark, F., & Adami, H. O. (2010). Effect of screening mammography on breast cancer mortality in Norway. *New England Journal of Medicine, 367*(13), 1203–1210.

Kosters, J. P., & Gotzsche, P. C. (2008). Regular self-breast examination or clinical examination for early detection of breast cancer. *Cochrane Database Systematic Review.* http://onlinelibrary.wiley.com/doi/10.1002/14651858.CD003373/abstract;jsessionid=D01FBED1514E1F3A9D78B541B0B05BE7.d02t04.

Mandel, J. S., & Smith, R. (2011). Principles of cancer screening. In V. T. Devita, T. S. Lawrence, S. A. Rosenberg, R. A. DePinho,

& R. A. Wineburg (Eds.), *Cancer: Principles and practice of oncology* (9th ed., pp. 582–587). Philadelphia, PA: Wolters Kluwer Health/Lippincott Williams & Wilkins.

National Cancer Institute. (2013). *Genetics of colorectal cancer PDQ.* http://www.cancer.gov/cancertopics/colorectal/health professionals#Section_12.

National Comprehensive Cancer Network (NCCN). (2012a). *NCCN clinical practice guidelines in oncology. Cervical cancer screening. Version 2.2012.* http://www.nccn.org/professionals/physician_gls/pdf/cervical_screening.pdf.

National Comprehensive Cancer Network (NCCN). (2012b). *NCCN clinical practice guidelines in oncology. Colorectal cancer screening. Version V.1.2012.* <http://www.nccn.org/professionals/physician_gls/pdf/colorectal_screening.pdf/>.

National Comprehensive Cancer Network (NCCN). (2012c). *NCCN guidelines. Version 2.2012. Prostate cancer early detection.* http://www.nccn.org/professionals/physician_gls/pdf/prostate_detection.pdf.

National Comprehensive Cancer Network (NCCN). (2013). *NCCN clinical practice guidelines. Breast cancer screening. Version 1:2013. Breast cancer screening and diagnosis.* http://www.nccn.org/professionals/physician_gls/pdf/ breast-screening.pdf.

National Comprehensive Cancer Network (NCCN). (2014). *NCCN clinical practice guidelines in oncology. Lung cancer screening. Version 1.2013.* Retrieved from, http://www.nccn.org/professionals/physician_gls/pdf/lung_screening.pdf.

Pox, C. (2011). Colon cancer screening: which non-invasive filter tests? *Digestive Diseases, 29*(Suppl. 1), 56–59.

Schroeder, F. H., Hugosson, J., Roobol, M. J., Tammela, T. L., Ciatto, S., Nelen, V., et al. (2012). Prostate-cancer mortality at 11 years of follow up. *New England Journal of Medicine, 366,* 981–990.

Solomon, D., Davey, D., Kurman, R., Moriarty, A., O'Conner, D., Prey, M., et al. (2002). The 2001 Bethesda system. Terminology for reporting results of cervical cytology. *Journal of the American Medical Association, 287*(16), 2114–2119.

U.S. Preventive Services Task Force Cancer. (2008). *Screening for colorectal cancer.* http://www.uspreventiveservicestaskforce.org/uspstf08/colocancer/colors.htm.

U.S. Preventive Services Task Force. (2009). *Screening for breast cancer.* http://www.uspreventiveservicestaskforce.org/uspstf/uspsbrca.htm.

U.S. Preventive Services Task Force. (2012a). *Screening for prostate cancer.* http://uspreventiveservicestaskforce.org/prostatecancerscreening.htm.

U.S. Preventive Services Task Force. (2012b). *Screening for cervical cancer.* <http://www.uspreventiveservicestaskforce.org/uspstf/uspscerv.htm/>.

U.S. Preventive Services Task Force. (2013). *Screening for lung cancer.* http://www.uspreventiveservicestaskforce.org/uspstf13/lungcan/lungcanfinalrs.htm.

CHAPTER 3
Carcinogenesis

Jennifer Alisangco Tschanz and Cathleen Sugarman

THEORY

I. What is cancer?
  A. Definition of cancer (Cancer, n.d.)
    1. "A neoplasm characterized by the uncontrolled growth of anaplastic cells that tend to invade surrounding tissue and metastasize to distant body sites."
    2. "Any of a larger group of malignant neoplastic disease characterized by the presence of malignant cells. Each cancer is distinguished by the nature, site, or clinical course of the lesion."
  B. Pathology of carcinogenic change: Cancer arises from the combination of multiple mutations in a cell's genes, genomic instability, and inflammation.
    1. Mutations in regulatory cells
      a. *Proto-oncogenes:* Proto-oncogenes are genes that code for proteins involved in normal cell growth. When mutated, they may enable a cancer cell to be self-sufficient in growth. A commonly used analogy is that these genes, when mutated, are like a car's gas pedal that is stuck.
        (1) *Ras* is a commonly mutated proto-oncogene, especially in pancreatic and colorectal cancers. A point mutation can change *Ras* from a proto-oncogene to an oncogene.
      b. *Tumor suppressor genes:* Tumor suppressor genes in normal cells control proliferation by preventing uncontrolled growth. When mutated in cancer cells, these genes no longer suppress proliferation. In the car analogy, these genes, when mutated, are like the brake pedal that does not work.
        (1) The *RB* gene normally inhibits cell division. This gene is mutated in childhood retinoblastoma and many lung, breast, and bone cancers (Virshup, 2012).
      c. Deoxyribonucleic acid (DNA) repair genes are needed in normal cells to correct mistakes that might be caused by carcinogens during replication. In some individuals, these genes may not be functional, which makes it easier for a mutation to result in cancer. These genes are sometimes referred to as the *caretaker genes.*
        (1) *BRCA1* and *BRCA2* are examples. When a person inherits a mutated copy of the gene, he or she is more susceptible to breast, ovarian, and prostate cancers (Latendresse & McCance, 2012).
      d. Epigenetic changes are just beginning to be appreciated in the field of cancer research. *Epigenetics* describes a mechanism that may change the activity of a gene without changing the sequence of DNA. An example of an epigenetic mechanism is DNA methylation. Adding or removing methyl groups from DNA affects the transcription of genes. The addition or subtraction of methyl groups may be affected by diet and the environment, among other things. If DNA is not transcribed, it is essentially silenced. Some kinds of cancer are associated with hypermethylation of the regulatory regions of genes. Other cancers are associated with lack of methylation, which makes it easier for these genes to be overexpressed. Hypomethylation may also contribute to cancer when it is a tumor suppressor gene that is not being transcribed (Stricker & Kumar, 2010).
      e. Chromosome translocations result when pieces of one chromosome move to another chromosome as the cell divides. This type of genetic alteration may activate an oncogene.
        (1) The *MYC* proto-oncogene is normally located on chromosome 8. In the Burkitt lymphoma cells, this portion of DNA is relocated to chromosome 14.
        (2) In chronic myeloid leukemia (CML), the *BCR* gene on chromosome 9 is fused to the *Abl* gene on chromosome 22. This

translation is also known as the *Philadelphia chromosome*. This fusion makes a protein called a *tyrosine kinase*, which promotes proliferation of myeloid cells. Imatinib, the original targeted tyrosine kinase inhibitor, was designed to specifically inhibit this pathway.

2. Genomic instability: Cancer cells have defects in the mechanisms that regulate genome replication and chromosomal segregation. This defective regulation results in an increased rate of genetic alterations compared with normal cells. In other words, the genetic make-up of cancer cells is less stable than that of normal cells. Clonal evolution describes the process of cells within a tumor accumulating genetic changes over time that are different from one cell to the next. This genomic instability is a hallmark of cancer cells and increases the pace of clonal evolution in tumors (Bunz, 2010).

   a. Hereditary nonpolyposis colon cancer syndrome (HNPCC) is characterized by microsatellite instability (MSI). Microsatellites are a series of tandem repeated nucleotides. The variation in the number of these tandem repeated nucleotides can be identified in pathology. Normal cells have a consistent length of nucleotides (Stricker & Kumar, 2010).

3. Inflammation may activate tumor bioactive molecules that enhance the process of carcinogenesis (Hanahan & Weinberg, 2011).

   a. An example is tumor necrosis factor (TNF). This cytokine may have an antitumor effect (in immune surveillance); however, it plays a role in carcinogenesis as well.

   b. Some chronic inflammatory conditions are associated with tumor formation (Table 3-1).

4. Interactions between tumor cells and the surrounding normal tissue's stroma or the environment contribute to the growth and evolution of cancer (Figure 3-1).

   a. The stroma consists of connective tissue, blood vessels, immune inflammatory cells such as macrophages and lymphocytes, and associated fibroblasts.

   b. Communication and signaling between tumor cells and normal stroma cells lead to tumor growth and metastasis through a multitude of reciprocal pathways that transform both the normal tissue and the tumor. For example, tumors may elicit immune and stromal responses to stimulate formation of new blood vessels (angiogenesis). These multiple and

Table 3-1

Chronic Inflammatory Conditions Associated with Tumor Formation

Pathologic Condition	Etiologic Agent	Associated Tumor(s)
Asbestosis, silicosis	Asbestos fibers, silica particles	Mesothelioma, lung carcinoma
Bronchitis (nitrosamines, peroxides)	Asbestos, silica, smoking	Lung carcinoma
Chronic pancreatitis	Genetic (mutation in trypsinogen gene on chromosome 7), alcoholism, smoking	Pancreatic carcinoma
Cystitis, bladder	Chronic indwelling, urinary inflammation catheters	Bladder carcinoma
Epidermolysis bullosa	Genetic, mechanical	Squamous cell carcinoma (SCC)
Gingivitis, lichen planus		Oral SCC
Hematochromatosis	Genetic	Liver
Inflammatory bowel disease, Crohn disease, chronic ulcerative colitis		Colorectal carcinoma, small intestine carcinoma
Lichen sclerosus		Vulvar SCC
Liver cirrhosis	Alcoholism	Hepatocellular carcinoma
Reflux esophagitis, Barrett esophagus	Gastric acid, alcoholism, smoking	Esophageal carcinoma
Severe thermal injury		Marjolin ulcer (SCC)
Sialadenitis		Salivary gland carcinoma
Sjögren syndrome, Hashimoto thyroiditis		Mucosa-associated lymphoid tissue, lymphomas
Sunburned skin, burn scar	Ultraviolet light	Basal cell carcinoma, SCC, melanoma

Adapted from Devita, V.T., Lawrence, T.S., Rosenberg, S.A., DePinho, R.A., Weinberg, R.A. (Eds.). (2011). *DeVita, Hellman, and Rosenberg's cancer: Principles and practice of oncology* (9th ed.). Philadelphia: Lippincott Williams & Wilkins.

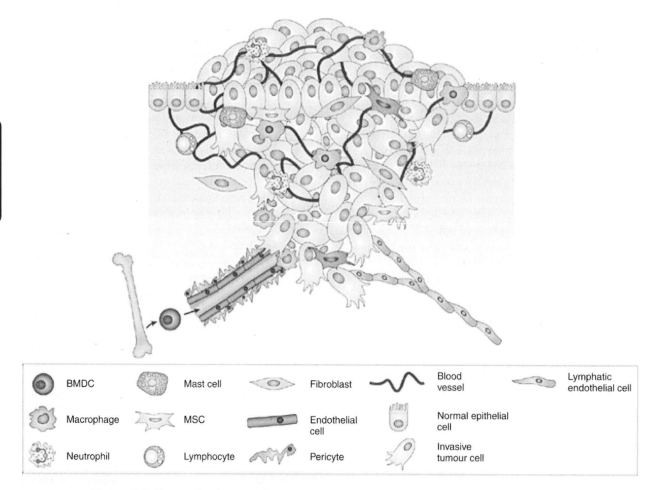

Figure 3-1 Cancers live in a complex microenvironment. From Joyce, J. A., Pollard, J. W. (2009). Microenvironmental regulation of metastasis. *Nature Review of Cancer, 9,* 239–252.

complex interactions are the focus of current cancer research (Hallahan & Weinberg, 2011).

c. For example, transforming growth factor alpha (TGF-α) or the epidermal growth factor receptor (EGFR) signaling pathway plays a role in some colon cancer metastases. Some metastatic colon cancer cells produce five times more EGFR compared with nonmetastatic cells. TGF-α initiates angiogenic processes in normal endothelial cells. The signal is mediated by EGFR in both the colon cancer and resident endothelial populations. When combined with vascular endothelial growth factor (VEGF) production, lymphangiogenesis is stimulated, and tumor cells may spread to regional lymph nodes. The use of cetuximab, a monoclonal antibody that blocks ligand binding to EGFR, has been used in EGFR-positive patients to reduce primary tumor size and lymphatic spread (Langley & Fidler, 2011).

C. Carcinogenesis is the process of initiating and promoting cancer through the action of biologic, chemical, or physical agents. *Carcinogenesis* is synonymous with the term *oncogenesis* (Carcinogenesis, n.d.; Oncogenesis, n.d.).

1. Several theories have been proposed to explain how and why cancer occurs. The theories continue to evolve as our understanding of cancer biology continues to grow. Some theories overlap (Table 3-2).

2. Nowell's theory of clonal evolution is an overarching theory that has three decades of evidence to support it (Nowell, 1976).

   a. Clonal cells are cells that can be traced to a single origin.

   b. Clonal cells have mutations that may give their cell lineage a survival advantage or disadvantage.

   c. With cumulative mutations, the hallmarks of cancer, or the characteristics that allow cancer cells to proliferate and spread, may be acquired.

   d. Different clones may arise from the same tumor, and clones change over time and in response to treatments.

Table 3-2

Key Points and Major Theories of Carcinogenesis

Theory of clonal expansion	All the cells in a tumor can be traced to a single origin. Mutations occur in these cells that give their lineage a survival advantage or disadvantage.
Multistep	Carcinogenesis is a multistep process that involves initiation, promotion, and progression steps.
Mutagenesis	Cancer is caused by changes in genetic information.
Epigenetics	Cancer may be caused by factors that do not change the DNA but change the way it is translated and expressed in proteins.
Oncogene hypothesis	All cells have genes that are involved in cell growth signaling and proliferation. Cancer may result in mutations to these genes.
Tumor suppressor gene	Genes that slow and prevent the growth of cells, if lost or mutated, may make a cell cancerous.
Knudsen's two-hit hypothesis	Two mutations, by deletion, epigenetics, or random mutation, are required for cancer to grow, one on each allele of a gene.
Cancer stem cell hypothesis	Within a tumor, some cells create new tumor cells and direct the growth of the tumor. They have self-renewal capacity like other stem cells, but are not derived from either stem cells or tissue of origin.
Immunosurveillance theory	Cells of the immune system patrol the body looking to destroy cancer cells and precancerous cells.
Cancer as speciation	Cancer cells represent a return to a more primitive unicellular organism distinct from their host.

Part 2

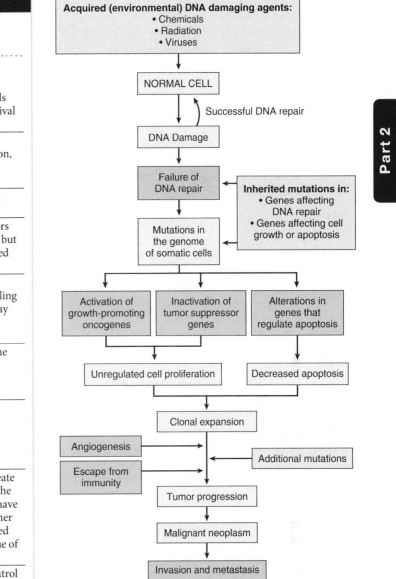

Figure 3-2 Flow chart depicting a simplified scheme of the molecular basis of cancer From Kumar et al. (Eds.) (2009). *Robbins and Cotran pathologic basis of disease* (8th ed.) Philadelphia: Saunders.

f. This spatial variation may explain disease progression and treatment response over time.

g. Future implications

(1) Genome sequencing over the life of the tumor may help direct treatment.

(2) Current studies are investigating the technique of locating circulating tumor DNA to identify the status of a tumor and its responsiveness to treatment (Aparicio & Caldes, 2013).

3. Process of carcinogenesis (Figure 3-2)

II. Characteristics of cancer cells

A. Microscopic studies show structural changes in cancer cells that are described in pathologic terms such as the following:

1. Pleiomorphism—cells variable in size and shape

2. Hyperchromatism—nuclear chromatin more pronounced on staining

3. Polymorphism—nucleus enlarged and variable in shape

4. Abnormal chromosome arrangements (Virshup, 2012)

a. Translocation—exchange of material between chromosomes

b. Deletions—loss of chromosome segments

c. Amplification—increase in the number of copies of a DNA sequence

d. Aneuploidy—abnormal number of chromosomes

B. Biochemical studies show differences in cell metabolism and products such as the following:

1. Cell membrane changes (Stricker & Kumar, 2010)

   a. Production of surface enzymes that may aid in invasion and metastasis

   b. Loss of glycoproteins that normally aid in cell-to-cell adhesion and organization

   c. Production of abnormal growth factor receptors that may independently "signal" the cell to grow and may cause the cell to be highly sensitive to presence of normal growth factors

   d. Abnormal receptors that may activate these signals without exposure to a growth factor and may persist in delivering signals to the cell

   e. Loss of antigens that otherwise label the cell as "self," and production of new tumor-associated antigens that mark the cell as "non-self"

      (1) Oncofetal antigens—antigens that are expressed by certain normal cells during fetal development but are subsequently suppressed; may reappear when cell becomes malignant—examples:

         (a) Carcinoembryonic antigen (CEA)—may be elevated in colorectal, breast, lung, liver, pancreatic, and gynecologic cancers

         (b) Alpha-fetoprotein (AFP)—may be elevated in hepatocellular, testicular, lung, pancreatic, and ovarian cancers

         (c) Placental antigens—antigens normally produced by the placenta; for example, human chorionic gonadotropin (HCG) and human placental lactogen (HPL), which usually are associated with gynecologic cancers

      (2) Prostate-specific antigen (PSA)—protein produced by prostate gland cells; elevation in PSA may indicate prostate cancer

      (3) Differentiation antigens, which are found in normal differentiating tissue; associated with acute lymphocytic leukemia (ALL), chronic lymphocytic leukemia (CLL), and lymphoblastic lymphoma

      (4) Lineage-associated determination antigens such as CA-125, which is associated with ovarian cancer

      (5) Viral antigens—appear in certain cancers associated with viral origins

   f. Clinical usefulness—certain tumor antigens may be used as *tumor markers*, which are biochemical substances synthesized and released by tumor cells (Table 3-3).

      (1) May be used as indicators of tumor presence

      (2) May also be present in a variety of benign conditions; many tumor markers lack specificity to cancer

      (3) Most often not used for screening but as a tool to monitor response to therapy

2. Abnormal glycolysis—higher rate of anaerobic glycolysis, making the cell less dependent on oxygen

---

Table 3-3

Examples of Tumor Markers

Marker Name	Nature	Type of Tumor
Alpha-fetoprotein (AFP)	70-kDa protein	Hepatic, germ cell
Carcinoembryonic antigen (CEA)	200-kDa glycoprotein	GI, pancreas, lung, breast
Beta-human chorionic gonadotropin (ß-HCG)	Glycopeptide hormone	Germ cell
Prostate-specific antigen (PSA)	33-kDa glycoprotein	Prostate
Catecholamines	Epinephrine and precursors	Pheochromocytoma (adrenal medulla)
Homovanillic acid/vanillylmandelic acid (HVA/VMA)	Catecholamine metabolites	Neuroblastoma
Urinary Bence Jones protein	Immunoglobulin (Ig) light chain	Multiple myeloma
Adrenocorticotropic hormone (ACTH)	Peptide hormone	Pituitary adenomas

GI, Gastrointestinal; *Ig*, immunoglobulin; *kDa*, kilodalton(s).

From Huether, S.E. & McCance, K.L. (Eds.). (2011). *Understanding pathophysiology* (5th ed.) (pp. 222-252). St. Louis: Elsevier.

3. Abnormal production of substances that give rise to paraneoplastic syndromes (signs or symptoms that occur in a client with cancer but are not due directly to the local effects of the tumor)

C. Cell kinetic growth and division

1. Increased mitotic index (the proportion of cells in a tissue that are in mitosis at any given time)
   a. Large numbers of mitotic cells reflect the higher proliferative activity of the tumor.
   b. A high mitotic index is not unique to cancer; normal cells in the gastrointestinal (GI) system, bone marrow, and hair follicles have a rapid rate of cell turnover and thus a high mitotic index.

2. Abnormal cell differentiation
   a. Differentiation—refers to the extent to which tumor cells resemble comparable normal cells, both morphologically and functionally
      (1) Grade—an evaluation of the degree of differentiation of the malignant cells
      (2) Grading criteria—vary greatly for different tumors; based on degree to which tumor cells resemble their normal counterpart
      (3) Tumors often characterized as grade I, II, III, or IV
          (a) Grade 1—well differentiated; also termed *low grade*
          (b) Grade II—moderately differentiated; also termed *intermediate grade*
          (c) Grade III—poorly differentiated; also termed *high grade*
          (d) Grade IV—undifferentiated; also termed *high grade*
      (4) Benign tumors composed of well-differentiated cells; tend to resemble the mature, functionally normal cells of the tissue of origin
      (5) Malignant tumors may be composed of cells that range from well-differentiated to undifferentiated, primitive cells
      (6) Anaplasia, or lack of differentiation—a hallmark of malignancy and the result of proliferation of transformed cells that do not mature
   b. Functional changes
      (1) The greater the degree of differentiation of a cell, the more likely it will have some part of the functional capabilities of its normal counterpart.
      (2) The more anaplastic the tumor, the less likely it is that any specialized function will be present.

3. Growth characteristics—the length of time required for a tumor to become clinically detectable is influenced by the following (Cooper & Cooper, 2001):
   a. Growth fraction—the fraction of proliferating cells in the tumor
      (1) Normal tissue—growth fraction varies depending on type of tissue. For example, intestinal epithelium contains approximately 16% actively proliferating cells; central nervous system (CNS) cells are nonproliferating.
      (2) Type of malignancy—growth fractions also vary, depending on type of cancer. For example, in many solid tumors, 1% to 8% of cells are actively proliferating.
   b. Tumor doubling, also called *doubling time*—the time within which the total cancer cell population doubles; influenced by tumor type because since most tumors have a high proportion of nonproliferating cells, and tumor vascularity
   c. Hormone levels—certain cancers arise from hormone-dependent tissues and require hormones for growth
      (1) Reduction in hormone levels reduces tumor growth.
      (2) Increased hormone levels promote growth.
   d. Gompertzian growth—refers to a hypothetical growth curve over the lifetime of an "average" tumor (Figure 3-3)

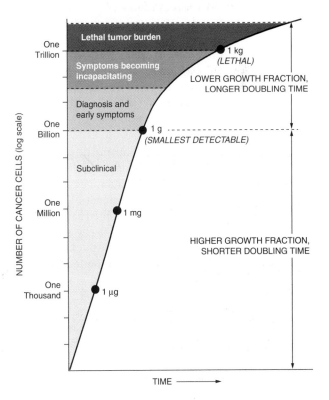

Figure 3-3 Gompertzian function. From Lehne, R. (2012). *Pharmacology for nursing care* (8th ed.). Philadelphia: Saunders.

(1) Growth increases exponentially at first (tumor growth doubles constantly over time).

(2) Growth then slows because of hypoxia, decreased availability of nutrients, and growth factors, toxins, and faulty cell-to-cell communication.

e. Wide variance in tumor growth rates

(1) Smallest clinically detectable mass equals 1 gram (g) in weight, 1 cubic centimeter (cm^3) in diameter, one billion cells, or approximately 30 tumor volume–doubling times.

(2) Tumors increase in size because the rate of cell production exceeds the rate of cell death.

D. Tumor growth patterns

1. Noncancerous and precancerous growth changes

a. *Hyperplasia*—an increase in the number of cells in a tissue

(1) May be a normal process (e.g., tissue hyperplasia that occurs in wound healing)

(2) May occur in cancer but is not a unique or defining characteristic

b. Metaplasia—potentially reversible process involving replacement of one mature cell type by another mature cell type not usually found in the involved tissue (Virshup, 2012)

c. Dysplasia—alteration in normal adult epithelial cells (Virshup, 2012)

(1) Loss of uniformity of cells; also characterized by variations in cell size, shape, organization (architecture)

2. Cancerous conditions

a. *Anaplasia*—most often used to describe malignancy

(1) Cytologic and positional disorganization of cells

(2) Varying degree of anaplastic changes

(3) Cells tend to be poorly differentiated and vary in sizes and shapes

(4) Cell nuclei disproportionately large

b. *Neoplasm* versus *tumor*—interchangeable terms

(1) Refers to abnormal growth of tissue that serves no function and continues to grow unchecked

(2) Can be benign or malignant

c. *Cancer*—common term for all malignancies

E. Hallmarks of cancer—refers to the biologic capabilities that a cancer cell acquires in a progressive multistep process that transforms a normal cell to a malignant cell, as described below (Hanahan & Weinberg, 2011). Tumors consist of tissues made up of distinct cell types with various mutations. When the tumor gains a variety of

clonally evolved and mutated cells that collectively have all the hallmarks of cancer, it is considered malignant (Figure 3-4).

1. Cancer cells sustain proliferative signaling.

a. Normal cells regulate proliferation with growth-promoting signals that start and stop mitosis.

b. Some cancer cells deregulate the signals through various means, including the following:

(1) Cancer cells may produce growth factors themselves.

(2) Cancer cells may send signals to stimulate normal cells to supply cancer cells with growth factors.

(3) Cancer cells may have mutations that disrupt negative feedback signaling.

c. Example: The Ras oncoprotein normally signals cells to stop proliferating. Mutated *ras* inactivates the negative feedback mechanism, and cancer cells consequently keep proliferating or producing. This is a prevalent mutation in many human cancers.

2. Cancer cells evade growth suppressors.

a. Normal cells regulate growth with tumor suppressor genes that lead to senescence (cellular aging) and apoptosis (programmed cell death). Cell growth is also limited by contact inhibition (cell growth and division stops on physical contact with other cells).

b. Some cancer cells have mutations that disable gatekeeper proteins controlling mitoses. Contact inhibition is inactivated.

3. Cancer cells resist cell death.

a. Normal cells experience apoptosis, or programmed cell death. A process called *autophagy* allows normal cells to be broken down during cellular stress so that organelles and cell contents can be reused in other cells.

b. It is still unclear how cancer cells evade programmed cell death. It is believed that cancer cells might use autophagy to survive in nutrient-deprived conditions. Necrotic cells may release proinflammatory signals that may promote growth of cancer cells.

4. Cancer cells enable replicative immortality.

a. Normal cells have a limited number of growth and division cycles because of senescence (a nonproliferative but viable state) and crisis (involves cell death).

b. Normal cells have limited amounts of telomerase, an enzyme that adds telomere repeat segments. Telomeres are protective DNA at the ends of chromosomes that shorten with repeated cell duplication. An analogy for the protective effects of telomere DNA is the protective coating at the end of shoelaces that prevent fraying. When the

Part 2

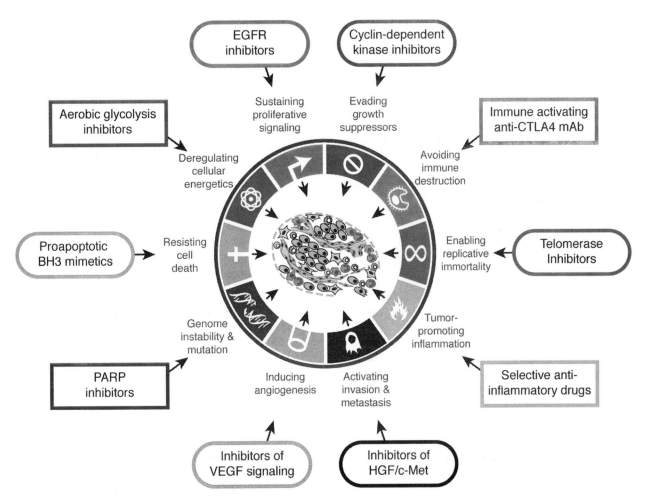

Figure 3-4 Therapeutic targets of the hallmarks of cancer. From Hanahan, D. & Weinberg, R. A. (2011). Hallmarks of cancer: The next generation. *Cell, 144,* 646–674.

shortened ends reach a critical level, they signal cell death (Virshup, 2012).

c. Cancer cells contain high amounts of telomerase, which adds protective telomeres and prevents the telomere segment from shortening. This process is believed to allow continued cell replication and contributes to immortalization wherein cells avoid or survive crises.

5. Cancer cells induce angiogenesis.

a. Angiogenesis is the creation of new blood vessels from existing ones to provide nutrients and remove waste products.

b. In normal tissues, angiogenesis takes place during embryogenesis with tissue and organ development. The process happens transiently in adulthood for wound healing and during female reproductive cycling. Otherwise, the process is dormant (Figure 3-5).

6. Cancer cells have the ability to secrete substances such as VEGFs, which stimulate angiogenesis to support continued tumor growth. The stimulation may lead to the creation of new

growing vessels that supply nutrients to tumors. Cancer cells activate invasion and metastasis.

a. Normal cells have a developmental regulatory program called *epithelial-mesenchymal transition* (EMT). This process causes epithelial cells to lose cell polarity and cell-cell adhesion and have invasive properties so that they can become mesenchymal cells. This process is involved in mesoderm formation and neural tube formation during embryogenesis. It has also been found to play a role in wound healing and organ fibrosis (Kalluri & Weinberg, 2009). Cancer cells appear to use this mechanism during invasion and metastasis. Little is understood about the way that cancer cells exploit this regulatory program.

7. Cancer cells have altered energy metabolism.

a. Normal cells in the presence of oxygen metabolize glucose to pyruvate and then carbon dioxide. In conditions where oxygen is limited, they favor glycolysis. Embryonic cells

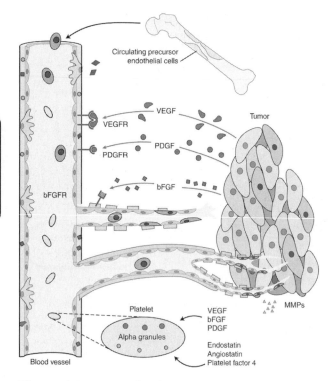

Figure 3-5 Tumor-induced angiogenesis. Adapted from Folkman, J. (2007). Angiogenesis: An organizing principle for drug discovery? *Nature Review of Drug Discovery, 6*(4), 273–286.

also use the glycolysis process in the presence of oxygen.

   b. Cancer cells use mostly glycolysis for energy production, even in the presence of oxygen.

   c. The mechanism of this change is unclear. It is not completely evident how using this less efficient method of adenosine triphosphate (ATP) production could be beneficial to the cancer cell.

8. Cancer cells evade immune destruction.

   a. Evidence indicates that deficiencies in T lymphocytes, T helper cells, and natural killer (NK) cells increase the risk of cancer development.

   b. Chronically immunosuppressed patients are more likely to get viral forms of cancer but not significantly more nonviral cancers compared with immunocompetent patients.

   c. Thus, successful cancer therapy may require a multitargeted approach.

III. Carcinogens

   A. Physical carcinogens

      1. Radiation

         a. Ionizing radiation contributes to carcinogenesis by damaging DNA.

         b. Ionizing radiation exposure in human is mostly from natural sources, the largest of which is radon (Krewski et al, 2005).

         c. Diagnostic radiography and computed tomography (CT) are medical sources of exposure.

         d. Environmental exposure can also come from atomic bombs or leaking nuclear energy plants (Ljungman, 2011).

         e. Thyroid cancer and acute and chronic myeloid leukemias are the most common cancers associated with radiation exposure.

         f. Breast, lung, and salivary gland tumors are also associated with radiation exposure.

         g. The age at exposure influences the likelihood of developing cancer after ionizing radiation, with younger children being more susceptible.

         h. Ultraviolet (UV) radiation from sunlight exposure and tanning beds is associated with an increased risk of skin cancer (melanoma, basal cell and squamous cell carcinomas).

         i. The UVB spectrum of light is carcinogenic because it forms pyrimidine dimers in DNA (Stricker & Kumar, 2010).

   B. Chemical carcinogens

      1. The first associations of chemicals causing cancer came from the observation that certain professions had a higher incidence of particular cancers. See Table 3-4 for some examples of chemical carcinogens and the cancers they cause.

      2. Generally, humans are protected from the effects of chemical carcinogens by DNA repair mechanisms.

      3. Genetic susceptibility to particular carcinogens may be inherited, but the interaction of the environment with the genome is rather complex and not fully understood.

      4. Emerging technology related to genomic and other related biologic systems in cells has begun to identify biomarkers that will potentially identify individuals or populations with increased risk associated with particular chemical carcinogens.

   C. Viruses, both ribonucleic acid (RNA) and DNA viruses, have been linked to human cancer, with DNA viruses being more prevalent. See Table 3-5 for a list of the most common viruses and the tumors they can cause (Yuspa & Shields, 2011).

IV. *Metastasis* is the spread of cancer cells from the site of the original tumor or organ to distant tissues and organs in the body.

   A. "Metastasis is regarded as a highly inefficient process in that less than 0.01% of circulating tumor cells eventually succeeds in forming secondary tumor growths. Studies examining the individual steps in the metastatic process determined that initiating cell growth in secondary organs is the

Table 3-4

Known or Suspected Chemical Carcinogens in Humans*

Target Organ	Agents	Tumor Type	Industries
Lung	Tobacco smoke, arsenic, asbestos, crystalline silica, benzo(a)pyrene, beryllium, bis(chloro) methyl ether, 1,3-butadiene, chromium VI compounds, coal tar and pitch, nickel compounds, soots, mustard gas, cobalt-tungsten carbide powders	Squamous large cell and small cell cancers, adenocarcinoma	Aluminum production, coal gasification, coke production, hematite mining, painting, grinding in oil and gas
Pleura	Asbestos, erionite	Mesothelioma	Insulation, mining
Oral cavity	Tobacco smoke, alcoholic beverages, nickel compounds	Squamous cell cancer	Boot and shoe production, furniture manufacturer, isopropyl alcohol production
Esophagus	Tobacco smoke, alcoholic beverages	Squamous cell cancer	
Gastric	Smoked, salted, and pickled foods	Adenocarcinoma	Rubber industry
Colon	Heterocyclic amines, asbestos	Adenocarcinoma	Pattern making
Liver	Aflatoxin, vinyl chloride, tobacco smoke, alcoholic beverages, thorium dioxide	Hepatocellular carcinoma, hemangiosarcoma	
Kidney	Tobacco smoke, phenacetin	Renal cell cancer	
Bladder	Tobacco smoke, 4-aminobiphenyl, benzidine, 2-napthylamine, phenacetin	Transitional cell carcinoma	Magenta manufacturing, auramine manufacturing
Prostate	Cadmium	Adenocarcinoma	
Skin	Arsenic, benzo(a)pyrene, coal tar and pitch, mineral oils, soots, cyclosporine A, Psoralen UV-A	Squamous cell cancer, basal cell cancer	Coal gasification, coke production
Bone marrow	Benzene, tobacco smoke, ethylene oxide, antineoplastic agents, cyclosporine A	Leukemia, lymphoma	Rubber industry

*These carcinogen designations do not imply proof of carcinogenicity in individuals. This table is not all-inclusive. For additional information, the reader is referred to agency documents and publications.

Adapted from Devita, V. T., Lawrence, T. S., Rosenberg, S. A., DePinho, R. A., & Weinberg, R. A. (Eds.). (2011). *DeVita, Hellman, and Rosenberg's cancer: Principles and practice of oncology* (9th ed.). Philadelphia: Lippincott Williams & Wilkins.

Table 3-5

Human Viruses with Oncogenic Properties

Virus Family	Type	Cofactors	Associated Human Tumors
Adenovirus	Types 2, 5, 12		Not associated with human cancer
Flaviviruses	HCV		Hepatocellular carcinoma
Hepadnavirus	HBV	Aflatoxin, alcohol, smoking	Hepatocellular carcinoma
Herpes viruses	EBV	Malaria Immunodeficiency Nitrosamines	Burkitt lymphoma Immunoblastic lymphoma Nasopharyngeal carcinoma Hodgkin lymphoma Leiomyosarcomas Gastric cancers
	KSHV (HSV8)	HIV infection HIV infection HIV infection	Kaposi sarcoma Pulmonary effusion lymphoma Castleman disease
Papillomaviruses	HPV-16, -18, -33, -39, others	Smoking, other factors	Anogenital cancers and some upper airway cancers
	HPV-5, -8, -17, others	EV, sunlight, immunosuppression	Non-melanoma skin cancer
Polyomavirus	Merkel cell virus SV40 (monkey virus) JC virus BK virus	Immunosuppression	Merkel cell carcinoma Brain tumors, non-Hodgkin lymphomas, mesotheliomas Brain tumors Prostate cancer
Retroviruses	HTLV-1	Uncertain	Adult T-cell leukemia or lymphoma

BK virus, a human polyomavirus discovered from the urine of a renal transplant recipient, whose initials were B.K.; *EBV*, Epstein-Barr virus; *EV*, epidermodysplasia verruciformis; *HBV*, hepatitis B virus; *HCV*, hepatitis C virus; *HIV*, human immunodeficiency virus; *HPV*, human papillomavirus; *HTLV*, human T-lymphotropic virus; *JC*, John Cunningham; *KSHV*, Kaposi sarcoma–associated herpesvirus; *SV40*, simian virus 20.

Adapted from Devita, V.T., Lawrence, T.S., Rosenberg, S.A., DePinho, R.A., Weinberg, R.A. (Eds.). (2011). *DeVita, Hellman, and Rosenberg's cancer: Principles and practice of oncology* (9th ed.) Philadelphia: Lippincott Williams & Wilkins.

most challenging step for disseminating cells. Some tumor cells exit the cell cycle and remain dormant in secondary organs, while others are incapable of triggering the angiogenic switch necessary for tumor expansion. The fate of the metastatic process is determined by a complex series of interactions between metastatic cells and their organ microenvironment." (Langley & Fidler, 2011)

1. Soil and seed hypothesis: Originally proposed in 1889, this hypothesis asserts that metastasis does not occur by chance. Metastasis thrives in organs and tissues where the environment is supportive to tumor survival and growth.

2. The presence of metastatic disease at diagnosis is an important prognostic factor because it indicates advanced disease.

B. Major factors of metastatic cascade (Figures 3-6 and 3-7)

1. Invasion of the extracellular matrix (ECM) by tumor cells

   a. Tumor cells downregulate cadhedrin glycoproteins that mediate cell-cell interactions.

   b. Tumor cells produce or stimulate stromal cells such as fibroblasts or inflammatory cells to secrete proteases that degrade the ECM.

   c. Tumor cells then attach to ECM proteins that can assist with mobility and interact with the ECM to create an environment conducive to migration of the tumor cells.

   d. Through a process called *locomotion*, which involves complex signaling involving proteases, cytokines, and motility factors, tumor cells are able to migrate through the ECM and gain access to the vascular basement membrane.

   e. This process occurs in reverse when tumor cell emboli reach and invade a distant site.

2. Survival in transport: Tumor cells in circulation are susceptible to destruction by mechanical stress, immune defenses, and apoptosis because of lack of cell-cell adhesion. To survive, tumor cells tend to travel in clumps, may combine with platelets to form platelet-tumor aggregates, and may interact with coagulation factors to create emboli.

3. Pathways of cancer dissemination

   a. Direct invasion to an adjoining organ

   b. Seeding throughout a body cavity such as the peritoneal cavity

   c. Dissemination through the lymphatic system

      (1) Entrapment at the first lymph node, or

      (2) "Skip metastasis," where cells bypass the first node and reach more distant sites

   d. Dissemination through the blood vessels

      (1) Arterial spread

         (a) Tumor cells may be spread through the pulmonary capillary beds or

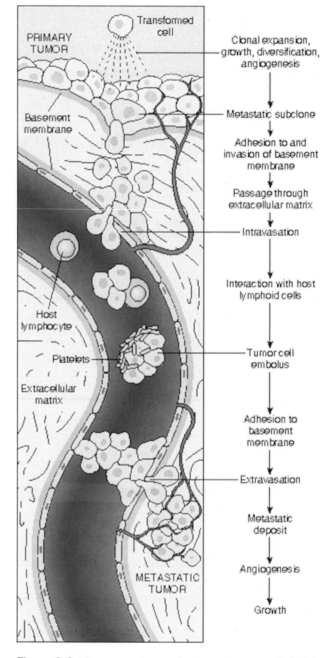

Figure 3-6 The metastatic cascade. From Kumar et al., (Eds.) (2009). *Robbins and Cotran pathologic basis of disease* (8th ed.) Philadelphia: Saunders.

pulmonary arteriovenous (AV) shunts or when pulmonary tumors metastasize and create tumor emboli.

         (b) Because arteries have thicker walls, they are less readily penetrated than veins (Stricker & Kumar, 2010).

      (2) Venous spread

         (a) Tumor cells often go to the first capillary bed encountered. Liver and lung are the most frequent sites of metastasis.

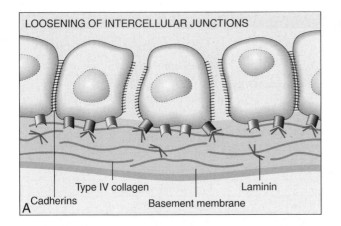

LOOSENING OF INTERCELLULAR JUNCTIONS

Type IV collagen

Laminin

Cadherins

Basement membrane

A

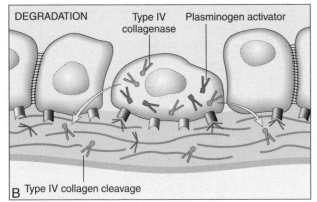

DEGRADATION

Type IV collagenase

Plasminogen activator

Type IV collagen cleavage

B

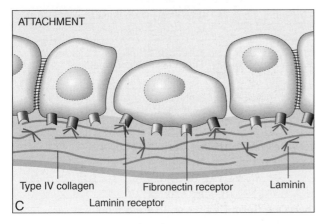

ATTACHMENT

Type IV collagen

Fibronectin receptor

Laminin

Laminin receptor

C

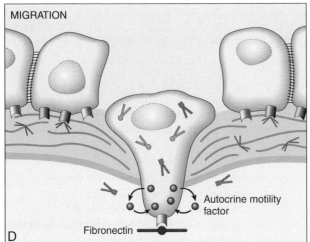

MIGRATION

Autocrine motility factor

Fibronectin

D

Table 3-6

Specific Cancers and Their Common Sites for Metastasis, Excluding Lymph Nodes

Cancer	Common Sites
Breast Cancer	Bone, lung, liver and brain
Colon Cancer	Liver, potentially lungs
Colorectal Cancer	Liver, lung and brain
Kidney Cancer	Liver, bone, brain, lungs
Lung cancer	Adrenal gland, liver, bone and brain
Melanoma (skin cancer)	Lung and Brain

Adapted from National Cancer Institute at the National Institute for Health. (2013). *Metastatic cancer.* http://www.cancer.gov/cancertopics/factsheet/Sites-Types/metastatic> Accessed 29 October 2013.

4. Common sites for metastasis include bones, the lungs, the liver, and the CNS (Table 3-6). Predilection for certain tumors to metastasize to specific sites may be influenced by the following:
   a. Patterns of blood flow
   b. Cell receptors and genes that direct the cell to travel to specific sites
   c. Tumor cell production of adhesion molecules that prefer certain distant organs
   d. Chemical signals and growth factors, which are found only in selected organs
   e. Inhibitor substances produced by organs that are not typically sites for metastatic growth
   f. Collectively, items b to e may be a result of "cross-talk" between cancer cells and normal host cells. That is, cancer cells may release cytokines that induce the host cells to produce substances that recognize receptors on the cancer cells. Hence, the cancer cells may have a "homing device" that attracts them to select host organs and may promote their growth in these distant tissues (Stricker & Kumar, 2010).

C. Clinical implications
   1. Metastasis contributes to the pain and suffering caused by cancer and is the major cause of death from cancer (Virshup, 2012).
   2. Understanding of the process of metastasis helps lead to therapies targeting the molecular changes associated with the disease.

V. Diagnosis and staging
   A. Diagnosis and staging are necessary to determine treatment.
   B. Information about the tissue of origin is used to select the appropriate treatment.

Figure 3-7 Invasion of the epithelial basement membrane. From Kumar et al. (Eds.) (2009). *Robbins and Cotran pathologic basis of disease* (8th ed.) Philadelphia: Saunders.

Table 3-7

Nomenclature of Tumors

Tissue of Origin	Benign	Malignant
Composed of One Parenchymal Cell Type—Tumors of Mesenchymal Origin		
Connective tissue and derivatives	Fibroma	Fibrosarcoma
	Lipoma	Liposarcoma
	Chondroma	Chondrosarcoma
	Osteoma	Osteogenic sarcoma
Endothelial and Related Tissues		
Blood vessels	Hemangioma	Angiosarcoma
Lymph vessels	Lymphangioma	Lymphangiosarcoma
Synovium		Synovial sarcoma
Mesothelium		Mesothelioma
Brain coverings	Meningioma	Invasive meningioma
Blood Cells and Related Cells		
Hematopoietic cells		Leukemias
Lymphoid tissue		Lymphomas
Muscle		
Smooth	Leiomyoma	Leiomyosarcoma
Striated	Rhabdomyoma	Rhabdomyosarcoma
Tumors of Epithelial Origin		
Stratified squamous	Squamous cell papilloma	Squamous cell carcinoma
Basal cells of skin or adnexa		Basal cell carcinoma
Epithelial lining of glands or ducts	Adenoma	Adenocarcinoma
	Papilloma	Papillary carcinomas
	Cystadenoma	Cystadenocarcinoma
Respiratory passages	Bronchial adenoma	Bronchogenic carcinoma
Renal epithelium	Renal tubular adenoma	Renal cell carcinoma
Liver cells	Liver cell adenoma	Hepatocellular carcinoma
Urinary tract epithelium (transitional)	Transitional cell papilloma	Transitional cell carcinoma
Placental epithelium	Hydatidiform mole	Choriocarcinoma
Testicular epithelium (germ cells)		Seminoma
		Embryonal carcinoma
Tumors of melanocytes	Nevus	Malignant melanoma
More Than One Neoplastic Cell Type—Mixed Tumors, Usually Derived from One Germ Cell Layer		
Salivary glands	Pleomorphic adenoma (mixed tumor of salivary origin	Malignant mixed tumor of salivary gland origin
Renal anlage		Wilms tumor
More Than One Neoplastic Cell Type Derived from More Than One Germ Cell Layer—Teratogenous		
Totipotential cells in gonads or in embryonic rests	Mature teratoma, dermoid cyst	Immature teratoma, teratocarcinoma

From Kumar, V., Abbas, A. K., Fausto, N., Aster, J. C. (Eds.). (2009). *Robbins and Cotran pathologic basis of disease* (8th ed.) (pp. 259-330). Philadelphia: Saunders.

1. Tumor nomenclature
   a. Benign tumors generally are named by the cell of origin with the *-oma* suffix (Table 3-7).
   b. Malignant tumors are generally named for the tissue layer that they arise from—that is, those of mesenchymal origin are sarcomas, and those of epithelial origin are carcinomas.
   c. Exceptions to these naming conventions do exist.

C. Staging also determines appropriate treatment options, monitoring response to treatment and prognosis.
D. The elements of diagnosis and staging are as follows:
   1. Physical examination and patient history
      a. Assessments of the general health of the patient and performance status are used in selecting appropriate treatment.

2. Laboratory studies
   a. Evaluation of the status of system functions—for example, those of the pulmonary, cardiac, renal, liver, and gastrointestinal (GI) systems.
   b. Tumor markers are tumor antigens released by tumor cells that can be measured to assess the presence of tumor and response to therapy. Most are nonspecific to cancer cells and are less useful in screening for cancer. See Table 3-3.
3. Imaging examinations
   a. Examples are radiography, CT, magnetic resonance imaging (MRI), ultrasonography, and positron emission tomography (PET).
4. Histology type and grade of cancer
   a. Pathologists examine tissue biopsies to determine the histology and grade of the cancer using tools such as immunohistochemistry (IHC), flow cytometry, and molecular diagnosis.
      (1) Incisional biopsy—aspiration, fine-needle biopsy, or punch biopsy
      (2) Excisional biopsy—removal of entire lesion
      (3) Cytology—examination of fluid-containing cells that have been shed
   b. Biomarkers have become increasingly more important in diagnosis and staging as we come to understand more about the biology of cancer (Edge & Compton, 2010). Some biomarkers provide prognostic information and directed treatment options.
   c. An advancement in the pathologist's technology is molecular profiling of tumors. This method is being used to determine possible treatments based on the genetics of the tumor. The genetic heterogeneity of tumors does present some challenges for the use of this technology, but techniques and strategies to address this challenge are being developed (Bunz, 2010).
5. Extent of disease or stage of cancer
   a. Knowledge of cancer patterns and spread determines the use of various tests in evaluation of staging.
   b. Tests to determine the extent of local disease and potential metastasis are as follows:
      (1) Noninvasive test procedures such as radiography, CT, MRI, ultrasonography, and PET
      (2) Invasive procedures such as exploratory surgery, bronchoscopy, and endoscopy are used either to determine the extent of disease or to obtain tumor biopsy.

6. Staging systems allow comparisons of tumors across individuals and are used to evaluate appropriate and standard therapy.
   a. TNM system—most widely used system for staging of solid tumors. *T* denotes the size or extent of the primary tumor; *N* denotes the absence or present of regional lymph node metastasis; *M* denotes the absence or presence of distant metastases.

References

Aparicio, S., & Caldas, C. (2013). Mechanisms of disease: The implications of clinical genome evolution for cancer medicine. *New England Journal of Medicine, 368*(9), 842–851.

Bunz, F. (2010). *Principles of cancer genetics.* Dordrecht, Netherlands: Springer Science + Business Media B.V.

Cancer. (n.d.). In *Mosby's dictionary of medicine, nursing & health professions.* http://www.nursingconsult.com/nursing/index. Accessed 29.10.13.

Carcinogenesis. (n.d.). In *Mosby's dictionary of medicine, nursing & health professions.* http://www.nursingconsult.com/nursing/index. Accessed 29.10.13.

Cooper, M. R., & Cooper, M. R. (2001). Systemic therapy. In R. E. Lenhard, R. T. Osteen, & T. Gansler (Eds.), *Clinical oncology* (pp. 175–215). Atlanta: American Cancer Society.

Edge, S. B., & Compton, C. C. (2010). The American Joint Committee on Cancer: the 7th edition of the AJCC cancer staging manual and the future of TNM. *Annals of Surgical Oncology, 17*, 1471–1474.

Hanahan, D., & Weinberg, R. A. (2011). Hallmarks of cancer: The next generation. *Cell, 144*, 646–674.

Kalluri, R., & Weinberg, R. A. (2009). The basics of epithelial-mesenchymal transition. *Journal of Clinical Investigation, 119*(6), 1420–1428.

Krewski, D., Lubin, J. H., Zielinski, J. M., Alavanja, M., Catalan, V. S., Field, R., et al. (2005). Residential radon and risk of lung cancer—a combined analysis of 7 North American case-control studies. *Epidemiology, 16*(2), 137–145.

Langely, R. R., & Fidler, I. J. (2011). The seed and soil hypothesis revisited—the role of tumor-stroma interactions in metastasis to different organs. *International Journal of Cancer, 128*(11), 2527–2535.

Latendresse, G., & McCance, K. L. (2012). Alterations of the reproductive systems, including sexual transmitted infection. In S. E. Huether & K. L. McCance (Eds.), *Understanding pathophysiology* (5th ed., pp. 799–866). St. Louis: Elsevier.

Ljungman, M. (2011). Physical factors. In V. T. Devita, T. S. Lawrence, S. A. Rosenberg, R. A. DePinho, & R. A. Weinberg (Eds.), *DeVita, Hellman, and Rosenberg's* cancer: *Principles and practice of oncology* (9th ed.). Philadelphia: Lippincott Williams & Wilkins.

Nowell, P. (1976). The clonal evolution of tumor population. *Science, 194*, 23–28.

Oncogenesis. (n.d.). In *Mosby's dictionary of medicine, nursing & health professions.* http://www.nursingconsult.com/nursing/index. Accessed 29.10.13.

Stricker, T. P., & Kumar, V. (2010). Neoplasia. In V. Kumar, A. K. Abbas, N. Fausto, & J. C. Aster (Eds.), *Robbins and Cotran's pathologic basis of disease* (8th ed., pp. 259–330). Philadelphia: Saunders Elsevier.

Virshup, D. M. (2012). Biology, clinical manifestations, and treatment of cancer. In S. E. Huether & K. L. McCance (Eds.), *Understanding pathophysiology* (5th ed., pp. 222–252). St. Louis: Elsevier.

Yuspa, S. H., & Shields, P. G. (2011). Chemical factors. In V. T. Devita, T. S. Lawrence, S. A. Rosenberg, R. A. DePinho, & R. A. Weinberg (Eds.), *DeVita, Hellman, and Rosenberg's cancer: Principles and practice of oncology.* (9th ed.). Philadelphia: Lippincott Williams & Wilkins.

Part 2

CHAPTER 4

Immunology

Kristi V. Schmidt and Tracy Webb Warren

OVERVIEW

I. Definition of immunology
- A. Study of detailed components involved in the recognition of cellular and tissue changes, invasion of microbes, development of infections, and process of malignant tumor growth (Liu & Zeng, 2012)
- B. Impairment or lack of these components keeps the body from adequately responding to allergens, antigens, infectious microbes, or tumor cells (Paul, 2013); key terms related to oncology include:
  1. Immunosurveillance—where the immune system can identify and control tumor cells (Vesely & Schreiber, 2013)
  2. Immune escape—the loss of recognition by cells within the immune system, which leads to tumor escape and cell proliferation (Devita, Lawrence, Rosenberg, DePinho, & Weinberg, 2011)

II. Basic concepts
- A. Hematopoiesis—regulation, production, and development of blood cells
  1. Hematopoiesis begins with a single cell, a self-renewing pluripotent stem cell.
  2. This cell divides into undifferentiated hematopoietic stem cells that are committed to one of two cell lineages or pathways; lymphoid or myeloid progenitor cells (Sompayrac, 2012). These include:
     - a. Lymphoid—B cell, helper T cell, killer T cell, natural killer (NK) cells
     - b. Myeloid—dendritic cell, macrophage, neutrophil, eosinophil, mast cell, megakaryocyte, red blood cells
- B. Protect against infection by recognizing and destroying pathogens
- C. Homeostasis—maintaining the balance of blood cell supply

III. Organ and tissue components of the immune system
- A. Primary lymphoid organs—allow for the maturation of lymphocytes, including the growth and expression of specific antigen receptors; include the following (Male, Brostoff, Roth, & Roitt, 2013):
  1. Bone marrow—location of B-cell differentiation and maturation
  2. Thymus—location of T-cell differentiation and maturation
- B. Secondary lymphoid organs and tissues
  1. Sites where foreign antigens encounter lymphocyte immune responses and activation of naïve B cells and T cells takes place (Sompayrac, 2012)
     - a. Waldeyer ring (tonsils and adenoids)—mucosa-associated lymphoid tissue
     - b. Bronchus-associated lymphoid tissue—mucosa-associated lymphoid tissue
     - c. Lymph nodes—initiate immune responses to antigens circulating in the lymph, skin, or mucosal surfaces
     - d. Spleen—responds to bloodborne antigens
     - e. Bone marrow—functions as both primary and secondary lymphoid organ
     - f. Lymphoid tissue—gastrointestinal mucosa–associated and urogenital lymphoid tissue

IV. Cellular components of the immune system
- A. Cells
  1. Lymphocytes are derived from the lymphoid stem cell lineage and key for all immune responses. Two types are:
     - a. B cells
       - (1) Develop in the bone marrow
       - (2) Multiplication of B cells on recognition of a specific antigen and further differentiation into plasma cells, which produce one of five types of immunoglobulins (IgG, IgA, IgM, IgE, IgD)
     - b. T cells
       - (1) T cells migrate to the thymus gland for development and play a role in immune surveillance.

(2) Before antigen recognition by T cells, antigens are processed by antigen-presenting cells (APCs) displayed on the cell surface as peptides.

(3) The different types of T cells include the following (Abbas, Lichtman, & Pillai, 2012):

(a) T helper cells (CD4+ cells): type 1 (Th1) secretes cytokines and interacts with mononuclear phagocytes to assist in their ability to destroy intracellular pathogens

(b) T helper cells (CD4+ cells): type 2 (Th2) interacts with B cells, enhancing cell division, differentiation, and antibody production

(c) T cytotoxic cells (CD8+ cells): also referred to as *Tc*, destroy host cells with the direction of CD4+ cells

2. Phagocytes—internalize (engulf) and consume pathogenic microorganisms and debris and function to engulf and destroy particles (Sompayrac, 2012)

a. Mononuclear phagocytes—fixed and mobile phagocytic cells associated with blood monocytes and tissue macrophages

b. Polymorphonuclear granulocytes

(1) Polymorphonuclear neutrophils (PMNs)

(a) Short-lived cells that migrate into tissues (inflammatory response), where they engulf and destroy material (Male et al., 2013)

(2) Eosinophil polymorphs—also known as *eosinophils*

(a) Attracted to large extracellular parasitic worms; cell kill done by the release of the contents of the intracellular granules close to them

(b) Release histamine and arylsulfatase to reduce an inflammatory response and granulocyte accumulation (Male et al., 2013)

(3) Basophils

(a) Circulating granulocytes that move to tissue sites where antigens are present and can create immediate hypersensitivity reactions

(b) Similar in function to mast cells, as described below (Abbas et al., 2012)

3. Dendritic cells (DCs)

a. Starfish-shaped cells that travel from tissue to secondary lymphoid organs to present antigen to T cells (Sompayrac, 2012)

b. Function as APCs that initiate T-cell–(CD4+, CD8+) as well as naive T-cell–dependent immune responses known as *priming* (Abbas et al., 2012)

c. Effective in stimulating both antiviral and antitumor immune responses in experimental animal and human models

d. Immature DCs found in peripheral tissue; possess phagocytic and macropinocytotic functions that express multiple receptors that enhance antigen uptake with low surface expression of class I and II MHC molecules (Devita et al., 2011)

(1) MHC molecules expressed on the surface of human cells are also known as *human leukocyte antigens* (HLAs) (Abbas et al., 2012).

(2) Class I MHC molecules bind to and display a cell's peptides to specific immune cells such as T cells (HLA-A, HLA-B, HLA-C).

(3) Class II MHC molecules have antigen presentation capabilities (HLA-DR, HLA-DP, HLA-DQ).

e. Mature DCs influenced by inflammatory stimuli that lead to decreased phagocytosis and increased cell surface expression of class I and II molecules

f. Mature DCs then able to migrate through the lymphatics to adjacent lymphoid tissue through specific molecular function to present antigen proteins to CD4+ and CD8+ T cells (Sompayrac, 2012)

4. Null cells

a. Represent a small portion of lymphocytes, which are a separate lineage of lymphoid cells that express neither T-cell nor B-cell surface markers

b. Early in cell differentiation, display T-cell markers but with further maturation acquire markers also found on macrophages and neutrophils (Mosby, 2012)

c. Two types

(1) NK cells

(a) Contain substances called *perforin*, serine proteases, and other enzymes that create a hole in the membrane of the cell resulting in cell death

(b) Activity increased with the addition of cytokines such as interleukin 2 (IL-2), IL-12, and interferon gamma (IFN-γ)

(c) Ultimate function—identification and destruction of virus-infected cells and certain tumor cells (Liu & Zeng, 2012)

(2) Lymphokine-activated killer (LAK) cells
   (a) Produced when lymphocytes are removed from a client's blood and cultured with IL-2 or alloantigens
   (b) LAK subset of cells creates cytotoxicity in a wide spectrum of targeted cells
   (c) Continued presence of IL-2 and LAK cells must have direct contact with target cell for cytotoxic effect (Male et al., 2013)

5. Mast cells
   a. Granulocytes with multiple mediators that produce inflammatory response within tissues
   b. Contain receptors on the surface that bind to the Fc region on IgE antibodies, leading to cellular degradation (Sompayrac, 2012)
   c. Located close to blood vessels in all tissues and are often indistinguishable from basophils
   d. Two kinds of mast cells
      (1) Mucosal mast cell (MMC)
      (2) Connective tissue mast cell (CTMC)

6. Platelets
   a. Have immunologic function that releases inflammatory mediators through the process of thrombogenesis or antigen-antibody complexes (Sompayrac, 2012)

B. Mediators of immune system function
   1. Complement system—an interactive network of approximately 20 unique serum and cell proteins present in plasma (Abbas et al., 2012)
      a. Complement cascade (McCance, Huether, Brashers, & Rote, 2010).
         (1) Classical pathway (acquired immunity) activated by antigen-antibody complexes
         (2) Lectin pathway activated by specific bacterial carbohydrates (mannose-binding lectin [MBL] plasma protein)
         (3) Alternative pathway activated by gram-negative bacteria and fungal polysaccharides
      b. Functions
         (1) Mast cell degranulation
         (2) Leukocyte chemotaxis
         (3) Opsonization—phagocytosis of antigen-antibody complexes when products of the complement cascade interact with neutrophils and macrophages
         (4) Cell lysis—destruction of targeted pathogen
   2. Cytokines
      a. Molecules that enhance communication and induce growth and differentiation of lymphocytes and other cells within the immune and neuroendocrine system (Male et al., 2013)
         (1) IFNs—limit the spread of certain viral infections, are produced early in response to infection, and offer first line of viral resistance.
         (2) ILs—produced mainly by T cells; however, some production in mononuclear phagocytes or tissue cells
         (3) Hematopoietic growth factors—guide and direct cell division and differentiation of bone marrow stem cells and leukocytes
         (4) Tumor necrosis factors (TNF-α or TNF-ß) and transforming growth factor-ß—play key roles in mediating inflammation and cytotoxic reactions
         (5) Chemokines—guide leukocyte movement around the body between blood and tissues and may activate cells to perform specialized immunologic functions (Abbas et al., 2012)

C. MHC
   1. MHC genes coded on chromosomes for presentation of peptides and key in immune surveillance (Sompayrac, 2012)

V. Immune system responses
   A. Innate immunity, which occurs naturally in almost all animals, does not rely on previous exposure or "memory" to be initiated.
      1. Natural barriers—in place at birth to prevent damage by environmental substances and thwart infection by pathogens (McCance et al., 2010)
         a. Physical—epithelial cells of intact skin and mucous membranes
         b. Mechanical—respiratory cilia movement, sneezing, coughing, vomiting, and urination to clear or wash the affected epithelial surface
         c. Biochemical—secretions such as mucus, sweat, saliva, tears, flora of gastrointestinal (GI) tract and earwax that trap and kill microorganisms
      2. Inflammatory response—results in the rapid activation of several plasma protein systems, mast cell degranulation, vascular changes, and the influx of leukocytes (McCance et al., 2010)
         a. Vascular response
            (1) Influx of fluid dilutes toxins released by bacteria and dying cells, and plasma proteins contain and destroy bacteria.
            (2) Influx of neutrophils and macrophages "eat" and destroy both cellular debris and pathogens.
            (3) Eosinophils, enzymes, and clotting factors prevent spread of response to healthy tissue.

(4) Interaction with the adaptive immune system when a more specific response is required through influx of macrophage and lymphocytes (McCance et al., 2010)

(5) This response removes debris and prepares for healing by using lymph drainage vessels and channels through the epithelium.

B. Acquired immunity reacts to specific molecules, is slower to respond, has "memory," and therefore is much longer lived than innate responses (McCance et al., 2010).

1. Begins with an unique antigen that is phagocytized by a macrophage and is presented to B or T lymphocytes and T helper cells (Male et al., 2013)

2. Need for the existence of two antigen characteristics to be recognized by a B or T lymphocyte as non-self:

a. High molecular weight (HMW) defined as greater than 8 to 10 kilodaltons (kDa); antigens associated with melanoma, breast cancer, and pancreatic tumor cells considered HMW (www.Millipore.com)

b. Consist of recurring molecules called epitopes; genes that pattern the epitope comprise the MHC

3. B-cell immunity (humoral immunity)

a. B lymphocytes wait for macrophages to bring antigens to them for processing within lymphoid tissue (Male et al., 2013).

b. Each B-cell lymphocyte recognizes only one type of antigen, called *specificity*.

(1) Three processes occur.

(a) Specific B-cell lymphocytes are produced at a fast pace.

(b) Some specific B-cell lymphocytes differentiate to become plasma cells. Each specialized plasma cell produces one specific antibody; these committed, highly differentiated cells are not phagocytic.

(c) Some become memory cells; these exist in the body capable of recognizing a particular antigen at future exposures and producing plasma cells to generate abundant antibody specific to the antigen.

C. Some antibodies circulate in the bloodstream in addition to gathering at the site of invasion.

D. Antibodies (immunoglobulins) protect the body from antigens and cells containing them by direct action via immune effector mechanisms such as neutralization, antibody-dependent cell-mediated cytotoxicity (ADCC),

complement-dependent cytotoxicity (CDC), and apoptosis (programmed cell death) (Sompayrac, 2012).

1. Neutralization occurs when cell growth is stopped because of interference of the immunoglobulin with the antigen.

2. ADCC occurs when the antibody binds to the antigen and forms a bridge to cause direct cell kill. Immunoglobulins, NK cells, and macrophages participate in this process.

3. Apoptosis occurs because of the attachment of the antibody to the antigen; this sends a complex, multistep signal that causes breakage of cells' DNA.

4. CDC is the interaction of serum and cell surface proteins along with other molecules via cascade mechanisms, as described earlier.

a. CDC is activated via the "classical pathway." The end result is cell lysis and recruitment of other components of the immune system to enhance the effector cell response (Sompayrac, 2012).

5. T-cell immunity (cell-mediated immunity)

a. Antigens are presented to T lymphocytes by macrophages via APCs (Male et al., 2013).

b. T lymphocytes specific to the presented antigen are produced (activated T cells).

c. Activated T cells are released into lymphatic fluid from the bloodstream and navigate back and forth.

d. T-lymphocyte memory cells are produced and respond by activating T lymphocytes when exposed to the same antigen in the future.

e. Cytotoxic T cells and NK cells are capable of directly attacking other cells and destroying them (Male et al., 2013).

f. T lymphocytes are also able to recognize and bind to antigens (Sompayrac, 2012).

(1) T lymphocytes cannot read epitopes until a molecule is phagocytized and digested and its antigens are linked with the MHC antigens on the surface of the NK T lymphocytes.

VI. Tumor immunology—it is hypothesized that the immune system can protect a host from cancer (Male et al., 2013).

A. Tumor protective antigens—proteins that can induce protective immunity against tumors

1. Part of a group of proteins called *heat shock proteins*

2. Seen in mouse sarcomas, melanomas, colon, lung carcinomas, and hematomas (Male et al., 2013)

B. Tumor-associated antigens (TAAs)—changes may occur in cell surface molecules when a cell transitions from normal to malignant; examples of TAAs include HER2/neu, CEA, CA 125, TAG-72, EGFR, PSA, and gangliosides (Male et al., 2013).

C. Examples of how tumor cells evade immune system effector functions include:

1. Hosts with T-cell immunodeficiencies are at higher risk of developing malignancies because of oncogenic viral invasion, such as Epstein-Barr virus (EBV). T cells play a critical role in immune surveillance.

2. Class I MHC expression may be deregulated on tumor cells so that they are not targeted by cytotoxic T cells.

3. Tumor cells are created from host cells and resemble or function similar to normal cells, except tumor cells lose expression of antigens that do the following:
   a. Ignite an immune response.
   b. Secrete cytokines that suppress immune cell responses.

4. Tumor cells fail to recruit cytotoxic T cells because the cells do not express co-stimulators that normally induce cytotoxic T cells or class II MHC molecules.

5. Cell turnover and rapid growth rates in malignant tumors may overpower immune system effector cell functions intending to destroy and eliminate the tumor cells.

D. Immune receptors and signal transduction—basic concepts in understanding mechanism of action for current immunologic and biologic therapy approaches in treating cancer (Male et al., 2013)

1. Cell surface receptors are located mostly on the plasma membrane. Specifically, cell surface receptors function to:
   a. Create a communication signal from the outside to the inside of the cell, which includes immune response
   b. Allow cells to attach to other cells or within a cellular matrix
      (1) Cellular receptors are classified based on signaling mechanisms and pathways they activate:
         (a) Non-receptor tyrosine kinases
         (b) Receptor tyrosine kinases
         (c) Nuclear receptors
         (d) Serpentine receptors
      (2) Immune receptors are membrane proteins in the immunoglobulin class the recognize ligands:
         (a) T and B cell antigen receptors
         (b) IgE receptor on mast cells
         (c) Fc receptors on innate immune cells and B lymphocytes that either activate or inhibit cell function

2. Signal transduction changes the way a cell responds after the binding of ligands to specific cellular receptors. As a result, a cell may acquire new functions, begin to differentiate, become a specific cell type, work to inhibit apoptosis, create immune reactions, and grow, proliferate, or die (Abbas et al., 2012).

References

Abbas, A., Lichtman, A., & Pillai, S. (2012). *Cellular and molecular immunology* (7th ed.). Philadelphia: Elsevier Saunders.

Devita, V., Lawrence, T., Rosenberg, S., DePinho, R., & Weinberg, R. (2011). *Devita, Hellman and Rosenberg's cancer: Principles and practice of oncology* (9th ed.). Philadelphia: Lippincot Williams & Wilkins.

Liu, Y., & Zeng, G. (2012). Cancer and innate immune system interactions: Traditional potentials for cancer immunotherapy. *Journal of Immunotherapy, 35*(4), 299–308.

Male, D., Brostoff, J., Roth, D., & Roitt, I. (2013). *Immunology* (8th ed.). Philadelphia: Elsevier Saunders.

McCance, K. L., Huether, S. E., Brashers, V. L., & Rote, N. S. (2010). *Pathophysiology: The biologic basis for disease in adults and children* (6th ed.). Maryland Heights, MO: Mosby Elsevier.

Mosby. (2012). *Mosby's medical dictionary* (9th ed.). Maryland Heights, MO: Mosby Elsevier.

Paul, W. (2013). *Fundamental immunology* (6th ed.). Philadelphia: Lippincott Williams & Wilkins.

Sompayrac, L. (2012). *How the immune system works* (4th ed.). West Sussex, England: John Wiley & Sons.

Vesely, M., & Schreiber, R. (2013). Cancer immunoediting: Antigens, mechanisms and implications to cancer immunotherapy. *Annals of the New York Academy of Sciences, 1284*(1), 1–5.

CHAPTER 5

Genetic Risk Factors

Kathleen A. Calzone and Julie Eggert

OVERVIEW

I. Organization and function of genetic material
   A. Chromosomes are threadlike structures that contain genetic information.
      1. The 46 chromosomes in the human body are made up of 23 chromosome pairs, one copy from each parent.
         a. The small arm of the chromosome is identified as the "petite" or "p" arm of the chromosome.
         b. The large arm is labeled the "q" arm, because "q" follows "p" (Figure 5-1).
      2. Autosomes represent the 22 chromosome pairs, numbered 1 to 22, which do not determine sex.
      3. Sex chromosomes are the X and Y chromosomes, which determine an individual's sex.
         a. Women have two X chromosomes.
         b. Men have one X chromosome and one Y chromosome.
   B. Nucleic acids consist of bases and a sugar and phosphate group. Two types of nucleic acids exist.
      1. Deoxyribonucleic acid (DNA) comprises two nucleotide chains, running in opposite directions and held together by hydrogen bonds, which are coiled around one another to form a double helix (Figure 5-2).
         a. In DNA, two types of bases are present: purines and pyrimidines.
            (1) Two types of purines: adenine (A) and guanine (G)
            (2) Two types of pyrimidines: thymine (T) and cytosine (C)
         b. DNA base pairs are complementary on the double strand; A attaches to T, and G attaches to C.
      2. Ribonucleic acid (RNA) consists of a single nucleotide chain, which represents a complimentary copy of a strand of DNA.
         a. In RNA, the bases are the same as DNA except the base uracil (U) replaces thymine (T).
         b. *Transcription* refers to the process of making RNA from DNA.
         c. *Translation* refers to the process of making proteins from RNA.
         d. Proteins consist of chains of amino acids. Sequences of the amino acids determine the function of the protein.
         e. Primary types of RNA (Figure 5-3)
            (1) Messenger RNA (mRNA) contains information about the order of the amino acids in a protein.
               (a) A codon is a chain of three mRNA nucleotides that specifies the production of one of 20 different amino acids.
               (b) More than one codon will code for a specific amino acid.
               (c) An mRNA nucleotide change in the third place of the codon rarely causes an amino acid change. A change in the first place of the codon usually will cause a different amino acid to be produced and an error in building the protein. These changes are the direct cause of polymorphisms and mutations.
               (d) Three "stop" codons and the associated RNAs stop the growth of the amino acid chain.
                  (i) Transfer RNA (tRNA) brings the amino acids to the site of protein synthesis.
                  (ii) Ribosomal RNA (rRNA) provides the structural support for the protein in addition to other functions.
                  (iii) Small silencing RNAs have important roles in gene regulation. These include microRNA (miRNA), Piwi-interacting RNA (piRNA) and small interfering RNA (siRNA) (Ghildiyal & Zamore, 2009).

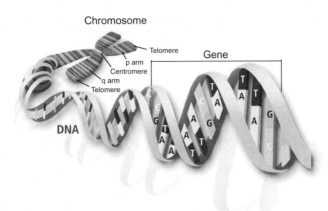

Figure 5-1 Chromosome and Gene Structure. Courtesy of the National Human Genome Research Institute, Bethesda, MD.

C. As seen in Figure 5-1, genes are individual units of hereditary information, which are located at a specific position on the chromosome.
   1. Genes consist of a sequence of DNA that codes for a specific protein (see Figure 5-1).
   2. Genes consist primarily of exons and introns.
      a. Exons are protein-coding segments of a gene.
      b. Introns are non–protein-coding segments or the sequence-interrupting piece of a gene.
II. Basic mechanisms of carcinogenesis, mutations, and heredity
   A. Cancer has a multifactorial etiology with several genetic, environmental, and personal factors interacting to produce a malignancy.

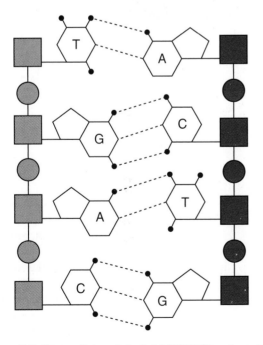

Figure 5-2 Deoxyribonucleic Acid (DNA) Structure. From Coed, J. & Dunstall, M. (2006). Anatomy and physiology for midwives (2*nd* ed.). New York: Churchill Livingstone.

B. Genetic mutations and genetic instability are at the very core of cancer development. Most cancers are not the result of inherited mutations.
   1. Most cancers are associated with genetic mutations that occur in single cells some time during the life of an individual.
   2. A malignant tumor arises after a series of genetic mutations have accumulated.
B. Genetic mutations that are acquired are associated with exogenous (environmental) or indigenous factors (biologic). For example, carcinogens are exogenous factors thought to operate by causing genetic mutations.
C. Mutations are disease-causing variations in the sequence of DNA.
   1. Genetic mutations are usually acquired over a lifetime. These are designated as somatic and are acquired genetic mutations in body cells that occur after conception.
   2. In a person with a genetic predisposition to cancer, a mutation has been inherited in the germline reproductive cells.
   3. Types of mutations
      a. Frameshift mutations occur when one or more bases are added or deleted from the normal sequence, resulting in an altered form of the protein.
      b. Missense mutations are single–base pair changes that result in the substitution of one amino acid for another in the protein being constructed. Some of the substituted amino acids may be critical to the function of the protein.
      c. Nonsense mutations change an amino acid signal into a signal to stop adding amino acids to a growing protein. Nonsense mutations result in a truncated, presumably nonfunctional, protein.
      d. RNA-negative mutations result in the absence of RNA transcribed from a gene copy.

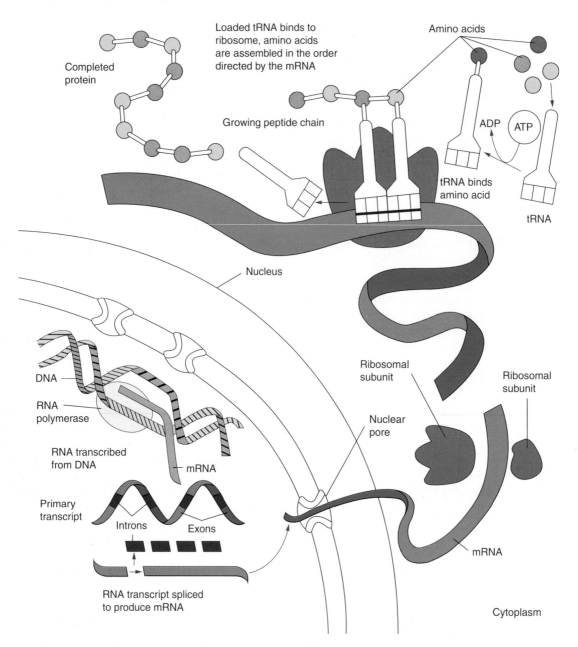

Loaded tRNA binds to ribosome, amino acids are assembled in the order directed by the mRNA

Completed protein

Growing peptide chain

Amino acids

ADP

ATP

tRNA binds amino acid

tRNA

Nucleus

DNA

RNA polymerase

RNA transcribed from DNA

mRNA

Ribosomal subunit

Ribosomal subunit

Nuclear pore

Primary transcript

Introns

Exons

RNA transcript spliced to produce mRNA

mRNA

Cytoplasm

Figure 5-3 Three Types of Ribonucleic Acid (RNA). Adkinson, N., Yunginger, J., Busse, W., Bochner, B., Holgate, S., & Simons, E. Middleton's allergy principles and practice online (6*th* ed.). St. Louis, MO: Elsevier.

e. Splicing mutations occur when DNA that should be removed from the coding sequence is retained or when DNA that should not be added is spliced in, resulting in frameshift mutations.

f. Polymorphisms are changes in the DNA sequence of a gene that often are not disease related, occur at variable frequency, and are associated with individualization in the general population. A single nucleotide polymorphism (SNP, pronounced "snip") is a DNA change in one nucleotide.

4. Chromosomal abnormalities
   a. Translocations refer to segments of one chromosome that break off and attach themselves to other chromosomes, resulting in altered protein production.
   b. Aneuploidy is an abnormal number of chromosomes.
   c. *Loss of heterozygosity* refers to the loss of a segment of both copies of a chromosome.
   d. Microsatellite instability (MSI) segments are repetitive pieces of DNA scattered throughout the genome in the noncoding

regions (introns). MSI is a marker of germline abnormality in mismatch repair genes in colorectal cancer, also known as *Lynch syndrome*. If MSI is identified in sporadic cases, it is referred to as *gene hypermethylation*.

D. A malignant tumor is derived from genetic instability and genetic mutations in genes that control cell growth and proliferation.

1. Types of regulatory genes
   a. Proto-oncogenes are normal genes essential for normal cell growth and regulation. Mutations occurring in proto-oncogenes convert to oncogene activation, which may result in uncontrolled cell division.
   b. Tumor suppressor genes function as regulators of cell growth. Some tumor suppressor genes appear to play a role in cell cycle regulation, whereas others have a role in DNA repair. Cells with mutation of a tumor suppressor gene may develop uncontrolled cell growth.
   c. DNA repair genes
      (1) Mismatch repair (MMR) genes are a type of DNA repair genes responsible for keeping the DNA free of "changes" during DNA synthesis. MMR genes are associated with microsatellite instability in Lynch syndrome.
      (2) Mutations in DNA repair genes may be inherited from a parent or acquired over time because of aging or carcinogens from the environment.

2. Mutator phenotype
   a. The mutator gene phenotype allows an increased mutation of genes because of poor proofreading or insertion of incorrect nucleotides left unrepaired. They seem to be efficient at acquiring mutations with both clonal and random mutations, allowing thousands of mutations versus lower rates seen with normal cells (Loeb, 2011).
   b. DNA damage that is overlooked by repair mechanisms may lead to incorrect messages in the DNA sequences, offering increased chance of oncogene mutations. If this occurs, "driver" mutations offer a growth advantage.
   c. "Passenger" mutations are those nucleotide changes that do not provide a growth advantage.

3. Control of cell growth and proliferation
   a. *Apoptosis* refers to the activation of a program that leads to normal, programmed cell death and often occurs in response to DNA damage. Malfunction results in uncontrolled cell proliferation of damaged and malignant cells.
   b. Telomerase plays a role in cellular aging through the telomeres, which are the ends of the chromosome.
      (1) As cells age, telomerase is normally repressed, and the telomeres are progressively lost.
      (2) In cancer, telomerase is reactivated, which keeps the telomeres intact, facilitating cell immortalization.

4. Cancer theories
   a. Knudson's two-hit damage hypothesis refers to the inactivation of both copies of a given regulatory gene. Because all individuals are born with two copies of almost every gene, Knudson originally theorized that both functioning copies of the gene must be inactivated for cancer to occur. Now, on the basis of molecular-level research, it is known that that one hit may exist, as seen with chronic myeloid leukemia (CML), that two hits cause retinoblastoma, and that many hits over time cause cancers, such as colorectal cancer (Knudson, 2001).
   b. Viral (retrovirus) infections copy a piece of RNA genome into the human DNA by using viral reverse transcriptase. Once the viral DNA or RNA (viral oncogene) is integrated into the human genome, it is transcribed by host RNA polymerase, causing mRNA to be translated into a nonfunctioning protein and resulting in cell proliferation (Rickinson & Kieff, 2001).
   c. The inflammation theory of cancer development notes that a variety of infectious agents and their relationships with inflammatory cells are the primary causes of cancer, proliferation, survival, and migration of cancer cells. From the innate immune system, selectins, chemokines (e.g., nuclear factor κB [NFκB]) and their receptors encourage invasion, migration, and metastasis (Coussens & Werb, 2002; Kawanishi, Hiraku, Pinlaor, & Ma, 2006).

E. Mendelian inheritance
   1. Autosomal dominant inheritance requires only one altered copy of a gene to result in disease expression (Figure 5-4).
   2. Autosomal recessive inheritance requires two altered copies of a gene, one from each parent, to result in disease expression (Figure 5-5).
   3. X-linked inheritance is associated with the inheritance of genes located on the X chromosome. Men carry one X and one Y chromosome, and genes on their X chromosome are hemizygous (having only one copy of a chromosome pair), so a mutation in a gene on an

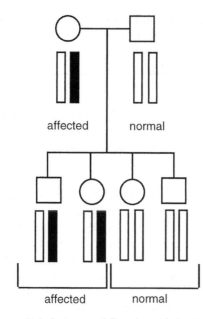

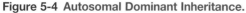

Figure 5-4 Autosomal Dominant Inheritance.

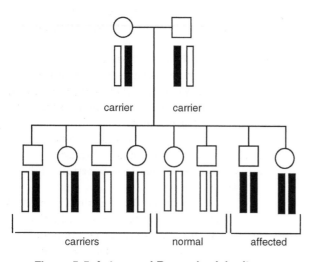

Figure 5-5 Autosomal Recessive Inheritance.

X chromosome in a man may result in disease expression.

III. Key technical characteristics of predisposition genetic testing and tumor profiling
   A. Techniques for identifying mutations
      1. Direct sequencing
         a. Determines the sequence of the gene being tested and detects sequence changes in the regions being analyzed
         b. Detects sequence changes in the regions being analyzed but may miss mutations outside the coding region or mutations that are large genomic rearrangements or large deletions

2. Allele-specific oligonucleotide (ASO)
   a. Detects one single specific mutation that involves a short sequence of DNA
3. Genome-wide association studies (GWAS)
   a. Survey the entire genome for small nucleotide alterations and do the following:
      (1) Detect SNPs or small mutations to determine association with disease (NCI Dictionary of Genetic Terms, n.d.)
      (2) Review for changes with specific disease (cancer type) versus people without the disease
      (3) Design high-throughput genome sequencing techniques to offer faster and cheaper ways to obtain genetic data, with potential impact on personalized profiling for diagnosis, pharmacogenomics, and disease monitoring (Soon, Hariharan & Snyder, 2013)
4. Single-strand confirmation polymorphism analysis (SSCP)
   a. A sequence change of DNA alters the size and shape of a DNA fragment, which is detected by SSCP on a gel.
   b. An altered gene produces a gel band different from that produced by a normal gene.
   c. SSCP easily detects insertions or deletions of four or more bases of DNA; however, mutations exchanging one base for another without altering the length of the DNA fragment are difficult to detect. In this technique, gel electrophoresis separates different conformations of the strands prior to sequencing.
5. Large genomic rearrangements (LGRs)
   a. Detect large rearrangements, deletions, and duplications (like pages or paragraphs missing or rearranged in a mystery novel)
   b. Found in *BRCA1* family mutations:
      (1) At least two persons younger than 50 years diagnosed with breast cancer
      (2) Family history of breast and ovarian cancers
      (3) Only ovarian cancer, with at least two members diagnosed with ovarian cancer
      (4) A single breast cancer case prior to the age of 36 years
      (5) None identified in only one breast cancer case prior to age 51 (Engert et al., 2008)
6. Microarray
   a. Technique attaches large numbers (hundreds to thousands) of DNA, RNA, protein, or tissue segments to slides specific locations on the slide, followed by application of a fluorescent label. The biosample is processed so that the genetic material of the sample

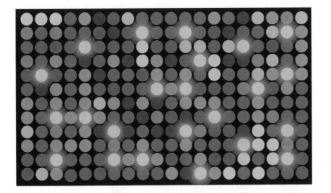

Figure 5-6 Microarray. Courtesy of the National Human Genome Research Institute, Bethesda, MD.

binds to the genetic material on the slide. The slide is scanned to measure the brightness of each fluorescent dot. The brighter the dot, the greater is the fluorescent activity (Figure 5-6).

   b. Microarray is used for mutation detection as well as gene expression.

  7. Next-generation DNA sequencing (second-generation sequencing)

    a. New, lower-cost, higher-efficiency techniques to target the whole genome, whole exome, and whole transcriptome

    b. Detect somatic cancer genome alterations of the nucleotide (substitutions, small insertions, deletions, variations in copy number)

  8. Whole-exome sequencing (WES) or targeted exome capture

    a. Low-cost alternative technique to sequence exon (gene to protein-coding regions) pieces of the genome

    b. Identifies area of protein function change in mendelian and common diseases

  9. Transcriptome sequencing

    a. Analyzes coding RNA molecules and non-coding RNA sequences in one or specific populations of cells (Meyerson, Gabriel, & Getz, 2010)

  10. Sequential analysis of gene expression (SAGE)

    a. Provides a picture of the mRNA population in a cancer sample

  11. Protein truncation assay

    a. Refers to an analysis of coding DNA, directly translated in the laboratory into protein

    b. Shortened proteins detected on a gel, based on mobility differences between larger and smaller proteins

    c. Sensitive for detection of mutations in which the sequence change results in a shortened form of the protein but does not detect other types of mutations

  B. Techniques to identify chemical modification or packaging of DNA

    1. Review methylation across entire genome (methylome)

      a. Addition of methyl groups to GC-rich region of DNA

      b. Hypomethylation with removal of methyl groups causing inactivation of a gene

    2. Methylation pattern of genes by tissue type

  C. Considerations in genetic testing laboratory selection

    1. Laboratories where genetic testing is performed should meet the following criteria:

      a. Clinical Laboratory Improvement Act (CLIA)–approved laboratory

      b. Does not evaluate proficiency of DNA testing

      c. Laboratory director certified by the American Board of Medical Genetics

    2. Research in which genetic research is performed in institutional laboratories with oversight to ensure meeting biosafety standards such as the NIH Guidelines for Research Involving Recombinant DNA Molecules (http://oba.od. nih.gov/oba/rac/Guidelines/NIH_Guidelines. htm)

IV. Use of genetic markers for diagnosis

  A. Cytogenetics focuses on the structure, function, and abnormalities of chromosomes (Jorde, 2009). It is commonly used to diagnose both solid and hematologic malignancies.

    1. Karyotype offers a view of the number and structural appearance of chromosomal structures in the cell nucleus (Lobo, 2008) (Figure 5-7).

      a. Balanced structural change in chromosomes with evenly exchanged genetic material; for example, Philadelphia chromosome translocation of 9;22, which yields an abnormal chromosome but genetic material amount remains constant although reshuffled (Figure 5-8)

        (1) Chromosomal rearrangement example: CML with the hybrid *bcr-abl* gene

        (2) Some thyroid cancers associated with rearrangements in the *RET* gene

      b. Nonreciprocal change of chromosomes with unequal genetic material to be lost or gained

        (1) Deletions or inactivation of a gene on a chromosome begin the process of accumulation of genetic variation, which then initiates cancer development. Tumor suppressor genes are an example of this type of nonreciprocal change.

        (2) Increases in the gene copy number contribute to cancer transformation.

Part 2

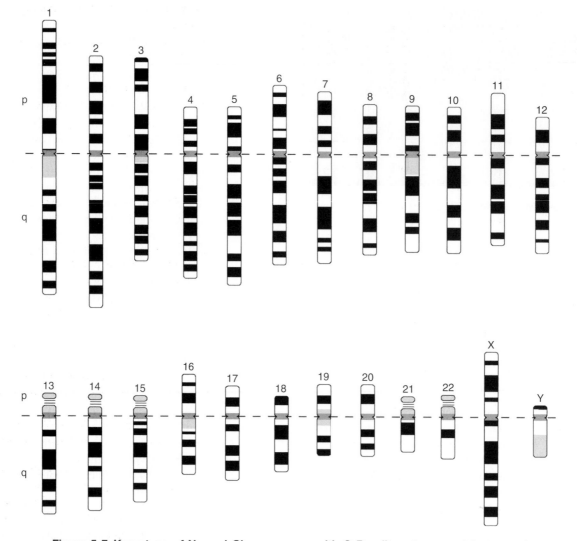

Figure 5-7 Karyotype of Normal Chromosomes with G-Banding. Courtesy of the National Human Genome Research Institute, Bethesda, MD.

In sarcomas, the chromosome 12q13-14 region is commonly amplified.

(3) Extra copies of the *ERBB2* (*HER2/neu*) gene cause overexpression of the epidermal growth factor protein, which is associated with aggressive breast cancer.

2. Nomenclature common to cytogenetic reports includes the modal number of chromosomes, the sex chromosome designation (XX or XY or aberrations of these chromosomes), the abnormality abbreviation, with the first chromosome separated with a semicolon from the second chromosome t(14;16), and then the arm and band number (q32; q23) (Table 5-1).

B. Gene expression (tumor) profiling uses multiple techniques (e.g., gene sequencing) to identify the expression (proteins) of tens to thousands of genes concurrently. It uses a personalized approach to cancer to diagnose, predict outcomes, or suggest the best treatment regimen for a person's cancer. Techniques such as a DNA microarray or serial analysis of gene expression (SAGE) are also used.

1. Colon cancer profiling examples include OncotypeDX and ColoPrint.

2. Breast cancer gene profiling examples include Mammaprint, Symphony, and OncotypeDX.

3. Myeloma Prognostic Risk Signature (MyPRS) measures the expression values (levels) of 70 risk-related genes.

V. Potential therapeutic interventions

A. Pharmacogenomics and pharmacogenetics (Klotz, 2007)

1. Pharmacogenetics identifies the genetic basis for differences in the metabolism of an agent and associated treatment response, which can be used to individualize therapy.

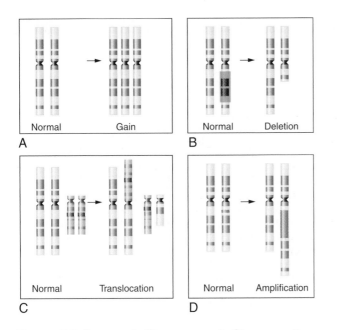

Figure 5-8 Types of Chromosomal Changes. *From Goldman,* L. & Schafer, A. *(2008). Cecil medicine (23rd ed.).* Philadelphia: Saunders.

Table 5-1

Common Cytogenetic Nomenclature

Nomenclature	Meaning
'	Separate of different elements of a cytogenetic report
( )	Surround structurally altered chromosomes
+	Gain of chromosome
-	Loss of chromosome
;	Separate rearranged chromosomes when >1 involved
cd	Cell or cluster of differentiation on surface of cell membrane
del	Deletion of chromosomal material
dn	New chromosomal abnormality; not inherited from parents
dup	Duplication of chromosomal material
ins	Insertion
inv	Inversion
mar	Unidentifiable piece of chromosome (marker)
t	Translocation or move of genetic material
tri	Trisomy
trp	Triplication of a chromosome piece
Example	46, XY, t(14;16)(q32;q23) = normal number of chromosomes, male, translocation of chromosome 4 and 16; specifically with position 32 on the long arm of chromosome 14 rearranging with position 23 on the long arm of chromosome 16

Data from *Basic nomenclature for cytogenetics.* <http://www.slh.wisc.edu/cytogenetics/abnormalities/nomenclature.dot> Accessed 11 September 2014.

a. A superfamily of enzymes, including the cytochrome P450 family, responsible for oxidation reactions for drug metabolism:
(1) Root symbol: CYP
(2) Arabic number for family
(3) Letter for subfamily
(4) Arabic numeral for specific gene
(5) Number 1 followed by an asterisk (*1) denotes the wild-type gene (most common)
(6) Additional number with (*) signifies a variant (*5)
(7) The enzyme (protein or gene product) identified as CYP2C19 and gene italicized (*CYP2C19*)
(8) Variances in specific allele frequencies among different populations; for example, the variant CYP2D6*4 occurs frequently in whites, whereas Asians have a higher frequency of CYP2D6*10

b. Pharmacodynamics—study of the biochemical and physiologic effects of drugs on the body

c. Pharmacokinetics—description of how the body absorbs, distributes, metabolizes, and excretes a drug

d. Genetic variation—affects differences in efficacy, toxicity, pharmacodynamics, and pharmacokinetics
(1) The DPD protein of the *DYPD* gene is involved in the metabolism of 5-fluorouracil (5-FU). DPD inactivates 80% of active 5-FU. Persons with a DYPD*2A variant have a greater risk of a grade 3 to 4 toxicity, most commonly neutropenia.
(2) The enzyme TPMT regulates 6-mercaptopurine (6-MP) for acute lymphoblastic leukemia (ALL). Persons with low TPMT activity may have high concentrations of 6-MP, leading to toxicities. Dosages are based on types of variants with TPMT*2, with TPMT*3A having low or intermediate TPMT activity. TPMT*1 (wild-type) has the highest TPMT activity, heterozygotes (*1/*3) with intermediate and (*3/*3) with the lowest activity.
(3) Drug transporters are responsible for pumping drug molecules across cell membranes. If these transporters are overactive, interference with drug effectiveness will occur. One of the transporters, P-glycoprotein, is encoded by the *ABCB1* gene. P-glycoprotein decreases intestinal absorption and brain

Table 5-2

Metabolizer Phenotypes and Anticipated Impacts on Active Drug and Prodrug

Genotype-Predicted Phenotype	Patient's Gene Pair	Anticipated Impact on Active Drug	Anticipated Impact on Prodrug
Poor or slow metabolizer	Homozygous for both variants with absent or nonfunctioning protein	Decreased efficiency in converting active drug to inactive metabolites Increases risk for higher levels of active drug and clinical toxicity	Inability to convert inactive prodrug to active metabolites If prodrug has no therepeutic properties, then patient will experience lack of efficacy despite drug dose increases
Intermediate metabolizer	Heterozygous variant of one gene results in absent or nonfunctioning protein variant of other member of gene pair results in protein with reduced function -or- Pair of genes, each with variant that results in protein with reduced function -or- One member of gene pair with variant results in protein reduced function other allele has sequence consistent with full functioning protein	Decreased efficiency in converting active drug to inactive metabolites Increases risk for higher levels of active drug and clinical toxicity If drug is normally dosed low and slowly titrated upward, effectiveness may be achieved sooner than in extensive metabolizers	Decreased efficiency in converting inactive prodrug to active metabolites Decreased effectivenss at standard maintenance doses may be anticipated
Extensive metabolizer	Homozygous with sequence for full-functioning protein	Active drug given at standard doses metabolized to inactive components, achieving effectiveness without or with minimal adverse drug reactions (ADRs)	Prodrug converted to active metabolites achieving effectiveness without or with minimal ADRs
Ultra-rapid metabolizer	Heterozygous with one locus consistent with full functioning protein, other locus has *two or more copies of gene sequence* resulting in full functioning protein Heterozygous with one member of gene pair has sequence consistent with full functioning protein and other member of gene pair has variant that causes increased amounts of full functioning protein to be produced	Increased efficiency in converting active drug to inactive metabolites Risk for decreased effectiveness at standard doses	Increased efficiency in converting prodrug to active metabolites Increased risk for toxicity from higher-than-expected levels of active metabolites

uptake while increasing drug excretion via the biliary intestinal and renal systems. High activity of *ABCB1* could increase removal of chemotherapy drugs, causing unsatisfactory treatment outcomes.

    e. Phenotypic responses of genotype that affect response to active and prodrug responses (Table 5-2).

2. Pharmacogenomic testing (Table 5-3) includes the following:

    a. Genetic testing is required for some cancer therapies. See Table 5-4 for a list of some of these cancer treatment agents (Whirl-Carrillo et al., 2012).

    b. Individualized treatment is based on the genetic characteristics of the individual and the tumor (see tumor profiling, section IV B, above) (Roses, 2000).

    c. Testing for use of drugs is specifically aimed at individualized genetic change and altered protein product of tumors.

Table 5-3

Some Genetic Variants and Their Effects on Pharmacotherapy*

Gene†	Molecular Effect	Polymorphism (Nucleotide Translation)	Drug	Effect on Therapy
Cytochrome P450 family	Decreased enzyme activity	Various polymorphism	Various	Interindividual variability in pharmacokinetics (PK)
TPMT2, 3A, 3C	Decreased enzyme activity	Various polymorphism	6-MP, thioguanine	Hematopoietic toxicity
UGT1A 28	Decreased enzyme activity	TA repeats in 5' promoter	Iriniotecan	Neutropenia toxicity
MDR1	Low expression	(C3435T)	Various	Drug resistance
TYMS	Increased enzyme activity	3 tandem repeats	5-FU, Methotrexate	Drug resistance
DPYD	Decreased enzyme activity	IVS14+1G	5-FU, Methotrexate	Neutropenia toxicity
DHFR	Increased enzyme activity	T91C	Methotrexate	Drug resistance
MTHFR	Decreased enzyme activity	(C677T) (A1298C)	5-FU, Methotrexate	Toxicity
c-KIT	Constitutive signal activation	D860 N567K	Imatinib	Desensitizes activity in GIST
K-RAS	Inhibition of the tyrosine kinase domain-binding drug	G12x G13D	Cetuximab Panitumomab	Desensitizes activity in colon-rectum
B-RAF	Inhibition of the tyrosine kinase domain-binding drug	V600E	Vemurafenib Gefitinib	Good response in melanomas
EGFR	Inhibition of the tyrosine kinase domain-binding drug	L858R	Erlotinib	Good response in NSCLC
BCR/ABL fusion gene	Constitutive signal activation	T(9;22) BCR/ABL	Imatinib Dasatinib Nilotinib	Good response in CML
ABL	Inhibition of the tyrosine Kinase domain-binding drug	T315I; M351T	Imatinib	Drug resistance in CML
PML/RARα fusion gene	Block of myeloid lineage cells	T(15;17) PML/RARα	All-Trans Retinoic acid (ATRA)	Good response in AML-M3 subtypes
ADRB1 ADRB2	G-protein altered	R389G	Beta-bloccants	Desensitizes activity
MHC class B 1	HLA-B~5701 aplotype	Several SNPs including codon K751Q	Abacavir	Hypersensitivity r
VKORC1	Associated with a higher/lower warfarin dose	Many, VKORC1 haplotypes including codon G3673A	Warfarin	Variable anticoagulant effect

5-FU, 5-Fluorouracil; 6-MP, 6-mercaptopurine; ADRB, adrenergic beta-receptors; AML, acute myeloid leukemia; CML, chronic myeloid leukemia; DHFR, dihydrofolate reductase; EGFR, epidermal growth factor receptor; GIST, gastrointestinal stromal tumor; MDR1, multidrug resistance 1; MTHFR, 5,10-methylene tetra hydrofolate reductase; NSCLC, non–small-cell lung cancer; PK, pharmacokinetics; TPMT, thiopurine methyl transferase; TYMS, thymidylate synthase; UGT1A1, UDP-glucuronosyl transferase 1A1; VKORC1, vitamin K epoxide reductase complex 1.

*The present list is not comprehensive.

†Genes are available for genotyping test or under consideration for clinical diagnostics.

Adapted from Di Francia, R., Valente, D., Catapano, O., Rupolo, M., Tirelli, U., & Berretta, M. (2012). Knowledge and skills needs for health professions about pharmacogenomics testing field. *European Review for Medical and Pharmacological Sciences*, 16(6), 781–788.

B. Proteomics
  1. Analysis of the structure, composition, and function of proteins
  2. Can aid in the diagnosis and enhance the understanding of the biologic basis of cancer
C. Somatic gene therapy
  1. Introduction of a functioning gene into the somatic cells to replace missing or defective genes or to provide a new cellular function
  2. Ongoing investigational trials using somatic gene therapy for a variety of cancers

Table 5-4

*Necessity of Pharmacogenetic Testing for Some Approved Oncologic Agents**

Pharmacogenetic Biomarker	Cancer Target	Oncologic Agent
Test Required Prior to Treatment		
BRAF (cobas 4800 *BRAF* V600 Mutation Test)	Unresectable or metastatic melanoma	Vemurafenib
EGFR expression	Metastatic colon cancer, Head and neck (testing not required) cancer	Cetuximab Panitumumab
Estrogen receptor (ER) and progesterone receptor (PR)	Breast cancer	Exemestane Fulvestrant Letrozole
K-ras	Colon cancer	Cetuximab Panitumumab Dasatinib
HER2/neu overexpression	Breast cancer	Trastuzumab Lapatinib
Presence of Philadelphia chromosome (Ph +)	Chronic myeloid leukemia (CML)	Imatinib Imatinib
PDGFRα	Gastrointestinal stromal tumors (GIST)	Tyrosine kinase inhibitors
FIP1L1-PDGFRα	Myelodysplastic//proliferative disorders	Imatinib
Tests Recommended for Treatment Decision		
EGFR	NSCLC	Erlotinib
G6PD	Tumor lysis syndrome	Rasburicase
Ph+	CML	Nilotinib
TPMT variants	Acute lymphocytic leukemia, acute nonlymphocytic leukemia	Mercaptopurine, thioguanine
UGT1A1 variants	Colorectal cancer	Irinotecan Nilotinib
Tests for Information Only		
CD-30	Hodgkin lymphoma Anaplastic large cell lymphoma	Brentuximab vedotin
c-Kit expression	Kit+gastrointestinal stromal tumors	Imatinib
DYPD deficiency	Colorectal or breast cancers	Capecitabine, 5-fluorouracil
Philadelphia chromosome deficiency (Ph-)	CML	Busulfan
PML/RAR gene expression	Promyelocytic leukemia	Arsenic Trioxide

*This information changes frequently and should be checked for current accuracy.

Data from U.S. Food and Drug Administration. (2013, June 19). *Table of valid genomic biomarkers in drug labels.* http://www.fda.gov/Drugs/ScienceResearch/ResearchAreas/Pharmacogenetics/ucm083378. Accessed 11 September 2014.; PharmGKB. (2013). *Genetic tests.* http://www.pharmgkb.org/views/viewGeneticTests.action. Accessed. 11 September 2014.

D. Germline gene therapy
1. Introduction of a functioning gene into the egg or sperm to prevent transmission of a genetic mutation
2. Germline gene therapy not available because it raises several ethical, legal, and social concerns

VI. Common hereditary cancer syndromes and cancer susceptibility genes
A. The common hereditary cancer syndromes, clinical manifestations, inheritance patterns, and genes are outlined in Table 5-5.
B. Features of hereditary cancer (Lindor, McMaster, Lindor & Greene, 2008)

1. Family member with a known germline deleterious mutation in a cancer susceptibility gene
2. Early age of cancer onset
3. Cancer of rare histology
4. Cancer in two or more close biologically related relatives
5. Bilateral cancer in paired organs (e.g., breast or ovary)
6. Multiple primary cancers in a single individual
7. Constellation of cancers in the family part of a known hereditary cancer syndrome

Table 5-5

Common Hereditary Cancer Syndromes and Cancer Susceptibility Genes

Syndrome	Clinical Manifestations	Gene	Mode of Inheritance
Ataxia-telangectasia	Cerebral ataxia, oculocutaneous telangectasias, radiation hypersensitivity, leukemia, lymphoma, breast cancer, and other solid tumors	*ATM*	Autosomal recessive
Basal cell nevus syndrome	Basal cell carcinoma, medulloblastoma, ovarian fibrosarcoma, odontogenic keratocyst, palmar or plantar pits, and ectopic calcification	*PTCH*	Autosomal dominant
Breast/ovarian cancer syndrome	Breast, ovary, fallopian tube, prostate, pancreas, and possibly gastric as well as other sites	*BRCA1*	Autosomal dominant
	Breast, ovary, fallopian tube, prostate, pancreas, melanoma, and possibly gastric as well as other sites	*BRCA2*	Autosomal dominant
Cowden syndrome	Multiple mucocutaneous lesions, vitiligo, angiomas, benign proliferative disease of multiple organ systems, macrocephaly, breast cancer, thyroid (nonmedullary) cancer, endometrial cancer, and renal cancer, as well as other possible sites	*PTEN*	Autosomal dominant
Familial adenomatous polyposis	Colon polyposis (adenomas), desmoid tumors, osteomas, thyroid cancer, and hepatoblastoma	*APC*	Autosomal dominant
Familial juvenile polyposis	Hamartomatous polyps of the stomach, small intestine, colon, and rectum Colon cancer as well as cancers of the stomach, duodenum, and pancreas	*BRIP1* *SMAD4*	Autosomal dominant
Fanconi anemia	Leukemia, hepatocellular carcinomas, squamous cell carcinomas of the head and neck, esophagus, cervix, vulva, anus, hepatic adenoma, myelodysplastic syndrome, aplastic anemia	*FANCA* *FANCB/FAAP95* *FANCC* *FANCD1?BRCA2* *FANCD2* *FANCE* *FANCF* *FANCG/XRCC* *(FANCI/KIAA1784* *FANCJ/BACH1/BRIP1* *FANCL/PHF9/* *FAAP43/POG* *FANCM/FAAP250/Hef* *FANCCN/PALB2*	Autosomal recessive
Gorlin syndrome	Basal cell carcinoma, brain tumors, and ovarian cancer	*PTCH*	Autosomal dominant
	Gastric cancer, lobular breast cancer, and signet ring colon cancer	*CDH1*	Autosomal dominant
Lynch syndrome (previously known as hereditary nonpolyposis colorectal cancer [HNPCC])	Cancers of the colon, rectum, stomach, small intestine, biliary tract, brain, endometrium and ovary, and transitional cell carcinoma of the ureters and renal pelvis	*MLH1* *MSH2* *MSH6* *MSH3* *PMS1* *PMS2*	Autosomal dominant
Li-Fraumeni syndrome	Breast cancer, sarcoma, brain tumors, leukemia, and adrenocortical carcinoma, as well as other possible cancers	*TP53*	Autosomal dominant
Melanoma	Melanoma, astrocytoma, pancreatic cancer, and ocular melanoma, as well as possibly breast cancer	*CDKN2A* *CDK4*	Autosomal dominant
Muir-Torre syndrome	Gastrointestinal and genitourinary cancers, skin, breast cancer, and benign breast tumors	*MSH2* *MLH1*	Autosomal dominant
Multiple endocrine neoplasia type 1	Pancreatic and neuroendocrine tumors, gastrinomas, insulinomas, parathyroid disease, and carcinoids, as well as adrenal cortical tumors, malignant schwannomas, ovarian tumors, pancreatic islet cell cancers, and gastrointestinal stromal tumors	*MEN1*	Autosomal dominant

Continued

Table 5-5

Common Hereditary Cancer Syndromes and Cancer Susceptibility Genes—cont'd

Syndrome	Clinical Manifestations	Gene	Mode of Inheritance
Multiple endocrine neoplasia type 2	Medullary thyroid cancer, pheochromocytoma, papillary thyroid cancer, and ganglioneuromas	*RET*	Autosomal dominant
MYH-associated polyposis (MAP)	Colon cancer and duodenal cancer, as well as colon, duodenal, and gastric fundic gland polyps, osteomas, sebaceous gland adenomas, and pilomatricomas	*MYH*	Autosomal recessive
Neurofibromatosis type 1	Malignant peripheral neural sheath tumors, neurofibromas, benign pheochromocytomas, meningiomas, hamartomatous intestinal polyps, gastrointestinal stromal tumors, optic gliomas, café-au-lait macules, axillary or inguinal freckles, iris hamartomas, and sphenoid wing dysplasia or congenital bowing or thinning of long bones, as well as other malignancies	*NF1*	Autosomal dominant
Neurofibromatosis type 2	Neurofibromas, gliomas, vestibular schwannoma, schwannomas of other cranial and peripheral nerves, meningioma, ependymonas, and astrocytoma	*NF2*	Autosomal dominant
Prostate cancer	Prostate and other cancers not established	*BRCA1* *BRCA2* *HOXB13* *RNASEL* *ELAC2/HPC2* *MSR1* *EMSY* *AMACR* *KLM6* *NBS1* *CHEK2* Mismatch repair genes (*MLH1, MSH2, MSH6, PMS2*) Several other loci under study	Varied: Autosomal dominant, Autosomal recessive, X-Linked
Retinoblastoma	Retinoblastoma, soft tissue sarcoma and osteosarcoma, melanoma, brain tumors, nasal cavity cancers, lung cancer, bladder cancer, retinomas, and lipomas	*RB1*	Autosomal dominant
Von Hippel-Lindau	Renal cell cancer, hemangioblastoma of brain, spinal cord, and retina, renal cysts, pheochromocytomas, endolymphatic sac tumors, and pancreatic islet cell tumors	*VHL*	Autosomal dominant
Wilms tumor	Wilm tumor and nephrogenic rests	*WT1*	Autosomal dominant
Xeroderma pigmentosum	Basal and squamous cell skin cancer, melanoma, and sarcoma, as well as brain, lung, breast, uterus, kidney, and testicle cancers, leukemia, conjunctival papillomas, actinic keratosis, lid epithiomas, keratoacanthomas, angiomas, fibromas	*XPA* *ERCC3* *XPC* *ERCC2* *DDB2* *ERCC4* *ERCC5* *POLH*	Autosomal recessive

From Lindor, N.M., McMaster, M.L., Lindor, C.J., Greene, M.H. (2008). Concise handbook of familial cancer susceptibility syndromes (2nd ed.). *Journal of the National Cancer Institute Monographs, 38,* 1–93.

C. Indications for cancer predisposition testing
  1. Criteria for predisposition genetic testing vary, depending on the suspected inherited cancer syndrome and mutations in the gene or genes associated with that syndrome
    a. Universal criteria for predisposition genetic testing include the following:

(1) Confirmed family history consistent with the hereditary cancer syndrome
(2) A test that can be interpreted once performed
(3) The test that will be used to assist in medical decision making or will assist in diagnosis of a condition

(4) Informed consent by the client to be tested

(5) Testing done in the context of pre- and post-test genetic counseling (American Society of Clinical Oncology, 2003; Robson, Storm, Weitzel, Wollins, & Offit, 2010).

    (a) The National Society of Genetic Counselors defines genetic counseling as "the process of helping people understand and adapt to the medical, psychological, and familial implications of genetic contributions to disease (National Society of Genetic Counselors' Definition Task Force, 2006).

    (b) Providers delivering genetic counseling may be physicians, nurses, or genetics counselors with specialized training in genetics. Table 5-6 summarizes some resources available for finding a health care provider trained in genetics.

2. The American Society of Clinical Oncology (ASCO) also recommends a review of the evidence of clinical utility for any genetic test (including multiplex tests, tests for low or moderate disease genes, and SNP tests) be considered when either ordering or making medical recommendations based on a test result (Robson et al., 2010).

3. Not every client is appropriate for predisposition genetic testing for inherited cancer susceptibility.

    a. Genetic tests, including those for cancer risk, are also available directly to the consumer, in which case ASCO also recommends a review of the clinical utility of the result before

making medical recommendations (Robson et al., 2010).

D. Outcomes for cancer predisposition testing

1. The predictive value of a negative test result varies, depending on whether a known genetic mutation exists in the family.

    a. A negative test result in the presence of a known genetic mutation indicates that the client is within the general population risk of cancer associated with that branch of the family.

        (1) However, family history from the other parent still influences the risk of developing cancer.

    b. A negative result with no known family genetic mutation may occur because of one of the following:

        (1) Identifying a mutation in a cancer susceptibility gene may not be possible because of the limited sensitivity of the techniques used.

        (2) The function of the gene may be affected by a mutation in a different gene.

        (3) The cancer in the family may be associated with a cancer susceptibility gene other than the one tested.

        (4) The cancer in the family is not the result of a germline genetic mutation.

    c. A mutation of uncertain clinical significance is identified. This refers to mutations in which the association with cancer risk cannot be established.

2. The predictive value of a positive test result varies, depending on the type of genetic mutation identified and the degree of certainty that the function of the gene has been affected.

    a. *Penetrance* refers to the proportion of all individuals with a specific genotype that express the specific trait such as cancer.

    b. *Expression* refers to the degree to which a single individual with a specific genotype will exhibit a specific trait (e.g., cancer).

        (1) Expression may be different for different genetic mutations in the same cancer susceptibility gene.

        (2) Expression may also be affected by other genetic variations as well as by the environment and other personal factors.

VII. Medical management issues associated with the care of individuals harboring a mutation in a cancer susceptibility gene

A. The management of cancer risk falls into five basic categories:

Table 5-6

Resources for Finding a Genetic Health Care Provider

Resource	Website
American Society of Human Genetics	http://www.ashg.org/
International Society of Nurses in Genetics	http://www.isong.org/
National Society of Genetic Counselors, Find a Genetic Counselor	http://www.nsgc.org/tabid/69/Default.aspx
National Cancer Institute Cancer Genetics Services Directory	http://www.cancer.gov/cancertopics/genetics/directory

1. Surveillance, which is monitoring to detect cancer as early as possible, when the chances for cure are greatest
2. Risk-reducing surgery (also called *prophylactic surgery*), which is the removal of as much of the tissue at risk as possible to reduce the risk of developing a cancer
3. Chemoprevention, which involves taking a medicine, vitamin, or other substance to reduce the risk of cancer
4. Risk avoidance, which is the avoidance of exposures that may increase the risk of certain cancers
5. Healthy behaviors, including diet and exercise

B. Cancer risk management strategies available to individuals at high risk for cancer because of a mutation in a cancer susceptibility gene vary according to the gene, specific gene mutation identified, or both. Each strategy has varying degrees of risks, benefits, and limitations, as well as varying levels of evidence supporting the specific intervention.

1. The National Cancer Institute Physician Data Query (PDQ) Cancer Information Summaries on Genetics at http://www.cancer.gov/cancertopics/pdq/genetics provide evidence-based reviews for many common cancer genetic syndromes and include a summary of cancer risk management strategies associated with that particular syndrome, as well as the associated levels of evidence.

VIII. Ethical, legal, and social issues associated with genetic information (Offit & Thom, 2007)

A. Predisposition genetic testing may have psychological consequences, some of which could impact subsequent health behaviors and family communication.

1. Survivor guilt is often observed in persons who have not inherited the genetic mutation that is present in other close family members.
2. Transmitter guilt is often observed when family members pass on the genetic mutation to one of their offspring.
3. Heightened anxiety may result when clients learn that they are at a substantially increased risk for developing cancer or another primary lesion.
4. Depression and anger may occur regardless of genetic status.
5. Personal identity issues result because genetic information involves the very essence of an individual.
6. Regret for previous decisions may be present in clients who have made major decisions based on their perceived cancer risk, and

testing results are inconsistent with what they had previously thought.

7. Uncertainty occurs because predisposition genetic testing does not provide information about if or when cancer develops. In many instances, no proven risk-reducing strategy exists.
8. Intrafamilial issues arise because predisposition genetic testing affects all family members. These issues include, but are not limited to, the following:
   a. Coercion regarding testing, disclosure of testing results to family members, and cancer risk management approaches
   b. Effect of the genetic information on the partner, who is not at risk physically but whose children may be impacted
9. Stigmatization both within the family and within the individual's social network.
10. Identification of an incidental finding if multiplex testing or some form of whole genome analysis (e.g., whole exome sequencing, whole genome sequencing) is performed

B. Predisposition genetic testing also has social implications.

1. Financial considerations
   a. Predisposition genetic testing may be very expensive. Some, but not all, insurers cover testing and counseling.
   b. Insurers may be reluctant to cover enhanced surveillance programs unless efficacy has been proven.
   c. Insurers may not be willing to cover the expense of prophylactic surgery unless it has proven benefit.
2. Quality assurance of laboratory testing is not certain because no regulation exists beyond approval for molecular laboratories that perform testing based on the CLIA.
3. Availability and quality assurance of genetic counseling are of concern, given the small number of trained providers in cancer genetics.

C. Legal issues for the client undergoing predisposition testing may involve the following:

1. Discrimination may occur for those harboring an altered cancer susceptibility gene because they may be considered as having a preexisting condition or may be too high a risk to insure or employ (Offit & Thom, 2007).
   a. Health insurance
   b. Life insurance
   c. Disability insurance
   d. Long-term care insurance
   e. Education
   f. Employment

2. State and federal legislative approaches have already been proposed or enacted, depending on the issue and state (National Cancer Institute PDQ Genetics Editorial Board, 2013).
   a. The Health Insurance Portability and Accountability Act (HIPAA), a federal law enacted in 1996, states that genetic information cannot be used as a pre-existing condition or to determine eligibility for insurance.
      (1) This protection only applies to group and self-funded plans.
      (2) This law does not protect against rate hikes, access of insurers to an individual's genetic information, or the insurer requiring genetic testing as a condition of insurance coverage.
   b. The Genetic Information Nondiscrimination Act (GINA), federal legislation enacted in 2008, applies to health insurance and employment discrimination based on genetic information (Baruch & Hudson, 2008; Hudson, Holohan, & Collins, 2008).
      (1) Health insurance protections include protections against accessing an individual's genomic information, requirements for an individual to undergo a genetic or genomic test, and using genomic information against a person during medical underwriting.
      (2) Employment protections include prohibiting employers from accessing an individual's genetic information, use of genomic information to deny employment, or collecting genomic information without consent.
      (3) The GINA does not supersede state legislation that provides for more extensive protections.
      (4) The GINA does not apply to active duty military personnel, Veterans Administration, or the Indian Health Service because the laws amended for GINA do not apply to these groups.
   c. The U.S. Equal Employment Opportunity Commission released guidelines in March 1995 on the definition of "disability" under the Americans with Disabilities Act (ADA), which is now extended to include discrimination based on genetic information. This set of guidelines is not law but simply is an interpretation of the language of the ADA and may be overturned in a court of law.

3. Self-insured employers may also be exempt from state laws and regulations on health insurance because of the Employee Retirement Income Security Act of 1974 (ERISA), which governs employer pension plans as well as other benefits.
D. Informed consent should precede genetic testing and include the following (Riley et al., 2012; Weitzel, Blazer, Macdonald, Culver, & Offit, 2011):
   1. Purpose of the genetic test
   2. Motivation for testing
   3. Risks of genetic testing
   4. Benefits of genetic testing
   5. Limitations of genetic testing
   6. Inheritance pattern of the gene(s) being tested
   7. Risk of misidentified paternity, if applicable
   8. Accuracy and sensitivity of genetic testing method
   9. Outcomes of genetic testing
   10. Confidentiality of genetic testing results
   11. Possibility of discrimination
   12. Alternatives to genetic testing
   13. How testing will impact health care decision making
   14. Cost of testing
   15. Right to refuse
   16. Testing in children (<18 years of age)
      a. Performed when clinical utility for testing in children has been established
   17. Management of incidental findings
E. Genetic technology raises legal liability issues for the health care provider.
   1. Privacy and confidentiality
      a. Genetic information of all types should be handled in a confidential manner to prevent unauthorized access.
   2. Genetic testing should be preceded by genetic counseling by a genetic health care professional, education, counseling, and informed consent.
   3. Health care providers may have a duty to inform clients regarding their potential for increased cancer risk from an inherited susceptibility and the availability of predisposition genetic testing (Offit, Groeger, Turner, Wadsworth, & Weiser, 2004).
F. Table 5-7 summarizes some available genetic and genomic resources.

NURSING IMPLICATIONS

I. Interventions to assist the client and family to understand cancer genetics and genetic testing
   A. Description of the organization and function of genetic material and the role of genetics in carcinogenesis

Table 5-7

Genomic Health Care Resources

Resource	Website
Essential Genetic and Genomic Competencies for Nurses with Graduate Degrees	http://nursingworld.org/MainMenuCategories/EthicsStandards/Genetics-1/Essential-Genetic-and-Genomic-Competencies-for-Nurses-With-Graduate-Degrees.pdf
Genetic and Genomic Nursing: Competencies, Curricula Guidelines and Outcome Indicators, 2nd edition	http://www.genome.gov/Pages/Careers/HealthProfessionalEducation/geneticscompetency.pdf
Genetics/Genomics Competency Center for Education (G2C2)	http://www.g-2-c-2.org
Genetic Home Reference	http://ghr.nlm.nih.gov/
Genetic Testing Registry	http://www.ncbi.nlm.nih.gov/gtr/
Global Genetics and Genomics Community (G3C)	http://www.g-3-c.org
National Cancer Institute Physician Data Query (PDQ) Cancer Information Summaries: Genetics	http://www.cancer.gov/cancertopics/pdq/genetics
Online Mendelian Inheritance in Man	http://www.omim.org/
Telling Stories: Understanding Real Life Genetics	http://www.tellingstories.nhs.uk/about_us.asp
Oncology Nursing Society. (2012). *Oncology nursing: The application of cancer genetics and genomics throughout the oncology care continuum*	http://www.ons.org/Publications/Positions/HealthCarePolicy
Pharmacogenomics Education Program (PharmGenEd)	https://pharmacogenomics.ucsd.edu/
U.S. Surgeon General's Family History Initiative	http://www.hhs.gov/familyhistory/

B. Assessment of the client's beliefs about the cause of cancer in the family and correct misconceptions
C. Description of the process for cancer risk evaluation and predisposition genetic testing
D. Discussion of the risks and benefits of predisposition genetic testing
E. Discussion of the risks and benefits of pharmacogenetic or genomic testing
F. Description of the rationale for the use of tumor profiling

II. Interventions to decrease perceived and actual barriers to cancer risk management
   A. Education and monitoring of the performance of self-examination techniques
   B. Education on the benefits of cancer risk management
   C. Facilitating reimbursement for cancer risk management procedures
   D. Encouragement of communication regarding fears and concerns
III. Interventions to enhance coping and adaptation
   A. Referral of the client, family, or both to community support services.
   B. Referral of the client, family, or both to professional counseling services, when indicated
   C. Encouragement of the use of coping strategies that have previously been effective

References

American Society of Clinical Oncology. (2003). American Society of Clinical Oncology policy statement update: Genetic testing for cancer susceptibility. *Journal of Clinical Oncology, 21*(12), 2397–2406.

Baruch, S., & Hudson, K. (2008). Civilian and military genetics: Nondiscrimination policy in a post-GINA world. *American Journal of Human Genetics, 83*(4), 435–444.

Coussens, L. M., & Werb, Z. (2002). *Nature, 420*(6917), 860–867. http://dx.doi.org/10.1038/nature01322.

Di Francia, R., Valente, D., Catapano, O., Rupolo, M., Tirelli, U., & Berretta, M. (2012). Knowledge and skills needs for health professions about pharmacogenomics testing field. *European Review for Medical and Pharmacological Sciences, 16*(6), 781–788.

Engert, S., Wappenschmidt, B., Betz, B., Kast, K., Kutsche, M., Hellebrand, H., et al. (2008). MLPA screening in the BRCA1 gene from 1,507 German hereditary breast cancer cases: Novel deletions, frequent involvement of exon 17, anad occurrence in single early-onset cases. *Human Mutation, 7*(7), 948–958. http://dx.doi.org/10.1002/humu.20723.

Ghildiyal, M., & Zamore, P. (2009). Small silencing RNAs: An expanding universe. *Nature Reviews Genetics, 10*(2), 94–108. http://dx.doi.org/10.1038/nrg2504.

Hudson, K. L., Holohan, M. K., & Collins, F. S. (2008). Keeping pace with the times–The Genetic Information Nondiscrimination Act of 2008. *New England Journal of Medicine, 358*(25), 2661–2663.

Jorde, L. B. (2009). Clinical cytogenetics: The chromosomal basis of human disease. In L. B. Jorde, & J. C. Carey (Eds.), *Medical genetics* (pp. 100–127): Mosby, Inc., an affiliate of Elsevier Inc.

Kawanishi, S., Hiraku, Y., Pinlaor, S., & Ma, N. (2006). Oxidative and nitrative DNA damage in animals and patients with inflammatory diseases in relation to inflammation-related carcinogenesis. *The Journal of Biological Chemistry, 387*, 365–372. http://dx.doi.org/10.1515/BC.

Klotz, U. (2007). The role of pharmacogenetics in the metabolism of antiepileptic drugs: Pharmacokinetic and therapeutic implications. *Clinical Pharmacokinetics, 46*(4), 271.

Knudson, A. G. (2001). Two genetic hits (more or less). *Cancer*, *1* (2), 157–162.

Lindor, N. M., McMaster, M. L., Lindor, C. J., & Greene, M. H. (2008). Concise handbook of familial cancer susceptibility syndromes - second edition. *Journal of the National Cancer Institute Monographs*, *38*, 1–93.

Lobo, I. (2008). Chromosome abnormalities and cancer cytogenetics. *Nature Education*, *1*(1). Retrieved from, http://www.nature.com/scitable/topicpage/chromosome-abnormalities-and-cancer-cytogenetics-879.

Loeb, L. A. (2011). Human cncers express mutator phenotypes: Origin, consequences and targeting. *Nature Reviews. Cancer*, *11*, 450–457.

Meyerson, M., Gabriel, S., & Getz, G. (2010). Advances in understanding cancer genomes through second-generation sequencing. *Nature Reviews Genetics*, *11*, 685–696. http://dx.doi.org/10.1038/nrg2841.

National Cancer Institute PDQ Genetics Editorial Board. (2013, 5/24/2013). *Risk assessment and counseling: Employment and insurance discrimination*. Retrieved 6/5/2013, 2011, from, http://www.cancer.gov/cancertopics/pdq/genetics/risk-assessment-and-counseling/HealthProfessional/page6#Section_386.

National Society of Genetic Counselors' Definition Task Force, Resta, R., Biesecker, B. B., Bennett, R. L., Blum, S., Hahn, S. E., Strecker, M. N., et al. (2006). A new definition of genetic counseling: National Society of Genetic Counselors' Task Force report. *Journal of Genetic Counseling*, *15*(2), 77–83.

NCI Dictionary of Genetic Terms. (n.d.). *Genome wide association study (GWAS)*. Retrieved from http://www.cancer.gov/geneticsdictionary?cdrid=636780.

Offit, K., Groeger, E., Turner, S., Wadsworth, E. A., & Weiser, M. A. (2004). The "Duty to Warn" a patient's family members about hereditary disease risks. *Journal of the American Medical Association*, *292*, 1469–1473.

Offit, K., & Thom, P. (2007). Ethical and legal aspects of cancer genetic testing. *Seminars in Oncology*, *34*, 435–443.

PharmGKB. (2013). *Genetic tests*. Retrieved from, http://www.pharmgkb.org/views/viewGeneticTests.action.

Rickinson, A. B., & Kieff, E. (2001). Epstein–Barr virus. In D. M. Knipe, & P. M. Howley (Eds.), *Fields virology: Vol. 2* (4th ed., pp. 2575–2623). Philadelphia: Lippincott Williams and Wilkins.

Riley, B. D., Culver, J. O., Skrzynia, C., Senter, L. A., Peters, J. A., Costalas, J. W., et al. (2012). Essential elements of genetic cancer risk assessment, counseling, and testing: Updated recommendations of the National Society of Genetic Counselors. *Journal of Genetic Counseling*, *21*(2), 151–161. http://dx.doi.org/10.1007/s10897-011-9462-x.

Robson, M. E., Storm, C. D., Weitzel, J., Wollins, D. S., & Offit, K. (2010). American Society of Clinical Oncology policy statement update: Genetic and genomic testing for cancer susceptibility. *Journal of Clinical Oncology*, *28*(5), 893–901.

Roses, A. D. (2000). Pharmacogenetics and the practice of medicine. *Nature*, *405*(6788), 857–865. http://dx.doi.org/10.1038/35015728 DOI:10.1038%2F35015728.

Soon, W. W., Hariharan, M., & Snyder, M. P. (2013). High-throughput sequencing for biology and medicine. High-throughput sequencing for biology and medicine. *Molecular Systems Biology*, *9*, 640. http://dx.doi.org/10.1038/msb.2012.61.

U.S. Food and Drug Administration. (2013, June 19). *Table of valid genomic biomarkers in drug labels. Retrieved from*, http://www.fda.gov/Drugs/ScienceResearch/ResearchAreas/Pharmacogenetics/ucm083378.

Weitzel, J. N., Blazer, K. R., Macdonald, D. J., Culver, J. O., & Offit, K. (2011). Genetics, genomics, and cancer risk assessment: State of the Art and Future Directions in the Era of Personalized Medicine. *CA: A Cancer Journal for Clinicians*, *61*, 327–351.

Whirl-Carrillo, M., McDonagh, E. M., Hebert, J. M., Gong, L., Sangkuhl, K., Thorn, C. F., et al. (2012). Pharmacogenomics knowledge for personalized medicine. *Clinical Pharmacology & Therapeutics*, *92*(4), 414–417.

CHAPTER 6

Research Protocols and Clinical Trials

Angela D. Klimaszewski

Research Protocols

OVERVIEW

I. Definition: *Research protocol*: a detailed written plan of a clinical research study (Clinical Trials.gov, 2012a, 2012b; National Cancer Institute [NCI]–Cancer Therapy Evaluation Program [CTEP], 2013a)

II. *Clinical research study* (Clinical Trials.gov, 2012a; Knoop & Carney, in press; NCI- CTEP, 2013a; Ness & Cusack, in press; National Institute of Health [NIH], 2013; World Health Organization [WHO], 2013)

A. Research with human subjects

B. Types of clinical research
1. Interventional (also called *experimental study*, or clinical trial [CT])
   a. Prevention
   b. Screening and early detection
   c. Improving diagnostics
   d. Quality of life and supportive care
   e. Treatment
2. Observational
   a. Epidemiologic

C. Interventional study (CT)
1. Purpose: to assess the safety, efficacy, and effectiveness of biomedical or behavioral interventions
2. Interventions—may be new treatment (pharmacologic agents, biologics [stem cell transplantation, gene therapies]), devices, or behavioral
   a. One, more than one, or none (control)
   b. Assignments defined by research protocol
3. Phase 0 to IV CTs (Table 6-1) (ClinicalTrials. gov., n.d.)
   a. CT categories for an investigational or known drug or combined modalities
   b. Describes the CT based on traits such as goal or number of subjects

D. Observational study
1. Purpose: to assess biomedical and health outcomes in groups of humans

2. Participants may be subgrouped by traits—that is, males, older than 65 years
3. No intervention

E. Review, approval, and monitoring (Code of Federal Regulations [CFR], 2012b; Filchner & Herman, in press; NCI-CTEP, 2013a; Mitchell & Smith, in press)
1. Each research study to be approved by an institutional review board (IRB) or an independent ethics committee (IEC) before participant enrollment begins
2. IRB
   a. Definition: any group formally designated by an institution to perform ethical review of proposed clinical research involving human subjects (CFR, 2012b; Department of Health and Human Services [DHHS]–Office for Human Research Protections [OHRP], 2011)
   b. Purpose: to protect and safeguard the rights and welfare of the human subjects in a CT by providing independent review and overview of, for example, the protocol and informed consent form, balancing the individuals' rights with generalizable knowledge (CFR, 2012b; Department of Health and Human Services [HHS] OHRP, 2011, n.d.)
   c. Criteria for IRB approval (CFR, 2009)
      (1) Minimal risk to subjects
      (2) Risks reasonable to expected benefits and knowledge
      (3) Unbiased subject selection
      (4) Informed and voluntary consent of each subject or legally authorized representative (LAR) to be sought and documented
      (5) Protocol provides data monitoring to ensure subjects' safety
      (6) Privacy and confidentiality of subject and data to be maintained
      (7) Vulnerable subjects to be protected from coercion or undue influence

Table 6-1

Overview of Phases of a Clinical Trial

Phase	Description	Goals	Subjects
0	• Exploratory study using small doses of investigational agent • Very limited drug exposure with limited duration of dosing (approx. ≤7 days) • No therapeutic (or diagnostic) intent • Conducted prior to traditional phase 1 study • Conducted under and exploratory investigational new drug (IND) application	• Provide human pharmacokinetic (PK) or pharmacodynamic (PD) data • Determine whether mechanism of action defined in preclinical models could be observed in humans • Refine biomarker assay using human tumor tissue, surrogate tissue, or both • Enhance efficiency and increase chance of success of subsequent development of the agent	• 10-12

I	• Traditional first-in-human (FIH) dose finding study for single agent
	• Dose finding study when using multiple agents or multiple interventions (e.g., drug+radiation)
		• Evaluate the safety and tolerability
		• Determine the maximum tolerated dose (MTD):
		  • Single agent
		  • Combination of agents
		  • Combination interventions
		• Determine dose limiting toxicity (DLT)
		• Define optimal biologically active dose (BAD)
		• Evaluate PK or PD data
		• Observe preliminary response (e.g., antitumor activity)
			• 20-100
			• Healthy volunteer
			• Patient volunteer
			• Usually many cancer types (e.g., solid tumors)
			• Refractory to standard therapy or no remaining standard therapy
			• Adequate organ function, specifically bone marrow, liver, kidney
			• Pediatric studies conducted after safety ad toxicity evaluation in adults

II	• Phase IIA
	  • Proof of concept study to provide initial information on activity of intervention to justify conducting a larger study
	• Phase IIB
	  • Optimal dosing study to target population
		• Phase IIA
		  • Demonstrate activity of the intervention in the intended patient condition or targeted population
		  • Establish proof of concept
		• Phase IIB
		  • Establish optimal dosing for the intended patient condition or targeted population to be used in phase III study
		  • Evaluate for safety
			• 80-300
			• More homogenous population deemed likely to respond based on:
			  • Phase I data
			  • Preclinical models, and/or
			  • Mechanisms of action
			• Subject needs to have disease that can be accurately and reproducibility measured
			• May limit number of prior treatments

III	Randomized controlled trial (RCT)	• Compare efficacy of intervention being studied to a control group • Evaluate for safety	• Hundreds to thousands • Homogenous population
IV	Postmarketing study	• Evaluate safety during postmarketing period • May or may not be required by the U.S. Food and Drug Administration (FDA) • Compare the drug to another similar product that is already being marketed • Monitor for long-term and additional safety, efficacy, and quality of life • Assess drug-food interactions • Assess effect in specific populations (e.g., pregnant women, children), or determine cost-effectiveness	• Hundreds to thousands • With the labeled indication of the newly marketed drug or biologic

Adapted from Ness, E. & Cusack, G. (In press). Types of clinical research: experimental. In Klimaszewski, A.D., Bacon, M., Eggert, J., Ness, E., Westendorp, J. & Willenberg K. (Eds.), *Manual for clinical trials nursing*. Pittsburgh: Oncology Nursing Society.

Table 6-2

Types of Institutional Review Boards (IRBs)

INTERNAL IRB	EXTERNAL IRB	
Local IRB	**Commercial IRB**	**Central IRB**
Affiliated with the institution or organization conducting the research	Paid by institution or sponsor to conduct review of research	Used with research that involves large, multisite clinical trials
Example: a university or hospital	Not affiliated with a specific institution	Conducts review on behalf of all study sites that agree to participate in the centralized review process
	Often used by industry to expedite activation of studies at sites May see use in physician practice setting May allow for rapid opening of a study for a specific patient as the study has already been centrally approved	May be commercial (overlap with commercial IRB information) May be established by public research organizations such as the National Cancer Institute (https://www.ncicirb.org/)

Reprinted from Filchner, K. (In press). Protocol review and approval process. In Klimaszewski, A.D., Bacon, M., Eggert, J., Ness, E., Westendorp, J. & Willenberg K. (Eds.), *Manual for clinical trials nursing.* Pittsburgh: Oncology Nursing Society.

---

3. Types of IRBs (Table 6-2)
4. External IRBs: central IRB (CIRB) or commercial IRB (Moon & Khin-Maung-Gyi, 2009)
   a. Not affiliated with a research institute or researcher; may therefore improve efficiency of review or speed trial conduct
   b. A means for researchers to conduct research in compliance with regulations when they are not affiliated with academic or federal medical systems
   c. NCI Central Institutional Review Board (NCICIRB)—provides IRB reviews for NCI CTEP–sponsored multicentered phase III adult CTs and pilot, phase II, and phase III pediatric CTs (NCI CIRB Initiative, 2013)
5. Data Safety and Monitoring Board (DSMB) (NIH, 2013)
   a. Independent of the primary investigator (PI); designed to ensure subject safety and the validity and integrity of the data
   b. Provides oversight and monitoring to confirm the safety of subjects and the validity and integrity of data for some NIH-supported clinical trials (may not be required in minimal risk studies; i.e., behavioral interventions)
   c. A detailed data and safety monitoring plan to be submitted to the applicant's IRB and institution for approval prior to the accrual of human subjects
   d. Reports interim results and intervention-specific toxicity to IRB
   F. Expanded access (U.S. Food & Drug Administration [FDA], 2013; Lindberg, in press)

1. Investigational new drugs (INDs) made available by manufacturers with FDA approval to patients who:
   a. Are too ill to participate in a CT (poor performance status).
   b. Have a disease for which no approved treatment is available.
   c. Have shown a therapeutic response at the end of a CT.
2. Regulated by the FDA
   a. Potential risks outweighed by potential benefit to patient
   b. Enrollment in CTs evaluating the drug not affected by the expanded availability
   c. Patients may be charged for expanded access use of most investigational drugs.
3. Types of expanded access protocols
   a. Individual patients, including emergency use (also called *compassionate use*)
   b. Intermediate-size patient populations with a similar disease but not enough patients to establish a treatment protocol
   c. Large numbers of patients under treatment with an IND—evidence of drug effectiveness; patients must not be eligible for other CTs
II. The protocol document
   A. More than one model for protocol documents available (only key components of the CTEP model outlined here); all elements presented in Section 7.2 of *A Handbook for Clinical Investigators Conducting Therapeutic Clinical Trials Supported by CTEP, DCTD, NCI* (version 1.1) found at http://ctep. cancer.gov/investigatorResources/docs/ InvestigatorHandbook.pdf (ClinicalTrials.gov,

2013; NCI-CTEP, 2013b; Mitchell & Smith, in press).

B. Created, proposed, activated, and executed according to the CTEP *Investigator Handbook* (NCI-CTEP, 2013b)
    1. Designed for interventional studies but essential features applicable to all clinical research protocols; slight differences may be found with industry-sponsored or other studies
    2. The same protocol version to be used at all multicenter research sites for consistency and communication among research team members and to ensure that ethical, procedural, and regulatory aspects of the protocol are executed in a comparable manner across all sites

C. Schema (CFR, 2012a; NCI-CTEP, 2013b) (Box 6-1)
    1. Summarizes the treatment regimen(s); specifies which intervention(s) will be administered, the length of time for each intervention (i.e., days, cycles), and the estimated number of patients exposed to the intervention, if applicable

D. Study objectives or aims
    1. Primary and secondary; may be presented as hypotheses

E. Background and rationale for conducting CTs
    1. Includes prior CTs that led to current hypothesis
    2. Evaluates correlations between disease and patient outcome—that is, therapeutic response, disease-free survival, overall survival
    3. Clarifies rationale—that is, unpublished data, techniques used
    4. Ancillary studies information—that is, quality of life, supportive care

F. Patient eligibility criteria (CFR, 2012a)
    1. Identifies conditions that subjects are to meet (examples not all-inclusive)
        a. Parameters: type and stage of cancer, age, gender
        b. Requirements: capacity to give informed consent, life expectancy, acceptable organ function
    2. Format: must be unbiased and measurable
        a. Inclusion criteria: must be met before registering a patient for a CT
        b. Exclusion criteria: clarifies who is to be excluded because of risk

G. Pharmaceutical information for investigational and commercial drugs
    1. Including, but not limited to, agent name, how supplied, stability, preparation instructions, storage requirements, route of administration, mechanism of action, formulation, and adverse events (NCI-CTEP, 2013b)

H. Treatment plan (e.g., IND) (CFR, 2012a; NCI-CTEP, 2013b)
    1. Dose and treatment regimens must be accurate, clear, easy to follow, and expressed consistently throughout the protocol document.⚠
    2. For CTEP-sponsored studies, dose and treatment regimens must follow the "Guidelines for Treatment Regimen Expression and Nomenclature," Appendix IX (NCI-CTEP, 2013b)

I. Procedures for patient entry on study (ClinicalTrials.gov, 2013; Simon, 2011)
    1. Details patient characteristics at registration and the randomization process, confirming eligibility and exclusion criteria for the patient
    2. Randomized design: patients assigned to an intervention group by chance—that is, computer generated using a mathematical model (Simon, 2011)
    3. Nonrandomized design—process whereby patient assignment to an intervention group is intentional—that is, physician's choice
    4. Patient characteristics: age, gender, race, education

Box 6-1

Examples of a Schema

For Phase 1 Single-Agent Protocols
Dose Escalation Schedule

Dose Level	Level 1	Level 2	Level 3	Level 4	Level 5
Dose of [CTEP IND Agent]*					

For Phase 1 Combination Protocols

Dose Level	Level 1	Level 2	Level 3	Level 4	Level 5
Agent X [units]					
Agent Y [units]					
Agent Z [units]					

*Doses are stated as exact dose in units (e.g., mg/m^2, mcg/kg) rather than as a percentage.

Adapted from NCI-CTEP. (2013b). *Generic protocol template*. http://ctep.cancer.gov/protocolDevelopment/docs/Generic_Protocol_Template_for_Cancer_Treatment_Trial.docx.

5. Stratification: process whereby subjects in a group are further subgrouped according specific factors—that is, prognostic factors

J. Adverse events (AEs) grading and reporting requirements (NCI, 2012b; NCI-CTEP, 2010; Ness & Lau Clark, in press.)
1. Definition of adverse event
   a. Any unfavorable or unintended sign (including an abnormal laboratory value), symptom, or disease temporally linked with the use of a medical treatment or procedure that may or may *not* be related to the treatment or procedure
   b. Represents a specific event used for medical documentation and scientific analyses (NCI-CTEP, 2010, p. 2)
2. Responsibility
   a. CTEP, the Cancer Imaging Program (CIP), and the Division of Cancer Prevention (DCP) ensure that research is conducted as directed under federal regulations (CFR, 2012a).
   b. The PI and the clinical investigators have the primary responsibility for AE identification, documentation, grading, and assignment of attribution to the agent or intervention, as well as reporting AEs.
   c. Expedited adverse events reporting for CTEP-sponsored CTs and DCP cancer prevention trials is done using CTEP's adverse events reporting system (CTEP-AERS) online at https://eapps-ctep.nci.nih.gov/ctepaers/pages/task?rand=1391472079519.
3. Assessment (NCI-CTEP, 2010; NCI-CTEP, 2013b)
   a. Grading: assessment of AE severity
      (1) Current version (4.03) of the Common Terminology Criteria for Adverse Events (CTCAE) used to grade AEs in CTs
      (2) CTCAE—consists of a numeric scale from 1 (mild toxicity) to 5 (death) (see Table 6-3)
   b. Expectedness
      (1) Expected: as stated in protocol, investigator's brochure, informed consent, or medical literature
      (2) Unexpected: all other AEs assessed

   c. Attribution: assessed relationship of investigational intervention and AE; observed AE may or may not be related to CT intervention
4. Dose modification for AEs: every dose change (dose holds, dose decrements, and treatment discontinuation) for AEs, described in NCI CTCAE terms, to be stated for each study agent in the CT

K. Criteria for response assessment (CFR, 2012a; Eisenhauer et al., 2009; Madsen, in press; NCI-CTEP, 2013b)
1. Endpoints: reproducible and consistent clinical and biologic measures of protocol objectives that minimize risk to subjects
   a. Most common: objective response rate or time to disease progression
   b. Others: progression-free, disease-free, and overall survival
2. Example: Response Evaluation Criteria in Solid Tumors (RECIST)
   a. Standardized approach to solid tumor measurement
   b. Specifies measurement and evaluation of disease
3. Response evaluation criteria for hematologic cancers are usually defined within the protocol document

L. Statistical considerations (CFR, 2012a; NCI-CTEP, 2013b)
1. How study design relates to objectives and plan for data evaluation including, but not limited to:
   a. Randomization and stratification methods
   b. Sample size calculation
   c. Estimated accrual rate and study duration
   d. Primary endpoint for interim and final analysis; stopping rules
   e. Plan for analysis of data

M. Informed consent (IC) (NIH, 2013; Klimaszewski, in press)⚠
1. Definition: a person's voluntary agreement, based on adequate knowledge and understanding, to participate in human subjects research or undergo a medical procedure

Table 6-3				
Common Terminology Criteria for Adverse Events (CTCAE) for Fever				
Adverse Event	**1**	**2**	**3**	**4**	**5**
Fever	38.0°-39.0°C (100.4°-102.2° F)	>39.0°-40.0°C (102.3°-104.0°F)	>40.0°C (>104.0°F) for ≤24 hours	>40.0°C (>104.0° F) for >24 hours	Death

Definition: A disorder characterized by elevation of the body's temperature above the normal limit. C, Celsius; F, Fahrenheit.

From NCI-CTEP. (2010). *Common terminology criteria for adverse events (CTCAE)* (version 4.03). http://evs.nci.nih.gov/ftp1/CTCAE/CTCAE_4.03_2010-06-14_QuickReference_8.5x11[1].pdf.

a. A process involving verbal and written (and other) communication to help people decide if they want to take part in a CT

2. Basic ethical principles to protect human subjects enrolled in clinical research studies—Belmont Report (National Commission for the Protection of Human Subjects of Biomedical and Behavioral Research, 1979):
   a. Respect for persons—that is, autonomy and protection of those with diminished autonomy
   b. Beneficence—that is, protection from harms; maximize benefits and minimize possible harms
   c. Justice—that is, benefits and burdens fairly distributed among subjects

3. Elements of Informed Consent Form (ICF); See Box 6-2.
   a. NCI IC template version (May 2013) available at http://ctep.cancer.gov/highlights/informed_consent_template_info.htm (NCI-CETP, 2013b)

4. IC Process (CFR, 2010; Klimaszewski, in press)
   a. Initial meeting to provide information and ICF to potential subject, answer questions, encourage note taking

Box 6-2

Required Elements of an Informed Consent Document

- A statement that the study involves research, its purpose, and the duration of the subject's participation
- Description of procedures, identifying those that are experimental
- Description of anticipated risks or discomforts to the subject
- Description of benefits to subject or others
- Disclosure of alternative procedures or treatments
- Description of the confidentiality of records that identify the subject
- Explanation of procedures (e.g., compensation, medical treatments) if injury occurs in research involving more than minimal risk and where more information is available
- Contact person for questions about research, subject's rights, and regarding an injury
- A statement that participation is voluntary; refusal to participate or withdrawal from participation at any time will not result in penalty or loss of benefits.

Adapted from Code of Federal Regulations. (2010). *General requirements for informed consent. Title 45: Public Welfare, Part 46: Protection of Human Subjects, Subpart A, Section 116.* http://www.hhs.gov/ohrp/humansubjects/guidance/45cfr46.html#46.116.

b. Allowing time for potential subject to read ICF and consider participation; discussion with family and trusted advisors; writing down questions
c. Answering questions and assessing understanding with interactive questioning, a written questionnaire, or having the patient explain parts of the ICF in his or her own words; documentation of potential participant's understanding and his or her decision to participate or decline
d. Affirming that subject's decision to participate in the CT is made without coercion or influence and having him or her sign the IC document
e. Affirming that patient knows he or she may withdraw consent at any time
f. Continuing IC process by encouraging subject to make a list of questions to bring to every visit; answering questions until patient is satisfied with his or her understanding
g. Affirming patient's consent immediately prior to administering therapy, as applicable
h. Reconsenting: providing subject with new information regarding CT, documentation of subject's understanding in the presence of family members, and giving a copy of the signed new IC document to them; reiterating that subject may withdraw at any time without loss of benefits
i. Using multiple communication techniques to provide IC information—that is, DVDs, CDs, interactive computer programs, written materials, and discussions

5. Vulnerable populations (CFR, 2010; Klimaszewski, in press)
   a. Children
      (1) Must provide assent and parents provide consent until child is 18 years old; failure of child to object does not indicate assent
      (2) Assent obtained from all children old enough to consider risks and benefits of participation
   b. Subjects with mental disabilities or dementia
      (1) Consent by subject's legally authorized representative (LAR) required
   c. Prisoners (Stiles, Epstein, Poythress, & Edens, 2012)
      (1) Protection from coercion
      (2) Protection for those who decline to participate
   d. Pregnant women, fetuses, and neonates
      (1) Consent by the subject, parent, or subject's LAR required

Clinical Trials

THEORY

I. Definition: a prospective research study of human subjects designed to answer specific questions about biomedical or behavioral interventions (drugs, treatments, devices, or new ways of using known drugs, treatments, or devices)

    A. Used to determine whether new biomedical or behavioral interventions are safe, efficacious, and effective

    B. Synonymous with interventional or experimental research (ClinicalTrials.gov, 2013; NIH, 2013; Ness & Cusack, in press; WHO, 2013).

II. Oversight (Good, 2013a, 2013b; NCI, 2012a)

    A. DHHS: general oversight of all research according to the Common Rule (codified elements of the Belmont Report [45 CFR part 46 subpart A])

    B. Office of Human Research Protections (OHRP), part of DHHS, provides guidance and clarification on ethical and regulatory issues in biomedical research and maintains regulatory oversight regarding compliance with the Common Rule (45CFR46).

    C. FDA regulates CTs that involve labeling claims of a drug or product.

    D. NCI (part of DHHS) sponsors

        1. NCI National Clinical Trials Network (NCTN) as of March 2014

        2. NCI Community Oncology Research Program (NCORP)—activated in 2014 and comprising the following former programs: DCP Research Bases, Community Clinical Oncology Program (CCOP) including Minority-Based CCOP (MBCCOP), and the NCI Community Cancer Centers Program (NCCCP)

        3. Division of Cancer Treatment and Diagnosis (DCTD): one of NCI's extramural divisions that funds clinical research

            a. CTEP: sponsors investigational anticancer drugs and biologics for CTs to advance understanding of molecular targets and mechanisms of drug effects

III. Comparative Effectiveness Research (CER) (Armstrong, 2012; Knoop & Carney, in press; Lyman & Levine, 2012)

    A. Definition: the process of generating, synthesizing, and comparing the benefit and harm of interventions (i.e., diagnostic, prognostic, and therapeutic) in typical patients to identify the most efficacious, safe, and cost-effective care for an individual (Armstrong, 2012; Lyman & Levine, 2012)

    B. Goal: "...identify, evaluate, and provide truly effective, safe, and cost-effective modern cancer care to all patients on the basis of equitable,

informed, and evidence-based clinical and national policy decisions" (Lyman & Levine, 2012, p. 4184)

        1. Generation of evidence through research studies

            a. Innovative designs to improve translation to practice

            b. Observational research to investigate differences across subgroups

        2. Synthesis of evidence with meta-analysis

IV. Role of the oncology nurse in CTs (Daugherty et al., 2009; Klimaszewski, in press)⚠

    A. Advocating for patient safety

        1. Promotes ethical care of CT subjects as per state standards of nursing practice

        2. Ensures that members of vulnerable populations enrolled in CTs are identified and that their rights are addressed

        3. Ensures ongoing communication with the clinical trials nurse (CTN)

        4. Promotes the informed consent (IC) process by validating that the patient understands the CT and that the IC document is signed and in the chart before treatment is initiated; notifies CTN or PI if patient has questions or misconceptions, or if the IC document is missing (Klimaszewski, in press)

        5. Affirms verbal consent from patient before each administration of the research drug, as applicable (Klimaszewski, in press)

        6. Delivers therapies in a safe and effective way according to the protocol document and oncology nursing best practices

        7. Assesses and monitors patient for AEs and manages them as warranted; documents presence and severity of symptoms and interventions accurately in the clinical record

        8. Seeks resources on an ongoing basis that provide oncology treatment and nursing practice updates

    B. Advocating for CT integrity

        1. Attends and participates in study initiation meetings, as applicable

        2. Ensures validity of research results through timely, accurate, and complete documentation of care for a patient participating in a research study

        3. Gathers blood samples and other outcome measures, according to the protocol

        4. Consults with CTN before administering any new medications to a patient enrolled in a CT

        5. Promotes patient, protocol, and scientific confidentiality by keeping research data and personal health information confidential

PROBLEM STATEMENTS AND OUTCOME IDENTIFICATION

I. Deficient Knowledge (NANDA-I)
   A. Expected outcome: patient and family describing their roles in CTs
II. Decisional Conflict (NANDA-I)
   A. Expected outcome: patient and family expressing satisfaction in decisions related to participation in CTs

PLANNING AND IMPLEMENTATION

I. Interventions to provide information related to clinical trials participation
   A. Reinforcing information received from PI, CTN, or members of the research team regarding the research study in which they are considering participation
   B. Discussing the risks and benefits of the research study
   C. Explaining that participating is voluntary and that refusal to participate or withdrawal at a later date will not result in penalty or loss of benefits to which the research participant is otherwise entitled
   D. Reviewing alternatives for treatment
II. Interventions to assist patient and family in decision making
   A. Encouraging patient to discuss the research study with family, friends, and a trusted non–family member advisor (i.e., pastor, attorney)
   B. Instructing patient and family to write down pros and cons of, and alternatives to, participation in the research study
   C. Reading and discussing with others the ICF and educational information provided by the principal investigator or CTN
   D. Instructing patient and family to write down questions for principal investigator or research nurse
   E. Encouraging patient and family to approach PI or CTN to ask questions
   F. Allowing patient and family time to make a decision

References

Armstrong, K. (2012). Methods in comparative effectiveness research. *Journal of Clinical Oncology*, *30*(34), 4208–4214. http://dx.doi.org/10.1200/JCO.2012.42.2659.

Clinical Trials.gov. (2012a). *Glossary of common site terms (select letter) (revised 08/2012)*. http://www.clinicaltrials.gov/ct2/about-studies/glossary.

Clinical Trials.gov. (2012b). *Learn about clinical studies (revised 08/2012)*. http://www.clinicaltrials.gov/ct2/about-studies/learn.

ClinicalTrials.gov. (2013). *ClinicalTrials.gov protocol data element definitions (draft)*. http://prsinfo.clinicaltrials.gov/definitions.html.

ClinicalTrials.gov. (n.d.). *Glossary-definition: Phase.* http://clinicaltrials.gov/ct2/help/glossary/phase.

Code of Federal Regulations (2009). *Criteria for IRB approval of research. Title 45: Public welfare, Part 46: Protection of human subjects, subpart A, section 111.* http://www.hhs.gov/ohrp/humansubjects/guidance/45cfr46.html#46.111.

Code of Federal Regulations. (2010). *General requirements for informed consent. Title 45: Public welfare, Part 46: Protection of human subjects, subpart A, section 116.* http://www.hhs.gov/ohrp/humansubjects/guidance/45cfr46.html#46.116.

Code of Federal Regulations. (2012a). *IND content and format. Title 21, Volume 5, Part 312: Investigational New Drug (IND) application.* http://www.accessdata.fda.gov/scripts/cdrh/cfdocs/cfCFR/CFRSearch.cfm?fr=312.23.

Code of Federal Regulations. (2012b). *Institutional review boards. Title 21, Vol. 1, Part 56.102.* http://www.accessdata.fda.gov/scripts/cdrh/cfdocs/cfcfr/CFRSearch.cfm?CFRPart=56&showFR=1&subpartNode=21:1.0.1.1.21.1.

Daugherty, P., Schmieder, L., Good, M., Leos, D., Weiss, P., Belansky, H., et al. (2009). *Oncology clinical trials nurse competencies.* http://ons.org/media/ons/docs/publications/ctncompetencies.pdf.

Department of Health and Human Services (DHHS) Office of Human Research Protections (OHRP). (n.d.). *IRBs and assurances.* http://www.hhs.gov/ohrp/assurances/index.html.

DHHS OHRP. (2011). *Guidance on written IRB procedures.* http://www.hhs.gov/ohrp/policy/irbgd107.html.

Eisenhauer, E. A., Therasse, P., Bogaerts, J., Schwartz, L. H., Sargent, D., Ford, R., et al. (2009). New response evaluation criteria in solid tumours: Revised RECIST guideline (version 1.1). *European Journal of Cancer*, *45*, 228–247. http://dx.doi.org/10.1016/j.ejca.2008.10.026.

Filchner, K., & Herman, P. (In press). Protocol review and approval process. In A. D. Klimaszewski, M. Bacon, J. Eggert, E. Ness, J. Westendorp, & K. Willenberg (Eds.), *Manual for clinical trials nursing* (3rd ed.). Pittsburgh: Oncology Nursing Society.

Good, M. (2013a). *Integrated program developed for clinical trials. Clinical Trial Nurses Special Interest Group Newsletter.* Pittsburgh: Oncology Nursing Society. January, p. 6.

Good, M. (2013b). *Programs combined into community oncology program. Clinical Trial Nurses Special Interest Group Newsletter* Pittsburgh: Oncology Nursing Society January, p. 7.

Klimaszewski, A. (In press). Informed consent. In A. D. Klimaszewski, M. Bacon, J. Eggert, E. Ness, J. Westendorp, & K. Willenberg (Eds.), *Manual for clinical trials nursing* (3rd ed.). Pittsburgh: Oncology Nursing Society.

Knoop, T., & Carney, P. (In press). Types of clinical research: Background. In A. D. Klimaszewski, M. Bacon, J. Eggert, E. Ness, J. Westendorp, & K. Willenberg (Eds.), Manual for clinical trials nursing. Pittsburgh, PA: Oncology Nursing Society.

Lindberg, D. A. (In press). Expanded access of investigational drugs. In A. D. Klimaszewski, M. Bacon, J. Eggert, E. Ness, J. Westendorp, & K. Willenberg (Eds.), *Manual for clinical trials nursing*. Pittsburgh: Oncology Nursing Society.

Lyman, G. H., & Levine, M. (2012). Comparative effectiveness research in oncology: An overview. *Journal of Clinical Oncology*, *30*(34), 4181–4184. http://dx.doi.org/10.1200/JCO.2012.45.9792.

Madsen, L. (In press). Protocol development and response assessment. In A. D. Klimaszewski, M. Bacon, J. Eggert, E. Ness, J. Westendorp, & K. Willenberg (Eds.), *Manual for clinical trials nursing*. Pittsburgh: Oncology Nursing Society.

Mitchell, W. & Smith, Z. (In press). Elements of a protocol. In A. D. Klimaszewski, M. Bacon, J. Eggert, E. Ness, J. Westendorp, & K. Willenberg (Eds.), *Manual for clinical trials nursing*. Pittsburgh: Oncology Nursing Society.

Moon, M. R., & Khin-Maung-Gyi, F. (2009, April). *The history and role of Institutional Review Boards*. http://virtualmentor.ama-assn.org/2009/04/pfor1-0904.html.

National Commission for the Protection of Human Subjects of Biomedical and Behavioral Research. (1979). *The Belmont report: Ethical principles and guidelines for the protection of human subjects of research*. http://www.fda.gov/ohrms/dockets/ac/05/briefing/2005-4178b_09_02_Belmont%20Report.pdf.

National Institute of Health (NIH). (2013). *Grants and funding: Glossary and acronym list*. http://grants.nih.gov/grants/glossary.htm#C.

NCI. (2012a). *National clinical trials network program guidelines, version 1.1*. http://ctep.cancer.gov/investigatorResources/default.htm.

NCI. (2012b). *NCI guidelines for investigators: Adverse event reporting requirements for DCTD (CTEP and CIP) and DCP INDs and IDEs*. http://ctep.cancer.gov/protocolDevelopment/electronic_application/docs/aeguidelines.pdf.

NCI CIRB Initiative. (2013). *NCI CIRB: Top 5 FAQs*. https://www.ncicirb.org/IM%20Top%205%20FAQs.pdf.

NCI CTEP. (2013). *A handbook for clinical investigators conducting therapeutic clinical trials supported by CTEP, DCTD, NCI (version 1.1)*. http://ctep.cancer.gov/investigatorResources/docs/InvestigatorHandbook.pdf.

NCI CTEP. (2013, May 15b). *Generic protocol template*. http://ctep.cancer.gov/protocolDevelopment/docs/Generic_Protocol_Template_for_Cancer_Treatment_Trial.docx.

NCI, Cancer Therapy Evaluation Program (CTEP). (2010). *Common terminology criteria for adverse events (CTCAE) (version 4.03)*. http://evs.nci.nih.gov/ftp1/CTCAE/CTCAE_4.03_2010-06-14_QuickReference_8.5x11[1].pdf.

Ness, E., & Cusack, G. (In press). Types of clinical research: Experimental. In A. D. Klimaszewski, M. Bacon, J. Eggert, E. Ness, J. Westendorp, & K. Willenberg (Eds.), *Manual for clinical trials nursing*. Pittsburgh: Oncology Nursing Society.

Ness, E., & Lau Clark, A. M. (In press). Adverse events and unanticipated problems. In A. D. Klimaszewski, M. Bacon, J. Eggert, E. Ness, J. Westendorp, & K. Willenberg (Eds.), *Manual for clinical trials nursing*. Pittsburgh: Oncology Nursing Society.

Simon, R. (2011). Design and analysis of clinical trials. In V. T. DeVita, T. S. Lawrence, S. A. Rosenberg, R. A. DePinho, & R. A. Weinberg (Eds.), *Cancer: Principles and practice of oncology* (9th ed.), ISBN: 9781451105452.

Stiles, P. G., Epstein, M., Poythress, N., & Edens, J. F. (2012). Protecting people who decline to participate in research: An example from a prison setting. *IRB: Ethics & Human Research*, 34 (2), 15–18.

U.S. Food & Drug Administration (FDA). (2013). *FDA expands access to investigational drugs*. http://www.fda.gov/ForConsumers/ConsumerUpdates/ucm176845.htm.

World Health Organization (WHO). (2013). *Clinical trials*. http://www.who.int/topics/clinical_trials/en/.

CHAPTER 7
Breast Cancer

Jan Petree

I. Anatomy and physiology
  A. Anatomy of the breast—both men and women develop breasts from the same embryologic tissues. At puberty, female sex hormones, mainly, estrogen, promote development of tissue, but this does not occur in men because of higher amounts of testosterone. Women's breasts become more prominent than those of men.
    1. Female adult breast tissue overlies the chest (pectoral) muscles; it lies between the sternum and the midaxillary line (axilla) from the second to the sixth ribs and below the clavicle (Dirbas & Scott-Conner, 2011).
    2. Breast consists of connective tissues (collagen and elastin), nerves (peripheral nerves, with front and side branches of the fourth, fifth, and sixth intercostal nerves, and T4 [thoracic spinal nerve, innervates the skin and dermatome of the nipple and areola complex]), blood vessels, lymphatic vessels, fat, lobules, ducts, suspensory Cooper ligaments, and nipple and areola (Dirbas & Scott-Conner, 2011).
    3. Two main aspects of the breast—functional breast and anatomic breast
      a. Functional breast—composed of glandular and adipose tissues
        (1) Glandular tissue—lobes (14 to 18) lactiferous lobes with lobules and milk ducts that are 2.0 to 4.55 mm in diameter, heading toward the nipple and surrounded by dense connective tissue, are called *terminal duct lobular units* (TDLUs), which produce fatty breast milk
        (2) Adipose tissue—becomes more prominent after menopause; 2:1 ratio of milk glands to fat in lactating breast; 1:1 ratio of milk glands to fat in nonlactating breast (Osborne & Boolbol, 2010)
      b. Anatomic breast
        (1) Size and shape of breasts vary from women to women and will change over course of her life.
        (2) Men may develop increased breast tissue; this condition is called *gynecomastia*.
    4. Lymphatic tissues—consist of lymph nodes and lymph channels; 75% of lymph fluid flows toward the axilla (pectoral, subscapular, humeral); 25% flows toward the parasternal lymph nodes, other breast, or abdomen (Osborne & Boolbol, 2010).
II. Epidemiology
  A. Most common cancer in women worldwide (International Agency for Research on Cancer and Cancer Research UK, 2011)
  B. In the United States, approximately 234,580 (232,340 women and 2240 men) new cases diagnosed; about 40,030 (39,620 women and 410 men) deaths reported from breast cancer in 2013 (American Cancer Society [ACS], 2013a)
  C. Second leading cause of cancer-related deaths in U.S. women
  D. Steady decrease in death rates since 1989, with 3% decrease in young women (<50 years old), and 2% decrease in women older than 50 years (ACS, 2013a)
  E. Trends in incidence rates
    1. Between 2002 and 2003, breast cancer incidence rate dropped by 7%, largely because of reduction in the use of hormone replacement therapy.
    2. From 2005 to 2009, incidence rates were stable.
    3. An estimated 64,640 U.S. women were newly diagnosed with in situ breast cancer in 2013 (ACS, 2013a).
      a. Increased incidence rate of 2.8% seen between 2005 and 2009 (ACS, 2013a)
      b. Two main types of in situ breast cancer
        (1) Ductal carcinoma in situ (DCIS)
          (a) Noninvasive breast cancer involving the duct cells
          (b) Make up 85% of in situ cases

(2) Lobular carcinoma in situ (LCIS)
   (a) Involves milk-producing lobule cells
   (b) Pleomorphic LCIS, an aggressive variant, more likely to develop into invasive lobular carcinoma (National Comprehensive Cancer Network [NCCN], 2014)

III. Risk factors (ACS, 2013b; Pegram, Takita, & Casciato, 2011)
  A. Gender—100 times more common in women than men
  B. Age—incidence higher with aging, particularly in women age 55 years or older; approximately 75% of all breast cancers in postmenopausal women
  C. Race and ethnicity
    1. 1 in 8 white women will develop breast cancer.
    2. 1 in 10 African American women will develop breast cancer.
      a. More African American women are diagnosed with breast cancer at a younger age (<45 years old).
  D. Early menarche (Anderson, Schwab, & Martinez, 2014)
  E. Late age of first full-term pregnancy: first child after age 30
  F. Number of births—lower risk seen in higher number of births
  G. Lactation or breast feeding—decreased risk of breast cancer in women who breastfed their babies, especially for long duration (Anderson et al., 2014)
  H. Older age at menopause
  I. Nulliparity—never pregnant
  J. Use of hormone replacement therapy, oral contraceptives, or both
  K. Post-thoracic radiation therapy to chest (e.g., radiation therapy to the chest for Hodgkin lymphoma and non-Hodgkin lymphoma)
  L. Family history—increased risk in women who have first-degree relative(s) (mother, father, sister, daughter) with breast cancer
  M. Genetic factors—hereditary breast cancer syndromes or mutations: account for 5% to 10% of all female breast cancers; 4% to 40% chance of genetic abnormality of all male breast cancers
    1. *BRCA1* gene mutation (Daly et al., 2010)
      a. Located in chromosome 17q21; accounts for 20% of all familial breast cancers
      b. 50% to 85% lifetime risk of developing breast cancer; 15% to 45% chance of developing ovarian cancer (Pegram et al., 2011)
      c. Increased risk of developing prostate cancer in males

      d. *BRCA1* gene mutations usually found in the following situations:
        (1) Breast cancer diagnosed before age 45
        (2) Diagnosed before age 50 with one or more first-degree relative(s) with breast cancer
        (3) Two primary tumors in the breast and first breast cancer diagnosed before age 50
        (4) Diagnosed in women younger 60 years of age with triple-negative breast cancer or first-degree male relative with breast cancer
        (5) Ashkenazi Jewish descent
        (6) Personal history of pancreatic cancer at any age with two or more first-degree relatives with breast, ovarian, or pancreatic cancer (NCCN, 2014).
    2. *BRCA2* gene mutation (Daly et al., 2010)
      a. Located in chromosome 13q12
      b. Lifetime risk of developing breast cancer as high as 80% (Pegram et al., 2011)
      c. Increased risk of breast, pancreatic, melanoma, and ovarian cancers with *BRCA2* gene mutation
      d. *BRCA1* gene mutations usually found in the following situations:
        (1) Ashkenazi Jewish descent
        (2) Personal history of epithelial ovarian cancer
        (3) Diagnosed with breast cancer before age 50 with limited family history.
        (4) Diagnosed with breast cancer at any age with two or more first-degree relatives with epithelial ovarian cancer at any age
        (5) Personal history of pancreatic cancer at any age with two or more close blood relatives with breast, ovarian, or pancreatic cancer (NCCN, 2014).
    3. *TP53* (tumor protein 53) gene—results in Li-Fraumeni syndrome, which increases the risk for breast cancer, soft tissue sarcomas, osteosarcomas, brain tumors, leukemia, and adrenocortical carcinoma (NCCN, 2014)
    4. *ATM* (ataxia telangiectasia mutated) gene—causes ataxia-telangiectasia disease, which is associated with higher rate of breast cancer
    5. *PTEN* mutation
      a. Causes Cowden disease, a rare disorder that increases the risk for benign or malignant breast cancers, hamartomas (benign abnormal formation of normal tissue) of the breast or gastrointestinal tract, cutaneous lesions of lips and mouth, thyroid abnormalities, follicular cancer, and

thyroid, kidney, and colorectal cancers (Pegram et al., 2011; NCCN, 2014)
  b. Lifetime risk of developing breast cancer 25% to 50%
6. *STK11/LKB*—can cause Peutz-Jeghers syndrome; is associated with an increased risk of developing cancers of the breast, gastrointestinal tract, ovary, testis, uterine, and cervix
7. *CHEK2*
  a. A cell cycle checkpoint kinase gene, which is an important component of the DNA cellular repair pathway
  b. Located on chromosome 22
  c. Mutation of gene increases risk of breast cancer in women (Pegram et al., 2011)
8. Lynch syndrome
  a. Often referred as *hereditary nonpolyposis colorectal cancer* (HNPCC)
  b. Associated with an increased risk of developing breast, ovarian, stomach, small bowel, pancreatic, prostate, urinary tract, liver, kidney, and bile duct cancers (Pegram et al., 2011)
9. *PALB2*
  a. Gene that provides instructions for making a protein called *partner* and *localizer* of *BRCA2*
  b. 2.3-fold increased risk of developing breast cancer
  c. 10 mutations in the *PALB2* gene identified in people with familial forms of breast cancer (National Institutes of Health [NIH], 2014)
10. *BRIP1*
  a. A *BRCA1* interacting protein gene
  b. Involved in making a protein that repairs damaged deoxyribonucleic acid (DNA) in the nucleus with the *BRCA1* gene and mends strands of damaged DNA seen in families with *BRCA1* and *BRCA2* mutations (NIH, 2014)

N. Diets high in fat, especially polyunsaturated fats
O. Monounsaturated fats such as olive oil may be protective.
P. Obesity
Q. Alcohol intake—risk increases with amount of alcohol consumed
R. Smoking—starting at a young age and continuing for more than 20 years

IV. Prevention of breast cancer
  A. Tamoxifen (Nolvadex)—first-generation selective estrogen receptor modulator (SERM)
    1. Results of the National Surgical Adjuvant Breast and Bowel Project (NSABP P1) showed a 49% overall reduction of breast cancer among women at high risk for the disease (Fisher et al., 1998; Sporn & Suh, 2000).
    2. Side effects include hot flashes, cognitive changes, increased triglyceride levels, thromboembolism, and endometrial cancer.
  B. Raloxifene (Evista)—second-generation SERM
    1. Approved by the U.S. Food and Drug Administration (FDA) for reducing risk of breast cancer in postmenopausal women and treatment of osteoporosis in postmenopausal women (Sporn & Suh, 2000)
    2. Side effects—hot flashes, leg cramps, arthralgias, headache, and flulike symptoms
    3. STAR (Study of Tamoxifen and Raloxifene) trial—a randomized, double-blinded, multicenter study comparing tamoxifen with raloxifene in over 19,000 postmenopausal women showed no statistically significant difference in the incidence of invasive breast cancer between the two groups; tamoxifen group had less noninvasive breast cancer (57 cases) compared with the raloxifene group (80 cases) (Vogel et al., 2006).
  C. Aromatase inhibitors (exemestane)
    1. Exemestane—showed benefit in reducing invasive breast cancers in postmenopausal women who were at moderate risk for breast cancer (Goss et al., 2011)
    2. Side effects—hot flashes, headache, vaginal bleeding, joint pain, bone loss

V. Screening and early detection (see Chapter 2: Early Detection of Cancer)
  A. Early detection—increases chance of survival if breast cancer is diagnosed at an early stage

VI. Diagnostic measures
  A. Biopsy—considerations based on location in breast or axilla; microscopic evaluation to make the diagnosis
    1. Gives the patient the opportunity to decide on type of surgery to receive
    2. Enough cells are needed for estrogen-receptor (ER), progesterone-receptor (PR), and HER-2/neu testing
    3. Types of biopsies
      a. Core needle biopsy
      b. Stereotactic vacuum-assisted breast biopsy
      c. Fine-needle aspiration (FNA)
      d. Incisional biopsy
      e. Excisional biopsy
    4. Magnetic resonance imaging (MRI), mammography, or ultrasonography may be used to better localize the site to be biopsied (Evers, 2010)

VII. Classic histopathologic classifications of breast cancer (Pegram et al., 2011)

A. Ductal adenocarcinoma—70% to 80% of breast cancer cases
1. Invasive ductal carcinoma (IDC)—most common type
2. Clinical prognosis highly variable; depends on cellular morphologic characteristics: ER, PR, Ki67 (marker of cell proliferation), and HER-2/neu
B. Lobular carcinoma—10% to 15% of breast cancer cases
1. Invasive lobular carcinoma (ILC)—capable of metastasis; has a range of prognosis similar to invasive ductal carcinoma
2. Difficult to diagnose because of radial pattern of spread, not easily detected on mammography, usually nonpalpable, and more likely to affect bilateral breasts compared with IDC
3. Metastasizes to unusual surfaces such as the pericardium, abdomen, ovary, uterus, stomach, and eye
C. Special subtypes with a favorable prognosis—less than 10% of cases
1. Includes papillary, tubular, mucinous, pure medullary carcinomas, and metaplastic carcinoma
D. Inflammatory breast cancer—1% of cases.
1. Aggressive subtype
2. Based on presence of dermolymphatic invasion with erythema, which mimics mastitis
3. Exhibits edema in skin (peau d'orange) with palpable border
E. Paget disease of the breast—characterized by unilateral eczematous changes in the nipple; frequently seen with ductal carcinoma in situ (DCIS)
F. Cystosarcoma phyllodes—less than 1% of breast neoplasms
1. 90% benign and 10% malignant
2. Rarely metastasizes but may recur locally
G. Rare tumors—include squamous cell carcinoma, lymphoma, and angiosarcoma
H. Nonmalignant tumors
1. Ductal carcinoma in situ (DCIS)—also referred to as intraductal carcinoma
a. Proliferation of cells inside the ducts
b. Staged as stage 0
c. May become invasive if not removed, so surgical excision recommended
d. Usually not palpable, often detected by mammography, and pleomorphic (broken glass dispersal pattern of calcifications) calcifications; highly suspicious of malignancy and need further evaluation; biopsy recommended—FNA or core biopsy

e. Architectural patterns—micropapillary, solid, comedo, papillary, cribiform
(1) Comedonecrosis often more aggressive and at higher risk of recurrence or becoming invasive
2. Lobular carcinoma in situ (LCIS)—also called *lobular neoplasia*
a. Often multicentric (more than one tumor) and multifocal (involves more than one quadrant of the breast)
b. Usually not detected on mammography or in physical examination but may be an incidental finding on pathology report
c. Staged as stage 0
d. Surgical excision recommended
3. Atypical ductal hyperplasia and atypical lobular hyperplasia
a. Surgical excision recommended (Pegram et al., 2011)
VIII. Molecular classification of breast cancer
A. Molecular classification of breast tumors may be based on:
1. Single gene arrays: ER, PR, HER-2/neu, Ki67, and proliferation index
2. Multigene expression:
a. Multigene transcript profiles use gene chip expression microarray (e.g., Oncotype DX Assay) or real-time polymerase chain reaction (RT-PCR) (e.g., Mammaprint).
3. Recent reports indicate distinct gene expression profiles for inflammatory breast cancer, HER2-positive breast cancer, lobular breast cancer, and *BRCA*-mutant breast cancer
B. Breast cancer has been divided into at least five subgroups with distinct clinical outcomes and biologic features (Pegram et al., 2011; Schnitt, 2010).
1. Luminal A tumors
a. Have the highest levels of ER expression: ER-positive, PR-positive, HER2-negative
b. Tend to be low grade
c. Most likely to respond to endocrine therapy and have a favorable prognosis
d. Tend to be less responsive to chemotherapy (Pegram et al., 2011)
2. Luminal B tumors
a. Tumor cells' gene patterns—ER-positive, PR-negative, HER2-positive
b. Prognosis worse than luminal A tumors
c. Tend to be high grade
d. May benefit from chemotherapy and targeted HER2 therapy (Pegram et al., 2011)

3. Normal-like breast tumors
   a. Gene expression profile similar to nonmalignant normal breast epithelium
   b. Prognosis similar to luminal B tumors (Pegram et al., 2011)
4. *HER2*-amplified
   a. Tumors have amplification of *HER2* gene on chromosome 17q and may have overexpression of other genes adjacent to *HER2*.
   b. *HER2*-positive cancers have decreased expression of ER and PR and upregulation of vascular endothelium growth factor (VEGF).
   c. Clinical prognosis of these tumors was poor, but with the advent of trastuzumab (Herceptin) therapy, clinical outcome has improved.
5. Basal tumors
   a. Tumors negative for ER, PR, and HER2, or "triple-negative."
   b. Tend to be high grade and express cytokeratins (5/6, and 17), vimentin, p63, CD10, smooth muscle actin, and epidermal growth factor receptor (EGFR)
   c. *BRCA1* breast cancers may fall into this group and often have poor prognosis; therefore, will likely benefit from chemotherapy (Pegram et al., 2011)

IX. Histologic grade
   A. Bloom-Richardson or Nottingham grading system most often used
      1. Grade 1: low grade or well differentiated
      2. Grade 2: intermediate grade or moderately differentiated
      3. Grade 3: high grade or poorly differentiated

X. Staging
   A. Staging workup includes the following:
      1. CT of chest (if pulmonary symptoms present). Abdominal pelvic ± CT or MRI (if there is elevated alkaline phosphatase, abnormal liver function test, abdominal symptoms, or clinical stage IIA or higher).
      2. Bone scan (if indicated for bone pain or elevated alkaline phosphatase)
      3. Positron emission tomography (PET) or CT (optional)—not recommended for all women
      4. Bilateral breast MRI (stages I-III optional)—not recommended for all women
      5. Blood work, including complete blood cell count (CBC), platelets (plts), liver and alkaline phosphatase (NCCN, 2014)
   B. Stages of breast cancer (Table 7-1)
   C. Metastatic pattern
      1. Most common organs involved in metastases in the local area are regional lymph nodes (axillary, internal mammary, inferior, supraclavicular lymph nodes) or in the skin
         a. Internal mammary nodes—involved in about 25% of patients with tumors in the upper inner quadrant and 15% with outer quadrant lesions
      2. Contralateral breast—most common in invasive lobular carcinomas
      3. Distant metastatic sites—include bone, skin, lung, liver, abdomen, eyes, bladder, brain, and spinal cord
         a. Hematogenous spread—to liver, lung, bone, brain, and abdomen
         b. Lymphatic spread—to intramammary lymph nodes, axillary nodes, mediastinal nodes, other lymphatics
      4. Unusual sites of distant metastasis—eye, bladder, ovary, peritoneum
         a. More common with invasive lobular cancers (NCI, 2014)

XI. Prognosis and survival rates
   A. 5-year survival rate by stage: stage 0 (100%), I (100%), II (93%), III (72%), and IV (22%) (ACS, 2013a)
   B. Factors affecting prognosis and treatment (Hortobagyi, Esserman, & Buchholz, 2010).
      1. Lymph node status—poorer prognosis with more lymph node involvement
      2. Tumor size—better prognosis with smaller tumors
      3. Histologic grade—more aggressive disease with higher grade tumors
      4. Hormone receptor status—better prognosis with ER- and/or PR-positive tumors
      5. Histologic tumor type—invasive tumors have the ability to metastasize.
      6. Ki-67 (*MIB1*) proliferation rate—Ki67 ratio in percentage of cells that are actively proliferating
      7. Oncogene *HER2/neu* and EGFR overexpression
      8. Breast cancer assay—Oncotype DX, MammaPrint
         a. Oncotype DX—a 21-gene assay used to predict chemotherapy benefit and estimate the 10-year risk of distant recurrence in women with early-stage, node-negative, estrogen receptor positive (ER+) invasive breast cancer (Dowsett et al., 2010; Genomic Health, 2014).
            (1) Ribonucleic acid (RNA) extracted from the breast cancer specimen is analyzed by RT-PCR assay.
            (2) Recurrence score result is calculated from the gene expression results.
               (a) Low risk: recurrence score of 0 to 17
               (b) Intermediate risk: recurrence score of 18 to 31
               (c) High risk: recurrence score ≥ 32
         b. MammaPrint—70-gene array used to identify women with early-stage breast cancer (either

Table 7-1

Staging of Breast Cancer

Primary Tumor (T)

TX	Primary tumor cannot be assessed
T0	No evidence of primary tumor
Tis	Carcinoma in situ
T1	Tumor $\leq$ 20 mm in greatest dimension
T1mi	Tumor $\leq$ 1 mm in greatest dimension
T1a	Tumor $>$ 1 mm but $\leq$ 5 mm in greatest dimension
T1b	Tumor $>$ 5 mm but $\leq$ 10 mm in greatest dimension
T1c	Tumor $>$ 10 mm but $\leq$ 20 mm in greatest dimension
T2	Tumor $>$ 20 mm but $\leq$ 50 mm in greatest dimension
T3	Tumor $>$ 50 mm in greatest dimension
T4	Tumor of any size with direct extension to the chest wall and/or to the skin (ulceration or skin nodules)
T4a	Extension to the chest wall, not including only pectoralis muscle adherence/invasion
T4b	Ulceration and/or ipsilateral satellite nodules and/or edema (including peau d'orange) of the skin, which do not meet the criteria for inflammatory carcinoma
T4c	Both T4a and T4b
T4d	Inflammatory carcinoma

Regional Lymph Nodes (N)

NX	Regional lymph nodes cannot be assessed
N0	No regional lymph node metastases
N1	Metastases to movable ipsilateral level I, II, axillary lymph node(s)
N2	Metastases in ipsilateral level I, II axillary lymph nodes that are clinically fixed or matted OR Metastases in clinically detected ipsilateral internal mammary nodes in the absence of clinically evident axillary lymph node metastases
N2a	Metastases in ipsilateral level I, II, axillary lymph nodes fixed to one another (matted) or to other structures
N2b	Metastases only in clinically detected ipsilateral internal mammary nodes and in the absence of clinically evident level I, II axillary lymph node metastases
N3	Metastases in ipsilateral infraclavicular (level III) axillary lymph node(s), with or without level I, II axillary lymph node involvement OR Metastases in clinically detected ipsilateral internal mammary lymph node(s) with clinically evident level I, II axillary lymph node metastases OR Metastases in ipsilateral supraclavicular lymph node(s) with or without axillary or internal mammary lymph node involvement
N3a	Metastases in ipsilateral infraclavicular lymph node(s)
N3b	Metastases in ipsilateral internal mammary lymph node(s) and axillary lymph node(s)
N3c	Metastases in ipsilateral supraclavicular lymph node(s)

Distant Metastasis (M)

M0	No evidence of distant metastases
cM0(i+)	No evidence of distant metastases, but deposits of molecularly or microscopically detected tumor cells in circulating blood, bone marrow, or other nonregional nodal tissue that are $\leq$ 0.2 mm in a patient without symptoms or signs of metastases
M1	Distant detectable metastases as determined by classic clinical and radiographic means and/or histologically proven as $>$0.2 mm

Anatomic Stage

Stage 0	Tis	N0	M0
Stage IA	T1	N0	M0
Stage IB	T0	N1mi	M0
	T1	N1mi	M0
Stage IIA	T0	N1	M0
	T1	N1	M0
	T2	N0	M0
Stage IIB	T2	N1	M0
	T3	N0	M0

Continued

Table 7-1

Staging of Breast Cancer—cont'd

Anatomic Stage—cont'd

Stage IIIA	T0	N2	M0
	T1	N2	M0
	T2	N2	M0
	T3	N1	M0
	T3	N2	M0
Stage IIIB	T4	N0	M0
	T4	N1	M0
	T4	N2	M0
Stage IIIC	Any T	N3	M0
Stage IV	Any T	any N	M1

Used with permission of the American Joint Committee on Cancer (AJCC), Chicago, Illinois. The original source for this material is the AJCC Cancer Staging Manual, Seventh Edition (2010) published by Springer Science and Business Media LLC, www.springer.com.

hormone receptor–positive or hormone receptor–negative) who are at risk of distant recurrence following surgery (Drukker, Bueno-de-Mesquita, & Retel, 2013).

  (1) 70 genes affect all the steps known to be important for metastasis, including cell cycle regulation, angiogenesis, invasion, cell migration, and signal transduction (Knauer et al., 2010).

  (2) Recurrence score is assigned as low risk or high risk.

    (a) No intermediate risk group

XII. Treatment

  A. Locoregional treatment of clinical stage I, IIA, or IIB disease or T3 N1 M0 (NCCN, 2014).

    1. Lumpectomy with surgical axillary staging followed by radiation therapy and possible chemotherapy, antihormonal therapy and antibody therapy (NCCN, 2014; Murphy & Sacchini, 2013; Mahmood et al., 2012)

    2. Total mastectomy with surgical axillary staging, with or without reconstruction

      a. Consider chemotherapy followed by radiation therapy for those with close margins (<1 mm), positive margins, and/or positive lymph nodes.

      b. Breast reconstruction for mastectomy can be performed at the same time as mastectomy or at some time after completion of cancer treatment (Strålman, Mollerup, Kristoffersen, & Elberg, 2008).

      (1) Options for breast reconstruction include the following:

        (a) Implants alone

        (b) Tissue expanders with implants later

        (c) Latissimus dorsi alone or with implants

        (d) TRAM (transverse rectus abdominus myocutaneous), DIEP (deep inferior epigastric perforator) tissue flap

        (e) Pedicle or gluteal flap

    3. Sentinel lymph node biopsy—preferred method of axillary lymph node staging (Mansel et al., 2006)

      a. Sentinel node—most likely the first lymph nodes to which cancer may spread from a primary tumor

    4. Axillary lymph node dissection—done if sentinel nodes positive, or if palpable or biopsy-proven positive lymph nodes in axilla

  B. Adjuvant endocrine therapy—ER- and/or PR-positive

    1. Premenopausal at diagnosis

      a. Tamoxifen for 5 years, with or without ovarian suppression or ablation

      (1) Potential side effects include hot flashes, uterine cancer, deep vein thrombosis, vaginal discharge, increased bone density, and depression (Hackshaw et al., 2011).

    2. Postmenopausal at diagnosis

      a. Aromatase inhibitor for 5 years, (Cuzick et al., 2010)

      (1) Potential side effects include hot flashes, joint aches, loss of bone density, dry skin, vaginal dryness, and decreased libido.

      b. May use tamoxifen for 5 years for women with contraindications or who are intolerant of aromatase inhibitors

  C. *HER2*-positive disease

    1. Trastuzumab (Herceptin)—a monoclonal antibody

a. Given intravenously

b. Potential side effects include allergic reaction, decreased left ejection fraction, pulmonary toxicity with interstitial pneumonitis, and pulmonary fibrosis.

2. Lapatinib (Tykerb)—a kinase inhibitor for use in metastatic *HER2*-positive disease in combination with chemotherapy agents (Blackwell et al., 2010; Frenel et al., 2009).

   a. Recommended dose 1250 mg orally daily.

   b. Must be taken at least 1 hour before or 1 hour after a meal

   c. Potential side effects include decreased left ejection fraction, hepatic toxicity, nausea, vomiting, diarrhea, interstitial lung disease or pneumonitis, Q-T interval prolongation, palmar and plantar erythrodysesthesia, rash, and fatigue

3. Pertuzumab (Perjeta)—a monoclonal antibody

   a. Given intravenously and in combination with trastuzumab and docetaxel for metastatic breast cancer (Baselga et al., 2012)

4. TDM-1 (Kadcyla, ado-trastuzumab emtansine)—an antibody drug conjugate with the monoclonal antibody trastuzumab, linked to a cytotoxic agent mertansine (DMI), which enters the cycle and destroys tubulin formation (LoRusso et al., 2011)

   a. Potential side effects include fatigue, headache, musculoskeletal pain, thrombocytopenia, nausea, constipation, and elevated liver enzyme levels (Verma et al., 2012)

D. Chemotherapy for locally advanced and metastatic disease

1. Non–trastuzumab-containing regimens

   a. Preferred regimens (NCCN, 2014)

      (1) TAC (docetaxel, doxorubicin, and cyclophosphamide)

      (2) Dose-dense AC (doxorubicin and cyclophosphamide) followed by paclitaxel every 2 weeks

      (3) AC (doxorubicin and cyclophosphamide) followed by weekly paclitaxel

      (4) TC (docetaxel and cyclophosphamide)

2. Trastuzumab-containing regimens

   a. Preferred regimens (NCCN, 2014)

      (1) AC followed by T plus concurrent trastuzumab (doxorubicin and cyclophosphamide followed by paclitaxel plus trastuzumab)

      (2) TCH (docetaxel, carboplatin, trastuzumab)

      (3) Traztuzumab, pertuzumab, and docetaxel—approved in metastatic disease and in neoadjuvant setting (Baselga et al., 2012; Gianni et al., 2012)

XIII. Nursing implications

A. Nurses play a vital role in educating patients regarding disease process, treatment options, side effects, and self-care.

1. Interventions to increase patient knowledge regarding disease process, treatment, and side effects

   a. Explaining disease process and treatment options in a nonjudgmental way and at the patient's level of understanding

   b. Encouraging discussion regarding potential physical and emotional changes resulting from treatment and exploration of personal values and beliefs as they relate to treatment options

   c. Facilitating patient's involvement in treatment decision making to the extent desired

   d. Providing education regarding the risk for lymphedema; teaching the patient how to measure the circumference of the affected arm and to notify the physician if it increases

      (1) Teaching the patient about precautions to take with regard to the affected arm to prevent trauma and infection, which could lead to lymphedema ⚠

   e. Informing the patient about altered arm and breast sensations (numbness and tingling of arm, lack of sensation on chest wall, phantom breast sensation after mastectomy) that may persist indefinitely following surgery

   f. Assessing for menopausal symptoms (hot flashes, vaginal dryness) that may be associated with adjuvant endocrine therapy or chemotherapy-induced ovarian failure

   g. Monitoring for and managing side effects of surgery, radiation, biotherapy, and chemotherapy

2. Interventions to promote self-care and enhance adaptation and rehabilitation

   a. Facilitating communication between patient and her health care providers; alerting the health care team to the patient's concerns about breast cancer and its treatment

   b. Assessing coping skills, support system, feelings about body image, sexually identity, role relationships

c. Providing the patient with information regarding community resources available for support, rehabilitation, and breast prostheses

d. Educating the patient on long-term follow-up, surveillance, and office visits

e. Teaching the patient about the important of practicing breast self-examination (BSE) and examining the axillary for any lymphadenopathy

f. Teaching about survivorship (see Chapter 42: Survivorship)

References

American Cancer Society. (2013a). *Cancer facts & figures, 2013.* Atlanta: Author.

American Cancer Society. (2013b). *What are the risk factors for breast cancer?* http://www.cancer.org/cancer/breastcancer/detailedguide/breast-cancer-risk-factors.

Anderson, K. N., Schwab, R. B., & Martinez, M. E. (2014). Reproductive factors and breast cancer subtypes: A review of the literature. *Breast Cancer Research and Treatment, 144*(1), 1–10.

Baselga, J., Cortes, J., Kim, S.-B., Im, S., Hegg, R., Im, Y., et al. (2012). Pertuzumab plus trastuzumab plus docetaxel for metastatic breast cancer. *New England Journal of Medicine, 366*(2), 109–119.

Blackwell, K. L., Burstein, H. J., Storniolo, A. M., Rugo, H., Sledge, G., Koehler, M., et al. (2010). Randomized study of Lapatinib alone or in combination with trastuzumab in women with ErbB2-positive, trastuzumab-refractory metastatic breast cancer. *Journal of Clinical Oncology, 28*(7), 1124–1130.

Cuzick, J., Sestak, I., Baum, M., Buzdar, A., Howell, A., Dowsett, M., et al. (2010). Effect of anastrozole and tamoxifen as adjuvant treatment for early-stage breast cancer: 10-year analysis of the ATAC trial. *Lancet Oncology, 11*(12), 1135–1141.

Daly, M. B., Axilbund, J. E., Buys, S., Crawford, B., Farrell, C. D., Friedman, S., et al. (2010). Genetic/familial high-risk assessment: Breast and ovarian. *Journal of the National Comprehensive Cancer Network, 8*(5), 562–594.

Dirbas, F. M., & Scott-Conner, C. E. H. (Eds.). (2011). *Breast surgical techniques and interdisciplinary management.* New York: Springer.

Dowsett, M., Cuzick, J., Wale, C., Forbes, J., Mallon, E., Salter, J., et al. (2010). Prediction of risk of distant recurrence using the 21-gene recurrence score in node-negative and node-positive postmenopausal breast cancer patients treated with anastrozole or tamoxifen: A transATAC study. *Journal of Clinical Oncology, 28*, 11.

Drukker, C. A., Bueno-de-Mesquita, J. M., & Retel, V. P. (2013). A prospective evaluation of a breast cancer prognosis signature in the observational RASTER study. *International Journal of Cancer*, 1–8.

Edge, S. B., Byrd, R. R., Compton, C. C., Fritz, A. G., Greene, F. L., & Trotti, A. (Eds.). (2010). *AJCC: Cancer staging manual* (p. XV).

Evers, K. (2010). Image-guided biopsy of nonpalpable breast lesions. In J. R. Harris, M. E. Lippman, M. Morrow, & C. K. Osborne (Eds.), *Diseases of the breast* (4th ed.). Philadelphia: Lippincott Williams & Wilkins.

Fisher, B., Costantino, J. P., Wickerham, D. L., Redmond, C. K., Kavanah, M., Cronin, W. M., et al. (1998). Tamoxifen for prevention of breast cancer: Report of the National Surgical Adjuvant Breast and Bowel Project P-1 Study. *Journal of the National Cancer Institute, 90*(18), 1371–1388.

Frenel, J. S., Bourbouloux, E., Berton-Rigaud, D., Sadot-Lebouvier, S., Zanetti, A., & Campone, M. (2009). Lapatinib in metastatic breast cancer. *Women's Health, 5*(6), 603–612.

Genomic Health. (2014). *Oncotype DX.* http://www.genomichealth.com/OncotypeDX.aspx#.UnLbpfmsigI.

Gianni, L., Pienkowski, T., Im, Y. H., Roman, L., Tseng, L. M., Liu, M. C., et al. (2012). Efficacy and safety of neoadjuvant pertuzumab and trastuzumab in women with locally advanced, inflammatory, or early HER2-positive breast cancer (NeoSphere): A randomised multicentre, open-label, phase 2 trial. *The Lancet Oncology, 13*(1), 25–32.

Goss, P. E., Ingle, J. N., Alés-Martínez, J. E., Cheung, A. M., Chlebowski, R. T., Wactawski-Wende, J., et al. (2011). Exemestane for breast-cancer prevention in postmenopausal women. *New England Journal of Medicine, 364*(25), 2381–2391.

Hackshaw, A., Roughton, M., Forsyth, S., et al. (2011). Long-term benefits of 5 years of tamoxifen: 10-year follow-up of a large randomized trial in women at least 50 years of age with early breast cancer. *Journal of Clinical Oncology, 29*(13), 1657–1663.

Hortobagyi, G. N., Esserman, L., & Buchholz, T. (2010). Neoplasms of the breast. In W. K. Hong, R. C. Bast Jr., W. N. Hait, D. W. Kufe, R. E. Pollock, & R. R. Weichselbaum, et al. (Eds.) *Cancer medicine* (pp. 1393–1458). Shelton, CT: People's Medical Publishing House-USA.

International Agency for Research on Cancer and Cancer Research UK (2011). *Cancer worldwide.* http://publications.cancerresearchuk.org/downloads/Product/CS_CS_WORLD.pdf.

Knauer, M., Mook, S., Rutgers, E. J., Bender, R. A., Hauptmann, M., Van de Vijver, M. J., et al. (2010). The predictive value of the 70-gene signature for adjuvant chemotherapy in early breast cancer. *Breast Cancer Research and Treatment, 120*(3), 655–661.

LoRusso, P. M., Weiss, D., Guardino, E., Girish, S., & Sliwkowski, M. X. (2011). Trastuzumab emtansine: A unique antibody-drug conjugate in development for human epidermal growth factor receptor 2–positive cancer. *Clinical Cancer Research, 17*(20), 6437–6447.

Mahmood, U., Morris, C., Neuner, G., Koshy, M., Kesmodel, S., Buras, R., et al. (2012). Similar survival with breast conservation therapy or mastectomy in the management of young women with early-stage breast cancer. *International Journal of Radiation Oncology, Biology, Physics, 83*(5), 1387–1393.

Mansel, R. E., Fallowfield, L., Kissin, M., Goyal, A., Newcombe, R. G., Dixon, J. M., et al. (2006). Randomized multicenter trial of sentinel node biopsy versus standard axillary treatment in operable breast cancer: The ALMANAC Trial. *Journal of the National Cancer Institute, 98*(9), 599–609.

Murphy, J. O., & Sacchini, V. S. (2013). New innovative techniques in radiotherapy for breast cancer. *Minerva Chirurgica, 68*(2), 139–154.

National Cancer Institue. (2014). *Metastatic breast cancer.* http://www.cancer.gov/cancertopics/metastaticdisease.

National Comprehensive Cancer Network. (2014). *NCCN practice guidelines in oncology: Breast cancer, [v.1.2014].* http://www.nccn.org/professionals/physician_gls/pdf/breast.pdf.

National Institutes of Health. (2014). *Genetics home reference.* http://www.ghr.nlm.nih.gov/gene/PALB2.

Osborne, M. P., & Boolbol, S. K. (2010). Breast anatomy and development. In J. R. Harris, M. E. Lippman, M. Morrow, & C. K. Osborne (Eds.), *Diseases of the breast* (4th ed.). Philadelphia: Lippincott Williams & Wilkins.

Pegram, M. D., Takita, C., & Casciato, D. A. (2011). Breast diseases. Breast cancer. In D. A. Casciato, & M. C. Territo (Eds.), *Manual of clinical oncology* (7th ed.). Philadelphia: Lippincott Williams & Wilkins.

Schnitt, S. J. (2010). Classification and prognosis of invasive breast cancer: From morphology to molecular taxonomy. *Modern Pathology, 23*, S60–S64.

Sporn, M. B., & Suh, N. (2000). Chemoprevention of cancer. *Carcingogenesis, 21*, 525–530.

Strålman, K., Mollerup, C. L., Kristoffersen, U. S., & Elberg, J. J. (2008). Long-term outcome after mastectomy with immediate breast reconstruction. *Acta Oncologica, 47*(4), 704–708.

Verma, S., Miles, D., Gianni, L., Krop, I. E., Welslau, M., Baselga, J., et al. (2012). Trastuzumab emtansine for HER2-positive advanced breast cancer. *New England Journal of Medicine, 367*(19), 1783–1791.

Vogel, V. G., Costantino, J. P., Wickerham, D. L., Cronin, W. M., Cecchini, R. S., Atkins, J. N., et al. (2006). Effects of tamoxifen vs raloxifene on the risk of developing invasive breast cancer and other disease outcomes. *Journal of the American Medical Association, 295*(23), 2727–2741.

CHAPTER 8

Lung Cancer

Marie Flannery

OVERVIEW

I. Pathophysiology
   A. Normal anatomy and function of lungs
      1. Located in the thorax
      2. Designed for air exchange, oxygen capture, and carbon monoxide exhalation
      3. Act to filter microparticles
      4. Trachea—provides the initial passageway into the bronchi, which subdivide into smaller bronchioles and end in alveoli
      5. An extensive blood vessel structure
      6. Pleura—a thin tissue that covers the lungs and lines the chest cavity
      7. Have an extremely large surface area, with tremendous reserve volume
      8. Separated into lobes (three on the right, two on the left), with further division into lobules
   B. Changes associated with cancer
      1. "Multihit" theory of carcinogen exposure resulting in deoxyribonucleic acid (DNA) damage and mutation
      2. Alterations and deregulation in the biology that control cell proliferation, vascular supply, and normal cell death
      3. Genetic alterations on chromosome 15 identified
      4. Long-term exposures to toxins, specifically cigarette smoking, damage the cells (American Thoracic Society [ATS], 2013).
      5. Specific pathways that lead to cancer are an active area of investigation.
II. Common metastatic sites (National Cancer Institute [NCI], 2013a; National Cancer Comprehensive Network [NCCN], 2013;)
   A. In part because of the large lung surface area, early signs and symptoms may be absent.
      1. Cancer may be incidentally diagnosed when a chest radiography is performed for some other reason.
      2. It is common for individuals to have both respiratory and constitutional symptoms.
   B. Local spread may cause obstruction, pleural effusion, and lymph node involvement.
      1. Symptoms may include dyspnea, hemoptysis, cough, and dysphagia.
   C. Systemic spread is common to the brain, liver, adrenal glands, and bone.
      1. Symptoms are variable and may include pain, weight loss, fatigue, anorexia, and neurologic symptoms.
   D. Affected individuals are at risk for paraneoplastic syndromes and oncologic emergencies such as hypercalcemia, syndrome of inappropriate antidiuretic hormone (SIADH), spinal cord compression (SCC), superior vena cava syndrome (SVC), cardiac tamponade, and uncontrolled pain (see Chapters 40 and 41). ⚠
III. Diagnostic measures (NCCN, 2013; NCI, 2013b)
   A. Complete history and physical examination to include:
      1. Identification of findings related to local or systemic spread
      2. Evaluation of pulmonary status and baseline status
      3. Identification of any comorbidities, all of which influence treatment options
   B. Laboratory evaluation, including complete blood cell count and chemistry panels
      1. To date, no specific tumor markers for disease status identified
   C. Pulmonary function tests to establish baseline and evaluate for treatment tolerance
   D. Imaging begins with a chest X-ray and CT of the chest, liver and adrenal glands.
      1. If spread is suspected, additional imaging may include positron emission tomography (PET) (particularly helpful for nodal evaluation and to identify metastatic sites) and additional imaging of suspicious sites (bone scan, abdominal imaging).

2. Because of the frequency of brain metastasis, head imaging with magnetic resonance imaging (MRI) performed if suspicion of advanced disease exists

E. Tissue sample to be obtained for diagnosis
    1. Involves targeting a readily accessible area (pleural fluid, lymph node) and a location that would establish the most advanced stage of disease
        a. The least invasive method likely to yield adequate tissue for evaluation preferred (Alberg, Brock, Ford, Samet, & Spivack, 2013)
    2. To adequately stage the tumor, additional molecular diagnostic testing for gene alterations conducted (for the epidermal growth factor receptor [*EGRF*] and anaplastic lymphoma kinase [*ALK*] genes)

IV. Prognosis (American Cancer Society [ACS], 2013)
    A. Leading cause of cancer-related deaths worldwide, in part because the disease is diagnosed at advanced stages and survival is poor
        1. Worldwide, lung cancer remains an epidemic, and deaths from lung cancer are four times more common than from any other cancer (NCCN, 2013).
        2. Overall survival rate for lung cancer at 5 years is only 16% in all clients.
        3. Improvements in the U.S. have been seen in the 1-year survival rates, which have increased to 44%.
        4. Survival rates depend on stage of disease:
            a. 5-year survival—52% for localized disease
            b. 25% for regional
            c. 3.7% for advanced
            d. Poorer survival rate for small cell lung cancer (ACS, 2013)
        5. Positive prognostic factors include early stage of disease, good performance status, less than 5% weight loss, and female gender. (NCCN, 2013).
    B. Epidemiology (ACS, 2013)
        1. As of 2013, the second most common cancer in both men and women in the United States
        2. Accounts for 14% of cases annually, with 228,190 new cases projected in 2013
        3. Leading cause of cancer mortality in the United States for both genders, accounting for 27% of cancer deaths, with 159,480 deaths projected for 2013
        4. Both incidence and mortality rates slowly declining in the United States for both genders, with changes correlating with decreased smoking
        5. Poorer outcomes and diagnosis at more advanced stage of disease among African Americans

V. Classification
    A. Cancer classification systems commonly in use include identification of the primary site or anatomic location in the body (lung) and the tissue of origin (histologic type) (NCI, 2013c).
        1. Establishment of lung cancer as the primary diagnosis may be challenging because the lung is a common metastatic site and lung cancer may first appear elsewhere in the body (e.g., brain).
        2. Determining the lungs as the primary site has been aided by the development of immunohistochemical staining (e.g., thyroid transcription factor 1 [TTF-1], multiple creatine kinase [CK] stains), which may assist in differentiating the histology and primary versus metastatic adenocarcinoma (NCCN, 2013).
    B. The two major types of lung cancer are non–small cell lung cancer (NSCLC), accounting for 85% of cases, and small cell lung cancer (SCLC).

VI. Staging
    A. Lung cancer is staged clinically on the basis of physical examination, imaging findings, and biopsy or after surgical resection.
        1. TNM (T = tumor size, N = nodal status, M = metastasis) staging was revised for lung cancer in the most recent edition of the TNM guidelines. (American Joint Commission on Cancer [AJCC], 2013; Edge, Byrd, Compton, Fritz, & Trotti, 2010).
            a. Changes were evidence-based.
            b. Based on analysis of a large multinational data set of lung cancer cases
            c. More accurately differentiate staging and prognosis
            d. Primary changes made in cutoff for tumor size and subdivisions in T staging
            e. Changes in M category made to include contralateral lung nodules and pleural effusions, with subdivisions added
        2. No changes to the N category, but a new lymph node map released for increased clarity and consistency (Figure 8-1); clinical staging system as follows:
            a. NSCLC—Ia, Ib, IIa, IIb, IIIa, IIIb, or IV with occult; stage 0 also identified
                (1) May be cross-walked with the TNM stage (see Table 8-1)
            b. SCLC—staged as either limited (confined to one lung and lymph nodes on same side) or extensive stage (spread widely in lung, to other lung, distant organs) (ACS, 2013)
                (1) Two thirds of cases diagnosed as extensive stage
        3. The new edition of the TNM guidelines recommends that TNM and clinical staging be

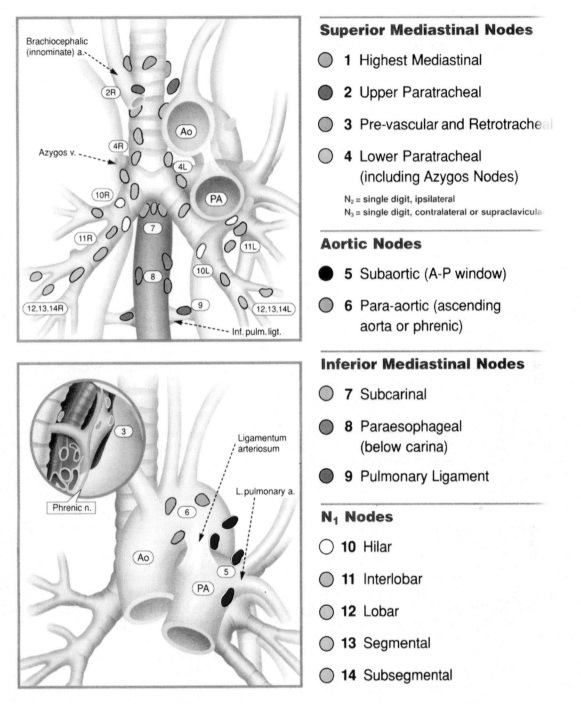

Figure 8-1 Nodal chart for lung cancer. *Top* courtesy the International Association for the Study of Lung Cancer and with permission of Aletta Frazier, MD. Copyright © 2009, 2010 Aletta Ann Frazier, MD. *Bottom* courtesy the International Association for the Study of Lung Cancer and with permission of Memorial Sloane-Kettering Cancer Center. Copyright © 2009, 2010 Aletta Ann Frazier, MD.

used for both NSCLC and SCLC staging (AJCC, 2013).

VII. Histology

    A. NSCLC is classified by the World Health Organization as squamous cell carcinoma, adenocarcinoma, and large cell carcinoma, with varying subtypes (NCI, 2013c).

        1. Categories of neuroendocrine, carcinoid, and mesothelioma have been defined.

        2. Although the World Health Organization (WHO) categories remain the standard, major revisions were proposed for NSCLC pathologic determination on the basis of a consensus international statement jointly released by three agencies: the International Association for the Study of Lung Cancer, the American Thoracic Society, and the European Respiratory Society (Travis et al., 2011).

Table 8-1

Lung Cancer: Anatomic Staging and TNM Staging

Anatomic Stage and Prognostic Groups

Occult Carcinoma	TX	N0	M0
Stage 0	Tis	N0	M0
Stage IA	T1a	N0	M0
	T1b	N0	M0
Stage IB	T2a	N0	M0
Stage IIA	T2b	N0	M0
	T1a	N1	M0
	T1b	N1	M0
	T2a	N1	M0
Stage IIB	T2b	N1	M0
	T3	N0	M0
Stage IIIA	T1a	N2	M0
	T1b	N2	M0
	T2a	N2	M0
	T2b	N2	M0
	T3	N1	M0
	T3	N2	M0
	T4	N0	M0
	T4	N1	M0
Stage IIIB	T1a	N3	M0
	T1b	N3	M0
	T2a	N3	M0
	T2b	N3	M0
	T3	N3	M0
	T4	N2	M0
	T4	N3	M0
Stage IV	Any T	Any N	M1a
	Any T	Any N	M1b

T, Tumor size; N, nodal status; M, metastasis.
Used with permission of the American Joint Committee on Cancer (AJCC), Chicago, Illinois. The original source for this material is the AJCC Cancer Staging Manual, Seventh Edition (2010) published by Springer Science and Business Media LLC, www.springer.com.

Changes were, in part, prompted by the development of targeted agents that are specific to certain histology:

a. Differentiating squamous and adenocarcinoma
b. Further standardizing the categories for adenocarcinoma (the most prevalent histology)
c. Classification systems made for both small biopsy or cytology and resection specimens
d. Additional recommendations, including molecular testing for both *EGFR* and *ALK* gene rearrangements (NCCN, 2013) to determine appropriate treatment recommendations:
  (1) Identification of EGRF mutations is critical, as these mutations are associated with sensitivity to tyrosine kinase inhibitor (TKI) responses.

  (2) *EGRF* mutations in adenocarcinomas occur in up to 50% of patients, being more common in Asians, women, and never-smokers.
  (3) *KRAS* mutations are associated with TKI resistance.
  (4) *ALK* gene rearrangements in NSCLC are associated with response to treatment with crizotinib.
  (5) However, not all individuals will have enough tissue available for multiple testing.
e. The proposed revisions are highlighted in Table 8-2.

VIII. Risk factors (NCCN, 2013)
  A. Tobacco smoking accounts for approximately 85% to 90% of lung cancers and is closely associated with all histologic types.
    1. Smoking is the greatest risk factor for developing lung cancer.
    2. Risk increases with number of years smoked and number of cigarettes per day. To quantify tobacco exposure, the number of packs of cigarettes a day is multiplied by the number of years smoked to obtain pack history.
    3. Exposure to secondhand smoke for nonsmokers is also a well-established risk.
    4. Tobacco smoke also promotes the carcinogenic effect of other carcinogens.
  B. Additional environmental and occupational factors that increase risk include asbestos exposure (especially for mesothelioma), radon gas, and additional toxic chemical exposure.
  C. Genetic risk factors have also been identified.
  D. Pre-existing pulmonary disease (chronic obstructive pulmonary disease [COPD], pulmonary fibrosis, tuberculosis) is associated with an increased incidence.
  E. Prevention and screening
    1. Recommended prevention measures are as follows:
      a. To not smoke, not to use any tobacco products, and if smoking to stop
        (1) Smoking cessation is associated with a gradual decrease in the risk of lung cancer.
        (2) Five or more years must elapse before an appreciable decrease in risk occurs.
        (3) Symptomatic improvements may be noted immediately on smoking cessation.
      b. Additional preventive measures— avoiding exposures to secondhand smoke, asbestos, radon, and other toxic chemicals

Table 8-2

Lung Cancer: Proposed IASLC Histology Classification

Proposed IASLC/ATS/ERS Classification for Small Biopsies and Cytology
SMALL BIOPSY AND CYTOLOGY: IASLC/ATS/ERS

Morphologic adenocarcinoma patterns clearly present: Adenocarcinoma—describe identifiable patterns present (including micropapillary pattern not included in 2004 WHO classification).
Comment: If pure lepidic growth—mention that an invasive component cannot be excluded in this small specimen.

Adenocarcinoma with lepidic pattern (if pure, add note: an invasive component cannot be excluded)

Mucinous adenocarcinoma (describe patterns present)

Adenocarcinoma with fetal pattern

Adenocarcinoma with colloid pattern

Adenocarcinoma with (describe patterns present) and signet ring features

Adenocarcinoma with (describe patterns present) and clear cell features

Morphologic adenocarcinoma patterns not present (supported by special stains):
Non–small cell carcinoma, favor adenocarcinoma

Morphologic squamous cell patterns clearly present:
Squamous cell carcinoma

Morphologic squamous cell patterns not present (supported by stains):
Non–small cell carcinoma, favor squamous cell carcinoma

Small cell carcinoma

Non–small cell carcinoma, not otherwise specified (NOS)

Non–small cell carcinoma with neuroendocrine (NE) morphology (positive NE markers), possible LCNEC

Non–small cell carcinoma with NE morphology (negative NE markers); see comment.
Comment: This is a non–small cell carcinoma where LCNEC is suspected, but stains failed to demonstrate NE differentiation.

Morphologic squamous cell and adenocarcinoma patterns present:
Non–small cell carcinoma, with squamous cell and adenocarcinoma patterns
Comment: This could represent adenosquamous carcinoma.

Morphologic squamous cell or adenocarcinoma patterns not present but immunostains favor separate glandular and adenocarcinoma components
Non–small cell carcinoma, NOS (specify the results of the immunohistochemical stains and the interpretation)
Comment: this could represent adenosquamous carcinoma.

Poorly differentiated NSCLC with spindle and/or giant cell carcinoma (mention if adenocarcinoma or squamous carcinoma are present)

ATS, American Thoracic Society; *ERS*, European Respiratory Society; *IASLC*, International Association for the Study of Lung Cancer; *LCNEC*, large cell neuroendocrine carcinoma; *NSCLC*, non–small cell lung carcinoma; *WHO*, World Health Organization.

Reprinted courtesy of the International Association for the Study of Lung Cancer. Copyright © 2011.

2. Recently completed trials of screening for high-risk individuals have resulted in new screening guidelines for current or former heavy smokers (>30 pack-year history).
   a. The largest trial (National Lung Screening Trial [NLST]) found fewer lung cancer deaths with spiral low-dose computed tomography (CT).
   b. Current screening guidelines are for current or former smokers (>30 pack-years or <15 years quit), apparently healthy, age 55 to 74, to have annual screening with low-dose chest CT (Wender et al., 2013).
   c. CT must be performed in settings that have expertise in lung cancer screening, diagnosis, and treatment (NCCN, 2013).
   d. Guidelines do not recommend routine use of chest radiography or sputum cytology.
   e. Screening does result in increased detection of early-stage lung cancer, which is more treatable; however, screening also results in the identification of many nodules that may be benign and may result in unnecessary procedures and psychological distress (Bach et al., 2012).
   f. Because early-stage lung cancer may be curable, effective population-based screening could decrease mortality rates.
   g. Results of ongoing trials may prompt further changes in the screening recommendations. Specifically, the U.S. Preventive Services Task Force has issued draft guidelines that expand the age range to 55 to 79 years (U.S. Preventive Services Task Force (USPSTF), 2013).
IX. Principles of medical management
   A. Considerations for treatment of NSCLC (accounts for 85% of all lung cancers)

1. Individuals with lung cancer often experience extensive delays and testing prior to diagnosis (Spiro, Gould, & Colice, 2007).
2. Individuals may have comorbid conditions that mask or complicate initial evaluation—for example, emphysema, COPD, bronchitis, pneumonia, or a combination of all these conditions.
3. Treatment decisions are influenced by stage of disease, histologic subtype, patient status (especially performance status), and patient preferences (NCCN, 2013).
4. Individualized treatment is recommended.
   a. Most are currently diagnosed in the advanced stage of the disease.
   b. The treatment goals vary widely.
   c. Treatment goals are highly context-dependent in individual cases, ranging from treating life-threatening emergencies, to palliation of major symptoms, to initiating maximal therapy.

B. Evidence-based treatment algorithms are readily available electronically from multiple national organizations.
1. These decision trees with detailed treatment options are routinely updated with new information and should be consulted because the range of options for treatments changes frequently.
2. These resources should be consulted for treatment recommendations specific to lung cancer type, stage, and individual context.
   a. Examples of available treatment guidelines include the websites of the following organizations:
      (1) American Society of Clinical Oncology (ASCO, 2013) (www.asco.org/guidelines/lung-cancer)
      (2) National Comprehensive Cancer Network (NCCN) (www.nccn.org/professionals/physician_gls/pdf/nscl.pdf)
      (3) National Cancer Institute (NCI) (www.cancer.gov/cancertopics/pdq/treatment/non-small-cell-lung/healthprofessional)
      (4) American College of Chest Physicians (ACCP) (www.chestnet.org/Publications/CHEST-Publications/Guidelines-Consensus-Statements)

C. Given the overall poor prognosis of lung cancer, participation in a clinical trial is often recommended.
1. Review of the NCI clinical trials database provides information on multiple active trials at any time (www.cancer.gov/cancertopics/types/lung).

D. Individuals with suspected lung cancer benefit from evaluation by a multidisciplinary team specializing in lung cancer (medical oncologist, radiation oncologist, thoracic surgeon, pulmonologist) (ACCP, 2013; NCCN, 2013).

E. Surgery
1. Surgery (ACCP, 2013; NCCN, 2013) is the primary treatment for the management of early-stage NSCLC (stages I and II).
   a. Surgery is the best option for curative therapy.
   b. Role of surgery in stage III disease is controversial and reserved for select cases.
   c. Only 25% to 35% of cases are candidates for surgical resection.
   d. Surgery also plays a major role in the establishment of the diagnosis by obtaining tissue and has a role in the palliation of symptoms.
   e. Multiple evidence-based algorithms have been developed for the following:
      (1) Surgical biopsy decision of a suspicious nodule
      (2) Techniques to obtain tissue for diagnosis
      (3) Techniques for resection
   f. Involvement of multidisciplinary thoracic team with experience in the most recent techniques and access to the most up-to-date technology improves outcomes. ⚠
   g. A complete evaluation and an individualized plan are necessary (Alberg, et al., 2013).
      (1) The least invasive technique that is likely to provide the highest yield of tissue for histopathology is preferred.
         (a) Newer techniques include radial endobronchial ultrasound (EBUS) and transthoracic needle aspiration (TTNA).
   h. As primary treatment, the surgical procedure selected depends on both the extent of the disease and the patient's cardiopulmonary status.
      (1) In general, lung-sparing resection is preferred, and lobectomy remains the standard approach.
      (2) Minimally invasive techniques such as video-assisted thoracic surgery (VATS) are recommended; this surgery may be done in conjunction with wedge resection and has been associated with decreased morbidity.

(3) Systematic lymphadenectomy is recommended (rather than complete lymph node dissection).

(4) Not all clients with lung cancer are candidates for surgery, and in those who are undergoing surgery, resection may be halted if evidence of metastasis is found.

(5) Surgery may also be indicated for metastatic sites of disease that are symptomatic (i.e., resection of a solitary brain metastasis).

F. Radiation therapy (RT) (NCCN, 2013)

1. May be the primary therapy used as an adjuvant treatment and for palliation of symptoms

2. May be used as the primary modality for stage I and stage II disease if the individual is not a surgical candidate

3. Postoperative radiation administered to those with positive surgical margins

4. May be administered for stage III and stage IV disease

5. May be particularly effective for palliation of symptoms and management of brain metastasis

6. Advanced techniques—conformal simulation and intensity-modulated radiotherapy, which reduce toxicity and increase survival

   a. Commonly prescribed dosing is 60 to 70 gray (Gy) in 2-Gy fractions.

   b. Treatment planning standard is a minimum of three-dimensional conformal RT.

   c. Stereotactic ablative radiotherapy (SRT) is used to treat inoperable early-stage disease and improves local control.

   d. Radiofrequency ablation (RFA) involves whole-brain RT and stereotactic radiosurgery for the management of brain metastasis and improves quality of life.

G. Chemotherapy (NCCN, 2013; NCI, 2013)

1. Chemotherapy may be administered as adjuvant therapy, concurrently with RT, or as single modality.

2. Rapid advancements in targeted therapy specific to the tumor histology have been developed to treat lung cancer; multiple changes have been made to therapy options and first-line recommendations. It is important to seek out the latest information and nationally recommended guidelines.

3. Findings on postoperative chemotherapy after surgical resection have had mixed results, and clinical trials continue.

4. For stage III disease, concurrent chemoradiation is the standard therapy.

5. For advanced disease, chemotherapy is the standard of care.

6. Chemotherapy is indicated for individuals with a good performance status and may be contraindicated in individual scenarios.

7. Chemotherapy is considered in as many as 80% of NSCLC cases.

   a. The current mainstay of chemotherapy is cisplatin-based doublets, which are used for neoadjuvant and adjuvant therapy in combination with RT.

   b. The side effects of these regimens include multiple toxicities: nausea and vomiting, neurotoxicity, potential kidney damage, and fatigue (see Chapter 22).

8. A cisplatin-based doublet is the standard regimen for treating advanced disease.

   a. Multiple regimens are in use, with many agents administered with cisplatin (e.g., etoposide, gemcitabine, docetaxel, vinorelibine, paclitaxel).

   b. Pemetrexed is the second agent to be considered for individuals with adenocarcinoma and is superior when the histology is nonsquamous.

   c. Individuals who cannot tolerate cisplatin (because of decreased kidney function, hearing loss, and neuropathies) are treated with carboplatin.

   d. Platinum-based chemotherapy improves survival, time to progression, and 1-year and 2-year survival rates and is superior to best supportive care (in good performance status [PS]).

9. Targeted therapy involves the following considerations:

   a. Effective in individuals with certain genetic mutations

   b. Holds promise for further development of targeted therapies for specific pathways of mutations

   c. EGRF-targeted therapies—include oral TKIs now indicated for treatment in selected cases

   d. Bevacizumab—in addition to chemotherapy, recommended in select patients with advanced NSCLC but increases risk of bleeding

   e. Erlotinib—first-line therapy for individuals with advanced, recurrent, or metastatic non–squamous NSCLC (NCCN, 2013)

   f. Crizotnib—first-line therapy for individuals with advanced disease and who are ALK-positive

10. In advanced disease, two drug regimens are preferred with good PS; for PS, two single agents are used.
11. The optimal duration of therapy is an area of active study; current options include close surveillance, maintenance, and switch therapy.

H. Palliative care (NCCN, 2013)
1. Early palliative care combined with standard therapy is recommended because it improves quality of life, mood and, in one study, survival (Temel et al., 2010).

I. Recurrent disease
1. The management of recurrent or progressive NSCLC is an area of active investigation, but few guidelines are available for the use of second- and third-line agents.
2. With systemic therapy, different agents are often tried, with disease response monitored after two cycles of therapy and careful attention paid to toxicities and tolerance (NCCN, 2013; NCI, 2013).
3. Treatment decisions need to be individualized to the specific context with chemotherapy, RT, and surgery all having a role in symptom relief, treatment of emergencies, and disease stabilization.
4. Maximization of palliative care, consideration of hospice care, or a combination of both is recommended.

J. Small cell lung cancer (NCCN, 2013; NCI, 2013d)
1. Accounts for approximately 15% of cases and is responsive to chemotherapy and RT
2. Prognosis poor with overall 5-year survival at 5% to 10%
3. Untreated median survival 2 to 4 months
4. Standard of care for individuals with limited disease—concurrent combined modality with chemotherapy or RT
5. Chemotherapy (cisplatin and etoposide) associated with increased survival (18 to 24 months) but is curative only in a minority
6. Prophylactic cranial RT indicated for individuals with complete response to chemotherapy or RT to reduce the risk of developing brain metastasis
7. Maintenance chemotherapy outside of a clinical trial not supported by current evidence
8. Standard therapy for individuals with extensive disease—a doublet chemotherapy regimen (cisplatin, etoposide).
   a. Carboplatin used if contraindications are present; duration of treatment generally four to six cycles

X. Nursing implications
A. Nursing implications related to patient or family understanding of diagnosis and treatment options
1. Establishing goals of care
2. Assessing coping with diagnosis and prognosis
3. Helping the family to allow the client to maintain roles and activities most important to him or her
4. Placing emphasis on short-term goals in daily care and priority setting
5. Referral to community resources, as appropriate and available
6. Teaching supportive care skills
7. Assisting to maintain realistic hope and yet prepare for changes in lifestyle if prognosis is poor
8. Recognizing needs related to anticipatory grieving
9. Assisting to resume previous roles and responsibilities if prognostic factors are favorable

B. Nursing implication specific to treatment
1. These include teaching, side effect prevention, and monitoring (see Chapters 19, 21, and 22).
2. Individuals who have had surgery may require wound care and pain and pleural catheter management and will need reinforcement of deep breathing exercises and increasing physical activity level.
3. Individuals who receive radiation therapy may experience localized skin reactions, esophagitis, fatigue, and symptoms specific to the treatment field.
4. Individuals who receive chemotherapy or targeted agents will have side-effect profiles specific to the regimen.
   a. In addition to risk for neutropenia, cisplatin-based regimens may cause nausea and vomiting and peripheral neuropathies, which require monitoring of kidney functioning.
   b. Some of the targeted therapies may cause rash, diarrhea, or both.

C. Nursing implications to decrease severity of symptoms associated with the disease, treatment, or both
1. Individuals diagnosed with lung cancer are known to be at high risk for pain and multiple other symptoms.
2. In studies including multiple cancer diagnoses, individuals with lung cancer have reported the highest number of symptoms, worst symptom severity, and highest levels of symptom distress (Cooley, Short & Moriarty, 2003).
3. Maximal palliative care interventions for all symptoms are necessary.

4. Refer to the following evidence-based guidelines for management:
   a. Oncology Nursing Society PEP resources (www.ons.org/Research/PEP/)(ONS, 2013)
   b. Guidelines for pain and symptom management available at NCCN (2013)
   c. See Chapters 27 to 34 in this text.
D. Care of individuals with lung cancer requires coordination because these clients are seeing multiple care providers and may experience frequent transitions in care (hospital to home to ambulatory). ⚠
E. Individuals with lung cancer are at high risk for the development of paraneoplastic syndromes and oncologic emergencies. See Chapters 40 and 41.

References

Alberg, A., Brock, M., Ford, J., Samet, J., & Spivack, S. (2013). Diagnosis and management of lung cancer, 3rd ed: American College of Chest Physicians evidenced-based practice guidelines. *Chest, 143*(5 Suppl.), e1S–e29S.

American Cancer Society [ACS]. (2013). *Cancer facts & figures 2013.* Atlanta: American Cancer Society.

American College of Chest Physicians [ACCP]. (2013). *Lung cancer.* www.chestnet.org/Publications/CHEST-Publications/Guidelines-Consensus-Statements.

American Joint Commission on Cancer [AJCC]. (2013). *Lung cancer staging.* www.cancerstaging.org.

American Society Clinical Oncology [ASCO]. (2013). *Lung cancer treatment guidelines.* www.asco.org/guidelines/lung-cancer.

American Thoracic Society [ATS]. (2013). *Lung cancer.* emedicine.medscape.com/article/279960-overview#aw2aab6b2b3.

Bach, P., Mirkin, J., Oliver, T., Azzoli, C., Berry, D., Brawley, O., et al. (2012). Benefits and harms of CT screening for lung cancer: A systematic review. *JAMA, 307,* 2418–2429. http://dx.doi.org/10.1001/jama.2012.5521.

Cooley, M. E., Short, T. H., & Moriarty, H. J. (2003). Symptom prevalence, distress, and change over time in adults receiving treatment for lung cancer. *Psychooncology, 12*(7), 694–708.

Edge, S., Byrd, D., Compton, C., Fritz, A., & Trotti, A. (Eds.). (2010). *AJCC cancer staging manual.* (7th ed.). New York: Springer.

National Cancer Institute [NCI]. (2013a). *Clinical trials for lung cancer.* www.cancer.gov/cancertopics/types/lung.

National Cancer Institute [NCI]. (2013b). *Non-small cell lung cancer treatment PDQ.* Retrieved from, www.cancer.gov/cancertopics/pdq/treatment/non-small-cell-lung/healthprofessional/page1/AllPages.

National Cancer Institute [NCI]. (2013c). *SEER training modules; Cancer classification.* Retrieved from, training.seer.cancer.gov/disease/categories/classification.html.

National Cancer Institute [NCI]. (2013d). *Small cell lung cancer treatment PDQ.* www.cancer.gov/cancertopics/pdq/treatment/small-cell-lung/healthprofessional/page4/AllPages.

National Comprehensive Cancer Network [NCCN]. (2013). *Non-small cell lung cancer. Version 2.2013, NCCCN clinical practice guidelines in oncology.* Retrieved from, www.nccn.org/professionals/physician_gls/f_guidelines.asp#site.

Oncology Nursing Society. (2013). *PEP resources.* www.ons.org/Research/PEP.

Spiro, S., Gould, M., & Colice, G. (2007). Initial evaluation of the patient with lung cancer: Symptoms, signs, laboratory tests and paraneoplastic syndromes: ACCP evidenced-based clinical practice guidelines. *Chest, 132*(3 Suppl.), 149S–160S. http://dx.doi.org/10.1378/chest.07-1358.

Temel, J., Greer, J., Muzikansky, A., Gallagher, E., Admane, M., Jackson, V., et al. (2010). Early palliative care for patients with metastatic non-small cell lung cancer. *New England Journal of Medicine, 363,* 733–742.

Travis, W., Brambilla, E., Noguchi, M., Nicholson, A., Geisinger, K., Yatabe, Y., et al. (2011). International Association for the Study of Lung Cancer/American Thoracic Society/European Respiratory Society International Multidisciplinary Classification of Lung Adenocarcinoma. *Journal of Thoracic Oncology, 6*(2), 244–285.

U.S. Preventive Service Task Force. (USPSTF). (2013). *Screening for lung cancer.* http://www.uspreventiveservicestaskforce.org/uspstf/uspslung.htm.

Wender, R., Fontham, E., Berrera, E. Jr., Colditz, G., Church, T., Ettinger, D., et al. (2013). American Cancer Society Lung cancer screening guidelines. *CA: A Cancer Journal for Clinicians, 63,* 106–117. http://dx.doi.org/10.3322/caac.21172.

CHAPTER 9

Cancers of the Gastrointestinal Tract

Christa Braun-Inglis

I. Introduction
   A. Cancers of the gastrointestinal (GI) tract include cancers of the esophagus, stomach, colon, rectum, anus, pancreas, and liver.
   B. The incidence, staging, treatment, and prognosis of these cancers depend on the specific location of the primary tumor.
   C. For the purpose of this chapter, the most common cancers of the GI tract will be reviewed: esophageal, gastric (adenocarcinoma), colorectal (adenocarcinoma), anal, hepatocellular, and pancreatic cancers.

II. Anatomy and physiology
   A. General
      1. The major functions of the GI tract are mechanical and chemical breakdown of food and the digestion of absorbed nutrients.
      2. GI tract begins at the mouth and ends at the anus.
      3. Accessory organs of digestion include the liver, gallbladder, and pancreas.
   B. Specific organs
      1. Esophagus
         a. Hollow, muscular tube measuring approximately 25 cm
         b. Swallowed food moved to stomach by peristalsis
         c. Each end of the esophagus opened and closed by a sphincter
      2. Stomach
         a. Hollow muscular organ that stores food during eating
         b. Secretes digestive juices
         c. Food mixes with digestive juices to form chime, which is propelled into the duodenum.
         d. Major anatomic boundaries—lower esophageal sphincter and pyloric sphincter
         e. Has three layers of smooth muscle
         f. Innervated by sympathetic and parasympathetic divisions of the autonomic nervous system

      3. Small intestine
         a. Approximately 5 m long
         b. Divided into three segments: duodenum, jejunum, and ileum
         c. Continuation of digestion in the proximal portion of the small intestine by the action of pancreatic and intestinal enzymes and bile salts
         d. Carbohydrates broken down into monosaccharides and dissacharides; proteins degraded into amino acids, and fats emulsified and reduced to fatty acids and monoglycerides
         e. Minerals and water-soluble vitamins absorbed by both active and passive transport
      4. Large intestine
         a. Approximately 1.5 m long
         b. Consists of cecum, appendix, colon (ascending, transverse, descending and sigmoid), rectum, and anal canal
         c. Massages fecal mass and absorbs water and electrolytes
         d. Defecation stimulated when the rectum is distended with feces (Wood, 2013).
      5. Liver
         a. Largest organ in the body
         b. Has digestive, metabolic, hematologic, vascular, and immunologic functions
         c. Divided into right and left lobes
         d. Hepatocytes—functional cells of the liver that initiate formation and secretion of bile
         e. Sinusoids—capillaries located between plates of hepatocytes
         f. Blood from portal vein and hepatic artery flows through the sinusoids to a central vein in each lobule, then to the hepatic vein and into the superior vena cava (SVC) (Rhodes, 2013)
      6. Pancreas
         a. Gland located behind the stomach
         b. Endocrine portion—produces glucagon and insulin that facilitate cellular uptake of glucose

c. Exocrine pancreas—secretes enzymes that digest proteins, carbohydrates, and fats (Rhodes, 2013)

III. Epidemiology and risk factors

A. Esophageal cancer

1. Estimated 17,990 new cases and 15,210 deaths in the United States in 2013 (American Cancer Society [ACS], 2013a).

2. Two major histologic types:

a. Adenocarcinoma—more common in North America and western European countries

b. Squamous cell carcinoma—more common in Asians and African Americans

3. Overall 5-year survival rate of 38% (ACS, 2013a)

4. Risk factors (ACS, 2013f; Tsottles, 2011):

a. Modifiable

(1) Smoking

(2) Alcohol

(3) Workplace exposure, especially among dry cleaning workers (Ruder, Ward, & Brown, 2001)

(4) Obesity

(5) Diet—low consumption of fruits and vegetables and high intake of nitrosamine

b. Nonmodifiable

(1) Male gender—more prevalent in men than in women

(2) Tylosis—an inherited autosomal dominant condition characterized by palmoplantar keratoderma (Blaydon et al., 2012)

(3) Achalasia—a rare disorder in which the muscle ring in the lower esophagus fails to relax during swallowing, resulting in decreased peristalsis of food into the stomach (Leeuwenburgh et al., 2010)

(4) Esophageal webs

(5) Human papilloma virus (HPV)

(6) History of other cancers

(7) Hiatal hernia

(8) Gastroesophageal reflux disease (GERD)

(9) Barrett esophagus Holmes & Vaughan, 2007)

B. Gastric cancer

1. Second most common cause of cancer-related death in the world

2. Difficult to cure, even in Western countries

3. Estimated 21,600 new cases and 10,990 deaths in the United States in 2013 (ACS, 2013a)

4. Higher incidence in Asians

5. Higher incidence in males compared with females

6. Invention of refrigeration—mark of a pivotal point of decline in incidence

7 Increase in absolute number despite decline in incidence

8. Five-year survival rate for stomach cancer approximately 27% (ACS, 2013a; ACS, 2013b).

9. Risk factors

a. Modifiable

(1) Diet

(2) Obesity

(3) Smoking

(4) Alcohol

b. Nonmodifiable

(1) *Helicobacter pylori*

(2) Epstein-Barr virus (EBV)

(3) Previous gastric surgery

(4) Gastric polyps

(5) Gastric ulcers

(6) Pernicious anemia

(7) Blood group A

(8) Family history

(9) Genetic polymorphisms (ACS, 2013b)

C. Colorectal cancer

1. Estimated 142,820 new cases and 50,830 deaths in the United States in 2013 (ACS, 2013a)

2. Fourth most common cause of cancer and second leading cause of cancer-related deaths in the United States.

3. Overall incidence declining

4. 72% of cases arise from colon and 28% from rectum (ACS, 2013a; ACS, 2013c).

5. Risk factors

a. Modifiable

(1) Smoking

(2) Alcohol

(3) High-fat diet or high intake of red meat

(4) Obesity

(5) Inadequate intake of fruits and vegetables

(6) Physical inactivity

b. Nonmodifiable

(1) Age older than 50 years

(2) Personal or family history of colon cancer or inflammatory bowel disease

(3) Hereditary polyposis syndrome—familial adenomatous polyposis (FAP), hereditary nonpolyposis colorectal cancer (HNPCC), Lynch syndrome

(4) Presence of edematous polyps (ACS, 2013c)

D. Anal cancer

1. Estimated 7060 new cases and 880 deaths in the United States in 2013 (ACS, 2013a)

2. Comprises 2.2% of GI malignancies

3. Incidence rates increasing (ACS, 2013a; ACS, 2013d)

4. Risk factors
   a. Modifiable
      (1) Smoking
      (2) Receptive anal intercourse
      (3) Sexually transmitted diseases—HPV, human immunodeficiency virus (HIV)
   b. Nonmodifiable
      (1) History of cervical, vulvar, or vaginal cancer
      (2) Immunosuppression
      (3) Hematologic malignancy (Minsky & Guillem, 2010)
E. Hepatocellular cancer (HCC)
   1. Estimated 30,640 new cases and 21,670 deaths in the United States in 2013 (ACS, 2013a)
   2. Incidence increasing because of increasing incidence of hepatitis C infection (ACS, 2013e)
   3. Third leading cause of cancer-related deaths worldwide
   4. Risk factors (Grenon, 2011)
      a. Modifiable
         (1) Alcohol
         (2) Smoking
         (3) Exposure to chemical carcinogens such as nitrites, hydrocarbons, pesticides, and solvents
      b. Nonmodifiable (ACS, 2013e)
         (1) Hepatitis B
         (2) Hepatitis C
         (3) Hemochromatosis
         (4) Alpha-1-antitrypsin deficiency
         (5) Cirrhosis
F. Pancreatic cancer
   1. Estimated 45,220 new cases and 38,640 deaths in the United States in 2013 (ACS, 2013a)
   2. Tenth most common cancer among men and ninth most common among women
   3. Most patient die within first year of diagnosis.
   4. Overall 5-year survival rate of 6% (ACS, 2013a; National Comprehensive Cancer Network [NCCN], 2013g)
   5. Risk factors (Hodgkin, 2011)
      a. Modifiable
         (1) Smoking
         (2) Obesity
         (3) Dietary factors—high consumption of cholesterol, meat, fried foods, refined sugar
         (4) Occupational exposures such as in chemists, coal gas workers, metal industries, leather tanning industry, and transportation workers
      b. Nonmodifiable
         (1) Advancing age
         (2) Male gender
         (3) African American ethnicity
         (4) Ashkenazi Jewish heritage

IV. Pathophysiology and histologic classification
   A. Esophageal cancer—related to exposure of its mucosa to noxious chemicals, resulting in a sequence of dysplasia to carcinoma in situ to invasive carcinoma
      1. Squamous cell carcinoma
         a. Arises from squamous cell epithelium
         b. More common in developing nations
      2. Adenocarcinoma
         a. Arises from glandular tissue
         b. Affects mostly the distal esophagus
         c. Appears to be related to GERD and Barrett esophagus (Swisher, Rice, Ajani, Komaki, & Ferguson, 2010).
   B. Gastric cancer
      1. Adenocarcinoma
         a. 95% arise from the glandular epithelium in the stroma
         b. Two types, intestinal or diffuse
            (1) Intestinal, expansive, epidemic-type gastric cancer
               (a) Associated with chronic atrophic gastritis, retained glandular structure, little invasiveness, and a sharp margin
               (b) Better prognosis
               (c) No family history
            (2) Diffuse, infiltrative, endemic gastric cancer
               (a) Consists of scattered cell clusters with poor differentiation and dangerously deceptive margins
               (b) Associated with genetic factors, blood type, and family history
      2. Lymphomas, carcinoid, and stromal tumors make up the remaining 5% of gastric malignancies (Yao, Crane, Sano, & Mansfield, 2010).
   C. Colorectal cancer
      1. Adenocarcinoma
         a. Accounts for 95% of all cases; originates from the glandular epithelium of the mucosa
      2. Lymphomas and squamous cell carcinomas
         a. Account for 5% of cases (Padussis, Beaseley, McMahon, Tyler, & Ludwig, 2010)
   D. Anal cancer
      1. Squamous cell carcinomas comprise 80% to 85% of cases.
      2. Anal canal lesions most common, usually poorly differentiated (Minsky & Guillem, 2010)
      3. Anal margin lesions usually well differentiated
   E. Hepatocellular cancer
      1. Arise from hepatocytes
      2. Nodular or infiltrative tumor (Sung & Thung, 2010)

F. Pancreatic cancer
  1. Adenocarcinoma
     a. Accounts for 95% of cases; arises from the exocrine pancreas
  2. Neuroendocrine tumors—rare (Wolff, Crane, Li, & Evans, 2010)
V. Clinical presentation
  A. Esophageal cancer
     1. Dysphagia or odynophagia
     2. Chest pain
     3. Hoarseness
     4. Hematemesis
     5. Chronic cough
     6. Black tarry stools, or melena
     7. Weight loss
     8. Fatigue (Holmes & Vaughan, 2007)
  B. Gastric cancer
     1. Usually nonspecific, leading to late diagnosis
     2. Indigestion
     3. Nausea and vomiting
     4. Dysphagia
     5. Anorexia
     6. Abdominal pain
     7. Early satiety
     8. Black tarry stools or melena
     9. Pallor secondary to anemia
     10. Weight loss (Yao et al., 2010)
  C. Colorectal cancer
     1. Early colorectal cancer is usually asymptomatic but patients may complain of the following:
        a. Bleeding—most common symptom (Padussis et al., 2010)
        b. Vague abdominal pain
        c. Flatulence
        d. Changes in bowel movement, with or without bleeding
     2. Advanced colorectal cancer—20% of patients present with distant metastases (Table 9-1).
        a. Presentation—depends on site
        b. Weight loss
        c. Fatigue

  d. Palpation of mass
  e. Right upper quadrant pain or hepatomegaly
  f. Abdominal distention
  g. Supraclavicular adenopathy
  h. Periumbilical nodules
  D. Anal cancer
     1. Bleeding from anal area—occurs in 45% of patients
     2. Anal pain or pressure
     3. Anal itching, discharge, or both
     4. Change in bowel habits
     5. Lump or swelling in anus
     6. Weight loss (Minsky & Guillem, 2010; NCCN, 2013e)
  E. Hepatocellular cancer
     1. Symptoms usually related to chronic liver disease
     2. Ascites
     3. Jaundice
     4. Encephalopathy
     5. Weight loss
     6. Abdominal pain
     7. Early satiety (Sung & Thung, 2010)
  F. Pancreatic cancer
     1. Weight loss
     2. Abdominal pain
     3. Indigestion or bloating
     4. Jaundice (may be painless in early disease)
     5. Nausea and vomiting (Wolff et al., 2010)
VI. Metastatic patterns
  A. Esophageal cancer
     1. Local through lymphatics
     2. Distant through lymphatics and bloodstream
        a. Most common—liver and lung
        b. Other possible sites—pleura, stomach, peritoneum, kidney, adrenal, bone, and brain (Swisher et al., 2010)
  B. Gastric cancer
     1. Direct extension to adjacent organs such as liver, diaphragm, pancreas, spleen, and colon
     2. Spread to lymphatics and distant nodes
     3. Hematogenously to the liver

Table 9-1

Signs and Symptoms of Advanced Colorectal Cancer by Tumor Site

Right (Ascending)	Transverse	Left (Descending)	Rectum
Vague abdominal aching	Blood mixed with stool	Constipation alternating with diarrhea	Changes in bowel movements
Weakness	Changes in bowel movement patterns	Abdominal pain	Rectal fullness, tenesmus
Weight loss	Bowel obstruction	Obstructive symptoms such as nausea and vomiting	Urgency
Changes in stool			Bleeding
Anemia resulting from chronic blood loss			Pelvic pain

4. Direct penetration into the peritoneum (Yao et al., 2010)
C. Colorectal cancer
   1. Local extension through penetration of the bowel
   2. Via lymphangitic spread
   3. Hematogenously to liver and lung (Padussis et al., 2010)
D. Anal cancer
   1. Direct extension into the pelvis
   2. Into lymph nodes—intrapelvic and extrapelvic
   3. Hematogenously into lung and liver—rare (Minsky & Guillem, 2010)
E. Hepatocellular cancer
   1. Rarely metastasizes because tumor itself carries very poor prognosis
   2. Metastases late in the disease—may develop in the lung, portal vein, periportal nodes, bone, or brain (Sung & Thung, 2010)
F. Pancreatic cancer
   1. Usually spread via lymph nodes
   2. Hematogenously into the liver and lung (Wolff et al., 2010)
VII. Screening, diagnostic measures, staging, and grading
A. Esophageal cancer
   1. Screening
      a. No standard screening
      b. Clinical trials in progress to evaluate screening
   2. Diagnostic measures
      a. Endoscopy and biopsy
      b. Computed tomography (CT) of chest and abdomen with oral and intravenous (IV) contrast
      c. Positron emission tomography–CT (PET-CT)
      d. Endoscopic ultrasonography
      e. Bronchoscopy
   3. Staging and grading
      a. American Joint Committee on Cancer (AJCC) staging and grading system (Table 9-2)
      b. Separate staging for adenocarcinoma versus squamous cell carcinoma
      c. Advanced cancer stage associated with poorer survival
B. Gastric cancer
   1. Screening
      a. Value of screening for gastric cancer remains controversial.
      b. In high-risk areas such as Japan, individuals are screened with simple risk interview and barium studies.
   2. Diagnostic measures
      a. Endoscopy with biopsy—six to eight biopsies recommended
      b. CT of chest and abdomen with IV and oral contrast

   c. Pelvic CT, as clinically indicated
   d. PET-CT—useful for predicting response to neoadjuvant chemotherapy
   e. Endoscopic ultrasound (EUS) recommended if M1 disease is not evident.
   3. Staging and grading
      a. AJCC staging and grading system (Table 9-3)
      b. Retrieval of at least 15 lymph nodes recommended to adequately stage nodal status (NCCN, 2013b)
C. Colorectal cancer
   1. Screening
      a. Begins at age 50 for both men and women
      b. Evidence that screening decreases mortality
      c. Patients at average risk
         (1) Age 50 years or older
         (2) No history of adenoma or colorectal cancer
         (3) No history of inflammatory bowel disease
         (4) Negative family history
            (a) Comparison of screening recommendations between the ACS and the NCCN for average-risk

Table 9-2

Staging of Esophageal Cancer

Stage	Description
Primary Tumor (T)	
TX	Primary tumor cannot be assessed
T0	No evidence of primary tumor
Tis	High-grade dysplasia
T1	Tumor invades lamina propria but not beyond submucosa.
T2	Tumor invades the muscularis propria
T3	Tumor invades adventitia
T4a	Resectable tumor invading the pleura, pericardium or diaphragm
T4b	Unresectable tumor invading other adjacent structures, such as the aorta, vertebral body, and trachea
Regional Lymph Nodes (N)	
NX	Regional nodes cannot be assessed
N0	No regional lymph node metastasis
N1	Metastasis in one or two regional lymph nodes
N2	Metastasis in three to six regional lymph nodes
N3	Metastasis in seven or more regional lymph nodes
Distant Metastasis (M)	
M0	No distant metastasis
M1	Distant Metastasis

Used with permission of the American Joint Committee on Cancer (AJCC), Chicago, Illinois. The original source for this material is the AJCC Cancer Staging Manual, Seventh Edition (2010) published by Springer Science and Business Media LLC, www.springer.com.

Table 9-3

Staging of Gastric Cancer

Stage	Description
Primary Tumor (T)	
TX	Primary tumor cannot be assessed
T0	No evidence of primary tumor
Tis	Carcinoma in situ: intraepithelial tumor without invasion of the lamina propria
T1	Tumor invades lamina propria but not beyond submucosa
T2	Tumor invades the muscularis propria
T3	Tumor penetrates subserosal connective tissue without invasion of visceral peritoneum or adjacent structures
T4	Tumor invades the serosa or adjacent structures
T4a	Tumor invades serosa (visceral peritoneum)
T4b	Tumor invades adjacent structures
Regional Lymph Nodes (N)	
NX	Regional lymph nodes cannot be assessed
N0	No regional lymph node metastasis
N1	Metastasis in one or two regional lymph nodes
N2	Metastasis in three to six regional lymph nodes
N3	Metastasis in seven or more regional lymph nodes
N3a	Metastasis in 7 to 15 regional lymph nodes
N3b	Metastasis in 16 or more regional lymph nodes
Distant Metastasis (M)	
M0	No distant metastasis
M1	Distant metastasis

Anatomic Stage Grouping

Stage	T	N	M
Stage 0	Tis	N0	M0
Stage IA	T1	N0	M0
Stage IB	T2	N0	M0
Stage IIA	T3	N0	M0
	T2	N1	M0
Stage IIB	T4a	N0	M0
	T3	N2	M0
	T2	N2	M0
	T1	N3	M0
Stage IIIA	T4a	N1	M0
	T3	N2	M0
	T2	N3	M0
Stage IIIB	T4b	N1	M0
	T4a	N2	M0
	T3	N3	M0
Stage IIIC	T4b	N2 or N3	M0
	T4a	N3	M0
Stage IV	Any T	Any N	M1

Used with permission of the American Joint Committee on Cancer (AJCC), Chicago, Illinois. The original source for this material is the AJCC Cancer Staging Manual, Seventh Edition (2010) published by Springer Science and Business Media LLC, www.springer.com.

Table 9-4

Comparison of Colon Cancer Screening between the American Cancer Society (ACS) and National Comprehensive Cancer Network (NCCN) for Average-Risk Patients

ACS	NCCN
• Colonoscopy every 10 years	• Colonoscopy every 10 years (preferred)
• Flexible sigmoidoscopy every 5 years	• Flexible sigmoidoscopy every 5 years
• Double contrast barium enema every 5 years	• Guaiac-based or immunochemical-based testing annually, with or without flexible sigmoidoscopy, every 5 years
• Virtual colonoscopy every 5 years	
• Fecal occult blood test (FOBT) every year	
• Fecal immunochemical test (FIT) every year	

patients (ACS, 2013c; NCCN, 2013c) (Table 9-4)

2. Diagnostic measures
   a. Colonoscopy
   b. Blood tests—complete blood cell count (CBC), chemistry, carcinoembryonic antigen (CEA)
   c. CT of chest, abdomen, and pelvis with IV and oral contrast
   d. PET-CT not routinely indicated
   e. All tumor samples to be tested for *KRAS* mutation to guide treatment (Tan & Du, 2012)
     (1) *KRAS* mutation in approximately 40% of persons diagnosed with colorectal cancer
3. Staging and grading
   a. AJCC staging and grading system (Table 9-5)

D. Anal cancer
  1. Screening
   a. No recommended screening
  2. Diagnostic measures
   a. Digital rectal examination (DRE)
   b. Inguinal lymph node evaluation with biopsy
   c. Anoscopy
   d. CT of chest, abdomen, and pelvis
   e. HIV testing to be considered
   f. PET-CT to be considered
  3. Staging
   a. AJCC staging system (Table 9-6)

E. Hepatocellular cancer (HCC)
  1. Screening
   a. High-risk patients—patients with liver cirrhosis from viral and nonviral causes and hepatitis B carriers without cirrhosis
   b. Periodic screening with ultrasonography and alpha-fetoprotein (AFP) every

Part 2

Table 9-5

Staging of Colorectal Cancer

Stage	Description
Primary Tumor (T)	
TX	Primary tumor cannot be assessed
T0	No evidence of primary tumor
Tis	Carcinoma in situ
T1	Tumor invades submucosa
T2	Tumor invades muscularis propria
T3	Tumor invades through the muscularis propria and into the pericolorectal tissues
T4a	Tumor penetrates to the surface of the visceral peritoneum
T4b	Tumor directly invades or is adherent to other structures
Regional Lymph Nodes (N)	
NX	Regional lymph nodes cannot be assessed
N0	No regional lymph node metastasis
N1	Metastasis in one to three lymph nodes
N2	Metastasis in four or more lymph nodes
N2a	Metastasis in four to six regional lymph nodes
N2b	Metastasis in seven or more regional lymph nodes
Distant Metastasis (M)	
M0	No distant metastasis
M1	Distant metastasis
M1a	Metastasis defined to one organ site
M1b	Metastases in more than one organ or site or in peritoneum

Anatomic Stage Groupings

Stage 0	Tis	N0	M0
Stage I	T1	N0	M0
	T2	N0	M0
Stage IIA	T3	N0	M0
Stage IIB	T4a	N0	M0
Stage IIIA	T1-2	N1	M0
	T1	N2a	M0
Stage IIIB	T3-4a	N1	M0
	T2-3	N2a	M0
	T1-2	N2b	M0
Stage IIIC	T4a	N2a	M0
	T3-4a	N2b	M0
	T4b	any N	M0
Stage IVA	Any T	any N	M1a
Stage IVB	Any T	any N	M1b

Used with permission of the American Joint Committee on Cancer (AJCC), Chicago, Illinois. The original source for this material is the AJCC Cancer Staging Manual, Seventh Edition (2010) published by Springer Science and Business Media LLC, www.springer.com.

Table 9-6

Staging for Anal Cancer

Stage	Description
Primary Tumor (T)	
TX	Tumor cannot be assessed
T0	No evidence of primary tumor
Tis	Carcinoma in situ
T1	Tumor ≤ cm in greatest dimension
T2	Tumor 2-5 cm in greatest dimension
T3	Tumor > 5 cm in greatest dimension
T4	Tumor invades any adjacent organs
Regional Lymph Nodes (N)	
NX	Regional lymph nodes cannot be assessed
N0	No regional lymph node metastasis
N1	Metastasis in the perirectal lymph nodes
N2	Metastasis in unilateral internal iliac and/or inguinal lymph nodes
N3	Metastasis in perirectal and inguinal lymph nodes and/or bilateral internal iliac and/or inguinal lymph nodes
Distant Metastasis (M)	
M0	No distant metastasis
M1	Distant metastasis

Anatomic Stage Groupings

Stage 0	Tis	N0	M0
Stage I	T1	N0	M0
Stage II	T2 or T3	N0	M0
Stage IIIA	T1-3	N1	M0
	T4	N0	M0
Stage IIIB	T4	N1	M0
	Any T	N2-N3	M0
Stage IV	Any T	any N	M1

Used with permission of the American Joint Committee on Cancer (AJCC), Chicago, Illinois. The original source for this material is the AJCC Cancer Staging Manual, Seventh Edition (2010) published by Springer Science and Business Media LLC, www.springer.com.

b. Four-phase dynamic contrast-enhanced magnetic resonance imaging (MRI)

c. Contrast-enhanced ultrasound (CEUS)

d. In tumor sizes greater than 2 cm, diagnosis made without a positive biopsy if both CEUS and MRI are conclusive (Forner et al., 2008; NCCN, 2013f)

e. Core needle biopsy preferred for tumors greater than 2 cm in size

f. CT of chest

g. Blood tests, including CBC, prothrombin time (PT) or international normalized ratio (INR), hepatitis panel, liver function, AFP

3. Staging and grading

a. AJCC staging system and grading (Table 9-7)

b. Child-Pugh and MELD (Model for End-Stage Liver Disease) scores also components of staging and evaluate aspects of liver function only

3 to 6 months recommended for patients at high-risk for HCC (ACS, 2013f); however, the NCCN recommends screening with ultrasonography and AFP every 6 to 12 months (NCCN, 2013f).

2. Diagnostic measures

a. Four-phase helical CT

Table 9-7

Staging for Hepatocellular Carcinoma

Stage	Description
Primary Tumor (T)	
TX	Primary tumor cannot be assessed
T0	No evidence of primary tumor
T1	Solitary tumor without vascular invasion
T2	Solitary tumor with vascular invasion or multiple tumors, none more than 5 cm
T3a	Multiple tumors > 5 cm
T3b	Single tumor or multiple tumors of any size involving a major branch of the portal or hepatic vein
T4	Tumor(s) with direct invasion of adjacent organs other than the gallbladder or with perforation of visceral peritoneum
Regional Lymph Node (N)	
NX	Regional lymph nodes cannot be assessed
N0	No regional lymph node metastasis
N1	Regional lymph node metastasis
Distant Metastasis (M)	
M0	No distant metastasis
M1	Distant metastasis

Anatomic Stage Groupings

Stage I	T1	N0	M0
Stage II	T2	N0	M0
Stage IIIA	T3a	N0	M0
Stage IIIB	T3b	N0	M0
Stage IIIC	T4	N0	M0
Stage IVA	Any T	N1	M0
Stage IVB	Any T	Any N	M1

Used with permission of the American Joint Committee on Cancer (AJCC), Chicago, Illinois. The original source for this material is the AJCC Cancer Staging Manual, Seventh Edition (2010) published by Springer Science and Business Media LLC, www.springer.com.

Table 9-8

Staging for Pancreatic Adenocarcinoma

Stage	Description
Primary Tumor (T)	
TX	Tumor cannot be assessed
T0	No evidence of primary tumor
Tis	Carcinoma in situ
T1	Tumor limited to the pancreas ≤ 2 cm in greatest dimension
T2	Tumor limited to the pancreas > 2 cm in greatest dimension
T3	Tumor extends beyond the pancreas but without involvement of the celiac axis or superior mesenteric artery
T4	Tumor involves the celiac axis or superior mesenteric artery (unresectable primary tumor)
Regional Lymph Node (N)	
NX	Regional lymph nodes cannot be assessed
N0	No regional lymph node metastasis
N1	Regional lymph node metastasis
Distant Metastasis (M)	
M0	No distant metastasis
M1	Distant metastasis

Anatomic Stage Groupings

Stage 0	Tis	N0	M0
Stage IA	T1	N0	M0
Stage IB	T2	N0	M0
Stage IIA	T3	N0	M0
Stage IIB	T1-3	N1	M0
Stage III	T4	Any N	M0
Stage IV	Any T	Any N	M1

Used with permission of the American Joint Committee on Cancer (AJCC), Chicago, Illinois. The original source for this material is the AJCC Cancer Staging Manual, Seventh Edition (2010) published by Springer Science and Business Media LLC, www.springer.com.

c. Patients generally stratified into one of four categories:
   (1) Potentially resectable or transplantable
   (2) Unresectable disease
   (3) Inoperable because of performance status or comorbidity
   (4) Metastatic disease

F. Pancreatic cancer
   1. Screening—no single reliable test for early detection of pancreatic cancer to date
   2. Diagnostic measures
      a. CT performed according to pancreas protocol—diphasic cross-sectional imaging and thin slices
      b. MRI—pancreas protocol emerging as alternative to CT
      c. EUS-guided fine needle aspiration (FNA) preferred over CT-guided FNA in patients with respectable disease; yield is better, safer, and decreased risk of seeding (NCCN, 2013g)

   3. Staging and grading
      a. AJCC staging and grading system (Table 9-8)

VIII. Principles of medical management
   A. Treatment of esophageal cancer
      1. Surgery
         a. Endoscopic mucosal resection—for carcinoma in situ (Tis) and stage I patients
         b. Esophagectomy— patients with stages I to III cancers
      2. Radiation therapy
         a. Concurrent with chemotherapy—usually in the neoadjuvant setting
         b. May be used with concurrent chemotherapy as definitive therapy if patient declines surgery or not a surgical candidate
         c. May be used with stage IV patients in palliative setting to alleviate obstruction, control pain, and restore swallowing

Table 9-9

Common Chemotherapy Regimens Used in Esophageal and Gastric Cancers

Type of Chemotherapy	Regimen
Preoperative chemoradiation	Paclitaxel and carboplatin; cisplatin and 5-fluorouracil (5-FU); oxaliplatin and 5-FU; cisplatin and capecitabine; oxaliplatin and capecitabine
Perioperative chemotherapy (3 cycles preoperative and 3 cycles postoperative)	Epirubicin, cisplatin and 5-FU (ECF); epirubicin, oxaliplatin, and 5-FU; epirubicin, cisplatin, and capecitabine; epirubicin, oxaliplatin, and capecitabine (EOX); 5-FU and cisplatin
Definitive chemoradiation	Cisplatin and 5-FU; oxaliplatin and 5-FU,; cisplatin and capecitabine; oxaliplatin and capecitabine; paclitaxel and carboplatin
Postoperative chemoradiation	Infusional 5-FU or capecitabine
Metastatic	Docetaxel, cisplatin, 5-FU (DCF); ECF, cisplatin and 5-FU or capecitabine; oxaliplatin and 5-FU or capecitabine; irinotecan and 5-FU

Data from National Comprehensive Cancer Network. (2013a). *Practice guidelines in oncology: Esophageal and esophagogastric junction cancers* [v.2.2013]. http://www.nccn.org/professionals/physician_gls/pdf/esophageal.pdf; and National Comprehensive Cancer Network. (2013b). *Practice guidelines in oncology: gastric cancer* [v.2.2013]. http://www.nccn.org/professionals/physician_gls/pdf/gastric.pdf.

3. Chemotherapy
   a. Used in combination with radiation as neoadjuvant or definitive therapy
   b. Used as primary treatment for stage IV disease (NCCN, 2013a)
   c. Common chemotherapy regimens used for esophageal cancer listed in Table 9-9.
B. Treatment of gastric cancer
   1. Surgery
      a. Endoscopic mucosal resection may be appropriate for Tis-T1b tumors
      b. Adequate gastric resection via subtotal or total gastrectomy preferred for T1b-T3 tumors
      c. Need for en bloc resection of involved structures in T4 tumors
      d. Controversy ongoing with regard to adequate sampling of lymph nodes
   2. Radiation therapy
      a. Used postoperatively with concurrent chemotherapy to decrease incidence of local recurrence
      b. Used preoperatively in clinical trials at present time

3. Chemotherapy
   a. Perioperative chemotherapy—pre- and postresection (see Table 9-9)
   b. Metastatic disease—provides palliation and improves survival and quality of life compared with the best supportive care (see Table 9-9)
4. Biotherapy
   a. Trastuzumab (Herceptin)—used in HER2+ tumors in metastatic setting in combination with chemotherapy (NCCN, 2013b)
C. Treatment of colorectal cancer
   1. Surgery (Figure 9-1, for colectomy sites)
      a. Right-sided colon cancer—right hemicolectomy
      b. Transverse colon cancers—extended right hemicolectomy
      c. Left-sided colon cancers—left hemicolectomy
      d. Sigmoid colon cancers—anterior sigmoid colectomy
      e. Rectal cancer
         (1) Local excision sometimes possible for early-stage tumors
         (2) Low anterior resection most common surgery for rectal cancers—allows for sphincter preservation
      f. Colostomy sometimes necessary—may be permanent or temporary (Padussis et al., 2010)
      g. Need to assess minimum of 12 lymph nodes for proper lymph node staging
      h. Liver and lung metastases sometimes eligible for resection to obtain remission and possible cure in stage IV disease
         (1) Dependent on amount and position of metastases
   2. Radiation therapy
      a. Used in neoadjuvant or adjuvant setting with concurrent chemotherapy to decrease local recurrence of rectal cancers
      b. May also be used in the palliative setting
   3. Chemotherapy
      a. Not indicated for stage I disease; unclear if it benefits patients with stage II disease
      b. Neoadjuvant setting
         (1) For unresectable tumors
         (2) With concurrent radiation for locally advanced rectal cancers
      c. Adjuvant setting for colorectal cancer
         (1) 5-Fluorouracil (5-FU)–based chemotherapy alone or in combination with oxaliplatin (Eloxatin)
      d. Metastatic setting

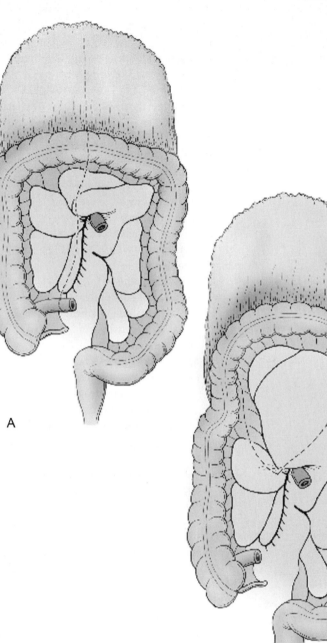

A   B

C

Figure 9-1 Extent of resection for colon cancer. A, Right colectomy. **B,** Left colectomy. **C,** Transverse colectomy. From Rothrock, J. (2011). *Alexander's care of the patient in surgery* (14th ed.). Philadelphia: Mosby.

(1) 5-FU–based chemotherapy alone or in combination with oxaliplatin (Eloxatin) or irinotecan (Camptosar)
(2) Irinotecan (Camptosar) may be used as a single agent
(3) Chemotherapy commonly used in conjunction with biotherapy in metastatic setting
4. Biotherapy—used for advanced or metastatic disease or as part of a clinical trial

(NCCN, 2013c; NCCN, 2013d; Roman & Whiteside, 2013)
a. Bevacizumab (Avastin)—used in combination with chemotherapy
b. Cetuximab (Erbitux)
   (1) Used in patients with *KRAS* mutation
   (2) Can be given in combination with chemotherapy or as single agent
c. Panitumumab (Vectibix)
   (1) Used in patients with *KRAS* mutation

(2) Can be given in combination with chemotherapy or as single agent in patients who cannot tolerate combination chemotherapy

d. Regorafenib (Stivarga)—used as single agent only

e. Ziv-alferbecept (Zaltrap)—used in combination with irinotecan

D. Treatment of anal cancer
  1. Radiation
     a. Definitive therapy with chemoradiation for stages I to III cancers
     b. Palliative treatment for stage IV cancers, if indicated (NCCN, 2013e)
  2. Chemotherapy
     a. Early stage—for definitive therapy, concurrent combination chemotherapy (5-FU and mitomycin) and radiation therapy
     b. Metastatic disease—cisplatin and 5-FU combination chemotherapy

E. Treatment of hepatocellular cancer
  1. Can be limited because of underlying liver disease
  2. Surgery
     a. Partial hepatectomy—potentially curative for patients with early-stage HCC
        (1) Optimal candidates—those with solitary tumors without vascular invasion
        (2) Evaluation of future liver remnant (FLR)
     b. Transplantation
        (1) Additional option for patients with early-stage HCC
        (2) Removes both detectable and undetectable tumor lesions and treats underlying cirrhosis
        (3) Avoids surgical complications associated with small FLR
        (4) Treatment before transplantation—may include bridge therapy, downstaging therapy, or ablative therapy
  3. Embolization
     a. Chemoembolization
     b. Bland embolization
     c. Radioembolization
  4. Radiation
     a. May be considered as alternative to ablation or chemoembolization
  5. Systemic chemotherapy
     a. Low response rates; no survival benefit (NCCN, 2013f)
  6. Targeted therapy
     a. Sorafenib (Nexavar)—approved by the U.S. Food and Drug Administration (FDA) for patients with unresectable HCC

F. Treatment of pancreatic cancer
  1. Surgery
     a. Pancreatoduodenectomy (Whipple)
     b. Distal pancreatectomy—left-sided resection
     c. Stenting—done with EUS for obstructive symptoms
  2. Radiation
     a. Palliative treatment
     b. Can be used concurrently with chemotherapy in different settings
        (1) Neoadjuvant—resectable
        (2) Borderline—resectable
        (3) Locally advanced—unresectable
        (4) Adjuvant (NCCN, 2013g)
  3. Chemotherapy
     a. Adjuvant setting
        (1) Clinical trial preferred, if available
        (2) Gemcitabine (Gemzar)
        (3) 5-FU or leucovorin
        (4) Capecitabine
     b. Metastatic or unresectable disease
        (1) Folfirinox—a combination of the chemotherapy drugs 5-FU, leucovorin, irinotecan, and oxaliplatin
        (2) Gemcitabine and abraxane (albumin-bound paclitaxel)
        (3) Gemcitabine and erlotinib
        (4) Gemcitabine and cisplatin
     c. Targeted therapy
        (1) Erlotinib may be used in conjunction with gemcitabine.

IX. Nursing implications
  A. Nurses play an important role in educating patients with GI malignancy about the disease process, diagnostic and treatment plans, and potential side effects.
     1. Interventions to increase patient knowledge about disease process, treatment, and side effects:
        a. Encouraging patient to verbalize feelings about disease and treatment
        b. Educating patient about treatment (rationale, type, and duration of treatment)
        c. Providing teaching on potential side effects and how to manage the side effects based on patient's learning style (written, verbal, audiovisual presentation, or combination of these)
        d. Discussing nonpharmacologic and pharmacologic interventions to manage side effects
  B. Nurses should continuously monitor for any alterations in GI function, fluid volume, and nutrition.

1. Interventions to maintain GI function and adequate fluid and nutritional intake include the following:
   a. Assessing for regular bowel function
   b. Assessing for factors (e.g., chemotherapy drugs) that may cause diarrhea or constipation
   c. Managing diarrhea or constipation, as appropriate
   d. Assessing for complications of diarrhea—for example, dehydration and electrolyte imbalance
   e. Assessing for complications of constipation—for example, nausea and bowel obstruction
   f. Providing nonpharmacologic and pharmacologic interventions to normalize bowel function
   g. Assessing and administering pain medications to relieve dysphagia, odynophagia, or both
   h. Assessing need for percutaneous endoscopic gastronomy (PEG) tube placement and feeding
   i. Administering tube feeding, as indicated
   j. Teaching patient how to administer tube feeding and care for PEG tube
   k. Instructing patient on adequate fluid intake
   l. Assessing for weight loss and orthostatic changes
   m. Administering IV fluids, as necessary
   n. Educating patient on proper caloric intake to maintain weight
   o. Educating patient on proper diet choices related to disease process
   p. Recommending nutritional supplements for additional caloric support
   q. Referral to dietician, swallow evaluation, or both, as needed
2. See Chapter 28 for more details on how to manage patients with alterations in GI function.
3. See Chapter 33 for more details on how to manage patients with alterations in nutritional status.

References

American Cancer Society. (2013a). *Cancer facts & figures, 2013.* Atlanta: Author.

American Cancer Society. (2013b). *Stomach cancer detailed guide.* http://www.cancer.org/cancer/stomachcancer/detailedguide/index.

American Cancer Society. (2013c). *Colorectal cancer detailed guide.* http://www.cancer.org/cancer/colonandrectumcancer/detailedguide/.

American Cancer Society. (2013d). *Anal cancer detailed guide.* http://www.cancer.org/cancer/analcancer/detailedguide/.

American Cancer Society. (2013e). *Liver cancer detailed guide.* http://www.cancer.org/cancer/livercancer/detailedguide/.

American Cancer Society. (2013f). *Esophagus cancer detailed guide.* http://www.cancer.org/cancer/esophaguscancer/detailedguide/index.

Blaydon, D. C., Etheridge, S. L., Risk, J. M., Hennies, H. C., Gay, L. J., Carroll, R., et al. (2012). RHBDF2 mutations are associated with tylosis, a familial esophageal cancer syndrome. *The American Journal of Human Genetics, 90*(2), 340–346.

Forner, A., Vilana, R., Ayuso, C., Bianchi, L., Solé, M., Ayuso, J. R., et al. (2008). Diagnosis of hepatic nodules 20 mm or smaller in cirrhosis: Prospective validation of the noninvasive diagnostic criteria for hepatocellular carcinoma. *Hepatology, 47*(1), 97–104.

Grenon, N. N. B. (2011). Liver cancer. In C. H. Yarbro, D. Wujcik, & B. H. Gobel (Eds.), *Cancer nursing: Principles and practice* (7th ed.). Sudbury, MA: Jones and Bartlett.

Hodgkin, M. B. (2011). Pancreatic cancer. In C. H. Yarbro, D. Wujcik, & B. H. Gobel (Eds.), *Cancer nursing: Principles and practice* (7th ed.). Sudbury, MA: Jones and Bartlett.

Holmes, R. S., & Vaughan, T. L. (2007). Epidemiology and pathogenesis of esophageal cancer. *Seminars in Radiation Oncology, 17*(1), 2–9.

Leeuwenburgh, I., Scholten, P., Alderliesten, J., Tilanus, H. W., Looman, C. W. N., Steijerberg, E. W., et al. (2010). Long-term esophageal cancer risk in patients with primary achalasia: A prospective study. *The American Journal of Gastroenterology, 105*(10), 2144–2149.

Minsky, B. D., & Guillem, J. G. (2010). Neoplasms of the anus. In K. Hong, R. Bast, W. Hait, D. Kue, R. Pollock, & R. Weichselbaum, et al. (Eds.), *Cancer medicine* (8th ed., pp. 1194–1203). Shelton, CT: People's Medical Publishing House-USA.

National Comprehensive Cancer Network. (2013a). *NCCN practice guidelines in oncology: Esophageal and esophagogastric junction cancers [v.2.2013].* http://www.nccn.org/professionals/physician_gls/pdf/esophageal.pdf.

National Comprehensive Cancer Network. (2013b). *NCCN practice guidelines in oncology: Gastric cancer [v.2.2013].* http://www.nccn.org/professionals/physician_gls/pdf/gastric.pdf.

National Comprehensive Cancer Network. (2013c). *NCCN practice guidelines in oncology: Colon cancer [v.3.2013].* http://www.nccn.org/professionals/physician_gls/pdf/colon.pdf.

National Comprehensive Cancer Network. (2013d). *NCCN practice guidelines in oncology: Rectal cancer [v.4.2013].* http://www.nccn.org/professionals/physician_gls/pdf/rectal.pdf.

National Comprehensive Cancer Network. (2013e). *NCCN practice guidelines in oncology: Anal carcinoma [v.2.2013].* http://www.nccn.org/professionals/physician_gls/pdf/anal.pdf.

National Comprehensive Cancer Network. (2013f). *NCCN practice guidelines in oncology: Hepatobiliary cancers [v.1.2013].* http://www.nccn.org/professionals/physician_gls/pdf/hepatobiliary.pdf.

National Comprehensive Cancer Network. (2013g). *NCCN practice guidelines in oncology (NCCN guidelines): Pancreatic adenocarcinoma [v.1.2013].* http://www.nccn.org/professionals/physician_gls/pdf/pancreatic.pdf.

Padussis, J. C., Beaseley, G. M., McMahon, N. S., Tyler, D. S., & Ludwig, K. A. (2010). Neoplasms of the small intestine, vermiform appendix and peritoneum, and carcinoma of the colon and rectum. In K. Hong, R. Bast, W. Hait, D. Kue, R.

Pollock, R. Weichselbaum, & E. Frei (Eds.), *Cancer medicine* (8th ed., pp. 1179–1188). Shelton, CT: People's Medical Publishing House-USA.

Rhodes, R. A. (2013). Gastrointestinal secretion, digestion and absorption. In R. Rhodes & D. Bell (Eds.), *Medical physiology: Principles for clinical medicine* (4th ed., pp. 511–517). Baltimore: Lippincott, Williams and Wilkins.

Roman, D., & Whiteside, R. (2013). Regorafenib: Adding to the armamentarium for refractory colorectal cancer and GIST. *Journal of the Advanced Practitioner in Oncology, 4*(2), 118–122.

Ruder, A. M., Ward, E. M., & Brown, D. P. (2001). Mortality in dry cleaning workers: An update. *American Journal of Industrial Medicine, 39*(2), 121–132.

Sung, M. W., & Thung, S. N. (2010). Primary neoplasms of the liver. In K. Hong, R. Bast, W. Hait, D. Kue, R. Pollock, & R. Weichselbaum, et al. (Eds.), *Cancer medicine* (8th ed., pp. 1124–1129). Shelton, CT: People's Medical Publishing House-USA.

Swisher, S. G., Rice, D. C., Ajani, J. A., Komaki, R. K., & Ferguson, M. K. (2010). Neoplasms of the esophagus. In K. Hong, R. Bast, W. Hait, D. Kue, R. Pollock, & R. Weichselbaum, et al.

(Eds.), *Cancer medicine* (8th ed., pp. 1074–1085). Shelton, CT: People's Medical Publishing House-USA.

Tan, C., & Du, X. (2012). KRAS mutation testing in metastatic colorectal cancer. *World Journal of Gastroenterology, 18*(37), 5171–5180.

Tsottles, N. D. (2011). Esophageal cancer. In C. H. Yarbro, D. Wujcik, & B. H. Gobel (Eds.), *Cancer nursing: Principles and practice* (7th ed.). Sudbury, MA: Jones and Bartlett.

Wolff, R. A., Crane, C. H., Li, D., & Evans, D. B. (2010). Neoplasms of the exocrine pancreas. In K. Hong, R. Bast, W. Hait, D. Kue, R. Pollock, & R. Weichselbaum, et al. (Eds.), *Cancer medicine* (8th ed., pp. 1144–1148). Shelton, CT: People's Medical Publishing House-USA.

Wood, J. D. (2013). Neurogastroenterology and motility. In R. Rhodes & D. Bell (Eds.), *Medical physiology: Principles for clinical medicine* (4th ed., pp. 487–489). Baltimore: Lippincott, Williams and Wilkins.

Yao, J. C., Crane, C. H., Sano, T., & Mansfield, P. F. (2010). Carcinoma of the stomach. In K. Hong, R. Bast, W. Hait, D. Kue, R. Pollock, & R. Weichselbaum, et al. (Eds.), *Cancer medicine* (8th ed., pp. 1086–1108). Shelton, CT: People's Medical Publishing House-USA.

CHAPTER 10
Cancers of the Reproductive System

Susan Vogt Temple

Cervical Cancer

I. Physiology and pathophysiology (Schiffman & Wentzensen, 2013)
  A. Anatomy of the cervix
    1. Consists of the lower portion of the uterus, which is contiguous with the upper portion of the vagina
    2. Composed of the exocervix and endocervix
    3. Surrounded by paracervical tissues rich in lymph nodes
  B. Changes associated with cancer of the cervix
    1. Cellular changes range from premalignant changes (mild to moderate to severe cervical intraepithelial neoplasia [CIN]) to carcinoma in situ (CIS) to invasive disease.
    2. Persistent infection with oncogenic human papillomavirus (HPV) is necessary for the development of cervical cancer.
      a. Certain genotypes of HPV are known to be oncogenic.
      b. Co-factors include a history of smoking, history of sexually transmitted disease, parity, contraceptive use, early age at onset of vaginal intercourse, large number of sexual partners, and chronic immunosuppression.
    3. Most cases of invasive cervical cancer arise in the transformation zone at the squamocolumnar junction.
      a. Exophytic, fungating, or cauliflower-like lesions
      b. Excavating or ulcerative necrotic lesions
      c. Endophytic lesions that extend within the cervical canal
    4. Two main histologic types
      a. Squamous carcinoma, which is most common (80%)
      b. Adenocarcinoma (approximately 20%)
  C. Trends in epidemiology (International Agency for Research on Cancer [IARC], 2013; Smith et al., 2014)
    1. Cervical cancer is the fourth most common cancer in women worldwide.
      a. Over 80% of cervical cancer cases occur in low-resource or developing nations (which lack the infrastructure to vaccinate, educate, screen, and treat).
      b. This is the fourth most frequent cause of cancer-related deaths in women worldwide.
    2. Incidence of invasive cervical cancer in the United States (U.S.) has decreased significantly since 1945 because of successful screening programs (Papanicolaou [Pap] smear test), with a concomitant increase in the diagnosis of preinvasive disease.
      a. Approximately half of the cervical cancers diagnosed in the U.S. are in women who have never been screened.
      b. An additional 10% occurs in women who have not been screened within the past 5 years.
II. Metastatic patterns
  A. Direct extension into the parametrium, vagina, lower uterine segment, abdomen, and other pelvic structures
  B. Lymph node metastases
  C. Metastasis to lung, liver, and bone through the hematologic route
III. Screening and diagnostic procedures
  A. Screening procedures (American Congress of Obstetricians and Gynecologists [ACOG], 2009a; Moyer, 2012; Saslow et al., 2012, Schiffman et al., 2011; Smith et al., 2014)
    1. Cervical liquid–based cytology (Pap test) with bimanual pelvic examination
    2. HPV deoxyribonucleic acid (DNA) testing for high-risk types of HPV; recommendations for average-risk individuals:
      a. Age younger than 21 years—no routine screening
      b. Screening to begin at age 21
      c. Age 21 to 29 years—liquid-based cytology every 3 years; HPV DNA testing not required unless Pap test is abnormal

d. Age 30 to 65 years—HPV testing and cytology (co-test) every 5 years (preferred) or cytology alone every 3 years

e. Age older than 65 years—no screening following adequate negative prior screening ($\geq$3 consecutive negative Pap tests or $\geq$2 consecutive negative HPV and PAP tests within the last 10 years, with the most recent test occurring within the last 5 years)

f. Women who have had a total hysterectomy—no cervical cancer screening to be performed if they no longer have a cervix and are without a history of CIN2 or more severe diagnosis in the past 20 years or have a history of cervical cancer

g. Tailored screening in case of higher risk for cervical cancer (e.g., history of long-term immunosuppression for organ transplantation, diethylstilbestrol [DES] exposure while in utero, chronic immunosuppression by chemotherapy or chronic corticosteroid treatment, or HIV-positive status)

(1) If cervix has been removed—no further screening unless a history of CIN2 or more severe diagnosis exists

(2) Screening recommendations for women age 30 to 65 (combination of HPV and cytology every 5 years or every 3 years with cytology alone) to be followed for at least 20 years, even if screening extends beyond 65 years, in women with a history of CIN2 or more severe diagnosis

(3) Women who are immunocompromised (organ transplantation, chemotherapy or chronic corticosteroid treatment, or HIV positive)—should be evaluated (co-test) twice during the first year after diagnosis and treatment and annually thereafter

B. Diagnostic procedures (ACOG, 2009a; Massad et al., 2013)

1. Colposcopy (examination of the cervix under magnification after application of a 3% to 5% acetic acid solution followed by colposcopically directed biopsies of all suspicious lesions)

2. Cervical biopsy—recommended when abnormalities are identified on the cervix by colposcopy

3. Endocervical curettage—recommended when the upper limits of cervical abnormalities are not visualized or the transformation zone within the endocervical canal is not visualized completely

4. Cone biopsy or loop electrosurgical excision procedure (LEEP)—may be recommended to obtain a larger wedge of tissue and to rule out invasive cancer

IV. Staging methods and procedures

A. The Bethesda System describing Pap results was revised in 2001. General categories include the following:

1. Negative for intraepithelial lesion or malignancy

2. Epithelial cell abnormalities (includes atypical squamous cells, squamous intraepithelial lesions, squamous cell carcinoma, atypical glandular cells)

3. Other malignant neoplasms (including melanoma, sarcomas, lymphoma)

B. Biopsy reports of cervical intraepithelial neoplasia include the following:

1. CIN1 (mild dysplasia [low-grade lesion])

2. CIN2 (moderate dysplasia [high-grade lesion])

3. CIN3 (severe dysplasia and carcinoma in situ [high-grade lesion])

4. Squamous cell cancer of the cervix

C. For invasive cervical cancer, examination is done with the client under anesthesia to evaluate extent of disease.

1. Extension of disease to the bladder or rectum is determined by cystoscopy, sigmoidoscopy, proctoscopy, or barium enema (Pecorelli, 2009).

D. Abdominal or pelvic computed tomography (CT), ultrasonography, magnetic resonance imaging (MRI), or positron emission tomography (PET) may be performed to evaluate the extent of the local lesion and metastasis to regional lymph nodes.

E. Chest radiography is used to rule out lung metastasis.

F. Invasive cervical cancer is clinically staged.

G. Surgical or pathology results guide treatment-related decisions.

V. Trends in survival

A. No change in survival rate has occurred for clients with invasive cervical cancer, although mortality rate has decreased because of decreased incidence.

B. Prognosis is related to stage of disease.

C. Cause of death from cervical cancer is associated most often with uremia, infection, or hemorrhage.

VI. Principles of medical management

A. Treatment strategies (ACOG, 2009a; National Comprehensive Cancer Network [NCCN], 2014a)

1. Preinvasive disease—biopsy, cauterization cryotherapy, laser therapy, conization, loop electrosurgical excision procedure (LEEP), or hysterectomy; treatment depends on the following:

a. Size and location of CIN visualized

b. Client's desire for preservation of childbearing capacity

c. Physician's skills and preference

2. Invasive disease—surgery, radiation, or both
    a. Treatment choice—depends on client's age, physical condition, body habitus, tumor volume, and desire to maintain fertility or ovarian function
    b. Primary surgical treatment—early-stage disease (Abu-Rustum & Sonoda, 2010; NCCN, 2014a; Rydzewska, Tierney, Vale, & Symonds, 2010)
        (1) For fertility sparing
            (a) Stage 1A1 and no lymphovascular space invasion (LVSI)—cone biopsy with negative margins
            (b) Stage 1A1 with LVSI or 1A2—cone biopsy with negative margins or radical trachelectomy (surgical removal of the cervix) and pelvic node dissection
            (c) Radical trachelectomy and pelvic node dissection
        (2) Non–fertility sparing
            (a) Stage 1A1 (no LVSI)—observation, if cone biopsy margins are negative and patient is not a surgical candidate; extrafascial hysterectomy if surgical candidate; extrafascial hysterectomy or modified radical hysterectomy if cone biopsy margins positive
            (b) Stage 1A1 with LVSI/stage 1A2—modified radical hysterectomy with pelvic lymphadenectomy; consider para-aortic lymph node sampling
            (c) Stage 1B1, 2A2—radical hysterectomy, pelvic lymph node dissection, para-aortic lymph node sampling
        (3) Bilateral salpingo-oophorectomy included for postmenopausal women and for those older than 40 years or no longer desirous of childbearing
    c. Primary radiation therapy (RT) treatment—early- or advanced-stage disease (Monk, Tewari, & Koh, 2007; NCCN, 2014a; Tewari & Monk, 2009)
        (1) Combination of external and either high-dose outpatient or conventional inpatient intracavitary brachytherapy implantation
        (2) Intracavitary implantation before or after external RT is completed
        (3) Radiosensitization with cisplatin-based chemotherapy weekly during radiation
    d. Combination of surgery and radiation or chemotherapy for advanced-stage disease or early-stage disease with positive lymph nodes or positive surgical margins
3. Recurrent disease (Monk et al., 2007; Tewari & Monk, 2009)
    a. Central recurrence only—anterior, posterior, or total pelvic exenteration
        (1) Triad of unilateral leg edema, sciatic pain, and ureteral obstruction is indicative of recurrent and unresectable disease.
        (2) Extensive preoperative workup is done to rule out extrapelvic disease.
        (3) Initial pelvic sidewall biopsy, lymph node evaluation, or frozen section is performed to rule out metastatic disease (intraoperatively).
        (4) Total pelvic exenteration includes removal of all pelvic viscera and creation of urinary and bowel diversions.
    b. Unresectable or disseminated disease
        (1) Chemotherapy or targeted therapies are palliative with single agents or combination therapy. Agents with known activity include cisplatin, carboplatin, paclitaxel, docetaxel, bevacizumab, 5-fluorouracil (5-FU), ifosfamide, cyclophosphamide, gemcitabine, topotecan, irinotecan, mitomycin, pemetrexed, and vinorelbine; response rates are low.
VII. Nursing implications
    A. Interventions related to prevention, screening, and early detection
        1. Assessment for pertinent personal and family history
            a. Average age between 45 and 55 years
            b. Presence of HPV oncogenic genotypes, including HPV 16, 18, 31, 33, 35, 39, 45, 51, 52, 56, 58, and 59; long-term use of oral contraceptives, high parity
            c. Multiple sexual partners and sexual partners who have had multiple sexual partners
            d. History of CIN
            e. Cigarette smoking (increases risk by twofold to fivefold)
            f. Immunosuppression (e.g., with acquired immunodeficiency disease [AIDS] or after transplantation)
    B. Interventions to maximize safety for the client
        1. Education about changes in lifestyle that can modify risks of cervical cancer
            a. HPV vaccine—prevents infection with certain subtypes of the HPV implicated in the cause of cervical, vaginal, vulvar, and anal cancers; data regarding number of

doses and timing of vaccination still accruing

b. Teaching about limiting the number of sexual partners

c. Providing information about the use of barrier-type contraceptives—diaphragm or condom, although not protective for HPV exposure, protective for other sexually transmitted diseases (STDs)

d. Discontinuation of cigarette smoking and tobacco use

e. Screening as recommended to detect premalignant changes; vaccination does not alter screening recommendations

C. Interventions to decrease the severity of symptoms associated with disease and treatment

1. Teaching the client about potential symptoms associated with treatment modality options

2. Primary symptoms related to surgery

a. Inability to void—innervation to the bladder is disrupted during radical hysterectomy, resulting in an inability to sense the need to void and an inability to empty the bladder completely

(1) A suprapubic catheter is placed postoperatively.

(2) Bladder training is initiated by clamping the catheter for 2 to 3 hours.

(3) The client is encouraged to drink fluids unless contraindicated by physiologic status.

(4) The catheter is removed after less than 50 mL of residual urine remains after voiding, as ordered.

(5) Alternatively, the client or the caregiver may be taught intermittent self-catheterization before discharge from the hospital.

b. Constipation—bowel is manipulated during radical surgery; peristalsis may not return for several days

c. Shortened vagina—approximately one third of the upper vagina may be excised with hysterectomy; remaining margins are sutured to form a vaginal cuff

d. Urinary and stool diversions with pelvic exenteration

3. Primary symptoms related to RT (see Chapter 21)

D. Interventions to monitor for sequelae of disease or treatment

1. Surgery

a. Assessment of changes in bowel pattern—constipation, bowel obstruction, rare fistula formation

b. Evaluation of changes in bladder pattern—recurrent urinary tract infection, fistula formation

2. Radiation therapy

a. Assessment of changes in bowel pattern—diarrhea, bowel obstruction, rectal ulcers, rectovaginal fistulas

b. Assessment of changes in bladder pattern—urinary retention, cystitis, vesicovaginal fistulas

c. Evaluation of changes in vaginal tissues—atrophy, stenosis, dryness

3. Recurrent disease

a. Assessment for history of vaginal bleeding

b. Evaluation of occurrence of new pain, particularly in hips or lower back

c. Evaluation of lower extremities for edema

d. Assessment for changes in appetite with weight loss

E. Interventions to incorporate the client and family in care

1. Encouraging open communication about the impact of disease and treatment on the client and significant others

2. Teaching the client and significant other new self-care skills required during or after treatment

3. Identifying concerns that the client and sexual partner may have about resuming sexual expression or intercourse after treatment; changes in sexual functioning or dyspareunia frequently occurs secondary to the following:

a. Decreased vaginal distensibility (radiation)

b. Shortened vagina (surgery, radiation therapy)

c. Lack of vaginal lubrication (radiation therapy)

d. Hormonal changes or altered libido

e. Altered self-concept or body image

4. Client education regarding the use of vaginal dilators, how to use vaginal lubricants, and, if an option, sexual positions that may be more comfortable during vaginal intercourse

Endometrial Cancer

I. Physiology and pathophysiology (Kitchener & Trimble, 2009; NCCN, 2014c)

A. Anatomy of the endometrium

1. Inner layer of the three layers of the uterus (endometrium, myometrium, parietal peritoneum)

2. Highly vascular

B. Primary functions of the endometrium—provides vascular and nutrient supply for developing fetus and responds to variations in estrogen and progesterone levels in a cyclic fashion

C. Changes associated with cancer of the endometrium
   1. Underlying cause of most endometrial cancers believed to be related to chronic endogenous or exogenous estrogen exposure
   2. Atypical hyperplasia that may evolve into or harbor an invasive cancer
   3. Histology—85% to 90% adenocarcinoma; rarer types include clear cell, uterine papillary serous, and sarcoma histologies
D. Trends in epidemiology (Kitchener & Trimble, 2009; Siegel, Ma, Zou, & Jemal, 2014)
   1. Most common gynecologic malignancy among women in the U.S.
   2. Fourth most common cancer in women in the U.S.
   3. Increase in incidence over the past several decades associated with the following:
      a. Increased use of estrogen replacement therapy (without progestin)
      b. Obesity (adipocytes convert androstenedione to estrone, thereby increasing circulating estrogen levels)
   4. Women with Lynch syndrome at higher risk for endometrial cancer (up to 60%) (NCCN, 2014c; Resnick, Hampel, Fishel, & Cohen, 2009)
II. Metastatic patterns
   A. Invades inner third of the endometrium and progresses to the full thickness of the endometrium
   B. Metastasis through local extension to adjacent structures such as the cervix and vagina and distantly to intra-abdominal sites and lung
   C. Metastasis in femoral, iliac, hypogastric, para-aortic, and obturator lymph nodes
   D. Hematologic metastasis uncommon in type I disease; more common in serous and sarcoma histologies
III. Screening and diagnostic procedures (Creasman, 2009; Frederick & Straughn, 2009; Kitchener & Trimble, 2009; Smith et al., 2014)
   A. Screening procedures
      1. Ultrasonography not been found to be cost-effective as a screening modality for endometrial cancer
      2. Bimanual pelvic examination to palpate the size and shape of the uterus
      3. Periodic testing or endometrial biopsy considered at age 35 in women at very high risk (Lynch syndrome, other genetic predisposition)
   B. Diagnostic procedures
      1. Endometrial aspiration or biopsy
      2. Endocervical curettage to rule out cervical cancer
      3. Fractional dilation and curettage (D&C) if previous endometrial biopsy results have been negative, stenosis makes endometrial biopsy impossible, and abnormal bleeding persists

IV. Staging methods and procedures (Creasman, 2009; Frederick & Straughn, 2009; Kitchener & Trimble, 2009; NCCN, 2014c)
   A. Procedures
      1. Genetic testing or counseling for suspected Lynch syndrome (significant family history of endometrial and/or colorectal cancer)
      2. Chest radiography
   B. Surgical staging based on findings from exploratory laparotomy, total hysterectomy–bilateral salpingo-oophorectomy (TH-BSO) and peritoneal washings; laparoscopy-assisted staging or robotic surgery appropriate in a subset of patients
   C. Results of staging reported as anatomic stage, histopathologic grade, depth of myometrial invasion, and peritoneal cytology results
V. Trends in survival
   A. Most curable gynecologic malignancy
   B. Prognostic factors—stage, grade, and depth of myometrial invasion, peritoneal cytology, and hormone receptor status
VI. Principles of medical management
   A. Treatment strategies (Kitchener & Trimble, 2009; May, Bryant, Dickinson, Kehoe, & Morrison, 2010; NCCN, 2014c).
      1. Treatment decisions based on stage of disease, grade, depth of myometrial invasion, presence or absence of prognostic features within the tumor specimen, and client characteristics
      2. Preinvasive disease—hormone therapy or simple hysterectomy
         a. For fertility sparing—if well-differentiated endometroid adenocarcinoma and limited to the endometrium (very early stage), with no evidence of extrauterine disease and no contraindications to medical therapy or pregnancy, can consider hormone therapy with interval endometrial sampling and close surveillance
         b. Must understand that option is not the standard of care for the treatment of endometrial cancer
   B. Invasive disease—surgery, radiation therapy, or both
      1. Surgery
         a. Surgical staging procedure (TH-BSO with peritoneal cytologic examination, pelvic and para-aortic lymph node dissection)—serves as primary treatment for endometroid disease confined to the uterus
         b. Cervical involvement—radical hysterectomy – BSO, pelvic and para-aortic lymph node dissection, and cytology
      2. RT—primary treatment for high-risk surgical candidates

3. Adjuvant RT
   a. Preoperative therapy for clients with extensive lesions involving the cervix or high-grade lesions
   b. Postoperative therapy for clients with risk factors for recurrent disease; high-grade lesions, deep myometrial invasion; or lower uterine segment or cervical involvement
   c. Techniques include intracavitary brachytherapy and external beam radiation
4. Disseminated disease (Dellinger & Monk, 2009; Moxley & McMeekin, 2010; NCCN, 2014c; Ray & Fleming, 2009).
   a. Hormonal agents, including progestational agents, tamoxifen, and aromatase inhibitors
   b. Single-agent and combination chemotherapy—agents with known activity, including cyclophosphamide, ifosfamide, doxorubicin, liposomal doxorubicin, docetaxel, paclitaxel, carboplatin, and cisplatin
5. Recurrent disease—surgery or RT to previously untreated areas, chemotherapy, bevacizumab, or hormone therapy

VII. Nursing implications
   A. Interventions related to prevention, screening, and early detection
      1. Assessment for pertinent personal and family history (Kitchener & Trimble, 2009)
         a. Age—peak incidence, 50 to 59 years
         b. Menopausal status—80% of clients are postmenopausal
         c. Socioeconomic status—higher status places women at increased risk
         d. Increased levels of estrogen—obesity, diabetes, high-fat diet, nulliparity, early age at menarche, late age at menopause, use of tamoxifen (estrogenic in the uterus), and estrogen replacement therapy without progestational agents
         e. Personal history of endometrial hyperplasia; breast, ovarian, or colorectal cancers
         f. Family history of hereditary nonpolyposis colorectal cancer, multiple endocrine-related cancers (NCCN, 2014c; Resnick et al., 2009).
         g. Significant increase in risk related to triad of obesity, diabetes, and hypertension
         h. Exposure to external carcinogens
   B. Interventions to maximize safety for the client
      1. Teaching changes in lifestyle that can modify risks of endometrial cancer
         a. Encouraging the client to maintain ideal body weight
         b. Encouraging the client to report any unexpected bleeding or spotting to physician

C. Interventions to decrease the severity of symptoms such as altered urinary and bowel function and pain, which are associated with disease and treatment from surgery and RT
   1. Venous stasis
      a. Encouraging turning in bed and ambulating as soon as possible
      b. Teaching isometric leg exercises to be done while in bed
      c. Applying antiembolic stockings
      d. Monitoring for discomfort in legs and thighs
      e. Avoiding use of a knee gatch in the bed
   2. Urinary retention
      a. Monitoring urinary output
      b. Assessment for bladder distention above the symphysis pubis
      c. Assessment for lower abdominal discomfort
   3. Assess for signs of recurrent disease
      a. Vaginal bleeding
      b. Change in bowel habits—constipation
      c. Pelvic pain

Ovarian Cancer

I. Physiology and pathophysiology (Fleming, Ronnett, & Seidman, 2009; NCCN, 2014b).
   A. Anatomy of the ovary
      1. Ovaries are located on each side of the uterus behind the fallopian tubes.
      2. Ovarian lymphatics drain into the iliac and periaortic lymph nodes.
   B. Primary functions of the ovary—production and release of ova and production of hormones to meet the needs of a female for development, growth, and function (estrogen, progesterone, testosterone)
   C. Trends in epidemiology (Fleming et al., 2009; Smith et al., 2014)—ovarian cancer is the leading cause of death from gynecologic cancer in the U.S. and the country's fifth most common cause of cancer mortality in women
II. Metastatic patterns
   A. Local extension to adjacent organs
   B. Exfoliation of the ovarian capsule
   C. Serosal seeding throughout the peritoneal cavity, including the omentum
   D. Lymphatic spread
   E. Hematologic spread is rare
III. Screening and diagnostic procedures
   A. Screening procedures (Buys et al., 2011; Clarke-Pearson, 2009; NCCN, 2014b).
      1. Bimanual pelvic examination
         a. Increase in size or irregularity of the ovary
         b. Palpable ovary in a postmenopausal woman

2. Serial cancer antigen 125 (CA-125) determinations in high-risk women supplemented by transvaginal ultrasonography
3. Routine screening for ovarian cancer in the general population not supported by randomized data; false-positive results may lead to unnecessary surgeries and serious complications

B. Diagnostic procedures
1. Laparoscopy or exploratory laparotomy to obtain tissue for diagnosis
2. Paracentesis of ascitic fluid

IV. Staging procedures and methods
A. CT of abdomen and pelvis
B. Barium enema or colonoscopy
C. Pulmonary involvement—chest radiography, cytologic evaluation of pleural fluid, if effusions present
D. Surgical staging laparotomy mandatory to evaluate pelvic and abdominal contents—total abdominal hysterectomy with bilateral salpingo-oophorectomy (TAH-BSO) or unilateral salpingo-oophorectomy in select patients desiring to maintain fertility; peritoneal cytology; omentectomy; lymph node biopsies or removal; multiple biopsies of bladder, bowel, liver, and diaphragm surfaces; appendectomy; and debulking cytoreduction of all visible tumor (Elattar, Bryant, Winter-Roach, Hatem, & Naik, 2011; Fleming et al., 2009)
E. Majority of clients with ovarian cancer diagnosed with late-stage disease
F. CA-125; other protein signatures continue to be evaluated as potential markers for early detection (Clarke-Pearson, 2009; NCCN, 2014b)

V. Trends in survival
A. In the majority of patients with advanced disease, the cancer is not curable; many patients will receive multiple lines of chemotherapy.
B. Stage, grade, and amount of residual disease following initial surgery (optimal versus suboptimal debulking) are important prognostic factors.
C. Abdominal carcinomatosis commonly occurs and results in intestinal obstruction, malabsorption, and fluid and electrolyte imbalances.

VI. Principles of medical management
A. Treatment strategies (Elattar et al., 2011; Fleming et al., 2009; NCCN, 2014b)
1. Primary surgical treatment
a. Best outcomes are achieved when surgery is performed by a gynecologic oncologist.
b. Optimal tumor debulking or cytoreduction and complete surgical staging, as well as removal of all tumor or tumors greater than 1 cm in size, so that minimal

residual disease remains, improve overall survival.
c. Surgery may be used alone to treat early-stage disease or borderline tumors with "low malignant potential."
d. In young women wishing to preserve fertility, a unilateral salpingo-oophorectomy may be sufficient in low-risk situations (select early stage or histologies).
e. Neoadjuvant chemotherapy may be considered in in patients who are not surgical candidates.

2. Adjuvant chemotherapy (Fleming et al., 2009)
a. For clients with early-stage or poorly differentiated disease or more advanced disease
b. Combination chemotherapy with a taxane and platinum doublet—now first-line therapy; recurrent progressive disease may be treated with a number of agents (either as single agents or in combination), including cisplatin, cyclophosphamide, bevacizumab, capecitabine, ifosfamide, irinotecan, pemetrexed, liposomal doxorubicin, paclitaxel, docetaxel, hexamethylmelamine, topotecan, etoposide, gemcitabine, oxaliplatin, melphalan, vinorelbine, and/or hormonal agents; choice of agents often determined by the progression-free interval or platinum sensitivity and comorbidities
c. Chemotherapy—may be administered orally, intravenously, or intraperitoneally (recommended for stage III patients who are optimally debulked); advantages of the intraperitoneal method are as follows:
(1) Higher concentrations of drug to the surface of the tumor
(2) Decreased systemic side effects
(3) Systemic tolerance of higher doses of drug
d. Hormone therapy (e.g., megestrol acetate [Megace], tamoxifen [Nolvadex])—may be used in clients unable to tolerate more aggressive regimens

VII. Nursing implications
A. Interventions related to prevention, early detection, and screening (ACOG, 2009b; Fleming et al., 2009; NCCN, 2014b; Shulman, 2010)
1. Assess pertinent personal and family history.
a. Age—occurs commonly in premenopausal women ages 40 to 65 years old; peak incidence at age 60 to 64 years
b. Germ cell tumors more common in children and adolescents
c. Infertility
d. Nulliparity

e. Personal history of breast, endometrial, or colon cancer

f. Family history of breast, endometrial, or colon cancer (*BRCA1* or *BRCA2* mutation, Lynch syndrome); hereditary ovarian cancer accounts for approximately 5% of all women with ovarian cancer

B. Interventions for management of symptoms related to disease, treatment modalities, and recurrent disease

1. Aggressive symptom management is necessary while women receive complex chemotherapy regimens (e.g., antiemetic control, prevention of neuropathies, and maintenance of fluid and electrolyte balance).

2. Coping issues need to be addressed because diagnosis is often delayed, therapy may be prolonged, and prognosis is poor.

3. Recurrence occurs in approximately 80% of patients, and many patients receive multiple lines of therapy. Patients need to be educated about surveillance, signs and symptoms of recurrence, and the chronic nature of ovarian cancer.

Gestational Trophoblastic Neoplasia

I. Physiology and pathophysiology of gestational trophoblastic neoplasia (GTN)

A. Spectrum of neoplasia, including invasive moles, choriocarcinomas, placental site trophoblastic disease, and epithelioid neoplasia associated with the products of conception

B. Chromosomal abnormalities involved in fertilization, differentiation and pronuclear cleavage, decidual implantation, and invasion under investigation

II. Metastatic patterns—most common sites of metastases are the lung, vagina, liver, and brain

III. Screening and diagnostic procedures

A. Diagnostic evaluation—history and physical examination, including pelvic examination; ultrasonography to evaluate suspected pregnancy if fetal abnormality or absence; quantitative serum beta–human chorionic gonadotropin (beta-HCG); and metastatic workup if necessary (complete blood cell count [CBC]; chemistries; CT or MRI of head, chest, abdomen)

IV. Staging methods and procedures, including ultrasonography; D&C with suction evacuation; metastatic evaluation of chest, abdomen, and brain, if appropriate

V. Trends in survival—cure in 90% of clients with metastatic disease

VI. Principles of medical management (Berkowitz & Goldstein, 2013)

A. Treatment strategies

1. Depend on classification and desired fertility

a. Suction evacuation of uterine contents eliminates mole and preserves childbearing.

b. Hysterectomy may be done if childbearing is not desired.

2. Invasive disease—removal of uterine contents with suction

3. Chemotherapy—extremely effective in management of GTN

a. Single-agent therapy with methotrexate (Mexate) or actinomycin-D (Cosmegen) for nonmetastatic or good-prognosis disease

b. Multiagent chemotherapy for clients with poor prognosis or resistant metastatic GTN

4. Surgical removal of isolated chemotherapy-resistant metastasis

5. RT of resistant metastatic sites

VII. Nursing implications

A. Interventions related to prevention, screening, and early detection

1. Assessment of pertinent personal and family history

a. Age—highest risk in women over 40 years of age becoming pregnant; some increased risk in women under 20 years

b. Previous molar pregnancy greatest risk factor

B. Interventions to decrease the severity of symptoms associated with disease and treatment

1. Patients need to understand the importance of staying on treatment and should endeavor to maintain treatment schedule.

2. High-dose chemotherapy requires expert knowledge and vigilance in administration and toxicity management.

C. Interventions to incorporate the client and family in care

1. Encouragement of open communication about the impact of disease and treatment on the client and significant others

2. Teaching the client and significant others new self-care skills required during and after treatment

3. Instructing the client to use oral contraceptives during treatment and follow-up:

a. Time frame variable; dependent on clinical situation

4. Identification of concerns the client and her sexual partner may have about future fertility

5. Teaching about the importance of beta-HGC monitoring, significance of results, and follow-up

Vulvar Cancer

I. Physiology and pathophysiology
  A. Anatomy of the vulva—comprises the external genital organs: mons pubis, labia majora and minora, clitoris, vaginal vestibule, perineal body, supporting subcutaneous tissue
  B. Changes associated with cancer of the vulva (Carter & Downs, 2012)
    1. Cellular changes on a continuum from premalignant changes to invasive carcinoma
      a. HPV-related changes
      b. Other changes, granulomatous changes
    2. Histology—85% squamous; rare—melanoma, sarcoma, basal cell carcinoma
  C. Trends in epidemiology—very rare cancer; comprises only 5% of all female cancers
II. Metastatic patterns
  A. Direct extension to adjacent structures
  B. Lymph node metastases (femoral and inguinal, iliac nodes)
  C. Hematogenous spread to distant sites, including lung
III. Screening and diagnostic procedures
  A. Screening procedures—careful visual and pelvic inspection and examination; acetic acid staining and colposcopy may be used to evaluate any suspicious lesions; cystoscopy and proctoscopy for advanced disease
  B. Diagnostic procedure—biopsy
IV. Staging methods and procedures—biopsy of suspected area and evaluation of lymph node involvement with CT, cystoscopy, and proctoscopy (Carter & Downs, 2012; Pecorelli, 2009)
V. Trends in survival
  A. Five-year survival rates of 80% to 90% reported for stages I and II disease
  B. Poor survival rates for clients with advanced disease: 60% for stage III and 15% for stage IV
  C. Prognosis related to inguinal nodal metastasis, tumor size, depth of invasion, and tumor thickness
VI. Principles of medical management
  A. Treatment strategies
    1. Stage 1A—surgical management with wide local excision
    2. Stages 1B and 2—surgery the major modality (i.e., radical excision or vulvectomy and nodal evaluation or dissection)
    3. Advanced disease—chemotherapy or RT as an adjunct preoperatively or postoperatively
VII. Nursing implications
  A. Interventions related to prevention, screening, and early detection
    1. Assessment of pertinent personal and family history:
      a. Age—peak incidence in postmenopausal women at ages ranging from 65 to 75 years; 15% of cases in women younger than 40 years
      b. Increased risk with history of HPV infection, vulvar inflammation, and other genitourinary (GU) cancers
  B. Interventions to decrease the severity of symptoms associated with disease and treatment
    1. Teaching client about possible symptoms associated with treatment
    2. Monitoring for the development of leg edema if lymph node dissection completed
    3. Identifying concerns the client and her sexual partner may have about resuming sexual functioning after treatment

Vaginal Cancer

I. Physiology and pathophysiology (Carter & Downs, 2012)
  A. Anatomy of the vagina—mucous membrane tube forming the passageway between the uterus and the vulva
  B. Associated changes—can be premalignant to invasive
  C. Pathology—squamous cell carcinoma 85%; rarely melanoma, adenocarcinoma, clear cell cancers
  D. Incidence—extremely rare cancer; comprises 1% to 2% of female GU cancers
II. Metastatic patterns
  A. Local extension and lymph node involvement
  B. More commonly a metastatic site for cervical cancer
III. Screening and diagnostic procedures
  A. Screening procedures
    1. Careful pelvic inspection and examination
    2. Cytologic washings, even after hysterectomy
  B. Diagnostic procedures
    1. Biopsy of lesion, usually an outpatient procedure
    2. Examination with client under anesthesia—cystoscopy, proctoscopy
    3. Chest radiography, CT of abdomen and pelvis
IV. Staging methods and procedures—FIGO staging system used (International Federation of Gynecology and Obstetrics [FIGO], 2009; Pecorelli, 2009).
  A. Stage I— carcinoma is limited to the vaginal wall
  B. Stage II— carcinoma has involved the subvaginal tissue but has not extended to the pelvic wall
  C. Stage III— carcinoma has extended to the pelvic wall
  D. Stage IV— carcinoma has extended beyond the true pelvis or has involved the mucosa of the

bladder or rectum; bullous edemas as such do not permit a case to be allotted to stage IV
1. IVa—tumor has invaded bladder and rectal mucosa, direct extension beyond the true pelvis, or both
2. IVb—spread to distant organs

V. Treatment strategies (Carter & Downs, 2012)
A. Preinvasive disease—vaginal intraepithelial neoplasia: localized treatments include application of topical agents, laser vaporization, brachytherapy, and surgical excision
B. Invasive disease—surgery, RT, or both
C. Recurrent disease—surgery or RT to previously untreated areas

VI. Nursing implications
A. Interventions related to prevention, early detection, and screening
1. Assessment of pertinent personal and family history
a. Age—primarily a disease of adults older than 60 years
b. Personal history of maternal DES use during pregnancy; should be screened for rare clear cell pathology
c. Increased risk with prior history of invasive cervical carcinoma (ICC)
B. Monitor for sequelae of disease and treatment
1. Side effects of chemotherapy—see Chapter 22
2. Vaginal stenosis and shortening—may manifest several months after radiation
3. Other complications—rectal ulceration, vaginal necrosis, small bowel obstruction, cystitis, leg edema, neuritis, and diverticulitis
C. Incorporate the client and family in care
1. Identification of concerns the client and her sexual partner may have about resuming sexual functioning after treatment

Testicular Cancer

I. Physiology and pathophysiology
A. Anatomy of the testes—ovoid glands located in the scrotal sac that descend from the abdomen through the inguinal canal during the seventh month of fetal life
B. Primary functions of the testes—spermatogenesis and production of a hormone (testosterone) for male development, growth, and function
C. Changes associated with cancer of the testes (Nallu, Mannuel, & Hussain, 2013; Viatori, 2012)
1. Arises from germinal epithelium
2. Usually occurs in only one testis
3. Cause unknown; risk factors include cryptorchidism, chromosomal abnormalities (e.g., Klinefelter syndrome), and abnormalities in reproductive tract development in utero

4. Behavior of testicular cancer varies with histologic subtype
a. Seminomas
(1) Occur in approximately 50% of cases
(2) Spread slowly, primarily through the lymphatics
(3) Are responsive to RT
b. Nonseminoma germ cell testicular tumors (NSGCTTs)—embryonal tumor (20%), teratoma, choriocarcinoma; yolk sac, interstitial cell, and gonadal stromal tumors
(1) More aggressive than pure seminomas; 60% to 70% have lymph node spread at diagnosis
(2) Embryonal tumors—invade the spermatic cord and metastasize to lung
(3) Embryonal tumors not responsive to RT
c. Mixed cell types fairly common
D. Trends in epidemiology
1. Very rare cancer; incidence approximately 1% in males in the U.S.
2. Most commonly occurring cancer among men ages 15 to 35 years
3. Incidence higher and is increasing among white males; incidence in African Americans increasing since the 1990s

II. Metastatic patterns
A. Direct extension to adjacent structures
B. Lymphatic spread
C. Hematologic metastasis to the lung, brain, bone, and liver

III. Screening and diagnostic procedures
A. Screening procedures
1. Monthly testicular self-examination
2. Annual bimanual palpation and examination of the testes by the health care provider
B. Diagnostic procedure—ultrasonography to diagnose mass; tissue diagnosis by radical inguinal orchiectomy

IV. Staging methods and procedures
A. CT of the abdomen and pelvis; chest if positive abdominal CT or abnormal chest radiography
B. MRI of brain if symptomatic; bone scan to be considered
C. PET in seminomas; teratomas are not PET-avid
D. Clinical evaluation and histologic determination required for clinical staging
E. Pathologic staging dependent on surgical findings
F. Alpha-fetoprotein (AFP), lactate dehydrogenase (LDH), and beta-HCG testing

V. Trends in survival
A. Survival from testicular cancer has increased dramatically.
B. Testicular cancer is almost always considered curable, and the prognosis for clients is excellent.

C. Prognosis depends on bulk of disease at diagnosis.

D. Recurrences usually occur within 2 years; however, recurrences beyond 5 years have been reported, and recurrent disease is also responsive to treatment.

VI. Principles of medical management (Nallu et al., 2013)

  A. Treatment strategies (vary by histology)

    1. Surgery

      a. Transinguinal orchiectomy—primary treatment for seminomas and nonseminomas

      b. Retroperitoneal lymph node dissection (RPLND)

      c. Surgery—may be used to resect residual disease and isolated metastatic lesions of lung, liver, and retroperitoneum

    2. Radiation therapy

      a. Primary or adjuvant treatment for early-stage seminomas

    3. Chemotherapy

      a. Primary chemotherapy regimens for germ cell tumors—includes etoposide and cisplatin (EP), etoposide, cisplatin, and bleomycin (BEP), and etoposide, mesna, ifosfamide, and cisplatin (VIP)

      b. Carboplatin AUC7 for one to two cycles recommended for patients with stage 1A or 1B pure seminoma

      c. Recurrent disease also responds to chemotherapy with active agents, including vinblastine, ifosfamide or mesna, paclitaxel, cisplatin, etoposide, and carboplatin; palliative chemotherapies, including doublets or triplets with gemcitabine, oxaliplatin, and paclitaxel; surgical resection of recurrent disease or isolated resistant metastasis may be done

VII.

  Nursing implications

A. Interventions related to prevention, early detection, and screening

  1. Assessment of pertinent personal and family history

    a. Age

      (1) Most commonly occurs in men ages 20 to 35 years

      (2) Decrease in incidence among men ages 40 to 60 years; increase seen after age 60 years

    b. Cryptorchidism (undescended testis)—increases risk 20-fold to 40-fold; protection lost if orchipexy is done after age 6 years

    c. Polythelia (multiple nipples) associated with increased risk

  2. Teaching adolescent males to perform monthly testicular self-examination (TSE)

B. Interventions to decrease severity of symptoms associated with disease and treatment

  1. Chemotherapy regimens are aggressive and require intensive nursing support and symptom management for fluid and electrolyte maintenance, monitoring renal function, antiemetic control, and prevention of constipation and neuropathies.

  2. Inguinal orchiectomy is performed as an outpatient procedure for both diagnostic and therapeutic purposes. Client education should be specific for pain management, activity, and incisional wound care.

  3. Other considerations include pulmonary, GI, quality of life, and fertility concerns (Viatori, 2012).

  4. Psychosexual issues require the following interventions:

    a. Discussion of sperm banking as an option before treatment begins

    b. Encouragement of open discussion about changes in body image between the client and his sexual partner; long-term sexual dysfunction reported in approximately 25% of testicular cancer survivors

C. Interventions to incorporate the client and family in care

  1. Identification of concerns the client and his sexual partner may have about resuming sexual functioning after treatment

Penile Cancer

I. Physiology and pathophysiology

  A. Anatomy of the penis

    1. Composed of the shaft and the glans

    2. Shaft—has three cylindric layers: bilateral corpus spongiosum, corpora cavernosa, and erectile tissues

  B. Primary functions of the penis—urination and copulation

  C. 50% to 80% of penile cancers associated with oncogenic HPV exposure; other risk factors include phimosis, poor penile hygiene, chronic inflammation, tobacco use, HIV, and lack of circumcision

II. Metastatic patterns

  A. Direct extension to adjacent tissues

  B. Metastasis to regional lymphatics—inguinal and iliac nodes

III. Screening and diagnostic procedures

  A. Diagnostic procedures—include incisional, punch, or excisional biopsy of the penile lesion

IV. Staging methods and procedures

  A. If appropriate, MRI or ultrasonography to evaluate depth of invasion

B. Nodal status most significant prognostic variable predicting survival
V. Trends in survival—accurate trends in survival not available because the disease is extremely rare in the U.S.
VI. Principles of medical management
  A. Treatment strategies
    1. Premalignant lesions—wide or limited local excision, imiquimod or 5-FU cream, or laser therapy
    2. Invasive cancer
      a. Surgery
        (1) Wide excision or partial penectomy
        (2) Glansectomy, partial or total penectomy
        (3) Total penectomy—requires creation of a perineal urostomy for urination
        (4) Inguinal lymph node dissection or sentinel node evaluation in high-risk or positive nodes
      b. Radiation therapy
        (1) Includes interstitial and external beam therapy
        (2) May also be used for palliative treatment
    C. Chemotherapy
      (1) Neoadjuvant therapy with cisplatin-based chemotherapy
      (2) Chemotherapy agents—paclitaxel, ifosfamide, and cisplatin; use of these agents followed by curative surgery improve progression-free survival and overall survival
      (3) Other agents with known activity in squamous cell cancers of the cervix and head and neck (cisplatin and 5-FU) may be useful
VII. Nursing implications
  A. Interventions related to prevention, early detection, and screening
    1. Assessment of pertinent personal and family history
      a. Age—60 years or older
      b. Penile hygiene practices—increased risk with poor hygiene
      c. Circumcision status—increased risk with no circumcision
  B. Interventions to maximize safety for the client
    1. Discussion of the option of circumcision before puberty for protective effect
    2. Instructing high-risk clients in penile self-examination
    3. Teaching penile hygiene practices
      a. Retraction of foreskin for cleansing
      b. Washing penis with mild soap and water

C. Interventions to enhance adaptation and rehabilitation
  1. Encouragement of open discussion of sexual concerns
    a. Reinforcement of information that clients with partial penectomy maintain sexual desire and the ability to penetrate, reach orgasm, and ejaculate
    b. Discussion of prosthetic options with clients who have had a total penectomy
  2. Discussion with the client and his sexual partner about alternative forms of sexual expression

List of Resources

Examples of Helpful Resources	Website/Title
National Comprehensive Care Network (NCCN) Guidelines (disease state, supportive care and screening guidelines for professionals)	http://www.nccn.org/professionals/default.aspx
Some patient information	http://www.nccn.org/patients/resources/default.aspx
National Cancer Institute (professional and patient versions)	www.cancer.gov/cancertopics/types/alphalist
Centers for Disease Control (information for professionals and patients)	
• Cervical cancer	www.cdc.gov/cancer/cervical
American Cancer Society	www.cancer.org/cancer
Women's Cancer Network/Foundation for Women's Cancers (general information on the more uncommon women's malignancies)	http://www.foundationforwomenscancer.org/types-of-gynecologic-cancers/
FORCE: Facing Our Risk of Cancer Empowered (a resource for hereditary cancers)	http://www.facingourrisk.org/

Fertility resources   http://www.myoncofertility.org/
www.fertilehope.org
www.nccn.org/patients/resources/
life_with_cancer/fertility.aspx

Sexuality   www.cancer.gov/cancertopics/
pdq/supportivecare/sexuality/
• Male   patient
• Female   www.cancer.org/treatment/
treatmentsandsideffects/
physicalsideeffects
Katz, A. (2010). *Man cancer sex.*
Pittsburgh: Hygeia Media.
Katz, A. (2010). *Women cancer sex.*
Pittsburgh: Hygeia Media.

References

Abu-Rustum, N. R., & Sonoda, Y. (2010). Fertility-sparing surgery in early-stage cervical cancer: Indications and applications. *Journal of the National Comprehensive Cancer Network (JNCCN), 8*(12), 1435–1438. http://www.ncbi.nlm.nih.gov/pubmed/21147906.

ACOG. (2009a). ACOG Practice Bulletin no. 109: Cervical cytology screening. *Obstetrics and Gynecology, 114,* 1409–1420. http://www.ncbi.nlm.nih.gov/pubmed/20134296.

ACOG. (2009b). ACOG Practice Bulletin no. 103: Hereditary breast and ovarian cancer syndrome. *Obstetrics and Gynecology, 113,* 957–966. http://www.ncbi.nlm.nih.gov/pubmed/19305347.

Berkowitz, R. S., & Goldstein, D. P. (2013). Current advances in the management of gestational trophoblastic disease. *Gynecology Oncology, 128*(1), 3–5.

Buys, S., Partridge, E., Black, A., Johnson, C., Lamerato, L., Issacs, C., et al.; PLCO Project Team. (2011). Effect of screening on ovarian cancer mortality; the Prostate, Lung, Colorectal, and Ovarian Screening Randomized Controlled Trial. *Journal of the American Medical Association (JAMA), 305*(22), 2295–2303.

Carter, J. S., & Downs, L. S., Jr. (2012). Vulvar and vaginal cancer. *Obstetrics and Gynecology Clinics of North America, 39*(2), 213–231.

Clarke-Pearson, D. L. (2009). Clinical practice. Screening for ovarian cancer. *New England Journal of Medicine, 361*(2), 170–177. http://www.ncbi.nlm.nih.gov/pubmed/19587342.

Creasman, W. (2009). Revised FIGO staging for carcinoma of the endometrium. *International Journal of Gynaecology and Obstetrics, 105*(2), 109. http://www.ncbi.nlm.nci.gov/pubmed/19345353.

Dellinger, T. H., & Monk, B. J. (2009). Systemic therapy for recurrent endometrial cancer: A review of North American Trials. *Expert Review of Anticancer Therapy, 9*(7), 905–916. http://www.ncbi.nlm.nih.gov/pubmed/19589030.

Elattar, A., Bryant, A., Winter-Roach, B. A., Hatem, M., & Naik, R. (2011). Optimal primary surgical treatment for advanced epithelial ovarian cancer. *Cochrane Database of Systematic Reviews,* CD007565. http://www.ncbi.nlm.nih.gov/pubmed/21833960

FIGO (International Federation of Gynecology and Obstetrics) Committee on Gynecologic Oncology. (2009). Current FIGO staging for cancer of the vagina, fallopian tube, ovary, and gestational trophoblastic neoplasia. *International Journal of Gynaecology and Obstetrics, 105*(1), 3–4.

Fleming, G. F., Ronnett, B., & Seidman, J. (2009). Epithelial ovarian cancer. In R. Barakat, M. Markman, & M. Randall (Eds.), *Principles and practice of gynecologic oncology* (5th ed., pp. 763–836). Philadelphia: Lippincott Williams & Wilkins.

Frederick, P. J., & Straughn, J. M., Jr. (2009). The role of comprehensive surgical staging in patients with endometrial cancer. *Cancer Control, 16*(1), 23–29. http://www.ncbi.nlm.nih.gov/pubmed/1907892.

International Agency for Research on Cancer (IARC). (2013). *Latest world cancer statistics.* (Press release no. 223.)

Kitchener, H. C., & Trimble, E. L. (2009). Endometrial cancer: State of the science meeting. *International Journal of Gynecological Cancer, 19*(1), 134–140. http://www.ncbi.nlm.nih.gov/pubmed/19258955.

Massad, S., Einstein, M., Huh, W., Katki, H., Kinney, W., Schiffman, M., et al. (2013). 2012 updated consensus guidelines for the management of abnormal cervical cancer screening tests and cancer precursors. *Journal of Lower Genital Tract Disease, 17*(5), S1–S27.

May, K., Bryant, A., Dickinson, H. O., Kehoe, S., & Morrison, J. (2010). Lymphadenectomy for the management of endometrial cancer. *Cochrane Database of Systematic Reviews,* CD007585. http://www.ncbi.nlm.nci.gov/pubmed/20091639.

Monk, B. J., Tewari, K. S., & Koh, W. J. (2007). Multimodality therapy for locally advanced cervical carcinoma: State of the art and future directions. *Journal of Clinical Oncology, 25*(20), 2952–2965. http://www.ncbi.nlm.nih.gov/pubmed/17617527.

Moxley, K. M., & McMeekin, D. S. (2010). Endometrial carcinoma: A review of chemotherapy, drug resistance, and the search for new agents. *The Oncologist, 15*(10), 1026–1033. http://www.ncbi.nlm.nih.gov/pubmed/20930101.

Moyer, V. A. (2012). Screening for cervical cancer: U.S. Preventive Services Task Force recommendation statement. *Annals of Internal Medicine, 156*(12), 880–891. http://www.ncbi.nlm.nih.gov/pubmed/22422943.

Nallu, A., Mannuel, A. D., & Hussain, A. (2013). Testicular germ cell tumors: Biology and clinical update. *Current Opinion in Oncology, 25*(3), 266–272.

National Comprehensive Cancer Network (NCCN). (2014a). *Clinical practice guidelines in oncology-cervical cancer. v.1.2014.* http//www.nccn.org/professionals/physician_gls/pDF/cervical.pdf.

National Comprehensive Cancer Network (NCCN). (2014b). *Clinical practice guidelines in oncology-ovarian cancer. v.1.2014.* http//www.nccn.org/professionals/physician_gls/pDF/ovarian.pdf.

National Comprehensive Cancer Network (NCCN). (2014c). *Clinical practice guidelines in oncology-uterine neoplasms. v.1.2014.* http//www.nccn.org/professionals/physician_gls/pDF/uterine.pdf.

Pecorelli, S. (2009). Revised FIGO staging for carcinoma of the vulva, cervix, and endometrium. *International Journal of*

Gynaecology and Obstetrics, 105(2), 103–104. http://www.ncbi.nlm.nih.gov/pubmed/19367689.

Ray, M., & Fleming, G. (2009). Management of advanced-stage and recurrent endometrial cancer. *Seminars in Oncology, 36*(2), 15–154. http://www.ncbi.nlm.nih.gov/pubmed/19332249.

Resnick, K. E., Hampel, H., Fishel, R., & Cohen, D. E. (2009). Current and emerging trends in Lynch syndrome identification in women with endometrial cancer. *Gynecologic Oncology, 114*(1), 128–134. http://www.ncbi.nlm.nih.gov/pubmed/19375789.

Rydzewska, L., Tierney, J., Vale, C. L., & Symonds, P. R. (2010). Neoadjuvant chemotherapy plus surgery versus surgery for cervical cancer. *Cochrane Database of Systematic Reviews,* CD007406. http://www.ncbi.nlm.nih.gov/pubmed/20091632.

Saslow, D., Solomon, D., Lawson, H. W., Killackey, M., Kulasingam, S. L., Cain, J., et al. (2012). American Cancer Society (ACS), American Society for Colposcopy and Cervical Pathology (ASCCP), and American Society for Clinical Pathology (ASCP) screening guidelines for the prevention and early detection of cervical cancer. *American Journal of Clinical Pathology, 137*(4), 516–542. http://www.ncbi.nlm.nih.gov/pubmed/20841605.

Schiffman, M., & Wentzensen, N. (2013). Human papillomavirus infection and the multistage carcinogenesis of cervical cancer. *Cancer Epidemiology, Biomarkers & Prevention, 22*(4), 553–560. http://www.ncbi.nlm.nih.gov/pubmed/23549399.

Schiffman, M., Wentzensen, N., Wacholder, S., Kinney, W., Gage, J. C., & Castle, P. E. (2011). Human papillomavirus testing in the prevention of cervical cancer. *Journal of the National Cancer Institute, 103*(5), 368–383. http://www.ncbi.nlm.nih.gov/pubmed/21282563.

Shulman, L. P. (2010). Hereditary breast and ovarian cancer (HBOC): Clinical features and counseling for BRCA1 and BRCA2, Lynch syndrome, Cowden syndrome, and Li-Fraumeni syndrome. *Obstetrics and Gynecology Clinics of North America, 37*(1), 109–133. http://www.ncbi.nlm.nih.gov/pubmed/20494261.

Siegel, R., Ma, J., Zou, Z., & Jemal, A. (2014). Cancer statistics, 2014. *CA: A Cancer Journal for Clinicians, 64*(1), 9–29.

Smith, R., Manassaram-Baptiste, D., Brooks, D., Cokkinides, V., Doroshenk, M., Saslow, D., et al. (2014). Cancer screening in the United States, 2014: A review of current American Cancer Society guidelines and current issues in cancer screening. *CA: A Cancer Journal for Clinicians, 64,* 30–51.

Tewari, K. S., & Monk, B. J. (2009). Recent achievements and future developments in advanced and recurrent cervical cancer: Trials of the Gynecologic Oncology Group. *Seminars in Oncology, 36*(2), 170–180. http://www.ncbi.nlm.nih.gov/pubmed/19332251.

Viatori, M. (2012). Testicular cancer. *Seminars in Oncology Nursing, 28*(3), 180–189.

CHAPTER 11

Cancers of the Urinary System

Sally L. Maliski[*]

Kidney Cancer

I. Physiology and pathophysiology
  A. Primary function
    1. Kidneys are a pair of organs, each measuring approximately 10 cm in length by 5.5 cm in width, positioned behind the peritoneum in a mass of fatty tissue.
    2. Urine production occurs in the renal lobes. Ducts within papillae drain urine into renal calyces, into the renal pelvis, and ultimately to the renal sinus, which is connected to the ureter. Urine drains from the ureter into the bladder.
    3. The nephron is the basic structural and functional unit of the kidney (Lote, 2012).
  B. Changes associated with cancer—excessive cell production results in growth into adjacent organs and gradual loss of function in the affected kidney.
  C. Major classifications of kidney cancer (Prino & Jonasch, 2012)
    1. Clear cell carcinoma, also known as conventional or nonpapillary
      a. Comprises 70% to 80% of cases
      b. Thought to arise from proximal renal tubule
      c. Hereditary and sporadic forms
    2. Papillary renal cell carcinoma (RCC)
      a. Comprises 10% of cases
      b. Thought to arise from proximal renal tubular epithelium
      c. Hereditary and sporadic forms
    3. Chromophobe renal cell carcinoma
      a. Comprises 5% of cases
      b. Arises from renal tubular epithelium; proposed to originate in collecting ducts
      c. Excellent prognosis—better than papillary or clear cell carcinoma
    4. Collecting duct carcinoma, or Bellini duct carcinoma of the kidney
      a. Comprises fewer than 1% of all cases
      b. Arises in medullary collecting ducts
      c. Aggressive with rapid metastasis
      d. Subtype of collecting duct carcinoma
        (1) Renal medullary carcinoma (RMC)
          (a) Occurs almost exclusively in African American men with sickle cell disease (Prino & Jonasch, 2012; Rini, Heng, Zhou, Novick, & Raghavan, 2010)
    5. Unclassified renal cell carcinoma
      a. Remains as diagnostic category for tumors that do not fit into other categories
      b. Sarcomatoid is no longer considered a distinct category but is viewed as a manifestation of high-grade carcinoma.
    6. Tumors of the renal pelvis (American Cancer Society [ACS], 2013)
      a. Very rare, 5% or less of all cases
      b. Urothelial or transitional cell carcinomas
      c. May occur at any site within the upper urinary collecting system
      d. Generally multifocal
      e. Decreased incidence over past decades (Howlader et al., 2013)
    7. Renal cell cancers—tend to grow toward the medullary portion of the kidney and spread via direct extrusion to the renal vein or the vena cava
    8. Metastasis at diagnosis in 30% of clients; recurrence in 40%, even among those with early-stage disease (Prino & Jonasch, 2012)
  D. Trends in epidemiology
    1. Kidney cancer relatively rare in the United States (U.S.), accounting for only 3% of all cancers (Siegel, Naishadham, & Jemal, 2013)
      a. Both incidence and death rates have been rising since 1998 (Howlader et al., 2013).
      b. Rising incidence may be related to common use of high-resolution imaging and incidental finding of tumors among asymptomatic persons (Sun et al., 2011).

---

[*]The author acknowledges prior authors of this chapter for their contributions, most recently Maureen O'Rourke, RN, PhD.

   c. Two thirds of renal carcinomas are now discovered incidentally during pelvic and abdominal scanning (Prino & Jonasch, 2012).

  2. Male predominance, 1.5:1 (Prino & Jonasch, 2012)

  3. Risk factors (Chow, Dong, & Devesa, 2010; Rini et al., 2010):

    a. Tobacco use, obesity, hypertension, unopposed estrogen use, diuretic treatment, prior radiation therapy (RT), occupational exposure to petroleum products or heavy metals, asbestos exposure, and dialysis-acquired cystic kidney disease

    b. Dietary factors also implicated: high-fat diets, high-protein diets, diets low in antioxidants

    c. Genetic predisposition, von Hippel-Lindau (VHL) disease, non-Hodgkin lymphoma, and sickle cell disease also linked to an increased risk of kidney cancer.

  4. Clear cell carcinomas strongly associated with loss or inactivation of the short arm of chromosome 3p

    a. Alterations found in 80% of clients (Morrissey et al., 2001)

    b. Association also found with von Hippel-Lindau disease

  5. Papillary renal cell carcinoma

    a. Normal 3p but often trisomies 3q, 8, 12, 17, and 20 noted

    b. Trisomies 7 and 17 and the loss of the Y chromosome also reported (Figlin, 2003; Hagenkord, Gatalica, Jonasch, & Monzon, 2011).

  6. Chromophobe renal cell carcinoma associated with loss of chromosomes 1, 2, 6, 10, 13, and 21 and alterations of chromosome 17 (Vera-Badillo, Conde, & Duran, 2012; Hagenkord et al., 2011)

 E. Common metastatic sites: lungs, abdominal and mediastinal lymph nodes, liver, and bone (Figures 11-1 and 11-2) (Rini et al., 2010)

II. Screening and diagnostic measures

 A. Screening—no screening tests available for kidney cancer

  1. Screening with ultrasonography would not be cost-effective because of the low prevalence of the disease.

  2. Patients with multiple affected relatives should be referred for genetic counseling and possible surveillance.

 B. Diagnostic measures (Table 11-1)

  1. Kidney, ureter, and bladder (KUB) radiography

  2. Intravenous pyelography (IVP; also referred to as *excretory urography*): commonly used to evaluate patients presenting with hematuria

  3. Renal ultrasonography

  4. Pelvic or abdominal computed tomography (CT)—diagnostic test of choice

  5. Renal angiography—less commonly performed; may be necessary because of large vascular mass if renal artery embolization is planned

  6. Magnetic resonance imaging (MRI)—especially important if vena cava involvement

  7. Retrograde urography

III. Grading and staging

 A. Grading

  1. Based on Fuhrman grading system on a scale of 1 (least aggressive) to 4 (most aggressive)

  2. Higher nuclear grade associated with a worse 5-year overall survival (Rini et al., 2010)

 B. Staging

  1. No known tumor or molecular marker to confirm diagnosis, remission, progression, or relapse (Prino & Jonasch, 2012; Figlin, 2003)

  2. Staging—based on tumor size, lymph node involvement, and distant metastasis

  3. American Joint Committee on Cancer (AJCC) staging system used for grading (Table 11-2) (Edge, Byrd, Compton, Fritz, & Greene, 2010)

IV. Prognosis

 A. Prognostic factors include patient age, histologic grade and type, disease stage, performance status, low hemoglobin level, elevated serum calcium and lactate dehydrogenase (LDH) levels, number and location of metastatic sites, time to appearance of metastasis, and prior nephrectomy (Prino & Jonasch, 2012; Rini et al., 2010).

 B. The production of antithyroid antibodies stimulated by interleukin-2 (IL-2) immunotherapy may be associated with improved survival (Prino & Jonasch, 2012; Figlin, 2003).

 C. The 5-year survival rate is determined by the stage of kidney cancer: stage I (81%), stage II (74%), stage III (53%), and stage IV (8%) (ACS, 2013).

V. Principles of medical management

 A. Surgery

  1. Radical nephrectomy—has been the primary treatment since 1960 (Prino & Jonasch, 2012)

  2. Partial nephrectomy—preferred whenever feasible, especially in a patient with limited renal function, bilateral tumors and in a patient with a solitary kidney (Rini et al., 2010)

  3. Open, laparoscopic, or robotic surgical techniques used to perform radical and partial nephrectomies

  4. Cryosurgery and radiofrequency ablation (RFA)

    a. Option for patients with clinical stage T1 lesions who are not surgical candidates (National Comprehensive Cancer Network [NCCN], 2013a)

  5. Active surveillance (stage 1A RCC)

    a. Option in selected patients and should be considered for patients with decreased life expectancy or extensive comorbidities that

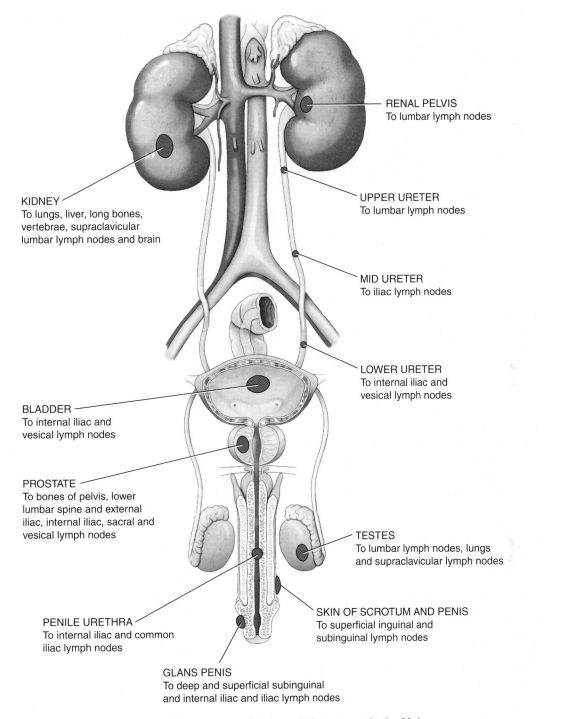

KIDNEY
To lungs, liver, long bones, vertebrae, supraclavicular lumbar lymph nodes and brain

RENAL PELVIS
To lumbar lymph nodes

UPPER URETER
To lumbar lymph nodes

MID URETER
To iliac lymph nodes

LOWER URETER
To internal iliac and vesical lymph nodes

BLADDER
To internal iliac and vesical lymph nodes

PROSTATE
To bones of pelvis, lower lumbar spine and external iliac, internal iliac, sacral and vesical lymph nodes

TESTES
To lumbar lymph nodes, lungs and supraclavicular lymph nodes

PENILE URETHRA
To internal iliac and common iliac lymph nodes

SKIN OF SCROTUM AND PENIS
To superficial inguinal and subinguinal lymph nodes

GLANS PENIS
To deep and superficial subinguinal and internal iliac and iliac lymph nodes

Figure 11-1 Sites of Tumor Origin and Metastases in the Male.

would place them at risk for more invasive treatment (NCCN, 2013a)

6. For patients with resectable solitary metastatic site, nephrectomy with surgical metastasectomy

7. Cytoreductive nephrectomy prior to systemic therapy an option for select patients with surgically resectable primary with multiple metastatic sites (NCCN, 2013a)

a. Patients most likely to benefit are those with lung-only metastases, good prognostic features, and good performance status.

B. Radiation therapy
  1. Renal cell cancers unresponsive to radiotherapy
  2. May be used for palliation (e.g., skeletal metastasis, brain metastasis)

C. Chemotherapy—has not been shown to improve survival

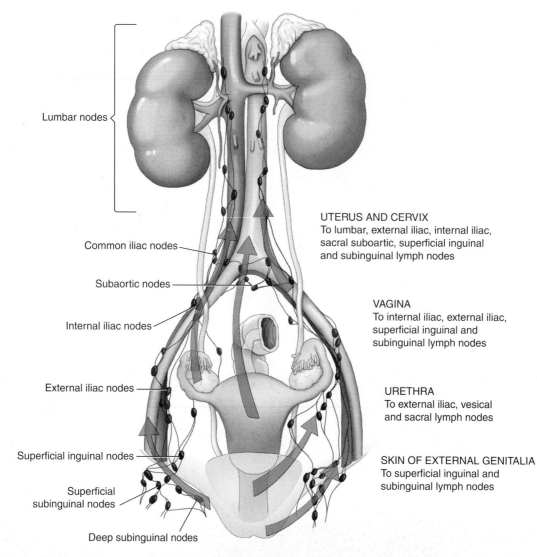

Lumbar nodes

Common iliac nodes

Subaortic nodes

Internal iliac nodes

External iliac nodes

Superficial inguinal nodes

Superficial subinguinal nodes

Deep subinguinal nodes

UTERUS AND CERVIX
To lumbar, external iliac, internal iliac, sacral suboartic, superficial inguinal and subinguinal lymph nodes

VAGINA
To internal iliac, external iliac, superficial inguinal and subinguinal lymph nodes

URETHRA
To external iliac, vesical and sacral lymph nodes

SKIN OF EXTERNAL GENITALIA
To superficial inguinal and subinguinal lymph nodes

Figure 11-2 Anatomic Relationships and Sites of Lymph Nodes for Urinary Tumors in Females.

D. Immunotherapy
  1. Interleukin-2 (IL-2)
    a. Overall response rate of 14%, with 5% complete responses
      (1) Majority of those who had complete response had durable complete remissions (Rini et al., 2010; Prino & Jonasch, 2012).
      (2) Patients receiving high-dose IL-2 should have good performance status and normal organ function.
  2. Interferon-alpha (IFN-α)
    a. Produced response rates of 10% to 15% given as single agent
    b. Can be given in combination with IL-2 or bevacizumab (Avastin) (Escudier et al., 2008)

E. Targeted therapies
  1. Agents approved by the U.S. Food and Drug administration (FDA)—everolimus (RAD001), axitinib (Inlyta), sorafenib (Nexavar), sunitinib (Sutent), temsirolimus (Torisel), bevacizumab (Avastin), pazopanib (Votrient) (National Cancer Comprehensive Network [NCCN], 2013a)
  2. Common side effects—fatigue, skin rash, diarrhea, hand-foot syndrome, increased glucose and cholesterol levels, and delayed wound healing

VI. Nursing implications
  A. Interventions to maximize safety postoperatively
    1. Pulmonary toiletry—teaching patients to perform cough and deep breathing exercises; use of incentive spirometry

Table 11-1

Urologic Diagnostic Tests and Nursing Interventions

Test	Preparation	Nursing Interventions
Radiographic examination of kidneys, ureter, bladder (KUB)	None—plain film of abdomen	Explain to the client the need to lie flat on examination table. Do not schedule after barium studies (will obscure kidneys).
Excretory urography	Dye excreted unchanged by kidneys, so hydration is important; should be followed by nothing by mouth for 6-8 hr before test. Dye injected intravenously; anaphylactic or allergic reaction to dye may occur; may need to premedicate with antihistamines	Assess history of allergy to iodine dyes or contrast media before test; pretesting may be indicated. Use of iodine dyes may be contraindicated in clients with severe renal or hepatic disease or clinical hypersensitivity (severe allergies, asthma). Have emergency equipment and personnel available before injection (anaphylaxis and cardiovascular reactions may occur) and 30-60 min after test (delayed reactions). Observe for adverse reactions to dye—angina, chest pain, arrhythmias, hypotension, dizziness, blurred vision, headache, fever, convulsions, dyspnea, rhinitis, laryngitis, and nausea.
Retrograde urography	General anesthesia or narcotic analgesia may be used; cystoscope is inserted; iodinated dye is injected via the urethral catheter. Laxatives at bedtime before test may be used to cleanse bowel.	Observe for reaction to anesthetic or analgesic. Monitor for bleeding, symptoms of urinary tract infections, dysuria, or difficulty voiding after test.

Table 11-2

AJCC (2010) Staging of Renal Cell Carcinoma

Primary Tumor (T)

TX	Primary tumor cannot be assessed
T0	No evidence of primary tumor
T1	Tumor $\leq$ 7 cm in greatest dimension, limited to kidney
T1a	Tumor $\leq$ 4 cm in greatest dimension, limited to kidney
T1b	Tumor > 4 cm but not > 7 cm in greatest dimension, limited to kidney
T2	Tumor > 7 cm in greatest dimension, limited to kidney
T2a	Tumor > 7 cm but $\leq$10 cm in greatest dimension, limited to kidney
T2b	Tumor > 10 cm, limited to kidney
T3	Tumor extends into major veins or perinephric tissues but not into the ipsilateral adrenal gland and beyond Gerota fascia
T3a	Tumor grossly extends into the renal vein or its segmental (muscle containing) branches, or tumor invades perirenal and/or renal sinus fat but not beyond Gerota fascia
T3b	Tumor grossly extends into the vena cava below the diaphragm
T3c	Tumor grossly extends into the vena cava above diaphragm or invades the wall of vena cava
T4	Tumor invades beyond Gerota fascia (including contiguous extension into the ipsilateral adrenal gland)

Regional Lymph Nodes (N)*

NX	Regional lymph nodes cannot be assessed
N0	No regional lymph node metastases
N1	Metastases in regional lymph node(s)

Distant Metastasis (M)

M0	No distant metastasis
M1	Distant metastasis

Stage Grouping

Stage I	T1	N0	M0
Stage II	T2	N0	M0
Stage III	T1	N1	M0
	T2	N1	M0
	T3	N0	M0
	T3	N1	M0
Stage IV	T4	Any N	M0
	Any T	Any N	M1

*Laterality does not affect the N classification.

Used with permission of the American Joint Committee on Cancer (AJCC), Chicago, Illinois. The original source for this material is the AJCC Cancer Staging Manual, Seventh Edition (2010) published by Springer Science and Business Media LLC, www.springer.com.

2. Observing for signs of hemorrhage
3. Monitoring vital signs, hemoglobin, hematocrit, kidney function tests, and urine output
4. Providing pharmacologic and nonpharmacologic pain relief measures
   B. Interventions related to the management of targeted therapies and biotherapies (see Chapter 23)
   C. Interventions related to educating the patient regarding follow-up care and surveillance
      1. Teaching patient to identify and manage symptoms (including potential late effects), and to report symptoms to health care providers
      2. Referral to mental health specialist, community resources (ACS), and support groups, as needed
      3. Providing education and cancer survivorship care plan, which includes treatment summary and follow-up plan

Bladder Cancer

I. Physiology and pathophysiology
   A. Primary function
      1. The bladder is a hollow muscular organ that serves as temporary reservoir for urine, which is then discharged through the urethra.
      2. In men, critical adjacent structures include the prostate, seminal vesicles, urethra, nerves at the base of the penis, and local lymph nodes (Figure 11-1).
      3. In women, critical adjacent structures include the uterus, ovaries, fallopian tubes, urethra, and local lymph nodes (Figure 11-2).
   B. Changes associated with cancer
      1. Proliferation of abnormal tissue in one or more places within the bladder
      2. Clinical manifestations—hematuria (especially if the tumor involves the bladder wall), dysuria, burning, frequency, and pelvic pain (Raghavan, Stein, Cote, & Jones, 2010)
   C. Major classifications of bladder cancer
      1. Urothelial carcinoma (formerly known as *transitional cell carcinoma*)
         a. Arises from the epithelial layer of the bladder, which rests on the basement membrane
         b. Comprises about 95% of bladder tumors (ACS, 2013)
         c. Can be further subdivided—carcinoma in situ (CIS), noninvasive papillary carcinoma, invasive papillary carcinoma, and solid tumors
            (1) 70% to 80% considered "superficial" disease (Lerner, Schoenberg, Coran, & Shernberg, 2006), although the World Health Organization (WHO) has

recommended that this term be abandoned; also referred to as non-muscle invasive bladder cancer (NMIBC)
            (2) Papillary tumors confined to the first two layers of the bladder but project toward the lumen (Lerner et al., 2006)
               (a) These tumors demonstrate changes to chromosome 9 and an overexpression of vascular endothelial growth factor, leading to angiogenesis (Lerner et al., 2006).
      2. Squamous cell carcinomas—make up approximately 1% to 2% of bladder cancer cases
      3. Adenocarcinomas—make up approximately 1% of bladder cancer cases
      4. Small cell tumors—make up approximately less than 1% of bladder cancer cases (ACS, 2013)
   D. Trends in epidemiology
      1. Incidence rates high in the United States and Africa, especially Egypt, where schistosomiasis is endemic (Raghavan et al., 2010)
      2. Estimated new cases in the U.S. in 2013—72,570 (ACS, 2013)
      3. Estimated deaths in the U.S. in 2013—15,210 (ACS, 2013); male-to-female ratio nearly 4:1
      4. Median age at diagnosis 65 years; rarely diagnosed before age 40 years (ACS, 2013)
      5. African Americans continuing to lag behind whites in 5-year survival rates for all stages of urinary bladder cancer (ACS, 2013)
      6. Risk factors
         a. Tobacco use
            (1) Most significant risk factor, accounting for 50% to 66% of all bladder tumors in men, 25% in women (ACS, 2013; Lerner et al., 2006)
         b. Diets high in consumption of fried meats and fats associated with increased risk (Lerner et al., 2006)
         c. Other important risk factors—work-related contact with cyclic chemicals, especially benzenes and arylamines, and heavy exposure to chemicals used in dyes, rubbers, textiles, paints, and leathers (Lerner et al., 2006)
         d. Diets high in consumption of vitamins A, E, and zinc suggested to be highly protective (Lerner et al., 2006; ACS, 2013)
   E. Common metastatic sites—lymph nodes, bones, lung, liver, and peritoneum (Shinagare et al., 2011)
II. Screening and diagnostic measures
   A. Screening—not currently recommended by any major preventive group in the U.S.
      1. No serologic tumor markers specific to bladder cancer (Raghavan et al., 2010)
      2. Urinary assays for bladder cancer

a. FDA-approved nuclear matrix protein 22 (NMP-22) assay—a noninvasive test used for the surveillance and monitoring of patients with bladder cancer (Lerner et al., 2006)

b. Other FDA-approved urinary assays for bladder cancer detection and monitoring—bladder tumor–associated antigen (BTA) assays, ImmunoCyt test, and UroVysion FISH assay (Goodison, Rosser, & Urquidi, 2013)

B. Diagnostic measures (Lerner et al., 2006)

1. Intravenous pyelography (IVP), also referred to as *excretory urography*—allows visualization of upper tracts to determine whether the source is intravesicular, within the bladder, or located elsewhere (see Table 11-1)

2. Cystoscopy with bladder washings and biopsies

3. Urinary cytology—for best results, specimens obtained from late-morning or early-afternoon urine

4. CT—aids in defining the extent of local tumor and in identifying pelvic lymph node metastasis

5. MRI—distinguishes the tumor from the normal bladder wall and identifies the presence of pelvic lymph node involvement

III. Grading and staging

A. Grading

1. Tumor grade (grades X, 1, 2, 3, 4)—refers to the degree of tumor cell differentiation and aggressive nature of the tumor cells

a. This grading system has changed to a low- and high-grade designation to match current WHO/International Society of Urologic Pathology (WHO/ISUP)–recommended grading system (Edge et al., 2010).

b. High-grade tumors tend to grow more quickly and are more likely to metastasize.

B. Staging

1. AJCC staging system is detailed in Table 11-3 (Edge et al., 2010).

IV. Prognosis

A. Prognostic indicators—tumor grade, size, location, biomarkers such as the p21 gene and ki67 antigen, cellular adhesion models, and response to therapy (Lerner et al., 2006)

B. 5-year survival rate by stage of bladder cancer— stage 0 (98%), stage I (88%), stage II (63%), stage III (46%), and stage IV (15%) (ACS, 2013)

V. Principles of medical management

A. NMIBC

1. Goal—to prevent disease progression and invasion, avoid loss of bladder, and increase survival (Lerner et al., 2006)

a. Primary mode of treatment—cystoscopy to confirm tumor presence, followed by transurethral resection of the bladder tumor

Table 11-3

AJCC (2010) Staging of Bladder Cancer

Primary Tumor (T)

TX	Primary tumor cannot be assessed
T0	No evidence of primary tumor
Ta	Noninvasive papillary tumor
Tis	Carcinoma in situ: "flat tumors"
T1	Tumor invades subepithelial connective tissue
T2	Tumor invades muscle
T2a	Tumor invades superficial muscularis propria (inner half)
T2B	Tumor invades deep muscularis propria (outer half)
T3	Tumor invades perivesicular tissue
T3a	Tumor invades perivesicular tissue microscopically
T3b	Tumor invades perivesicular tissue macroscopically (extravesicular mass)
T4	Tumor invades any of the following: prostate, uterus, vagina, pelvic wall, abdominal wall
T4a	Tumor invades prostate, uterus, vagina
T4b	Tumor invades pelvic wall, abdominal wall

Regional Nodes (N)*

NX	Regional lymph nodes cannot be assessed
N0	No regional lymph node metastasis
N1	Single regional lymph node metastasis in the true pelvis (hypogastric, obturator, external iliac, or presacral lymph node)
N2	Multiple regional lymph node metastases in the true pelvis (hypogastric, obturator, external iliac, or presacral lymph node)
N3	Lymph node metastasis to the common iliac lymph nodes

Distant Metastasis (M)

MX	Distant metastasis cannot be assessed
M0	No distant metastasis
M1	Distant metastasis

Stage Grouping

Stage	T	N	M
Stage 0a	Ta	N0	M0
Stage 0is	Tis	N0	M0
Stage I	T1	N0	M0
Stage II	T2a	N0	M0
	T2b	N0	M0
Stage III	T3a	N0	M0
	T3b	N0	M0
	T4a	N0	M0
Stage IV	T4b	N0	M0
	Any T	N1-N3	M0
	Any T	Any N	M1

*Regional nodes are those within the true pelvis; all other nodes are distant lymph nodes.

Used with permission of the American Joint Committee on Cancer (AJCC), Chicago, Illinois. The original source for this material is the AJCC Cancer Staging Manual, Seventh Edition (2010) published by Springer Science and Business Media LLC, www.springer.com.

Part 2

(TURBT); tumor removal achieved by fulguration (burning with electrical current) or laser therapy (Lerner et al., 2006)

(1) Most common side effects—bleeding and infection

(2) Perforation of surrounding tissues also risk of treatment

2. Intravesical therapy—includes both intravesical chemotherapy and intravesical immunotherapy

a. Indications for intravesical therapy are based on probability of recurrence and progression to muscle-invasive disease such as size, number, and grade (NCCN, 2013c).

b. Intravesicular chemotherapy has been found to be more effective than TUR alone in preventing tumor recurrence (Shen, Shen, Wientjes, O'Donnell, & Au, 2008).

c. Most common agents are mitomycin C (MMC), Bacillus Calmette-Guerin (BCG) (TheraCys, TICE BCG), thiotepa (Thioplex), valrubicin, and doxorubicin (Adriamycin).

(1) Combination of above drugs has also been used.

(2) Thiotepa is infrequently used in clinical practice due to higher systemic side effects, such as myelosuppression (Johnson, Pruthi, & Woods, 2013).

B. Treatment of muscle invasive disease

1. Radical cystectomy with urinary diversion

a. Removal of the bladder and prostate in men

b. Hysterectomy in women

c. Bilateral pelvic lymphadenectomy, including at a minimum common, internal iliac, external iliac, and obturator nodes in both men and women

d. Potential complications—infection, bleeding, and sexual dysfunction

e. Presurgical chemotherapy using MVAC (methotrexate [Mexate], vinblastine [Velban], doxorubicin [Adriamycin], cisplatin [Platinol]) demonstrated to double survival rates in clients with advanced bladder cancer compared with surgery alone (Grossman et al., 2003)

f. Cisplatin-based combination chemotherapy strongly recommended by NCCN guidelines (NCCN, 2013c)

g. Types of urinary diversions (see Chapter 29)

(1) Ileal conduit (Figure 11-3)—well-known urinary diversion performed with cystectomy

(a) A portion of the terminal end of the ileum is isolated, the proximal end is closed, and the distal end is brought out through an opening in the

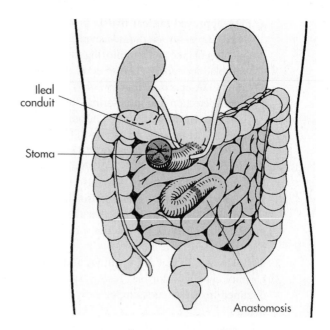

Figure 11-3 Urinary Diversion Using a Segment of Ileum. As short a segment as possible is used and positioned in the right lower quadrant of the abdomen in an isoperistaltic direction. *From Christensen, B. L., & Kockrow, E. O. (2010). Adult health nursing care (6th ed.). St. Louis: Mosby.*

abdominal wall and sutured to the skin, creating a stoma.

(b) Ureters are implanted into the ileal segment, urine flows into the conduit, and peristalsis propels urine out through the stoma.

(2) Continent ileal reservoir (Figure 11-4)—technique that provides an intra-abdominal pouch for storage of urine

(a) Typically, the stoma has a nipple valve to prevent ureteral reflux. The stoma is generally placed below the undergarment line.

(b) No external collecting device is needed; urine remains in the reservoir until client self-catheterizes through stoma, approximately every 6 hours (Hautman et al., 2007).

(3) Orthotopic neobladder—a technique that provides a creation of a new bladder that is made from the intestine

(a) A health-related, quality-of-life–based comparison between ileal conduit and neobladder following a cystectomy revealed better quality of life and a more active lifestyle with orthotopic substitution versus ileal conduit diversion (Philip, Manikandan, Venugopal, Desouza, & Javle, 2009).

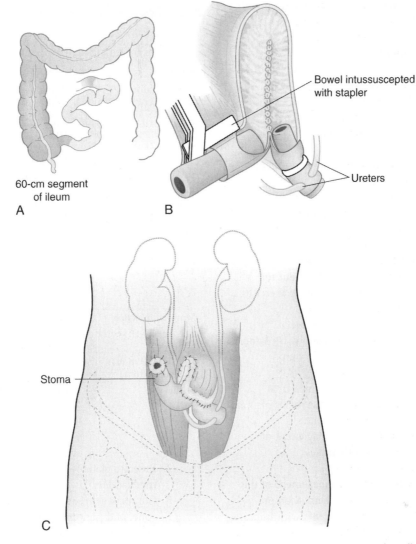

60-cm segment
of ileum

A

Bowel intussuscepted
with stapler

Ureters

B

Stoma

C

Figure 11-4 Kock Pouch Urinary Reservoir. A, Shaded area indicates section of small intestine selected for reservoir construction. **B,** Afferent (nonrefluxing) limb for ureteral implantation and efferent limb (with nippled valve) for stoma are created by using stapling devices. **C,** Completed reservoir with the efferent limb drawn through the abdominal wall and stoma created. In *Tanagho, E.A., & McAninch, J.W. (Eds.) (1992). Smith's general urology (13th ed.). San Mateo, CA: Appleton & Lange.*

2. Bladder preservation therapy
   a. Although radical cystectomy is the current primary treatment modality, some clients cannot tolerate cystectomy or are unwilling to undergo the procedure
   b. Bladder preservation strategies include the following:
      (1) External beam radiation therapy (XRT)
      (2) Trimodality therapy—transurethral resection (TUR), radiation therapy, and systemic chemotherapy (Lerner et al., 2006)
3. Chemotherapy
   a. Advanced bladder cancer is often treated with single-agent or combination systemic chemotherapy.

   (1) On the basis of NCCN guidelines (2013c), first-line combination chemotherapy for metastatic disease include the following:
      (a) Dose-dense MVAC (methotrexate, vinblastine, doxorubicin [Adriamycin], cisplatin) with growth factor support
      (b) Gemcitabine and cisplatin
   (2) For second-line therapy, depending on first-line treatment received, single-agent taxane or gemcitabine is preferred.
   (3) For concurrent treatment with radiation therapy, radiosensitizing chemotherapy regimens include the following:
      (a) Cisplatin alone or in combination with 5-fluorouracil (5-FU)

(b) Mitomycin C in combination with 5-FU

(c) Clinical trial

4. Radiation therapy

a. Useful in the management of invasive disease

b. Linear accelerator with multiple fields, daily or twice daily

c. An empty bladder required for both simulation and treatment

d. Radiation usually preceded by TUR

e. Often used as combined modality therapy with chemotherapy

f. Dose range to whole bladder—40 to 55 gray (Gy), with an additional boost of 9 to 11 Gy, for a total of 49 to 66 Gy (NCCN, 2013c).

VI. Nursing implications

A. Interventions to maximize safety postoperatively

1. Pulmonary toiletry—teaching patient to perform cough and deep breathing exercises; use of incentive spirometry

2. Observing for signs of hemorrhage

3. Monitoring vital signs, hemoglobin, hematocrit, kidney function tests, and urine output

4. Providing pharmacologic and nonpharmacologic pain relief measures

B. Interventions related to the management of radiation therapy (see Chapter 21)

C. Interventions related to the management of targeted therapies and biotherapies (see Chapter 23)

D. Interventions related to the management of the patient receiving intravesical chemotherapy

1. BCG—contraindicated in clients with immune system compromise because of human immunodeficiency virus (HIV) or steroid use, urinary tract infection, or past reactions to tuberculosis strains; systemic tuberculosis may develop.

2. Thiotepa—low molecular weight leads to high rates of systemic absorption, leading to severe myelosuppression.

3. Mitomycin C—may cause dysuria, frequency, and, less commonly, allergic reactions and myelosuppression (Lerner et al., 2006; Shen et al., 2008)

E. Interventions related to the management of common ileal conduit problems (see Table 11-4).

Prostate Cancer

I. Physiology and pathophysiology

A. Primary function

1. Located posterior to the symphysis pubis, inferior to the bladder, and in front of the rectum (see Figure 11-1)

Table 11-4

Management of Common Ileal Conduit Problems

Problem	Interventions
Urinary odor	Avoid use of rubber pouch. Soak appliance in vinegar and water, 1:4
Rash around stoma or under pouch	Dry and powder skin except under adhesive. Use a skin barrier (e.g., Stomahesive).
Macerated skin around stoma	Dry skin, and apply a hydroponic skin barrier. Decrease size of pouch opening.
Crystals on or around stoma	Apply vinegar compresses on stoma and inside pouch.
Ulcerated stoma	Enlarge pouch opening. Consult enterostomal therapist if not partially healed in 1 week.
Monilial infection following antibiotic therapy	Dry skin, and apply nystatin (Mycostatin) powder. Encourage oral fluids.
Hyperplasia of skin around stoma	Decrease pouch-opening size.
Fistula	Revise stoma at new site.

2. Prostate gland—encircles the urethra as it leaves the bladder

3. Comprises three zones—transitional zone, central zone, and peripheral zone

4. Functions as a secondary sex organ that secretes a component of seminal fluid

B. Changes associated with cancer

1. Most cancers develop in the peripheral zone (Logothetis et al., 2010).

2. Malignant cell growth spreads locally to the seminal vesicles, bladder, and peritoneum (see Figure 11-1).

3. Lymphatic and hematogenous spread is also common.

a. Pelvic lymph node invasion

C. Major classifications of prostate cancer

1. 95% adenocarcinomas

2. Remaining 5% sarcomas, mucinous or signet ring tumors, adenoid cystic carcinomas, and small cell undifferentiated cancers (Logothetis et al., 2010)

D. Trends in epidemiology

1. National trend in prostate cancer incidence—increased rates from 1988 to 1992 coinciding with the advent of widespread prostate-specific antigen (PSA) testing; sharp declines from 1992 to 1995, followed by a leveling off from 1995 to 2013

2. Approximately 238,590 men estimated to be newly diagnosed in 2013 and 29,720 to die from the disease (ACS, 2013)
3. Accounts for one third of all male cancers
4. Five-year survival rates—steady improvement since 1974 for both whites and African Americans; however, continuing lower 5-year survival rates for all stages of prostate cancer among African Americans (ACS, 2013)
5. Risk factors
   a. Age
      (1) More than 75% of prostate cancers are diagnosed in men 65 years or older.
      (2) Autopsy studies have shown that 30% of men aged 50 years have evidence of adenocarcinoma of the prostate, and by age 90 years that percentage rises to 57% (Mydlo & Godec, 2003).
   b. Ethnicity
      (1) Higher mortality rates in Western countries compared with non-Western countries (e.g., developing countries such as in Asia and the Middle East) (Haas, Delongchamps, Brawley, Wang, & de la Roza, 2008)
      (2) Highest incidence and mortality rates in the world among African Americans (ACS 2013; Haas et al., 2008).
   c. Dietary factors
      (1) Possible role of high-fat diets in promotion of prostate cancer
      (2) Diets high in vitamins E, D, and selenium possibly inhibit or prevent prostate cancer.
      (3) Diets high in lycopene linked to a low incidence of prostate cancer (Vance, Su, Fontham, Koo, & Chun, 2013)
   d. Occupational exposures
      (1) Farming and cadmium exposure through welding and battery manufacturing associated with increased risk (Mydlo & Godec, 2003)
   e. Genetic factors
      (1) Prostate cancer susceptibility locus, called HPC1, located on chromosome 1—thought to be responsible for 33% of all hereditary prostate cancer and 3% of cases overall (Haiman et al., 2011; Mydlo & Godec, 2003)
      (2) Mutations of *BRCA1* and *BRCA2* genes—implicated in breast cancer, as well as in prostate cancer (Mydlo & Godec, 2003)
      (3) Having a single first-degree relative with prostate cancer—increases risk twofold to threefold; having a first- and second-degree relative affected increases risk sixfold (Mydlo & Godec, 2003)
   E. Common metastatic sites—lung, liver, adrenal glands, kidneys, and bones
II. Screening and diagnostic measures
   A. Screening
      1. High level of controversy continues at the national level with regard to routine screening for prostate cancer with PSA testing.
         a. Central issue—PSA testing may reveal clinically insignificant tumors; ensuing treatment causes significant side effects, resulting in diminished quality of life.
      2. Following U.S. Preventive Service Task Force (USPSTF) recommendations, the American Urological Association (AUA) published new guidelines for prostate cancer screening in 2013 (Carter et al., 2013).
         a. PSA screening in men younger than 40 years not recommended
         b. Routine screening in men 40 to 54 years at average risk not recommended; at-risk men may benefit from shared decision making at this earlier age.
         c. Shared decision making about PSA screening for men ages 55 to 69 years; greatest screening benefit in this age group
         d. Screening interval of 2 or more years for those deciding on screening
         e. PSA screening not recommended for men 70 years or older or for those with less than a 10- to 15-year life expectancy
      3. Normal range for PSA varies by age, race, and prostate size—0 to 4 ng/mL is considered the standard norm. Other important markers include PSA density and PSA velocity (Carter et al., 2013).
   B. Diagnostic tests
      1. Digital rectal examination (DRE)—assess for size, lesions, symmetry, texture
         a. Simple and inexpensive, but only the posterior and lateral areas can be palpated
      2. Transrectal ultrasound (TRUS)—evaluation of the prostate volume
      3. Biopsy
         a. Performed with TRUS for guidance
         b. Transrectal route preferred; six specimens obtained from both sides of the prostate
      4. Pelvic MRI to evaluate capsular penetration, seminal vesicle involvement, and lymph node metastasis
      5. Bone scans—to evaluate possible bone metastasis; generally not performed unless PSA level is above 10 ng/mL or client complains of skeletal symptoms (NCCN, 2013b)

6. Laboratory studies
   a. PSA—increased levels may be significant as an adjunct in differential diagnosis or as a marker for disease progression
      (1) Men should avoid ejaculation for 48 hours before test.
      (2) Finasteride (Propecia), androgen receptor blockers, PC-SPES may also affect PSA levels (NCCN, 2013b).

III. Grading and staging
   A. Grading—based on the Gleason score (Table 11-5) (NCCN, 2013b)
      1. Primary grade—based on evaluation of architecture of malignant glands in the largest portion of the specimen; most common cell grade seen
      2. Secondary grade—assigned to the next largest area of malignant growth; second most common cell grade seen
      3. Score computed by adding the primary and secondary grades together; order reveals most common cell grade (i.e., $3+4=7$ versus $4+3=7$)
      4. Scores of 2 to 10 possible; higher scores indicate aggressive disease, with a poor prognosis
   B. Staging
      1. AJCC staging system (see Table 11-5)

Table 11-5

AJCC (2010) Staging of Prostate Cancer

Primary Tumor (T)
Clinical

TX	Primary tumor cannot be assessed
T0	No evidence of primary tumor
T1	Clinically inapparent tumor neither palpable nor visible by imaging
T1a	Tumor incidental histologic finding in 5% or less of tissue resected
T1b	Tumor incidental finding in more than 5% of tissue resected
T1c	Tumor identified by needle biopsy (e.g., because of elevated PSA)
T2	Tumor confined within prostate*
T2a	Tumor involves half of one lobe or less
T2b	Tumor involves more than half of one lobe but not both lobes
T2c	Tumor involves both lobes
T3	Tumor extends though the prostate capsule†
T3a	Extracapsular extension (unilateral or bilateral)
T3b	Tumor invades seminal vesicle(s)
T4	Tumor is fixed or invades adjacent structures other than seminal vesicles: bladder neck, external sphincter, levator muscles, and/or pelvic wall

Continued

Table 11-5

AJCC (2010) Staging of Prostate Cancer—cont'd

Pathologic

pT2‡	Organ confined
pT2a	Unilateral, involving half of one lobe or less
pT2B	Unilateral, involving more than half of one lobe but not both lobes
pT2c	Bilateral disease
pT3	Extraprostatic extension
pT3a	Extraprostatic extension¶
pT3b	Seminal vesicle invasion
pT4	Invasion of bladder, rectum

Regional Lymph Nodes (N)

NX	Regional nodes not sampled
N0	No regional node metastasis
N1	Metastasis in regional node(s)

Distant Metastasis (M)

MX	Distant metastasis cannot be assessed (not evaluated by any modality)
M0	No distant metastasis
M1	Distant metastasis
M1a	Nonregional lymph node(s)
M1b	Bone(s)
M1c	Other site(s) with or without bone disease

Histologic Grade

GX	Grade cannot be assessed
G1	Well differentiated (slight anaplasia) (Gleason 2-4)
G2	Moderately differentiated (moderate anaplasia) (Gleason 5-6)
G3-4	Poorly differentiated/undifferentiated (marked anaplasia) (Gleason 7-10)

Stage Grouping

Stage I	T1a	N0	M0	G1
Stage II	T1a	N0	M0	G2, 3-4
	T1b	N0	M0	Any G
	T1c	N0	M0	Any G
	T1	N0	M0	Any G
	T2	N0	M0	Any G
Stage III	T3	N0	M0	Any G
Stage IV	T4	N0	M0	Any G
	Any T	N1	M0	Any G
	Any T	Any N	M1	Any G

PSA, Prostate-specific antigen.

*Tumor found in one or both lobes by needle biopsy but not palpable or reliably visible by imaging is classified as T1c.

†Invasion into the prostatic apex or into (but not beyond) the prostatic capsule is classified not as T3 but as T2.

‡No pathologic T1 classification.

¶Postsurgical margin to be indicated by an R1 descriptor (residual microscopic disease).

Used with permission of the American Joint Committee on Cancer (AJCC), Chicago, Illinois. The original source for this material is the AJCC Cancer Staging Manual, Seventh Edition (2010) published by Springer Science and Business Media LLC, www.springer.com.

IV. Prognosis
   A. 5-year survival rate by stage of prostate cancer—local (100%), regional (100%), and distant disease (29%)
   B. 5-year survival for all stages combined—89.9% for whites, 65.5% for African Americans
V. Principles of medical management
   A. Early-stage disease
      1. Treatment options—active surveillance, observation or expectant management, radical prostatectomy with lymph node dissection, three-dimensional conformal radiotherapy (3D-CRT), or brachytherapy
         a. Radical prostatectomy—complete removal of prostate; lymph node sampling
            (1) Alternative approaches—laparoscopic prostatectomy and robotic laparoscopic prostatectomy (Logothetis et al., 2010)
         b. 3D-CRT—radiation doses to prostate greater than 81 Gy (NCCN, 2013b); intensity-modulated radiation therapy (IMRT) replacing 3D in major cancer centers
         c. Brachytherapy—guided by TRUS, radioactive seed placement into the prostate gland via the perineum through a grid template (NCCN, 2013b)
            (1) Isotopes used—iodine-125 or palladium-103
         d. Active surveillance, expectant management—careful follow-up monitoring with PSA testing, needle biopsy and DRE, followed by active treatment if disease progression is noted (Klotz, Zhang, Lam, Mamedov, & Loblaw, 2009; NCCN, 2013b)
         e. Cryosurgery—direct application of freezing temperatures to the prostate via percutaneously inserted cryogenic probes (NCCN, 2013b)
      2. Complications of treatment
         a. Incontinence—conflicting data because of imprecise measurement; estimated to range from 3% to 87% after radical prostatectomy, 3% to 7% for external beam radiotherapy, and 6% for brachytherapy; other complications include urethral stricture, urethral sloughing, and bladder outlet obstruction (Mydlo & Godec, 2003).
         b. Erectile dysfunction—nerve-sparing prostatectomy techniques lessen incidence; comparisons difficult because of imprecise definitions and measurement; high rates reported after surgery, and some form of impotence seen in 6% to 61% of cases after brachytherapy (Simmons, 2011)
         c. Gastrointestinal dysfunction—diarrhea, proctitis, and rectal bleeding associated with both radiation therapy and brachytherapy (Logothetis et al., 2010)
      3. Treatment for advanced prostate cancer
         a. Hormonal manipulation—accepted standard for management of metastatic prostate cancer and also used in management of patients at high risk for relapse; also used in neoadjuvant setting
            (1) Orchiectomy—surgical removal of testicles; produces rapid response; indicated for patients who are unreliable in taking medication or for whom estrogen is contraindicated
               (a) Not acceptable as an option for many men
               (b) Psychological trauma as a result of surgical castration
            (2) Luteinizing hormone-releasing hormones (LHRH analogues; such as leuprolide [Lupron], goserelin [Zoladex])—decrease production of testosterone; may produce fewer side effects compared with estrogens; used with flutamide (Eulexin) to reduce "flare," which is the sudden exacerbation of symptoms (Simmons, 2011)
               (a) Flare can be life-threatening, with spinal cord compression and ureteral obstruction (Simmons, 2011)
               (b) Other side effects include hot flashes, loss of libido, erectile dysfunction, and gynecomastia.
            (3) Antiandrogens (flutamide[Eulexin], megestrol acetate [Megace])—interfere with intracellular androgen activity; effects may be delayed 1 to 2 months
            (4) Estrogen therapy—generally, diethylstilbestrol (DES)
               (a) Used in castration-resistant prostate cancer
               (b) Results in decreased pain, decreased tumor size, decreased urinary symptoms (Simmons, 2011)
               (c) Complications—gynecomastia, sodium retention, weight gain, and severe cardiovascular and thrombotic complications
               (d) Associated with relapse within 2 to 3 years; at the time of relapse, disease often becomes resistant to further hormone treatment.
            (5) Ketoconazole (Nizoral)—suppresses adrenal testosterone production
               (a) Used in castration-resistant prostate cancer

(b) Administered with hydrocortisone to reduce risk of adrenal insufficiency (NCCN, 2013b; Simmons, 2011)

(6) Abiraterone (Zytiga)—used in combination with prednisone for castration-resistant prostate cancer (NCCN, 2013b)

4. Radiation therapy—for local extension and distant metastases
   a. May be primary treatment for stage D lesions if hormone manipulation is ineffective or contraindicated; may be used as a component of combined-modality therapy
   b. Used for palliation of pain from bone metastasis or spinal cord compression
   c. Radium-223 for symptomatic bone metastases

5. Chemotherapy
   a. Optimal timing of initiation of chemotherapy in men with castration-resistant prostate cancer undetermined (Logothetis et al., 2010)
   b. Docetaxel (Taxotere) preferred (NCCN, 2013b)
   c. Other options—sipuleucel-T, mitoxantrone, cyclophosphamide, estramustine, vinblastine, and vinorelbine; cabazitaxel preferred following docetaxel

VI. Nursing implications
   A. Interventions to decrease physical, emotional, psychological, social, and spiritual distress during and after treatment
      1. Encouraging patient to verbalize feelings about disease and treatment
      2. Referral to mental health specialist, community resources, support groups (e.g., ACS, UsToo), as needed
      3. Teaching patient to identify and manage symptoms and to report symptoms to health care providers
      4. Providing pharmacologic and nonpharmacologic interventions to manage pain and other side effects
   B. Interventions to promote optimal sexual functioning
      1. Facilitating discussion among the physician, nurse, patient, and significant other about the potential impact of treatment on sexual functioning and interventions to minimize effects
         a. Obtain permission, before and after treatment, to discuss functional and anatomic changes with treatment and resultant sexual concerns.

b. Respect the patient's reticence in discussing sexual concerns.
      2. Use of terminology appropriate to social and cultural level
      3. Providing written information and anatomic drawings, as indicated, for clarifications and to reinforce teaching
      4. Providing specific suggestions related to treatment used and alternatives
         a. Teach patient and partner about available options for the treatment of impotence—pharmacologic, mechanical, surgical.
         b. Initiate referral for physical therapy, sexual counseling, or both, if indicated (Simmons, 2011).

References

American Cancer Society. (2013). *Cancer facts & figures, 2013.* Atlanta: Author.

Carter, H. B., Albertsen, P. C., Barry, M. J., Etzioni, R., Freedland, S. J., Greene, K. L., et al. (2013). Early detection of prostate cancer: AUA guideline. *The Journal of Urology, 190*(2), 419–426.

Chow, W. H., Dong, L. M., & Devesa, S. S. (2010). Epidemiology and risk factors for kidney cancer. *Nature Reviews. Urology, 7*(5), 245–257.

Edge, S. B., Byrd, D. R., Compton, C. C., Fritz, A. G., & Greene, F. L. (Eds.), (2010). *AJCC cancer staging manual* (7th ed.). New York: Springer.

Escudier, B., Pluzanska, A., Koralewski, P., Ravaud, A., Bracarda, S., Szczylik, C., et al. (2008). Bevacizumab plus interferon alfa-2a for treatment of metastatic renal cell carcinoma: A randomised, double-blind phase III trial. *The Lancet, 370*(9605), 2103–2111.

Figlin, R. A. (Ed.), (2003). *Kidney cancer treatment and research.* Norwell, MA: Kluwer Academic.

Goodison, S., Rosser, C. J., & Urquidi, V. (2013). Bladder cancer detection and monitoring: Assessment of urine- and blood-based marker tests. *Molecular Diagnosis & Therapy, 17,* 71–84.

Grossman, H. B., Natale, R. B., Tangen, C. M., Speights, V. O., Vogelzang, N. J., Trump, D. L., et al. (2003). Neoadjuvant chemotherapy plus cystectomy compared with cystectomy alone for locally advanced bladder cancer. *New England Journal of Medicine, 349*(9), 859–866.

Haas, G. P., Delongchamps, N., Brawley, O. W., Wang, C. Y., & de la Roza, G. (2008). The worldwide epidemiology of prostate cancer: Perspectives from autopsy studies. *The Canadian Journal of Urology, 15*(1), 3866–3871.

Hagenkord, J. M., Gatalica, Z., Jonasch, E., & Monzon, F. A. (2011). Clinical genomics of renal epithelial tumors. *Cancer Genetics, 204*(6), 285–297.

Haiman, C. A., Chen, G. K., Blot, W. J., Strom, S. S., Berndt, S. I., Kittles, R. A., et al. (2011). Characterizing genetic risk at known prostate cancer susceptibility loci in African Americans. *PLoS Genetics, 7*(5), e1001387. http://dx.doi.org/10.1371/journal.pgen.1001387.

Hautman, R. E., Abol-Emain, H., Halez, K., Haro, I., Mansson, W., Millis, R. D., et al. (2007). Urinary diverion. *Urology, 69*(1 Suppl.), 17–49.

Howlader, N., Noone, A. M., Krapcho, M., Garshell, J., Neyman, N., & Altekruse, et al. (Eds.). (2013). *SEER cancer statistics review, 1975–2010*. Bethesda, MD: National Cancer Institute.

Johnson, D. C., Pruthi, R. S., & Woods, M. E. (2013). Perioperative chemotherapy: When to use it, what to use, and why. *The Urologic Clinics of North America, 40*(2), 183–195.

Klotz, L., Zhang, L., Lam, A., Mamedov, A., & Loblaw, A. (2009). Clinical results of long-term follow-up of a large, active surveillance cohort with localized prostate cancer. *Journal of Clinical Oncology, 28*(1), 126–131.

Lerner, S. P., Schoenberg, M. P., Coran, S., & Shernberg, M. D. (Eds.), (2006). *Textbook of bladder cancer*. Boca Raton, FL: Taylor & Francis.

Logothetis, C. J., Kim, J., Davis, J., Kuban, D., Mathew, P., & Aparicio, A. (2010). Neoplasms of the prostate. In W. K. Hong, R. C. Bast, Jr., W. N. Hait, D. W. Kufe, R. E. Pollock, R. R. Weichselbaum, & E. Frei, III., (Eds.), *Cancer medicine* (pp. 1228–1254). Shelton, CT: People's Medical Publishing House-USA.

Lote, C. J. (Ed.). (2012). *Principles of renal physiology*. (5th ed.). New York: Springer.

Morrissey, C., Martinez, A., Zatyka, M., Agathanggelou, A., Honorio, S., Astuti, D., et al. (2001). Epigenetic inactivation of the RASSF1A 3p21. 3 tumor suppressor gene in both clear cell and papillary renal cell carcinoma. *Cancer Research, 61* (19), 7277–7281.

Mydlo, J. H., & Godec, C. J. (Eds.). (2003). *Prostate cancer: Science and practice*. Oxford, UK: Elsevier.

National Comprehensive Cancer Network. (2013a). *NCCN guidelines version 1.2013: Kidney cancer*. http://www.nccn.org/professionals/physician_gls/pdf/kidney.pdf.

National Comprehensive Cancer Network. (2013b). *NCCN guidelines version 4.2013: Prostate cancer early detection*. http://www.nccn.org/physician_gls/prostate.pdf.

National Comprehensive Cancer Network. (2013c). *NCCN guidelines version 1.2013: Bladder cancer*. http://www.nccn.org/professionals/physician_gls/pdf/bladder.pdf.

Philip, J., Manikandan, R., Venugopal, S., Desouza, J., & Javle, P. (2009). Orthotopic neobladder verus ileal conduit urinary diversion after cystectomy—a quality-of-life based comparison. *Annals of the Royal College of Surgeons of England, 91*(7), 565–569. http://www.ncbi.nlm.nih.gov/pmc/articles/PMC2966160/.

Prino, L. N., & Jonasch, E. (2012). *Kidney cancer: Principles and practice*. New York: Springer Verlag.

Raghavan, D., Stein, J. P., Cote, R., & Jones, J. S. (2010). Bladder cancer. In W. K. Hong, R. C. Bast, Jr., W. N. Hait, D. W. Kufe, R. E. Pollock, R. R. Weichselbaum, & E. Frei, III, (Eds.), *Cancer medicine* (pp. 1219–1227). Shelton, CT: People's Medical Publishing House-USA.

Rini, B. I., Heng, D. Y. C., Zhou, M., Novick, A., & Raghavan, D. (2010). Renal cell carcinoma. In W. K. Hong, R. C. Bast, Jr., W. N. Hait, D. W. Kufe, R. E. Pollock, R. R. Weichselbaum, & E. Frei, III., (Eds.), *Cancer medicine* (pp. 1204–1211). Shelton, CT: People's Medical Publishing House-USA.

Shen, Z., Shen, T., Wientjes, M. G., O'Donnell, M. A., & Au, J. L. S. (2008). Intravesicular treatments of bladder cancer: Review. *Pharmacological Research, 25*(7), 1500–1510. http://dx.doi.org/10.1007/511095-007-9566-7.

Shinagare, A. B., Ramaiya, N. H., Jagannathan, J. P., Fennessy, F. M., Taplin, M. E., & Van den Abbeele, A. D. (2011). Metastatic pattern of bladder cancer: Correlation with the characteristics of the primary tumor. *American Journal of Roentgenology, 196*(1), 117–122.

Siegel, R., Naishadham, D., & Jemal, A. (2013). Cancer statistics, 2013. *CA: A Cancer Journal for Clinicians, 63*(1), 11–30.

Simmons, M. W. (2011). A practical guide to prostate cancer diagnosis and management. *Cleveland Clinic Journal, 78*(5), 321–331.

Sun, M., Thuret, R., Abdollah, F., Lughezzani, G., Schmitges, J., Tian, Z., et al. (2011). Age-adjusted incidence, mortality, and survival rates of stage-specific renal cell carcinoma in North America: A trend analysis. *European Urology, 59*(1), 135–141.

Vance, T. M., Su, J., Fontham, E. T., Koo, S. I., & Chun, O. K. (2013). Dietary antioxidants and prostate cancer: A review. *Nutrition and Cancer, 65*(6), 793–801.

Vera-Badillo, F. E., Conde, E., & Duran, I. (2012). Chromophobe renal cell carcinoma: A review of an uncommon entity. *International Journal of Urology, 19*(10), 894–900.

Part 2

CHAPTER 12
Skin Cancer

Krista M. Rubin

OVERVIEW

I. Pathophysiology of skin cancer
- A. Anatomy of the skin (Kolarsick, Kolarsick, & Goodwin, 2009)
  1. Epidermis—outermost layer
     a. Stratified epithelium layer made of keratinocytes and dendritic cells
     b. Contains melanocytes, Langerhans cells, and Merkel cells
  2. Dermis—underlying layer
     a. Comprises the bulk of the skin and provides pliability, elasticity, and tensile strength
     b. Principal component—collagen (protein that provides structure)
- B. Primary organ function (Asrani & Wanner, 2011)
  1. Protection from elements—wind, cold, heat, and ultraviolet radiation (UVR)
  2. Defense against infection
  3. Regulation of temperature, sensation, and excretion; prevention of water loss from the body to the environment
- C. Pathogenesis of skin cancer (Gordon, 2013; Skin Cancer Foundation, 2013; Tran, 2011; Tsao & Gabree, 2013;)
  1. Uncontrolled growth of abnormal skin cells that occurs when unrepaired deoxyribonucleic acid (DNA) damage to skin cells triggers mutations, or genetic defect; this leads to the development of malignant cells, which multiply rapidly to form malignant tumors
  2. Primary causative—UVR (in sunlight and artificial tanning beds); two main types of UVR rays:
     a. Ultraviolet A (UVA)—passes deeper into skin; damage is indirect, mediated by free radical formation and damage to cellular membranes
     b. Ultraviolet B (UVB)—causes erythema or sunburn and directly damages DNA
  3. Genetics—inherited predisposition for skin cancer
     a. Xeroderma pigmentosum (XP)
     b. Oculocutaneous albinism
     c. Basal cell nevus syndrome (Gorlin syndrome)
     d. Familial atypical mole melanoma syndrome (dysplastic nevus syndrome)

II. Epidemiology
- A. Incidence and prevalence (Skin Cancer Foundation, 2013)
  1. Skin cancer commonly categorized as melanoma and nonmelanoma skin cancer (NMSC) (Gordon, 2013)
     a. Basal cell carcinoma (BCC)
        (1) A malignant neoplasm arising from the basal cell layer of the epidermis
        (2) Typically caused by a combination of cumulative UV exposure and intense, occasional UV exposure
        (3) Most common form of skin cancer; approximately 2.8 million cases per year in the United States (U.S.)
        (4) More common in older people; average age at time of diagnosis steadily decreasing
     b. Squamous cell carcinoma (SCC) (Lazareth, 2013; Skin Cancer Foundation, 2013)
        (1) A malignant neoplasm arising from the squamous cells layer of the epidermis
        (2) Primarily caused by cumulative UV exposure over the lifetime
        (3) Second most common form of skin cancer; approximately 700,000 cases per year in the U.S.
        (4) Increased incidence among women younger than 40 years by almost 700% in the last 30 years
     c. Melanoma (Lazareth, 2013; Siegel, Naishadham, & Jemal, 2013)
        (1) Arises from malignant proliferation of melanocytes; pigment-producing cells that originate from the neural crest and

migrate to the skin, meninges, mucous membranes, upper esophagus, and eyes; most melanoma arise on the skin but may occur anywhere melanocytes are found.

    (2) Primarily caused by intense, occasional UV exposure (frequently leading to sunburn)

    (3) Fifth most common cancer in men, fourth in women in U.S.

    (4) Most common form of cancer for young adults 25 to 29 years old and the second most common form of cancer for those 15 to 29 years old, with approximately 76,690 new U.S. cases per year, 9480 deaths

B. Characteristics
  1. BCC (Table 12-1)
  2. SCC (Box 12-1)
  3. Melanoma (Table 12-2)

Table 12-1

Subtypes and Characteristics of Basal Cell Carcinoma (BCC)

Subtype	Characteristics
Nodular	• 50%-80% of all basal cell carcinomas • Most likely to occur on the head and neck • Typically presents as a round, pink, pearly, flesh-colored papule with a central depression • Telangiectasia (dilation of small blood vessels) often seen within the lesion • May or may not be crusted, ulcerated, or bleeding
Superficial	• 15% of all basal cell carcinomas • Most commonly found on the trunk • Typically presents as a bright red to pink patch; often scaly • Lesions are slowly progressive
Micronodular	• Aggressive subtype • May appear yellow-white when stretched • Firm to touch
Pigmented	• Uncommon variant of nodular BCC • Common in darker pigmented individuals

---

Box 12-1

Features of Squamous Cell Carcinoma (SCC)

• Typically slow-growing, but some may enlarge rapidly
• Often presents as a new or enlarging lesion that may bleed, weep, be tender or painful
• May be indurated, rounded, superficial, or discrete with hyperkeratotic (thickened) scale
• Invasive SCCs tend to be more nodular with ulceration
• Numbness, tingling, or muscle weakness may indicate perineural invasion

---

C. Metastatic incidence and pattern (Tran, 2011)
  1. BCC
    a. Rarely metastasizes; if untreated, may become ulcerated and locally invasive
    b. Perineural invasion possible, resulting in deep and extensive invasion of tumor and loss of nerve function
  2. SCC
    a. Recurrence rates—vary depending on tumor and patient risk factors (Table 12-3)
    b. Local recurrences—may sometimes lead to distant metastasis and death (2%-6% of patients)
  3. Melanoma (Rubin, 2009)
    a. Most important prognostic features in localized melanoma
      (1) Breslow depth (depth of invasion measured in millimeters [mm])
      (2) Ulceration of the primary lesion (defined as absence of an intact epidermal layer)
    b. Metastasizes to regional lymph nodes and commonly to distant skin, subcutis, lung, liver, and brain; risk of metastases dependent on stage at time of diagnosis

III. Principles of management
  A. Diagnostic procedures
    1. NMSCs (Tran, 2011)
      a. Biopsy types—shave, punch, incisional, excisional; shave biopsy most commonly used for nonpigmented lesions
    2. Melanoma (Jarrell & Schalock, 2011; Tran, 2011)
      a. Choice of biopsy technique—depends on size, location, and shape of lesion
      b. Full epidermal or dermal thickness biopsy down to subcutaneous fat required
  B. Staging (Tran, 2011)
    1. NMCS (Lazareth, 2013; Nolen, Beebe, King, Bryn, & Limaye, 2009)
      a. Staging seldom needed because most do not metastasize
      b. When appropriate, American Joint Committee on Cancer (AJCC) tumor-node-metastasis (TNM) staging system most commonly used to plan treatment and monitor progress
    2. Melanoma (Rubin, 2013)
      a. AJCC's TNM staging system most commonly used to plan treatment and monitor progress of disease (Table 12-4)
      b. Sentinel lymph node biopsy (SLNB)—a staging procedure to evaluate for regional node involvement
        (1) Recommended for primary melanomas greater than 1 mm thick or those less than 1 mm thick that demonstrate adverse pathologic features such as ulceration or mitosis

Table 12-2

Subtypes and Characteristics of Melanoma

Type	Frequency	Site	Features
Superficial spreading melanoma (SSM)	60%-70%	Any site; preference for lower extremities in females, and back (both sexes)	• Most common type in fair-skinned individuals • Begins as an asymptomatic brown to black macule with color variations • Typically asymmetric, poorly circumscribed • Notching and scalloping common • 25% found in association with a pre-existing nevus; the remainder arise de novo
Nodular melanoma (NM)	15%-30%	Any site; primarily in sun-exposed areas on the head, neck and trunk Males more than in females	• Does not have a recognizable radial growth phase • Usually presents as a deeply invasive lesion; most commonly dark brown-black to blue nodules, but may sometimes be pink to red
Lentigo maligna melanoma (LMM)	~5%	Sun-exposed areas: face and neck	• Occurs as a large hyperpigmented macule or plaque with irregular borders and variable pigmentation • Approximately 5% will progress to invasive melanoma
Acral lentiginous melanoma (ALM)	Uncommon in whites; most common in persons of African, Asian, and Hispanic descent	Palms, soles, nail unit, mucous membranes	• Often an enlarging hyperpigmented macule or plaque on the palms and soles • Lesions under the nails may present as longitudinal melanonychia (brown or black pigmentation of the nail plate) or as hyperpigmentation extending beyond the proximal nail • Often mistaken for a benign lesion
Desmoplastic	1.7%	Head and neck	• Rare variant of vertical growth phase melanoma • Frequently mistaken for a scar, fibroma, fibromatosis, or BCC because it presents as an amelanotic, pale, fleshy nodule or plaque

Data from Longo, D.L., Fauci, A.S., Kasper, D.L., Hauser, S.L., Jameson, J.L., & Loscalzo, J. (2011). *Harrison's principles of internal medicine* (18th ed.). New York: McGraw Hill.

Table 12-3

Tumor-Related and Patient-Related Risk Factors in Squamous Cell Carcinoma (SCC)

Tumor-Related Risk Factors	Patient-Related Risk Factors
Location: lip, ear, or within a scar	Chronic immunosuppression (e.g., human immunodeficiency virus [HIV]), hematologic malignancy
Lesions > 2 cm in size	Organ transplantation
Recurrent tumor	
Poor differentiation	
Perineural invasion	
Invasion to subcutaneous fat	

(2) Has replaced elective node dissection

(3) Completion node dissection of the involved lymph node basin(s) usually recommended if positive sentinel node(s) are identified

IV. Treatment (Tran, 2011)

  A. NMSC—depends on multiple factors, including location and size of the lesion, histology, primary or recurrent tumor, perineural invasion, aggressive biologic behavior of the lesion, immune status and general condition of the patient, as well as patient wishes (Nolen et al., 2009; Tran, 2011)

    1. Surgery—treatment of choice for majority of lesions

      a. Electrodessication and curettage (ED&C)—uses a curette to scrape off friable tumor cells until normal, then destroys any remaining tissue with electrocautery (Lazareth, 2013)

      b. Excision—most often used for lesion in non–cosmetically sensitive areas

Table 12-4

AJCC Criteria for Melanoma Staging

Clinical Staging*				Pathologic Staging[†]			
Stage 0	Tis	N0	M0	0	Tis	N0	M0
Stage IA	T1a	N0	M0	IA	T1a	N0	M0
Stage IB	T1b	N0	M0	IB	T1b	N0	M0
	T2a	N0	M0		T2a	N0	M0
Stage IIA	T2b	N0	M0	IIA	T2b	N0	M0
	T3b	N0	M0		T3a	N0	M0
	T4a	N0	M0				
Stage IIB	T3b	N0	M0	IIB	T3a	N0	M0
	T4a	N0	M0		T4a	N0	M0
Stage IIC	T4b	N0	M0	IIC	T4b	N0	M0
Stage III	Any T	N1	M0	IIIA	T1-4a	N1a	M0
					T1-4a	N2a	M0
				IIIB	T1-4b	N1a	M0
					T1-4b	N2a	M0
					T1-4a	N2b	M0
					T1-4a	N2c	M0
				IIIC	T1-4b	N1b	M0
					T1-4b	N2b	M0
					T1-4B	N2c	M0
					Any T	N3	M0
Stage IV	Any T	Any N	M1	IV	Any T	Any N	M1

*Includes microstaging of the primary melanoma and clinical or radiologic evaluation for metastases. By convention, it should be used after complete excision of the primary melanoma with clinical assessment for regional and distant metastases.

[†]Includes microstaging of the primary melanoma and pathologic information about the regional lymph nodes after partial or complete lymphadenectomy. Pathologic stage 0 or stage IA patients are the exception; they do not require pathologic evaluation of their lymph nodes.

Used with permission of the American Joint Committee on Cancer (AJCC), Chicago, Illinois. The original source for this material is the AJCC Cancer Staging Manual, Seventh Edition (2010) published by Springer Science and Business Media LLC, www.springer.com.

c. Moh micrographic surgery—removes tissue in multiple, progressive thin layers; preserves maximum amount of tissue
2. Topical therapy
   a. Cryotherapy—tissue destruction with liquid nitrogen to freeze clinically apparent tissue
   b. 5-fluorouracil (5-FU) and imiquimod (an immune response modifier)
3. Radiotherapy—recommended for patients who are not surgical candidates with lesions between 1 and 10 cm in size
4. Systemic therapy
   a. Unresectable or metastatic SCC, or for recurrence after surgery or radiation
      (1) Capecitabine (an oral 5-FU) as a single agent, or combined with interferon for metastatic SCC; cisplatin, bleomycin, cyclophosphamide, vinblastine, and doxorubicin have been used (Nolen et al., 2009; Tran, 2011).
   b. Unresectable or recurrent BCC
      (1) Vismodegib, a first-in-class Hedgehog pathway inhibitor, recently approved

5. Photodynamic therapy (PDT)—combines photosensitizing medications with light or lasers to induce cell death; used primarily to treat large numbers of actinic keratosis (AK) lesions in a single session (Nolen et al., 2009)

B. Melanoma
1. Surgery for primary melanoma (Wong et al., 2012)
   a. Wide local excision preferred treatment for primary melanoma
   b. Appropriate surgical margins determined by tumor thickness (Table 12-5)

Table 12-5

Recommended Surgical Margins for Melanoma

Tumor Thickness	Recommended Margin*
In situ	0.5 cm
≤1.0 mm	1.0 cm
1.01-2 mm	1-2 cm
2.01-4 mm	2.0 cm
>4 mm	2.0 cm

*Margins may be modified to accommodate individual anatomic or functional considerations.

Data from National Comprehensive Cancer Network (NCCN). (2014). www.nccn.org.

2. Surgery for advanced melanoma (Rubin, 2013)
   a. Elective lymph node dissection for clinically palpable nodal metastasis
   b. Isolated limb perfusion or infusion, most commonly with melphalan and moderate hyperthermia for recurrent or unresectable in-transit metastasis of an extremity (method for intravascular delivery of chemotherapy)
   c. Metastasectomy for a certain subset of patients (Leung, Hari, & Morton, 2012)
      (1) Those with solitary metastasis involving skin, lungs, distant lymph nodes, or gastrointestinal (GI) tract
      (2) Those with long disease-free interval between disease recurrences
      (3) Those in whom the metastatic focus can be completely resected
3. Palliative surgery (Leung et al., 2012)
   a. Considered for symptomatic distant metastases (e.g., a GI bleed) or large brain metastases
   b. For metastases that, if left untreated, are likely to lead to significant symptoms such as pain
4. Radiotherapy (Wazer, 2013)
   a. Not generally used as a primary modality
   b. May be used as adjuvant therapy in certain cases to increase regional control
   c. Often used as palliation for patients with bone or brain metastases, particularly spinal cord metastases (Leung et al., 2012)
5. Systemic therapy
   a. Immunotherapy (Sosman, 2013a)
      (1) Adjuvant setting—interferon alpha-2b (IFN-α), the only approved treatment for high-risk melanoma; limited use and efficacy
      (2) Advanced setting—no standard treatment for stage IV melanoma; recent treatment advances have changed the landscape for treating advanced disease
         (a) Ipilimumab—anticytotoxic T-lymphocyte antigen (CTLA)-4 antibody
         (b) Interleukin-2 (IL-2)—T-cell growth factor; 10% to 20% response rates, with 4% to 6% of patients achieving a durable complete remission
      (3) Advanced setting—investigational agents showing promise, as demonstrated by data from recent clinical trials (Rubin, 2013)
         (a) Anivolumab, lambrolizumab—anti–PD-1 antibodies
         (b) Anti–PDL-1 antibodies
         (c) Combinations of immunotherapeutic agents

   b. Targeted therapy (Rubin, 2013; Sosman, 2013b)—agents that inhibit key cancer-promoting enzymes and pathways; effective only if the specific mutation is identified within the tumor⚠
      (1) BRAF inhibitors (BRAFi)—vemurafenib and dabrafenib; often produce rapid and dramatic tumor regression but responses usually transient; typically used as first-line agents in symptomatic patients
      (2) MEK inhibitors (MEKi)—mekinist; approved for monotherapy in patients with *BRAF*-mutated melanoma
      (3) CKIT inhibitors (CKITi)—imatinib, dasatinib, and nilotinib for *CKIT*-mutated melanoma, a rare mutation seen in mucosal or acral melanomas (these agents are currently in clinical trials; not yet approved)
      (4) Combinations, including BRAFi+MEKi, for *BRAF*-mutated melanomas (currently in clinical trials; not yet approved)
   c. Chemotherapy—limited efficacy, no survival advantage; less favored treatment modality
      (1) Dacarbazine (dimethyl triazeno imidazole carboxamide [DTIC])—the only chemotherapeutic agent approved by the U. S. Food and Drug Administration (FDA) for the treatment of melanoma
      (2) Temozolomide—oral analog of DTIC, but not FDA approved for use in melanoma

V. Nursing implications
   A. Risk factors
      1. Skin cancer
         a. Multiple risk factors exist for all skin cancers (Gordon, 2013) (Box 12-2)
            (1) Endogenous factors—phototype, skin and eye color, number or nevi, and individual or family history of skin cancer
            (2) Exogenous factors—type and degree of cumulative sun exposure, history of sunburns, sun protection behaviors

---

Box 12-2

Risk Factors for Melanoma

- Personal history of melanoma
- Family history of melanoma
- Number of moles (typical and atypical)
- Exposure to ultraviolet rays
- Fair skin, red or blond hair, freckling
- Immunosuppression
- Age (increasing risk with age)
- Gender: Males more than females
- Genetics

    b. UVR exposure is chief environmental risk

    c. Hereditary conditions

    d. Immunosuppression associated with more aggressive tumors

  B. Nursing interventions

    1. Prevention of skin cancer

      a. Reviewing factors that place an individual at risk for skin cancer

      b. Describing specific health-promotion activities to minimize UVR exposure (Box 12-3)

        (1) Discussing the role of sunscreen and demonstrating proper application

          (a) Sunscreen sun protection factor (SPF)—a measurement of how long unprotected skin can be exposed to UV rays before burning compared with how long it takes to burn without protection

          (b) Must be properly applied for full protection

          (c) Broad spectrum advised to filter both UVA and UVB rays

    2. Early detection

      a. Obtaining a history of any recent changes in lesions

      b. Teaching systematic assessment of skin lesion for changes; teaching high-risk patients to perform monthly self-skin examination stressing importance and rationale

      c. Discussing the warning signs of early melanoma (Table 12-6)

Table 12-6

ABCDEs of Melanoma Recognition

Warning Sign	Description
A: Asymmetry	One half unlike the other half
B: Border	Irregular, scalloped, or uneven border
C: Color	Color varied (more than one color present within the lesion)
D: Diameter	Larger than 6 mm
E: Enlarging	Enlarging or evolving

        (1) Describing the importance of assessing for early signs of change in nevi or development of new lesions

      d. Use of educational resources (Table 12-7)

    3. Therapeutic measures

      a. Oncology nurses must have a comprehensive understanding of skin cancer behavior, in particular advanced melanoma.

      b. Oncology nurses must be well versed in the disease process of advanced melanoma, the recent advances in tumor immunology and tumor genetics, and the unique and vast toxicity profile, in particular of the newer immunotherapy agents, as well as the targeted agents.

      c. Oncology nurses must provide anticipatory guidance regarding intervention and what to expect for treatment recommendations using an open, optimistic approach.

      d. Oncology nurses must provide ongoing assessment of patient understanding of the disease process, treatment effects and recommendations.

      e. Oncology nurses must manage both the disease and the treatment effects.

    4. Rehabilitative measures

Box 12-3

Skin Cancer Prevention Measures

- Minimize exposure to sunlight between the hours of 10 AM and 4 PM
- Do not allow skin to burn.
- Avoid tanning and use of ultraviolet tanning booths.
- Use clothing with built-in sun protection factor (SPF), or wear long-sleeved shirt, long pants, and wide-brimmed hat, during times of sun exposure.
- Use sunscreen and lip balm: physical (blockers) or chemical (absorbers) with an SPF of 15+, and reapply every 1.5 to 2 hours.
- Use broad-spectrum eye protection.
- Keep infants younger than 6 months out of the sun.

Data from Skin Cancer Foundation. (2013). http://www.skincancer.org/skin-cancer-information; American Cancer Society. (2013). *Skin cancer prevention and early detection.* http://www.cancer.org/cancer/skincancer-melanoma/moreinformation/skincancerpreventionandearlydetection/index; American Academy of Dermatology. (2013). *Skin cancer prevention.* http://www.aad.org/spot-skin-cancer/understanding-skin-cancer/how-do-i-prevent-skin-cancer/skin-cancer-prevention-tips.

Table 12-7

Resources for Information on Skin Cancer

American Academy of Dermatology (AAD), Spot Skin Cancer	http://www.aad.org/spot-skin-cancer
American Cancer Society (ACS)	http://www.cancer.org/cancer/cancercauses/sunanduvexposure/skin-cancer-facts
Skin Cancer Foundation	http://www.skincancer.org/
National Cancer Institute	http://www.cancer.gov/cancertopics/types/skin
Aim for Melanoma	http://www.aimatmelanoma.org
SunAWARE	http://www.sunaware.org/

a. Assessment of the impact of the treatment for skin cancer

b. Stressing the importance of evaluation at regular intervals for potential recurrence

c. Stressing the importance of lifestyle changes in relation to sun exposure in high-risk individuals and families to minimize risk for development of other skin cancers

5. Psychological measures

a. Discussing the potential psychosocial issues associated with the diagnosis of skin cancer

b. Assessment of the patient's coping strategies related to the diagnosis

c. Exploring with the patient the impact of change in recreational activities or work because of skin cancer and changes in lifestyle as a result of a diagnosis

d. Consideration of psychological screening in patients with melanoma

References

American Academy of Dermatology. (2013). *Skin cancer prevention.* http://www.aad.org/spot-skin-cancer/understanding-skin-cancer/how-do-i-prevent-skin-cancer/skin-cancer-prevention-tips.

American Cancer Society. (2013). *Skin cancer prevention and early detection.* http://www.cancer.org/cancer/skincancer-melanoma/moreinformation/skincancerprevention andearlydetection/index.

Asrani, F., & Wanner, M. (2011). Care and maintenance of normal skin. In P. C. Schalock, J. T. S. Hsu, & K. Arndt (Eds.), *Lippincott's primary care dermatology* (pp. 28–36). Philadelphia: Lippincott, Williams & Wilkins.

Gordon, R. (2013). Skin cancer: An overview of epidemiology and risk factors. In P. Rieger (Ed.), *Seminars in oncology nursing: Skin cancer, 29*(3), 160–169.

Jarrell, A., & Schalock, P. S. (2011). Procedures in dermatologic diagnosis and therapy. In P. C. Schalock, J. T. S. Hsu, & K. Arndt (Eds.), *Primary care dermatology* (pp. 20–27). Philadelphia: Lippincott, Williams & Wilkins.

Kolarsick, P. A., Kolarsick, M. A., & Goodwin, C. (2009). Anatomy and physiology of the skin. In P. Muehlbauer & C. McGowan (Eds.), *Site-specific cancer series: Skin cancer* (pp. 1–11). Pittsburgh: Oncology Nursing Society.

Lazareth, V. (2013). Management of non-melanoma skin cancer. Rieger, P. (Ed.), *Seminars in Oncology Nursing: Skin Cancer, 29*(3), 182–194.

Leung, A. M., Hari, D. M., & Morton, D. L. (2012). Surgery for distant melanoma metastasis. *Cancer Journal, 18*(2), 176–184.

National Comprehensive Cancer Network. (2013). http://www.nccn.org.

Nolen, M. E., Beebe, V. R., King, J. M., Bryn, N., & Limaye, K. M. (2009). Nonmelanoma skin cancer. In P. Muehlbauer & C. McGowan (Eds.), *Site-specific cancer series: Skin cancer* (pp. 13–49). Pittsburgh: Oncology Nursing Society.

Rubin, K. M. (2009). Melanoma staging: A review of the revised American Joint Committee on Cancer guidelines. *Journal of the Dermatology Nurses' Association, 2,* 254–259.

Rubin, K. M. (2013). Management of primary cutaneous and metastatic melanoma. *Seminars in Oncology Nursing: Skin Cancer, 29*(3), 195–205.

Siegel, R., Naishadham, D., & Jemal, A. (2013). Cancer statistics. *Cancer Journal for Clinicians, 63,* 11–30.

Skin Cancer Foundation. (2013). http://www.skincancer.org/skin-cancer-information.

Sosman, J. A. (2013a). Advanced melanoma: Anti-CTLA-4 antibodies and other immune checkpoint strategies. M. B. Atkins (Ed.), *UpToDate,* Waltham, MA.

Sosman, J. A. (2013b). Molecularly targeted therapy for metastatic melanoma. In M. B. Atkins (Ed.), *UpToDate.* Waltham, MA.

Tran, T. N. (2011). Premalignant and malignant skin lesions. In P. C. Schalock, J. T. S. Hsu, & K. Arndt (Eds.), *Primary care dermatology* (pp. 68–90). Philadelphia: Lippincott, Williams & Wilkins.

Tsao, H., & Gabree, M. J. (2013). Inherited susceptibility to melanoma. In M. B. Atkins (Ed.), *UpToDate.* Waltham, MA.

Wazer, D. (2013). *Role of radiation therapy in the management of melanoma.* In M. B. Atkins (Ed.), *UpToDate.* Waltham, MA.

Wong, S. L., Balch, C. M., Hurley, P., Agarwala, S. S., Akhurst, T. J., Cochran, A., et al. (2012). Sentinel lymph node biopsy for melanoma: American Society of Clinical Oncology and Society of Surgical Oncology joint clinical practice guideline. *Journal of Clinical Oncology, 30,* 2912–2918.

CHAPTER 13

Head and Neck Cancers

Ellen Carr

I. Introduction
   A. Include cancers of the oral cavity, oropharynx, nasal cavity, paranasal sinuses, nasopharynx, larynx, hypopharynx, and salivary glands; also cancers of the thyroid and parathyroid
   B. Incidence small in number (approximately 3% to 5% of all cancers) (National Cancer Institute [NCI], 2013e, f); patient coping with dysfunction and body image requires adaptation and support from nursing
      1. Incidence, staging, and treatment of cancer in this area depend on the specific location of the tumor.
      2. Most head and neck tumors occur in the oral cavity, larynx, and oropharynx (American Cancer Society [ACS], 2013a; Carr, 2011).
      3. Smoking cessation programs are encouraged to successfully help at-risk patients (for head and neck cancers) quit smoking (ACS, 2013a; NCI, 2013a).
   B. Epidemiology
      1. Usually occur in the 50- to 70-year age group (ACS, 2013a; Estrada, Van Waes, Moni, & Conley, 2010; NCI, 2013a)
      2. More men than women diagnosed with these cancers; exception: more women than men diagnosed with thyroid cancer; three of four thyroid cancers occur in women (NCI, 2013f).
      3. Risk factors for specific head and neck cancers (Box 13-1):
         a. Tobacco use increases the risk of developing head and neck cancers 25-fold; excessive alcohol intake increases the risk of developing oral or pharyngeal cancer ninefold (ACS, 2013a; Carr, 2011).
         b. Smokeless tobacco (snuff, chew), pipes, and cigars are also risk factors for head and neck cancers (ACS, 2013a; Carr, 2011).
         c. Infection with cancer-causing types of human papillomavirus (HPV), especially HPV-16, is a risk factor for some types of head and neck cancers, particularly oropharyngeal cancers (involving tonsils or the base of the tongue) (ACS, 2013a).
            (1) In the United States (U.S.), the incidence of oropharyngeal cancers caused by HPV infection is increasing, whereas the incidence of oropharyngeal cancers related to other causes is falling (NCI, 2013a).
   C. Histology classification of head and neck tumors— 90% squamous cell; 10% adenocarcinoma (salivary glands), melanoma, sarcoma, or lymphoma (Carr, 2011; Estrada et al., 2010)
      1. Rapid cell turnover in head and neck tumors affects their initial development and growth. The relatively high mitotic rate of tumor cells also provides the basis for treatment strategies (i.e., high-dose cancer therapies) (Mendenhall, Werning, & Pfister, 2011).
      2. The oral mucosa has a high cell turnover rate and is home to diverse and complex microflora. Therefore the mucosa, when treated with chemotherapy or radiation, is highly susceptible to treatment-related toxic side effects (NCI, 2013a).
   D. Developments in care and treatment—reduced deformities and improved cosmetic effect because of prosthetic devices and surgical flaps (myocutaneous and free flaps)
      1. Since the early 1970s, more conservative surgical technique and reconstruction have resulted in increased quality of life—decreasing dysfunctions (airway, communication, swallowing).
   E. Metastatic patterns
      1. Head and neck cancer is a locally aggressive disease that can spread regionally to the lymphatics of the neck (Figure 13-1).
      2. Most patients present with stage III or IV disease (tumor is very large, has invaded adjacent tissue, or is a primary tumor that has spread to the lymphatics) (Carr, 2011) (Figure 13-2).

Box 13-1

Risks for Specific Head and Neck Cancers

- Oral cavity—sun exposure (lip); human papillomavirus (HPV) infection.
- Salivary glands—radiation to the head and neck. This exposure can come from diagnostic x-rays or from radiation therapy (RT) for noncancerous conditions or cancer.
- Paranasal sinuses and nasal cavity—certain industrial exposures, such as wood or nickel dust inhalation. Tobacco and alcohol use may play less of a role in this type of cancer.
- Nasopharynx—Asian, particularly Chinese, ancestry; Epstein-Barr virus infection; occupational exposure to wood dust; consumption of certain preservatives or salted foods
- Oropharynx—poor oral hygiene, mechanical irritation such as from poorly fitting dentures, and use of mouthwash that has a high alcohol content

- Hypopharynx—Plummer-Vinson syndrome (also called *Paterson-Kelly syndrome*), a rare disorder that results from nutritional deficiencies. This syndrome is characterized by severe anemia and leads to difficulty swallowing because of webs of tissue that grow across the upper part of the esophagus.
- Larynx—exposure to airborne particles of asbestos, especially in the workplace
- *Note:* Those with previously diagnosed head and neck cancers are at risk to develop a new primary cancer, usually in the head and neck, esophagus, or lungs. Those who smoke are at higher risk for head and neck cancers.

Data from National Cancer Institute. (2013b). *Head and neck cancer: treatment.* http://www.cancer.gov/cancertopics/treatment/head-and-neck; and National Institutes of Health, National Institute of Dental and Craniofacial Research. (2011). *Detecting oral cancer: A guide for health care professionals.* http://www.nidcr.nih.gov/OralHealth/Topics/OralCancer/DetectingOralCancer.htm.

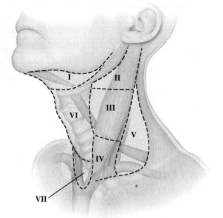

Figure 13-1 A, Regional lymphatic pattern in the head and neck. **B,** Neck levels of the head and neck. *From Friedman, M., Kelley, K., & Maley, A. (2011). Central neck dissection. Operative Techniques in Otolaryngology—Head and Neck Surgery 22(2): 169-172.*

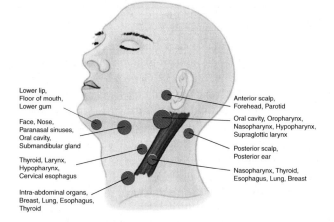

Figure 13-2 Likely sites of metastasis from various sites of the head and neck.

3. At the time of initial diagnosis, 43% have nodal involvement and 10% have distant metastasis (Carr, 2011; NCI, 2013a).
4. Head and neck cancers tend to recur locally; can also develop second primary head and neck cancers; depend on original cancer site and if patients continue to use tobacco and drink alcohol (Carr, 2011)
5. Most common sites of distant metastasis are the lung, liver, and bone.

F. Prognosis and trends in survival
  1. Several specific cancer categories grouped as head and neck cancers, with each category having its own incidence and survival rates.
  2. Survival rates
     a. Oral and pharyngeal cancers somewhat better; 1-year survival = 84%; 5-year survival = 62% (ACS, 2013a)
     b. For laryngeal cancer (all stages), 5-year survival if disease is local when detected, 60% to 90%; if regional, when detected, 60% to 75%; if distant metastases present when detected, 32% to 44% (ACS, 2013b)

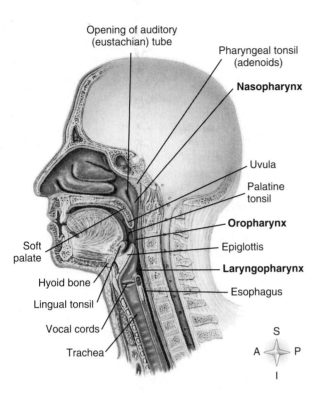

Opening of auditory (eustachian) tube

Pharyngeal tonsil (adenoids)

Nasopharynx

Uvula

Palatine tonsil

Oropharynx

Epiglottis

Laryngopharynx

Esophagus

Soft palate

Hyoid bone

Lingual tonsil

Vocal cords

Trachea

S

A ✦ P

I

Figure 13-3 Anatomy of the head and neck. *From Thibodeau, G, & Patton, K. (2003). Anatomy and physiology (6th ed.). St. Louis: Mosby.*

    c. Thyroid cancer overall 5-year survival rate 98% (ACS, 2013a)

  3. Increased risk of developing recurrent disease with smoking and drinking alcohol

  4. The rate of new cases of laryngeal cancer decreasing by about 2% to 3% a year, most likely because fewer people are smoking (ACS, 2013a)

II. Anatomy of the head and neck (Figure 13-3)

  A. Oral cavity—extends from the lips to the hard palate above and the circumvallate papillae below; structures include lips, buccal mucosa, floor of the mouth, upper and lower alveoli, retromolar trigone, hard palate, and anterior two thirds of the tongue

  B. Oropharynx—extends from the circumvallate papillae below and hard palate above to the level of the hyoid bone; structures include the base of tongue (posterior one third), soft palate, tonsils, and posterior pharyngeal wall

  C. Nasal cavity and paranasal sinuses—include nasal vestibule; paired maxillary, ethmoid, and frontal sinuses; and a single sphenoid sinus

  D. Nasopharynx—located below the base of skull and behind the nasal cavity; continuous with the posterior pharyngeal wall

  E. Larynx—extends from the epiglottis to the cricoid cartilage; protected by the thyroid cartilage, which encases it; subdivided into three areas

    1. Supraglottis—below the base of tongue, extending to but not including the true vocal cord; includes epiglottis, aryepiglottic folds, arytenoid cartilages, and false vocal cords

    2. Glottis—area of the true vocal cord

    3. Subglottis—below the true vocal cord, extending to the cricoid cartilage

  F. Hypopharynx—extends from the hyoid bone to the lower border of the cricoid cartilage; structures include pyriform sinuses, postcricoid region, and the lower posterior pharyngeal wall

  G. Thyroid—at base of neck, below Adam's apple; provides thyroid hormones to the system (NCI, 2013e)

  H. Parathyroid—located on the posterior thyroid; four glands (ranges from two to eight glands) in most people; glands provide parathyroid hormone to the system (NCI, 2013e)

  I. Critical adjacent structures (Carr, 2011; Estrada et al., 2010; Mendenhall et al., 2011)

    1. Regional lymph nodes of the neck drain the anatomic structures of the head and neck; the area includes submental submaxillary, upper and lower jugular, posterior triangle (spinal accessory), and preauricular nodes (see Figure 13-1).

    2. Head and neck structures are contiguous with the lower aerodigestive tract—trachea, lungs, and esophagus.

    3. The nasopharynx and paranasal sinuses are close to the brain.

III. Primary functions of the head and neck (Carr, 2011; Mendenhall et al., 2011)

  A. Respiration—the upper respiratory tract is passageway for transporting air into the lungs. The respiratory process is as follows:

    1. The diaphragm descends, increasing intrathoracic pressure.

    2. Negative pressure results in air entering the mouth and nose, where it is warmed, filtered, and humidified.

    3. Air enters the upper air passageways of the pharynx, larynx, and trachea and then enters the lung.

    4. The olfactory membrane lies along the superior part of each nostril as well as along the septum and superior turbinates. The olfactory cells within the membrane serve as receptors for the sense of smell.

  B. Speech is formed from sound waves created as air is expelled from the lungs, passing through the vocal cords. Speech is mechanically perfected through the following processes:

    1. Phonation—achieved by the larynx

    2. Articulation—achieved by the lips, tongue, and soft palate

3. Resonation— tone and quality of speech created by resonators (pharynx, mouth, nose, paranasal sinuses)
C. Swallowing—26 muscles and six cranial nerves orchestrate the transport of food from the mouth to the stomach in four phases of swallowing (Carr, 2011; Mendenhall et al., 2011).
   1. Oral preparatory—in the oral cavity, bolus of food is chewed and combined with saliva.
      a. Taste receptors are on the tongue, soft palate, glossopalatine arch, and posterior wall of the pharynx.
   2. Oral—the tongue, using front and back movement, propels bolus into the pharynx.
   3. Pharyngeal—the bolus moves through the pharynx and is propelled toward the esophagus; the vocal cords close, and the larynx moves upward and forward, preventing aspiration.
   4. Esophageal—the bolus moves through the esophagus and enters the stomach.
D. Hormone regulation
   1. Thyroid—thyroid hormones serve as a growth factor in bone formation and regulate metabolism (NCI, 2013f).
   2. Parathyroid—parathyroid hormone regulates the body's calcium level (NCI, 2013d).
IV. Functional changes associated with cancers of the head and neck (Carr, 2011; Mendenhall et al., 2011)
   A. Respiration
      1. Head and neck cancers affect the structures of the upper airway, which transports warmed, filtered, and humidified air into the lungs.
      2. When disease and treatment affect this area, the natural air-conditioning function of the upper air passageways is bypassed. The effect—cooling and dryness of the trachea and lungs—may lead to infection.
      3. When the upper airway is altered, the sense of smell changes (e.g., inability to sniff).
   B. Speech
      1. When the larynx is removed (all or part), it results in loss of vibrating component for speech; thus sound waves cannot be produced (total laryngectomy) or are diminished (partial).
      2. Surgery to the mouth, tongue, or palate causes changes in the person's ability to articulate clear, understandable speech.
      3. Cancer or treatment of the nose or paranasal sinuses influences the tone and quality of the speech.
   C. Swallowing
      1. Supraglottic laryngectomy affects the pharyngeal phase of swallowing, undermining the protection of the glottis. Until swallowing techniques are mastered, aspiration is a risk.

2. When the structures in the oral cavity and oropharynx undergo extensive resections (requiring flap reconstruction), swallowing phases (oral preparatory and oral) change and may result in the following:
   a. Drooling of saliva
   b. Decreased mastication
   c. Aspiration
   d. Pooling of food and fluids
3. Radiation therapy (RT) to this area causes decreased saliva production (xerostomia), with loss of lubrication of food bolus and taste changes.
   a. Thorough dental care is necessary before RT treatment begins.
   b. With RT, the risk for dental caries or osteoradionecrosis is increased.
   c. With RT, it is important to adhere to fluoride treatment protocol.
D. Trismus (restriction in opening the mouth)—may be a side effect of RT (NCI, 2013b).
   1. This condition may affect the client's ability to eat a regular diet. It also may affect the following:
      a. Speech
      b. Swallowing
      c. Mastication
      d. Adequate oral hygiene
   2. Jaw exercises to increase opening of the mouth may help reduce the stiffness of trismus.
      a. Specially trained speech pathologist can provide therapy and instruction
V. Principles of medical management
   A. Screening and diagnostic measures
      1. For early detection, no definitive screening examination established. However, thorough oral examination is recommended (ACS, 2013b).
         a. Every 3 years for 20- to 40-year-olds
         b. Every year for people older than 40 years
      2. Those diagnosed with head and neck cancers are at an increased risk of development other primary tumors because of prolonged exposure of the mucosal surface to carcinogens (NCI, 2013a).
         a. The initial workup includes evaluation to rule out multiple primary tumors.
   B. Evaluation of suspected head and neck tumors includes the following (Carr, 2011; Mendenhall et al., 2011):
      1. Thorough history and examination of all structures of the upper aerodigestive tract
      2. History of specific risk factors (see Box 13-1)
      3. Signs and symptoms of disease (Box 13-2)
      4. Physical examination
         a. Visualization

Box 13-2

Signs and Symptoms of Head and Neck Cancers*

Common Symptoms of Several Head and Neck Cancer Sites
- A lump or sore that does not heal
- A sore throat that does not go away
- Difficulty swallowing
- A change or hoarseness in the voice

Other Possible Symptoms
- Oral cavity
  - White or red patch on the gums, tongue, or lining of the mouth
  - Swelling of the jaw that causes dentures to fit poorly or become uncomfortable
  - Unusual bleeding or pain in the mouth
- Nasal cavity and sinuses
  - Sinuses that are blocked and do not clear
  - Chronic sinus infections that do not respond to treatment with antibiotics
  - Bleeding through the nose
  - Frequent headaches
  - Swelling or other trouble with the eyes
  - Pain in the upper teeth
  - Problems with dentures
- Salivary glands
  - Swelling under the chin or around the jawbone
  - Numbness or paralysis of the muscles in the face
  - Pain that does not go away in the face, chin, or neck
- Oropharynx and hypopharynx
  - Ear pain
- Nasopharynx
  - Trouble breathing or speaking
  - Frequent headaches
  - Pain or ringing in the ears, or trouble hearing
- Larynx
  - Pain when swallowing
  - Ear pain
  - Metastatic squamous neck cancer
  - Pain in the neck or throat that does not go away

*These symptoms may be caused by cancer or by other, less serious conditions. It is important to check with a physician or dentist about any of these symptoms.

Data from National Cancer Institute. (2013b). *Head and neck cancer: treatment.* http://www.cancer.gov/cancertopics/treatment/head-and-neck; Accessed 03/14/13; and National Institutes of Health, National Institute of Dental and Craniofacial Research. (2011). *Detecting oral cancer: A guide for health care professionals.* http://www.nidcr.nih.gov/OralHealth/Topics/OralCancer/DetectingOralCancer.htm.

---

   b. Mirror examination of the pharynx and larynx

   c. Palpation via a bimanual examination to assess the oral cavity and upper neck

5. Radiologic studies (Table 13-1)
   a. Computed tomography (CT)—to assist in determining the extent of the primary tumor and to identify metastasis to the cervical lymph nodes
   b. Chest radiography—to identify disease in the lung, a second primary tumor, or distant metastasis
   c. Panorex (radiography)—panoramic views to evaluate mandibular invasion from oral cavity and oropharyngeal lesions
   d. Magnetic resonance imaging (MRI)—superior to CT in staging nasopharyngeal primaries
   e. Cine-esophagography with barium swallow—to identify the extent of lesions in the oropharynx that may extend into the hypopharynx
   f. Positron emission tomography (PET) with CT (PET-CT)—helps pinpoint the location of cancer and detect distant metastasis
6. Laboratory studies—complete blood cell count, chemistry studies, liver function tests

7. Histologic diagnosis from the following:
   a. Fine-needle aspiration from suspicious neck nodes
   b. Excisional biopsy of the lesion—to diagnose or to cure
      (1) On small oral cavity, lip, or skin lesions
      (2) As a rule, an open or excisional biopsy of suspicious neck nodes contraindicated (to avoid seeding of the tumor)
         (a) Exception—when all other examinations fail to identify a primary site or when lymphoma is suspected
   c. Incisional biopsy—taking a small sample of tumor along with adjoining normal tissue.
   d. Panendoscopy (passing an endoscope along the entire mucosa of the upper aerodigestive tract)—to examine and perform a biopsy on suspicious areas, determine the full extent of disease, and identify synchronous primary tumors
8. Pathology or histologic diagnosis based on molecular pathway expression and targeted markers
   a. Identification of p16 and p53 protein expression and high-risk HPV (HPV-HR) types have been associated with survival in

Part 2

Table 13-1

Diagnostic Procedures in Evaluation of Head and Neck Tumors

Description	Time Required	Sensations Experienced	Potential Side Effects and Complications	Self-Care Measures	Symptoms to Report to Health Care Team
Panoramic Radiography (Panorex)					
Examination of an entire dental arch viewed on one film To evaluate mandibular invasion	10 min	None	None	None	N/A
Cine-esophagography					
Video radiography of oral and pharyngeal stages of swallowing To identify extension of lesions into hypopharynx	30 min	Vary, depending on degree of dysphagia	Aspiration	None	Temperature elevation Productive cough
Barium Swallow and Radiography of Upper Gastrointestinal Tract					
To evaluate tumor invasion of hypopharynx and cervical esophagus	15 min	Chalky taste	Constipation secondary to use of barium	Assess bowel function Take laxative, as needed Force fluids	No bowel movement for 3 days Abdominal distention
Panendoscopy					
Surgical procedure in which a lighted scope is passed along the upper aerodigestive tract to inspect and obtain biopsy specimens from areas of the entire mucosa (includes bronchoscopy, esophagoscopy, laryngoscopy) To detect metastasis or second primary tumor	1 hr	Related to general anesthesia	Reactions to general anesthesia Airway obstruction Tracheoesophageal fistula Sore throat Aspiration Hemorrhage from biopsy site Pneumothorax	Deep-breathe, turn, ambulate	Difficulty breathing Excessive bleeding Inability to swallow (nurse should check for return of gag reflex) Increased temperature, cough, or sputum production

N/A, Not applicable.

Data from Yarbro, C.H., Wujcik, D., Gobel, B.H. (Eds.) (2011). *Cancer nursing: principles and practice* (7th ed.). Sudbury, MA: Jones and Bartlet; and DeVita, V.T., Lawrence, T.S., & Rosenberg, S.A. (Eds.) (2011). *Cancer: principles and practice of oncology* (9th ed.). Philadelphia: Lippincott Williams & Wilkins.

---

head and neck malignancies. Evidence suggests that multiple molecular pathways better predict the outcomes and potentially the type of treatment targeted to those markers (Smith, Rubenstein, Hoffman, Haugen, & Lubomir, 2010).

C. Staging—TNM (tumor–node–metastasis) classification system for specific diagnoses developed by the American Joint Committee on Cancer (Edge et al., 2010) (Table 13-2; Figure 13-4)

D. Histologic grading (Edge et al., 2010)
1. GX—grade cannot be assessed
2. G2—well differentiated
3. G3—poorly differentiated
4. G4—undifferentiated

E. Treatment strategies
1. Surgery and radiation—the primary treatment modalities for managing malignant head and neck tumors; adjuvant chemotherapy for recurrent and metastatic disease (Estrada et al., 2010)
   a. Best to implement interdisciplinary (interprofessional) approach to managing the patient and family with head and neck cancers on admission (e.g., nurses, various physicians, dental, social worker, nutritionists, physical therapist [PT], occupational therapist [OT])
2. Treatment—based on the TNM classification
   a. For T1 and T2 lesions of the oral cavity, larynx, nose, and paranasal sinuses, treatment is surgery or radiation.

Table 13-2

Overview of Selected TNM Staging of Cancers of the Head and Neck*

Classification

T = Primary Tumor

General: for All Sites

TX	Primary tumor cannot be assessed
T0	No evidence of primary tumor
Tis	Carcinoma in situ

Oral Cavity, Oropharynx

T1	Greatest diameter of primary tumor ≤2 cm
T2	>2 cm or ≤4 cm
T3	>4 cm
T4a or T4b	Moderately to very advanced local disease, with invasion deep or to adjacent structures

Hypopharynx

T1	Tumor limited to one subsite of hypopharynx and ≤2 cm in greatest dimension
T2	Tumor invades more than one subsite of hypopharynx or an adjacent site, or measures >2 cm or ≤4 cm without fixation of the hemilarynx
T3	Tumor measures >4 cm or with fixation of hemilarynx or extension to esophagus
T4a or T4b	Moderately to very advanced local disease; involves adjacent structures (e.g., cartilage or soft tissues of neck)

Nasopharynx

T1	Tumor confined to nasopharynx or tumor extends to oropharynx and/or nasal cavity without parapharyngeal extension.
T2	Tumor with parapharyngeal extension
T3	Tumor involves bony structures of skull base and/or paranasal sinuses
T4a or T4b	Invasion into skull and/or cranial nerve(s)

Larynx

Glottic

T1	Limited to true vocal cords; normal vocal cord mobility; may include anterior or posterior commissure
T2	Supraglottic or subglottic extension; normal or impaired mobility
T3	Confined to larynx proper; vocal cord fixation
T4a or T4b	Moderately to very advanced local disease, cartilage destruction and/or extension out of larynx to adjacent structures

Supraglottic

T1	Limited to subsite of supraglottis; normal vocal cord mobility
T2	Extension to glottis or adjacent supraglottic subsite; normal vocal cord mobility
T3	Confined to larynx proper; cord fixation and/or extension into hypopharynx or pre-epiglottic space
T4a or T4b	Moderately to very advanced local disease, invasion of adjacent structures cartilage destruction, and/or extension out of larynx

Subglottic

T1	Limited to subglottic region
T2	Extension to vocal cord(s) with normal or impaired mobility
T3	Limited to larynx; vocal cord fixation
T4a or T4b	Moderately to very advanced local disease, invasion of adjacent structures, cartilage destruction and/or extension out of larynx

N = Nodal Metastasis

NX	Nodes cannot be assessed
N0	No regional lymph node metastasis
N1	Single, ipsilateral node: ≤3 cm
N2A	Single, ipsilateral node: >3 cm or ≤6 cm
N2B	Multiple, ipsilateral nodes: all ≤6 cm
N2C	Metastasis in bilateral or contralateral lymph nodes, none more than 6 cm in greatest dimension
N3	Metastasis in a lymph node > 6 cm in dimension

M = Distant Metastasis

M0	No distant metastasis
M1	Distant metastasis present

Continued

Part 2

Table 13-2

Overview of Selected TNM Staging of Cancers of the Head and Neck—cont'd*

Stage Groupings

Stage 0	Tis, N0, M0
Stage I	T1, N0, M0
Stage II	T2, N0, M0
Stage III	T3, N0, M0; T1, T2, or T3 with N1, M0
Stage IVA	T4a or T4b, N0 or N1, M0 T1, T2 or T3, T4a, N2, M0
Stage IVB	T4b, Any N, M0 Any T, N3, Mo
Stage IVC	Any T, any N, M1

*Changes to system include subcategories for T4 lesions (T4a: resectable; T4b: unresectable).

Used with permission of the American Joint Committee on Cancer (AJCC), Chicago, Illinois. The original source for this material is the AJCC Cancer Staging Manual, Seventh Edition (2010) published by Springer Science and Business Media LLC, www.springer.com.

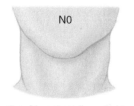

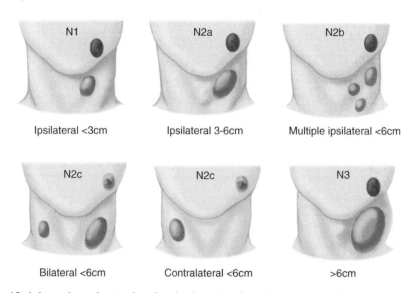

Figure 13-4 Lymph node staging for the head and neck. *From Som, P. M., & Curtin, H. D. (2002). Head and neck imaging (4th ed.). St. Louis: Mosby.*

b. For T3 and T4 tumors, treatment is combination therapy.

c. For N1, N2, and N3, see Table 13-2.

d. For clinically negative neck nodes and a large primary lesion (T2, N0) of the oral cavity, oropharynx, hypopharynx, or larynx, treatment is either lymphadenectomy or radiation (because tumor cells can spread) (Mendenhall et al., 2011).

3. Surgery

a. Common surgical procedures used in treating head and neck malignancies (Table 13-3).

4. Radiation therapy (see Chapter 21 for nursing diagnoses and interventions related to RT)

a. Primary treatment to control the primary tumor and adjacent lymph nodes while maintaining structure and

Table 13-3

Surgical Procedures for Head and Neck Cancers

Procedure	Physical Alteration	Nursing Implications
Laser	Little to none	Minimal bleeding
Composite resection	Resection of oral cavity, oropharyngeal lesion in continuity with neck dissection Portion of mandible is resected Reconstruction with myocutaneous flaps is usually required, with resections of large amounts of tissue	May experience problems with speech (decreased articulation with tongue involvement), swallowing (impaired mastication, salivary drooling, aspiration), altered facial contour
Supraglottic laryngectomy	Resection of structures above the false vocal cords, including the epiglottis (preserves the true vocal cords)	Aspiration until swallowing techniques are learned Maintains a relatively normal voice
Hemilaryngectomy	Vertical excision of one true and one false cord and underlying cartilage	Hoarse voice Minimal or no swallowing problems
Total laryngectomy	Excision of the entire larynx from the hyoid bone to the second tracheal ring	Permanent tracheostomy Aphonia Decreased sense of smell Unable to perform Valsalva maneuver
Maxillectomy	Partial or total en bloc resection of the cavity May include the ethmoid sinus, lateral nasal wall, palate, and floor of orbit	Preoperatively, maxillofacial prosthodontist makes dental obturator to fill the large surgical defect and to facilitate swallowing Requires daily care to cavity and placement of obturator
Orbital exenteration	Resection of orbit secondary to extension of maxillary sinus tumor or recurrent disease	Facial defect Unilateral vision loss Requires daily care and cleansing of cavity
Craniofacial, skull base resection	Surgical approach to inaccessible midfacial and extensive paranasal sinus and nasopharyngeal lesions	May have facial defect and cranial nerve (III, IV, V) deficits
Radical neck dissection	Resection of sternocleidomastoid muscle, jugular vein, spinal accessory nerve, and cervical lymph nodes	Shoulder droop Concave contour of neck
Modified neck dissection	Radical neck dissection with preservation of the sternocleidomastoid muscle, jugular vein, or spinal accessory nerve	Shoulder droop if spinal accessory nerve resected Concave contour of neck
Lymphadenectomy	Resection of lymph nodes in neck	Surgical scars

Data from American Cancer Society (ACS). (2013b). *Laryngeal and hypopharyngeal cancer.* http://www.cancer.org/cancer/laryngealandhypopharyngealcancer/detailedguide/index; American Cancer Society (ACS). (2013c). *Surgery for laryngectomy.* http://www.cancer.org/cancer/laryngealandhypopharyngealcancer/detailedguide/laryngeal-and-hypopharyngeal-cancer-treating-surgery; and National Cancer Institute. (2013b). *Head and neck cancer: Treatment.* http://www.cancer.gov/cancertopics/treatment/head-and-neck.

function—external beam dose range 6000 to 7000 centigray (cGy) (Carr, 2011; Foote & Ang, 2012; Mendenhall et al., 2011)

b. Adjuvant treatment for stages III and IV disease and tumors that can spread toward the midline (e.g., oropharyngeal lesions)—external beam dose approximately 5000 cGy (Foote & Ang, 2012; Mendenhall et al., 2011)

c. External beam RT performed approximately 4 to 6 weeks after surgery

d. Preoperative radiation or permanently placed iodine-125 seeds used to debulk large or unresectable lesions

   (1) Advantage—fewer wound complications

(2) Need to have preoperative dental evaluations, removal of diseased teeth, and prophylactic fluoride treatment

(3) Postoperative radiation started after wounds heal (3 to 6 weeks); treatment is for 6 to 7 weeks.

e. Treatment for nasopharyngeal cancer primarily radiation

   (1) Surgery avoided because area is close to vital structures of the brain

   (2) Carefully selected clients who experience treatment failure with RT treated with base-of-skull resection of tumor

---

f. Brachytherapy—treatment for lesions of the anterior and posterior tongue, floor of mouth, and nasal vestibule (implanted iridium-192 or cesium-137)

  (1) Maximizes dose to the tumor bed and minimizes exposure to surrounding tissue

g. For metastatic thyroid cancer, iodine-191 ablation treatment after thyroidectomy (NCI, 2013f)

5. Chemotherapy (see Chapter 22 for nursing diagnoses and interventions related to chemotherapy)

  a. Chemotherapy alone not curative

    (1) Reduces tumor volume or rids clinically detectable squamous cell carcinomas

    (2) Treatment for recurrent or metastatic disease

  b. As adjuvant and neoadjuvant therapy, single-agent or combination chemotherapy regimens—cisplatin (Platinol), bleomycin (Blenoxane), fluorouracil (5-Fluorouracil, 5-FU), paclitaxel (Taxol), and methotrexate (Mexate); also for palliative therapy for recurrent or unresectable lesions (Carr, 2011; Estrada et al., 2010; Mendenhall et al., 2011)

  c. Combination protocols of chemotherapy with RT used because of sensitizing effect of chemotherapy

    (1) Example—RADPLAT (protocol for mouth cancers; strategy is concurrent RT and cisplatin infusion to the tumor) (Mendenhall et al., 2011)

6. Targeted therapies

  a. Treatment for those diagnosed with HPV-positive oropharyngeal cancer may be different from that for those with oropharyngeal cancers that are HPV-negative. Recent research has shown that patients with HPV-positive oropharyngeal tumors have a better prognosis and may do just as well on less intense treatment (NCI, 2013a; Smith et al., 2010).

  b. Strategies for targeted therapy include blockage of growth factor–based cellular signaling and interference with angiogenesis-related pathways (ACS, 2013b).

  c. Examples of targeted therapies treatments are as follows:

    (1) EGFR inhibitors (cetuximab, panitumumab, zalutumumab)

    (2) EGFR tyrosine kinase inhibitors (gefitinib, erlotinib)

    (3) VEGFR inhibitors (bevacizumab, vandetanib)

  d. Targeted therapies may be combined with radiation therapy.

7. Palliative therapy

  a. Surgery, radiation, chemotherapy, or combination therapy is used for unresectable lesions or recurrent tumors or when surgery is considered high risk.

  b. To relieve pain, bleeding, or obstruction, treatment may include short courses of radiation (3000 cGy over 2 to 3 weeks) (Erickson et al., 2011; Foote & Ang, 2012; Mendenhall et al., 2011).

VI. Nursing implications

A. Preoperative preparation (Baehring & McCorkle, 2012; Carr, 2011)

1. Initiation of patient and family preoperative teaching; discussion about disease, treatment, side effects, and anticipated postoperative changes

2. Providing instruction about equipment (tracheostomy tube, drains, nasogastric tube, tonsil-tip suction catheter)

3. Providing counseling and support, as needed

4. Discussing economic and rehabilitation resources

5. Preoperatively determining the reading ability and planning for postoperative communication

  a. Paper and pencil

  b. Magic slate

  c. Picture board

  d. Nonverbal cues

  e. Electronic communication board or device

B. Postoperative interventions to maximize safety for client (Carr, 2011; NCI, 2013b)

1. Placement of patient in proximity to nurses' station to monitor client with altered airway

2. For tracheotomy patients, ensuring that the tracheotomy is securely held in place

  a. Keeping an extra tracheostomy tube of the same size (inner and outer cannulas and obturator), scissors, cotton-free gauze, and a tracheal dilator at the bedside

3. Keeping the call bell within reach at all times

4. Identifying a method of communication if patient has a tracheostomy

5. Observing for signs and symptoms of delirium tremens in patients with recent history of alcohol abuse

6. Observing for aspiration in patients who have had a supraglottic laryngectomy (includes resection of structures in the oropharynx, or cranial nerve [IX, X, XII] deficits)

7. For patients at risk for carotid rupture, implementing carotid precautions

C. Postoperative interventions to decrease severity of symptoms

1. Managing the airway (tracheostomy) (ACS, 2013c; Carr, 2011; Mendenhall et al., 2011)
   a. Permanent tracheostomy (total laryngectomy)
      (1) Airway
         (a) Use of a cuffed tracheostomy tube when client needs mechanical ventilation; may be removed by postoperative day 2 or 3
      (2) Laryngectomy tube used if stoma begins to narrow
   b. Humidity
      (1) Humidified air or oxygen provided via a tracheostomy collar to prevent mucosa drying and crusting of secretions
      (2) Application of moistened 4 × 4 gauze pads over stoma to provide humidity
      (3) Providing advice that a stoma bib worn over the stoma helps lessen drying of mucosa
      (4) Teaching about symptoms of inadequate humidity—thick, tenacious secretions that are difficult to expectorate
   c. Stoma care
      (1) Cleansing stoma with 50% peroxide and 50% normal saline solution
      (2) Removal of all mucous crusting twice each day and as needed
      (3) Removal of visible mucous plugs with a Kelly clamp
      (4) Application of a thin layer of prescribed ointment around the stoma twice each day
2. Temporary tracheostomy (ACS, 2013c; NCI, 2013e)
   a. If mechanical ventilation is needed or if the patient is at risk for aspiration, a cuffed tube is kept inflated. (The tube is usually placed in the operating room and maintained for 5 days.)
   b. The physician usually changes initial tracheostomy tube to a noncuffed tube. (If the patient is aspirating, the cuffed tube is maintained.)
   c. As edema decreases, the patient may be able to breathe without the tracheostomy tube.
      (1) The tube is downsized to a no. 4 or 5 or fenestrated tube.
      (2) The tube is plugged for 24 hours.
      (3) If the patient can breathe with the tube plugged for a prolonged time and can expectorate secretions through the mouth, the patient's cannula can be removed.
      (4) Stoma care—mucous crustings around stoma (opening in neck) are removed. Care must be taken in cleaning rim area around stoma so that patient does not aspirate debris or saline used when cleaning. The dressing (small gauze pad, affixed with tape) over the stoma is changed every day or as needed. Once healed, stoma cover (small bandana-like fabric) can cover stoma to protect it from debris from room air.
      (5) Until the wound has sealed, the patient must be taught to place a finger over stoma dressing when coughing or speaking.
   d. For all tracheostomies, suctioning is based on the need for airway clearance.
      (1) To prevent hypoxemia and arrhythmia, the lungs are hyperoxygenated, hyperinflated, or both before and after suctioning.
      (2) To precipitate coughing and mobilize secretions if needed, 2 to 5 mL of normal saline solution is instilled into the tracheostomy for lavage and the trachea and bronchi are stimulated.
      (3) To mobilize secretions and prevent atelectasis, an incentive spirometer is attached via a female adapter to a plastic tracheostomy tube, chest physical therapy is provided (as indicated), or both.
      (4) The color, amount, and odor of sputum produced and how frequently suctioning is required are recorded.
3. Tracheostomy care (Carr, 2011; Eadie & Bowker, 2012; Mendenhall et al., 2011; NCI, 2013b)
   a. The inner cannula is removed and cleansed of all mucus and crusts initially with a solution of 50% peroxide and 50% normal saline every 4 to 8 hours, then twice daily and as needed.
   b. The soiled tracheostomy ties are replaced, as needed. To determine tightness, one fingerbreadth should be allowed underneath the ties.
4. Wound care (Carr, 2011)
   a. Every 3 to 4 hours, the surgical wounds are assessed, noting color (pink versus cyanotic), temperature, and capillary refill (immediately after blanching) of skin and muscle flaps.
   b. Excessive pressure that interferes with flap perfusion and viability (e.g., tight tracheostomy ties, oxygen collars, hyperextension of the neck, and the client lying on the flap) should be avoided.
   c. The integrity of suture lines, both external and intraoral (if applicable) is assessed; breakdown may be the first sign of wound infection or fistula formation.
   d. The external suture lines are cleaned with a solution of 50% peroxide and 50% normal

saline; then the prescribed ointment is applied every 4 to 8 hours.

  e. If the patient has had nasal surgery, a maxillectomy, an orbital exenteration, or a combination of all these, as ordered by the physician, the cavities are gently cleansed to remove accumulated crusts.

    (1) A solution of 50% normal saline and 50% sodium bicarbonate or normal saline solution alone is used.

  f. Wound drains are assessed for color, amount, and odor of drainage, and drain patency is maintained.

    (1) If not prevented or treated early, clotting and air leaks may lead to wound infections.

5. Oral care (ACS, 2013b; Li & Trovato, 2012; NCI, 2013c; Song, Twumasi-Ankrah, & Salcido, 2012)

  a. Prevention—thorough and frequent mouth care

    (1) As ordered by physician, systematic oral care is performed at least every 4 hours with soft toothbrush and a rinse of normal saline or a solution of 50% normal saline and 50% baking soda. Nonabrasive (waxed) dental floss should be used.

    (2) A fluoridated toothpaste or a fluoride treatment recommended by the dentist should be used.

    (3) To gently cleanse the cavity, a gravity gavage or jet-spray dental cleansing system is used.

D. Nutrition (ACS, 2013b; Jack, Dawson, Reilly, & Shoaib, 2012)

1. The patient's nutritional status should be assessed before surgery; 60% of head and neck patients initially present with malnutrition.

  a. Nutrition should be protein-rich, easy to swallow (e.g., protein shakes, soups, pudding), given in small and frequent meals (if needed) to meet daily caloric requirements, and promote adequate, continuous hydration.

2. It is important to identify patients who have nutritional deficiencies and require oral, enteral, or parenteral nutritional supplements.

  a. Greater than 10% body weight loss during any treatment phase

  b. More than 20% below ideal body weight

3. The physician should be consulted about the methods of nutritional support—enteral tube feedings, other methods.

4. The client should be assessed after surgery for swallowing dysfunction.

E. Mobility

1. Neck dissection—the spinal accessory nerve and the sternocleidomastoid muscles may be resected; physical therapy referral needed to evaluate and treat

  a. Could result in shoulder droop, atrophy of the trapezius muscle, forward curvature of the spine, and limited range of motion (approximately 90 degrees) of the shoulder

  b. Treatment—after wound drains removed and patient has progressed to resistive exercises, initiate passive and active range of motion shoulder exercises; optimal goal is functional range of 150 degrees.

F. Body image changes (Eadie, Day, Sawin, Lamvik, & Doyle, 2013; Scarpa et al., 2011).

1. Promoting control of secretion and odors; teaching wound, oral, and tracheostomy care

2. Encouraging self-care activities (e.g., tracheostomy care, tube feeding, suctioning) and activities of daily living (e.g., grooming, hair combing, shaving, applying makeup)

3. Encouraging resocialization: progressive ambulation, social interactions, support group participation (e.g., Voice Masters, Lost Chord Club, I Can Cope, CanSurmount)

4. On admission and ongoing during period of care, consultation with the social worker to assist with counseling and financial, vocational, and adjustment issues

5. Informing the patient of resources to purchase tracheostomy covers, scarves, makeup, or other cosmetic assistance; consulting with the ACS Look Good, Feel Better programs (e.g., hair care, scarves)

6. Supporting patients and their families to grieve; allowing them to voice concerns, fears, and anxieties

G. Interventions to enhance adaptation and rehabilitation

1. Communication (Luckett, Britton, Clover, & Rankin, 2011)

  a. Cancers in the oral cavity affect the function of articulation; therapy includes the following:

    (1) Exercises to increase strength, range of motion, coordination, and accuracy of tongue movement

    (2) Use of oral prostheses to compensate for tissue loss and allow for greater contact of the tongue with the palate, creating more intelligible speech

  b. Cancers in the larynx affect phonation; therapy includes the following:

    (1) After a partial laryngectomy, exercises to improve voice quality, pitch, and loudness

(2) After a total laryngectomy
(a) Use of artificial larynx that transmits sound into the vocal tract
(b) Use of esophageal speech—air is swallowed and trapped in the esophagus, then released, allowing air to vibrate against the walls of the esophagus
(c) Use of tracheoesophageal prosthesis—placement of a prosthesis in a surgically created tracheoesophageal fistula; sound is formed by air from the lungs, creating a better quality of esophageal speech (NCI, 2013e; Carr, 2011).

2. Swallowing (Carr, 2011)
a. Surgeries in the head and neck may affect swallowing.
b. A thorough clinical evaluation of the oral preparatory and pharyngeal stages of swallowing should be performed.
c. To assess the oral and pharyngeal stages of the swallow, a barium swallow and radiography or cine-esophagography are performed.
d. A swallowing plan for the patient includes the following (Carr, 2011):
(1) Compensatory strategies—postural changes that facilitate passage of food into the oral cavity and pharynx (head elevated, upper body upright positioning); changes in food consistency (i.e., thin versus thick fluids, semisolid versus pureed foods)
(2) Indirect swallowing therapy—jaw and tongue range of motion exercises; adduction of tongue exercises to improve laryngeal closure
(3) Direct swallowing therapy using supraglottic swallow, with the following instructions to the patient:
(a) Prepare the bolus of food in the oral preparatory phase.
(b) Before initiating the swallow, hold breath to close vocal cords.
(c) Swallow while still holding breath.
(d) Cough while exhaling after the swallow to expectorate remaining food or fluids on top of vocal cords.
(e) Repeat steps c and d (swallow and cough).
(4) To avoid aspiration, the cuff on the tracheostomy tube is partially or totally inflated during meals and 30 minutes afterward.
(5) With some patients, removal of the tracheostomy tube improves swallowing by allowing the larynx to elevate.
(6) Until the patient can take adequate amounts by mouth, enteral tube feedings are used to maintain nutritional requirements.

References

American Cancer Society (ACS). (2013a). *Cancer facts & figures 2013.* http://www.cancer.org/research/cancerfactsfigures/cancerfactsfigures/cancer-facts-figures-2013.

American Cancer Society (ACS). (2013b). *Laryngeal and hypopharyngeal cancer.* http://www.cancer.org/cancer/laryngealandhypopharyngealcancer/detailedguide/index.

American Cancer Society (ACS). (2013c). *Surgery for laryngectomy.* http://www.cancer.org/cancer/laryngealandhypopharyngealcancer/detailedguide/laryngeal-and-hypopharyngeal-cancer-treating-surgery.

Baehring, E., & McCorkle, R. (2012). Postoperative complications in head and neck cancer. *Clinical Journal of Oncology Nursing,* 16(6), E203–E209. http://dx.doi.org/10.1188/12.CJON.E203-E209.

Carr, E. (2011). Head and neck malignancies. In C. H. Yarbro, D. Wujcik, & B. H. Gobel (Eds.), *Cancer nursing: Principles and practice.* (7th ed., pp. 1334–1368). Sudbury, MA: Jones and Bartlett.

Eadie, T. L., & Bowker, B. C. (2012). Coping and quality of life after total laryngectomy. *Otolaryngology: Head and Neck Surgery, 146* (6), 959–965. http://dx.doi.org/10.1177/0194599812437315.

Eadie, T. L., Day, A. M., Sawin, D. E., Lamvik, K., & Doyle, P. C. (2013). Auditory-perceptual speech outcomes and quality of life after total laryngectomy. *Otolaryngology: Head and Neck Surgery,* 148(1), 82–88. http://dx.doi.org/10.1177/0194599812461755.

Edge, S. B., Byrd, D. R., Compton, C. C., Fritz, A. G., Greene, F. L., & Trotti, A. (2010). *AJCC cancer staging manual* (7th ed., pp. 21–99). New York: Springer.

Erickson, B. A., Demanes, D. J., Ibbott, G. S., Hayes, J. K., Hsu, I. C., Morris, D. E., et al. (2011). American Society for Radiation Oncology (ASTRO) and American College of Radiology (ACR) practice guideline for the performance of high-dose-rate brachytherapy. *International Journal of Radiation Oncology, Biology, Physics, 79*(3), 641–649. http://dx.doi.org/10.1016/j.ijrobp.2010.08.046.

Estrada, D. T., VanWaes, C., Moni, J., & Conley, B. A. (2010). Head and neck cancer. In J. Abraham, J. L. Gulley, & C. J. Allegra (Eds.), *Bethesda handbook of clinical oncology.* (3rd ed., pp. 3–32). Philadelphia: Lippincott Williams & Wilkins.

Foote, R. L., & Ang, K. K. (2012). Head and neck tumors. In L. L. Gunderson & J. E. Tepper (Eds.), *Clinical radiation oncology: Expert consult.* (3rd ed., pp. 543–782). Philadelphia: Elsevier Saunders.

Jack, D. R., Dawson, F. R., Reilly, J. E., & Shoaib, T. (2012). Guideline for prophylactic feeding tube insertion in patients undergoing resection of head and neck cancers. *Journal of Plastic, Reconstructive & Aesthetic Surgery, 65*(5), 610–615. http://dx.doi.org/10.1016/j.bjps.2011.11.018.

Li, E., & Trovato, J. A. (2012). New developments in management of oral mucositis in patients with head and neck cancer or receiving targeted anticancer therapies. *American Journal of Health System Pharmacy, 69,* 1031–1037.

Luckett, T., Britton, B., Clover, K., & Rankin, N. M. (2011). Evidence for interventions to improve psychological outcomes in people with head and neck cancer: A systematic review of the literature. *Support Care Cancer, 19*(7), 871–881. http://dx.doi.org/10.1007/s00520-011-1119-7.

Mendenhall, W. M., Werning, J. W., & Pfister, D. G. (2011). Treatment of head and neck cancers. In V. T. DeVita, T. S. Lawrence, & S. A. Rosenberg (Eds.), *Cancer: Principles and practice of oncology.* (9th ed., pp. 662–731). Philadelphia: Lippincott Williams & Wilkins.

National Cancer Institute. (2013a). *Head and neck cancer.* http://www.cancer.gov/cancertopics/factsheet/Sites-Types/head-and-neck.

National Cancer Institute. (2013b). *Head and neck cancer: Treatment.* http://www.cancer.gov/cancertopics/treatment/head-and-neck.

National Cancer Institute. (2013c). *Oral complications of chemotherapy and head/neck radiation.* http://www.cancer.gov/cancertopics/pdq/supportivecare/oralcomplications/HealthProfessional.

National Cancer Institute. (2013d). *Parathyroid cancer.* http://www.cancer.gov/cancertopics/types/parathyroid.

National Cancer Institute. (2013e). *Throat (laryngeal and pharyngeal) cancer.* http://www.cancer.gov/cancertopics/types/throat.

National Cancer Institute. (2013f). *Thyroid cancer.* http://www.cancer.gov/cancertopics/types/thyroid.

National Institutes of Health (NIH) National Institute of Dental and Craniofacial Research. (2011). *Detecting oral cancer: A guide for health care professionals.* http://www.nidcr.nih.gov/OralHealth/Topics/OralCancer/DetectingOralCancer.htm.

Scarpa, M., Valente, S., Alfieri, R., Cagol, M., Diamantis, G., Ancona, E., et al. (2011). Systematic review of health-related quality of life after esophagectomy for esophageal cancer. *World Journal of Gastroenterology, 17*(42), 4660–4674. http://dx.doi.org/10.3748/wjg.v17.i42.4660.

Smith, E., Rubenstein, L., Hoffman, H., Haugen, T., & Lubomir, P. (2010). Human papillomavirus, p16 and p53 expression associated with survival of head and neck cancer. *Infect Agent Cancer, 5,* 4. http://dx.doi.org/10.1186/1750-9378-5-4.

Song, J. J., Twumasi-Ankrah, P., & Salcido, R. (2012). Systematic review and meta-analysis on the use of honey to protect from the effects of radiation-induced oral mucositis. *Advances in Skin & Wound Care, 25*(1), 23–28. http://dx.doi.org/10.1097/01.ASW.0000410687.14363.a3.

CHAPTER 14

Cancers of the Neurologic System

Mady C. Stovall, Nanette C. Fong, Carrie Graham, Stacey Danielle Green, and Gabriele Brunhart Tsung

OVERVIEW

I. Brain
  A. Anatomy (Crossman & Neary, 2010)
    1. Main structures of the brain
      a. Cerebrum—large outer part of the brain, two hemispheres comprising four lobes: frontal, occipital, parietal, and temporal
      b. Cerebellum—located in the posterior fossa at the back of the head
      c. Brainstem—located at the base of the brain and top of the spinal cord, connects cerebrum with the spinal cord; consists of midbrain, pons, medulla oblongata and reticular formation
    2. Critical adjacent structures
      a. Meninges—three membranes that cover the brain and spinal cord; outermost layer is the dura, a thick, whitish, inelastic covering
      b. Ventricles—connected cavities that contain cerebral spinal fluid (CSF); two lateral ventricles, third ventricle, and fourth ventricle
        (1) CSF—clear watery fluid made in the choroid plexus that nourishes and protects the brain
      c. Cerebral blood vessels
        (1) Two vertebral arteries and two internal carotid arteries supply blood to the brain.
        (2) The circle of Willis connects the anterior and posterior arteries to provide alternative routes if blood flow to single vessel is blocked.
        (3) Venous drainage occurs via the dural sinuses, which are vascular channels between the two layers of the dura.
      d. Blood-brain barrier
        (1) Tight junction among cells of the brain capillaries that selectively allows substances to cross neuronal membranes
        (2) Maintains brain's metabolic balance and keeps harmful toxins from getting into the brain
        (3) Movement across barrier depends on particle size, lipid solubility, chemical dissociations, and protein-binding potential
      a. Skull—acts as protective framework
      b. Cranial nerves—12 pairs; 10 arise from brainstem and two from the cerebrum (Figure 14-1)
    3. Cells of interest
      a. Glial cells (three types of supportive cells of the brain)
        (1) Astrocytes—connective tissue for supporting and nourishing neurons
        (2) Oligodendrocytes—produce myelin, a fatty substance that surrounds and insulates the nerve cells axons of the brain and spinal cord
        (3) Ependymal cells—line the ventricles and form a pathway through which CSF flows
      b. Other pertinent cells of consideration
        (1) Meninges—cover or protect brain and spinal cord
        (2) Neurons—important for cognitive functioning
        (3) Lymphocytes—immune mediation
  B. Functions of the brain (Crossman & Neary, 2010; National Brain Tumor Society, 2013) (Figure 14-2)
    1. Frontal lobe—personality, higher-order functioning, planning, reasoning, judgment, impulse control, memory, speech (in left frontal lobe for most right-handed people)
      a. Broca region—functions in understanding of language, speech, and control of facial neuron
    2. Motor strip—at junction of frontal and parietal lobes; right hemisphere motor strip controls left side body motor function; left hemisphere motor strip controls right side body motor function
    3. Parietal lobe—integrates sensory input; visual and tactile perception, coordinating input from

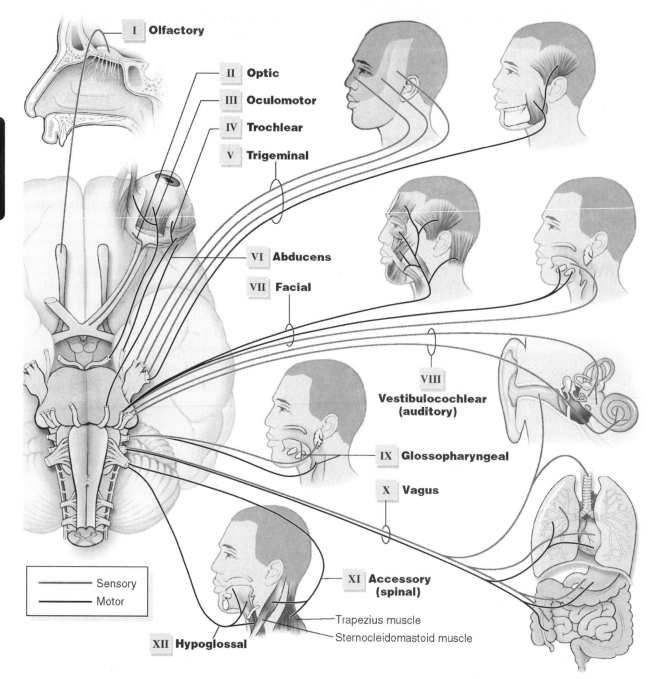

Figure 14-1 Cranial Nerves (Motor and Sensory Distribution): Schema *From Thibodeau, G.A., & Patton, K.T. (2005). The human body in health and disease (4th ed.). St. Louis: Mosby.*

senses, sensory control of body, body positioning, stereognosis and graphesthesia, verbal and nonverbal memory

4. Occipital lobe—interpreting visual images, reading and writing, finding objects, identifying color, recognizing words, drawn objects, and whether object is moving

5. Temporal lobe—hearing, memory of what is seen and heard, recognizing words; Wernicke's area essential for understanding and formulating speech

6. Cerebellum—coordination and balance, muscle tone

7. Thalamus—processes and relays sensory information, regulates motor function

8. Hypothalamus—regulates sleep cycle, body temperature, water balance, appetite, blood pressure, coordination of overall patterns of activity

9. Brainstem—heart rate, blood pressure, breathing, swallowing, level of alertness, vomiting

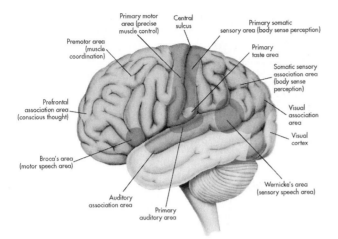

Figure 14-2 Cerebral Cortex Functions and Associated Pathways. *From Christenson, B., & Kockrow, E. (2010). Foundations and adult health nursing (6th ed.). St. Louis: Elsevier.*

II. Spine
  A. Anatomy (Hickey, 2011; Snell, 2010) (Figure 14-3)
    1. Cord—begins as a continuation of the medulla oblongata and extends through the foramen magnum of the occipital bone, usually to the upper border of L2, although it may terminate between the T12 and L3
    2. 31 pairs of spinal nerves attached by the anterior (motor) roots and the posterior (sensory) roots
    3. Critical adjacent structures
      a. Vertebral column
        (1) 33 vertebrae joined by ligaments
        (2) Bony structure encasing and protecting the cord; divisions—seven cervical, 12 thoracic, five lumbar, five sacral (fused), four coccygeal (fused)
      b. Intravertebral disks—cartilage pad separating vertebrae, allowing flexion of the cord
      c. Meninges—layers of tissue that surround the spinal cord and brain
      d. CSF—fluid that bathes and cushions the spinal cord; contained within the meninges
      e. Vertebral blood vessels—supply blood from vertebral and spinal arteries
    4. Consist of same cell types as brain
    5. Malignant primary tumors—tend to arise from intramedullary (within the spinal cord) support cells
      a. Astrocytes
      b. Ependymal cells
  B. Functions of the spinal cord
    1. Motor function of the body from neck to toes
    2. Sensory function of the body from the back of the head to the toes

3. Loss of function depends on the following:
    a. Site of tumor
      (1) Cervical—neck, arms, hands
      (2) Thoracic—chest to umbilicus
      (3) Lumbar—hips to toes
    b. Size of tumor
  C. Changes in function with spinal tumors
    1. Compression created by growth of tumor as it enlarges
    2. Spinal nerves and occluded blood vessels may also be compressed
III. Pathophysiology of central nervous system (CNS) cancers
  A. Primary CNS tumors
    1. Primary brain tumors (PBTs)
      a. Arise from cells within the CNS
      b. Brain tumors the most common solid tumor of childhood
        (1) Gliomas and medulloblastomas are the most prevalent, with an incidence of 3.2 per 100,000 (Ries et al., 2007).
        (2) Leukemia (blood cell cancers) and tumors of the brain and spinal cord account for over 50% of all newly diagnosed pediatric malignancies.
      c. Incidence
        (1) All primary malignant and nonmalignant brain or CNS tumors (Central Brain Tumor Registry of the United States [CBTRUS], 2005-2009)
          (a) 20.6 cases per 100,000
          (b) 7.3 cases per 100,000 for malignant tumors
          (c) 13.3 cases per 100,000 for nonmalignant tumors.
          (d) Rate higher in females (22.3 per 100,000) than males (18.8 per 100,000)
          (e) Estimated 69,720 new cases of primary malignant and nonmalignant brain and CNS tumors expected to be diagnosed in the United States in 2013
        (2) Primary malignant brain and CNS tumors (CBTRUS, 2005-2009)
          (a) 6.5 cases per 100,000
          (b) Rate higher in males (7.7 per 100,000) than in females (5.4 per 100,000)
          (c) Excludes lymphomas, leukemias, tumors of pituitary and pineal glands, and olfactory tumors of the nasal cavity (Howlader et al., 2012)
          (d) Estimated 24,620 new cases of primary malignant brain and CNS

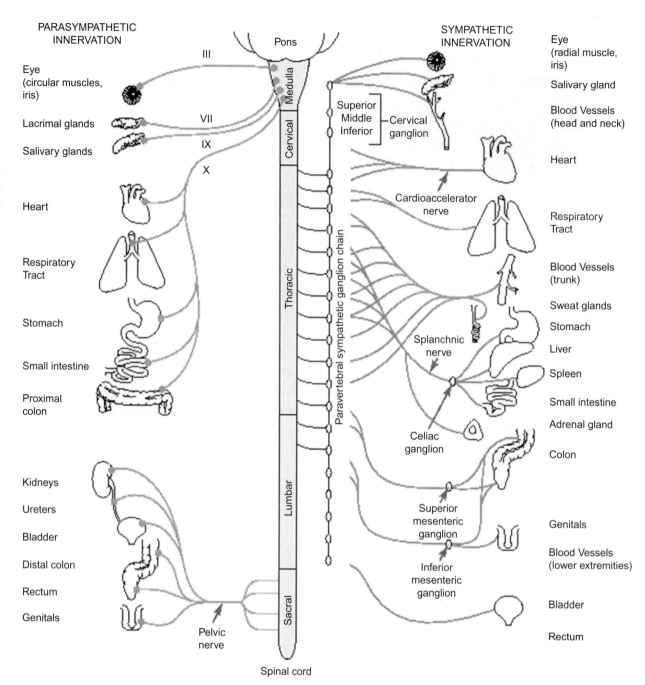

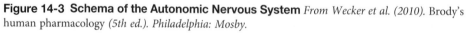

Figure 14-3 Schema of the Autonomic Nervous System *From Wecker et al. (2010).* Brody's human pharmacology *(5th ed.). Philadelphia: Mosby.*

system tumors expected to be diagnosed in the United States (U.S.) in 2013 (13,630 in males and 10,990 in females) (CBTRUS, 2005-2009)

(3) Lifetime risk (National Cancer Institute (NCI), SEER 2013)

(a) Males—0.69% lifetime risk of being diagnosed with a primary malignant brain or CNS tumor and 0.32% chance of dying from a brain or CNS tumor

(b) Females—0.55% lifetime risk of being diagnosed with a primary malignant brain or CNS tumor and a 0.4% chance of dying from a brain or CNS tumor

d. Most common histologies of primary brain tumors

(1) Gliomas—astrocytomas, oligodendrogliomas, mixed gliomas (Figure 14-4)

(2) Ependymomas

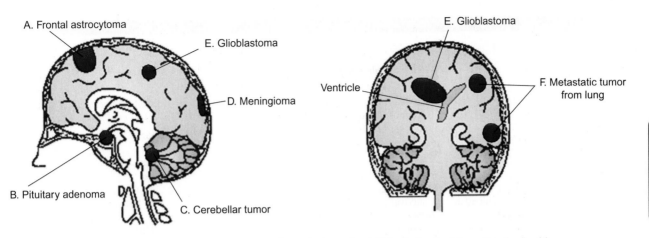

Figure 14-4 *Location of From Gould, B. & Dyer, R. (2011). Pathophysiology for the health professions (4th ed.). St. Louis: Saunders.*

(3) Primitive neuroectodermal cells (PNETs)
   (a) Medulloblastomas
   (b) Ependymoblastomas
   (c) Pinealoblastomas
(4) Primary CNS lymphoma
(5) Meningiomas
(6) Neuromas
e. Epidemiology of primary brain tumors (Table 14-1)

f. Grading and staging of primary brain tumors
   (1) TNM (tumor-node-metastasis) classification not used in this setting (two of three indicators not applicable in brain tumors; no nodes, and extracranial metastases extraordinarily rare)
   (2) Grading based on histologic appearance with criteria established by the World Health Organization (WHO) (Table 14-2)

Table 14-1	
Central Nervous System (CNS) Tumor Risk Factors	
Known intrinsic risk factors	Age—children and older adults Gender—men, glioma; women, meningioma Race/ethnicity—Caucasian northern European; meningioma more common in African American populations
Known situational risk factors	History of viral infection—Epstein-Barr virus increases risk of CNS lymphoma Immunocompromised—human immunodeficiency virus/acquired immunodeficiency syndrome (HIV/AIDS), immunosuppressive medical therapies, post-transplantation lymphoproliferative disorder (PTLD), CNS, often donor-derived Injury—history of head trauma associated with meningiomas Personal history of cancer
Known extrinsic risk factors	Ionizing radiation (IR)—causal relationship between therapeutic irradiation of doses > 2500 cGy and development of brain tumors; risk higher for nerve sheath tumors and meningiomas than gliomas Children with leukemia—risk highest if treated prior to age 5 years Panorex radiography prior to age 10 years associated with increased risk of meningioma Prior radiation for treatment of *Tinea capitus*—common in the 1950s
Genetic/inherited risk factors (5%-10% of primary brain tumors associated with genetic disorders)	Neurofibromatosis 1 (*NF1* gene), neurofibromatosis 2 (*NF2* gene) Turcot syndrome (*APC* gene) Gorlin syndrome (*PTCH* gene) Tuberous sclerosis (*TSC1* and *TSC2* genes) Li-Fraumeni syndrome (*TP53* gene) Von Hippel-Lindau (*VHL* gene) Brain cancer "clusters" in families without known genetic cause
Unproven risk factors currently under investigation	Late menarche in females Obesity Exposures—pesticides, vinyl chloride, petrochemicals, electromagnetic fields (high-power lines), inks and solvents, dietary N-nitroso compounds, long-term use of black or brown hair dyes, cell phones

Table 14-2

Biomarkers in Glioma

Biomarker/Description	Clinical Significance	Source
MGMT O6-methylguanine-DNA-methyltransferase DNA repair protein Protective against effects of alkylating chemotherapies	Methylation (destruction) of MGMT a favorable prognostic indicator (FPI) in glioblastoma (GBM) Predicts ⇑ benefit from alkylating agent	Reifenberger et al., 2011; Hegi et al., 2008
IDH1 Isocitrate dehydrogenase 1 Enzyme mutation (IDH1m) found in multiple human cancers ⇑ In the young and in secondary GBM versus primary GBM	FPI for longer progression-free survival (PFS) and overall survival (OS) in GBM Presence of mutation predicts improved sensitivity of glioma to radiation	National Center for Biotechnology Information, 2013; Ohgaki & Kleihues, 2011; Li et al., 2013; Vancheri, 2011
1p19q Co-deletion of chromosomal arms 1p and 19q Associated with oligodendrogliomas	Presence of mutation predicts: ⇑ Chemosensitivity FPI in oligodendrogliomas Slower tumor growth	Chang & Newton, 2010; van den Bent, 2013
EGFR Epidermal growth factor receptor Tyrosine kinase ligand Exists on cell surface Activated by various growth factors which leads to cell proliferation	EGFR Expression Amplified ~50% of primary GBM Associated with poor prognosis EGFRvIII expression associated with worse prognosis than wild-type EGFR expression (amplification) alone	National Center for Biotechnology Information, 2013; Dunn et al., 2012
PTEN Phosphatase and tensin homolog Protein encoded by PTEN gene Plays roll in cancer suppression	PTEN loss (mutation) associated with proliferation of GBM	National Center for Biotechnology Information, 2013; Chang & Newton, 2010

g. Size of lesion (single versus multifocal), location, and degree of malignancy best prognostic indicators

2. Spine
   a. Benign primary spinal tumors—more likely to occur inside the dura but outside the spinal cord (extramedullary); examples include meningiomas, neurofibromas, schwannomas

3. Metastatic patterns of primary CNS tumors
   a. Rare for PBT to metastasize outside of CNS
   b. PBT may invade dura and adjacent structures
   c. PBT may have drop metastases to spine
   d. Primary spine tumors
      (1) Intradural or intramedullary tumors—ependymomas and gliomas
      (2) Extradural or extramedullary tumors—nerve sheath tumors

B. Metastatic CNS tumors
   1. Spread to the CNS through hematogenous seeding, direct extension or invasion, and seeding in the CSF

2. Most common metastatic histologies to brain (Fox, Cheung, Patel, Suki, & Rao, 2011)
   a. Lung
      (1) Most frequent source of brain metastases
      (2) Small cell and adenocarcinoma most common
      (3) >90% of patients with lung cancer diagnosed with brain metastases within 1 year of initial diagnosis
   b. Breast
      (1) Most common type of brain metastases in women
      (2) Tends to metastasize later in the disease (2 to 3 years after initial diagnosis)
   c. Melanoma
      (1) Highest predilection to metastasize to CNS
      (2) Typically associated with poorer prognosis than other types of brain metastases
   d. Renal
   e. Colorectal

3. Most common malignant histologies to spine (Sciubba et al., 2010)
    a. Reflection of prevalence of tumor type and tendency to metastasize to bone
    b. Metastatic tumors more likely to occur in the vertebral bodies or epidural space
        (1) Breast
        (2) Lung
        (3) Prostate
        (4) Multiple myeloma (Roodman, 2008)
4. Staging metastatic CNS tumors
    a. Metastatic CNS disease indicative of TNM stage 4
    b. Size, location, and number of metastatic lesions often used in stratification for treatment decision making and as prognostic indicators

IV. Diagnostic imaging examinations
    A. Computed tomography (CT) of brain and spine (Drevelegas & Papanikolaou, 2011; Herholz, Langen, Schiepers, & Mountz, 2012)
        1. Without contrast—helpful in emergency room at initial presentation to evaluate stroke versus intracranial lesions in persons with new-onset neurologic symptoms
            a. Superior for detecting hemorrhage and calcification
            b. Readily available in the community
            c. Less expensive than magnetic resonance imaging (MRI)
        2. With intravenous radiocontrast for some surgical and radiation planning or for surveillance of patients not able to get MRI
        3. CT is modality of choice for patients with metallic devices (e.g., cochlear implants or pacemakers because of potential magnetic damage to the implanted device) and critically ill patients.
        4. Malignant tumors best visualized with contrast-enhanced scans
        5. CT is test of choice for evaluating spinal bony metastases.
    B. MRI of brain and spine
        1. Without gadolinium—helpful in evaluating edema, nonenhancing tumors, radiation-induced leukoencephalopathy, or acute blood products
        2. With intravenous gadolinium—test of choice for visualizing brain and spine lesions and for ongoing disease surveillance
        3. Modality of choice in persons with symptoms of brain tumor
            a. Superior contrast resolution
            b. Multiplanar capability
        4. High-grade tumors best visualized with contrast
            a. When to use imaging

(1) Preoperatively—to identify patterns of cerebral edema and location of mass or disease
(2) Postoperatively, within 24 hours—to assess residual tumor volume and as a new baseline to measure treatment effect
(3) Follow-up examinations—every 3 to 4 months is typical standard practice outside of clinical trials unless clinically indicated (Stupp, Tonn, Brada & Pentheroudakis, 2010).
        5. MRI test of choice for evaluating soft tissue tumors involving the spine
        6. MRI CSF flow study for evaluating the flow of CSF around the brain, brainstem, and spinal cord when concern about obstruction exists
    C. Functional MRI—for identifying areas of eloquent brain preoperatively
    D. Spectroscopy—to differentiate normal versus abnormal tissues
    E. Nuclear medicine studies—provide physiologic picture as opposed to structural picture
        1. Positron emission tomography (PET)—high sensitivity to high-grade malignancies and radiation necrosis but low specificity
        2. Octreotide scan—may be useful in evaluating malignant meningioma or PNET tumors
        3. Bone scan—indicated for staging medulloblastoma
    F. Radiography (spine)
    G. Myelography—aids in finding source of spinal compression
    H. Electromyography—detects muscular innervation dysfunctions peripherally

V. Diagnostic lumbar puncture
    A. Cell count and differential
    B. Glucose level
    C. Protein concentration
    D. Gram stain
    E. Culture and sensitivity
    F. Tumor markers
    G. Cytopathology

VI. Diagnostic serum blood tests
    A. Serum tests—vary according to primary diagnosis
    B. Tumor markers—may include beta-human chorionic gonadotropin (beta-HCG), alpha-fetoprotein (AFP), placental isoenzyme of alkaline phosphatase (PLAP) for germinoma tumors or teratomas
    C. No serum evaluation for diagnosis of gliomas

VII. Treatment options or modalities for CNS malignancies
    A. Surgery
        1. Surgical management of brain tumors (Bergsneider & Barkhoudarian, 2012)
            a. Stereotactic brain biopsy

(1) Method of tissue diagnosis if tumor near eloquent areas, difficult to access, or patient is poor surgical candidate because of comorbidities

(2) Sampling error possible because of small tissue sample; may result in underdiagnosis

b. Brain surgical resection—goal of surgical procedures: provide tissue diagnosis and improve outcomes (survival and neurologic functioning)

(1) Obtain diagnostic tissue sample

(2) Provide symptom relief: reduction in mass effect

(3) Primary treatment modality (or restaging in recurrence)

(a) Subtotal resection—removal of a portion of the tumor; preferred resection type if tumor near eloquent areas and an aggressive surgical approach could result in worse neurologic deficits

(b) Gross total—removal of all visible tumor tissue; theoretically improves response to treatment because of smaller tumor burden

(4) Second or third craniotomy performed for restaging (lower-grade tumors often become more malignant over time) in the recurrent setting or to provide symptom relief

(5) Postoperative imaging with CT or MRI recommended within 24 hours of surgical resection to assess residual tumor volume and establish new baseline

2. Surgical management of spinal tumors

a. Biopsy

(1) If tumor difficult to access without risk of worsening neurologic deficits

b. Spinal surgical resection

(1) Extradural tumors

(a) If tumor is not radiosensitive

(b) If neurologic status is deteriorating

(c) If tumor type is not known

(d) If surgery will not put the client at risk for more severe neurologic deficit or other life-threatening complications

(2) Intradural or extramedullary—best managed with surgery

(3) Intradural or intramedullary—surgical resection, if possible

3. Ventricular access devices

a. Ventriculoperitoneal (VP) shunt—placed for management of hydrocephalus

(1) Programmable VP shunt—may be affected by magnetic fields during MRI; therefore, patient will require plain film within 4 hours of MRI to assess valve settings. ⚠

(2) Nonprogrammable VP shunt

b. Ommaya reservoir—placed for delivery of intrathecal chemotherapy

c. Ventriculostomy—performed to relieve pressure within the CNS

B. Radiation—use of photons or other forms of energy to treat brain and spinal cord tumors

1. Brain

a. Conventional radiation therapy uses photon beams (x-ray directed at tumor target, plus defined margin

(1) External beam radiation therapy (EBRT)

(2) Three-dimensional conformal radiotherapy

(3) Intensity-modulated radiation therapy (IMRT)

b. Stereotactic radiosurgery or stereotactic radiotherapy

c. Conformal proton beam radiotherapy— uses protons (positive part of atoms) to target the tumor tissue; allows minimal radiation exposure upon entry into or exit from the brain

d. Whole-brain radiation therapy

e. Craniospinal radiation therapy

2. Spinal cord tumors

a. Three-dimensional conformal radiotherapy

b. IMRT

c. Radiosurgery

3. General side effects of radiation therapy to CNS

a. Acute effects (during and immediately following radiation therapy)

(1) Causes

(a) Inflammation caused by disruption of blood-brain barrier

(b) Early radiation-induced demyelination

(2) Toxicities

(a) Global—headaches, neurocognitive changes, seizures, and somnolence

(b) Focal—specific neurologic deficits based on tumor location

b. Subacute effects (within weeks to 4 to 6 months following radiation)

(1) Causes

(a) Radiation-induced demyelination

(b) Inflammation

(c) Altered capillary permeability

(d) Radionecrosis

(2) Toxicities—somnolence and exacerbation of tumor-related symptoms (based on tumor location)

(3) Imaging features (evaluable on MRI)

   (a) During this subacute period, MRI findings show increased enhancement, vasogenic edema, and mass effect.

   (b) It is difficult to distinguish between tumor progression and pseudoprogression (seen in 20% of high-grade gliomas receiving combination chemoradiotherapy; 50% of these cases with imaging features are pseudoprogression versus true tumor progression).

     (i) Defined criteria exist for evaluating pseudoprogression for high-grade gliomas (HGGs) and metastatic brain tumors following SRT.

     (ii) Failure to this subacute reaction may lead to premature discontinuation of potentially beneficial therapy.

  c. Late radiation effects (occurring more than 6 months to several years following radiotherapy)

   (1) Radiation necrosis

   (2) Diffuse white matter changes

   (3) Neurocognitive effects

   (4) Cerebrovascular events

   (5) Optic nerve toxicities

   (6) Endocrine toxicities

   (7) Secondary malignancies

     (a) Most common—meningiomas, gliomas, and nerve sheath tumors

     (b) Risk greatest with cranial radiation given to young children

C. Chemotherapy (National Comprehensive Cancer Network [NCCN], 2013)

  1. General principles (Michaud & Chang, 2011)—since the 1960s, only four drugs (temozolomide, lomustine, carmustine, and bevacizumab) approved by the U.S. Food and Drug Administration (FDA) for specific use in treating primary brain tumors

   a. Used to control growth or reduce tumor burden, but benefit often limited because of the following:

    (1) Resistance of tumor cells

    (2) Inadequate drug delivery across the blood-brain barrier (which is a lipid membrane, so smaller lipophilic drugs are more able to penetrate)

   b. Positive prognostic genetic markers—include 1p19q co-deletion (often seen in anaplastic oligodendrogliomas) and protein O6-alkylguanine DNA alkyltransferase (AGT) silencing (AGT is encoded in humans by the O-6-methylguanine-DNA methyltransferase [*MGMT*] gene); hence, patient's whose tumors are MGMT promoter methylation-positive more sensitive to alkylating chemotherapy because of epigenetic silencing of the *MGMT* gene, thereby preventing AGT synthesis; conversely, glioma tumors that are MGMT promoter methylation-negative have a poorer prognosis because of expression of AGT.

  2. Gliomas

   a. First-line glioma treatment (Stupp et al., 2005)

    (1) Temozolomide (Temodar)—an oral, second-generation alkylating agent, which can permeate the blood-brain barrier

     (a) Approved by the FDA in 1999 for refractory grade III anaplastic astrocytoma and in 2005 for newly diagnosed glioblastoma

     (b) Myelosuppression minimal and noncumulative; good quality of life during this treatment described by clients

     (c) Temozolomide in combination with radiation therapy—standard of care in the treatment of high-grade gliomas; may be used as monotherapy in lower-grade tumors

    (2) Gliadel wafers

     (a) FDA approved in 1997 as an adjunct to surgery and radiation for newly diagnosed high-grade glioma

     (b) Questionable whether this adds survival benefit when added to standard treatment described above (Bock et al., 2010; DeBonis et al., 2012; Michaud & Chang, 2011)

     (c) Because of difficulty with imaging evaluation, use of wafers often an exclusion criterion for clinical trials and rarely used in first-line treatment settings; may be a consideration for persons with underlying bone marrow toxicities or as a salvage therapy for patients undergoing a second or later surgical resection

b. Second-line glioma treatment (Beal, Abrey, & Gutin, 2011; NCCN, 2013)
  (1) No established standard regimen; consider clinical trial
  (2) Bevacizumab shown to have survival benefit (Cai et al., 2013; Friedman et al., 2009; Wen & Brandes, 2009)
    (a) Monoclonal antibody targeting the vascular endothelial growth factor
    (b) Approved by the FDA as second-line treatment for glioblastoma in 2009
    (c) May be used in combination with chemotherapy or as monotherapy
    (d) Decreases corticosteroid requirement
    (e) Generally well tolerated; risks may include hypertension, proteinuria, vascular events such as stroke and intracranial bleed ⚠
  (3) Other agents used in the recurrent setting: nitrosoureas (lomustine [CCNU, CeeNu]), platinums (cisplatin, carboplatin), etoposide
3. Metastatic CNS lesions
  a. Systemic chemotherapy for underlying primary disease site
4. Medulloblastoma
  a. Unclear role for adjuvant chemotherapy in the adult population
  b. Cisplatin-based regimen
  c. Adult first-line cytotoxic regimens are generally formulated using pediatric treatment protocols.
5. CNS lymphoma
  a. High-dose methotrexate-based regimen
  b. If CSF or spinal MRI positive, intra-CNS chemotherapy to be considered
  c. If eye examination positive, intraocular chemotherapy to be considered
D. Biotherapy
E. Blood and marrow transplantation
  1. Used for treatment of recurrent medulloblastoma
F. Investigational modalities
  1. Current standard therapies treat all malignant primary brain tumors the same.
  2. Limited options exist for treating recurrent disease.
    a. Investigational agents are one treatment option.
    b. The diagnosis of glioblastoma multiforme encompasses a wide range of tumor types with varying gene mutations and heterogenous molecular characteristics.

c. Investigational therapies aim to identify molecular targets for personalized therapy. Future treatment will ultimately differ among tumor types.
3. Several targeted therapies have been successfully used for malignancies outside of the brain.
  a. Tyrosine kinase inhibitors—block proteins involved in tumor cell growth and production
  b. mTOR inhibitors—target other enzymes involved in cell growth and replication
4. Immunotherapy—the patient's endogenous immune response is stimulated to kill tumor cells.
  a. Monoclonal antibodies—block receptors at cell surface or attach to receptor and deliver cytotoxic agents into the tumor cell
  b. Vaccines—derived from patient's own leukocytes, cultured with various antigens, modifying dendritic cells to recognize tumor antigens as targets
  c. Immunotoxins
5. Gene therapy
  a. Delivery of retroviral "suicide" gene transferring vectors directly into tumor tissue
  b. Gene transfer using modified stem cells either intravascularly or directly into tumor tissue
G. Symptom management with medical therapy
  1. Glucocorticoids
    a. High dose to manage acute cerebral edema
    b. High dose to manage extradural spinal lesions causing compression of spinal cord
    c. Doses high as 16 mg per day or even higher likely to be used; ideally, using the lowest possible dose for the shortest time possible to reduce serious steroid-related complications such as myopathy, diabetes, infections, and other comorbid conditions
  2. Mannitol—generally used only in emergency situations to capitalize on the osmotic properties of mannitol effects on brain edema resulting from leakage of plasma into the brain parenchyma through dysfunctional cerebral capillaries; only administered in intensive care unit (ICU) setting; likely only to be a last resort effort for management of cerebral edema if bevacizumab is not an option
  3. Bevacizumab—used to manage cerebral edema related to radiation necrosis (Levin et al., 2011) or progressive tumor; ideally, reducing vascular endothelial growth factor (VEGF)–induced dysfunction of tight junction proteins leading to development of vasogenic edema

VIII. Nursing implications
  A. Interventions related to screening
    1. No population screening for neurologic tumors
    2. Genetic testing considered for hereditary cancer syndromes
  B. Interventions related to oncologic emergencies ⚠ (see Chapter 41)
    1. CSF leak
    2. Spinal cord compression
    3. Increased intracranial pressure
    4. Seizures
      a. Seizure risk—risk highest with cortical tumors, with temporal tumors tending to be the most epileptogenic
      b. Possible seizure triggers
        (1) Tumor or edema causing abnormal electrical stimulation
        (2) Metabolic derangement
        (3) Chemotherapy toxicities
        (4) Medication
        (5) Infection
      c. Management of seizures
        (1) Levetiracetam (Keppra)—first drug of choice in neuro-oncology because this drug is not metabolized by the p450 enzyme system and thus has low risk of fluctuating levels
        (2) Other frequently encountered antiepileptic drug (AED) options— include phenytoin (Dilantin), lamotrigine (Lamictal), valproic acid (Depakote), carbamazepine (Tegretol), oxcarbazepine (Trileptal), and topiramate (Topamax)
        (3) AED options at end of life—include phenobarbital (not recommended for active, alert individuals because of sedation)
        (4) Risks and benefits with each seizure medication; thus AED therapy must be individualized
        (5) Enzyme-inducing antiepileptic medication use frequently an exclusion criteria for pharmacologic clinical trials
    5. Venous thromboembolism (VTE) (Perry, 2010)
      a. Deep vein thrombosis (DVT) or pulmonary embolism (PE)
      b. Clinically significant VTE in 20% to 30% of patients with malignant glioma
      c. Therapeutic anticoagulation indicated in most patients with DVT or PE, including those patients receiving treatment with antiangiogenic agents
  C. Interventions related to quality of life
    1. Research tools to measure health-related quality of life (QOL)—no single gold standard tool (Taphoorn, Sizoo, & Bottomley, 2010)
      a. MD Anderson Symptom Inventory—Brain Tumors (MDSI-BT)
      b. European Organization for Research and Treatment of Cancer Quality of Life Questionnaire—Brain Cancer Module (EORTC QLQ-BN20)
      c. Functional Assessment of Cancer Therapy—Brain Tumor subscale (FACT-Br)
    2. Common QOL issues—include fatigue, cognitive disturbance, mood disturbance, sleep disturbance (Liu, Page, Solheim, Fox, & Chang, 2009)
  D. Interventions related to survivorship issues
    1. Trends in survival with primary brain tumors
      a. Treatment is palliative, and survival is dependent on tumor factors (histology, extent of surgical excision [dependent on tumor location, size, and accessibility]) and patient factors (age, functional status) (Nicolato et al., 1995; Stupp et al., 2010). Range may be from several months to several years; generally, long-term prognosis for high-grade gliomas is very poor.
    2. Trends in survival with primary spine tumors
      a. Life expectancy is normal for patients with benign tumors that can be completely resected.
      b. Treatment is palliative for patients with primary malignant spine tumors, and life expectancy is predictive by location, volume, multifocality, surgical accessibility, radiosensitivity, and chemosensitivity. Range may be from a few months up to 1 to 2 years.
    3. Trends in survival with metastatic brain or spine cancer
      a. Survival is directly related to the volume of disease at CNS diagnosis, whether or not systemic control of the underlying malignant disease has been achieved, and the sensitivity of the tumor to treatments such as surgery, radiation, or chemotherapy. Survival may be as little as a few weeks for patients with leptomeningeal carcinomatosis to years, as in some patients with breast cancer whose CNS cancers are diagnosed early and treated aggressively.

References

Beal, K., Abrey, L., & Gutin, P. (2011). Antiangiogenic agents in the treatment of recurrent or newly diagnosed glioblastoma: Analysis of single-agent and combined modality approaches. *Radiation Oncology*, 6(2), 2. http://www.ro-journal.com/content/6/1/2.

Bergsneider, M., & Barkhoudarian, G. (2012). Principles of neurosurgery. In R. B. Daroff, G. M. Fenichel, J. Jankovic, & J. C. Mazziotta (Eds.), *Bradley's neurology in clinical practice* (6th., pp. 820–827). Philadelphia, PA: Elsevier Saunders.

Bock, H., Puchner, M., Lohmann, F., Schutze, M., Koll, S., Ketter, R., et al. (2010). First-line treatment of malignant glioma with carmustine implants followed by concomitant radiochemotherapy: A multicenter experience. *Neurosurgery Review*, 33(4), 441–449.

Cai, L., Li, J., Lai, M., Shan, C., Lian, Z., Hong, W., et al. (2013). Bevacizumab rescue therapy extends the survival in patients with recurrent malignant glioma. *Clinical Journal of Cancer Research*, 25(2), 206–211.

Central Brain Tumor Registry of the United States (CBTRUS). (2005-2009). *Analyses of the NPCR and SEER data.* www.cbtrus.org/.

Chang, S., & Newton, H. (2010). Glioma survival and prognosis, E version. In *Principles and practice of neuro-oncology: A multidisciplinary approach* (pp. 57–111). New York: Demos Medical.

Crossman, A., & Neary, D. (2010). *Neuroanatomy. An illustrated colour text* (4th ed.). London: Churchill Livingstone Elsevier.

DeBonis, P., Anile, C., Pompucci, A., Fiorentino, A., Bladucci, M., Chiesa, S., et al. (2012). Safety and efficacy of Gliadel wafers for newly diagnosed and recurrent glioblastoma. *Acta Neurochirurgica*, 154(8), 1371–1378.

Drevelegas, A., & Papanikolaou, N. (2011). Imaging modalities in brain tumors. In A. Drevelegas (Ed.), *Imaging of brain tumors with histological correlations* (pp. 13–22). Berlin-Heidelberg: Springer.

Dunn, G., Rinne, M., Wykosky, J., Genovese, G., Quayle, S., Dunn, I., et al. (2012). Emerging insights into the molecular and cellular basis of glioblastoma. *Genes & Development*, 26(8), 756–784.

Fox, B., Cheung, V., Patel, A., Suki, D., & Rao, G. (2011). Epidemiology of metastatic brain tumors. *Neurosurgery Clinics of North America*, 22(1), 1–6.

Friedman, H., Prados, M., Wen, P., Mikkelsen, T., Schiff, D., Abrey, L., et al. (2009). Bevacizumab alone and in combination with irinotecan in recurrent glioblastoma. *Journal of Clinical Oncology*, 27(28), 4733–4740.

Hegi, M., Liu, L., Herman, J., Stupp, R., Wick, W., Weller, M., et al. (2008). Correlation of O6-methylguanine methyltransferase (MGMT) promoter methylation with clinical outcomes in glioblastoma and clinical strategies to modulate MGMT activity. *Journal of Clinical Oncology*, 26(25), 4189–4199.

Herholz, K., Langen, K., Schiepers, C., & Mountz, J. (2012). Brain tumors. *Seminars in Nuclear Medicine*, 42(6), 356–370.

Hickey, J. (2011). *Clinical practice of neurological and neurosurgical nursing* (6th ed.). Philadelphia: Lippincott Williams and Wilkins.

Howlader, N., Noone, A., Krapcho, M., Neyman, N., Aminou, R., & Altekruse, S., et al. (Eds.). (2012). *SEER cancer statistics review, 1975–2009 (Vintage 2009 Populations)*. Bethesda, MD: National Cancer Institute. http://seer.cancer.gov/csr/1975_2009_pops09/.

Levin, V., Bidaut, L., Hou, P., Kumar, A., Wefel, J., Bekele, B., et al. (2011). Randomized double-blind placebo-controlled trial of bevacizumab therapy for radiation necrosis of the central nervous system. *International Journal of Oncology, Biology, and Physics*, 79(5), 1487–1495.

Li, S., Chou, A., Lou, J., Everson, R., Wu, K., Cloughesy, T., et al. (2013). Overexpression of isocitrate dehydrogenase mutant proteins renders glioma cells more sensitive to radiation. *Neuro-Oncology*, 15(1), 57–68.

Liu, R., Page, M., Solheim, K., Fox, S., & Chang, S. (2009). Quality of life in adults with brain tumors: Current knowledge and future directions. *Neuro-Oncology*, 11(3), 330–339.

Michaud, K., & Chang, S. (2011). Principles of chemotherapy. In H. R. Winn (Ed.), *Youmans neurological surgery*, (6th ed. pp. 1236–1242), Philadelphia: W.B. Saunders.

National Brain Tumor Society. (2013). *Frankly speaking about cancer: Brain tumors*. Washington, D.C: Cancer Support Community.

National Cancer Institute (NCI). (2013). *Surveillance epidemiology and end results (SEER) cancer statistics review, 1975-2010. Devcan version 6.7.0*. http://surveillance.cancer.gov/devcan/.

National Center for Biotechnology Information. (2013). IDH1 isocitrate dehydrogenase 1 (NADP+), soluble [*Homo sapiens* (human)]. http://www.ncbi.nlm.nih.gov/gene?cmd=retrieve&list_uids=3417.

National Comprehensive Cancer Network (NCCN). (2013). *Clinical practice guidelines in oncology-central nervous system cancers. version 2.* http//www.nccn.org/professionals/physician_gls/pDF/cns.pdf.

Nicolato, A., Gerosa, M., Fina, P., Iuzzolino, P., Giorgiutti, F., & Bricolo, A. (1995). Prognostic factors in low-grade supratentorial astrocytomas: A uni-multivariate statistical analysis in 76 surgically treated adult patients. *Surgical Neurology*, 44(3), 208–223.

Ohgaki, H., & Kleihues, P. (2011). Genetic profile of astrocytic and oligodendroglial gliomas. *Brain Tumor Pathology*, 28(3), 177–183.

Perry, J. (2010). Anticoagulation of malignant glioma patients in the era of novel antiangiogenic agents. *Current Opinion in Neurology*, 23(6), 592–596.

Reifenberger, G., Hentschel, B., Loeffler, M., Weller, M., Felsberg, J., Schackert, G., et al. (2011). Predictive impact of MGMT promoter methylation in glioblastoma of the elderly. *International Journal of Cancer*, 131(6), 1342–1350.

Ries, L., Melbert, D., Krapcho, M., Mariotto, A., Miller, B., & Feuer, E., et al. (2007). *SEER cancer statistics review, 1975-2004*. Bethesda, MD: National Cancer Institute. http://seer.cancer.gov/csr/1975_2004/.

Roodman, G. (2008). Skeletal imaging and management of bone disease. *Hematology American Society of Hematology Education Program*, 2008(1), 313–319.

Sciubba, D., Petteys, R., Dekutoski, M., Fisher, C., Fehlings, M., Ondra, S., et al. (2010). Diagnosis and management of metastatic spine disease. *Journal of Neurosurgery: Spine*, 13(1), 94–108.

Snell, R. (2010). *Clinical neuroanatomy* (7th ed.). Lippincott Williams & Wilkins.

Stupp, R., Mason, W., van den Bent, M., Weller, M., Fisher, B., Taphoorn, M., et al. (2005). Radiotherapy plus concomitant and adjuvant temozolomide for glioblastoma. *New England Journal of Medicine, 352*(10), 987–996.

Stupp, R., Tonn, J., Brada, M., & Pentheroudakis, G. (2010). High-grade malignant glioma: ESMO clinical practice guidelines for diagnosis, treatment, and follow-up. *Annals of Oncology, 21* (Suppl. 5), v190–v193.

Taphoorn, M., Sizoo, E., & Bottomley, A. (2010). Review on quality of life issues in patients with primary brain tumors. *The Oncologist, 15*(6), 618–626.

van den Bent, M. (2013). How to use molecular markers when caring for a patient with brain cancer: 1P/19Q as a predictive and prognostic marker in the neuro-oncology clinic. *American Society of Clinical Oncology Educational Book. 2013*: 114–116.

Vancheri, C. (2011). New data on nonmalignant brain tumors could spur research efforts. *Journal of the National Cancer Institute, 103*(9), 706–713.

Wen, P., & Brandes, A. (2009). Treatment of recurrent high-grade gliomas. *Current Opinion in Neurology, 22*(6), 657–664.

Part 2

CHAPTER 15
Leukemia

Dawn Hew and Francisco A. Conde

I. Pathophysiology and classification of leukemia (Grigoropoulos, Petter, Van't Veer, Scott & Follows, 2013; Kurtin, 2010).
  A. Leukemia—malignant disorder of blood cells and lymphatic tissue, most commonly involving the white blood cells (WBCs)
    1. Leukemic or malignant cells excessively proliferate, resulting in overcrowding of bone marrow and inability to produce normal-functioning hematopoietic cells.
    2. Leukemic cells are capable of infiltrating and accumulating in other organs (e.g., spleen, liver, central nervous system [CNS], lymph nodes).
    3. Leukemias are classified according to cell type (myeloid or lymphoid) and divided into acute and chronic types.
      a. Acute leukemias—characterized by excessive proliferation of immature blast cells
        (1) Onset usually acute
        (2) Two main classifications of acute leukemias
          (a) Acute myeloid leukemia (AML)—see Box 15-1 for classification.
          (b) Acute lymphoblastic leukemia (ALL)—see Box 15-2 for classification.
      b. Chronic leukemias—characterized by excessive proliferation of functionally incompetent cells
        (1) Onset gradual and diagnosis often incidental
        (2) Two main classifications of chronic leukemias: chronic myeloid leukemia (CML) and chronic lymphocytic leukemia (CLL).
II. Epidemiology
  A. Estimated 48,610 new cases and 23,720 deaths in the United States (U.S.) in 2013 (American Cancer Society [ACS], 2013); 2013 incidence and mortality figures for each category of leukemia as follows:
    1. AML—14,590 new cases and 10,370 deaths
    2. CML—5920 new cases and 610 deaths
    3. ALL—6070 new cases and 1430 deaths
    4. CLL—15,680 new cases and 4580 deaths
  B. Almost 90% of leukemia cases diagnosed in adults (ACS, 2013)
  C. In adults, most common types of leukemia are CLL (38%) and AML (30%).
  D. In children and teens, ALL most common, accounting for 75% of leukemia cases
  E. From 2005 to 2009, overall leukemia incidence rates increased by 0.4% per year.
III. Risk factors
  A. Exposure to radiation
    1. Previous treatment with radiation therapy (RT)
    2. Exposure to radiation among atomic bomb survivors of Hiroshima and Nagasaki (Kato & Schull, 1982)
    3. Exposure to radiation in the work setting
  B. Exposure to chemicals
    1. Previous treatment with antineoplastic agents such as alkylating agents and topoisomerase inhibitors (Schiffer & Stone, 2010)
    2. Previous treatment with medications such as chloramphenicol and phenylbutazone
    3. Accidental or work-related exposure to chemicals such as benzene and formaldehyde and to pesticides such as Agent Orange, phenoxy herbicides, triazine herbicides, arsenic-containing pesticides, atrazine, lindane, dichlorodiphenyltrichloroethane (DDT) (Polychronakis, Dounias, Makropoulos, Riza, & Linos, 2013)
  C. Exposure to viruses
    1. Human T-cell leukemia virus type 1 (HTLV-1)—associated with adult T-cell leukemia

BOX 15-1

World Health Organization (WHO) Classification of Acute Myeloid Leukemia

- Acute myeloid leukemia with recurrent genetic abnormalities
  - AML with t(8;21)(q22;q22); RUNX1-RUNX1T1
  - AML with inv(16)(p13.1q22) or t(16;16)(p13.1;q22); CBFB-MYH11
  - APL with t(15;17)(q22;q12); PML-RARA
  - AML with t(9;11)(p22;q23); MLLT3-MLL
  - AML with t(6;9)(p23;q34); DEK-NUP214
  - AML with inv(3)(q21q26.2) or t(3;3)(q21;q26.2); RPN1-EVI1
  - AML (megakaryoblastic) with t(1;22)(p13;q13); RBM15-MKL1
  - Provisional entity: AML with mutated NPM1
  - Provisional entity: AML with mutated CEBPA
- Acute myeloid leukemia with myelodysplasia-related changes
- Acute myeloid leukemia, not otherwise specified
  - AML with minimal differentiation
  - AML without maturation
  - AML with maturation
  - Acute myelomonocytic leukemia
  - Acute monoblastic/monocytic leukemia
  - Acute erythroid leukemia
    - Pure erythroid leukemia
    - Erythroleukemia, erythroid/myeloid
  - Acute megakaryoblastic leukemia
  - Acute basophilic leukemia
  - Acute panmyelosis with myelofibrosis
- Therapy-related myeloid neoplasms
- Myeloid sarcoma
- Myeloid proliferations related to Down syndrome
  - Transient abnormal myelopoiesis
  - Myeloid leukemia associated with Down syndrome
- Blastic plasmacytoid dendritic cell neoplasm

From Vardiman, J. W., Thiele, J., Arber, D. A., Brunning, R. D., Borowitz, M. J., Porwit, A., et al. (2009). The 2008 revision of the World Health Organization (WHO) classification of myeloid neoplasms and acute leukemia: Rationale and important changes. *Blood, 114*(5), 937–951.

BOX 15-2

World Health Organization (WHO) Classification of Acute Lymphoblastic Leukemia

- T lymphoblastic leukemia/lymphoma
- B lymphoblastic leukemia/lymphoma
  - B lymphoblastic leukemia/lymphoma, NOS
  - B lymphoblastic leukemia/lymphoma with recurrent genetic abnormalities
  - B lymphoblastic leukemia/lymphoma with t(9;22) (q34;q11.2);BCR-ABL 1
  - B lymphoblastic leukemia/lymphoma with t (v;11q23);MLL rearranged
  - B lymphoblastic leukemia/lymphoma with t(12;21) (p13;q22) TEL-AML1 (ETV6-RUNX1)
  - B lymphoblastic leukemia/lymphoma with hyperdiploidy
  - B lymphoblastic leukemia/lymphoma with hypodiploidy
  - B lymphoblastic leukemia/lymphoma with t(5;14) (q31;q32) IL3-IGH
  - B lymphoblastic leukemia/lymphoma with t(1;19) (q23;p13.3);TCF3-PBX1

From Vardiman, J. W., Thiele, J., Arber, D. A., Brunning, R. D., Borowitz, M. J., Porwit, A., et al. (2009). The 2008 revision of the World Health Organization (WHO) classification of myeloid neoplasms and acute leukemia: Rationale and important changes. *Blood, 114*(5), 937–951.

B. Symptoms related to bone marrow failure—recurrent infections from neutropenia and bleeding; easy bruising from thrombocytopenia; symptoms of anemia (e.g., fatigue, weakness, shortness of breath)

C. Symptoms related to organ and lymphatic infiltration by leukemic cells:
  1. Lymphadenopathy
  2. Bone pain from increased pressure in bone marrow
  3. Early satiety, fullness and abdominal discomfort secondary to splenomegaly and hepatomegaly
  4. Seizure caused by central nervous system (CNS) involvement

V. Diagnostic measures
  A. For all leukemias:
    1. Medical history and physical examination
    2. Complete blood cell count (CBC), with differential, chemistry profile, disseminated intravascular coagulation (DIC) panel (prothrombin time [PT], partial thromboplastin time [PTT], fibrinogen, D-dimer)
    3. Computed tomography (CT) or magnetic resonance imaging (MRI) and lumbar

D. Inherited genetic disorders—Down syndrome, Turner syndrome, Bloom syndrome, Klinefelter syndrome, Fanconi anemia, ataxia telangiectasia (Faderl, Pui, O'Brien, Kantarjian, 2010)

E. Cigarette smoking—increased risk of AML and CML (Musselman, et al., 2013)

IV. Signs and symptoms (Simpson, 2009)
  A. Patients with chronic leukemias possibly asymptomatic

puncture (LP), if symptomatic for neurologic signs or symptoms

  a. LP is contraindicated in patients with meningeal disease, CNS bleeding, and uncorrected coagulopathy such as DIC and thrombocytopenia.

4. Cardiac scan or echocardiography for patients who will receive an anthracycline chemotherapy, had prior anthracycline use, history of cardiac disease, and any clinical symptoms of cardiac dysfunction

5. Human leukocyte antigen (HLA) typing, except in patients with a major contraindication to hematopoietic stem cell transplantation (HSCT)

6. Early evaluation for alternative donor search for patients with poor risk features who lack a sibling donor

7. Central venous access device of choice

B. Additional diagnostic tests for AML (National Comprehensive Cancer Network [NCCN], 2013a)

  1. Bone marrow aspirate and biopsy with cytogenetics

  2. Presence of more than 20% myeloid blasts in bone marrow

  3. Immunophenotyping and cytochemistry

  4. Evaluation for c-KIT, FMS-like tyrosine kinase 3–internal tandem duplication (FLT3-ITD), NPM, and CEBPA mutations

C. Additional diagnostic tests for CML (NCCN, 2013c)

  1. Bone marrow aspirate and biopsy with cytogenetic analysis

    a. Cytogenetic analysis—presence of the Philadelphia chromosome (Ph chromosome); translocation between chromosomes 9 and 22, resulting in *BCR-ABL1* fusion gene

  2. Fluorescence in situ hybridization (FISH), if collection of bone marrow is not feasible.

  3. Quantitative reverse transcriptase polymerase chain reaction RT-PCR (QPCR) using international scale (IS) (blood or bone marrow)

D. Additional diagnostic tests for ALL (NCCN, 2013b)

  1. Bone marrow aspirate and biopsy with cytogenetic analysis

    a. Presence of more than 20% lymphoblasts in bone marrow

    b. Cytogenetic analysis:

      (1) Presence of the Philadelphia chromosome

        (a) Positive Ph chromosome seen in 25% of adults with ALL and in 3% of children with ALL (NCCN, 2013b)

      (2) Other recurrent genetic abnormalities—hyperdiploidy (DNA index >1.16; 51 to 65 chromosomes); hypodiploidy (<46 chromosomes); t(v;11q23), MLL

rearrangement; t(12;21)(p13;q22), TEL-AML1; t(1;19)(q23;p13.3), E2A-PBX1; and t(5;14)(q31;q32), IL3-IGH

2. Tumor lysis syndrome (TLS) panel—lactate dehydrogenase (LDH), uric acid, potassium, calcium, phosphorus

  a. High risk of TLS seen in patients with elevated WBC count, pre-existing elevated uric acid level, renal disease, or all of these conditions

3. Chest CT (for T-cell ALL)

4. Testicular examination

E. Additional diagnostic tests for CLL (Hallek et al., 2008)

  1. Blood—presence of greater than 5×10^9/L B-lymphocytes (5000/μL) in peripheral blood for the duration of at least 3 months

  2. Immunophenotype—T-cell antigen CD5 and B-cell surface antigens CD19, CD20, and CD23

  3. Cytogenetic analysis

    a. Deletions in chromosome 13 [del(13q14.1)], chromosomes 11 [del(11q)] and 6 [del(6q)], chromosome 12, and chromosome 17 [del(17p)]

VI. Staging

  A. No staging system for AML

  B. No staging system for CML

Table 15-1

World Health Organization (WHO) Criteria: Phases of Chronic Myelogenous Leukemia

Phase	Description
Chronic phase	Blasts <10% of white blood cells (WBCs) in peripheral and/or nucleated bone marrow cells
Accelerated phase	Blasts 10%-19% of WBCs in peripheral and/or nucleated bone marrow cells Peripheral blood basophils ≥ 20% Persistent thrombocytopenia (<100 × 10⁹/L) unrelated to therapy or persistent thrombocytosis (>1000 × 10⁹/L) unresponsive to therapy Increasing spleen size and increasing WBC count unresponsive to therapy Cytogenetic evidence of clonal evolution
Blast crisis	Blasts ≥ 20% of WBCs in peripheral and/or nucleated bone marrow cells Extramedullary blast proliferation Large foci or clusters of blasts in the bone marrow biopsy

Data from National Comprehensive Cancer Network. (2013). *NCCN practice guidelines in oncology: Chronic myelogenous leukemia* [v.2.2014]. http://www.nccn.org/professionals/physician_gls/pdf/cml.pdf.

1. CML is categorized into three phases—chronic, accelerated, and blastic phases (Table 15-1).
C. No staging system for childhood and adult ALL; risk stratification used to plan treatment
   1. Risk stratification for childhood ALL (NCCN, 2013b)
      a. Standard (low) risk
         (1) B-cell ALL
         (2) Children from 1 to 10 years of age
         (3) WBC count of less than 50,000/μL at diagnosis
      b. High risk
         (1) T-cell ALL (regardless of age or WBC count)
         (2) Children younger than 1 year or older than 10 years and children who have a WBC count of 50,000/μL or more at diagnosis
      c. Very high risk
         (1) Ph chromosome–positive ALL, presence of BCR-ABL fusion protein, or both
         (2) Hypodiploidy (<44 chromosomes)
         (3) Failure to achieve remission with induction therapy
   2. Risk stratification for adult ALL (NCCN, 2013b)
      a. Low risk
         (1) Ph chromosome–negative ALL
         (2) Older than 65 years
         (3) None of the following—hypodiploidy; t(v;11q23) or MLL rearrangements; t(9;22) or BCR-ABL; or complex karyotype (>five chromosomal abnormalities)
      b. High risk
         (1) Ph chromosome–positive ALL
         (2) Older than 65 years
         (3) Has any of the following—hypodiploidy; t(v;11q23) or MLL rearrangements; t(9;22) or BCR-ABL; or complex karyotype (>five chromosomal abnormalities)
D. Staging for CLL
   1. Two common staging systems used
      a. Rai staging system—commonly used in the U.S. (Table 15-2) (Rai, 1987)
      b. Binet staging system—commonly used in Europe
VII. Prognosis
   A. Overall 5-year relative survival rate (Howlader et al., 2013a)
      1. AML—25.7%
         a. Children and adolescents (ages 0 to 19 years) with AML—63.9% (Howlader et al., 2013b)
      2. CML—62.7%
      3. ALL—67.3%
         a. Children and adolescents (ages 0 to 19 years) with ALL—90% (Howlader et al., 2013b)
      4. CLL—80.5%
VIII. Principles of medical management
   A. AML—Treatment divided into induction chemotherapy and post-remission (or consolidation) therapy
      1. Induction—initial treatment with chemotherapy agents given at high doses to eradicate leukemia and achieve complete remission (CR) resulting in bone marrow repopulation with normal cells (<5% blasts) and normal blood counts
         a. Induction regimen for AML includes cytarabine (cytosine arabinoside, AraC, Cytosar-U) plus an anthracycline (idarubicin or daunorubicin) (NCCN, 2013a).
            (1) "7 + 3" regimen—most common; cytarabine (Ara-C) given as a 24-hour continuous infusion × 7 days with idarubicin or daunorubicin ×3 days
      2. Post-remission (or consolidation) therapy—given to reduce leukemic cell population and achieve long-term, disease-free survival (DFS)

Table 15-2		
Modified Rai Staging System for Chronic Lymphocytic Leukemia		
Risk	**Extent of Disease**	
Low	Lymphocytosis (lymphoid cells >30%) No lymphadenopathy, splenomegaly, hepatomegaly Red blood cell and platelet counts near normal	
Intermediate	Lymphocytosis Lymphadenopathy in any site, splenomegaly, and/or hepatomegaly Red blood cell and platelet counts near normal	
High	Lymphocytosis Presence of anemia (hemoglobin <11 g/dL) or thrombocytopenia (platelet count $<100 \times 10^9$/L) With or without lymphadenopathy, splenomegaly, hepatomegaly	

From Rai, K. R. (1987). A critical analysis of staging in CLL. In R.P. Gale & K.R. Rai (Eds.). *Chronic lymphocytic leukemia: Recent progress and future direction.* New York: Alan R. Liss.

a. Better risk cytogenetics or molecular abnormalities
   (1) One or two cycles of the same chemotherapy agents used in the induction therapy, followed by maintenance therapy or autologous HSCT
   (2) Clinical trial
b. Intermediate risk—options include the following:
   (1) Matched sibling or unrelated donor HSCT
   (2) One or two cycles of high-dose, cytarabine-based consolidation, followed by autologous HSCT
   (3) Three to four cycles of high-dose cytarabine
   (4) Clinical trial
c. Poor risk—options include the following:
   (1) Matched sibling or alternative donor HSCT
   (2) One or two cycles of high-dose, cytarabine-based consolidation, followed by autologous HSCT, if no allogeneic transplantation option available
3. Surveillance (NCCN, 2013a)
   a. CBC every 1 to 3 months for 2 years, then every 3 to 6 months for up to 5 years
   b. Bone marrow aspirate if peripheral smear abnormal or cytopenias develop
   c. Initiation of sibling or alternative donor search at first relapse
B. CML—goal for treatment: return to hematologic values to normal and reduction or elimination of BCR/ABL transcripts
   1. Primary treatment options (NCCN, 2013c)
      a. Tyrosine kinase inhibitors (TKI)—imatinib (Gleevec), nilotinib (Tasigna), dasatinib (Sprycel)
      b. HSCT
      c. Clinical trial
   2. Supportive care for leukocytosis and thrombocytosis
      a. Symptomatic leukocytosis—hydroxyurea, apheresis, imatinib, dasatinib, nilotinib, or clinical trial
      b. Symptomatic thrombocytosis—hydroxyurea, antiaggregants, anagrelide, or apharesis
C. ALL—treatment divided into induction, consolidation, maintenance, and CNS prophylaxis or treatment
   1. Disease-related and patient-specific prognostic factors—include age, WBC count,

immunophenotypic or cytogenetic subtype, and response to induction therapy
2. Induction therapy for Ph chromosome–positive ALL
   a. Adult patients older than 40 years (NCCN, 2013b)
      (1) Patients older than 65 years
         (a) Clinical trial
         (b) TKIs (imatinib or dasatinib) + hyper-CVAD (hyperfractionated cyclophosphamide, vincristine, doxorubicin, and dexamethasone, alternating with high-dose methotrexate and cytarabine)
         (c) TKIs (imatinib) with multi agent chemotherapy (daunorubicin, vincristine, prednisone, and cyclophosphamide)
      (2) Patients older than 65 years
         (a) Clinical trial
         (b) TKIs with corticosteroids for patients older than 65 years or with significant comorbidities
         (c) TKI + chemotherapy with consideration for dose modifications based on comorbidities and performance status
   b. Adolescent and young adult (AYA) patients aged 15 to 39 years (NCCN, 2013b)
      (1) Multi agent chemotherapy—vincristine, prednisone (or dexamethasone), pegaspargase ± daunomycin
      (2) TKIs (imatinib) + hyper-CVAD
      (3) TKIs with multi agent chemotherapy
      (4) Clinical trial
3. Consolidation therapy for Ph chromosome–positive ALL
   a. Adult patients older than 40 years (NCCN, 2013b)
      (1) Allogeneic HSCT, if a donor available
      (2) Continuation of TKI + multi agent chemotherapy if an allogeneic HSCT donor not available
      (3) Continuation of TKI with corticosteroids for patients older than 65 years or with significant comorbidities
   b. AYA patients aged 15 to 39 years (NCCN, 2013b)
      (1) Allogeneic HSCT, if a donor available
      (2) Continuation of TKI + multi agent chemotherapy

4. Maintenance therapy for Ph chromosome–positive ALL
   a. Lasts 2 to 3 years
   b. Commonly used agents—include methotrexate (MTX), 6-mercaptopurine (6-MP), vincristine, prednisone, TKIs
5. Induction therapy for Ph chromosome-negative ALL
   a. Adult patients older than 40 years (NCCN, 2013b)
      (1) Multi agent chemotherapy—daunorubicin, vincristine, prednisone, pegaspargase, and cyclophosphamide
      (2) Hyper-CVAD ± rituximab (Rituxan)
      (3) Corticosteroids for patients older than 65 years or with significant comorbidities
      (4) Clinical trial
   b. AYA patients aged 15 to 39 years (NCCN, 2013b)
      (1) Multi agent chemotherapy—daunorubicin, vincristine, prednisone pegaspargase, and cyclophosphamide
      (2) Clinical trial
6. Consolidation therapy for Ph chromosome-negative ALL
   a. Adult patients older than 40 years (NCCN, 2013b)
      (1) Continued multi agent chemotherapy
      (2) Allogeneic HSCT to be considered, if a donor is available
      (3) Continued corticosteroids for patients older than 65 years or with significant comorbidities
   b. AYA patients aged 15 to 39 years (NCCN, 2013b)
      (1) Continued multi agent chemotherapy.
      (2) Consideration of allogeneic HSCT, if a donor is available
7. Maintenance therapy for Ph chromosome-negative ALL
   a. Weekly methotrexate + daily 6-mercaptopurine + monthly vincristine or prednisone pulses for 2 to 3 years
8. CNS prophylaxis and treatment for Ph chromosome–positive and negative patients
   a. Common intrathecal agents used
      (1) Methotrexate alone
      (2) Methotrexate + cytarabine and corticosteroids (triple intrathecal regimen)
9. Patients with CNS involvement at diagnosis—may be treated with either intrathecal chemotherapy or cranial irradiation
   a. Intrathecal chemotherapy started during induction chemotherapy (Linker et al., 1987)
   b. Cranial irradiation therapy—generally reserved for salvage therapy
D. CLL (Hallek et al., 2008; Simpson, 2009)
   1. Monitoring of patients with low or moderate risk who are asymptomatic, with observation until symptoms develop or disease progresses
   2. Common drugs used
      a. Purine analogues—fludarabine (Fludara), pentostatin (Nipent), cladribine (2-CdA)
      b. Alkylating agent—bendamustine (Treanda), chlorambucil (Leukeran), cyclophosphamide (Cytoxan)
      c. Monoclonal antibodies—rituximab (Rituxan), alemtuzumab (Campath)
      d. Corticosteroids—prednisone, methylprednisolone, dexamethasone
         (1) Leukocytosis and immune-mediated cytopenias—can be controlled with corticosteroids
      e. Phosphoinositide 3-kinase delta isoform (PI3Kδ) inhibitor
         (1) Idelalisib (Idela)—first, oral inhibitor of PI3Kδ
            (a) Results of phase 3 clinical trial comparing idelalisib + rituximab versus placebo + rituximab in patients with pretreated, relapsed CLL showed that those who received idelalisib + rituximab had significant improvement in progression-free survival, overall response rate, and overall survival compared with the placebo + rituximab group (Furman et al., 2013).
   3. Splenectomy—may be used for symptom relief when steroids are no longer effective
   4. RT—effective treatment for symptomatic lymphadenopathy, splenomegaly, or both
IX. Nursing implications
   A. An individualized and holistic plan of care developed and implemented in cooperation with the patient, family, and multi disciplinary team
   B. Interventions related to physical, emotional, psychological, social, and spiritual distress during extensive diagnostic testing and treatment regimen
      1. Encouraging the patient to verbalize feelings about disease and treatment

2. Exploring coping options with the patient and family and validating effective mechanisms
3. Referral to a mental health specialist, community resources, support groups (Leukemia and Lymphoma Society, American Cancer Society), as needed
4. Teaching the patient to identify and manage symptoms and to report symptoms to health care providers
5. Providing pharmacologic and nonpharmacologic interventions to managing side effects

C. Interventions related to the prevention of complications
1. It is important for nurses to conduct ongoing assessment for potential disease and treatment-related complications, such as tumor lysis syndrome, myelosuppression (neutropenia, anemia, thrombocytopenia), electrolyte imbalance, infection, cerebellar and neurologic toxicity, cardiac toxicity, steroid-related toxicities, coagulation disorders, hyperviscosity, and graft-versus-host disease

D. Fertility counseling, as indicated
E. Management of vascular access devices

References

American Cancer Society. (2013). *Cancer facts and figures—2013.* Atlanta: Author.

Faderl, S., Pui, C. -H., O'Brien, S., Kantarjian, H. M., et al. (2010). Acute lymphoblastic leukemia. In K. Hong, R. Bast, W. Hait, D. Kue, R. Pollock, & R. Weichselbaum (Eds.), *Cancer medicine* (8th ed., pp. 1591–1603). Shelton, CT: People's Medical Publishing House-USA.

Furman, R. R., Sharman, J. P., Coutre, S. E., Cheson, B. D., Pagel, J. M., Hillmen, P., et al. (2013). A phase 3, randomized, double-blind, placebo-controlled study evaluating the efficacy and safety of idelalisib and rituximab for previously treated patients with chronic lymphocytic leukemia (CLL). *Blood, 122*(21), LBA-6.

Grigoropoulos, N. F., Petter, R., Van't Veer, M. B., Scott, M. A., & Follows, G. A. (2013). Leukaemia update. Part 1: Diagnosis and management. *BMJ [British Medical Journal], 346,* f1932.

Hallek, M., Cheson, B. D., Catovsky, D., Caligaris-Cappio, F., Dighiero, G., Döhner, H., et al. (2008). Guidelines for the diagnosis and treatment of chronic lymphocytic leukemia: A report from the International Workshop on Chronic Lymphocytic Leukemia updating the National Cancer Institute–Working Group 1996 guidelines. *Blood, 111*(12), 5446–5456.

Howlader, N., Noone, A. M., Krapcho, M., Garshell, J., Neyman, N., Altekruse, S. F., et al. (2013a). *SEER cancer statistics review, 1975-2010.* http://seer.cancer.gov/csr/1975_2010/.

Howlader, N., Noone, A. M., Krapcho, M., Garshell, J., Neyman, N., & Altekruse, S. F., et al. (Eds.). (2013b). *Childhood cancer by site, incidence, survival and mortality, 1975-2010.* http://seer.cancer.gov/csr/1975_2010/results_merged/sect_28_childhood_cancer.pdf.

Kato, H., & Schull, W. J. (1982). Studies of the mortality of A-bomb survivors: 7. Mortality, 1950-1978: Part I. Cancer mortality. *Radiation Research, 90*(2), 395–432.

Kurtin, S. E. (2010). Leukemia and myelodysplastic syndromes. In C. H. Yarbro, D. Wujcik, & B. H. Gobel (Eds.), *Cancer nursing: Principles and practice* (pp. 1370–1399, 7th ed.). Sudbury, MA: Jones and Bartlett.

Linker, C. A., Levitt, L. J., O'Donnell, M., Ries, C. A., Link, M. P., Forman, S. J., et al. (1987). Improved results of treatment of adult acute lymphoblastic leukemia. *Blood, 69*(4), 1242–1248.

Musselman, J. R., Blair, C. K., Cerhan, J. R., Nguyen, P., Hirsch, B., & Ross, J. A. (2013). Risk of adult acute and chronic myeloid leukemia with cigarette smoking and cessation. *Cancer Epidemiology, 37*(4), 410–416.

National Comprehensive Cancer Network. (2013a). *NCCN practice guidelines in oncology: Acute myeloid leukemia, [v.2.2013].* http://www.nccn.org/professionals/physician_gls/pdf/aml.pdf.

National Comprehensive Cancer Network. (2013b). *NCCN practice guidelines in oncology: Acute lymphoblastic leukemia, [v.1.2013].* http://www.nccn.org/professionals/physician_gls/pdf/all.pdf.

National Comprehensive Cancer Network. (2013c). *NCCN practice guidelines in oncology: Chronic myelogenous leukemia, [v.2.2014].* http://www.nccn.org/professionals/physician_gls/pdf/cml.pdf.

Polychronakis, I., Dounias, G., Makropoulos, V., Riza, E., & Linos, A. (2013). Work-related leukemia: A systematic review. *Journal of Occupational Medicine and Toxicology, 8*(1), 14.

Rai, K. R. (1987). A critical analysis of staging in CLL. In R. P. Gale & K. R. Rai (Eds.), *Chronic lymphocytic leukemia: Recent progress and future directions.* New York: Alan R. Liss.

Schiffer, C. A., & Stone, R. M. (2010). Acute myeloid leukemia in adults: Mast cell leukemia and other mast cell neoplasms. In K. Hong, R. Bast, W. Hait, D. Kue, R. Pollock, & R. Weichselbaum. et al. (Eds.). *Cancer medicine* (pp. 1559–1581, 8th ed.). Shelton, CT: People's Medical Publishing House-USA.

Simpson, J. K. (2009). The leukemias. In S. Newton, M. Hickey, & J. Marrs (Eds.), *Oncology nursing advisor* (pp. 100–107). St. Louis.

Vardiman, J. W., Thiele, J., Arber, D. A., Brunning, R. D., Borowitz, M. J., Porwit, A., et al. (2009). The 2008 revision of the World Health Organization (WHO) classification of myeloid neoplasms and acute leukemia: Rationale and important changes. *Blood, 114*(5), 937–951.

CHAPTER 16
Lymphoma and Multiple Myeloma

Judy Petersen

I. Physiology of the lymphoid system
   A. The primitive or pluripotent stem cell—located in the bone marrow; is the progenitor for both myeloid and lymphoid cell lines with the capacity for continuous self-renewal (Friedberg, Mauch, Rimsza, & Fisher, 2011; Koury & Lichtman, 2010)
   B. Primary lymphoid tissues—bone marrow and the thymus
      1. Lymphocytes develop from committed lymphoid stem cells in the bone marrow.
      2. A portion migrates to the thymus.
         a. These cells proliferate and mature into T lymphocytes (T cells).
         b. In adults, T cells continue to proliferate peripherally.
      3. Lymphoid cells maturing in the bone marrow become B cells.
         a. Mature B cells (plasma cells) produce immunoglobulins (antibodies).
   C. Secondary lymphoid tissues where antigen-specific reactions occur:
      1. Lymph nodes, spleen, Waldeyer ring (oropharyngeal lymphoid tissue)
      2. Groups of cells in the gut, called *Peyer patches.*
      3. Lymphoid cells in the epithelium of the gut and respiratory tract called *mucosa-associated lymphoid tissue* (MALT)
      4. Distributed in interstitium and in most tissues, except in the central nervous system (CNS)
   D. Cells of the lymphoid system:
      1. T cells and B cells
      2. Reticular supporting cells, which form the lymph node structure
      3. Dendritic (Langerhans) cells, found in the skin as well as lymph nodes
II. Malignancies of the lymphoid system
   A. Hodgkin lymphoma (HL) (also referred to as *Hodgkin disease* [HD])
      1. Epidemiology
         a. Estimated 9290 new cases diagnosed and 1180 deaths from HL in 2013 (American Cancer Society [ACS], 2013)
         b. Age-related bimodal incidence—most common among teens and adults aged 15 to 35 years and adults aged 55 years and older
      2. Risk factors
         a. The exact cause of HL unknown
         b. Factors that increase the risk of HL (Engert, Eichenauer, Harris, Mauch, & Diehl, 2011; Mauch, Weiss, & Armitage, 2010):
            (1) Age—most often diagnosed in people between ages 15 and 35 years and in those 55 years or older
            (2) Infection with the Epstein-Barr virus (EBV) and human immunodeficiency virus (HIV)
            (3) Family history of lymphoma
            (4) Primary immunodeficiencies, prior solid organ and allogeneic bone marrow transplantation, and HIV
            (5) Prior treatment with cytotoxic chemotherapy drugs for other diseases
            (6) Early exposure to infections may be protective against HL (Engert et al., 2011).
      3. Pathophysiology
         a. The two distinct types of HL are classic HL (cHL) and nodular lymphocyte-predominant HL (NLPHL).
         b. Malignant cell in both types is Hodgkin/Reed-Sternberg (HRS) cell; these giant multinucleated cells are a minority (1% to 2%) in the involved tissue that is surrounded by activated immune cells (Engert et al., 2011; Mauch et al., 2010).
         c. Although clinically uniform, HL may be a group of related diseases.
      4. Clinical presentation (Engert et al., 2011; Manson & Porter, 2011)
         a. Enlarged lymph nodes, spleen, or other immune tissue, with or without systemic symptoms
         b. cHL—half of patients present with localized disease (stage I or II) in cervical and supraclavicular nodes and mediastinal lymph node

    c. NLPHL—more than 80% present with localized disease in cervical, axillary, or inguinal nodes

    d. Tends to spread first to adjacent lymph nodes

    e. Systemic symptoms (B symptoms)—fever, weight loss, fatigue, and night sweats; present in approximately 40% of patients

    f. NLPHL—earlier stage disease at presentation, longer survival, and fewer treatment failures than with classic HL (Nogová et al., 2008)

5. Diagnostic measures (Engert et al., 2011; Manson & Porter, 2011; National Comprehensive Cancer Network [NCCN], 2013)

    a. Excisional lymph node biopsy required

    b. Presence of Reed-Sternberg cells on pathologic examination

    c. Radiographic studies (contrast CT of the chest, abdomen, and pelvis) to assess disease burden

    d. Bone marrow biopsy may be required for accurate staging

    e. Immunohistochemistry and cytogenetic evaluation

    f. HIV testing and additional testing based on recommended treatment plan (e.g., evaluation of ejection fraction, pulmonary function tests)

    g. Fertility counseling

6. Classification (Engert et al., 2011; Manson & Porter, 2011; National Cancer Institute [NCI], 2013a)

    a. Two major subtypes recognized—cHL and LPHL (Box 16-1)

      (1) 95% HL are cHL, which includes four subtypes: nodular sclerosis HL, mixed cellularity HL, lymphocyte depletion HL, and lymphocyte-rich cHL.

        (a) The typical immunophenotype for cHL is CD15+, CD20−, CD30+, CD45−.

      (2) Patients with NLPHL have earlier stage disease, longer survival, and fewer treatment failures than those with cHL.

        (a) Clinicopathologic entity of B cell origin that is distinct from cHL

        (b) A common immunophenotype is CD15−, CD20+, CD30−, CD45+.

7. Staging

    a. The Ann Arbor Staging System is used. Staging is based on the extent of disease and the presence of systemic symptoms (B symptoms) (Box 16-2) (American Joint Committee on Cancer [AJCC], 2010a).

    b. The clinical staging system divides patients into four major prognostic groups that support treatment decisions (Box 16-3) (NCCN, 2013; NCI, 2013a).

8. Prognosis.

    a. Combination chemotherapy and/or radiation therapy (RT) cures more than 80% of all newly diagnosed HL patients.

    b. U.S. death rate has decreased more rapidly for adult HL than for any other malignancy in the last 5 decades (Manson & Porter, 2011).

9. Principles of medical management (Engert et al., 2011; NCCN, 2013; NCI, 2013a).

    a. Choice of therapy influenced by clinical stage and prognostic group more than histology

    b. Standard treatment approaches being defined for the different prognostic groups

    c. Early favorable stages—limited amount of chemotherapy (typically two or three cycles) plus involved field radiation

    d. Early unfavorable stages—moderate amount of chemotherapy (typically four cycles) plus involved field radiation

    e. Advanced stages—extensive chemotherapy (typically eight cycles), with or without consolidation RT (usually to residual tumors)

    f. Relapse after treatment

      (1) Chemotherapy with the same or another regimen followed by high-dose chemotherapy and autologous bone marrow or peripheral stem cell or allogeneic bone marrow transplantation for patients who meet transplantation criteria

    g. Survivorship issues and monitoring for long-term effects (see Chapter 42)

B. Non-Hodgkin lymphoma (NHL)

1. Epidemiology

    a. Estimated 69,740 new cases diagnosed and 29,020 deaths from NHL in 2013; overall incidence rates stable among men and women from 2005 to 2009; however, NHL encompasses a wide variety of disease subtypes for which incidence patterns may vary (ACS, 2013).

    b. Incidence—increased over the past 3 decades but has remained relatively steady since 2004 (Howlader et al., 2013)

    c. Mortality rates—began decreasing in the late 1990s; decrease by 3% per year from 2005 to 2009 (ACS, 2013)

    d. From 2006 to 2010, median age at diagnosis was 66 years (Howlader et al., 2013).

2. Risk factors

    a. Cause of most cases of NHL unknown

    b. Risk factors for NHL (Freedman, 2010; Friedberg et al., 2011)

      (1) Immunodeficiency—inherited, acquired, solid organ transplantation.

Box 16-1

2008 WHO Classification of Mature B-Cell, T-Cell and NK Cell Neoplasms*

Mature B-Cell Neoplasms

- Chronic lymphocytic leukemia, small lymphocytic lymphoma
- B-cell prolymphocytic leukemia
  - Splenic marginal zone lymphoma*
  - Hairy cell leukemia
- Lymphoplasmacytic lymphoma*
  - Waldenstrom macroglobinemia*
- Heavy-chain disease
  - Alpha heavy-chain disease
  - Gamma heavy-chain disease
  - Mu heavy-chain disease
- Plasma cell myeloma (multiple myeloma)
- Solitary plasmacytoma of bone
- Extraosseous plasmacytoma
- Extranodal marginal zone lymphoma of mucosa-associated lymphoid tissue (MALT type)
- Nodal marginal zone lymphoma (MZL)*
- Follicular lymphoma*
- Primary cutaneous follicle center lymphoma
- Mantle cell lymphoma
- Diffuse large B-cell lymphoma (DLBCL), not otherwise specified (NOS)
  - T-cell/histiocyte-rich large B-cell lymphoma
  - DLBCL associated with chronic inflammation
  - Primary cutaneous DLBCL, leg type
- Lymphomatoid granulomatosis
- Primary mediastinal (thymic) large B-cell lymphoma
- Intravascular large B-cell lymphoma
- ALK-positive large B-cell lymphoma
- Plasmablastic lymphoma
- Primary effusion lymphoma
- Large B-cell lymphoma arising in HHV8-associated multi centric Castleman disease
- Burkitt lymphoma
- B-cell lymphoma, unclassifiable, with features intermediate between diffuse large B-cell lymphoma and Burkitt lymphoma

- B-cell lymphoma, unclassifiable, with features intermediate between diffuse large B-cell lymphoma and classic Hodgkin lymphoma

Hodgkin Lymphoma

- Classic Hodgkin lymphoma
- Nodular lymphocyte-predominant Hodgkin lymphoma (NLPHL)
  - Nodular sclerosis HL
  - Mixed-cellularity HL
  - Lymphocyte depletion HL
  - Lymphocyte-rich classic HL

Mature T-Cell and NK Cell Neoplasms

- T-cell prolymphocytic leukemia
- T-cell large granular lymphocytic leukemia
- Aggressive NK cell leukemia
- Systemic EBV-positive, T-cell lymphoproliferative disorder of childhood
- Hydroa vacciniforme-like lymphoma
- Adult T-cell leukemia, lymphoma
- Extranodal NK cell and T-cell lymphoma, nasal type
- Enteropathy-type T-cell lymphoma
- Hepatosplenic T-cell lymphoma
- Subcutaneous panniculitis-like T-cell lymphoma
- Mycosis fungoides
- Sézary syndrome
- Primary cutaneous CD30-positive T-cell lymphoproliferative disorders
  - Lymphomatoid papulosis
  - Primary cutaneous anaplastic large cell lymphoma*
- Primary cutaneous gamma-delta T-cell lymphoma
- Peripheral T-cell lymphoma, NOS
- Angioimmunoblastic T-cell lymphoma
- Anaplastic large cell lymphoma, ALK-positive

*Several histologic types were newly identified as provisional in the 2008 WHO classification system. They have been left out of this box.

Data from Swerdlow, S.H., Campo, E., Harris, N.L., Jaffe, E.S., Pileri, S.A., Stein, H., et al. (Eds.). (2008). *World Health Organization classification of tumours of the haematopoietic and lymphoid tissues* (4th ed.). Lyon, France: IARC Press; National Comprehensive Cancer Network. (2013). *NCCN clinical practice guidelines in oncology* [v.2.2013]; Jaffe, E.S. (2009). The 2008 WHO classification of lymphomas: Implications for clinical practice and translational research. *Hematology*, 1, 523–531.

(2) Infectious agents
    (a) Infection with EBV—associated with Burkitt lymphoma
    (b) Infection with the HTLV-1—increases risk for T-cell lymphoma
    (c) HIV

    (d) *Helicobacter pylori* bacterial infection linked to MALT lymphoma in the stomach
(3) Environmental and occupational exposure to radiation, chemicals, pesticides, and solvents

Part 2

Box 16-2

Ann Arbor Staging System

Stage I
- Involvement of single lymph node region (I), or
- Localized involvement of a single extralymphatic organ or site (Ie)

Stage II
- Involvement of two or more lymph node regions, same side of diaphragm (II), or
- Localized involvement of a single associated extralymphatic organ or site and its regional lymph node(s), with or without involvement of other lymph node regions on the same side of the diaphragm (IIe)

Stage III
- Involvement of lymph nodes on both sides of diaphragm (III), which may also be accompanied by
- Localized involvement of an associated extralymphatic organ or site (IIIe), or
- Involvement of the spleen (IIIs), or
- Both (IIIe+IIIs)

Stage IV
- Disseminated involvement of extralymphatic organs, with or without associated lymph node involvement, or isolated extralymphatic organ involvement with distant nodal involvement

If the patient has fever, night sweats, or weight loss (>10% of body weight), the B designation is added to the stage. If the patient does not have these symptoms, this is designated with the letter "A."

Box 16-3

Hodgkin Lymphoma Prognostic Categories by Stage and Clinical Features

- **Early favorable:** Clinical stage I or II without any risk factors
- **Early unfavorable:** Clinical stage I or II with one or more of the following risk factors:
  - Large mediastinal mass (>33% of the thoracic width on the chest radiography; ≥10 cm on CT)
  - Extranodal involvement
  - Three or more lymph node areas' involvement
  - Elevated erythrocyte sedimentation rate (>30 mm/hr for B stage, >50 mm/hr for A stage)
  - B symptoms
- **Advanced favorable:** Clinical stage III or IV with zero to three adverse risk factors

- **Advanced unfavorable:** Clinical stage III or IV with four or more of the following risk factors:
  - Male gender
  - Age ≥ 45 years
  - Albumin level < 4.0 g/dL
  - Hemoglobin level < 10.5 g/dL
  - Stage IV disease
  - White blood cell (WBC) count ≥ 15,000/mm^3
  - Absolute lymphocytic count < 600/mm^3 or lymphocyte count that was <8% of the total WBC count

---

3. Pathophysiology
   a. A heterogeneous group of lymphoproliferative cancers with wide range of histologic appearances, clinical features, behavior, and response to treatment
   b. 85% to 90% arising from B lymphocytes, rest from T lymphocytes or natural killer (NK) lymphocytes (Shankland, Armitage, & Hancock, 2012)
4. Clinical presentation (Friedberg et al., 2011; Manson & Porter, 2011; Shankland et al., 2012)
   a. Dependent on site of involvement and natural history of the subtype
   b. Painless lymphadenopathy more generalized, less predictable than HL, more commonly spreads to extranodal sites
   c. Other possible symptoms—pruritus, fatigue, abdominal pain (enlarged spleen or liver; bulky adenopathy), bone pain
   d. Involvement of bone marrow, liver, or other extranodal site common; most often presents as disseminated disease
5. Diagnostic measures (Manson & Porter, 2011; NCCN, 2013).
   a. Excisional lymph node biopsy required

b. Radiographic studies (contrast CT of the chest, abdomen, and pelvis) to assess disease burden

c. Bone marrow biopsy may be required for accurate staging.

d. Immunohistochemistry and cytogenetic evaluation

e. HIV testing and additional testing based on recommended treatment plan (i.e., evaluation of ejection fraction, pulmonary function tests)

6. Classification (AJCC, 2010a; Freedman, 2010; NCCN, 2013)

a. New diseases and subtypes added in the revised 2008 World Health Organization (WHO) classification system (see Box 16-3)

b. Cell of origin (B, T, or NK) considered; further refinement based on immunophenotype and genetic and clinical features; B-cell neoplasms, T-cell or (NK) cell neoplasms, HL

7. Staging

a. Ann Arbor Staging System—based on the extent of disease and the presence of systemic symptoms (B symptoms) (see Box 16-2) (AJCC, 2010a)

b. Most patients with advanced (stage III or stage IV) disease at presentation

c. Additional factors not included in the staging system important to consider for prognosis and treatment; age, performance status, tumor size, lactate dehydrogenase (LDH) values, and number of extranodal sites

8. Prognosis

a. Depends on grade or aggressiveness of lymphoma and responsiveness to treatment

b. Low-grade lymphomas—have an indolent course with prolonged survival (10 to 15 years) without aggressive therapy; not considered curable and characterized by recurrences, especially in advanced stages; occasionally, can transform into high-grade NHL

c. Prognosis of high-grade lymphomas—depends on tumor bulk, responsiveness to therapy, and patient's ability to tolerate treatment; majority of patients with localized disease curable with radiation plus chemotherapy or combination chemotherapy alone; 50% of patients with advanced-stage disease cured with doxorubicin-based combination chemotherapy and rituximab

d. International prognostic index (IPI) (The International Non-Hodgkin's Lymphoma Prognostic Factors Index [INHLPFP], 1993)

(1) Assigns patients to a risk group and predict outcome

Table 16-1		
International Prognostic Index (IPI)		
IPI Risk Factors	**Unfavorable (1 Point)***	**Favorable (0 Points)**
Age (yr)	>60	≤60
Ann Arbor tumor stage	III or IV	I or II
Number of extranodal sites	>1	≤1
Performance status (ECOG)	≥2	0 or 1
Serum LDH level	Abnormal	Normal
IPI Risk		
Low	0-1	
Intermediate	2	
High intermediate	3	
High	4-5	

ECOG, Eastern Cooperative Oncology Group; *LDH*, lactate dehydrogenase.

*The sum of the unfavorable risk factors determines the overall risk level.

Data from the International Non-Hodgkin's Lymphoma Prognostic Factors Project. (1993). A predictive model for aggressive non-Hodgkin's lymphoma. *New England Journal of Medicine, 329*(14), 987–994.

(2) Five risk factors identified; predict lower complete response, relapse-free survival, and overall survival (Table 16-1)

e. Relapse—may occur; requires biopsy and restaging

9. Principles of medical management (Friedberg et al., 2011; Manson & Porter, 2011; NCI, 2013b; NCCN, 2013)

a. Therapeutic choices are increasingly tailored to the immunologically classified lymphoma.

b. The most common NHL types are indolent (follicular lymphoma [FL] 20%) and aggressive (diffuse large B-cell lymphoma [DLBCL] 30%) NHL; treatment plans are representative for NHL.

c. Standard treatment options for indolent FL include the following:

(1) For stage I or II disease:

(a) RT (loco-regional treatment)

(b) Monoclonal antibodies (rituximab [Rituxan] alone or combination with chemotherapy (single-agent or combination therapy)

(c) Observation until symptomatic

(2) For stage III or IV disease

(a) Observation recommended if no symptoms, cytopenias, or end-organ dysfunction

(b) Monoclonal antibodies (rituximab [Rituxan]) alone or combination with chemotherapy (single-agent or combination therapy)

(c) Radiation therapy for palliation of symptomatic disease

d. Intermediate and high-grade DLBCL are considered systemic disease. Standard treatment options include the following:

(1) For stage I or contiguous II disease

(a) Chemotherapy with or without involved-field radiation therapy (IF-XRT)

(b) R-CHOP (rituximab [Rituxan], cyclophosphamide, doxorubicin [Adriamycin], vincristine, prednisone)

(2) Treatment for aggressive, noncontiguous stage II/, III, or IV disease:

(a) R-CHOP or other combination chemotherapy

e. Recurrent NHL

(1) Other chemotherapy regimens (single agent or combination)

(2) Autologous peripheral blood stem cell (PBSC), allogeneic PBSC, or bone marrow transplantation for aggressive NHL, under investigation for indolent NHL

(3) Palliative radiation therapy

f. Supportive care

(1) Management of infections, tumor lysis syndrome, use of myeloid growth factors and blood product transfusions (NCCN, 2013b)

C. Multiple myeloma

1. Epidemiology

a. Estimated 22,350 new cases diagnosed and 10,710 deaths from multiple myeloma in 2013 (ACS, 2013)

b. Second most common hematologic malignancy in the United States; constitutes approximately 1% of all cancers (ACS, 2013)

2. Risk factors

a. Risk factors for multiple myeloma (De Roos, Baris, Weiss, & Herrinton, 2006)

(1) Environmental exposure to ionizing radiation

(2) Exposure to low-level radiation (e.g., radiologists, those employed in the nuclear industry or who handle radioactive materials)

(3) Exposure to metals (especially nickel), agricultural chemicals, benzene, and petroleum products, aromatic hydrocarbons, and silicone

(4) Family history

(5) History of monoclonal gammopathy of undetermined significance (MGUS)

(6) Ethnicity—higher incidence among African Americans

(7) Older age—most patients diagnosed with this disease in their 60s (Munshi & Anderson, 2011; Tariman & Faiman, 2011)

3. Pathophysiology

a. Multiple myeloma is the most common of the several types of plasma cell neoplasms. These diseases are all associated with a monoclonal (or myeloma) protein (M protein).

b. Although a solitary plasmacytoma could occur, multiple myeloma, by definition, is a systemic disease.

c. This malignant plasma cell is a B cell that has differentiated to produce abnormally high blood levels of a monoclonal immunoglobulin or M protein.

(1) Not effective in immune function

(2) Growth influenced by cytokines (e.g., interleukin-6 [IL-6], vascular endothelial growth factor [VEGF])

d. Myeloma cells also produce osteoclast-activating factor.

(1) Produces lytic bone lesions, resulting in a "punched-out" appearance on radiographs and often in pathologic fractures

(2) Increases bone resorption, which may cause hypercalcemia

4. Clinical presentation (Munshi & Anderson, 2011; Tariman & Faiman, 2011)

a. Commonly presents with bone pain from lytic lesions (back and chest)

b. Multiple lytic bone lesions, high serum M protein, and extensive bone marrow plasmacytosis (>30%) common presentation

c. Multiple systemic symptoms—anemia, uremia, recurrent infections, hypercalcemia, hyperviscosity, polyneuropathy, and spinal cord compression

5. Diagnostic measures (De Roos et al., 2006; Munshi & Anderson, 2011; NCCN, 2013)

a. Bone marrow biopsy—demonstrates presence of more than 10% plasma cells

b. Serum protein immunoelectrophoresis—demonstrates increased levels of heavy-chain M proteins. Urine protein immunoelectrophoresis demonstrates increased levels of light-chain

c. M proteins (Bence Jones proteins)

d. Myeloma-related organ dysfunction (CRAB criteria)

(1) **C**alcium elevation in blood—calcium level greater than 10.5 ng/L or upper limit of normal

(2) **R**enal insufficiency—serum creatinine level greater than 2 mg/dL

(3) **A**nemia—hemoglobin less than 10 g/dL

(4) **B**one lytic lesions

e. Serum albumin and beta-2-microglobulin levels; level of beta-2-microglobulin reflects tumor mass, standard measure for tumor burden

  (1) Beta-2-microglobulin is used as a marker for multiple myeloma but is not specific to myeloma.

f. Additional blood studies, biologic assessment to differentiate symptomatic and asymptomatic myeloma (i.e., decreased kidney function indicated by increased blood urea nitrogen [BUN] and creatinine levels)

6. Classification (AJCC, 2010b; Munshi & Anderson, 2011; NCCN, 2013).

a. Multiple myeloma (plasma cell myeloma or plasmacytoma) is included in the REAL/WHO classification system (see Box 16-1).

7. Staging

a. Historical Durie-Salmon staging system (stages I to III)—quantifies tumor volume on the basis of the amount of M proteins in urine and blood, along with clinical parameters, hemoglobin, serum calcium level, and presence of bone lesions (AJCC, 2010b; Durie & Salmon, 1975).

b. More recently developed International Staging System (ISS)—stages I to III based on the levels of beta-2-microglobulin and albumin in blood; these factors are better predictors of patient survival (Greipp et al., 2005).

c. Genetic factors and risk groups—support individualized treatment strategies

  (1) Genetic abnormalities identified by fluorescence in situ hybridization (FISH) have defined prognostic groups in retrospective and prospective analyses (Avet-Loiseau et al., 2007).

    (a) Risk stratification based on genetic translocations (Chesi & Bersagel, 2011)

      (i) Standard risk—t(11;14) and t(6;14) translocations

      (ii) Intermediate risk—t(4;14) translocation

      (iii) High risk—del17p, t(14;16), and t(14;20) translocations

d. Resultant risk group stratification; standard versus high risk (NCI, 2013)

8. Prognosis

a. No cure exists for multiple myeloma. Improvements in survival continue with newer therapies, and median survival now exceeds 45 to 60 months (NCI, 2013c).

9. Principles of medical management (Munshi & Anderson, 2011; NCCN, 2013; NCI, 2013c; Tariman & Faiman, 2011;)

a. Diagnostic challenge—identification of stable, asymptomatic patients who do not require treatment versus those with symptomatic myeloma, which requires immediate treatment

b. Treatment choices for symptomatic myeloma based on therapy for transplantation candidate versus nontransplantation candidate

  (1) For nontransplantation candidates

    (a) Melphalan and prednisone (MP)—a standard treatment since 1960; MP results in a 60% response rate and overall survival of 24 to 36 months (Gregory, Richards, & Malpas, 1992)

    (b) Combination of melphalan, prednisone, and thalidomide (Thalomid) (MPT)—has better response rates and progression-free survival compared with MP alone (Kapoor et al., 2011)

      (i) MPT considered category 1 primary treatment for nontransplantation candidates (NCCN, 2013)

      (ii) Need to use thromboprophylaxis because of significant risk of deep venous thrombosis (DVT) with thalidomide

    (c) Other preferred regimens (NCCN, 2013)

      (i) Bortezomib (Velcade) and dexamethasone

      (ii) Lenalidomide (Revlimid) and low-dose dexamethasone

      (iii) Melphalan, prednisone, and bortezomib

  (2) For transplantation candidates, alkylating agents (e.g., melphalan) avoided during induction therapy to prevent compromise of stem cell collection

    (a) Introduction of new drugs (immunomodulatory, proteasome inhibitor drugs) has significantly prolonged survival, but no therapy is curative.

    (b) Preferred regimens include the following (NCCN, 2013):

      (i) Bortezomib and dexamethasone

      (ii) Bortezomib, doxorubicin, and dexamethasone

      (iii) Bortezomib, thalidomide, and dexamethasone

      (iv) Lenalidomide and dexamethasone

c. No clear choice of induction therapy at this time; options include several categories:

steroids (e.g., dexamethasone and prednisone), antiangiogenesis agents and immunomodulating agents (e.g., thalidomide, lenalidomide), proteasome inhibitors (e.g., bortezomib), alkylating agents (e.g., melphalan and cyclophosphamide), and other cytotoxic drugs (e.g., vincristine, doxorubicin, liposomal doxorubicin)

  (1) Steroids usually given in high doses

    (a) Given the median age of patients with multiple myeloma, it is important to monitor for potential toxicities: hyperglycemia, hypokalemia, sodium and water retention, weight gain, cushingoid changes, mood changes, euphoria, psychosis, and insomnia (Wilkes & Barton-Burke, 2013).

    (b) It may be necessary to adjust the warfarin (Coumadin) and insulin doses.

  d. Stem cell transplantation (SCT)—important component for eligible, newly diagnosed patients

    (1) Types of SCT

      (a) Autologous SCT—standard of care after primary therapy for eligible patients

      (b) Tandem SCT—planned second course of high-dose therapy and SCT within 6 months of the first course

        (i) May be an option as salvage therapy for relapse or progressive disease

      (c) Allogeneic SCT—an option as part of a clinical trial or salvage therapy in patients with progressive disease

  e. Different maintenance therapies studied to sustain remission; modest improvements have been shown, but role of maintenance therapy remains unclear

  f. Eventual relapse in all patients; treatment with alternative chemotherapy; choice dependent on prior treatment used for induction and toxicities (e.g., neuropathy, cytopenias, DVT)

  g. Supportive care

    (1) Bisphosphonates—for all patients receiving myeloma therapy

    (2) RT—for painful lytic lesions, spinal cord compression

    (3) Ongoing treatment for disease complications—hypercalcemia, hyperviscosity, renal impairment, anemia, infection, coagulation disorders

III. Nursing implications

  A. An individualized and holistic plan of care needed when caring for the patient with a lymphoid malignancy

  B. The plan of care developed and implemented in cooperation with the patient, family, and multidisciplinary team

  C. Interventions related to physical, emotional, psychological, social, and spiritual distress during extensive diagnostic testing and treatment regimen

    1. Encouraging patient to verbalize feelings about disease and treatment

    2. Exploring the coping options with the patient and family and validating effective mechanisms

    3. Referral to a mental health specialist, community resources, support groups (Leukemia and Lymphoma Society, American Cancer Society, International Myeloma Foundation), as needed

    4. Teaching the patient to identify and manage symptoms, and to report symptoms to health care providers

    5. Providing pharmacologic and nonpharmacologic interventions to managing side effects

  D. Interventions related to the prevention of complications

    1. Ongoing assessment for potential disease and treatment-related complications: tumor lysis syndrome, superior vena cava syndrome, hypercalcemia, hyperviscosity, renal impairment, skeleton-related events, anemia, infection, and coagulation disorders

References

American Cancer Society. (2013). *Cancer facts & figures, 2013.* http://www.cancer.org/research/cancerfactsstatistics/cancerfactsfigures2013/index.

American Joint Committee on Cancer. (2010a). Hodgkin and non-Hodgkin lymphomas. In S. B. Edge, D. R. Byrd, C. C. Compton, A. G. Fritz, F. L. Greene, & A. Trotti (Eds.), *AJCC cancer staging manual* (7th ed.). New York: Springer.

American Joint Committee on Cancer. (2010b). Multiple myeloma and plasma cell disorders. In S. B. Edge, D. R. Byrd, C. C. Compton CC, A. G. Fritz, F. L. Greene, & A. Trotti (Eds.), *AJCC cancer staging manual* (7th ed.). New York: Springer.

Avet-Loiseau, H., Attal, M., Moreau, P., Charbonnel, C., Garban, F., Hulin, C., et al. (2007). Genetic abnormalities and survival in multiple myeloma: The experience of the Intergroupe Francophone du Myélome. *Blood, 109*(8), 3489–3495.

Chesi, M., & Bergsagel, P. L. (2011). Many multiple myelomas: making more of the molecular mayhem. *Hematology, 2011*(1), 344–353.

De Roos, A., Baris, D., Weiss, N. S., & Herrinton, L. J. (2006). Multiple myeloma. In D. Schottenfeld & J. F. Fraumeni (Eds.), *Cancer epidemiology and prevention*. (3rd ed.). New York, NY: Oxford University Press.

Durie, B. G. M., & Salmon, S. E. (1975). A clinical staging system for multiple myeloma. *Cancer, 36*(9), 842–854.

Engert, A., Eichenauer, D. A., Harris, N. L., Mauch, P. M., & Diehl, V. (2011). Hodgkin lymphoma. In V. DeVita, Jr., T. Lawrence, & S. Rosenberg (Eds.), *Cancer: principles and practice of oncology*. (11th ed.). Philadelphia: Lippincott Williams & Wilkins.

Freedman, A. S. (2010). Non-Hodgkin lymphoma. In W. K. Hong, R. C. Bast, Jr., W. N. Hait, D. W. Kufe, R. E. Pollock, R. R. Weichselbaum, & E. Frei, III., (Eds.), *Cancer medicine* (pp. 1646–1658). Shelton, CT: People's Medical Publishing House-USA.

Friedberg, J. S., Mauch, P. M., Rimsza, L., & Fisher, R. I. (2011). Non-Hodgkin lymphomas. In V. DeVita, Jr., T. Lawrence, & S. Rosenberg (Eds.), *Cancer: principles and practice of oncology*. (11th ed.). Philadelphia: Lippincott Williams & Wilkins.

Gregory, W. M., Richards, M. A., & Malpas, J. S. (1992). Combination chemotherapy versus melphalan and prednisolone in the treatment of multiple myeloma: An overview of published trials. *Journal of Clinical Oncology, 10*, 334–342.

Greipp, P. R., San Miguel, J., Durie, B. G., Crowley, J. J., Barlogie, B., Blade, J., et al. (2005). International staging system for multiple myeloma. *Journal of Clinical Oncology, 23*(15), 3412–3420.

Howlader, N., Noone, A. M., Krapcho, M., Garshell, J., Neyman, N., Altekruse, S. F., & Cronin, K. A. (Eds.) (2013). *SEER cancer statistics review, 1975-2010*. Bethesda, MD: National Cancer Institute.

Jaffe, E. S. (2009). The 2008 WHO classification of lymphomas: Implications for clinical practice and translational research. *Hematology, 2009*(1), 523–531.

Kapoor, P., Rajkumar, S. V., Dispenzieri, A., Gertz, M. A., Lacy, M. Q., Dingli, D., et al. (2011). Melphalan and prednisone versus melphalan, prednisone and thalidomide for elderly and/or transplant ineligible patients with multiple myeloma: A meta-analysis. *Leukemia, 25*(4), 689–696.

Koury, M. J., & Lichtman, M. A. (2010). Structure of the marrow and the hematopoietic microenvironment. In K. Kaushansky, M. A. Lichtman, E. Beutler, T. J. Kipps, U. Seligsoh, & J. T. Prchal (Eds.), *Williams hematology* (8th ed.). New York: McGraw-Hill.

Manson, S., & Porter, C. (2011). Lymphomas. In C. H. Yarbro, D. Wujcik, & B. H. Gobel (Eds.), *Cancer nursing: principles and practice* (7th ed.). Sudbury, MA: Jones and Bartlett.

Mauch, P. M., Weiss, L., & Armitage, J. O. (2010). Hodgkin Lymphoma. In W. K. Hong, R. C. Bast, Jr., W. N. Hait, D. W. Kufe, R. E. Pollock, R. R. Weichselbaum, & E. Frei, III. (Eds.), *Cancer medicine* (pp. 1622–1644). Shelton, CT: People's Medical Publishing House-USA.

Munshi, N., & Anderson, K. (2011). Plasma cell neoplasms. In V. DeVita, Jr., T. Lawrence, & S. Rosenberg (Eds.), *Cancer: principles and practice of oncology* (11th ed.). Philadelphia: Lippincott Williams & Wilkins.

National Cancer Institute. (2013a). *PDQ adult Hodgkin lymphoma treatment*. http://cancer.gov/cancertopics/pdq/treatment/adulthodgkins/HealthProfessional.

National Cancer Institute. (2013b). *PDQ adult non-Hodgkin lymphoma treatment*. http://www.cancer.gov/cancertopics/pdq/treatment/adult-non-hodgkins/HealthProfessional.

National Cancer Institute (2013c). *PDQ adult Hodgkin lymphoma treatment*. http://www.cancer.gov/cancertopics/pdq/treatment/myeloma/healthprofessional/page1/AllPages#Section_53.

National Comprehensive Cancer Network. (2013). *NCCN clinical practice guidelines in oncology [v.2.2013]*. http://www.nccn.org/professionals/physician_gls/f_guidelines.asp.

Nogová, L., Reineke, T., Brillant, C., Sieniawski, M., Rudiger, T., Josting, A., et al. (2008). Lymphocyte-predominant and classical Hodgkin's lymphoma: A comprehensive analysis from the German Hodgkin Study Group. *Journal of Clinical Oncology, 26*(3), 434–439.

Shankland, K. R., Armitage, J. O., & Hancock, B. W. (2012). Non-Hodgkin lymphoma. *Lancet, 380*, 848–857.

Swerdlow, S. H., Campo, E., Harris, N. L., Jaffe, E. S., Pileri, S. A., Stein, H., & Vadiman, J. W. (Eds.), (2008). *World Health Organization classification of tumours of the haematopoietic and lymphoid tissues* (4th. ed.). Lyon, France: IARC Press.

Tariman, J., & Faiman, B. (2011). Multiple myeloma. In C. H. Yarbro, D. Wujcik, & B. H. Gobel (Eds.), *Cancer nursing: principles and practice* (7th ed.). Sudbury, MA: Jones & Bartlett.

The International Non-Hodgkin's Lymphoma Prognostic Factors Project. (1993). A predictive model for aggressive non-Hodgkin's lymphoma. *New England Journal of Medicine, 329*(14), 987–994.

Wilkes, G. M., & Barton-Burke, M. (2013). *2013 Oncology nursing drug handbook*. St. Louis: Jones & Bartlett.

CHAPTER 17

Bone and Soft Tissue Cancers

Ellen Carr

OVERVIEW

I. Pathophysiology

A. Bone cancer

1. From mesoderm and ectoderm; pseudocapsule contains tumor, then breaks through to surrounding tissue (called skip metastasis)

2. Patterns of growth (Samuel, 2011)
   a. Compression of normal tissue
   b. Resorption of bone by reactive osteoclasts
   c. Destruction of normal tissue (when malignant).

3. Staging based on biologic behavior and tumor aggressiveness
   a. "A" stage lesions—present as intracompartmental
   b. "B" stage lesions—present as extracompartmental

4. Common malignant bone and soft tissue cancers (with cell or tissue of origin) (Samuel, 2011) (Tables 17-1, 17-2, and 17-3)
   a. Osteosarcoma (osteogenic sarcoma, osseous tissue)—56% of all bone tumors (National Cancer Institute [NCI], 2013e)
      (1) Most often affects adolescents
      (2) Males affected more frequently than females (Samuel, 2011)
      (3) Tumor cells—spindle-shaped, from bone-forming mesenchyma in the medullary cavity; reactive osteoclasts interact with normal bone to destroy it.
      (4) Starts in metaphysis of long bones (area of highest growth), especially in cases in knee region (Samuel, 2011)
      (5) Metastasizes to the lung first; at diagnosis, 10% treated with surgery alone have 5-year survival; with adjuvant chemotherapy, 55% to 80% have 5-year survival (Malawer, Helman, & O'Sullivan, 2011; Samuel, 2011)
   b. Chondrosarcoma (cartilaginous tissue) (Singer, Nielsen, & Antonescu, 2011)
      (1) Occurs most often in adults aged 30 to 60 years (Samuel, 2011)
      (2) Occurs more often in men (Samuel, 2011)
      (3) Origin—malignant cartilaginous tumor cells from medullary canal or outside bone, destroying the bone
      (4) Commonly affects pelvis, femur, and shoulder
      (5) Often slow-growing but may metastasize distantly
   c. Fibrosarcoma (fibrous tissue)
      (1) Most often seen in adolescents and young adults
      (2) Commonly affects the femur and tibia
      (3) Arises from the medullary cavity, affects the metaphyseal area
      (4) Constitutes fewer than 7% of all primary malignant bone cancers (Samuel, 2011)
   d. Ewing family of tumors (EFT, reticuloendothelial tissue) (NCI, 2013d)
      (1) Constitutes approximately 6% of all primary malignant bone cancers (Samuel, 2011)
      (2) 80% of patients diagnosed when 5 to 15 years old (Samuel, 2011)
         (a) Occurs mainly during childhood; mean age, 15 years (NCI, 2013d)
      (3) Highly malignant (20% to 30% with metastases at time of diagnosis) (NCI, 2013d); origin in nonmesenchymal area of bone marrow; from shaft of long bones, pelvic bone, or chest wall
      (4) Most often affects pelvis and lower extremities; femoral diaphysis is the most common site
         (a) Primary sites of bone disease—lower extremity (41%), pelvis (26%), chest wall (16%), upper extremity (9%), spine (6%), skull (2%)

Table 17-1

Cancers of the Bone

Types of Cancer	Tissue of Origin	Common Locations	Common Ages (yr)
Osteosarcoma	Osteoid	Knees, upper legs, upper arms	10-25
Chondrosarcoma	Cartilage	Pelvis, upper legs, shoulders	50-60
Ewing sarcoma	Immature nerve tissue, usually in bone marrow	Pelvis, upper legs, ribs, arms	10-20

Data from *National Cancer Institute (2013d). Ewing sarcoma.* http://nci.nih.gov/cancertopics/types/ewing; *National Cancer Institute (2013b). Bone cancer.* http://nci.nih.gov/cancertopics/types/bone.

Table 17-2

Major Types of Soft Tissue Sarcomas in Adults

Tissue of Origin	Type of Cancer	Usual Location in the Body
Fibrous tissue	Fibrosarcoma	Arms, legs, trunk
	Malignant fibrous histiocytoma	Legs
	Dermatofibrosarcoma	Trunk
Fat	Liposarcoma	Arms, legs, trunk
Muscle Striated muscle Smooth muscle	Rhabdomyosarcoma Leiomyosarcoma	Arms, legs Uterus, digestive tract
Blood vessels	Hemangiosarcoma	Arms, legs, trunk
	Kaposi sarcoma	Legs, trunk
Lymph vessels	Lymphangiosarcoma	Arms
Synovial tissue (linings of joint cavities, tendon sheaths)	Synovial sarcoma	Legs
Peripheral nerves	Neurofibrosarcoma	Arms, legs, trunk
Cartilage and bone-forming tissue	Extraskeletal chondrosarcoma	Legs
	Extraskeletal osteosarcoma	Legs, trunk (not involving the bone)

Data from *National Cancer Institute. (2013d). Ewing sarcoma treatment (PDQ).* http://www.cancer.gov/cancertopics/pdq/treatment/ewings/HealthProfessional; *National Cancer Institute. (2013c). Childhood rhabdomyosarcoma.* http://nci.nih.gov/cancertopics/types/childrhabdomyosarcoma.

Table 17-3

Major Types of Soft Tissue Sarcomas in Children

Tissue of Origin	Type of Cancer	Ages: Most Common (yr)	Usual Location in the Body
Muscle Striated muscle	Rhabdomyosarcoma Embryonal Alveolar	Infant to adolescent	Head and neck, genitourinary tract Arms, legs, head and neck
Smooth muscle	Leiomyosarcoma	15-19	Trunk
Fibrous tissue	Fibrosarcoma	15-19	Arms, legs
	Malignant fibrous histiocytoma	15-19	Legs
	Dermatofibrosarcoma	15-19	Trunk
Fat	Liposarcoma	15-19	Arms, legs
Blood vessels	Infantile hemangiopericytoma	Infant to adolescent	Arms, legs, trunk, head, neck
Synovial tissue*	Synovial sarcoma	15-19	Legs, arms, trunk
Peripheral nerves	Malignant peripheral nerve sheath tumors (also called *neurofibrosarcomas, malignant schwannomas, neurogenic sarcomas*)	15-19	Arms, legs, trunk
Muscular nerves	Alveolar soft part sarcoma	Infant to adolescent	Arms, legs
Cartilage and bone-forming tissue	Extraskeletal myxoid chondrosarcoma	10-14	Legs
	Extraskeletal mesenchymal	10-14	Legs

*"Synovial tissue" includes linings of structures such as joint cavities, tendon sheaths.

Data from *National Cancer Institute. (2013a). Adult soft tissue sarcoma treatment (PDQ).* http://nci.nih.gov/cancertopics/pdq/treatment/adult-soft-tissue-sarcoma/HealthProfessional; *National Cancer Institute. (2013c).* Childhood rhabdomyosarcoma. http://nci.nih.gov/cancertopics/types/childrhabdomyosarcoma; *National Cancer Institute. (2013f). Soft tissue sarcoma.* http://nci.nih.gov/cancertopics/types/soft-tissue-sarcoma.

(b) With extraosseous Ewing (EOE) sarcoma—primary tumors, trunk (32%), extremity (26%), head and neck (18%), retroperitoneum (16%), other sites (9%)

(5) Spreads to adjacent tissue via many round cells; indistinct borders; necrotic and hemorrhagic areas common

(6) Metastasizes to lungs, lymph nodes, and other bones (NCI, 2013d)

(7) Associated with retinoblastoma and skeletal anomalies

(8) Disease-free survivors—40% to 70% (because of multimodality therapies, precision in surgery [wide resections]) (Samuel, 2011)

e. Soft tissue sarcomas

(1) Classified or staged by cell type, origin— connective tissue (fat, muscle, tendons, fibrous tissue) (American Joint Committee on Cancer [AJCC], 2010; Demetri et al., 2010; NCI, 2013f) (Table 17-4)

(a) Identifying cell type, through careful pathology, is key (NCI, 2013a)

(b) Specific and nonspecific genetic alterations (Brennan, Singer, Maki, & O'Sullivan, 2011)

(2) May appear anywhere because of the body's widespread connective tissue; most found in the lower extremities or trunk

(3) Prognosis depends on tumor size, grade, resection margin (NCI, 2013f)

(4) Prognosis poor with metastasis

(5) Miscellaneous types (Singer et al., 2011)

(a) Liposarcoma (adipose tissue)—most develop in thigh or inside back of abdomen (American Cancer Society [ACS], 2013b)

(b) Leiomyosarcoma (involuntary smooth muscle)

(c) Rhabdomyosarcoma (skeletal muscle)

(d) Angiosarcoma (vascular tissue)

(e) Malignant fibrous histiocytoma (histiocytic origin)

(f) Malignant peripheral nerve sheath tumors (nerve)

(g) Kaposi sarcoma (immunosuppression, human herpesvirus type 8 [HHV-8])

(h) Synovial sarcomas (synovial; joint)

(i) Extraskeletal chondrosarcoma (extraskeletal cartilage; osseous tumor)

B. Epidemiology

1. Low incidence of primary malignant bone and soft tissue tumors (ACS, 2013a)

a. Bone

Table 17-4

Staging System for Sarcoma

Primary Tumor (T)

TX	Primary tumor cannot be assessed
T0	No evidence of primary tumor
T1	Tumor ≤ 5 cm in greatest dimension
T2	Tumor > 5 cm in greatest dimension
T2a	Superficial tumor—near the surface of the skin
T2b	Deep tumor—deep in limb or abdomen

Histologic Grade

G1	Looks like normal tissue; tends to be slow growing
G2	Looks less like normal tissue; faster growing
G3	Only slightly looks like normal tissue; faster growing
G4	Does not look at all like normal tissue; fastest growing

Lymph Nodes (N)

N0	No regional lymph node metastasis
N1	Regional lymph node metastasis

Metastasis (M)

M0	No distant metastases
M1	Distant metastases

Anatomic Stage

Stage IA	G1-G2	T1a or T1b	N0	M0
Stage IB	G1-G2	T2a	N0	M0
Stage IIA	G1-G2	T2b	N0	M0
Stage IIB	G3-G4	T1a or T1b	N0	M0
Stage IIC	G3-G4	T2a	N0	M0
Stage III	G3-G4	T2b	N0	M0
Stage IVA	Any G	Any T	N1	M0
Stage IVB	Any G	Any T	Any N	M1

To assign a stage, information about the tumor, its grade, lymph nodes, and metastasis is combined by a process called stage grouping. The stage is described by Roman numerals from I to IV with the letters A or B.

Used with permission of the American Joint Committee on Cancer (AJCC), Chicago, Illinois. The original source for this material is the AJCC Cancer Staging Manual, Seventh Edition (2010) published by Springer Science and Business Media LLC, www.springer.com.

(1) 2013 estimates—3010 new cases; deaths, 1440 (NCI, 2013b)

(2) Accounts for fewer than 1% of all malignant tumors in the United States (U.S.) (NCI, 2013b)

(3) Between 1975 and 2002, increase in the 5-year survival rate for Ewing sarcoma from 59% to 76% for children younger than 15 years and from 20% 49% for adolescents aged 15 to 19 years (NCI, 2013d)

b. Soft tissue

(1) 2013 estimates—10,000 new cases; incidence slightly higher for men (ACS, 2013a, b)

II. Metastatic disease
   A. Spread from primary lesions to lung, breast, colon, pancreas, kidney, thyroid, prostate, stomach, testes (ACS, 2013b; Mayo Clinic, 2011).
   B. To evaluate spread—computed tomography (CT) of chest and regional lymph nodes
   C. Frequent metastasis of sarcomas to the lungs
   D. Other early metastatic sites—spine, ribs, pelvis (90% in axial skeleton) (ACS, 2013b)
   E. Presents as dull aching pain, increasing at night
   F. Palliative therapies—surgery, radiotherapy, chemotherapy

III. Diagnostic measures
   A. Osteosarcoma (Singer et al., 2011)
      1. Clinical symptoms
         a. Pain—onset, location, duration, quality; may be radicular; gradual onset, worse at night, increases with tumor burden
         b. Swelling in affected area
         c. Bone—injury has to be ruled out
         d. If pathologic fracture, acute, sudden pain may be present
      2. Physical examination
         a. Mass visible, palpable; may be firm, nontender, warm
         b. Size noted, bilateral comparison
         c. Limited range of motion
      3. Diagnostic data
         a. Laboratory
            (1) Elevated serum alkaline phosphatase level because of increased osteoblastic activity (45% to 50% of clients) (Samuel, 2011; Singer et al., 2011)
            (2) Radiography (cannot see changes until tumor is advanced)—three patterns of tumor (may occur isolated or together)
               (a) Slow-growing tumor meets nontumor tissue
               (b) Moderately aggressive—extends into soft tissue
               (c) Aggressive, infiltrating—perpendicular striated (sunburst pattern)
            (3) Other tests—magnetic resonance imaging (MRI), CT, fluoroscopy
            (4) Bone scan—shows additional skeletal lesions
      4. Staging
         a. Staging to identify subcategories, size, or depth of tumors (Edge et al., 2010) (see Table 17-4)
   B. Chondrosarcoma
      1. Clinical symptoms
         a. Dull, aching pain (as in arthritis)
      2. Physical examination
         a. Firm, swollen area; high-grade tumor may appear soft, viscous
      3. Diagnostic data
         a. Similar diagnostic studies as for osteosarcoma
   C. Fibrosarcoma (Singer et al., 2011)
      1. Clinical symptoms
         a. Pain in affected area
      2. Physical examination
         a. Swelling in affected area
      3. Diagnostic data
         a. On radiographs, usually seen within the bone; low-grade lesions have well-defined margins, high-grade lesions have poorly defined margins with a more moth-eaten pattern.
         b. Similar strategies as for osteosarcoma
   D. EFT (NCI, 2013d; Singer et al., 2011)
      1. Clinical symptoms
         a. Symptom report can be vague; pain progressing, lump progressing; sometimes feel heat over lump
         b. Flu like symptoms, fever, fatigue
         c. Anemia
      2. Physical examination
         a. Swelling, progressing in affected area
      3. Diagnostic data
         a. Appear onion like on radiographs from multiple layers of subperiosteal new bone reacting to tumor invading the bone cortex
         b. Diagnosed after ruling out other malignant cell possibilities (e.g., rhabdomyosarcoma, lymphoma, neuroblastoma)
         c. Similar diagnostic studies as for osteosarcoma
   E. Soft tissue (NCI, 2013f; Singer et al., 2011).
      1. Clinical symptoms
         a. Starts as painless, swollen mass (>5 cm) unless affecting blood vessels or nerves
         b. Only 50% of soft tissue sarcomas found in early stages (Mayo Clinic, 2011)
         c. Tumor infiltrates—may be distant from the site of origin
         d. Pain (worsening) in one third of cases (Mayo Clinic, 2011); in time, variety of presenting symptoms—peripheral neuralgias, vascular ischemia, paralysis, bowel obstruction, but often no symptoms reported
      2. Physical examination
         a. Depending on origin—lung, nerve, mobility affected
      3. Diagnostic data
         a. Tissue or cells from incisional, frozen, needle biopsies
         b. MRI, CT
         c. New technologies that offer more precision—electron microscope examination, immunohistochemical staining,

deoxyribonucleic acid (DNA) analysis, ultrasonography (for size and density)
  d. Smaller lesions usually benign (ACS, 2013b)
  e. Recurrence of lesions after resection, reappearing deeper and larger, more aggressive with metastasis
  f. Staging not standard; grading system based on mitotic activity (ACS, 2013b)

IV. Classification
  A. Classification of sarcoma subtypes by cell histology rather than by location—more accurate (previously, classification systems were based on site differences) (Demetri et al., 2010)
  B. No clear cause for all sarcomas; subtyping tissue of origin now possible; sarcomas share mesodermal cellular origin (Singer et al., 2011)
    1. Originate from many tissue types—fat, nerve, muscle, joint, deep skin tissue; arise in any of the mesodermal tissues of the extremities (50%), trunk and retroperitoneum (40%), or head and neck (10%) (NCI, 2013a)
    2. Locations (Singer et al., 2011) (Figure 17-1)

V. Principles of medical management
  A. Overview (Singer et al., 2011)
    1. No standard set of guidelines; require multidisciplinary management
    2. Goals
      a. Removal of tumor
      b. Avoidance of amputation
      c. Preservation of functioning
      d. For metastatic disease, palliative care
    3. Improvements in treatments because of development of better histologic assays via chromosomal translocations (Michelucci et al., 2013)
  B. Surgery
    1. Surgical strategies for treatment based on histology, size, location, tumor grade, extent of disease, resectability (Demetri et al., 2010)
    2. Surgical strategies also depend on the following factors (Singer et al., 2011):
      a. Treatment of choice with osteosarcoma, fibrosarcoma, chondrosarcoma

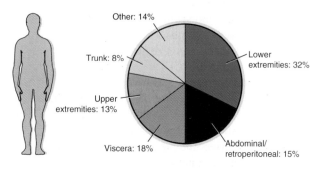

Other: 14%
Trunk: 8%
Upper extremities: 13%
Viscera: 18%
Lower extremities: 32%
Abdominal/retroperitoneal: 15%

Figure 17-1 Sites of soft tissue sarcomas.

      b. Amputation versus limb salvage issues—increased effort to salvage rather than amputate; issues that affect the decision (Singer et al., 2011) include the following:
        (1) Acceptable surgical margins
        (2) Blood vessels and nerves involved with the tumor
        (3) Age (in children younger than 10 years, surgery affects limb growth)
        (4) If limb salvage, radiation therapy (RT) follows (typical strategy)
        (5) Amputation issues
          (a) When tumor extends to incisional surface
          (b) When location necessitates (e.g., tumor extends to vertebral body and pelvis)
          (c) Infection, skeletal immaturity
          (d) Major neurovascular involvement (Singer et al., 2011)
      c. For bone cancer—dramatic increase in overall survival with adjuvant chemotherapy (55% to 80%) (Singer et al., 2011)
      d. Reconstruction (Samuel, 2011)
        (1) Bone autografts, allografts
        (2) After soft tissue resection, three common methods:
          (a) Arthrodesis or fusion (with implants or grafts)
          (b) Arthroplasty for joints
          (c) Allografts (since the 1960s)—bone, tendon, ligament, connective tissue
        (3) Tested for match, viral and bacterial contamination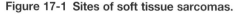
        (4) Method—bone frozen to accept graft
        (5) Intercalary allograft placed between two segments of host bone; used for long bone grafts
        (6) Issues—nonunion, infections, healing
  C. Adjuvant radiotherapy
    1. Soft tissue tumors can be radiosensitive and radioresponsive (Singer et al., 2011).
    2. Usually, external-beam RT, before or after surgery
      a. Used when tumor localized
      b. Used after surgical debulking or tumor removal
    3. In some cases, adjuvant brachytherapy used alone or with external-beam RT
  D. Chemotherapy or immunotherapy
    1. Used as an adjuvant or neoadjuvant with surgery (Brennan et al., 2011; Sarcoma Meta-analysis Collaboration [SMAC], 2011)
    2. Dramatic increase in disease-free periods with the addition of chemotherapy and immunotherapy as part of the multimodality approach to treatment

a. Studies are small, and conclusions are difficult to generalize (Brennan, et al., 2011; Demetri et al., 2010).

b. Outcomes show better local control, increased time to treatment failure, especially in EFT, rhabdomyosarcoma, and osteosarcomas (Demetri et al., 2010; NCI, 2013c, d).

c. In advanced tumors, sequential, single-agent protocols are more effective than complicated combination protocols (Demetri et al., 2010).

(1) Exception—highly active antiretroviral therapy (HAART) for Kaposi sarcoma (Deeken et al, 2012; NCI, 2013f; Pinzone et al., 2012)

d. To date, localized administration to tumor site (cryoablation radiofrequency) has not been shown to be effective (Demetri et al., 2010).

e. Targeted molecular therapies are promising (oncogene activation triggered by viruses or antibodies) (Demetri et al., 2010).

(1) Example—identification of CD117 expression associated with activation of C-kit receptors in gastrointestinal stromal tumors

3. Common chemotherapeutic agents—doxorubicin (Adriamycin), cisplatin (Platinol), cyclophosphamide (Cytoxan), dacarbazine (DTIC-Dome), ifosfamide (Ifex), methotrexate (Mexate), vincristine (Oncovin) (Brennan et al., 2011; Demetri et al., 2010; Singer et al., 2011).

4. Also, studies with topotecan (Hycamtin), vinblastine (Velban), paclitaxel (Taxol), docetaxel (Taxotere), gemcitabine (Gemzar), carboplatin (Paraplatin), dactinomycin (Cosmegen) (Demetri et al., 2010)

5. Early studies of systemic treatment using molecular and cell biology (antiangiogenesis, monoclonal antibodies, vaccines, T cells) (Brennan et al., 2011)

6. Also used in palliation

E. Treatment of common malignant bone and soft tissue tumors

1. Osteosarcoma
   a. Surgery
   b. Multimodality
      (1) Surgery
      (2) Adjuvant radiotherapy (when tumor in axial location; for palliation)
      (3) Adjuvant chemotherapy and immunotherapy (NCI, 2013d)

2. Chondrosarcoma
   a. Surgery

3. Fibrosarcoma
   a. Surgery
      (1) Radical surgery
      (2) Amputation
   b. Radiotherapy only for inoperable tumors

4. EFT
   a. Multimodality
      (1) Surgery (for local control)
      (2) Radiotherapy (4500 to 5600 cGy for metastatic disease) (NCI, 2013d)
      (3) Chemotherapy (vincristine, doxorubicin, cyclophosphamide, ifosfamide/etoposide [Ifex/VP-16, Etopophos, VePesid]) (Singer et al., 2011)

5. Miscellaneous soft tissue sarcomas (e.g., liposarcoma, leiomyosarcoma, rhabdomyosarcoma, angiosarcoma, malignant fibrous histiocytoma)
   a. Surgery
      (1) Resection (thoracotomy) when spread to lung, provided that the primary tumor is controlled
   b. Radiotherapy
   c. Chemotherapy

VI. Nursing implications

A. Interventions related to phantom limb pain or sensation (Samuel, 2011)

1. 1 to 4 weeks postoperatively; usually resolves in a few months

2. Client aware of itching, pressure, tingling, severe cramping, throbbing, burning pain

3. Usually triggered by fatigue, stress, excitement, other stimuli

4. Greater when the amputation site is more proximal

B. Interventions related to preoperative care when client will lose limb

1. For anticipated amputation, many psychological needs (especially with adolescents); issues to address include anxiety, depression; grief about lost limb—physical as well as emotional and social losses; altered body image; fear of disability; coping with deformity; short-term loss of independence and self-sufficiency

2. Rehabilitation plan after surgery—awareness of possible symptoms after surgery include phantom limb sensation, pain (throbbing, burning), itching pressure, tingling, and severe cramping

3. Visit from another amputee—can be helpful; shares how to master his or her prosthesis and deal with emotional issues and change

C. Interventions related to postoperative care when client has lost limb

1. Immediate postoperative management

a. Observation of drainage from site; also for redness, hemorrhage, increased pain, tenderness and swelling, blisters, abrasions
b. If need for stump care
   (1) Elevation of stump (usually at least 24 hours) to prevent edema and promote venous return
   (2) Frequent wrapping of stump with elastic bandages or stump shrinkers
   (3) Dangling and transfer to chair after day of surgery
c. Assisting client into prone position three or four times per day for 15 minutes minimum to prevent hip contractures
d. Teaching client and family measures such as self-care of stump, prosthesis
e. Coordination of collaborative services (e.g., physical therapy, social services, occupational therapy)
D. Interventions related to postoperative management of limb salvage
  1. Neurovascular checks distal to surgical site
  2. Monitoring for blood loss and anemia from extensive tumor resection and reconstruction
  3. Monitoring wound site for signs of infection
  4. Management of pain
  5. Coordination of rehabilitation plan

References

American Cancer Society. (2013a). *Cancer facts & figures 2013.* http://www.cancer.org/research/cancerfactsfigures/cancerfactsfigures/cancer-facts-figures-2013.

American Cancer Society. (2013b). *References: Soft tissue sarcoma detailed guide.* http://www.cancer.org/cancer/sarcoma-adultsofttissuecancer/detailedguide/sarcoma-adult-soft-tissue-cancer-references.

American Joint Committee on Cancer. (2010). Musculoskeletal sites (bone; soft tissue sarcoma). In *AJCC cancer staging manual.* (6th ed., pp. 281–300). New York: Springer.

Brennan, M., Singer, S., Maki, R., & O'Sullivan, B. (2011). Soft tissues sarcoma. In V. T. DeVita, T. S. Lawrence, & S. A. Rosenberg (Eds.), *Cancer: Principles and practice of oncology.* (9th ed., pp. 1581–1637). Philadelphia: Lippincott Williams & Wilkins.

Deeken, J. F., Tjen-A-Looi, A., Rudek, M. A., Okuliar, C., Young, M., Little, R. F., & Dezube, B. J. (2012). The rising challenge of non-AIDS-defining cancers in HIV-infected patients. *Clinical Infectious Diseases, 55*(9), 1228–1235.

Demetri, G. D., Antonia, S., Benjamin, R. S., Bui, M. M., Casper, E. S., Conrad, E. U., et al. (2010). Soft tissue sarcoma. *Journal of the National Comprehensive Cancer Network (JNCCN), 8*(6), 630–674.

Edge, S. B., Byrd, D. R., Compton, C. C., Fritz, A. G., Greene, F. L., & Trotti, A. (2010). *AJCC cancer staging manual* (7th ed., pp. 291–299). New York: Springer.

Malawer, M., Helman, L., & O'Sullivan, B. (2011). Sarcoma of bone. In V. T. DeVita, T. S. Lawrence, & S. A. Rosenberg (Eds.), *Cancer: Principles and practice of oncology* (9th ed., pp. 1638–1686). Philadelphia: Lippincott Williams & Wilkins.

Mayo Clinic. (2011). *Soft tissue sarcoma.* http://www.mayoclinic.com/health/soft-tissue-sarcoma/DS00601/METHOD=print.

Michelucci, A., Chiappetta, C., Cacciotti, J., Veccia, N., Astri, E., Leopizzi, M., et al. (2013). The KIT exon 11 stop codon mutation in gastrointestinal stromal tumors: What is the clinical meaning? *Gut and Liver, 7*(1), 35–40.

National Cancer Institute. (2013a). *Adult soft tissue sarcoma treatment (PDQ).* http://nci.nih.gov/cancertopics/pdq/treatment/adult-soft-tissue-sarcoma/HealthProfessional.

National Cancer Institute. (2013b). *Bone cancer.* http://nci.nih.gov/cancertopics/types/bone.

National Cancer Institute. (2013c). *Childhood rhabdomyosarcoma.* http://nci.nih.gov/cancertopics/types/childrhabdomyosarcoma.

National Cancer Institute. (2013d). *Ewing sarcoma treatment (PDQ).* http://www.cancer.gov/cancertopics/pdq/treatment/ewings/HealthProfessional.

National Cancer Institute. (2013e). *Osteosarcoma and malignant fibrous histiocytoma of bone treatment (PDQ).* http://nci.nih.gov/cancertopics/pdq/treatment/osteosarcoma/HealthProfessional.

National Cancer Institute. (2013f). *Soft tissue sarcoma.* http://nci.nih.gov/cancertopics/types/soft-tissue-sarcoma.

Pinzone, M. R., Fiorica, F., Di Rosa, M., Malaguarnera, G., Malaguarnera, L., Cacopardo, B., et al. (2012). Non-AIDS-defining cancers among HIV-infected people. *European Review for Medical and Pharmacological Sciences, 16*(10), 1377–1388.

Samuel, L. C. (2011). Bone and soft tissue sarcomas. In C. H. Yarbro, D. Wujcik, & B. H. Gobel (Eds.), *Cancer nursing: Principles and practice.* (7th ed., pp. 1052–1079). Sudbury, MA: Jones & Bartlett.

Sarcoma Meta-analysis Collaboration (SMAC). (2011). *Adjuvant chemotherapy for localized resectable soft tissue sarcoma in adults.* http://dx.doi.org/10.1002/14651858.CD001419.

Singer, S., Nielsen, T., & Antonescu, C. R. (2011). Sarcomas of soft tissue and bone. In V. T. DeVita, T. S. Lawrence, & S. A. Rosenberg (Eds.), *Cancer: Principles and practice of oncology.* (9th ed., pp. 1522–1609). Philadelphia: Lippincott Williams & Wilkins.

CHAPTER 18
HIV-Related Cancers

Brenda K. Shelton

OVERVIEW

I. Pathophysiology
  A. Definition of human immunodeficiency virus (HIV)
    1. Cytopathic retrovirus member of retroviridae, genus *Lentivirus* (Moss, 2013; Relf, Shelton, & Jones, 2013)
      a. Two species of HIV—HIV-1 (more virulent), HIV-2
      b. Long incubation and gradual progression typical
        (1) Average time from HIV infection to symptomatic disease depends on inoculation method, exposure, pre-existing health, and prompt initiation of treatment for antiretroviral disease.
        (2) Average time from infection to active acquired immunodeficiency syndrome (AIDs) is 2 to 3 years.
        (3) Average life expectancy is 11 to 14 years.
    2. Method of transmission (Moss, 2013; Relf et al., 2013)
      a. Transmission through body fluids (blood, semen, vaginal secretions, breast milk)
      b. Virus entry via the bloodstream; infection occurs with transmission across mucosal barriers, attaching to dendritic or Langerhans cells
      c. Surface antigen gp120—attracted to host CD4 surface marker
      d. Human cells with most abundant CD4—T lymphocytes; CD4 cell surface marker also found on macrophages, monocytes, microglial cells, Langerhans and dendritic cells
      e. Initial occurrence in partially activated CD4 cells, followed by spread via the CD4 cells in gut-associated lymphoid tissue
      f. For replication—HIV uses reverse transcriptase, an enzyme that mediates transcription of viral RNA to deoxyribonucleic acid (DNA) in infected CD4 cell.
      g. Viral protein integrated into the cells by integrase
      h. After incorporation into the cells' deoxyribonucleic acid (DNA), cellular components broken down into functional infectious virions by the enzyme protease
      i. Components for more virions made by host cells
      j. Process called *coating* undergone by the new virions, which are then expelled from the host cell by budding
      k. Daughter cells disseminate in the bloodstream, infecting new cells
      l. Approximately 30% of the viral burden in HIV-positive patients regenerated daily, weakening cellular stability of normal CD4 and progenitor cells, causing apoptosis and reduced circulating CD4 cells (Relf et al., 2013)
  B. Normal immunologic structures (see Chapter 4)
  C. Physiologic basis of HIV infection
    1. HIV effect on CD4 lymphocytes—apoptosis and reduced quantity
    2. May remain dormant for variable period, or immediate viral production by infected cell may occur
    3. HIV effect on immune system
      a. Progressive infection—leads to qualitative and quantitative T4-lymphocyte dysfunction, with resultant defect in both cellular and humoral immunity as immunoregulatory function of T4 cells is gradually impaired (Relf et al., 2013)
      b. Cofactors in disease progression (Relf et al., 2013)
        (1) Definitive role of specific co-factors in disease progression controversial; may be difficult to distinguish between comorbid infection and true causal relationship
        (2) Infectious cofactors including presence of cytomegalovirus (CMV), EBV, hepatitis C virus, human papillomavirus (HPV),

herpes simplex 6 (HSV-6), herpes simplex 8 (HSV-8), and other viruses (Alfitano, Barbaro, Perretti, & Barbarini, 2012).

c. Lifestyle factors—for example, inadequate nutrition, general poor health, smoking, activities that may result in infection with other strains of HIV, may also influence course of infection.

   (1) Over 50% of cases in gay, bisexual, and other men who have sex with men, comprising half of newly infected HIV infections and half of people living with the disease (Centers for Disease Control [CDC], 2013)

   (2) Increased risk of infection in uncircumcised males related to dendritic cells on foreskin (Tobian & Gray, 2011)

4. Clinical staging and classification of HIV infection

   a. Clinical status—may change rapidly in either direction

   b. Disease stage—guides therapeutic intervention and support

   c. Two major systems for classifying HIV disease—CDC system and Walter Reed system

      (1) CDC classification system (Table 18-1) (CDC, 2013)

      (2) Walter Reed staging system (Table 18-2)

D. Pathophysiology of malignancy with HIV (Carr, 2013)

   1. Impaired immune surveillance function and chronically stimulated B cells may result in growth of malignantly transformed cells.

   2. Patients may experience abnormal sites of presentation and poor duration of response to therapy (Carr, 2013; Malfitano, Barbaro, Perretti, & Barbarini, 2012).

II. Incidence and risk

A. HIV

   1. Estimated 33.2 million people living with HIV (Carr, 2013)

   2. 56,000 Americans newly infected with HIV every year

   3. Up to 20% unaware of their diagnosis (DeFreitas et al., 2013)

   4. African Americans, other blacks, and Hispanics disproportionately affected (Moss, 2013)

   5. Heterosexual women approximately 15% of the HIV cases diagnosed per year (CDC, 2013)

   6. Those older than 40 years the fastest growing HIV-positive population and at increased risk for diseases and cancers not defining acquired immunodeficiency syndrome (AIDS) (Carr, 2013)

B. Malignancy risks

   1. Cancer is most common cause of death among HIV-infected individuals (Malfitano et al., 2012).

   2. HIV-infected women are at increased risk for cervical dysplasia that rapidly progresses to cervical cancer; histology is often more aggressive (Zeier et al., 2012).

   3. Proportional decreases in HIV-related cervical cancers may have not matched other AIDS-related cancers because of the link to HPV.

   4. HIV-infected patients are also at risk for other age- and behavior-associated malignancies related to smoking and alcohol intake.

   5. Average onset of malignancies has increased by 9 years as a result of combined antiretroviral therapy (cART), also known as *highly active antiretroviral therapy* (HAART) (Yanik et al., 2013).

Table 18-1

Surveillance Case Definition for HIV Infection among Adults and Adolescents (Aged ≥13 yr)—United States, 2008

Stage	Laboratory Evidence	Clinical Evidence
Stage 1	Laboratory confirmation of HIV infection *and* CD4+ T-lymphocyte count ≥ 500 cells/μL *or* CD4+ T-lymphocyte percentage ≥ 29%	None required (but no AIDS–defining condition)
Stage 2	Laboratory confirmation of HIV infection *and* CD4+ T-lymphocyte count 200-249 cells/μL *or* CD4+ T-lymphocyte percentage of 14%-28%	None required (but no AIDS-defining condition)
Stage 3 (AIDS)	Laboratory confirmation of HIV infection *and* CD4+ T-lymphocyte count of <200 cells/μL *or* CD4+ T-lymphocyte percentage < 14%	Or documentation of an AIDS-defining condition (with laboratory confirmation of HIV infection)
Unknown	Laboratory confirmation of HIV infection *and* no information on CD4+ T-lymphocyte count or percentage	And no information on presence of AIDS-defining conditions

AIDS, Acquired immunodeficiency syndrome; *HIV*, human immunodeficiency virus.

From the Centers for Disease Control and Prevention. (2008). Revised surveillance case definitions for HIV infection among adults, adolescents, and children aged 18 months to less than 13 years—United States. *MMWR, Morbidity and Mortality Weekly Report 57*(RR10), 1–8.

Table 18-2

Walter Reed Staging System for HIV Infection

Stage	HIV Antibody Status	Chronic Lymphadenopathy	CD4 Count	Skin Test	Oral Thrush	Opportunistic Infections
0	Negative	—	>400	WNL	—	—
1	Positive	—	>400	WNL	—	—
2	Positive	Present	>400	WNL	—	—
3	Positive	±	<400	WNL	—	—
4	Positive	±	<400	Partial anergy	—	—
5	Positive	±	<400	Complete anergy	Yes	—
6	Positive	±	<400	Partial or complete anergy	±	Yes

HIV, Human immunodeficiency virus; *WNL,* within normal limits; ±, may or may not be present.

C. AIDS-defining malignancies—malignancies related specifically to HIV infection and the subsequently altered immune system
  1. AIDS-defining cancers include non-Hodgkin lymphoma (NHL), Burkitt lymphoma, Kaposi sarcoma, and cervical cancer.
  2. AIDS-defining malignancies are more common shortly after initiation of active retroviral therapy, particularly among patients with low CD4 counts.
  3. Decreased incidence is attributed to antiretroviral therapy (Cuttrell & Bedimo, 2013; Phatak et al., 2010).
  4. B-cell lymphoma is the most frequently diagnosed AIDS-defining malignancy
     a. Found equally in all subpopulations of HIV-infected persons; reflects same epidemiology as non–HIV-related lymphoma
  5. Since the advent of highly active combination antiretroviral therapy, the incidence of Kaposi sarcoma has declined dramatically (Malfitano et al., 2012; Shiels et al., 2011).
D. Non–AIDS-defining malignancies (Table 18-3)
  1. Cancers classified as non–AIDS defining—cancers of the anus, head and neck, kidney, liver, and lung and Hodgkin lymphoma
  2. Others with possible association— acute myelogenous leukemia colon, esophageal, and gastric cancers; melanoma; squamous cell skin cancer
  3. Increased incidence of non–AIDS-defining malignancies with extended time living with the disease
     a. Longer life expectancy with antiretroviral therapy; chronic immune suppression leads to late lymphoproliferative cancers.
     b. May be related to lifestyle commonalities in the population—higher incidence with sexually transmitted diseases, hepatitis, and smoking has led to emergence of other cancers

  c. Increased incidence of non–AIDS-defining malignancies—disproportionate compared with incidence in the normal population (Deeken et al., 2012; Winstone, Man, Hull, Montaner, & Sin, 2013)
  4. Malignancies associated with viral infection (e.g., hepatitis B and C and hepatocellular cancer, Epstein-Barr virus [EBV], Hodgkin disease)—more accelerated conversion to malignancy in HIV-infected individuals
     a. Comprise 58% of all cancers in HIV (in 1990 was 31%)
     b. Less likely to be related to viral load or CD4 count compared with AIDS-defining malignancies
     c. More likely to present with aggressive disease and higher risk of metastasis compared with other non–HIV-infected patients
     d. More common in whites, males
     e. Occur at younger age compared with same cancers in non-HIV malignancies.
E. General principles of HIV-related malignancies (Phatak et al., 2010)
  1. The co-existence of cancer and HIV may be related to the presence of HIV or other co-factors or lifestyle factors.
  2. Staging and diagnosis of HIV-associated cancers are the same as with non–HIV-related cancers of the same pathology.
  3. The treatment of cancer usually follows the same therapy plan as would be used even in the absence of HIV.
  4. Every attempt should be made to continue cART through antineoplastic therapy because a temporary reduction in CD4+ lymphocyte counts is likely to occur during antineoplastic therapy.
     a. Interactions between antiretroviral and antineoplastic agents may be caused by disruption of the CYP pathways (see Table 18-4).

Table 18-3

Non–AIDS-Defining Cancers (NADCs)—Common Features

Cancer	Cancer Risk In HIV (Standardized Incidence Ratios)	Association With Low CD4 Counts	Unique Risk Groups	Features Unique In HIV Disease	Management Implications
Anal cancer	28-60.9	Strong, consistent	Males having anal-receptive sex Human papilloma virus (HPV) co-infection	None known	Combined antiretroviral therapy (cART) likely to enhance remission when given in conjunction with antineoplastic therapy
Colon cancer					More right-sided cancers
Esophageal cancer	2-3	Unclear	Possible HPV infection		Upper esophagus more common
Head and neck cancer, oropharyngeal cancer	1.0-4.1	Moderate risk, similar to HPV-related cancers	HPV infection		Better prognosis than common nonhuman immunodeficiency virus (HIV)–related head and neck cancer Radiotherapy tolerance similar to non-HIV disease
Hepatic cancer	5.0-7.7	Uncertain, conflicting evidence	Hepatitis B and hepatitis C virus infection	Younger age at onset Higher rates of infiltrating or metastatic disease	
Hodgkin lymphoma	11-31.7	Risk highest if CD4 between 225 and 249 cells/mm^3	Epstein-Barr virus (EBV) infection Injection drug users higher	Aggressive clinical presentation with B symptoms, extranodal involvement, and bone marrow involvement Higher incidence of lymphocyte depleted and mixed cellularity	Treatment similar to non–HIV-associated Hodgkin lymphoma
Laryngeal	1.5	Not likely			
Leukemia	2.2-2.5	Uncertain, conflicting evidence		Usual cytogenetic markers with prognostic implications not true in HIV-related leukemia	Usually acute myeloid leukemia (AML) subtype
Lung cancer	2.2-6.6	Uncertain, conflicting evidence	Injection drug users—higher incidence Smoking association inconclusive Possible higher incidence with chronic lung inflammation (e.g., pneumonias, oncogenic viruses)	Younger age Higher mortality of HIV-associated cancers Higher among men	Increased risk esophagitis during radiation therapy Attempt to continue cART during chemotherapy
Melanoma	1.1-2.6			Invasive at smaller depth	
Renal cancer	1.7-2.2				Sorafenib dose 37.5 mg daily instead of 50 mg daily
Squamous cell skin cancer	3.2	Moderate evidence that lower CD4 is more common	Chronic ultraviolet (UV) light exposure Hispanic, nonwhite (light pigmentation)	Aggressive phenotypes Younger age Higher recurrence rates Conjunctival involvement	

Table 18-4

CYP Pathway Interactions Between Antiretroviral and Antineoplastic Agents

Enzyme or Metabolic Concern	Antiretroviral Inhibitor	Antiretroviral Inducer	Chemotherapy Effects
CYP 3A4	Amprenavir, atazanavir, delaviridine, indinavir, lopinavir, nelafinavir, ritonavir, saquinavir, zidovodine	Efavirenz, nevirapine	Cyclophosphamide, docetaxel, erolotinib, etoposide, paclitaxel, sorafenib, sunitinib, vinblastine, vincristine
CYP 2C9	Efavirenz, ritonavir		Cyclophosphamide
CYP 2C19	Amprenavir, efavirenz		Cyclophosphamide, ifosfamide, thalidomide
CYP 2D6	Ritonavir		Tamoxifen
CYP 2B6	Efavirenz, nelafanivir Ritonavir	Nevirapine	Cyclophosphamide, isfosfamide, thalidomide
CYP 2E1	Ritonavir		Etoposide, dacarbazine
UGT 1A1	Atazanavir, indinavir		Doxorubicin, etoposide, imatinib, irinotecan, paclitaxel, sorafenib, vincristine, vorinostat

b. Even when the metabolism is not disrupted by concomitant antiretroviral and antineoplastic medications, overlapping toxicities may be problematic with combination therapy (Table 18-5).

c. Non-oncologic medications may also be affected by cART (DeFreitas et al., 2013).

   (1) Frequent and thorough assessment of concomitant medications that result in inadequate absorption or altered effectiveness is recommended.

   (2) Nononcologic medications have adverse interactions with antiretroviral agents such as amiodarone, anticonvulsants, antihyperlipidemics, antimicrobials (metronidazole, rifabutin, rifampin), azole antifungals (posaconazole, voriconazole), benzodiazepines, contraceptives, dexamethasone, digitalis derivatives, histamine-2 receptor agonists, proton pump inhibitors, and warfarin.

III. HIV-related lymphoma (Brower, 2010; Carr, 2013; Phatak et al., 2010)

   A. Pathophysiology—traditionally considered a late manifestation of HIV infection, occurring in the setting of significant immune suppression

      1. Characteristics specific to HIV include lower CD4 counts (below 200/mm^3), older age, lack of CD20+ marker, and lack of cART-related lymphoma (Kaplan, 2012).

      2. Systemic lymphomas seem to have more complex pathophysiology (Bibas & Antinori, 2009; Kaplan, 2012).

      3. EBV is present in 33% to 67% of HIV lymphomas.

      4. Those without EBV have other genetic abnormalities, including *BCL6* and *C-myc* rearrangement, and *p53* mutations (Bibas & Antinori, 2009).

      5. Genetic analyses of patient cohorts have begun to reveal host-related factors relevant to the risk of lymphoma.

      6. Tat protein is an HIV gene product implicated in the pathogenesis of Burkitt and Burkitt-like lymphomas (Bibas & Antinori, 2009).

   B. Common presentation and metastatic sites

      1. In systemic disease, extranodal involvement is common; the most commonly affected sites are the gastrointestinal (GI) tract, central nervous system (CNS), and bone marrow (Kaplan, 2012).

      2. The presentation of primary effusion lymphoma (body cavity lymphoma) is associated with human herpesvirus type 8 (HHV-8) (Kaplan, 2012).

         a. Multifocal lesions are common; ocular involvement occurs in 20%.

         b. *BCL6* mutation is common (Bibas & Antinori, 2009; Gerstner & Batchelor, 2010).

      3. Metastasis— CNS, GI tract, and bone marrow involvement more frequent in HIV-infected persons; every organ system may be involved

      4. Primary CNS involvement—only the CNS involved; no other organs or tissues involved

         a. Primary CNS lymphoma (PCNSL) highly associated with HIV and EBV; linked to lower CD4+ counts

Table 18-5

Overlapping Toxicities between Antiretroviral and Antineoplastic Agents

Toxicity Concern	Antiretrovirals	Antineoplastic Interactions	Altered Chemotherapy Plan
Diarrhea	Darunavir, fosamprenavir, lopinavir, saquinavir, tipranavir	When given with antineoplastic agents such as fluoropyrimidines, irinotecan, may produce intolerable diarrhea	Consider changing antiretroviral
Hepatotoxicity	Didanosine, miraviroc, ralegravir, stavudine, tipranavir, zidovudine	Do not administer concomitantly with antineoplastic agents that have hepatic metabolism at standard doses	Consider changing antiretroviral
Hyperbilirubinemia	Didanosine, stavudine, zidovudine	Overlapping toxicities with chemotherapy may produce confusion about source of elevated bilirubin and premature discontinuation of antineoplastic therapies	Consider changing antiretroviral
Hyperglycemia	Atazanavir, darunavir, fosamprenavir, indinavir, ritonavir, saquinavir, tipranavir	Exacerbated hyperglycemia with mTOR inhibitors	Consider changing antiretroviral
Myelosuppression, neutropenia	Zidovudine	Approximately 8% of patients will develop severe neutropenia, so may be discontinued if antineoplastic therapy is also myelosuppressive. Antineoplastics that have been associated with exacerbated neutropenia when given with zidovudine include bevacizumab, etoposide, gemcitabine, irinotecan, pemetrexed, platinols, taxanes, topotecan	Consider changing antiretroviral. Close monitoring of laboratory values. Consider hematopoietic growth factor
Pancreatitis	Didanosine, stavudine	Avoid concomitant administration with antineoplastics such as L-asparaginase	Consider changing anti-retroviral
Peripheral neuropathy	Didanosine, stavudine	May want to discontinue if preferred antineoplastic therapy includes platinum, taxanes, vinca agents	Consider changing antiretroviral. Consider dose reduction of antineoplastic agents
Prolonged QT segment	Atazanavir, ritonavir, lopinavir, saquinavir	May be altered if given concomitantly with antineoplastics causing prolonged QT segment—anthracyclines, arsenic trioxide, dasatanib, lapatinib, nilotinob, sunitinib, tamoxifen	Consider changing antiretroviral
Renal toxicity	Tenofovir, zidovudine	Platinols	Close renal function monitoring
Vasculitis	Atazanavir, darunavir, fosamprenavir, indinavir, ritonavir, saquinavir, tipranavir	May enhance radiosensitivity, but may also enhance hypertension and idiosyncratic bleeding tendency of vascular endothelial growth factor (VEGF) inhibitors such as bevacizumab, lenalidamide, and thalidomide	Consider changing antiretroviral

C. Diagnostic measures
1. Need to confirm HIV positivity—diagnosis of HIV infection usually made on basis of positive antibody test
   a. Enzyme-linked immunosorbent assay (ELISA) for antibody to HIV used for screening—high sensitivity and specificity in populations at risk
   b. If ELISA test positive, test repeated; if second test positive, confirmatory Western blot conducted on same specimen
   c. Other tests to demonstrate infection with HIV—polymerase chain reaction (PCR; a gene amplification technique) or viral culture
2. Diagnosis of HIV-related lymphoma—similar to testing for non–HIV-related infection; because of wide variance in presenting symptoms, workup in HIV-infected person may have more aggressive disease
   a. Brain biopsy may be performed to establish a diagnosis of PCNSL versus opportunistic infection; night sweats may be related to

infection with *Mycobacterium avium-intracellulare*, and CNS symptoms are related to cerebral toxoplasmosis (Gerstner & Batchelor, 2010).

   b. In the absence of brain biopsy, diagnosis of PCNSL is by exclusion. Response to treatment for toxoplasmosis may indicate infection. Lack of response presumes PCNSL (Bibas & Antinori, 2009).

  3. Presentation factors to consider with diagnosis

   a. CNS lesions may cause changes in cognitive function, memory loss, decreased attention span, headaches, personality change, focal neurologic deficits, or generalized seizure activity.

   b. GI tract lesions may cause malabsorption, diarrhea, constipation, or focal or diffuse abdominal discomfort or may present as an asymptomatic abdominal mass.

   c. Patients with primary effusion lymphomas present with effusions (pericardial, pleural, or ascites) and no discrete mass.

   d. Involvement of the oral cavity is linked to HIV disease, low CD4+ counts (<100 μL), associated with EBV (Hansra et al., 2010).

   e. Blood counts are usually normal despite bone marrow involvement.

D. Prognosis (Brower, 2010; Kaplan, 2012)

  1. Survival depends on multiple factors, including cART, degree of immunosuppression, presence of opportunistic infection(s), nutritional status, presenting lesion location, lifestyle, and accessibility of adequate care.

  2. Factors associated with shorter survival include CD4 cell count below 100 cells/mm³, stage III or IV disease, age older than 35 years, history of intravenous drug use, and elevated lactate dehydrogenase (LDH). The International Prognostic Index (IPI) for aggressive lymphoma has also been validated in patients with AIDS-related lymphoma.

  3. Median survival time ranges from 4 to 10 months. Shortest survival time is with CNS primary tumor (median, 1 to 2 months); longest survival time is with low-grade lymphomas (1 to 4 years).

E. Classification of HIV-related lymphomas (Bibas & Antinori, 2009)

  1. Histology same as immunocompetent hosts—Burkitt, Burkitt-like, diffuse large cell, peripheral T-cell, extranodal marginal zone

  2. Lymphomas specific to HIV—primary effusion lymphoma, plasmablastic lymphoma of the oral cavity or other variants

  3. Lymphomas occurring in other patients with immune suppression; for example, polymorphic B-cell lymphoma (post-transplant lymphoproliferative disorder)

  4. Hodgkin disease, multiple myeloma, and B-cell acute lymphocytic leukemia examples of other lymphoid malignancies diagnosed in HIV-infected persons

  5. Although strongly suspected, no causal relationship identified as yet

F. Staging

  1. Staging for HIV-related lymphoma typically follows the same schema as that for non–HIV-related lymphoma (see Chapter 16).

  2. Because HIV-related malignancies may occur at abnormal sites, diagnostic imaging, endoscopic examinations, or both may be more extensive than in HIV-negative persons.

G. Histologic grading

  1. Majority intermediate or high-grade B-cell tumors

  2. Large cell lymphomas mostly found in the GI tract; small cell lymphomas more likely to involve the bone marrow and meninges

  3. Aggressive disease, poor prognosis; better outcomes with early clinical stage and complete response to therapy (Castillo et al., 2010)

   a. Lesions painful and rapidly proliferative; occasionally mistaken for KS (Kaplan, 2012)

   b. May be preceded by Castleman disease or plasmacytoma (Qing et al., 2011).

H. Risk

  1. PCNSL (González-Aguilar & Soto-Hernández, 2011)

   a. Typically a CD4 count less than 100 cells/mm³, often less than 50 cells/mm³; less common since the advent of cART

   b. Uniformly associated with EBV

  2. Systemic NHL (Phatak et al., 2010)

   a. Less dramatically reduced by cART; overall estimated twofold to sevenfold decline in incidence

   b. Declines in specific subsets of NHL, specifically immunoblastic lymphoma and PCNSL; incidence of Burkitt lymphoma and Hodgkin disease unchanged, suggesting the possible variable involvement of immune function in tumor development

I. Principles of medical management (Kaplan, 2012; Spina, Gloghini, Tirelli, & Carbone, 2010)—treatment based on approaches used for uninfected persons; underlying immune deficiency, presence of opportunistic infections, polypharmacy, and generalized poor health status may require dose reduction, scheduling modifications, and selection of alternative approaches.

1. Antiretroviral therapy
   a. Continuation of cART therapy during anticancer treatment is desirable, if tolerated by patient; ability to treat cancer while continuing cART therapy associated with reduced incidence of opportunistic infections and higher complete response rates (Kaplan, 2012)
   b. Increased risk if resistance with inconsistent administration or absorption of cART; sometimes influences response to entire categories of cART medications (Kaplan, 2012; Spina et al., 2010)
   c. cART delayed in patients with simultaneously diagnosed HIV and malignancy because of risk of severe immune reconstitution syndrome (IRIS) (Rudek, Flexner, & Ambinder, 2011)
   d. IRIS
      (1) A brisk inflammatory response when the white blood cell (WBC) count rapidly increases
      (2) More often occurs with initial cART therapy or with severe inflammatory or infectious reactions; has occurred with toxoplasmosis, pneumocystis, other opportunistic infections in HIV disease, and EBV reactivation
      (3) More often reported with lymphoma compared with other cancer; has been linked to administration of rituximab

2. Surgery—rarely used; exceptions include excisional or incisional biopsy in patients with HIV-related NHL.

3. Chemotherapy (Kaplan, 2012; Spina et al., 2010)
   a. Dose adjustment indicated on the basis of CD4 count, treatment-related side effects, response, concomitant infections
   b. HIV-related lymphoma treated with combination chemotherapy, using agents such as cyclophosphamide (Cytoxan), vincristine (Oncovin), methotrexate (Mexate), etoposide (VP-16, Vepesid), cytosine arabinoside (Ara-C, Cytosar), bleomycin (Blenoxane), and steroids; methotrexate, bleomycin, doxorubicin (Adriamycin), cyclophosphamide, vincristine (Oncovin), and dexamethasone (M-BACOD) regimen common (Dunleavy & Wilson, 2012)
   c. Burkitt lymphoma common in HIV disease; outcomes equivalent to those in other patients (Molyneux et al., 2012)
   d. PCNSL usually resistant to systemic chemotherapy because few agents cross the blood-brain barrier; exceptions are high-dose methotrexate (>3 g/m^2) and high-dose cytarabine (Ara-C) (>2 g/m^2) (Gerstner & Batchelor, 2010); rituximab recommended and usually well-tolerated (Dunleavy & Wilson, 2012; Gerstner & Batchelor, 2010)
   e. Intrathecal administration of chemotherapy considered to treat lymphomatous meningitis; not useful in bulky disease (Dunleavy & Wilson, 2012)
   f. Use of concomitant cART plus chemotherapy to be used cautiously when giving chemotherapy with zidovudine (AZT) because of significant bone marrow compromise (Makinson, Pujol, Le Moing, Peyriere, & Reynes, 2010; Park et al., 2012); increased risk for febrile neutropenia with older age and lower CD4 counts
   g. Ongoing studies evaluating usefulness of stem cell transplantation in HIV-positive patients with NHL or Hodgkin disease (Michieli, Mazzucato, Tirelli, & De Paoli, 2011)

4. Radiotherapy
   a. Used for palliation or consolidation (e.g., involved-field radiotherapy after chemotherapy)
   b. May be used to attempt to control otherwise unresponsive disease
   c. Response short lived in high-grade tumors; in low-grade tumors, good control of symptoms, often with longer duration of response (Mallik, Talapatra, & Goswami, 2010)

5. Biologic response modifiers—the addition of rituximab a standard therapy for HIV-related non-Hodgkin lymphoma; no dose adjustments appear to be necessary, but increased incidence of hemophagocytic syndrome has been noted (Dunleavy & Wilson, 2012).

6. Combined-modality treatment not well documented; synergistic therapeutic effects and side effects must be weighed carefully.

IV. HIV-related Kaposi sarcoma (KS) (Thomas, Sindhu, Sreekumar, & Sasidharan, 2011; Uldrick & Whitby, 2011)
   A. Pathophysiology—soft tissue malignancy characterized by malignant growth of reticuloendothelial cell origin in HIV-infected persons
      1. Before HIV, KS endemic in geographic regions such as the Mediterranean basin and sub-Saharan Africa
      2. Persons receiving immunosuppressive agents after organ transplantation
      3. Malignantly transformed cells reproducing as a result of underlying immune defect in patients with HIV-related KS (epidemic KS)

a. Disproportionate risk for KS among select immunodeficient populations raised suspicion of secondary infectious factor (Mesri, Cesarman, & Boshoff, 2010).

   (1) Confirmed by identification of HHV-8, also known as KS herpesvirus (KSHV)

   (2) Causative association of KSHV with KS

   (3) KSHV infection necessary but not sufficient for KS; malignant potential appears to be quite low outside the setting of immune compromise

b. KSHV genome—encodes a number of gene products; host response to the virus critical in determining outcome of infection and tumor development

c. HIV-associated tat gene product—may enhance KSHV replication, increase expression of various chemokines, potentiate KSHV effects, and indirectly contribute to oncogenesis

B. Metastatic sites

1. Presentation—includes skin lesions, ranging from pink to purple to brownish, flat or raised, usually painless (unless in a sensitive area), and do not blanch with pressure; body organ lesions usually nodular and hemorrhagic (Rashidi, Dorfler, & Goodman, 2012)

2. Common locations—lower extremities or face, oral cavity and palate, GI tract, respiratory tract (especially endobronchial)

C. Diagnostic measures (Rashidi et al., 2012)

1. Similar to testing done when not related to HIV infection

2. Once tissue diagnosis of KS lesions confirmed, biopsy of new skin lesions not always performed; biopsy of visceral lesions may be performed.

D. Prognosis

1. Survival—depends on cART, degree of immunosuppression, presence of opportunistic infection(s), nutritional status, presenting lesion location, lifestyle, care accessibility (Thomas et al., 2011; Uldrick & Whitby, 2011)

2. Dramatic increase in survival in the era of cART

3. Survival for several years possible; shorter in patients with GI tract lesions or B symptoms (fever, night sweats, unintentional weight loss); worse with prior or comorbid major opportunistic infection, with median survival time of less than 1 year

E. Classification

1. Endemic KS—loco-regional and related to viral cause

2. Classic KS—rare angiogenic malignancy

3. Pediatric (lymphadenopathic) KS—occurs in children in developing countries

4. Epidemic KS (AIDS-related)

F. Staging

1. All schemas include parameters of cutaneous, lymph node, and visceral involvement and the occurrence of B symptoms (Thomas et al., 2011).

G. Histologic grading

1. Classic KS is typically indolent, whereas HIV-related KS may be very aggressive and progress rapidly.

H. Risk (Phatak et al., 2010; Thomas et al., 2011)

1. The spectrum of tumors varies by risk group and has been dramatically influenced by HAART.

2. The incidence of KS is already on the decline in the United States (U.S.) even before introduction of cART; since then KS has become a relative rarity in the U.S.

3. Estimates of reduction of KS in HIV-infected persons are as much as 80-fold; in areas where cART is not available (sub-Saharan Africa), KS remains a major problem, and in some areas, it is the major cancer diagnosis.

4. Risk stratification into good risk and poor risk is helpful.

   a. Good risk—confined to skin or lymph nodes or minimal oral disease, CD4 greater than 200/μL, no oral thrush or B symptoms; Karnofsky performance status greater than 70

   b. Poor risk—edema or ulceration of tumor; extensive oral, GI, non-node visceral tumors; CD4 less than 200 μL, history of oral thrush or B symptoms, poor performance status, other HIV-related illness

I. Principles of medical management

1. Treatment based on approaches used for uninfected persons; treatment adjustment required for underlying immune deficiency, presence of other opportunistic infections, polypharmacy, and poor health status

2. Surgery—rarely used in the treatment of KS; exceptions include removal of lesions that interfere with function or cause significant pain

3. Chemotherapy (Carr, 2013; Kaplan, 2012; Uldrick & Whitby, 2011)

   a. Dose adjustment possibly indicated on the basis of CD4 count, treatment-related side effects, response, concomitant infections

   b. HIV-related KS treated with cART (up to 86% response rate, durable responses); if recurrent or persistent, may be treated with single-agent therapy (liposomal doxorubicin, paclitaxel) or combination chemotherapy (vincristine, doxorubicin, and bleomycin)

c. mTOR inhibition—reduces tumor angiogenesis and leads to tumor regression (Roy, Sin, & Lucas, 2013)

d. Because of the vascular nature of KS lesions, antiangiogenic compounds a natural strategy for treatment; ongoing trials include thalidomide (Thalomid), fumagillin, metastat (a matrix metalloproteinase inhibitor) (Sullivan & Pantanowitz, 2010)

4. Radiotherapy—may be given as photon radiotherapy or superficial electron beam (Mallik et al., 2010; See, Zeng, Tran, & Lim, 2011)

a. Doses from 10 to 30 Gy by 45 to 70 kV x-ray or 4-MV photon

b. Better response rates with multiple fractions

c. Effective short to moderate local control may be achieved, especially for cosmetic effects or relief of lymphedema caused by lymphatic lesions; response rates 92% for cutaneous lesions, 100% for oral lesions, and 89% for eyelids, conjunctiva and genitals (Mallik et al., 2010)

d. Permanent alteration in the radiated skin and lymphatics, with subsequent persistent edema and tissue breakdown (See et al., 2011)

5. Biologic response modifiers

a. Interferon-alpha (IFN-α), with or without concomitant zidovudine, approved as treatment for HIV-related KS

V. Other malignancies

A. Cervical cancer (Carr, 2013) (see also Chapter 10)

1. Squamous cell carcinoma (SCC) of the cervix was added to HIV-related malignancies in 1993 because of the incidence of HPV and cervical dysplasia found in women infected with HIV.

2. HPV increases risk of development of or rapid progression to cervical cancer.

3. HIV infection increases risk for cervical cancer recurrence after treatment.

4. Lesions may regress or be controlled with antiretroviral therapy alone.

a. Colposcopy—primary therapy if lesions persist on cART

b. Cryotherapy—for persistent lesions (World Health Organization [WHO], 2011)

c. Radiation therapy—in form of brachytherapy; may be administered for locally advanced disease; radiation toxicity increased in the population receiving antiretroviral agents (See et al., 2011)

B. Anal cancer (Salati & Al Kadi, 2012) (see also Chapter 9)

1. Incidence normally 1.5% of GI malignancies, increased in HIV-infected persons (Castor, da Silva, Gondim Martins, & de Mello, 2012)

2. More common among men practicing anal-receptive intercourse

3. Like cervical cancer, has been highly associated with HIV infection with HPV

4. No regression with cART (Chiao, Hartman, El-Serag, & Giordano, 2013)

5. Management—combined chemotherapy and radiation (Mallik et al., 2010)

C. Hepatocellular carcinoma (HCC) (see also Chapter 9)

1. Four times increased incidence of HCC in HIV-infected patients; contributes to longevity of survival epidemiologically (Curry, 2013)

2. More common in hepatitis C and HIV dual infection than in hepatitis B and HIV infection (Curry, 2013; Nunnari et al., 2012)

3. More likely in HIV-1 disease (Nunnari et al., 2012)

4. Increased risk with advanced age and hepatic cirrhosis, suggesting contribution of progressive liver dysfunction (Yopp et al., 2012)

5. HCC with HIV more aggressive and refractory to treatment, with shorter life expectancy compared with HCC from other causes (Puoti, Rossotti, Garlaschelli, & Bruno, 2011)

6. Highly responsive to sorafenib

D. Lung cancer (Lambert, Merlo, & Kirk, 2013; Mani, Haigeentz, & Aboulafia, 2012; Winstone et al., 2013) (see also Chapter 8)

1. Third most common malignancy in patients with HIV

2. Presentation usually at younger age compared with lung cancer; mean age 46 years

3. Highest incidence of mortality among HIV-related cancers

4. Average life expectancy 6 to 7 months after diagnosis; usually diagnosed at late stage with significant symptoms (cough, chest pain, dyspnea, hemoptysis)

5. Lung infection, which often precedes diagnosis, delaying diagnosis because of overlapping symptoms; up to 30% of one cohort had radiographic changes more typical of lung infection (Ruiz, 2010)

6. Possible link to chronic pulmonary inflammation and infection unclear

7. Increased survival with concomitant cART

8. Significant hematologic toxicity in most patients receiving concomitant cART (Mani, Haigeentz, & Aboulafia, 2012)

E. Hodgkin disease (Martis & Mounier, 2012; Sissolak, Sissolak, & Jacobs, 2010) (see also Chapter 16)

1. Most common non–AIDS-defining malignancy; relative risk 11 to 31.7 times that for normal population
2. Often occurs within 1 year of diagnosis and cART initiation (Gotti et al., 2013)
3. Common pathology—mixed cellularity and lymphocyte depleted subtypes; most express herpesvirus (Sissolak, Sissolak, & Jacobs, 2010)
4. More aggressive and less responsive than non-HIV Hodgkin disease (Xicoy et al., 2013)
   a. Late-stage presentation
   b. Common for multiple node groups
   c. Less sensitive to chemotherapy or radiotherapy compared with de novo Hodgkin disease

VI. Nursing implications
   A. Interventions to maximize patient safety ⚠️
      1. Ensuring environmental safety for patients experiencing sensorimotor changes (e.g., adequate lighting, especially at night) (Theroux, Phipps, Zimmerman, & Relf, 2013)
         a. Assessment for peripheral neuropathies that may occur from HIV, antiretroviral, or antineoplastic therapy
         b. Assessment for balance and strength because cachexia and muscle wasting are common in combined HIV and cancer cluster; referral to physical and occupational therapy, as indicated by functional deficits
      2. Instructing patient about avoidance of potential environmental sources of opportunistic infection—for example, animal waste from pets; or uncooked, undercooked, or improperly stored food (Relf et al., 2011).
      3. Teaching techniques to reduce possibility of HIV transmission (Moss, 2013; Perry, 2013; Relf et al., 2011)
         a. Providing education about the use of latex condom with a water-based lubricant to reduce risk (petroleum-based lubricants or cosmetic creams weaken the condom, increasing the chance of breakage during use) during every episode of vaginal, rectal, or oral intercourse
         b. Providing information about avoidance of sharing toothbrushes, razors, personal care items
         c. Wearing gloves and using a solution of one part household bleach to 10 parts water during cleanup of emesis or other body fluid spills
         d. Use of Universal Precautions as recommended by the CDC to reduce the risk of occupational exposure to HIV (Table 18-6)
   B. Interventions to decrease incidence and severity of symptoms

Table 18-6

Body Fluids in Universal Precautions from Centers for Disease Control and Prevention (CDC)

Body Fluids for Which Universal Precautions Apply	Body Fluids for Which Universal Precautions DO NOT Apply (Unless Contaminated by Blood)
Blood; any secretion or excretion contaminated with blood	Urine
Cerebrospinal fluid	Feces
Semen; vaginal secretions	Vomitus
Synovial fluid	Perspiration
Amniotic fluid	Nasal secretions
Pericardial fluid	Tears
Pleural fluid	Sputum or saliva (except in dental practice)
Peritoneal fluid	

Data from Centers for Disease Control and Prevention. (2013). www.cdc.gov.

1. Teaching (or referral for teaching) about ways to enhance appearance—for example, use of covering cosmetics to hide KS lesions in cosmetically sensitive areas; use of scarves or other clothing to cover swollen lymph nodes; use of clothing appropriate to changing body mass with weight loss
2. Instructing the patient to avoid aspirin because it may interfere with platelet function, and recommending use of acetaminophen instead to control fevers and pains
3. Assessment for opportunistic infections that occur from HIV but are compounded in patients undergoing cancer treatment
4. Monitoring for jaw pain in patients receiving vinca alkaloids; this neuropathy seems to occur more frequently in the HIV population
5. Palliative care referral—particularly helpful for patients experiencing significant physical symptoms or distress (Huang, 2013; Relf et al., 2011)
   a. Helps patients with multiple or overlapping symptoms
   b. Assists with management of complexities of polypharmacy
   c. Pain complex in this population because of multiple causes
   d. May help patients explore and rally support systems and informal care resources
   e. Sensitive assessment and interventions for spiritual distress

f. Support and consistent caregivers helpful in recognizing psychosocial distress or mental incapacity related to disease

C. Interventions to enhance nutritional status
   1. Teaching techniques to enhance nutritional intake (e.g., use of supplements, keeping ready-to-eat foods available, smaller and more frequent meals)
   2. Providing or encouraging frequent oral hygiene

D. Interventions to monitor for sequelae of disease and treatment that may be different from those for non–HIV-related malignancies
   1. The overlapping toxicities between antiretroviral therapy and chemotherapy must be considered in determining the best treatment plan and supportive measures (see Table 18-5).
      a. Diarrhea—lopinavir, tenofovir
      b. Hepatotoxicity—non-nucleoside reverse transcriptase inhibitors, nucleoside reverse transcriptase inhibitors, protease inhibitors
      c. Myelosuppression—zidovudine
      d. Neuropathy—didanosine, stavudine
      e. Nephrotoxicity—indinavir, tenofovir
      f. Nausea and vomiting—didanosine, protease inhibitors, zidovodine
   2. Many antiretroviral medications affect the CYP pathway enzymes and may interfere with chemotherapy therapeutic or toxic effects (see Table 18-4) (Deeken et al., 2012).
      a. CYP inhibitors may require dose reductions.
      b. CYP inducers may require lead to reduced benefit of specific chemotherapy agents, but insufficient research is available with most malignancies to make recommendations. Changes in antiretroviral therapy may be preferable in these situations.
   3. Immunosuppressive effects of chemotherapy are associated with up to 50% temporary reduction in CD4 counts, even if lymphopenia is not a normal adverse effect of that chemotherapy agent (Park et al., 2012).
      a. CD4 counts should be monitored during chemotherapy.
      b. Administration of appropriate antimicrobial prophylaxis is based on CD4 counts, if indicated.
      c. Counts are monitored more frequently in high-risk groups (e.g., older age).
      d. Concomitant administration of hematopoietic growth factors is based on increased risk of HIV-related cancer.

E. Interventions to monitor response to medical management
   1. Assessment and document of location, appearance, size of KS lesions, lymphadenopathy, organomegaly, or other tumor effects (e.g., abdominal masses, oral lesions, ascites)
   2. Monitoring for changes in size or appearance of the abnormalities
   3. Monitoring for tumor lysis syndrome in patients with HIV-related NHL as presentation, with bulky disease common and highly responsive to treatment (Kaplan, 2012)
   4. Assessment of neurologic status frequently as neurologic symptoms may signal advanced HIV disease, chemotherapy toxicity, or opportunistic infections (Theroux et al., 2013)

F. Interventions for cancer screening and disease prevention (Deeken et al., 2012; Momplaisir, Mounzer, & Long, 2014)
   1. Organizational recommendations for cancer screening—not delineated for HIV-infected patients despite clear risks for specific cancers
   2. Papanicolaou (Pap) testing—every 6 to 12 months for early detection of cervical cancer
   3. Anal screening with cytology or high-resolution anoscopy for early detection of squamous cell cancer—has not been adopted by professional organizations, but a growing body of literature suggests that at-risk individuals can benefit from screening (Cachay & Matthews, 2013); digital anal examination also a proven cost-effective method to screen for this cancer in high-risk individuals (Read et al., 2013).
   4. Computed tomography (CT) of the chest—as indicated, to assess high-risk individuals for lung cancer
   5. Sigmoidoscopy—controversy about value in patients with HIV disease, because most cancers are right-sided; full colonoscopy required to assess for colon cancer
   6. Periodic oral or dental examination—to detect early oropharyngeal masses that can signal HPV-related squamous cell head and neck cancers
   7. Vaccines (Moss, 2013)
      a. Hepatitis vaccines are recommended to prevent hepatitis and associated cancers.
      b. HPV vaccines have been proven safe in HIV-infected men.

G. Interventions to address the psychosocial issues of HIV and its malignancies
   1. Thorough psychosocial assessment of all patients (Carr, 2013)
   2. Assessment of health literacy and ability to comply with complex therapies, multiple appointments with medical specialists (Drainoni et al., 2008)
      a. Low literacy associated with only 17% to 40% maintaining regular medical care

    b. Low literacy associated with lack of understanding of CD4 counts, viral load, medications

    c. Studies of antiretroviral adherence reflect low rates of medication adherence among individuals with low health literacy.

    d. Low health literacy associated with English not being the first language, mental health disorder, lack of understanding of how to access care and support

    3. Assessment of self-image in patients with KS who have visible lesions that may contribute to distress and social isolation

H. Interventions to incorporate patient and significant other in care (Relf et al., 2011)

    1. Recognizing that the patient's family of choice may not be the biologic family of origin

    2. Determination of past experience with HIV disease; in areas of high incidence, multiple losses may occur without adequate time for effective grieving

    3. Recognizing that a significant other not infected with HIV may experience feelings of guilt, uncertainty about own health, concern for the future

    4. Monitoring for indications of maladaptive coping strategies, especially if history of substance use disorder is present; assisting with learning alternative behaviors to manage stress and cope

    5. Inclusion of persons identified by the patient as significant others in teaching and care decisions, when appropriate.

References

Alfitano, A., Barbaro, G., Perretti, A., & Barbarini, G. (2012). Human immunodeficiency virus-associated malignancies: A therapeutic update. *Current HIV Research*, *10*, 123–132. http://dx.doi.org/10.2174/157016212799937227.

Bibas, M., & Antinori, A. (2009). *Mediterranean Journal of Hematology and Infectious Disease*, *1*(2), e2009032. http://dx.doi.org/10.4084/MJHID.2009.032.

Brower, V. (2010). Clues emerge on how HIV increases lymphoma risk. *Journal National Cancer Institute*, *102*(14), 1002–1004. http://dx.doi.org/10.1093/jnci/djq274.

Cachay, E. R., & Matthews, W. C. (2013). Human papillomavirus, anal cancer, and screening considerations among HIV-infected individuals. *AIDS Review*, *15*(2), 122–133.

Carr, E. R. (2013). HIV- and AIDS-associated cancers. *Clinical Journal of Oncology Nursing*, *17*(2), 201–204.

Castillo, J. J., Winer, E. S., Stachurski, D., Perez, K., Jabbour, M., Milani, C., et al. (2010). Prognostic factors in chemotherapy-treated patients with HIV-associated plasmablastic lymphoma. *The Oncologist*, *15*(3), 293–299. http://dx.doi.org/10.1634/theoncologist.2009-0204.

Castor, M. D., da Silva, H. J., Gondim Martins, D. B., & de Mello, R. J. (2012). HPV and precancerous lesions of anal canal in women: Systematic review. *International Journal Colorectal Disease*, *27*(3), 271–276. http://dx.doi.org/10.1007/s00384-011-1298-1.

Centers for Disease Control. (2013). http://www.cdc.gov/hiv/statistics/index.html.

Chiao, E. Y., Hartman, C. M., El-Serag, H. B., & Giordano, T. P. (2013). The impact of HIV viral control on the incidence of HIV-associated anal cancer. *Journal of Acquired Immune Deficiency Syndromes*, *63*(5), 631–638.

Curry, M. P. (2013). HIV and hepatitis C virus: Special concerns for patients with cirrhosis. *Journal Infectious Disease*, *207* (Suppl. 1), S40–S44. http://dx.doi.org/10.1093/infdis/jis763.

Cuttrell, J., & Bedimo, R. (2013). Non-AIDS-defining cancers among HIV-infected patients. *Current HIV/AIDS Report*. http://dx.doi.org/10.1007/s11904-013-0166-8.

Deeken, J. F., Tjen-A-Looi, A., Rudek, M. A., Rudek, M. A., Okuliar, C., Little, R. F., et al. (2012). The rising challenge of non-AIDS-defining cancers in HIV-infected patients. *Clinical Infectious Diseases*, *55*, 1228–1235.

DeFreitas, A. A., D'Souza, T. L. M., Lazaro, G. L., Windes, E. M., Johnson, M. D., & Relf, M. V. (2013). Pharmacological considerations in human immunodeficiency virus-infected adults in the intensive care unit. *Critical Care Nurse*, *33*(2), 46–57.

Drainoni, M., Rajabiun, S., Rumptz, M., Welles, S. L., Relf, M., Rebholz, C., et al. (2008). Health literacy of HIV-positive individuals enrolled in an outreach intervention: Results of a cross-site analysis. *Journal of Health Communication*, *13*, 287–302.

Dunleavy, K., & Wilson, W. H. (2012). How I treat HIV-associated lymphoma. *Blood*, *119*, 3245–3255.

Gerstner, E. R., & Batchelor, T. T. (2010). Primary central nervous system lymphoma. *Archives Neurology*, *67*(3), 291–297. http://dx.doi.org/10.1001/archneurol.2010.3.

González-Aguilar, A., & Soto-Hernández, J. L. (2011). The management of primary central nervous system lymphoma related to AIDS in the HAART era. *Current Opinion in Oncology*, *23*(6), 648–653. http://dx.doi.org/10.1097/CCO.0b013e32834b6adc.

Gotti, D., Danesi, M., Calabresi, A., Ferraresi, A., Albini, L., Donato, F., et al. (2013). Clinical characteristics, incidence, and risk factors of HIV-related Hodgkin lymphoma in the era of combination antiretroviral therapy. *AIDS Patient Care and STDs*, *27*(5), 259–265.

Hansra, D., Montague, N., Stefanovic, A., Akunyili, I., Harzand, A., Natkunam, Y., et al. (2010). Oral and extraoral plasmablastic lymphoma: Similarities and differences in clinicopathologic characteristics. *American Journal Clinical Pathology*, *134*(5), 710–719. http://dx.doi.org/10.1309/AJCPJH6KEUSECQLU.

Huang, Y. (2013). Challenges and responses in providing palliative care for people living with HIV/AIDS. *International Journal of Palliative Nursing*, *19*(5), 218–225.

Kaplan, L. D. (2012). HIV-associated lymphoma. *Best Practice & Research. Clinical Haematology*, *25*, 101–117.

Lambert, A. A., Merlo, C. A., & Kirk, G. D. (2013). Human immunodeficiency virus-associated lung malignancies. *Clinical Chest Medicine*, *34*, 255–272.

Makinson, A., Pujol, J. L., Le Moing, V., Peyriere, H., & Reynes, J. (2010). Interactions between cytotoxic chemotherapy and antiretroviral treatment in human immunodeficiency virus-infected patients with lung cancer. *Journal of Thoracic Oncology*, *5*(4), 562–571.

Malfitano, A., Barbaro, G., Perretti, A., & Barbarini, G. (2012). Human immunodeficiency virus-associated malignancies: A therapeutic update. *Current HIV Research*, *10*, 123–132. http://dx.doi.org/10.2174/157016212799937227.

Mallik, S., Talapatra, K., & Goswami, J. (2010). AIDS: A radiation oncologist's perspective. *Journal of Cancer Research and Therapeutics*, *6*(4), 432–441.

Mani, D., Haigeentz, M., Aboulafia, D. M. (2012). Lung cancer in HIV infection. *Clinical Lung Cancer*, *13*(1), 6–13.

Martis, N., & Mounier, N. (2012). Hodgkin lymphoma in patients with HIV infection: A review. *Current Hematology Malignancy Report*, *7*, 228–234.

Mesri, E. A., Cesarman, E., & Boshoff, C. (2010). Kaposi's sarcoma and its associated herpes virus. *National Review Cancer*, *10* (10), 707–719. http://dx.doi.org/10.1038/nrc2888.

Michieli, M., Mazzucato, M., Tirelli, U., & De Paoli, P. (2011). Stem cell transplantation for lymphoma patients with HIV infection. *Cell Transplantation*, *20*, 351–370.

Molyneux, E. M., Rochford, R., Griffin, B., Newton, R., Jackson, G., Menon, G., et al. (2012). Burkitt's lymphoma. *Lancet*, *379*(9822), 1234–1244. http://dx.doi.org/10.1016/S0140-6736(11)61177-X.

Momplaisir, F., Mounzer, K., & Long, J. A. (2014). Preventive cancer screening practices in HIV-positive patients. *AIDS Care*, *26* (1), 87–94.

Moss, J. A. (2013). HIV/AIDS review. *Radiologic Technology*, *84* (3), 247–270.

Nunnari, G., Berretta, M., Pinzone, M. R., Di Rosa, M., Berretta, S., Cunsolo, G., et al. (2012). Hepatocellular carcinoma in HIV positive patients. *European Review Medical Pharmacology Science*, *16*(9), 1257–1270.

Park, J., Kim, T. M., Hwang, J., Kim, N., Choe, P. G., Song, K., et al. (2012). Risk factors for febrile neutropenia during chemotherapy for HIV-related lymphoma. *Journal Korean Academy Medical Sciences*, *27*, 1468–1471.

Perry, N. (2013). Preventing the spread of HIV infection. *Nursing Times*, *109*(22), 12–15.

Phatak, U. A., Joshi, R., Badakh, D. K., Gosavi, V. S., Phatak, J. U., & Jagdale, R. V. (2010). AIDS-associated cancers: An emerging challenge. *Journal Association Physicians India*, *58*, 159–162.

Puoti, M., Rossotti, R., Garlaschelli, A., & Bruno, R. (2011). Hepatocellular carcinoma in HIV hepatitis C virus. *Current Opinions in HIV & AIDS*, *6*(6), 534–538. http://dx.doi.org/10.1097/COH.0b013e32834bd2b7.

Qing, X., Sun, N., Chang, E., French, S., Ji, P., & Yue, C. (2011). Plasmablastic lymphoma may occur as a high-grade transformation from plasmacytoma. *Experimental Molecular Pathology*, *90*(1), 85–90. http://dx.doi.org/10.1016/j.yexmp.2010.10.007.

Rashidi, A., Dorfler, K. R., & Goodman, B. M. (2012). Diffuse Kaposi's sarcoma. *International Journal of Dermatology*, *51*, 964–965.

Read, T., Vodstrcil, L., Grulich, A., Farmer, C., Bradshaw, C., Chen, M., et al. (2013). Acceptability of digital anal screening examinations in HIV-positive homosexual men. *HIV Medicine*. http://dx.doi.org/10.1111/hiv.12035.

Relf, M. V., Mekwa, J., Chasokela, C., Nhlengethwa, W., Letsie, E., Mtengezo, J., et al. (2011). Essential nursing competencies related to HIV and AIDS. *Journal of Association Nurses and AIDS Care*, *22*(1 Suppl.), e5–e40. http://dx.doi.org/10.1016/j.jana.2010.07.007.

Relf, M. V., Shelton, B. K., & Jones, K. M. (2013). Common immunological disorders. In P. G. Morton, & D. K. Fontaine (Eds.), *Critical care nursing* (pp. 1094–1132). Philadelphia: Elsevier.

Roy, D., Sin, S. H., & Lucas, A. (2013). mTOR inhibitors block Kaposi sarcoma growth by inhibiting essential autocrine growth factors and tumor angiogenesis. *Cancer Research*, *73*, 2235–2246.

Rudek, M. A., Flexner, C., & Ambinder, R. F. (2011). Use of antineoplastic agents in patients with cancer who have HIV/AIDS. *Lancet Oncology*, *12*, 905–912.

Ruiz, M. (2010). Lung cancer in HIV-infected patients: The experience in an urban clinic. *Journal of the International Association Physicians in AIDS Care*, *9*, 214–217.

Salati, S. A., & Al Kadi, A. (2012). Anal cancer—a review. *International Journal Health Science (Qassim)*, *6*(2), 206–230.

See, A. P., Zeng, J., Tran, P. T., & Lim, M. (2011). Acute toxicity of second-generation HIV protease-inhibitors in combination with radiotherapy: A retrospective case series. *Radiation Oncology*, *6*, 25–33.

Shiels, M. S., Pfeiffer, R. M., Gail, M. H., Hall, H. I., Li, J., Chaturvedi, A. K., et al. (2011). Cancer burden in the HIV-infected population in the United States. *Journal of the National Cancer Institute*, *103*, 753–762. http://dx.doi.org/10.1093/jnci/djr076.

Sissolak, G., Sissolak, D., & Jacobs, P. (2010). Human immunodeficiency and Hodgkin lymphoma. *Transfusion and Apheresis Science*, *42*(2), 131–139.

Spina, M., Gloghini, A., Tirelli, U., & Carbone, A. (2010). Therapeutic options for HIV-associated lymphomas. *Expert Opinions Pharmacotherapy*, *11*(15), 2471–2481. http://dx.doi.org/10.1517/14656566.2010.502528.

Sullivan, R. J., & Pantanowitz, L. (2010). New drug targets in Kaposi sarcoma. *Expert Opinion Therapeutic Targets*, *14*(12), 1355–1366. http://dx.doi.org/10.1517/14728222.2010.532336.

Theroux, N., Phipps, M., Zimmerman, L., & Relf, M. V. (2013). Neurological complications associated with HIV and AIDS: Clinical implications for nursing. *The Journal of Neuroscience Nursing*, *45*(1), 5–13. http://dx.doi.org/10.1097/JNN.0b013e318275b1b2.

Thomas, S., Sindhu, C. B., Sreekumar, S., & Sasidharan, P. K. (2011). AIDS-associated Kaposi's sarcoma. *The Journal of the Association of Physicians of India*, *59*, 387–389.

Tobian, A. A., & Gray, R. H. (2011). The benefits of male circumcision. *Journal of the American Medical Association*, *306*(13), 1479–1480. http://dx.doi.org/10.1001/jama.2011.1431.

Uldrick, T. S., & Whitby, D. (2011). Update on KSHV epidemiology, Kaposi sarcoma pathogenesis, and treatment of Kaposi sarcoma. *Cancer Letters*, *305*(2), 150–162. http://dx.doi.org/10.1016/j.canlet.2011.02.006.

Winstone, T. A., Man, S. F. P., Hull, M., Montaner, J. S., & Sin, D. D. (2013). Epidemic of lung cancer in patients with HIV infection. *Chest*, *143*(2), 305–314.

World Health Organization. (2011). *WHO guidelines: Use of cryotherapy for cervical intraepithelial neoplasia*. Geneva: WHO.

Xicoy, B., Miralles, P., Morgades, M., Rubio, R., Valencia, M. E., & Ribera, J. M. (2013). Long-term follow up of patients with human immunodeficiency virus infection and advanced stage Hodgkin's lymphoma treated with doxorubicin, bleomycin, vinblastine and dacarbazine. *Haematologica*, *98*(8), e85–e86. http://dx.doi.org/10.3324/haematol.2012.079921.

Yanik, E. L., Napravnik, S., Cole, S. R., Achenbach, C. J., Gopal, S., Olshan, A., et al. (2013). Incidence and timing of cancer in HIV-infected individuals following initiation of combination antiretroviral therapy. *Clinical Infectious Diseases, 57*(5), 756–764.

Yopp, A. C., Subramanian, M., Jain, M. K., Mansour, J. C., Schwarz, R. E., Balch, G. C., et al. (2012). Presentation, treatment, and clinical outcomes of patients with hepatocellular carcinoma, with and without human immunodeficiency virus infection. *Clinical Gastroenterology Hepatology, 10*(11), 1284–1290. http://dx.doi.org/10.1016/j.cgh.2012.08.010.

Zeier, M. D., Botha, M. H., van der Merwe, F. H., Eshun-Wilson, I., van Schalkwyk, M., la Grange, M., et al. (2012). Progression and persistence of low-grade cervical squamous intraepithelial lesions in women living with human immunodeficiency virus. *Journal Lower Genital Tract Disease, 16*(3), 243–250. http://dx.doi.org/10.1097/LGT.0b013e3182403d18.

Part 2

CHAPTER 19
Nursing Implications of Surgical Treatment

Gail Wych Davidson

OVERVIEW

I. Principles of cancer surgery (Rosenberg, 2011)
   A. Surgery is the oldest form of cancer treatment.
   B. The cancer surgeon has an important role in prevention, diagnosis, treatment, palliation, and rehabilitation in cancer care.
   C. Advances in technology continue to expand the ability of the surgeon—anesthesia options, microsurgery, minimally invasive surgery, reconstruction options, postoperative and critical care management.

II. Role of surgery in the oncology patient
   A. Surgical measures for diagnosis and staging—histologic examination of tissue necessary for the diagnosis of most cancers; normal tissue and future resection planes must be free of contamination (Rosenberg, 2011).
      1. Aspiration biopsy—a fine needle is guided to the suspicious tissue and tissue fragments are aspirated to obtain a sample.
      2. Needle or core biopsy—a larger needle is guided to the suspicious area and a core or small piece of tissue is removed.
      3. Incisional biopsy—an incision is made, and a piece of tissue is removed from a larger mass.
      4. Excisional biopsy—the entire suspicious mass is removed through an incision.
      5. Thoracoscopic or laparoscopic staging—this is used for staging via direct visualization of tumor and lymph nodes to obtain washings for cytology and to evaluate resectability (Hosoya & Lefor, 2011).
   B. Surgery for prevention—prophylactic surgery to decrease risk of cancer linked to genetic traits or underlying conditions
      1. Examples—familial breast cancer: mastectomy; familial ovarian cancer: oophorectomy; familial colon cancer, polyposis coli, or ulcerative colitis: colectomy (Rosenberg, 2011)
   C. Surgical resection for cure—to completely remove a primary tumor with negative tumor margins,

regional lymph nodes, and adjacent affected organs, biopsy tracts, and tumor sinuses (Niederhuber, 2008)
   D. Surgical palliation—to enhance comfort when curative resection is not possible
      1. Cytoreduction—to remove the bulk of the disease to decrease tumor burden and improve the effect of chemotherapy or radiation therapy
      2. Decompression or diversion—to place a tube, stent, or ostomy or to remove a metastatic deposit causing morbidity (e.g., colostomy placement when intestinal obstruction occurs, spine surgery for metastasis to relieve pressure and stabilize)
   E. Surgical rehabilitation or reconstruction—to improve the function and appearance of a surgical deficit, improving quality of life (Stubblefield, 2011)
      1. Dependent on anatomic site, extent of procedure, and comorbidities
      2. Example—following resection of mandible and floor of mouth, creating a mandible to allow chewing (function) and improve appearance by placing a microvascular flap to fill a floor of the mouth and neck tissue deficit (appearance)
   F. Multimodality treatment—to improve resectability, spare additional tissue or organ resection, decrease tumor burden, or improve postsurgical outcomes
      1. Chemotherapy, biologics, or immunotherapy
         a. Preoperative— for pathologic downsizing; may affect wound healing
         b. Intraoperative—direct treatment to affected tissue (e.g., heated intraperitoneal chemotherapy, intraperitoneal liver perfusion)
         c. Postoperative—placement of infusion devices (e.g., ports, central venous lines, intrathecal or intra-arterial catheters, hepatic arterial infusion pump placement)
      2. Radiation therapy—50% of all cancer patients will have radiation therapy at some point in their disease trajectory (Stubblefield, 2011).

    a. Preoperative radiation—to downsize tumor; may affect wound healing; fibrosis to organs within the field of treatment may affect surgery.

    b. Intraoperative radiation—delivered directly to tissue via an open incision when cancer-free margins cannot be attained (e.g., beam, seed implants)

    c. Postoperative radiation support—placement of brachytherapy catheters, fiducials to guide postoperative treatment

  3. Interventional radiology

    a. Preoperative—biopsy, tissue sampling, central line placement

    b. Procedural treatments—percutaneous ablation, embolization

    c. Postoperative supportive care—drain or stent placement, kyphoplasty to treat compression fracture in the spine

G. Oncologic emergencies requiring surgical intervention—organ perforation, hemorrhage, drainage and washout of abscesses, cord compression (Rosenberg, 2011)

III. Surgical and procedural techniques and approaches

  A. Surgical techniques

    1. Local excision—removal of cancer and a small margin of surrounding tissue

    2. Wide excision—removal of cancer with some adjacent tissue and lymph nodes

    3. En bloc resection—removal of bulky cancer with contiguous tissues, nodes, vascular structures required to attain safe margins

    4. Debulking resection—removal of a significant part of a tumor to decrease overall tumor burden with the intention of greater chemosensitivity of remaining cancer

    5. Ablation—use of thermal-based energy (e.g., cryoablation, radiofrequency ablation, microwave) to destroy small lesions via direct application of energy for cellular destruction

  B. Surgical approaches—open, laparoscopic, robotic, endoscopic, laser, and percutaneous methods

    1. Open—large incision to allow complete exposure of target organs and associated structures for gross visual inspection and extensive manipulation of organs

    2. Laparoscopic—use of approximately 1-cm incisions for instruments and a camera or light to remove tumor with decreased blood loss, pain, and scarring

    3. Robotic—remote, computer-controlled robotic arms with instruments that can turn nearly 360 degrees through small, approximately 1-cm incisions with operative site magnification to allow delicate surgery with little scarring, blood loss, or postprocedure pain

    4. Endoscopic, single-port laparoscopy or natural orifice transluminal endoscopic surgery (NOTES)—surgical tools passed through existing orifices (e.g., mouth, anus, nares, urethra) for surgery without a scar

    5. Laser—used alone or in combination with photosensitive agents to apply precise beams to damage tumor cells at a cellular level (e.g., photodynamic therapy)

    6. Percutaneous—fine instruments (needles) placed through the skin directed by imaging equipment to treat small tumors (e.g., ablation, kyphoplasty)

C. Anesthesia

  1. Many types of regional and general anesthesia are available, with the choice matched to the specific patient need to best tolerate a procedure.

  2. The American Society of Anesthesiologists (ASA) Classification System (Box 19-1) is a tool used by the anesthesiologist to describe preoperative health status and operative mortality risk.

  3. Anesthetic agents alter the biochemical environment, potentially causing bone marrow suppression, immunosuppression, and a change in macrophage activity (Rosenberg, 2011) (Table 19-1).

IV. Safety measures related to surgical and procedural interventions⚠

  A. General safety interventions (see Box 19-2 for perioperative priorities)

    1. Informed consent

Box 19-1

Classes of Operative Risk

American Society of Anesthesiologists (ASA) Classification System

ASA Physical Status 1—A normal healthy patient

ASA Physical Status 2—A patient with mild systemic disease

ASA Physical Status 3—A patient with severe systemic disease

ASA Physical Status 4—A patient with severe systemic disease that is a constant threat to life

ASA Physical Status 5—A moribund patient who is not expected to survive without the operation

ASA Physical Status 6—A declared brain-dead patient whose organs are being removed for donor purposes

ASA Physical Classification System is reprinted with permission of the American Society of Anesthesiologists, 520 N. Northwest Highway, Park Ridge, Illinois.

Table 19-1

Types of Anesthesia

Name	Description	Agent (Noninclusive)
Regional Anesthesia—Reversible Loss of Sensation to a Specific Area or Region of the Body		
Topical	Application of agent to the skin or mucous membranes	Viscous lidocaine, lidocaine/prilocaine (EMLA)
Field block	Injection of agent directly into the operative field, covering the area with a continuous pool of anesthesia	Lidocaine, 0.% to 1.0%
Peripheral nerve block	Injection of agent around major nerve trunks	Lidocaine ± steroid or epinephrine, alcohol, phenol
Epidural anesthesia	Injection of agent into the extradural space within the vertebral canal without puncturing the dura or entering cerebrospinal fluid (CSF)	Lidocaine, bupivacaine, ropivacaine, chloroprocaine, morphine, fentanyl, sufentanil, clonidine, ketamine
Spinal anesthesia	Injection of agent into CSF; can use on abdominal, pelvic, lower extremity surgeries, but patient is awake and may become agitated, increasing myocardial stress	
General Anesthesia—Reversible Unconscious State with Amnesia, Analgesia, Decreased Reflexes, and Muscle Relaxation with Rapid Onset and Reversal		
Intravenous anesthesia	Neuromuscular blocks paralyze respiratory muscles (require oxygenation via ventilator support)	Intravenous (IV) anesthetics: sodium thiopental, ketamine, propofol, etomidate, midazolam IV neuromuscular blocks: rocuronium, succinylcholine
Inhalation anesthesia	Inhalation agent allows rapid onset and reversal of anesthesia	Nitrous oxide, isoflurane, sevoflurane, desflurane + narcotics and muscle relaxers
Monitored anesthesia care	Anesthesia without intubation Local anesthetic ± analgesic ± amnestic	Fentanyl, midazolam, propofol
Conscious sedation	Depressed consciousness while maintaining patent airway; anesthesiologist not required	Diazepam, midazolam, fentanyl

Data from DeVita, L., Lawrence, T., & Rosenberg, S. (Eds). *DeVita, Hellman, and Rosenberg's Cancer: principles and practice of oncology* (9th ed.), Philadelphia: Lippincott William and Wilkins; and Rothrock, J., & McEwen, D., & Allen, S. (Eds.). *Alexander's care of the patient in surgery* (14th ed.). St. Louis: Mosby.

Box 19-2

Priority Patient Safety Issues Identified by Perioperative Nurses

Wrong site or procedure of surgery
Retained surgical items
Medication errors
Failures in instrument reprocessing
Pressure injuries
Specimen error
Surgical fires
Hypothermia
Burns from energy devices
Airway emergencies
Venous thromboembolism

Adapted from Steelman, V., Graling, P., & Perkhounkova, Y. (2013). Priority patient safety issues identified by perioperative nurses. *AORN Journal, 97* (4), 402-418.

2. Surgical Safety Checklist (see IV.B below)
3. Asepsis
4. Proper patient positioning, padding, and restraint

5. Electrical safety—grounding of patient and equipment
6. Equipment availability, function, processing
B. National Patient Safety Goals from The Joint Commission (2013)
1. Surgical Safety Checklist—initiated by the World Health Organization (WHO, 2009); describes the three critical phases in the perioperative setting and safety checks at each time frame (Figure 19-1)
a. "Sign in" occurs before induction of anesthesia; at this time, patient identity, planned procedure, and monitoring equipment are checked.
b. "Time out" occurs before the skin incision and includes introductions of the operative team and review of the planned surgery and each person's role.
c. "Sign out" occurs after the first closing count to ensure that proper documentation is completed, counts are complete, specimens are labeled, and any operational issues are discussed.

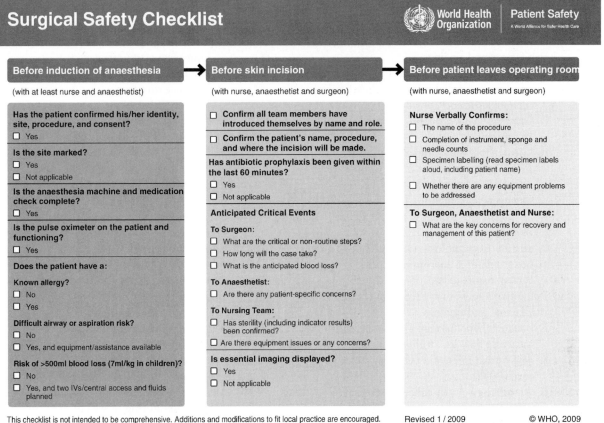

Figure 19-1 Surgical Safety Checklist. *From Johnson, K., & Barach, P. (2011). Quality improvement methods to study and improve the process and outcomes of pediatric cardiac care. Progress in Pediatric Cardiology, 32(2), 147-153.*

2. Time out or Universal Protocol—first mandated in 2003 by The Joint Commission; a team moment when all focus to make sure that all are prepared to begin
   a. Determining that the correct patient is prepared
   b. Review of the site or laterality of the operation
   c. Review of the planned procedure
   d. Ensuring that no questions remain about the plan
   e. Completed and documented prior to any surgical and nonsurgical invasive procedure (The Joint Commission, 2014)
C. Surgical Care Improvement Plan (SCIP)—National Quality Partnership, which consists of multiple quality-minded organizations, including Centers for Medicare and Medicaid, The Joint Commission, American Hospital Association, Centers for Disease Control and Prevention, Institute for Healthcare Improvement, and others
   1. SCIP—based on outcomes from Surgical Infection Prevention (SIP), a 2003 Medicare initiative and Joint Commission Core Measure

to evaluate antibiotic adherence standards and rate of surgical wound infections
2. Established in 2006 to decrease surgical site infections (SSIs) by 25% by 2010
3. Decrease in SSIs achieved by implementation of SIP processes
4. Performance measures expanded for SCIP to include glucose control, hair removal, normothermia in patients with colorectal cancer (Rosenberger, Politano, & Sawyer, 2011)

ASSESSMENT

I. Patient preparation prior to surgery
   A. History
      1. Pre-existing conditions
      2. Previous surgery, reactions to anesthesia and blood products
      3. Previous chemotherapy or radiation exposure
      4. Current medications, herbal and vitamin supplements
      5. Allergies
      6. Pertinent family and social histories (e.g., smoking, alcohol, drug use), including ability to

care for self, potential caregivers, plans for postdischarge care
B. Physical examination
1. Cardiovascular—thorough cardiac testing with risk factors and findings
   a. Increased cardiac risk if history of stroke, angina, myocardial infarction, heart failure, renal insufficiency, or diabetes (Guyatt, Aki, Crowther, Gutteermann, & Schunermann, 2012)
   b. Greater risk for venous thromboembolism (VTE) in the presence of previous VTE; immobility; hormone therapy; use of angiogenesis inhibitors, thalidomide, and lenalidomide (Lyman et al., 2013); and obesity
   c. History of cardiotoxic chemotherapy (e.g., doxorubicin, 5-fluorouracil [5-FU], cyclophosphamide)
2. Pulmonary—pulmonary function testing with risk factors and findings
   a. Anemia, hypothermia, anesthesia, and analgesia may lead to hypoxia and myocardial infarction (Deveraux et al., 2005).
   b. Aerodigestive tract cancers increase the risk of aspiration or postobstructive pneumonia.
   c. Preoperative chemotherapy (e.g., bleomycin, methotrexate, alkylating agents) and torso radiation are associated with interstitial pneumonitis and pulmonary fibrosis.
1. Hematologic—anemia, coagulopathy, malnutrition, liver, kidney or bone marrow disease, and recent chemotherapy or radiation therapy may increase risk profile for surgery.
2. Gastrointestinal, hepatic—malnutrition, coagulopathy, liver, and kidney or bone marrow disease may increase surgical risk.
3. Renal—fluid and electrolyte balance should be stable prior to surgery.
4. Endocrine—octreotide infusion during neuroendocrine or carcinoid procedures, glycemic control, and thyroid function should be optimized.
5. Integumentary—diabetes, malnutrition, inflammatory or connective tissue disease, previous surgery, or radiation exposure may affect wound healing.
C. Psychosocial evaluation and caregiver readiness
1. Psychosocial stressors and coping mechanisms
2. Appropriate care and recovery site
3. Caregiver access and readiness
   a. Patient and caregiver learning style, needs, barriers
   b. Insurance coverage or ability to obtain posthospital services
   c. Access to potential services (outpatient or home health, e.g., RN, health aid, physical therapy, occupational therapy, durable medical equipment, skilled nursing facility, long-term acute care facility)
   d. Emotional readiness
   e. Advance directives—documentation of patient wishes
II. Perioperative care
A. Surgical Safety Checklist (see Figure 19-1), patient identification
B. Patient skin preparation and antisepsis (Association of Perioperative Registered Nurses [AORN], 2013)
1. Preoperative showers twice with 4% chlorhexidine gluconate (CHG)
2. Hair removal by clipping, as needed; removal of jewelry
3. Procedure-dependent antimicrobial prophylaxis
4. Maintenance of sterile surgical field
C. Patient positioning, padding, and restraint (Heizenroth, 2011)
III. Postsurgical care
A. Hemodynamic and cardiopulmonary stability
1. Vital signs, oxygen saturations, intake and output, monitoring of weight
2. Laboratory value stability
B. Pain management (see Chapter 34)
1. Acute pain—surgery-related pain management
2. Chronic pain—preoperative medication use and triggers
C. Pulmonary toilet to decrease atelectasis, pneumonia (Kulayat & Dayton, 2012)
1. Most common postoperative respiratory complication is atelectasis.
2. Most common reason for a fever in the first 48 hours is atelectasis.
3. Pneumonia is the most common nosocomial infection.
D. Venous thromboembolism—prophylaxis to prevent deep vein thrombosis (DVT) or pulmonary embolism (PE) (Kulayat & Dayton, 2012)
1. Serious preventable morbidity; 50% silent
2. Responsible for 5% to 10% of hospital deaths
3. Fatal in one in four surgical patients
E. Skin integrity or wound healing (McEwen, 2011)
1. Primary intention—clean wounds with closure at skin level using glue, staples, stitches
2. Secondary intention—inability to approximate or significant tissue loss results in open wound requiring packing or dressing or negative pressure device
3. Tertiary intention (delayed primary closure)—intentionally delayed (>2 days after surgery) because of wound contamination or unstable patient condition

F. Nutrition—malnutrition and weight loss negatively affect surgical outcomes and survival (Huhmann & August, 2012).
   1. Impact based on pre-existing condition and surgical procedure
   2. Moderate glycemic control (140 to 180 mg/dL)
   3. Early initiation of nutrition—promotes wound healing, gut function, and gut immune function
G. Bowel function—return of function affected by decompression, hydration, activity, narcotic and antiemetic use, diet, and gastrointestinal, abdominal, or pelvic surgery
H. Tubes or drains—care and teaching dependent on the following:
   1. Purpose and temporary versus permanent
   2. Active or passive system
   3. Input (flushing) and output (drainage)—amount, color, viscosity, odor
   4. Insertion site care—open to air, dressing type, or pouch
I. Patient and caregiver education
   1. Wound care
   2. Activity
   3. Nutrition
   4. Discharge medication—review for changes in home medications, teaching related to new medications, pain, nausea, symptom management
   5. Follow-up appointment and plan
IV. Discharge and oncology rehabilitation plans
   A. Psychosocial options related to safe discharge destination and caregivers
   B. Level of care options; durable medical equipment and care supplies
   C. Payer limitations
   D. Rehabilitation needs for return to work; return to work potential

PROBLEM STATEMENTS AND OUTCOME IDENTIFICATION

I. Risk for Perioperative-Positioning Injury (NANDA-I)
   A. Expected outcome—the patient will be free of injury after surgery, as evidenced by no skin changes, paresthesia, or anesthesia related to operative positioning.
II. Impaired Gas Exchange (NANDA-I)
   A. Expected outcome—the patient will demonstrate effective pulmonary toilet with clear bilateral breath sounds and oxygen saturation level returned to pre-procedure level without atelectasis or pneumonia.
III. Impaired Physical Mobility (NANDA-I)
   A. Expected outcome—the patient will demonstrate return of mobility to pre-procedure ability.

IV. Acute Pain, Chronic Pain (NANDA-I)
   A. Expected outcome—the patient will verbalize manageable discomfort with minimal effect on activities of daily living.
V. Imbalanced Nutrition: Less than Body Requirements (NANDA-I)
   A. Expected outcome—the patient will demonstrate improving nutritional intake with caloric and protein intake greater than losses.
VI. Impaired Skin Integrity (NANDA-I)
   A. Expected outcome—the patient will demonstrate wound healing without redness, ecchymosis, edema, or drainage, with approximation of wound edges.
VII. Risk for Venous Thromboembolism
   A. Expected outcome—the patient will experience no intravascular blood clots or pulmonary embolism.
VIII. Risk for Impaired Resilience (NANDA-I)
   A. Expected outcome—the patient and family or caregivers will verbalize understanding of the disease process, surgical treatment, recovery expectations, and plan of care.

PLANNING AND IMPLEMENTATION

I. Interventions to decrease Perioperative Injury
   A. Proper positioning; padding and restraint
   B. Reassessment with repositioning; length of time in the operating room
   C. Surgical Safety Checklist (sign in, time out, sign out)
   D. Maintaining antisepsis of environment, surgical field, antibiotic administration
II. Interventions to improve Impaired Gas Exchange
   A. No smoking at least 1 week before surgery; optimization of treatments for asthma, chronic obstructive pulmonary disease (COPD), and congestive heart failure (CHF)
   B. Auscultation of lung sounds periodically
   C. Cough and deep-breathe, incentive spirometry, percussion, as needed
   D. Turning or repositioning; early ambulation (postoperative day [POD] 0)
   E. Checking oxygenation saturation and administering oxygen, as ordered
III. Interventions to improve Impaired Physical Mobility
   A. Early ambulation; encouragement for personal care
   B. Physical and occupational therapy
   C. Durable medical equipment (DME), as needed, to support rehabilitation
IV. Interventions to decrease Acute Pain, Chronic Pain
   A. Frequent assessment; reassessment with medication administration
   B. Ensuring adequate medication to meet preoperative and postoperative needs

C. Medications to facilitate activity; pulmonary toilet

D. Offering nonpharmaceutical comfort measures (e.g., repositioning, massage, warm or cool cloths, distraction, imagery)

V. Interventions to improve Inadequate Nutritional Intake

A. Early initiation of enteral nutrition, as appropriate

B. Allowing choices of foods and timing of meals and snacks

C. Providing parenteral nutrition if patient unable to meet caloric needs for 7 to 14 days

VI. Interventions to prevent Impaired Skin Integrity

A. Frequent full body assessment for skin integrity

B. Surgical wound dressing changed every 48 hours unless soiled

C. Dressing changes to wound, drains, and appliances

D. Keeping bed linens free from moisture and folds

E. Protection of pressure areas by positioning and use of skin care products

VII. Interventions to decrease Risk of Venous Thromboembolism

A. Prophylactic medication—heparin, low-molecular-weight heparin (Table 19-2)

B. Lower extremity sequential compression

C. Early ambulation; calf pumping

VIII. Interventions to eliminate Risk for Compromised Resilience

A. Patient and family education related to disease and surgery

B. Patient and family education related to recovery expectations and future plan

C. Facilitating verbalizations of interests, desires, life plans, and goals

D. Enhancing patient and caregiver perception of new-normal, postoperative goals

E. Facilitating realistic goal setting

EVALUATION

The oncology nurse identifies the unique aspects in the care of the patient undergoing cancer surgery and intervenes cognizant of the impact of multimodal therapies involved in the continuum of care.

Table 19-2

Prophylaxis of Venous Thromboembolism for the Surgical Patient with Cancer

Dosing Regimens for Pharmacologic Prophylaxis of Venous Thromboembolism (VTE)

Drug	Regimen
Unfractionated heparin	5000 units 2-4 hr preoperatively and once every 8 hr thereafter or 5000 units 10-12 hr preoperatively and 5000 U once daily thereafter
Dalteparin	2500 units 2-4 hr preoperatively and 5000 units once daily thereafter or 5000 units 10-12 hr preoperatively and 5000 units once daily thereafter
Enoxaparin	20 mg 2-4 hr preoperatively and 40 mg once daily thereafter or 40 mg 10-12 hr preoperatively and 40 mg once daily thereafter
Fondaparinux	2.5 mg, four times a day, beginning 6-8 hr postoperatively

All doses are administered by subcutaneous injections.
Fondaparinux is not approved by the U.S. Food and Drug Administration (FDA) for this indication.

When neuraxial anesthesia or analgesia is planned, prophylactic doses of once-daily low-molecular-weight heparin (LMWH) should not be administered within 10 to 12 hours before the procedure or instrumentation (including epidural catheter removal). After the surgery, the first dose of LMWH may be administered 6 to 8 hours postoperatively. After catheter removal, the first dose of LMWH may be administered no earlier than 2 hours afterward. Clinicians should refer to their institutional guidelines and the American Society of Regional Anesthesia Guidelines for more information.

Depending on significant renal clearance, avoid in patients with creatinine clearance ≤ 30 mL/min or adjust dose based on anti-factor Xa levels.

Optimal dose unclear in patients weighing more than 120 kg.

Twice-daily dosing may be more efficacious than once-daily dosing for enoxaparin based on post hoc data.

Adapted from Lyman, G. H., Khorana, A. A., Kuderer, N. M., Lee, A. Y., Arcelus, J. I., Balaban, E. P., et al. (2013). Venous thromboembolism prophylaxis and treatment in patients with cancer: American Society of Clinical Oncology clinical practice guideline update. *Journal of Clinical Oncology, 31*(17), 2189–2204.

References

Association of Perioperative Registered Nurses (AORN). (2013). Recommended practices for preoperative patient skin antisepsis. In *Perioperative standards and recommended practices* (pp. 75–90). Denver: AORN.

Deveraux, P. J., Goldman, L., Cook, D. J., Gilbert, K., Leslie, K., & Guyatt, H. G. (2005). Perioperative cardiac events in patients undergoing noncardiac surgery: A review of the magnitude of the problem, the pathophysiology of the events and methods to estimate and communicate risk. *Canadian Medical Association Journal, 173*(6), 627–634. http://dx.doi.org/10.1503/cmaj.050011.

Guyatt, H. G., Aki, E. A., Crowther, M., Gutteermann, D. D., & Schunermann, H. I. (2012). Executive summary: Antithrombic therapy and prevention of thrombus (9th ed.). American College of Chest Physicians evidence-based clinical practice guidelines. *Chest, 141*(Suppl. 2), S7–S47. http://dx.doi.org/10.1378/chest.1412S3.

Heizenroth, P. A. (2011). Positioning the patient for surgery. In J. C. Rothrock & D. R. McEwen (Eds.), *Alexander's care of the patient in surgery.* (14th ed., pp. 144–173). St. Louis: Elsevier Mosby.

Hosoya, Y., & Lefor, A. T. (2011). Surgical oncology: Laparoscopic surgery. In V. T. DeVita, S. Hellman, & S. Rosenberg (Eds.), *Cancer: Principles and practice of oncology* (9th ed., pp. 277–288). Philadelphia: Lippincott Williams and Wilkins.

Huhmann, M. B., & August, D. A. (2012). Perioperative nutrition support in cancer patients. *Nutrition in Clinical Practice, 27*(5), 586–592. http://dx.doi.org/10.1177/0884533612455203.

Kulayat, M. N., & Dayton, M. T. (2012). Surgical complications. In C. M. Townsend, R. D. Beauchamp, B. M. Evers, & K. L. Mattox (Eds.), *Sabiston textbook of surgery: The biological basis of modern surgical practice* (19th ed., pp. 281–309). Philadelphia Pennsylvania: Elsevier Saunders.

Lyman, G. H., Khorana, A. A., Kuderer, N. M., Lee, A. Y., Arcelus, J. I., Balaban, E. P., et al. (2013). Venous thromboembolism prophylaxis and treatment in patients with cancer: American Society of Clinical Oncology clinical practice guideline update. *Journal of Clinical Oncology, 18*(12), 1321–1329. http://dx.doi.org/10.1200/JCO.2013.491118.

McEwen, D. R. (2011). Wound healing, dressings, and drains. In J. C. Rothrock & D. R. McEwen (Eds.), *Alexander's care of the patient in surgery* (14th ed., pp. 250–253). St. Louis, MO: Elsevier Mosby.

Niederhuber, J. E. (2008). Surgical interventions in Cancer. In M. D. Abeloff, J. O. Armitage, J. E. Niederhuber, M. B. Kastan, & W. G. McKenna (Eds.), *Clinical oncology* (4th ed., pp. 407–416). Philadelphia: Churchill Livingston Elsevier.

Rosenberg, S. (2011). Surgical oncology: General issues. In V. T. DeVita, S. Hellman, & S. Rosenberg (Eds.), *Cancer: Principles and practice of oncology* (9th ed., pp. 268–276). Philadelphia: Lippincott Williams and Wilkins.

Rosenberger, L. H., Politano, A. D., & Sawyer, R. G. (2011). The surgical care improvement project and prevention of post-operative infection, including surgical site infection. *Surgical Infections, 12*(3), 163–168. http://dx.doi.org/10.1089/sur.2010.083.

Rothrock, J. C. (2011). Anesthesia. In J. C. Rothrock, & D. R. McEwen (Eds.), *Alexander's care of the patient in surgery* (14th ed., pp. 117–119). St. Louis: Elsevier Mosby.

Steelman, V. M., Graling, P. R., & Perkhounkova, Y. (2013). Priority patient safety issues identified by perioperative nurses. *AORN Journal, 97*(4), 402–418. http://dx.doi.org/10.1016/jaorn.2012.06.0116.

Stubblefield, M. D. (2011). Rehabilitation of the cancer patient. In V. T. DeVita, S. Hellman, & S. Rosenberg (Eds.), *Cancer: Principles and practice of oncology* (9th ed., pp. 2500–2522). Philadelphia: Lippincott Williams and Wilkins.

The Joint Commission. (2012). *National patient safety goals.* www.jointcommission.org/standards_information/npsgs.aspx.

The Joint Commission. (2014). *National patient safety goals.* http://www.jointcommission.org/assets/1/6/HAP_NPSG_Chapter_2014.pdf.

World Health Organization. (2009). *Surgical safety checklist 2009 edition.* http://www.who.int/patientsafety/safesurgery/en/.

Part 3

CHAPTER 20

Nursing Implications of Blood and Marrow Transplantation

Terry Wilke Shapiro

OVERVIEW

I. Principles of hematopoietic stem cell transplantation (HSCT) (Appelbaum, Forman, Negrin, & Blume, 2009; Brown, 2010; Ezzone, 2013; Forman & Nakamura, 2011; Gratwohl et al., 2010; Harris, 2010; Ljungman et al., 2009; Niess, 2013)

A. A dose-related response to chemotherapy or radiation therapy (RT) exhibited by many malignancies
   1. Increasing the dose raises the number of cells that are destroyed.
   2. Dose of chemotherapy or RT that can be delivered is limited by the degree of marrow toxicity.
   3. High-doses chemotherapy or RT may be administered to treat more aggressive, higher risk diseases.

B. Process of bone marrow transplantation (Appelbaum et al., 2009; Ezzone, 2013; Forman & Nakamura, 2011; Harris, 2010; Niess, 2013; Perumbeti & Sacher, 2012) (Figure 20-1)
   1. Marrow source is identified. Bone marrow or stem cells from either the patient (autograft) or a donor (allograft) are infused, and they engraft to "rescue" the patient's hematopoietic function from the toxic effects of antineoplastic therapy or RT. Box 20-1 outlines sources of autografts and allografts.
   2. Stem cell source—type of transplant is based on stem cell source (see Box 20-1).
      a. Autologous—patient receives own bone marrow or peripheral blood stem cells (PBSCs) that were harvested or collected before pretransplantation conditioning.
      b. Allogeneic—patient receives bone marrow, PBSCs, or umbilical cord blood (UCB) from a healthy, related or unrelated donor.
      c. Syngeneic—patient receives bone marrow or PBSCs from a genetically identical twin.

3. Factors affecting source of donor marrow
   a. Primary disease to be treated
   b. Availability of a histocompatible donor
   c. Age of the patient

C. Allografting
   1. Allografting involves transplanting marrow PBSCs or UCB to a recipient who is genetically different.
      a. The human leukocyte antigen (HLA) system is used to determine the best possible stem cell source for transplantation.
      b. HLA is a protein—or marker—found on most cells in the body, including white blood cells (WBCs).
      c. The immune system uses HLA markers to recognize "self" versus "non-self."
      d. Half of the HLA antigens (HLA type) are inherited from the mother and half from the father.
      e. Ten HLA antigens (markers) are used in HLA typing for allogeneic transplant recipients.
   2. Allografting using a monozygotic twin as a donor is termed *syngeneic transplantation*.
      a. The most common and preferred situation is for hematopoietic stem cells (HSCs) to be donated by a ten-out-of-ten (10/10) antigen, HLA-matched sibling.
      b. Partially matched family members or matched unrelated donors from a volunteer pool may also be used as donors.
      c. Within certain limitations, UCB may be used as a source of allogeneic stem cells in the related, matched sibling, as well as in the unrelated donor situations.
      d. Allografts are indicated for some congenital abnormalities of bone marrow function or in disease involving marrow that is not amenable to cure with standard treatment (e.g., leukemias). Box 20-2 shows diseases treated with allogeneic transplantation.

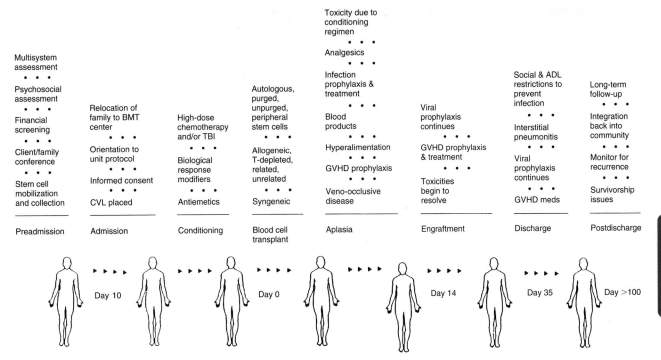

Figure 20-1 Usual stages of the inpatient transplantation process. *ADL*, Activities of daily living; *BMT*, bone marrow transplantation; *CVL*, central venous line; *GVHD*, graft-versus-host disease; *TBI*, total body irradiation.

Part 3

Box 20-1

Sources of Marrow or Stem Cells

Allografts
- Matched sibling donor
  - Bone marrow
  - Peripheral blood stem cells
  - Umbilical cord blood
- Identical twin donor
  - Bone marrow
  - Peripheral blood stem cells
- Partially matched family member
  - Bone marrow
  - Peripheral blood stem cells
  - Umbilical cord blood
- Matched unrelated donor
  - Bone marrow
  - Peripheral blood stem cells
  - Umbilical cord blood

Autografts
- Autologous bone marrow
- Autologous peripheral blood stem cells
- Autologous umbilical cord blood (rare)

e. "Mini," or nonmyeloablative (reduced intensity), HSCTs are used in the allogeneic transplantation setting when the patient is older, has pre-existing comorbidities, and has a

disease that will benefit from the graft-versus-tumor (GVT) immunologic effect (Forman & Nakamura, 2011).

(1) The patient receives lower doses of chemotherapy as immunotherapy, and this is often followed by total body irradiation and then transplantation of marrow or peripheral blood stem cells from an allogeneic donor.

(2) The objective is to induce an immunologic response known as the *GVT effect*, whereby the donor stem cells and host stem cells coexist in a state of mixed chimerism.

(3) This treatment is usually reserved for older patients (>60 years) or those with comorbidities (limited organ function), because the risk of acute toxicities from the lowered doses of chemotherapy and radiotherapy is less.

3. Allografting requires the use of post-transplantation immunosuppression to prevent graft-versus-host disease (GVHD), a condition in which donor T lymphocytes mount an immune response against the patient.

D. Autografting (Appelbaum et al., 2009; Beckers et al., 2010; Ezzone, 2013; Forman & Nakamura, 2011; Gratwohl et al., 2010; Harris, 2010; Jantunen & Sureda, 2012; Perumbeti & Sacher, 2012; Rajkumar, 2013)

Box 20-2

Diseases Treated with Allografting of Hematopoietic Stem Cells

Leukemias—Syndromes
Acute myelogenous leukemia
Acute lymphoblastic leukemia
Chronic myelogenous leukemia
Myelodysplastic syndromes
Acute myelofibroids

Immunodeficiencies
Severe combined immunodeficiency
Wiskott-Aldrich syndrome
Miscellaneous immunodeficiencies

Hematologic Disorders
β-Thalassemia
Sickle cell anemia
Congenital neutropenia
Osteopetrosis

Bone Marrow Failure
Severe aplastic anemia
Fanconi anemia
Reticular dysgenesis

Nonhematologic Genetic Disorders
Inclusion cell (I-cell) disease
Mucopolysaccharidosis
Adrenal leukodystrophy
Glycogen storage diseases
Miscellaneous metabolic disorders

Lymphoproliferative Disorders
Hodgkin disease
Non-Hodgkin lymphoma
Multiple myeloma
Chronic lymphocytic leukemia

Box 20-3

Diseases Treated with Autografting of Hematopoietic Stem Cells

Lymphoproliferative Disorders
Hodgkin disease
Non-Hodgkin lymphoma
Multiple myeloma

Solid Tumors
Neuroblastoma
Ewing sarcoma
Hepatoblastoma
Testicular cancer
Osteosarcoma
Cerebral tumors

Others
Autoimmune diseases
Systemic lupus erythematosus
Rheumatoid arthritis
Juvenile-onset diabetes

1. Autografting involves transplanting marrow or PBSCs back into the person from whom the blood cells originated.

2. Because marrow or stem cell sources for allografting cannot always be found, or because it may be too risky, autologous bone marrow or PBSC transplantation is used as a method for treating a number of malignant disorders.

3. Using autologous marrow or PBSCs is not feasible in patients who have a deficiency of their functional bone marrow, as is the case with aplastic anemia, inborn errors of metabolism, and immunodeficiency states.

4. Autografting may be used in circumstances in which autologous marrow or PBSCs are preferable to using an allogeneic source of stem cells (e.g., to avoid GVHD, in situations in which marrow contamination with malignant cells is unlikely, and when no evidence of an immunologic antitumor effect [GVT] with allogeneic transplantation exists).

5. In older patients (>50 years of age), autografting may also be considered more desirable because of the high morbidity and mortality associated with allografting and GVHD (William & de Lima, 2013).

6. Autografting is most frequently used for the treatment of multiple myeloma and lymphoma. Autologous stem cell transplantation (ASCT) is also being investigated for use in the treatment of other malignancies (e.g., sarcoma, neuroblastoma, brain tumors) in which the chance for cure is relatively low with standard or conventional doses of chemotherapy. In this case, autografting is considered a marrow or stem cell "rescue." Box 20-3 shows diseases treated with autologous transplantation.

7. In some autografting situations, it is debated whether a low (undetectable) level of tumor cells persisting in the infused cells may promote relapse. However, routine purging, even in diseases that involve bone marrow, is unproven. Using PBSCs instead of bone marrow is known to lower the risk of tumor infusion (DiPersio, Ho, Hanrahan, Hsu, & Fruehauf, 2010; Ossenkoppele, Janssen, & Huijgens, 2013).

8. PBSCs are most commonly used as an autografting source but are especially used in cases of prior pelvic irradiation, marrow fibrosis, unacceptable anesthesia risk, or when early engraftment is desired.

9. Autologous HSCT has recently been found to be effective in treating some autoimmune diseases, because it allows for high doses of immunosuppressive therapy to be administered (Alchi et al., 2013).

E. Bone marrow aspiration and biopsy are performed on the patient before HSCT to determine if the patient is in remission or has malignant cells present in bone marrow.
   1. Optimally, transplantation is performed in the interval as close to complete remission as possible, when the disease is considered "chemoresponsive," the patient is in a state of "minimal residual disease," or both (Zhao et al., 2012).
   2. In the case of autologous donation, marrow with malignant cells should not be used; PBSCs may be used instead, but the risk of post-transplantation relapse is high.
   3. Autologous PBSCs may also be harvested as a backup for patients whose risk of allogeneic rejection is high—for example, patients undergoing UCB transplantation (Shenoy, 2013).

F. In the patient receiving an allogeneic transplant, histocompatibility testing must be done to determine if the patient and donor are genetically compatible (Devine, 2013; National Marrow Donor Program [NMDP] website).
   1. HLA testing—major histocompatibility complex encoded by genes (one pair from each parent) present on chromosome 6
      a. Major loci of importance when using allogeneic stem marrow or PBSC donors are HLA-A, -B, -C, DRB1, and DQB1 (10 antigens). Only HLA-A, HLA-B, and DRB1 antigens (six antigens) are tested when using an umbilical cord blood unit (Stavropoulos-Giokas, Dinou, & Papassavas, 2012).
      b. The success of allogeneic transplantation is related to the degree of histocompatibility between the donor and recipient.
      c. Patients have a one-in-four chance of having a 10/10 antigen–matched donor among their full siblings.
      d. Patients without an HLA-matched sibling donor have approximately a 66% to 70% chance (depending on race or ethnicity) of finding an HLA-matched unrelated volunteer donor or donated UCB donor from the National Marrow Donor Registry. A minority of patients are less likely to find an HLA-compatible donor. Use of matched unrelated donors carries more risk because of higher incidence of GVHD and delay in immune reconstitution
   2. Further deoxyribonucleic acid (DNA) testing of HLA-DR—performed to determine the degree of histocompatibility between donor and recipient

G. Hematopoietic stem cell recipient is prepared with dose-intense (marrow ablative) therapy (McAdams & Burgunder, 2013) (Figures 20-2 and 20-3).
   1. The conditioning protocol is established on the basis of the primary disease and type of transplant.
   2. The goals of a pretransplantation conditioning regimen are as follows:
      a. To eradicate remaining malignancy in the recipient
      b. To suppress the immune system of the recipient to allow for marrow engraftment (allografts only)
      c. To open spaces within the marrow compartment for newly infused PBSCs or marrow to engraft
   3. The conditioning regimen may include high-dose chemotherapy alone or in combination with total lymph node or total body irradiation.
   4. Immunosuppressive therapy may also be used as part of the conditioning regimen in the allogeneic transplantation setting.
   5. Conditioning regimen is usually completed prior to marrow transplantation or infusion.

H. Marrow, PBSCs, or UCB from the donor (allogeneic) or the patient (autologous) is harvested and processed (Appelbaum et al., 2009; Ezzone, 2013; Forman & Nakamura, 2011; Gratwohl et al., 2010; Harris, 2010; Ljungman, 2009; Niess, 2013).
   1. Bone marrow harvesting is performed with the patient under general or regional anesthesia.
      a. Two to four punctures are made in the posterior iliac crests bilaterally.
      b. Approximately 10 mL/kg of the recipient's body weight is aspirated.
      c. Marrow is then filtered to remove bone and fat particles.
      d. Processed marrow is placed in a blood administration bag for cryopreservation (autologous) or immediate infusion (allogeneic).
      e. Matched, unrelated donor marrow is generally processed at the donor's closest NMDP collection center and then transported to the recipient's transplantation center for infusion.
   2. PBSCs are generally collected following stem cell mobilization with hematopoietic growth factors, chemotherapy, or both. Immunomodulators such as plerixafor may also be used prior to stem cell collection.
      a. Cells are collected, usually via a centrally placed pheresis catheter, using a special cell separator. After processing, autologous PBSCs are cryopreserved in small aliquots.
      b. A minimum of 2.5×10^6 CD34+ cells are required to ensure successful engraftment. ⚠
      c. Patients undergo the conditioning regimen at least 30 days after mobilization, at which point

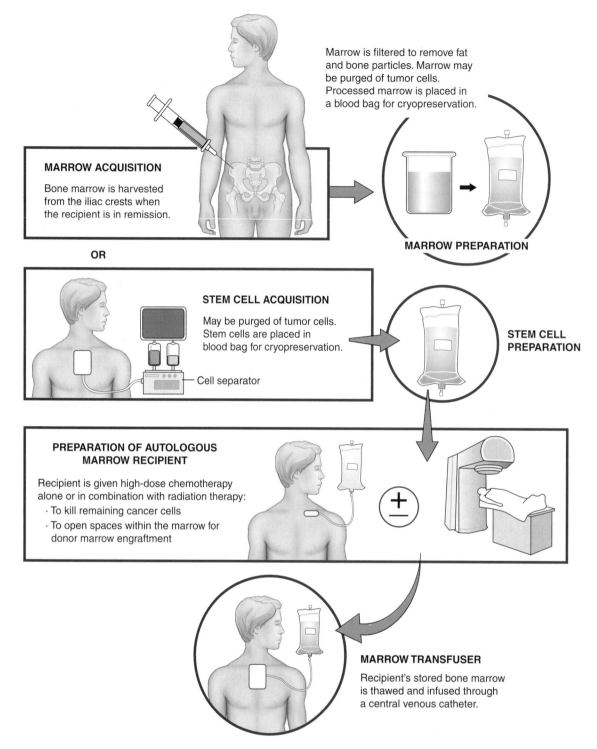

MARROW ACQUISITION

Bone marrow is harvested from the iliac crests when the recipient is in remission.

Marrow is filtered to remove fat and bone particles. Marrow may be purged of tumor cells. Processed marrow is placed in a blood bag for cryopreservation.

MARROW PREPARATION

OR

STEM CELL ACQUISITION

May be purged of tumor cells. Stem cells are placed in blood bag for cryopreservation.

Cell separator

STEM CELL PREPARATION

PREPARATION OF AUTOLOGOUS MARROW RECIPIENT

Recipient is given high-dose chemotherapy alone or in combination with radiation therapy:
· To kill remaining cancer cells
· To open spaces within the marrow for donor marrow engraftment

MARROW TRANSFUSER

Recipient's stored bone marrow is thawed and infused through a central venous catheter.

Figure 20-2 Preparation of the recipient for autologous hematopoietic stem cell transplantation (HSCT).

the cells are thawed and reinfused. Fresh allogeneic PBSCs are infused as soon as possible but generally not sooner than 24 hours after the high-dose therapy is completed.

3. Stem cells from an umbilical cord may be used as a source, although UCB is generally reserved for patients weighing less than 60 kg. Studies are currently underway using multiple matched cord blood units for larger patients (Stavropoulos-Giokas et al., 2012; Ustun et al., 2013).

a. Related and unrelated UCB cells are harvested at birth from volunteer maternal donors and are cryopreserved at a designated cord blood bank. Donated cord blood is accessible via the NMDP's Cord Blood Registry (Shenoy, 2013).

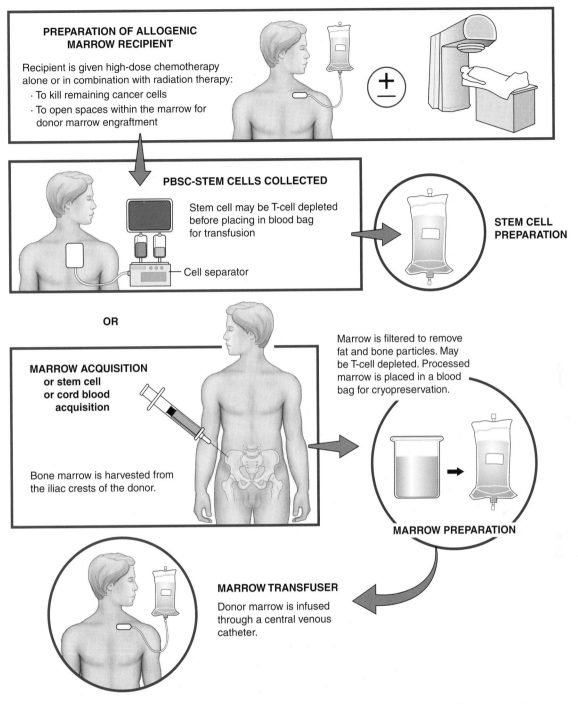

PREPARATION OF ALLOGENIC MARROW RECIPIENT

Recipient is given high-dose chemotherapy alone or in combination with radiation therapy:
· To kill remaining cancer cells
· To open spaces within the marrow for donor marrow engraftment

PBSC-STEM CELLS COLLECTED

Stem cell may be T-cell depleted before placing in blood bag for transfusion

— Cell separator

STEM CELL PREPARATION

OR

MARROW ACQUISITION or stem cell or cord blood acquisition

Bone marrow is harvested from the iliac crests of the donor.

Marrow is filtered to remove fat and bone particles. May be T-cell depleted. Processed marrow is placed in a blood bag for cryopreservation.

MARROW PREPARATION

MARROW TRANSFUSER

Donor marrow is infused through a central venous catheter.

Figure 20-3 Preparation of the recipient for allogeneic hematopoietic stem cell transplantation (HSCT). *PBSC*, Peripheral blood stem cell.

b. The cells are transported to the recipient's transplantation center, thawed, and infused on the day of transplantation.
4. Some centers are using a variety of experimental techniques to purge autologous marrow of possible tumor contaminants.
    a. Purging may be performed using monoclonal antibodies, chemotherapy, or physical means (centrifugation).

b. Purging may damage the stem cells, thus increasing the risk of delayed engraftment or rejection.
I. Marrow HSCs are infused through a central venous catheter.
    1. Autologous marrow and PBSCs are thawed at the patient's bedside and reinfused via a central venous line.

2. Freshly harvested marrow or PBSCs are brought to the patient's room and infused in a similar fashion to a unit of packed red blood cells (RBCs).
3. If allogeneic cord blood is used, the cells are thawed at the patient's bedside and reinfused.

J. The patient is supported through the period of marrow aplasia (10 to 30 days), and preventive measures to decrease potential complications (e.g., infection, GVHD) are instituted. See Table 20-1 for preventive measures for bone marrow transplantation–associated complication control practices. ⚠

II. Role of bone marrow transplantation
   A. Cure—because of the aggressive nature of the therapy, each patient is evaluated with curative intent.

Table 20-1

Preventive Measures for Bone Marrow Transplantation–Associated Complications

Complication	Infection	Preventive and Treatment Measures	Nursing Implications

Graft-versus-host disease (GVHD), acute and chronic	• Results from engraftment of immunocompetent donor T lymphocytes reacting against immunoincompetent recipient tissues (skin, gastrointestinal [GI] tract, liver)
	• Occurs in 30%-60% of all allogeneic bone marrow transplant recipients
	• Risk is increased when donor is not a 6/6 HLA antigen match or when a matched unrelated donor is used.
	• May be either acute or chronic
		• Depletion of T cells from marrow
		• Preventive immunosuppressive agents
		• Cyclosporine A (Gengraf, Sandimmune oral: Neoral)
		• FK 506 (Tacrolimus)
		• High-dose steroids:
		  • Antithymocyte globulin
		  • Alemtuzumab (Campath)
		  • Muromonab-CD3 (OKT-3/Ontak)
		  • Thalidomide (Thalomid)
		• Monoclonal antibodies
		• Polyclonal antibodies
		• Mycophenolate mofetil (MMF) (Cellcept)
		• Methotrexate (Mexate)
		• Rapamycin (Sirolimus)
		• Mesenchymal stem cells
			• Monitor for delayed marrow engraftment.
			• Monitor for prolonged lymphopenia and neutropenia.
			• Evaluate cyclosporine or tacrolimus levels, and notify practitioner of significant abnormalities.
			• Monitor side effects of immunosuppressive agents.
			• Monitor for signs of infection.
			• Monitor weekly infection markers (viral polymerase chain reactions [PCRs], galactomanin).
			• Maintain skin integrity.
			• Maintain patient's functional capacity.
			• Monitor for signs of hemolytic-uremic syndrome.

Idiopathic pulmonary interstitial pneumonitis (infectious and noninfectious)	• Occurs most frequently in patients > 30 yr, with history of chest irradiation or previous bleomycin therapy; allogeneic transplantation, and CMV-positive with CMV-negative donor • Causative agents infectious • Cytomegalovirus • *Aspergillus* species • *Pneumocystis jiroveci* • Other infections 15% • Noninfectious cause • Diffuse alveolar hemorrhage (DAH) • Chemotherapy-related • GVHD • Radiation therapy	• Use of cytomegalovirus (CMV)—seronegative blood products • Use of filtered air system (HEPA) • Antimicrobial therapy • Ganciclovir (Cytovene) • Foscarnet (Foscavir) • Intravenous immunoglobulin • Trimethoprim and sulfamethoxazole • Aerosolized or intravenous (IV) pentamidine (NebuPent, Pentacarinat, Pentam 300) • Azoles (voriconazole, posaconazole) • Amphotericin B (Abelcet, AmBisome)	• Monitor for side effects of antimicrobial therapy. • Implement turning, coughing, and deep-breathing routine. • Encourage activity. • Provide transfusion therapy (DAH).
Hepatic sinusoidal obstruction syndrome	• Damage to the small sinusoids of the liver from pretransplantation conditioning regimen • Occurs in 5%-54% of patients; most common in patients undergoing matched, unrelated donor transplants and those with pretransplantation liver enzyme elevations or previous radiation to abdomen	• Defibrotide • Ursodiol (Actigall) • Heparin • Diuretics • Renal dose of dopamine • Strict fluid management	• Monitor liver function studies. • Monitor for weight gain. • Evaluate abdominal pain. • Use caution when administering drugs that are cleared via hepatic system because increased toxicity may occur. • Monitor renal function.

Adapted from Becze, E. (2011). Veno-occlusive disease is the most common hepatic complication in stem cell transplants. *ONS Connect 11*, 16–17; Ezzone, S. A. (Ed.). (2013). *Hematopoietic stem cell transplantation: A manual for nursing practice* (2nd ed.). Pittsburgh: Oncology Nursing Society.

B. Disease control (palliation)—in some patients, notably those with multiple myeloma, autologous transplantation is used as a means of increasing the patient's progression-free survival.

ASSESSMENT

I. Pertinent medical history
  A. Diagnosis (see Boxes 20-2 and 20-3 for conditions commonly treated with HSCT) (Appelbaum et al., 2009; Ezzone, 2013; Forman & Nakamura, 2011; Gratwohl et al., 2010; Harris, 2010; Ljungman, 2009; Niess, 2013; Pasquini & Wang, 2011)
  B. Potential candidates for bone marrow transplantation—patients with malignancies that are at high risk for recurrence after standard therapy; however, malignancies must demonstrate a response to either antineoplastic therapy or RT.
  C. Factors that may increase the incidence of complications of marrow transplantation (Damiani et al., 2012; Estey, 2013; Slack et al., 2013)
    1. Amount of previous cancer therapy, length of time since last therapy, response to past therapy, and length of disease-free interval
    2. Underlying kidney, lung, liver, or cardiac dysfunction
    3. Previous infections and response to therapy
    4. Age—older patients (>17 years) more likely to develop transplantation-related complications
    5. Psychosocial dysfunction
II. Physical examination
  A. Pulmonary—respiratory rate, depth, and rhythm; lung expansion; adventitious breath sounds, oxygen saturation
  B. Renal—color and odor of urine and urinary output, edema, weight gain
  C. Mobility—muscle strength and endurance, range of motion, gait, activity level
  D. Nutrition—weight; skin turgor; amount, content, and patterns of nutritional intake.
  E. Comfort level—pain rating, anxiety, ability to rest or engage
  F. Cardiovascular—heart rate and rhythm, heart sounds, blood pressure, perfusion
  G. Gastrointestinal (GI)—volume, color, consistency, and caliber of stool; abdominal pain; distention; bowel sounds
  H. Genitourinary—color of urine, suppleness of bladder, condition of perineum
  I. Integumentary—color and intactness of skin, condition of oral mucous membranes, dental evaluation, condition of perineum and rectum
  J. Neurologic—mental status, orientation, sensation, reflexes
III. Psychosocial examination
  A. Psychological evaluation
    1. Feelings on decision to undergo bone marrow transplantation

2. Understanding of aggressiveness of treatment, goals of therapy, and chances of survival
    3. Number, type, effectiveness of coping mechanisms used in past stressful situations (before transplantation therapy) by patient and family members
    4. Perceptions of patient and family about isolation, prolonged hospitalization, living will, use of life-support technology, and potential death or survival
    5. Caregiver's ability to comprehend role
  B. Social evaluation
    1. Previous roles and responsibilities in the family and community
    2. Type, number, and history of use of support systems in the family and community
    3. Financial status—employment, insurance coverage, resources for daily living needs
    4. Eligibility for community resources
IV. Critical laboratory and diagnostic data unique to marrow transplantation (Ezzone, 2013)
  A. Hematologic—complete blood cell count, differential, platelet count, coagulation studies, type and cross-match with marrow donor, donor chimerism, minimal residual disease markers (Ezzone, 2013; Kim et al., 2013)
  B. Hepatic—liver transaminases (aspartate aminotransferase [AST] and alanine aminotransferase [ALT]), lactic acid dehydrogenase (LDH), bilirubin levels, coagulation studies; liver duplex ultrasonography (Anderson-Reitz, 2013)
  C. Renal—electrolytes, blood urea nitrogen (BUN), serum creatinine level, creatinine clearance, cyclosporine A levels, tacrolimus (FK-506) levels, animoglycoside levels, vancomycin levels, viral urine cultures, BK virus polymerase chain reaction (PCR), electron microscopy, renal ultrasonography (Anderson-Reitz, 2013; Lekakis, Macrinici, Baraboutis, Mitchell, & Howard, 2009)
  D. Cardiovascular—electrocardiography (ECG), cardiac ejection fraction or shorting fractions (in children), venography
  E. Pulmonary—chest radiography, computed tomography (CT) of chest or sinuses, pulmonary function tests (e.g., diffusing capacity of carbon monoxide [DLCO]), arterial blood gases [ABGs], oxygen saturation (pulse oximetry)
  F. Immune—antibody titers for cytomegalovirus (CMV) and herpesviruses (pretransplantation), Epstein-Barr virus (EBV) by quantitative PCR, hepatitis B surface antigen, immunoglobulin levels, human immunodeficiency virus (HIV) antibody, hepatitis C PCR, T-cell subsets (enumeration)
  G. Infectious disease—blood cultures for bacteria and fungi; urine and stool cultures for bacteria, fungi, and viruses; CMV quantitative PCR studies, adenovirus quantitative PCR studies, human

herpesvirus type 6 (ribonucleic acid [RNA]) studies, herpesvirus titers and cultures, toxoplasmosis antigenemia studies, respiratory and sputum cultures for bacteria, fungi, viruses, *Legionella*, acid-fast bacilli (AFB); stool and urine for electron microscopy cultures, stool for *Clostridium difficile* toxin, stains for *Pneumocystis carinii* pneumonia (PCP), multiviral respiratory panel.

PROBLEM STATEMENTS AND OUTCOME IDENTIFICATION

(Cohen et al., 2012; Cooke, Grant, & Gemmill, 2012; Ezzone, 2013; Livadiotti et al., 2012; Schoulte, Lohnberg, Tallman, & Altmaier, 2011; Williams, 2012)

I. Anxiety (NANDA-I)
   A. Expected outcome—patient and family describe the rationale for HSCT.
   B. Expected outcome—patient and family discuss the rationale, schedule, and procedures required for continued follow-up care after bone marrow transplantation.
II. Risk for Infection (NANDA-I)
   A. Expected outcome—patient and family states symptoms of infection to watch out for.
III. Impaired Oral Mucous Membrane (NANDA-I)
   A. Expected outcome—patient and family describe measures to prevent complications from impaired oral mucous membranes.
IV. Impaired Social Interaction (NANDA-I)
   A. Expected outcome—patient and family describe recommended changes in self-care, lifestyle, and social interactions to minimize the effects of bone marrow transplantation on health.
   B. Expected outcome—patient and family discuss strategies to maintain valued roles and relationships during the transplantation and post-transplantation periods.
   C. Expected outcome—patient and family list community resources available for assistance and support.
V. Diarrhea (NANDA-I)
   A. Expected outcome—patient maintains rectal area free of irritation.

PLANNING AND IMPLEMENTATION

I. Interventions to maximize safety for the patient and family
   A. Maintaining aseptic techniques and the level of protective isolation identified by the HSCT program (see Table 20-1 for general guidelines)
   B. Implementation of the conditioning regimen ordered by the physician or other provider
   C. Teaching the patient and family strategies to decrease risk of infection, bleeding, and injury during period of aplasia following bone marrow or stem cell or cord blood infusion

II. Interventions to decrease the incidence and severity of complications unique to bone marrow transplantation
   A. Anxiety
      1. Assessment of changes in and perceived contributing factors to anxiety levels in patient and family
      2. Providing a thorough orientation to the inpatient and outpatient bone marrow transplantation units and procedures common to bone marrow transplantation
      3. Implementation of strategies to encourage the patient and family to express concerns about bone marrow transplantation demands
      4. Consultation with an occupational therapist to develop a plan for diversional activities during isolation
      5. Teaching new anxiety-relieving strategies, as desired or needed by patient and family
      6. Assessment of the caregiver's ability to implement care demands
   B. Risk for infection (see Chapter 27)—common opportunistic infections and their time of occurrence after transplantation (Table 20-2) (Barrell, et al., 2012; Fisher et al., 2012; Livadiotti et al., 2012; Rosselet, 2013; Sohn et al., 2012)
      1. Notifying the advanced practice nurse (APN), physician's assistant (PA), or physician of initial temperature greater than 101° F (38.3° C) or other symptoms indicative of infection
      2. Teaching the patient and family strategies to decrease the risk of endogenous infections
         a. Meticulous hand washing
         b. Routine oral and perineal care
         c. Skin care
      3. Teaching the patient and family strategies to decrease risk of exogenous infections (Fisher et al., 2012)
         a. Restriction of visitors with suspected or known infections.
         b. Limiting visits by children (especially school-age children)
         c. Placing the patient on a low-microbial, stem cell transplantation (SCT) diet
         d. Avoidance of invasive procedures (e.g., peripheral intravenous [IV] catheter, intramuscular injections, urinary catheterization, rectal examinations, rectal temperatures)
         e. Recommendation for influenza vaccination for all close-contact individuals
         f. Proper care of central venous catheter
      4. Administration of prophylactic antimicrobial therapy, as ordered (Barrell et al., 2012; Fisher et al., 2012; Livadiotti et al., 2012; Rosselet, 2013; Sohn et al., 2012; Wingard, Hsu, & Hiemenz, 2011)

Table 20-2

Infectious Complications and Sites of Occurrence in Hematopoietic Stem Cell Transplantation (HSCT) Recipients

Type	Organism, Disease	Common Site
First Month after Transplantation		
Viral	Herpes simplex virus (HSV)	Oral, esophageal, skin, gastrointestinal (GI) tract, and genital
	Respiratory syncytial virus (RSV)	Sinopulmonary
	Epstein-Barr virus (EBV)	Oral, esophageal, skin, GI tract
	Human herpesvirus type 6 (HHV6)	Pulmonary, central nervous system (CNS), GI tract
Bacterial	Gram-positive organisms (*Staphylococcus epidermidis, S. aureus,* streptococci)	Skin, blood, sinopulmonary
	Gram-negative organisms (*Escherichia coli, Pseudomonas aeruginosa, Klebsiella*)	GI tract, blood, oral, perirectal
Fungal	*Candida (C. albicans, C. glabrata, C. krusei)*	Oral, esophageal, skin
	Aspergillus fumigatus, A. flavus	Sinopulmonary, skin
1-4 Months after Transplantation		
Viral	Cytomegalovirus (CMV)	Pulmonary, hepatic, GI tract
	Enteric viruses (rotavirus, coxsackie virus, adenovirus)	Pulmonary, urinary, GI tract, hepatic
	RSV	Sinopulmonary
	Parainfluenza virus	Pulmonary
	BK human polyoma virus	Genitourinary
Bacterial	Gram-positive organisms	Sinopulmonary, skin, venous access devices
Fungal	*Candida* species	Oral, hepatosplenic, integument, venous access devices
	Aspergillus species	Sinopulmonary, CNS, skin
	Mucormycosis	Sinopulmonary
	Coccidioidomycosis	Sinopulmonary
	Cryptococcus neoformans	Pulmonary, CNS
Protozoa	*Pneumocystis jiroveci (carinii)*	Pulmonary
	Toxoplasma gondii	Pulmonary, CNS
4-12 Months after Transplantation		
Viral	CMV, echoviruses, RSV, varicella-zoster virus (VZV), human polyoma virus	Integument, pulmonary, hepatic, genitourinary
Bacterial	Gram-positive organisms (*Streptococcus pneumoniae*),	Sinopulmonary, blood
	Haemophilus influenzae (pneumococci)	Sinopulmonary
Fungal	Aspergillosis	Sinopulmonary
	Coccidioidomycosis	Sinopulmonary
Protozoa	*P. jiroveci (carinii)*	Pulmonary
	Toxoplasma gondii	Pulmonary, CNS
12 Months After Transplantation		
Viral	VZV	Integument
	CMV	Pulmonary, hepatic
Bacterial	Gram-positive organisms (streptococci, *H. influenzae,* encapsulated bacteria)	Sinopulmonary, blood

Data from Ezzone, S.A. (Ed.). (2013). *Hematopoietic stem cell transplantation: A manual for nursing practice* (2nd ed., pp. 155–172). Pittsburgh: Oncology Nursing Society.

Part 3

a. Antibacterial prophylaxis with fluoroquinolones, third-generation cephalosporins (Simondsen, Reed, Mably, Zhang, & Longo, 2012; Sohn et al., 2012)

b. Amphotericin B by nebulation, caspofungin, fluconazole (Diflucan), posaconazole, voriconazole (Vfend), clotrimazole (Lotrimin, Mycelex), or nystatin (Mycostatin) to prevent fungal infection (Rosselet, 2013; Xu, Shen, Tang, & Feng, 2013).

(1) Obtaining and monitoring therapeutic drugs levels of posaconazole and voriconazole

c. Trimethoprim-sulfamethoxazole (Septra, Bactrim), IV or inhaled pentamidine (NebuPent, Pentacarinat, Pentam 300), or dapsone for prevention of PCP

d. Acyclovir (Aciclovir, Zovirax) for prevention of herpesvirus infection

e. Ganciclovir (Cytovene), foscarnet (Foscavir), or cidofovir for prevention of CMV and other viral infections

f. IV immunoglobulin for prevention of CMV and other viral infections

g. Ciprofloxacin (Cipro) for prophylaxis of bacterial infections

5. Administration of hematopoietic growth factors, as ordered

6. Routine surveillance cultures for bacteria, fungi, and viruses, antigenemia/PCR studies, and *Aspergillus* antigen study

7. Transfusion of irradiated, CMV-seronegative blood products or leukopoor-filtered blood products for all patients

C. Risk for injury

1. For patients receiving high-dose cyclophosphamide (Cytoxan), hemorrhagic cystitis is a potential complication (Reitz & Clancy, 2013).

a. Administration of mesna (Mesnex), a uroprotectant, as ordered, with IV hyperhydration; frequent voiding, with accurate urine output, necessary following high-dose cyclophosphamide

b. If mesna not used, continuous bladder irrigation (CBI), as ordered; administration of antispasmodics and analgesics, as ordered

c. Checking of urine specific gravity with each void on days of high-dose cyclophosphamide, and for 24 hours following the last dose, as required in some centers

d. Monitoring for cyclophosphamide-induced hyponatremia caused by syndrome of inappropriate antidiuretic hormone (SIADH) secretion

D. Alteration in oral mucous membranes

1. Cryotherapy (ice chips) for patients receiving melphalan

2. Encouragement for maintaining good oral hygiene (see Chapter 28 for general information)

E. Alteration in skin integrity

1. Instruction to patient to bathe four times daily while receiving thiotepa, because drug is excreted via the integumentary system and may lead to skin problems

F. Alteration in cardiovascular status

1. Monitoring of blood pressure and heart rate frequently with high-dose etoposide

2. Assessment for orthostatic hypotension with cyclophosphamide and high-dose etoposide

3. Assessment for decreased level of consciousness related to alcohol content in high-dose etoposide

G. Altered oral mucous membranes (see Chapter 28)

H. Nausea and vomiting (see Chapter 28)

III. Interventions to monitor for unique complications after bone marrow transplantation

A. GVHD (Table 20-3) (Brown, 2010; Mitchell, 2013)

1. Monitoring of condition of skin (erythema, rash), especially on the palms of hands and soles of feet

2. Evaluation of changes in liver function study results

3. Monitoring of amount, consistency, frequency, and color of stool

4. Administration of immunosuppressive therapy, cyclosporin, tacrolimus, sirolimus, mycofenolate, and anti-thymocyte globulin, systemic steroids, alemtuzumab (Campath), or others.

a. Obtaining and monitoring cyclosporin or tacrolimus levels

b. Monitoring for viral and fungal infection

B. Hepatic sinusoidal obstruction syndrome or hepatic veno-occlusive disease (Box 20-4) (Becze, 2011; Richardson et al., 2013)

1. Weighing the patient every day; notifying the medical practitioner of weight gain more than 5% of pretransplantation weight

2. Monitoring the location of pain (right upper quadrant)

3. Evaluation for elevation in serum bilirubin level

4. Evaluation for bleeding, poor response to platelet transfusions, and abnormal coagulation factors

5. Evaluation for changes in mental status

6. Measurement of abdominal girth every day if other parameters indicate possible veno-occlusive disease

Table 20-3

Clinical Staging and Grading of Acute GVHD Extent of Organ Involvement

Organ	Stage	Parameters
Rash*		
Skin	I	<25% BSA
	II	25%-50% BSA
	III	Rash on >50% BSA
	IV	Generalized erythroderma with bullous formation
Total Bilirubin		
Liver	I	2–3 mg/dL
	II	3–6 mg/dL
	III	6–15 mg/dL
	IV	>15 mg/dL

Volume of Diarrhea

		Adult	Pediatric
Gut	I	>500 mL/day	10–15 mL/kg/day
	II	>1000 mL/day	15–20 mL/kg/day
	III	>1500 mL/day	20–30 mL/kg/day
	IV	Adult and pediatric: Severe abdominal pain with or without an ileus	

Overall Clinical Grade

Grade	Description
I	Stage I-II clinical skin GVHD
II	Stage III clinical skin GVHD *or* Stage I liver and/or stage I gut GVHD Only one system stage III or greater
III	Stage II-III liver and/or stage II-IV gut GVHD Only one system stage III or greater
IV	Stage IV clinical skin GVHD (with grade 2 or higher histology) *and* Stage IV clinical liver and/or gut GVHD

*Use Rule of Nines or burn chart to determine extent of rash.

BSA, Body surface area; *GVHD*, Graft-versus-host disease.

Adapted from Dignan, F. L., Clark, A., Amrolia, P., et al. (2012). Diagnosis and management of acute graft-versus-host disease. Haemato-oncology Task Force of British Committee for Standards in Haematology; British Society for Blood and Marrow Transplantation. *British Journal of Haematology 158*(1), 30–45; and Ezzone, S. A. (Ed.). (2013). *Hematopoietic stem cell transplantation: A manual for nursing practice* (2nd ed., pp. 103–154). Pittsburgh: Oncology Nursing Society.

Box 20-4

Risk Factors for the Development of Hepatic Sinusoidal Obstruction Syndrome

- Pretransplantation chemotherapy (conditioning regimens containing cyclophosphamide, with or without busulfan)
- Abdominal radiation
- Pretransplantation hepatotoxic drug therapy (e.g., gemtuzumab ozogamicin [Mylotarg])
- Elevated transaminases before conditioning regimen
- Human leukocyte antigen (HLA)–mismatched or unrelated allogeneic transplantation
- Viral hepatitis
- Metastatic liver disease
- Karnofsky score < 90% before transplantation
- Second transplantation
- Older age recipient
- Female gender

IV. Interventions to enhance adaptation and rehabilitation
   A. Implementation of a program of range-of-motion and isometric exercises during the isolation period, especially if the patient is taking high-dose steroids
   B. Initiation of patient and family teaching about care of the central venous catheter early in the course of hospitalization
   C. Encouraging the patient, donor, and significant other to express concerns related to the transplant experience
   D. Discussion about potential changes in lifestyle and social interaction required immediately after discharge from the hospital
   E. Long-term follow-up (Syrjala, Martin, & Lee, 2012; Tierney & Robinson, 2013)
      1. Educating patient and family members on common outpatient problems after HSCT
      2. Common problems—fatigue, weight loss, sexual dysfunction, cataracts, chronic GVHD, chronic lung disease, herpes zoster virus, endocrinopathies, depression, isolation
      3. Ensuring that survivorship issues are addressed through long-term follow-up program
         a. Lifelong evaluation of allogeneic recipient for chronic GVHD
         b. Post-transplantation vaccinations
         c. Fertility issues
         d. Re-entry into community and work
         e. Delayed organ dysfunction (pulmonary, cardiac, renal, adrenal dysfunction)

      7. Skin care for patients with hyperbilirubinemia
      8. Evaluation of level of abdominal pain
      9. Administration of defibrotide, analgesics, vitamin K, fresh-frozen plasma, and other blood products
   C. Idiopathic pulmonary interstitial pneumonitis—infectious and noninfectious (Stephens, 2013)
      1. Monitoring temperature
      2. Assessment for presence of cough, chest pain, adventitious breath sounds, diminished oxygen saturation
      3. Evaluation of activity tolerance

Part 3

EVALUATION

The oncology nurse systematically and regularly evaluates the patient and the family's responses to interventions to determine progress toward the achievement of expected outcomes. Relevant data are collected, and actual findings are compared with expected findings. Nursing diagnoses, outcomes, and plans of care are reviewed and revised, as necessary.

References

Alchi, B., Jayne, D., Labopin, M., Kotova, O., Sergeevicheva, V., Alexander, T., et al., EBMT Autoimmune Disease Working Party members. (2013). Autologous haematopoietic stem cell transplantation for systemic lupus erythematosus: Data from the European Group for Blood and Marrow Transplantation registry. *Lupus, 22*(3), 245–253.

Anderson-Reitz, L. (2013). Hepatorenal complications. In S. A. Ezzone (Ed.), *Hematopoetic stem cell transplantation: A manual for nursing practice* (2nd ed., pp. 191–200). Pittsburgh: Oncology Nursing Society.

Appelbaum, F., Forman, S. J., Negrin, R. S., & Blume, K. G. (Eds.). (2009). *Thomas' hematopoietic cell transplantation* (4th ed.). Malden, MA: Blackwell Scientific.

Barrell, C., Dietzen, D., Jin, Z., Pinchefsky, S., Petrillo, K., & Satwani, P. (2012). Reduced-intensity conditioning allogeneic stem cell transplantation in pediatric patients and subsequent supportive care. *Clinical Journal of Oncology Nursing, 39*(6), E451–E458.

Beckers, M. M., Verdonck, L. F., Cornelissen, J. J., Schattenberg, A. V., Janssen, J. J., Willemze, R., et al. (2010). Autologous stem cell transplantation in haematological disorders, 1980–2002. *Nederlands Tijdschrift voor Geneeskunde, 154*, A2025; English translation.

Becze, E. (2011). Veno-occlusive disease is the most common hepatic complication in stem cell transplants. *ONS Connect,* (11), 16–17.

Brown, M. (2010). Nursing care of patients undergoing allogeneic stem cell transplantation. *Nursing Standards, 25*(11), 47–56.

Cohen, M. Z., Rozmus, C. L., Mendoza, T. R., Padhye, N. S., Neumann, J., Gning, I., et al. (2012). Symptoms and quality of life in diverse patients undergoing hematopoietic stem cell transplantation. *Journal of Pain and Symptom Management, 44*(2), 168–180.

Cooke, L., Grant, M., & Gemmill, R. (2012). Discharge needs of allogeneic transplantation recipients. *Clinical Journal of Oncology Nursing, 16*(4), 142–149.

Damiani, D., Tiribelli, M., Geromin, A., Cerno, M., Sperotto, A., Toffoletti, E., et al. (2012). Donor compatibility and performance status affect outcome of allogeneic haematopoietic stem cell transplant in patients with relapsed or refractory acute myeloid leukaemia. *Annals of Hematology, 91*(12), 1937–1943.

Devine, H. (2013). Overview of hematopoesis and immunology: Implications for hematopoetic stem cell transplantation. In S. A. Ezzone (Ed.), *Hematopoetic stem cell transplantation: A manual for nursing practice* (2nd ed., pp. 1–11). Pittsburgh: Oncology Nursing Society.

DiPersio, J. F., Ho, A. D., Hanrahan, J., Hsu, F. J., & Fruehauf, S. (2010). Relevance and clinical implications of tumor cell mobilization in the autologous transplant setting. *Biology of Blood and Marrow Transplantation, 17*(7), 943–955.

Estey, E. H. (2013). Acute myeloid leukemia: 2013 update on risk-stratification and management. *American Journal of Hematology, 88*(4), 318–327.

Ezzone, S. A. (Ed.). (2013). *Hematopoetic stem cell transplantation: A manual for nursing practice* (2nd ed.). Pittsburgh: Oncology Nursing Society.

Fisher, B. T., Alexander, S., Dvorak, C. C., Zaoutis, T. E., Zerr, D. M., & Sung, L. (2012). Epidemiology and potential preventative measures for viral infections in children with malignancy and those undergoing hematopoietic cell transplantation. *Pediatric Blood and Cancer, 59*(1), 11–15.

Forman, S. J., & Nakamura, R. (2011). *Hematopoietic cell transplantation.* http://www.cancernetwork.com/cancermanagment/hematopoetic-celltransplantation/article/10165/1802824?pageNumber=1.

Gratwohl, A., Baldomero, H., Alijurf, M., Pasquini, M., Bouzas, L. F., Yoshimi, A., et al. (2010). Hematopoietic stem cell transplantation: A global perspective. *JAMA, 303*(16), 1617–1624.

Harris, D. J. (2010). Transplantation. In J. Eggert (Ed.), *Cancer basics* (pp. 317–342). Pittsburgh: Oncology Nursing Society.

Jantunen, E., & Sureda, A. (2012). The evolving role of stem cell transplants in lymphomas. *Biology of Blood Marrow Transplantation, 18*(5), 660–673.

Kim, H. O., Oh, H. J., Lee, J. W., Jang, P. S., Chung, N. G., Cho, B., et al. (2013). Immune reconstitution after allogeneic hematopoietic stem cell transplantation in children: A single institution study of 59 patients. *Korean Journal of Pediatrics, 56*(1), 26–31.

Lekakis, L. J., Macrinici, V., Baraboutis, I. G., Mitchell, B., & Howard, D. S. (2009). BK virus nephropathy after allogeneic stem cell transplantation: A case report and literature review. *American Journal of Hematology, 84*(4), 243–246.

Livadiotti, S., Milano, G. M., Serra, A., Folgori, L., Jenkner, A., Castagnola, E., et al. (2012). A survey on hematology-oncology pediatric AIEOP centers: Prophylaxis, empirical therapy and nursing prevention procedures of infectious complications. Infectious Diseases Working Group of the Association of Italian Pediatric Oncology. *Haematologica, 97*(1), 147–150.

Ljungman, P., Bregni, M., Brune, M., Cornelissen, J., de Witte, T., Dini, G., et al. (2009). Allogeneic and autologous transplantation for haematological diseases, solid tumors and immune disorders: Current practice in Europe 2009. *Bone Marrow Transplantation, 45*(2), 219–234.

McAdams, F. W., & Burgunder, M. R. (2013). Transplantation treatment course and complications. In S. A. Ezzone (Ed.), *Hematopoetic stem cell transplantation: A manual for nursing practice* (2nd ed., pp. 47–66). Pittsburgh: Oncology Nursing Society.

Mitchell, S. A. (2013). Acute and chronic graft versus host disease. In S. A. Ezzone (Ed.), *Hematopoetic stem cell transplantation: A manual for nursing practice* (2nd ed., pp. 103–154). Pittsburgh: Oncology Nursing Society.

National Marrow Donor Program (NMDP) website. (2014). www.bethematch.org.

Niess, D. (2013). Basics concepts of transplantation. In S. A. Ezzone (Ed.), *Hematopoetic stem cell transplantation: A manual for nursing practice* (2nd ed., pp. 13–21). Pittsburgh: Oncology Nursing Society.

Ossenkoppele, G. J., Janssen, J. J., & Huijgens, P. C. (2013). Autologous stem cell transplantation in elderly acute myeloid leukemia. *Mediterranean Journal of Hematology and Infectious Disease, 5*(1), 77–81.

Pasquini, M. C., & Wang, A. (2011). *Current use and outcome of hematopoetic stem cell transplantation: CIBMTR summary slides.* http://www.cibmtr.org.

Perumbeti, A., & Sacher, R. (2012). Hematopoetic stem cell transplantation. http://emedicine.medscape.com/article/208954-overview#a1.

Rajkumar, S. V. (2013). Multiple myeloma: 2013 update on diagnosis, risk stratification, and management. *American Journal of Hematology, 88*(3), 226–235.

Reitz, L. A., & Clancy, C. (2013). Hepatorenal complications. In S. A. Ezzone (Ed.), *Hematopoetic stem cell transplantation: A manual for nursing practice* (2nd ed., pp. 191–200). Pittsburgh: Oncology Nursing Society.

Richardson, P. G., Ho, V. T., Cutler, C., Glotzbecker, B., Antin, J. H., & Soiffer, R. (2013). Hepatic veno-occlusive disease after hematopoietic stem cell transplantation: Novel insights to pathogenesis, current status of treatment, and future directions. *Biology of Blood and Marrow Transplantation, 19*(1 Suppl.), 88–90.

Rosselet, R. M. (2013). Hematologic effects. In S. A. Ezzone (Ed.), *Hematopoetic stem cell transplantation: A manual for nursing practice* (2nd ed., pp. 155–172). Pittsburgh: Oncology Nursing Society.

Schoulte, J. C., Lohnberg, J. A., Tallman, B., & Altmaier, E. M. (2011). Influence of coping style on symptom interference among adult recipients of hematopoietic stem cell transplantation. *Oncology Nursing Forum, 38*(5), 582–586.

Shenoy, S. (2013). Umbilical cord blood: An evolving stem cell source for sickle cell disease transplants. *Stem Cells in Translational Medicine, 2*(5), 337–340.

Simondsen, K. A., Reed, M. P., Mably, M. S., Zhang, Y., & Longo, W. L. (2012). Retrospective analysis of fluoroquinolone prophylaxis in patients undergoing allogeneic hematopoietic stem cell transplantation. *Journal of Oncology Pharmacology Practice, 19*(4), 291–297.

Slack, J. L., Dueck, A. C., Fauble, V. D., Sproat, L. O., Reeder, C. B., Noel, P., et al. (2013). Reduced toxicity conditioning and allogeneic stem cell transplantation in adults using fludarabine, BCNU, melphalan, and antithymocyte globulin (FBM-A): Outcomes depend on disease risk index but not age, comorbidity score, donor type, or HLA mismatch. *Biology of Blood and Marrow Transplantation, 19*(8), 1167–1174.

Sohn, B. S., Yoon, D. H., Kim, S., Lee, K., Kang, E. H., Park, J. S., et al. (2012). The role of prophylactic antimicrobials during autologous stem cell transplantation: A single-center experience. *European Journal of Clinical Microbiology and Infectious Disease, 31*(7), 1653–1661.

Stavropoulos-Giokas, S., Dinou, S., & Papassavas, A. (2012). The role of HLA in cord blood transplantation. *Bone Marrow Research, 2012,* 1–9.

Stephens, J. (2013). Cardioplumonary complications. In S. A. Ezzone (Ed.), *Hematopoetic stem cell transplantation: A manual for nursing practice* (2nd ed., pp. 201–229). Pittsburgh: Oncology Nursing Society.

Syrjala, K. L., Martin, P. J., & Lee, S. J. (2012). Delivering care to long-term adult survivors of hematopoietic cell transplantation. *Journal of Clinical Oncology, 30*(30), 3746–3751.

Tierney, D. K., & Robinson, T. (2013). Long-term care of hematopoetic cell transplant survivors. In S. A. Ezzone (Ed.), *Hematopoetic stem cell transplantation: A manual for nursing practice* (2nd ed., pp. 251–267). Pittsburgh: Oncology Nursing Society.

Ustun, C., Bachanova, V., Shanley, R., Macmillan, M. L., Majhail, N. S., Arora, M., et al. (2014). Importance of donor ethnicity/race matching in unrelated adult and cord blood allogeneic hematopoietic cell transplantation. *Leukemia & Lymphoma, 55*(2), 358–364.

William, B. M., & de Lima, M. (2013). Advances in conditioning regimens for older adults undergoing allogeneic stem cell transplantation to treat hematologic malignancies. *Drugs and Aging, 30*(6), 373–381.

Williams, B. J. (2012). Self-transcendence in stem cell transplantation recipients: A phenomenologic inquiry. *Oncology Nursing Forum, 39*(1), 41–48.

Wingard, J. R., Hsu, J., & Hiemenz, J. W. (2011). Hematopoietic stem cell transplantation: An overview of infection risks and epidemiology. *Hematology Oncology Clinics of North America, 25*(1), 101–116.

Xu, S. X., Shen, J. L., Tang, X. F., & Feng, B. (2013). Newer antifungal agents for fungal infection prevention during hematopoietic cell transplantation: A meta-analysis. *Transplant Proceedings, 45*(1), 407–414.

Zhao, X. S., Liu, Y. R., Zhu, H. H., Xu, L. P., Liu, D. H., Liu, K. Y., et al. (2012). Monitoring MRD with flow cytometry: An effective method to predict relapse for ALL patients after allogeneic hematopoietic stem cell transplantation. *Annals of Hematology, 91*(2), 183–192.

Part 3

CHAPTER 21

Nursing Implications of Radiation Therapy

Michelle Lynne Russell[*]

OVERVIEW

I. Principles of radiation—energy emitted and transferred through matter or space
   A. Radiation physics is the study of radiation energy and its effect on cellular biology.
      1. Ionizing radiation—used in the treatment of cancer based on the ability of radiation to interact with the atoms and molecules of the tumor cells to produce specific harmful biologic effects to the molecules of the cell or the cell environment (Gosselin, 2011)
      2. X-rays, gamma rays, protons, and cosmic radiation used in ionizing radiation (Hall, 2012)
      3. Forms of ionizing radiation
         a. Electromagnetic—radiation in the form of energy waves; includes photons (x-rays, gamma rays)
         b. Particulate—radiation in the form of subatomic particles; includes electrons, protons, neutrons, alpha particles, and beta particles
   B. Radiobiology—the study of the action of ionizing radiations on living things (Hall & Garcia, 2012)
      1. Biologic effects of ionizing radiation
         a. Cellular targets—the most important target for radiation damage is deoxyribonucleic acid (DNA). Radiation-induced DNA damage includes single- and double-strand breaks, as well as the formation of cross-links. This is a direct effect on the cell. Radiation also causes ionization of water and creates free radicals that damage DNA; this is an indirect effect (Murshad, 2010).
         b. Biologic response to radiation is affected by the level of DNA damage, oxygen effect (well-oxygenated tumors show greater response),

and sensitivity of the cell to the radiation (McBride & Withers, 2008).
      2. Normal tissue and tumor are both affected by ionizing radiation. The time in which biologic changes appear and the nature and severity of effects depend on the amount of radiation absorbed, fractionation, and rate at which it is administered. Acute- and late-responding tissues are affected differently by the biologic effect and radiosensitivity.
         a. Biologic effect of fractionation on tumors and normal tissue depends on four factors known as the four Rs of radiobiology.
            (1) Repair—normal tissue recovers with divided doses because it has greater repair of sublethal damage and repopulation abilities than dosed tumor tissue.
            (2) Redistribution—brings more of the cells into mitosis, the most sensitive phase of the cell cycle (after G2), with each successive radiation dose; theoretically, more tumor cells are delayed in the cycle and reach mitoses with the next dose, thereby increasing cell kill (Gosselin, 2011).
            (3) Repopulation—involves the replacement of dead or dying cells through cell multiplication; tumor cells that do divide usually do not survive because of radiation effect (Gosselin, 2011).
            (4) Reoxygenation—occurs because the decreased tumor burden (tumor shrinkage) leads to better blood flow patterns in the tumor, rendering it more radiosensitive.
         b. Radiosensitivity—all normal and cancer cells are vulnerable to effects of radiation and may be injured or destroyed by radiation therapy (RT).
            (1) Cells vary in sensitivity to radiation.

[*]The author would like to acknowledge Mary Ellen Witt, the previous author in the last edition, and Ellen Sitton, who was the original author of this chapter in the early editions. This fifth edition is an update of their previous work.

Table 21-1

Relative Radiosensitivity of Various Tumors and Tissues

Tumors	Relative Radiosensitivity	Tissues of Origin
Lymphoma, leukemia, seminoma, dysgerminoma	High	Lymphoid, hematopoietic (marrow), spermatogenic epithelium, ovarian follicular epithelium
Squamous cell cancer of the oropharyngeal, glottis, bladder, skin, and cervical epithelia; adenocarcinomas of the alimentary tract	Fairly high	Oropharyngeal stratified epithelium, sebaceous gland epithelium, urinary bladder epithelium, optic lens epithelium, gastric gland epithelium, colon epithelium, breast epithelium
Breast, salivary gland tumors, hepatomas, renal cancer, pancreatic cancer, chondrosarcoma, osteogenic sarcoma	Fairly low	Mature cartilage of bone tissue, salivary gland epithelium, renal epithelium, hepatic epithelium, chondrocytes, osteocytes
Rhabdomyosarcoma, leiomyosarcoma, ganglioneurofibrosarcoma	Low	Muscle tissue, neuronal tissue

Modified from Rubin, P. & Williams, J.P. (2001). Principles of radiation oncology and cancer radiotherapy. In Rubin, P. & Williams, J.P. (Eds.). *Clinical oncology: A multidisciplinary approach for physicians and students* (8th ed.). Philadelphia: Saunders.

(a) Generally, rapidly dividing cells, both normal and cancer cells, are most sensitive (e.g., mucosa) and are referred to as *radiosensitive*.

(b) Nondividing or slowly dividing cells are generally less radiosensitive, or *radioresistant* (e.g., muscle cells, neurons) (Table 21-1).

C. Principles behind treatment of cancer with radiation and control of side effects

1. A course of RT is planned to deliver a dose high enough to destroy the tumor in the primary site and surrounding lymph nodes at risk for cancer while not exceeding the tolerance of the normal tissues in the radiation field (or portal).

2. Side effects and sequelae of RT are generally the result of the effect of radiation on normal tissues. All normal tissues have a limit with regard to the amount of radiation they can receive and still remain functional.

   a. Early side effects occur during RT or immediately after and generally heal after the RT course (Ma, 2012). They are usually exhibited first by tissues with rapidly proliferating cells (e.g., gastrointestinal [GI] mucosa, bone marrow, and skin). These tissues are considered acute responding tissues and generally demonstrate early side effects. The severity of this early response to irradiation is not a predictor of the severity of a late response.

   b. Subacute responding tissues show few, if any, early effects but demonstrate damage in weeks to months after RT.

   c. Late effects occur months to years after RT and are permanent. Tissues composed of slowly proliferating cells develop injury slowly (e.g., central and peripheral nervous systems, kidney, dermis, cartilage, bone).

   d. Late responding tissues (e.g., spinal cord, peripheral nerves, kidney, dermis, cartilage, bone) generally demonstrate little evidence of early effects and show late effects months to years after RT (Ma, 2012) (Table 21-2). The risk of a second malignancy following radiation is low. Sarcoma is the most common radiation-induced second primary malignancy (Marcus, 2008).

   e. Combined treatment modality with concurrent chemotherapy and RT increases the risk of late effects on normal tissue and varies with drug and by anatomic location (Constantine et al., 2008).

Table 21-2

Response to Radiation: Acute or Late Responding

Acute-Responding Tissues	Subacute-Responding Tissues	Late-Responding Tissues
Bone marrow, ovary, testis, lymph node, salivary gland, small bowel, stomach, colon, oral mucosa, larynx, esophagus, arterioles, skin, bladder, capillaries, vagina	Lung, liver, kidney, heart, spinal cord, brain	Lymph vessels, thyroid, pituitary, breast, bone cartilage, pancreas, uterus, bile ducts

Adapted from Hall, E.J. & Cox, J.D. (2009). Physical and biologic basis of radiation therapy. In Cox, J.D. & Ang, K.K. (Eds.). *Radiation oncology: rationale, technique, results* (9th ed.). Philadelphia: Mosby.

D. Tissue response to fractionation
   1. External beam irradiation—a total dose tolerated by the tissues in the irradiated field is prescribed and is fractionated, or divided, into daily doses (usually 180 to 200 cGy/day). High dose per fraction and large total doses have been shown to be related to increased severity of late effects (McBride & Withers, 2008).
   2. Radioactive source therapy—a total dose tolerated by the tissues in the irradiated area is prescribed. This dose may be given over several days as a continuous application (low dose rate [LDR]) or in a single or several doses over several minutes (high dose rate [HDR]).
   3. Excessive prolongation of treatment or interruption in treatment schedule allows surviving tumor cells to proliferate during treatment.

II. RT fundamentals
   A. Approximately 60% of patients treated for cancer are treated with RT at some point during the course of their disease (Gosselin, 2011).
   B. The goal of RT is to destroy or inactivate malignant cells while minimizing damage to normal tissue within the treatment volume (Ma, 2012).
   C. Purpose and goals of radiation treatments
      1. Definitive—RT as the primary cancer treatment modality with or without chemotherapy; purpose—kill all cells in a malignant tumor capable of cell division while limiting the dose to the normal tissues (e.g., early prostate cancer, lung, and Hodgkin disease)
      2. Neoadjuvant—RT given before definitive treatment (e.g., surgery); purpose is to shrink tumor and facilitate complete resection (e.g., esophageal, some colon cancers)
      3. Adjuvant—RT given after definitive surgery or chemotherapy; purpose is to ensure local control (e.g., breast radiation after lumpectomy)
      4. Prophylaxis—RT given to asymptomatic, high-risk areas; purpose is to prevent future spread of disease in areas known to be vulnerable (e.g., whole-brain RT in leukemia and small cell lung cancer)
      5. Control—RT given at any point along the treatment continuum; purpose is to limit the growth and spread of disease (e.g., advanced non–small cell lung cancer); patient expected to have a period of symptom-free time
      6. Palliation—purpose is to improve quality of life by reducing or relieving symptoms or impending complications (e.g., relief of pain from bony metastasis, treatment of impending cord compression, relief of superior vena cava syndrome, decreasing obstruction, reduction or relief of symptoms from brain metastasis); life span not expected to be extended (Gosselin, 2011; Ma, 2012)

D. Methods of delivery of RT
   1. Local treatment
      a. External beam treatment machines in radiation oncology (teletherapy)
         (1) Linear accelerator (may treat with x-rays, electrons, or both)
            (a) X-rays—intermediate to deep treatment (depth of penetration varies with energy)
            (b) Electron beam—shallow treatment (spares deeper tissues; depth of penetration varies with energy; high skin doses)
         (2) Cobalt-60
            (a) Radioactive source—emission of gamma rays
      b. Radioactive source therapy—brachytherapy.
         (1) Beta particles and gamma rays from sealed radioactive sources (Table 21-3)
   2. Systemic treatment
      a. Radioactive source therapy—radiopharmaceutical therapy
         (1) Beta particles and gamma rays from unsealed radioactive sources (U.S. Nuclear Regulatory Committee, 2013) (see Table 21-3)
E. Treatment advances and innovative technologies in radiation
   1. Combined-modality treatment
      a. RT and chemotherapy (pre-RT, concurrent, post-RT)
      b. RT and concurrent biologic therapies (e.g., cetuximab)
      c. Intraoperative RT
         (1) Source-based RT
         (2) Electronic-based RT (XOFT)
      d. Radioimmunotherapy (RIT)—yttrium-90
      e. Hyperthermia and RT

Table 21-3

Radioisotopes and Their Properties

Radioisotope	Symbol	Half-Life	Type of Radiation
Cesium-137	^{137}Cs	30 yr	Beta, gamma
Gold-198	^{198}Au	2.7 days	Beta, gamma
Iodine-125	^{125}I	60 days	Beta, gamma
Iodine-131	^{131}I	8 days	Beta, gamma
Iridium-192	^{192}Ir	74.4 days	Beta, gamma
Phosphorus-32	^{32}P	14.3 days	Beta
Radium-226	^{226}Ra	1620 yr	Alpha, gamma
Strontium-90	^{90}Sr	28.1 yr	Beta

From National Council on Radiation Protection and Measurements. (1972). *Protection against radiation from brachytherapy sources. Report no. 40.* Bethesda, MD: National Council on Radiation Protection and Measurements.

2. Three-dimensional-conformal RT (e.g., six-field conformal prostate RT)
3. Intensity-modulated RT (IMRT)
4. Image-guided RT (IGRT)
5. Radiopharmaceuticals for metastatic bone pain (e.g., strontium-89)
6. HDR and LDR brachytherapy
7. Arc RT (e.g., rotational gantry with IMRT)
8. Gamma knife
9. Altered fractionation (e.g., hypo- and hyperfractionation, HDR)
10. Total body irradiation
11. Total skin electron irradiation
12. Particle beam therapy (e.g., neutron therapy, proton therapy); few machines available in the United States (U.S.)
13. Chemical modification (radiosensitizers, radioprotectors): 5-fluorouracil, a chemotherapy agent and a radiosensitizer; amifostine (Ethyol), a radioprotector
14. Intravascular brachytherapy for restenosis of cardiac stent
15. Accelerated partial breast irradiation (APBI) (Shah et al., 2013)
16. Selective internal RT (SIRT, SIRT-spheres)
17. Three-dimensional (3-D) surface imaging—real-time movement tracking
18. CyberKnife—frameless robotic radiosurgery system

III. Teletherapy (external beam RT)
   A. Precise dose delivered to the patient from outside the body
   B. Treatment process
     1. Patient consultation—with radiation oncologist and nurse
     2. Simulation—x-ray examination (scans) performed to create an image of the defined treatment volume; facilitates decisions for treatment position and treatment field(s); potential issues should be identified prior to treatment; treatment marks placed on skin or immobilization device (e.g., mask, Vac-Lok); computed tomography (CT), magnetic resonance imaging (MRI), and other modalities used for tumor localization to plan fields
     3. Treatment planning—done by radiation oncologist, dosimetrist, and physicist; based on pathology of tumor, location, radiosensitivity of tumor and normal tissue in treatment volume; CT or MRI from simulation used to plan and prescribe treatment; prescription will include daily and total dose of radiation, specific instructions on beam delivery, and number of radiation fields to be treated

4. Patient education—expectations of treatment and side effects
5. Treatment performed by radiation therapists
6. Weekly management evaluation—also referred to as *status check* or *on-treatment visit* (OTV); patients seen every week while undergoing therapy by a radiation oncologist and radiation nurse; evaluation of patient status and side effects as they occur during treatment course
7. Long-term follow-up—to evaluate the patient's response to treatment and monitor and manage long-term or late side effects

IV. Radioactive source therapy
   A. Radioactivity
     1. Definition—radioactivity, or radioactive decay, is the spontaneous emission of highly energetic particles (alpha and/or beta) or rays (gamma) from the nuclei of an element (radioisotope)
       a. Alpha (α) particles—large particles, shallow penetration; cause greater amount of damage; rare in the past, now seen with the emergence of radiolabeled monoclonal antibodies
       b. Beta (β) particles—deeper penetration; when ingested or injected, the body provides adequate shielding
       c. Gamma (γ) rays—Wide range of energy and penetration; more like x-rays with regard to shielding needed (Bucholtz, 2012)
     2. Energy—each radioactive element radiates energy as particles, rays, or both, characteristic for that element; some elements emit particles, rays, or both with energies that are more penetrating than others and therefore require more shielding to absorb the radiation; shielding measured in millimeters of lead (Pb) needed to block half of the radiation—the half-value layer (HVL)
     3. Half-life—predictable proportion of atoms that disintegrate in a given time; physical half-life, the time required for half of the atoms of a given quantity of radioactive material to decay; important in unsealed source RT (see Table 21-3)
     4. Units of measurement (Box 21-1)
       a. RT—radiation-absorbed dose; gray (Gy), rad
         (1) Gray—initially used in Europe, becoming more universal, absorbed dose; centigray (cGy)—unit of absorbed radiation dose equal to one hundredth of a gray
         (2) Rad—historically more common unit used in U.S., now being replaced by the more universal gray or centigray
         (3) 1 Gy = 100 cGy = 100 rad

Box 21-1

Units of Measurement

Absorbed Dose (gray, centigray, rad)

1 Gy = 100 rad

100 cGy = 100 rad

Therapeutic doses are prescribed in Gy or cGy.

Dose Equivalent (sievert, rem)

1 Sv = 100 rem

Badge readings are in mrem (millirem).

Activity (becquerel, curie)

$1 Bq = 2.7 \times 10^{-11} Ci = 1$ dps

$1 Ci = 3.7 \times 10^{10}$ dps

dps, Disintegrations per second.

b. Radiation protection—measurement of dose equivalent; sievert (Sv) measure, roentgen equivalent in man (rem); 100 rem = 1 Sv

c. Radioactivity of material—measured in becquerel (Bq) or curie (Ci) (U.S. Nuclear Regulatory Committee, 2013)

B. Treatment with radioactive sources (Figure 21-1)

1. Selection of type and method—depends on patient and disease factors

a. Sealed sources (brachytherapy)

(1) Dose rate—LDR, HDR

(2) Type—intracavitary, interstitial, intraluminal

b. Unsealed sources (radiopharmaceutical therapy)

(1) Dose—therapeutic dose (higher than tracer dose used in diagnostic tests)

2. Sealed sources (brachytherapy)—treatment of tumors with radioactive sources placed either temporarily or permanently adjacent to the

tumor (intracavitary or surface application), into the tumor (interstitial application), or into a lumen (intraluminal)

a. Primary advantage—ability to deliver high dose of radiation to small volume of tumor while delivering limited dose to adjacent normal tissues; can be delivered over a period of several days (e.g., LDR) or in a few minutes (e.g., HDR)

b. Radioactive material—sealed in a delivery device and never comes in direct contact with the patient

(1) The energy of radiation penetrates through device to treat the patient.

(2) When the sealed source is removed from the patient, the patient no longer requires radiation precautions.

(3) Sealed sources are used for LDR and HDR brachytherapy.

c. LDR remote afterloading machine—uses computer-controlled loading and unloading of sources from the patient from outside the patient's room

(1) Exposure to staff is reduced to a negligible amount, near zero.

(2) The physician prescribes treatment in the number of hours that the sources are loaded in the patient.

(3) Each treatment generally lasts several days.

d. HDR remote afterloading machines—generally use one highly radioactive computer-controlled source to treat patients

(1) This source may be used only where adequate shielding is available.

(2) Each treatment lasts only a few minutes.

(3) Patient is not radioactive after source is removed.

e. Principles of time, distance, and shielding used to minimize exposure to the staff and visitors (U.S. Environmental Protection Agency, 2013)

3. Unsealed sources (radiopharmaceutical therapy)—radioactive materials administered intravenously (IV), orally, or into a body cavity; result in uptake of radioactive element into various parts of the body, depending on element and form in which administered; radioactivity may be distributed fairly uniformly over the body or may concentrate in specific organs (Bucholtz, 2012).

a. Therapeutic dose—a dose of radiation high enough to treat the tumor; purpose is to deliver a predetermined dose to an organ or area of the body to treat the area with radiation

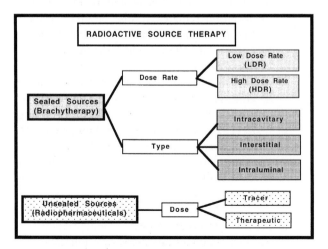

Figure 21-1 Radioactive source therapy.

Table 21-4

Recommendations Regarding Limits for Exposure to Ionizing Radiation

Class of Individual	Effective Dose Limits
Occupational Workers*	
Annual	50 mSv
Cumulative	10 mSv × age
Public (annual)	
Continuous or frequent exposure*	1 mSv
Infrequent exposure*	5 mSv
Embryo-Fetus Exposures (monthly)	
Equivalent dose limit	0.5 mSv
Negligible individual dose (annual)*	0.01 mSv

*Sum of external and internal exposures, but excluding doses from natural sources.

mSv, Millisievert.

From National Council on Radiation Protection and Measurements. (1972). *Protection against radiation from brachytherapy sources. Report no. 40.* Bethesda, MD: National Council on Radiation Protection and Measurements.

    b. Tracer dose—used for diagnostic tests (e.g., bone, liver, thyroid scans); dose very low and patient generally released from the hospital after the test
V. Radiation safety and protection
  A. Dose limitation—radiation protection (Table 21-4)
    1. Dose limits are applied to all individuals. Different limits are applied to workers who are occupationally exposed to radiation.
      a. ALARA (as low as reasonably achievable)—the best radiation protection guide is to keep radiation exposure as low as reasonably achievable. Radiation should be continually monitored and controlled.
      b. EDE (effective dose equivalent)—exposure to ionizing radiation from artificial sources is controlled by law.
  B. Radiation monitoring
    1. Personnel monitoring—individuals working in a restricted area should wear a personal monitor to measure radiation dose (e.g., film badge or dosimeter).
      a. Film badge—contains small photographic film; worn on the trunk of the body
        (1) Badges are read and exchanged monthly.
        (2) Workers should never wear a badge belonging to someone else because doing so does not allow determination of how much exposure each person received.
      b. Dosimeter (e.g., Luxel dosimeter)—worn in same manner, but measures radiation exposure from x-ray, beta, and gamma radiation through a thin layer of aluminum oxide

        (1) Dosimeters are available to measure radiation exposure; they can be read at the time of exposure.
    2. Survey meters (e.g., Geiger counter)—used for surveying, for example, the patient, room, trash, and linens, after brachytherapy or radiopharmaceutical therapy
  C. Radiation safety
    1. Essential considerations in minimizing exposure to radiation—time, distance, shielding
      a. Time—need to minimize the amount of time spent near radioactive sources; work quickly and efficiently; and rotate staff responsibilities.
      b. Distance—rapid decrease in intensity of radiation as the distance increases
        (1) Doubling the distance decreases exposure to one fourth the exposure received at the original distance (e.g., exposure of 40 mrem/hr at 1 m is 10 mrem/hr at 2 m).
        (2) Staff should work as far away from the source as possible and never touch a source (use long-handled forceps for dislodged sources).
      c. Shielding—type of shielding and its thickness dependent on type and energy of radioactive source

ASSESSMENT

I. Factors that influence effective communication
  A. Barriers to learning (e.g., language, hearing deficit, visual problems)
  B. Cultural issues
  C. Developmental stage
  D. Acute physical problems (e.g., pain or dyspnea)
II. History and physical assessment
  A. Cancer history (personal and family)
  B. Previous and current cancer treatment—prior radiation treatment
  C. Comorbidities—especially any condition involving tissues included in the radiation treatment volume
  D. Implanted devices (e.g., automatic implantable cardioverter-defibrillator [AICD], pacemakers, insulin pumps)
  E. Relevant laboratory data (e.g., complete blood cell count [CBC], tumor markers) and diagnostic data (e.g., results of CT, pathology examination, staging)
  F. Current symptoms and other medical conditions (e.g., pregnancy, restricted range of motion)
  G. Weight
  H. Current medications
III. Psychosocial assessment
  A. Coping patterns
  B. Support systems and patient's ability to meet transportation and care needs during treatment and follow-up care

Part 3

C. Knowledge and perceptions regarding treatment

IV. Factors influencing side effects of RT
   A. Site of radiation field (tissues to be irradiated)
   B. Time-dose-volume relationship (length of treatment, fractionation, volume of tissue irradiated)
   C. Radiosensitivity of tissues in treatment volume and potential early and late side effects
   D. Radiation type and energy, including depth of treatment prescribed
   E. Nutritional status
   F. Patient adherence to recommended care during RT
   G. Individual differences among patients

NURSING DIAGNOSES

I. Risk for Injury (NANDA)
   A. Expected outcomes
      1. Patient and family participate in measures to prevent unnecessary exposure to radiation.
      2. Patient demonstrates motivation to learn.
      3. Patient verbalizes understanding of potential side effects of RT.

II. Nursing diagnoses based on site of radiation therapy
   A. See Table 21-5.

PLANNING AND IMPLEMENTATION

I. Interventions to maximize radiation protection and safety with sealed and unsealed source RT
   A. Minimizing exposure—utilization of principles of time, distance, and shielding (United States Environmental Protection Agency [USEPA], 2013).
      1. Remote afterloading—sources automatically withdrawn from the patient and kept in a safe in the machine while staff and visitors are present; negligible radiation exposure to staff and visitors
      2. Unsealed sources—blood and body fluids become radioactive.
         a. Inpatient rooms specially prepared by radiation safety staff; plastic covers and absorbent floor coverings
         b. Radiation contamination—everything exposed to the patient's body fluids potentially contaminated by radiation; use of disposable dishes recommended; linens and wastes kept in containers in the room and monitored for radiation before being removed
         c. Patient to flush toilet three times after each use to dilute radioactive urine, stool, or vomitus.
         d. Staff precautions—gowns and gloves; washing hands, with the gloves on and then again after they are removed, before leaving room
      3. Sealed sources—accountability for all sources must be maintained.
         a. Shielded container is placed in room in the event of a dislodged source. Long forceps are used to place sources in the lead container.

Table 21-5

Potential Nursing Diagnoses for Specific Sites

Site of Irradiation	Potential Nursing Diagnoses
Skin	Impaired Skin Integrity, related to radiation-induced changes Disturbed Body Image, related to treatment lines, radiation-induced changes, tattoos
Head and neck	Impaired Oral Mucous Membranes, related to radiation-induced changes Imbalanced Nutrition: Less Than Body Requirements, related to mucositis, xerostomia, altered taste sensation, radiation caries Impaired Physical Mobility (temporomandibular joint), related to trismus Impaired Verbal Communication, related to vocal cord irradiation, mucositis, xerostomia
Central nervous system	Risk for Injury, related to radiation-induced increased intracranial edema Disturbed Body Image, related to alopecia
Chest	Imbalanced Nutrition: Less Than Body Requirements, related to esophagitis Risk for Infection, related to leukopenia Risk for Injury, related to thrombocytopenia Ineffective Breathing Pattern, related to radiation pneumonitis, fibrosis, or both Decreased Cardiac Output, related to cardiotoxicity Impaired Physical Mobility (shoulder joint), related to radiation fibrosis
Abdomen	Imbalanced Nutrition: Less Than Body Requirements, related to gastritis, nausea, vomiting Diarrhea Risk for Infection, related to leukopenia Risk for Injury, related to thrombocytopenia Acute Pain, related to radiation hepatitis Risk for Deficient Fluid Volume, related to radiation nephritis
Pelvis	Diarrhea Risk for Infection, related to leukopenia Risk for Injury, related to thrombocytopenia Impaired Urinary Elimination, related to radiation cystitis Sexual Dysfunction Ineffective Sexuality Patterns

b. Dressings at implant site are changed by the physician only.
c. Linens and wastes are kept in containers in the room and surveyed by a survey meter (e.g., Geiger counter) for radiation before being removed.

d. Patient and room are surveyed on removal of the sources.

4. Shielding—room designation for brachytherapy and radiopharmaceutical therapy dependent on facility and radioactive material being used; specially shielded rooms in many institutions; patients generally placed in a private room

5. Shielding (portable)—portable shields placed by radiation safety officer (RSO) or designee at the bedside; staff to stand behind the shield if possible when radioactive sources are placed in the patient

6. Exposure rate
    a. Measurements of exposure rate are generally done at 1 m from the patient, on the non patient side of a portable shield, and at the door of the room by the RSO or designee.
    b. Measurement of exposure rates in uncontrolled areas (e.g., room next door) may also be done.

7. Patient movement within the room—may be restricted during the procedure
    a. Unless specifically ordered by the physician, the patient is to remain in the room.
    b. Some patients may be out of bed but may be instructed to stay behind the shields unless using the bathroom. Patients may remain in bed when visitors are present.

8. Postradiation signs and instructions—radiation warning signs posted on the door, chart, and patient's armband; information regarding source, exposure rate, specific instructions to nurses and visitors generally placed in the chart

9. Contamination or lost sealed source—in the event of possible contamination or loss of a source, the RSO and radiation oncologist or nuclear medicine physician to be immediately notified

10. Time—amount of time personnel are in room to be minimized
    a. Personnel are also rotated when radioactive sources cannot be remotely afterloaded.
    b. Visitors are restricted in the amount of time spent in room.

11. Distance—visitors and personnel (when possible) to remain 6 feet from patient and behind the shield

12. Children (younger than 18 years), pregnant visitors, and staff not to enter the room when radioactivity is present.

13. Patient discharge
    a. Release of patient containing radioactive elements is very carefully controlled.
    b. The quantity of radioactivity and exposure should be limited at 1 m.
    c. Discharge instructions are provided to the patient, family, and significant others (Behrend, 2011).

II. Interventions related to deficit knowledge
    A. Determining who will be the learner: patient, family, significant other, or caregiver
    B. Assessment of motivation and willingness of patient and caregivers to learn
    C. Determining cultural influences on health teaching
    D. Providing teaching on potential side effects and how to manage the side effects based on patient's learning style (written, verbal, audiovisual presentation, or combination of these) (Table 21-6)
    E. Providing community resources and referral to support groups, as needed (Reinhard, Given, & Petlick, 2008).

Table 21-6

Side Effects of Radiation Therapy

Site	Potential Early Effects	Potential Intermediate or Late Effects	Nursing Considerations
Skin	Erythema, pigmentation, dry desquamation, moist desquamation, alopecia	Fibrosis, atrophy, telangiectasis, altered pigmentation, slow healing of trauma, carcinogenesis	*Early effects:* Nonmoist reaction: wash with mild soap and water and use calendula or hyaluronic-based cream. Use only electric razor, per institution guidelines. Moist desquamation: Wash with mild cleanser and use hydrocolloid or Silver leaf dressing. Observe for increased reaction in skin folds and with electrons. Observe for increased expected reaction if patient has had chemotherapy that enhances skin reaction (e.g., doxorubicin [Adriamycin], dactinomycin [Actinomycin D, Cosmegen]). *Early and late effects:* Protect skin from chemical, mechanical, thermal irritants and injury and from sun (see Chapter 30).

Continued

Table 21-6

Side Effects of Radiation Therapy—cont'd

Site	Potential Early Effects	Potential Intermediate or Late Effects	Nursing Considerations
Bone marrow	Myelosuppression (especially leukopenia, thrombocytopenia)		Large treatment areas covering significant amounts of bone marrow → increased myelosuppression (see Chapter 27)
Spine		Lhermitte sign; significantly damages growth in axial spine in children	*Late:* Radiation to growing bone decreases growth; monitor growth and development patterns after RT in children; assess neurologic and sensory functions.
Brain	Alopecia, somnolence	Hypothyroidism (if pituitary gland is in field)	*Early:* Use mild shampoo. Use moisturizing skin creams only as needed. Plan for alopecia (generally temporary) (see Chapter 30). *Late:* Assess neurologic and sensory function.
Head and Neck			
Mucosa	Mucositis	Pale mucosa, telangiectasia	Pretreatment dental evaluation Avoid chemical, thermal, and mechanical irritants to mucosa. Establish oral protocol with saline and bicarbonate rinses, soft toothbrushing at least twice daily (Harris, Eilers, Harriman, Cashvelly, & Maxwell, 2008).
Salivary glands	Xerostomia	Xerostomia, dental caries	Dental prophylaxis and fluoride program—assess for signs and symptoms of hypothyroidism.
Teeth		Radiation dental caries	See Chapter 33 for mucositis, xerostomia, and taste alterations and interventions.
Tongue, taste buds	Changes in taste		
Larynx	Laryngitis		
Thyroid		Hypothyroidism	
Bone (mandible)		Osteoradionecrosis	
Chest			
Lung	Radiation pneumonitis	Radiation pneumonitis, pulmonary fibrosis	Assess breathing. Assess nutritional status (see Chapter 33). See Chapter 31 for pulmonary toxicity.
Heart		Pericarditis, pancarditis, myocardial infarction	See Chapter 32 for cardiovascular toxicity.
Esophagus	Esophagitis, dysphagia	Stricture, fistula	See Chapter 33 for dysphagia.
Abdomen			
Small bowel	Diarrhea, fat malabsorption, nausea and vomiting	Small bowel obstruction, stricture	Antidiarrheal and antiemetic use Assess nutritional status. Low-residue diet Adequate fluids (see Chapter 28 for diarrhea, bowel obstruction)
Stomach	Gastritis, nausea and vomiting 1-2 hr after treatment		See Chapter 28 for nausea, vomiting.
Pelvis			
Bladder	Radiation cystitis	Fibrosis	Assess bladder function, bladder analgesic use.
Large bowel, rectum	Diarrhea, nausea and vomiting, inflammation of hemorrhoids, tenesmus	Bowel ulceration, inflammation	Antidiarrheal use (see Chapter 28)

Continued

Table 21-6

Side Effects of Radiation Therapy—cont'd

Site	Potential Early Effects	Potential Intermediate or Late Effects	Nursing Considerations
Ovaries	Premature menopause	Ovarian failure, especially if older than 25 years; altered sexuality	Family planning issues; before treatment, suggest consultation with fertility specialist regarding current methods of egg preservation.
Testes		Azoospermia	Discuss sperm banking before treatment if azoospermia anticipated; evaluate impact on patient (see Chapter 39).
Vagina	Inflammation, dryness, dyspareunia	Dryness, stenosis, vaginal shortening, dyspareunia	Water-based lubricants (women) Vaginal dilator after treatment
Penis	Inflammation	Erectile dysfunction, urethral stenosis	Assess potency before RT (men).
All Sites	Fatigue	Carcinogenesis	Fatigue reduction strategies; follow-up assessment (see Chapter 34 for fatigue interventions)

Adapted from Feight, D., Baney, T., Bruce, S., & McQuestion, M. (2011). Putting evidence into practice: Evidence-based interventions for radiation dermatitis. *Clinical Journal of Oncology Nursing* 15(5), 481–492; Dendaas, N. (2012). Toward evidence- and theory-based skin care in radiation oncology. *Clinical Journal of Oncology Nursing*, 16(5), 520–525.

Part 3

EVALUATION

The oncology nurse plays an active and critical role in the evaluation of a patient's physical response to radiation therapy, as well as the patient and family's psychosocial response to the radiation therapy process. Continuous assessment of the patient's status is performed, and relevant data are collected. An individualized plan of care is developed on the basis of the area being treated. Evidence-based interventions are performed to address the specific physical and psychosocial needs of the patient and family members. The oncology nurse evaluates the interventions on the basis of achievement of expected outcomes and makes revisions to the plan of care as necessary.

ADDITIONAL RESOURCES

1. American Cancer Society
1-800-ACS-2345
website: www.cancer.org
2. American Society for Therapeutic Radiology and Oncology (ASTRO)
1-800-962-7876
website: www.astro.org
3. National Cancer Institute
1-800-4-CANCER
website: http://cancernet.nci.nih.gov

References

Behrend, S. W. (2011). Radiation therapy treatment planning. In C. H. Yarbro, D. Wujcik, & B. H. Gobel (Eds.), *Cancer nursing: Principles and practice* (pp. 269–311). Sudbury, MA: Jones and Bartlett.

Bucholtz, J. D. (2012). Radiation protection and safety. In R. R. Iwamoto, M. L. Haas, & T. K. Gosselin (Eds.), *Manual for radiation oncology nursing practice and education* (pp. 29–43). Pittsburgh: Oncology Nursing Society.

Constantine, L. S., Milano, M. T., Friedman, D., Morris, M., Williams, J. P., Rubin, P., et al. (2008). Late effects of cancer treatment on normal tissues. In E. C. Halpern, C. A. Perez, & L. W. Brady (Eds.), *Principles and practice of radiation oncology* (pp. 320–355). Philadelphia: Lippincott Williams and Wilkins.

Dendaas, N. (2012). Toward evidence- and theory-based skin care in radiation oncology. *Clinical Journal of Oncology Nursing, 16* (5), 520–525.

Feight, D., Baney, T., Bruce, S., & McQuestion, M. (2011). Putting evidence into practice: Evidence based interventions for radiation dermatitis. *Clinical Journal of Oncology Nursing, 15*(5), 481–492.

Gosselin, T. K. (2011). Principles of radiation therapy. In C. H. Yarbro, D. Wujcik, & B. H. Gobel (Eds.), *Cancer nursing: principles and practice* (pp. 249–268). Sudbury, MA: Jones and Bartlett.

Hall, E. J., & Cox, J. D. (2009). Physical and biologic basis of radiation therapy. In J. D. Cox & K. K. Ang (Eds.), *Radiation oncology: Rationale, technique, results* (9th ed.). Philadelphia: Mosby.

Hall, E. J., & Garcia, A. J. (Eds.). (2012). *Radiobiology for the radiation oncologist* (7th ed.). Philadelphia: Lippincott Williams and Wilkins.

Harris, D. J., Eilers, J., Harriman, A., Cashvelly, B. J., & Maxwell, C. (2008). Putting evidence into practice: evidence based interventions for the management of oral mucositis. *Clinical Journal of Oncology Nursing, 12*(1), 141–152.

Ma, C.-M. C. (2012). The practice of radiation oncology. In R. R. Iwamoto, M. L. Haas, & T. K. Gosselin (Eds.), *Manual for radiation oncology nursing practice and education* (pp. 17–26). Pittsburgh: Oncology Nursing Society.

Marcus, R. B., Jr. (2008). Ewing tumor. In E. C. Halpern, C. A. Perez, & L. W. Brady (Eds.), *Principles and practice of radiation oncology* (pp. 1886–1891). Philadelphia: Lippincott Williams and Wilkins.

McBride, W. H., & Withers, H. R. (2008). Biologic basis of radiation therapy. In E. C. Halpern, C. A. Perez, & L. W. Brady (Eds.), *Principles and practice of radiation oncology* (pp. 76–108). Philadelphia: Lippincott Williams and Wilkins.

Murshad, H. (2010). *Clinical fundamentals for radiation oncologists.* Madison, WI: Medical Physics Publishing.

National Council on Radiation Protection and Measurements. (1972). *Protection against radiation from brachytherapy sources.* Report no. 40. Bethesda, MD: National Council on Radiation Protection and Measurements.

Reinhard, S. C., Given, B., & Petlick, N. H. (2008). Supporting family caregivers in providing care. In R. G. Hughes (Ed.), *Patient safety and quality: An evidence-based handbook for nurses.* Rockville, MD: Agency for Healthcare Research and Quality.

Rubin, P., & Williams, J. P. (2001). Principles of radiation oncology and cancer radiotherapy. In P. Rubin, & J. P. Williams (Eds.), *Clinical oncology: A multidisciplinary approach for physicians and students* (8th ed). Philadelphia, PA: W.B. Saunders Company.

Shah, C., Vicini, F., Wazer, D. E., Arthur, D., & Patel, R. R. (2013). The American brachytherapy society consensus statement for accelerated partial breast irradiation. *Brachytherapy*, *12*(4), 267–277.

U.S. Environmental Protection Agency. (2013). *Radiation protection basics.* http://www.epa.gov/radiation/understand/protection_basics.html.

U.S. Nuclear Regulatory Committee. (2013). *Glossary.* http://www.nrc.gov/reading-rm/basic-ref/glossary.html.

Part 3

CHAPTER 22
Nursing Implications of Chemotherapy

Susan Vogt Temple

OVERVIEW

I. Principles of cancer chemotherapy (Chu & DeVita, 2013)
  A. Cancer chemotherapy remains an integral component of systemic therapy in both hematologic and solid tumors.
  B. The use of chemotherapy is based on concepts of cellular kinetics, which includes cell cycle, time, growth fraction, and tumor burden.
    1. Cell cycle—a highly regulated five-stage process of reproduction that occurs in both normal and malignant cells (Reed, 2011b)
      a. Gap 0 (G0), or quiescent phase
        (1) Cells are not dividing; cellular activity continues but with a reduced rate of protein synthesis.
        (2) Entry into and out of quiescence is influenced by growth factors and mitogen interaction with cell surface receptors.
      b. Gap 1 (G1): postmitotic phase, or interphase
        (1) As cells are activated to proliferate they enter the cell cycle at the G1 phase.
        (2) Enzymes necessary for deoxyribonucleic acid (DNA) synthesis are produced.
        (3) Protein and ribonucleic acid (RNA) synthesis occurs.
      c. Synthesis (S)
        (1) Cellular DNA is replicated in preparation for DNA division.
      d. Gap 2 (G2), or premitotic phase
        (1) Further protein and RNA synthesis occurs.
        (2) Precursors of the mitotic spindle apparatus are produced.
      e. Mitosis (M)—cellular division occurs in five phases: prophase, prometaphase, metaphase, anaphase, telophase
        (1) Prophase—nuclear membrane breaks down, chromosomes clump, microtubule spindle assembled
        (2) Prometaphase—chromosomes attach to the microtubule spindle.
        (3) Metaphase—chromosomes align in the middle of the cell.
        (4) Anaphase—chromosomes separate to the centriole.
        (5) Telophase—nuclei reassemble, protein production resumes, and cellular division occurs with the production of two daughter cells during cytokinesis.
    2. Cell cycle time—the amount of time required for a cell to move from one mitosis to the next mitosis (Chu & DeVita, 2013; Shelburne, 2009)
      a. The length of the total cell cycle varies with the specific type of cell.
      b. A shorter cell cycle time results in higher cell kill with exposure to cell cycle–specific agents.
      c. Continuous infusion of cell cycle specific agents results in exposure of a greater number of cells and in a higher cell kill in tumors with short cell cycle times.
    3. Growth fraction of tumor—the percentage of cells actively dividing at a given point in time
      a. A higher growth fraction results in a higher cell kill with exposure to cell cycle–specific agents.
      b. Tumors with a greater fraction of cells in G0 are more sensitive to cell cycle–nonspecific agents.
    4. Tumor burden—volume of cancer present
      a. Cancers with a small tumor burden are usually more sensitive to antineoplastic therapy.
      b. As the tumor burden increases, the growth rate slows, and the number of cells actively dividing decreases.

c. The higher the tumor burden, the greater is the heterogeneity of tumor cells, which in turn increases the likelihood of drug-resistant clone development.

C. Approaches to chemotherapy (Chu & DeVita, 2013; Shelburne, 2009)
1. Single-agent chemotherapy
   a. Most common application is in the recurrent setting.
   b. Persistent use of single-agent chemotherapy increases the probability that drug-resistant clones will emerge.
2. Combination chemotherapy—use of two or more antineoplastic agents to produce additive or synergistic results against tumor cells
   a. Agents with actions in different phases of the cell cycle combine to increase the number of cells exposed to cytotoxic effects during a given treatment cycle.
   b. One agent modulates the toxicity of another agent.
   c. May decrease the incidence and severity of side effects of therapy
   d. Effective in large tumors containing a small number of proliferating cells; agents kill a high proportion of tumor cells and stimulate (recruits) remaining tumor cells to enter the proliferative phase; additional agents kill newly proliferating cells.
   e. Emergence of drug resistance forestalled by combining agents.
   f. Chemotherapy given in combination with target-specific agents (e.g., monoclonal antibodies)
   g. Criteria for selection of antineoplastic agents for combination therapy
      (1) Demonstration of cytotoxic activity when used alone to treat a specific cancer
      (2) Different, nonoverlapping toxicities
      (3) Toxicities that occur at different points of time from the treatment
      (4) Biologic effects that result in enhanced cytotoxicity
3. Regional chemotherapy—method of delivering doses of chemotherapy to the specific site of the tumor—for example, the liver, bladder, peritoneal cavity, pleural space—while reducing the intensity of systemic toxicity
4. High-dose chemotherapy administered with supportive therapy (e.g., colony-stimulating factors) or with an antidote to diminish toxicity (e.g., high-dose methotrexate with leucovorin rescue, ifosfamide with mesna)

D. Factors influencing the response to antineoplastic agents
1. Characteristics of the tumor
   a. Location
   b. Size or tumor burden
   c. Growth rate or fraction
   d. Resistance (inherent or acquired)
   e. Ratio of sensitivity of malignant cells and normal affected cells
   f. Genotype (e.g., molecular characteristics or hormone receptor status)
   g. Adequate blood supply with adequate drug uptake
2. Characteristics of the patient
   a. Physical status, performance status, age, comorbidities, physiologic deficits, prior therapies
   b. Psychosocial status
3. Administration or schedule
4. Routes—see Table 22-1
   a. Oral
   b. Subcutaneous
   c. Intramuscular
   d. Intrapleural
   e. Intravesicular
   f. Intraperitoneal
   g. Intrathecal or intraventricular
   h. Intra-arterial
   i. Intravenous
      (1) Intravenous push
      (2) Short infusion
      (3) Continuous infusion
      (4) Combined modality therapy

II. Role of chemotherapy in cancer care
A. Cure
1. Single-treatment modality (use of chemotherapy or biotherapies with curative intent)
2. Combined-treatment modality
B. Control
1. Goal—to extend the length and quality of life when cure is not realistic
C. Palliation
1. Improvement of comfort when neither cure nor control is possible
2. Relief of tumor-related symptoms

III. Types and classifications of chemotherapy (Box 22-1)—antineoplastic agents classified according to the phase of action during the cell cycle, mechanism of action, biochemical structure, or physiologic action (Chu & DeVita, 2013; Shelburne, 2009) (Table 22-2 lists potential side effects secondary to chemotherapy administration)
A. Phase of action during the cell cycle
1. Cell cycle–specific agents
   a. Major cytotoxic effects are exerted on cells actively dividing at specific phases throughout the cell cycle.

Table 22-1

Routes of Administration of Antineoplastic Agents

Route	Advantages	Disadvantages	Complications	Nursing Implications
Oral	Ease of administration	Inconsistency of absorption Potential for drug-drug or food- or herbal-drug interactions	Drug-specific complications	Teach adherence with medication schedule. Teach patient techniques for handling drugs, use gloves for handling chemotherapy; bring unused oral chemotherapy back to the facility for disposal. Follow same guidelines or policies and procedures for prescribing oral and IV chemotherapies.
Subcutaneous or intramuscular	Ease of administration Decreased side effects	Requires adequate muscle mass and tissue for absorption Inconsistent absorption	Infection Bleeding	Evaluate platelet count before administration. Use smallest gauge needle possible. Prepare injection site with an antiseptic solution. Assess injection site for signs and symptoms of infection.
Intravenous	Consistent absorption; most common method of chemotherapy administration Required for vesicants	Sclerosing of veins over time	Infection Phlebitis	Check for blood return before, during, and after drug administration.
Intra-arterial	Increased doses to tumor with decreased systemic side effects	Requires surgical procedure or special radiography for catheter and/or port placement	Bleeding Embolism Pain	Monitor for signs and symptoms of bleeding Monitor prothrombin time (PT), activated partial thromboplastin time (aPTT). Monitor catheter site.
Intrathecal or intraventricular *Note:* Vinca alkaloids are never given intrathecally because of the potential for lethal neurotoxicity or necrosis.	More consistent drug levels in cerebrospinal fluid	Requires lumbar puncture or surgical placement of reservoir or implanted pump Pump occlusion or malfunction Requires additional education for nurse, patient, family Nurse Practice Act may not allow nurse to administer agents via intrathecal or intraventricular route.	Increased intracranial pressure Headaches Confusion Lethargy Nausea or vomiting Seizures Infection	Observe site for signs of infection. Monitor reservoir or pump functioning. Assess patient for headache or signs of increased intracranial pressure.
Intraperitoneal	Direct exposure of intra-abdominal surfaces to drug	Requires placement of Tenckhoff catheter or intraperitoneal port	Abdominal pain Abdominal distention Bleeding Ileus Intestinal perforation Infection Nausea	Warm chemotherapy solution to body temperature. Check patency of catheter (note if no blood return) or port. Instill drug or solution according to protocol—infuse, dwell, and drain or continuous infusion.

Continued

Table 22-1

Routes of Administration of Antineoplastic Agents—cont'd

Route	Advantages	Disadvantages	Complications	Nursing Implications
Intravesicular	Direct exposure of bladder surfaces to drug	Requires insertion of indwelling catheter	Urinary tract infection Cystitis Bladder contracture Urinary urgency Allergic drug reactions	Maintain sterile technique when inserting indwelling catheter. Instill solution, clamp catheter for 1 hr, and unclamp to drain according to protocol.
Intrapleural	Sclerosing of pleural lining	Requires insertion of a thoracotomy tube Nurse Practice Act may not allow nurse to administer drug via intrapleural route.	Pain Infection	Monitor for complete drainage from pleural space before instillation of drug. Following instillation, clamp tubing, and reposition patient every 10 to 15 min × 2 hr for adequate distribution of the drug. Attach tubing to suction according to protocol. Assess patient for pain; provide analgesia. Assess patient for anxiety; provide emotional support.

Adapted from DeVita, V., Lawrence, T., Rosenberg, S., et al. (2011). *DeVita, Hellman, and Rosenberg's cancer: Principles & practice of oncology* (9th ed., pp. 375–421). Philadelphia: Lippincott Williams & Wilkins; Chu, E. & DeVita, V. (2013). *Physicians' cancer chemotherapy drug manual 2013*. Burlington, MA: Jones & Bartlett Learning; Whitford, J., Olsen, M., Polovich, M. (2009). *Chemotherapy and biotherapy guidelines and recommendations for practice* (3rd ed., pp. 25–34). Pittsburgh: Oncology Nursing Society.

Box 22-1

Classifications of Antineoplastic Agents*

Antimetabolites

Antifolates

Methotrexate (Mexate, Amethopterin)
Pemetrexed (Alimta)
Pralatrexate (Folotyn)

5-Fluoropyrimidines

5-Fluorouracil (5-FU, Efudex)
Capecitabine (Xeloda)
Floxuridine (FUDR)

6-Thiopurines

6-Thioguanine (6-TG, thioguanine)
6-Mercaptopurine (6-MP, Purinethol)
Azathioprine

Cytidine Analogues

Cytosine arabinoside (Ara-C, Cytosar, cytarabine)
Cytarabine liposomal (DepoCyt)
5-Azacytidine (Vidaza)
Decitabine (Dacogen)
Gemcitabine (Gemzar)

Adenosine Analogues

Fludarabine (Fludara)
Deoxycoformycin (pentostatin, Nipent)
Cladribine (2CdA, Leustatin)

Alkylating Agents—Platins

Carboplatin (Paraplatin)
Cisplatin (Platinol)
Oxaliplatin (Eloxatin)

Alkylating Agents—Nonplatins

Alkyl Sulfonates

Busulfan (Myleran, Busulfex)

Ethyleneimines, Methylmelamines

Altretamine (hexamethylmelamine, Hexalen)
Triethylenethiophosphoramide (Thiotepa)

Nitrogen Mustards

Mechlorethamine (nitrogen mustard, Mustargen)
Chlorambucil (Leukeran)
Cyclophosphamide (Cytoxan)
Melphalan (Alkeran)
Ifosfamide (Ifex)
Bendamustine (Treanda)

Nitrosoureas

Carmustine (BCNU, bischloroethylnitrosurea)
Streptozocin (Zanosar)
Lomustine (CeeNU, CCNU)

Triazenes

Dacarbazine (DTIC)
Temozolomide (Temodar)

Continued

Box 22-1

Classifications of Antineoplastic Agents—cont'd

Topoisomerase-Targeting Agents
Topoisomerase I Inhibitors—Camptothecins
Irinotecan (Camptosar, CPT-11)
Topotecan hydrochloride (Hycamtin)

Anthracyclines
Daunorubicin (Cerubidine, Daunomycin, Rubidomycin)
Daunorubicin citrate liposomal (DaunoXome)
Doxorubicin (Adriamycin)
Doxorubicin liposomal (Doxil)
Epirubicin (Ellence)
Idarubicin (Idamycin)
Valurubicin (Valstar)

Actinomycins
Dactinomycin (actinomycin D, Cosmegen)

Anthracenediones
Mitoxantrone (Novantrone)

Topoisomerase II Inhibitors—Epipodophyllotoxins
Etoposide (VP-16, VePesid, Etopophos)
Teniposide (VM 26, Vumon)

Antimicrotubule Agents
Vinca Alkaloids
Vinblastine (Velban)
Vincristine (Oncovin)
Vindesine
Vinorelbine (Navelbine)

Taxanes
Paclitaxel (Taxol)
Docetaxel (Taxotere)
Albumin-bound paclitaxel (Abraxane)
Cabazitaxel (Jevtana)

Epothilone, Antimicrotubule
Ixabepilone (Ixempra)

Nontaxane, Antimicrotubule
Eribulin (Halaven)

Glucocorticoids
Prednisone
Hydrocortisone
Methylprednisolone (Solu-Medrol)
Dexamethasone (Decadron)

Hormones
Estrogens
Chlorotrianisene (TACE)
Diethylstilbestrol (DES)
Estramustine (Emcyt)
Estratab
Estradiol

Nonsteroidal Aromatase Inhibitor
Anastrozole (Arimidex)

Steroidal Aromatase Inactivator
Exemestane (Aromasin)

Nonsteroidal Selective Aromatase Inhibitor
Letrozole (Femara)

Antiestrogen
Tamoxifen (Nolvadex)
Toremifene (Fareston)

Estrogen Antagonist
Fulvestrant (Faslodex)

Gonadotropin-Releasing Hormone (GnRH) Antagonist
Degarelix (Firmagon)

Progestins
Medroxyprogesterone acetate (Depo-Provera)
Megestrol acetate (Megace)

Luteinizing Hormone–Releasing Hormone (LHRH) Analogues
Leuprolide (Lupron)
Goserelin acetate (Zoladex)

Nonsteroidal Antiandrogens
Bicalutamide (Casodex)
Flutamide (Eulexin)
Nilutamide (Nilandron)

Adrenal Steroid Inhibitor
Aminoglutethimide (Cytadren)
Abiraterone acetate (Zytiga)

Miscellaneous Agents
Amsacrine (m-AMSA)
Arsenic trioxide (Trisenox)
Asparaginase (Elspar, L-asparaginase)
Bleomycin (Blenoxane)
Pegaspargase (Oncaspar)
Procarbazine (Matulane)
Tretinoin (ATRA, Vesanoid)

*This is not a comprehensive list.

Adapted from DeVita, V., Lawrence, T., Rosenberg, S., et al., (2011). *DeVita, Hellman, and Rosenberg's cancer: Principles & practice of oncology* (9th ed., pp. 375-421). Philadelphia: Lippincott Williams & Wilkins; Chu, E., & DeVita, V. (2013). *Physicians' cancer chemotherapy drug manual 2013*. Burlington, MA: Jones & Bartlett Learning; Whitford, J., Olsen, M., Polovich, M., (2009). *Chemotherapy and biotherapy guidelines and recommendations for practice* (3rd ed., pp. 25–34). Pittsburgh: Oncology Nursing Society.

Part 3

Table 22-2

Potential Side Effects of Chemotherapy

System	Side Effects
Hematopoietic	Neutropenia Thrombocytopenia Anemia
Gastrointestinal	Anorexia Nausea Vomiting Mucositis Stomatitis Diarrhea Constipation Pancreatitis Hepatic toxicity
Integumentary	Dermatitis Hyperpigmentation Alopecia Nail changes Radiation recall Photosensitivity Rash, urticaria
Genitourinary	Cystitis Hemorrhagic cystitis Acute renal failure Chronic renal insufficiency
Cardiovascular	Decreased ejection fraction Altered cardiac conduction Angina Venous fibrosis Phlebitis Extravasation
Neurologic	Cerebellar or central neurotoxicity Ototoxicity Metabolic encephalopathy Peripheral neuropathy
Pulmonary	Fibrosis Pneumonitis Edema
Reproductive	Infertility Changes in libido Erectile dysfunction Dyspareunia Amenorrhea
Mood alterations	Anxiety Depression Euphoria
Metabolic alterations	Hypocalcemia Hypercalcemia Hypoglycemia Hyperglycemia Hyperphosphatemia Hyperuricemia Hypokalemia Hyperkalemia Hypomagnesemia
Latent effects	Cognitive dysfunction Learning disabilities Changes in memory

Continued

Table 22-2

Potential Side Effects of Chemotherapy—cont'd

System	Side Effects
Secondary malignancies	
Other	Hypersensitivity Fatigue Ocular toxicity

Adapted from DeVita, V., Lawrence, T., Rosenberg, S., et al. (2011). *DeVita, Hellman, and Rosenberg's cancer: Principles & practice of oncology* (9th ed., pp. 375–421). Philadelphia: Lippincott Williams & Wilkins; Chu, E. & DeVita, V. (2013). *Physicians' cancer chemotherapy drug manual 2013.* Burlington, MA: Jones & Bartlett Learning; Whitford, J., Olsen, M., Polovich, M. (2009). *Chemotherapy and biotherapy guidelines and recommendations for practice* (3rd ed., pp. 25–34). Pittsburgh: Oncology Nursing Society.

    b. Agents are not active against cells in the resting phase (G0).

    c. Agents are schedule dependent and most effective if administered in divided doses or by continuous infusion.

    d. Cytotoxic effects occur during the cell cycle and are expressed when cell repair or division is attempted.

  2. Cell cycle–nonspecific agents

    a. Major cytotoxic effects are exerted on cells at any phase, including G0, in the cell cycle.

    b. Agents are dose dependent and most effective if administered by bolus doses because the number of cells affected is proportional to the amount of drug given.

    c. Cytotoxic effects occur during the cell cycle and are expressed when cell division is attempted.

  B. Biochemical structure, mechanism of action, or derivation

    1. Alkylating agents (Tew, 2011)

      a. Among the first antineoplastic drugs developed

      b. Mechanisms of action—interfere with DNA replication through cross-linking of DNA strands, DNA strand breaking, and abnormal base pairing of proteins

      c. Most agents cell cycle nonspecific; react in all phases of the cell cycle and have short half-lives

      d. Major toxicities, often directly related to the administered dose, occur primarily in the hematopoietic, gastrointestinal (GI), and reproductive systems

      e. Six major subgroups—nitrogen mustards, aziridines, alkyl sulfonates, epoxides, nitrosureas, and triazine compounds

    2. Antimetabolites (Chu & DeVita, 2013)

      a. Includes antifolates, 5-fluoropyrimidines, and thiopurines

b. Mechanisms of action—inhibit protein synthesis, substitute erroneous metabolites or structural analogues during DNA synthesis, and inhibit DNA synthesis

c. Most agents cell cycle–specific (S phase)

d. Major toxicities in the hematopoietic and GI systems

3. Platinum compounds (subgroup of alkylating agents) (Reed, 2011a)

a. Includes platins

b. Mechanism of action—form covalent bi functional DNA adducts

c. Most cell cycle–nonspecific

d. Major toxicities—hematopoietic, GI, neurologic systems (and genitourinary [GU] for cisplatin) affected

4. Topoisomerase targeting agents (Rasheed & Rubin, 2011)

a. Topoisomerase I–directed agents—include the camptothecins

(1) Mechanism of action—prevent realigning of DNA strands, maintaining single-strand DNA breaks

(2) Major toxicities affecting the hematopoietic and GI systems

b. Topoisomerase II–targeting agents—anthracyclines, anthracenediones, actinomycins, and epipodophyllotoxins

(1) Two main classes—inhibitors and poisons

(2) Major toxicities in the hematopoietic and GI systems

5. Microtubule targeting agents (Abu-Khalaf & Harris, 2011)

a. Mechanism of action—mitotic spindle poisons

b. Include taxanes and vincas

c. Most agents cell cycle–specific, primarily late G2 and M phases

d. Major toxicities in the hematopoietic, integumentary, neurologic, and reproductive systems

6. Miscellaneous agents (Chu & DeVita, 2013)

a. Mechanisms of action—poorly understood

b. Variety of toxic effects

IV. Chemoprotective agents

A. Agents designed to protect against specific toxic effects of chemotherapy

1. Dexrazoxane (Zinecard)

2. Amifostine (Ethyol)

3. Mesna (Mesnex)

V. Routes of administration—advantages of each route, potential complications, and nursing implications presented in Table 22-2

ASSESSMENT

I. Pertinent personal and family history

A. Documentation—should include pathology, stage, cytogenetic findings (when relevant), family and personal medical histories, co-morbidities, hematologic results, chemistries, and physical examination

B. Prior therapy or therapies

1. Attitudes of the patient and family toward prior and current therapies

2. Side effects experienced and their severity

3. Self-care measures and their effectiveness in reducing severity and incidence of side effects

C. Allergies or history of hypersensitivity reactions (note cycle of therapy)

1. Reactions to paclitaxel and docetaxel occur most frequently in the first or second infusion.

2. Reactions to platinum agents occur most often during the fifth (oxaliplatin), sixth, or later infusion (carboplatin).

D. Dietary intake, current weight, unintentional weight loss

E. Use of nutriceuticals, supplements, complementary therapies

F. Knowledge of, rationale for, and goals of treatment; agents to be given; potential side effects, management, risks and benefits, schedule, emotional, spiritual, and cultural considerations, other concerns

II. Physical examination

A. Thorough review of cardiopulmonary, GI, renal, reproductive, and neurologic functioning

B. Assess for pre-existing deficits, comorbidities, behavioral and cognitive functioning, functional ability, and performance status.

C. Presence of signs and symptoms of infection, other complications, or both

III. Psychosocial examination

A. Previous responses to stressors and effective coping mechanisms

B. Level of independence and responsibility, ability for self-care

C. Support systems and personnel available to the patient and family

IV. Laboratory and diagnostic data

A. Complete blood cell count with differential

B. Creatinine, blood urea nitrogen (BUN), liver function tests (LFTs)

C. Electrolytes

D. Other pertinent data (e.g., tumor marker, ejection fraction)

NURSING DIAGNOSES

I. Deficient Knowledge (NANDA-I), related to chemotherapy protocol, names of agents, potential side effects

Part 3

A. Expected outcome—patient describes the chemotherapy protocol: names of agents, routes, methods, schedules of administration, and schedules for routine laboratory and physical examination follow-up visits

B. Expected outcome—patient and family states potential immediate and long-term side effects of the antineoplastic agents.

C. Expected outcome—patient and family describe self-care measures to decrease the incidence and severity of complications of therapy.

D. Expected outcome—patient and family list changes that should be reported immediately to the health care team.
1. Signs and symptoms of infection—for example, temperature of 100.5° F (38.1° C) or higher, pain, swelling, redness, pus, chills, rigors, cough, change in cough, sore throat, diarrhea
   a. Risk of infection—directly related to duration and severity of neutropenia
   b. Typical signs and symptoms of infection will be muted in patients with severe neutropenia. ⚠
2. Nausea or vomiting that persists and is unrelieved by usual methods; inability to maintain oral intake
3. Unusual bleeding or bruising
4. Stomatitis or mucositis
5. Reduced urine output
6. Acute changes in mental or emotional status
7. Diarrhea or constipation unrelieved by usual control methods

E. Expected outcome—patient and family identify community resources to meet potential demands of treatment and rehabilitation.

F. Expected outcome—patient and family demonstrate competence in self-care skills demanded by the treatment plan.

II. Imbalanced Nutrition: Less Than Body Requirements (NANDA-I)
A. Expected outcome—patient weight stabilizes or is maintained during treatment.

III. Risk for Infection or Impaired Oral Mucous Membrane (NANDA-I)
A. Expected outcome—patient understands risks associated with mucositis and implements measures to facilitate healing and reduce the risk of infection.

IV. Sexual Dysfunction (NANDA-I)
A. Expected outcome—patient articulates altered sexual function and integrates strategies to maintain intimacy and self-image.

V. Fatigue (NANDA-I)
A. Expected outcome—patient incorporates prioritizes activities and seeks assistance, as appropriate.

VI. Constipation (NANDA-I)
A. Expected outcome—patient maintains normal bowel function.

VII. Diarrhea (NANDA-I)
A. Expected outcome—patient maintains normal bowel function.

VIII. Nausea (NANDA-I)
A. Expected outcome—patient is able to maintain adequate nutritional and fluid intake.

PLANNING AND IMPLEMENTATION

I. Interventions to maximize safe administration of chemotherapy to patient (Eisenberg, 2011; Neuss et al., 2013; Polovich, 2009; Power, 2011)
A. Review of orders
1. Comparing with formal drug protocol or reference source; ensuring accuracy and completeness (e.g., schedule, route, admixture solution) ⚠
2. Orders to be regimen-specific, preprinted, or electronic and list all agents and calculations in the regimen
3. Verbal orders not to be allowed except to hold or stop chemotherapy administration
4. Complete orders to include the patient's full name and a second patient identifier, date, diagnosis, regimen name and cycle number, criteria to treat, allergies, height and weight, full generic names of the agents or dosage calculations, route and rate of administration, supportive care agents or treatments, sequence, and time specifications

B. Determination of drug dosage
1. Verification of actual height and weight on day of administration
2. Calculation of body surface area (BSA) or appropriate dose calculation (e.g., area under the curve [AUC])
3. Recalculation of drug dosage and checking against order

C. Review of drugs to be administered and potential side effects and toxicities

D. Reviewing and obtaining orders for other medications, intravenous fluids (e.g., antiemetics; premedications, if indicated, for hypersensitivity reactions. prehydration and posthydration)

E. Verification of previous and current laboratory test values or need for dosage adjustment, if indicated

F. Verification that informed consent is documented according to practice or institution policies and procedures

G. Assessment of the patient
1. Previous experience with chemotherapy
2. Understanding and acceptance of the treatment plan
3. Resolution of prior cycle toxicities or side effects

H. Conducting patient and family teaching (e.g., chemotherapy administration procedures, antiemetic schedule, self-care measures for potential side effects)

I. Preparing drugs, as appropriate, following safe handling policies and procedures (Eisenberg, 2011; Glynn-Tucker, 2011; Polovich, 2009; Power, 2011)
  1. Plethora of data accumulated regarding risks of hazardous drug exposures and means of decreasing occupational exposures
  2. Many chemotherapies considered hazardous drugs and may evidence one or more of the following characteristics:
     a. Carcinogenic
     b. Teratogenic (fetal malformation or defects)
     c. Associated with adverse reproductive outcomes
     d. Genotoxic (damage genetic material)
     e. Other organ or system evidence of exposure or toxicity
     f. Similar in structure or toxicity to other agents known to be hazardous
  3. Potential risks for occupational exposures to hazardous drugs
     a. Increased risk for malignancies
     b. Embryofetal toxicities
     c. Chromosomal damage
     d. Other evidence of exposures (skin injury, alopecia, dermatitis)
  4. Mixing or compounding chemotherapy
     a. Guidelines and recommendations derived from the Oncology Nursing Society (ONS, 2011), the Occupational Safety and Health Administration (OSHA), and the American Society of Health-Systems Pharmacists (ASHP)
        (1) ONS published guidelines regarding special precautions for handling chemotherapies or hazardous drugs.
        (2) National Institute for Occupational Safety and Health (NIOSH) Alert on Preventing Occupational Exposure to Antineoplastic and Other Hazardous Drugs in Health Care Settings, 2004
        (3) U.S. Pharmacopeia (USP), General Chapter 797— "Pharmaceutical Compounding—Sterile Preparations," 2008
     b. Potentially high risk for exposure if proper procedures and guidelines are not followed
     c. Correct use of personal protective equipment (PPE) can significantly reduce exposure to hazardous drugs.
     d. All chemotherapy preparations, including crushing oral chemotherapies, to take place in a primary engineering control (PEC) setting — biologic safety cabinet or a compounding aseptic containment isolator
        (1) Uses vertical unidirectional air flow
        (2) Is vented to the outside (optimal) with exhaust emitted through a high-efficiency particulate air (HEPA) filter
        (3) Is set with the fan operating continuously
        (4) Is housed in an area with negative pressure
        (5) Is inspected and serviced as per manufacturer's recommendations and recertified if moved, repaired, when the filter is replaced, and every 6 months
        (6) Requires training to use techniques that minimize interference with air flow
     e. Washing of hands and donning PPE appropriate for use with chemotherapy
     f. Gathering necessary supplies for compounding; limit items housed in the PEC to reduce both contamination of items and interference with air flow
     g. Use of closed-system transfer devices to reduce environmental contamination during drug preparation
     h. Use of double glove for all handling; change every 30 minutes and whenever contamination occurs.
     i. Use of tubing and syringes with Luer-Lock fittings
     j. Avoidance of overfilling syringes
     k. Intravenous fluid (IVF)—should be spiked and tubing primed before chemotherapy is added to minimize exposure
     l. Damp-wiping outside of product (syringe, IVF) before placing in transport container; container should be identifiable as hazardous according to policy and procedures
     m. Transport containers or bags—should be labeled to ensure awareness of contents; contamination of the outside of the transport container or bags should be avoided.
     n. Disposal of all contaminated compounding materials in a sealed container within the PEC and placment in to a puncture-proof container located adjacent to the PEC
     o. Removing and discarding outer gloves, followed by the gown and the inner gloves, taking care not to contaminate self
     p. Washing hands with soap and water

J. Drugs to be labeled with the patient's full name and a second identifier, full generic drug name, route of administration, total dose, total volume required, date of administration or date and time of preparation and expiration, handling requirements

K. Double-checking chemotherapy order with second registered nurse (RN), pharmacist, or other licensed health care provider; BSA or dose calculation; and appropriate laboratory values

L. Obtaining appropriate supplies or pump
   1. Emergency equipment
   2. Agents for management of extravasation and/or anaphylaxis, as indicated
   3. Spill kit
   4. PPE
M. Donning PPE or applying principles of safe handling throughout administration of chemotherapy
   1. Potential routes of exposure
      a. Absorption—documented environmental exposures in areas where the drug is prepared and administered and in patient care areas
      b. Inhalation
      c. Ingestion
      d. Injection
   2. Guidelines regarding PPE
      a. Gloves—powder-free disposable gloves that have been tested for use with hazardous drugs
         (1) Double-glove for drug preparation, administration, and handling of contaminated waste.
         (2) Inspect for defects prior to use; remove and discard immediately after use, damage, drug spill, or 30 minutes of wear.
         (3) Do not reuse.
      b. Gowns—should be disposable, lint-free, low-permeability, with a solid front, long sleeves, tight cuffs, and back closure
         (1) Discard if visibly contaminated, after handling hazardous drugs, or after leaving the area.
         (2) Do not reuse.
      c. Respirators—National Institute for Occupational Safety and Health (NIOSH)–approved protective respirator when aerosolization, if possible
         (1) Check the material safety data sheet for appropriate respiratory protection.
         (2) Surgical masks are not respirators and do not protect against vapors or aerosols.
      d. Eye and face protection—plastic face shield to be worn when splashing is possible; surgical masks do not provide protection for eye and face exposures.
N. Selection of site for venipuncture if peripheral administration is to be performed
   1. Select distal sites before proximal sites.
   2. Evaluate general condition of veins.
   3. Note type of medications to be infused.
   4. Avoid sites where damage to underlying tendons or nerves is more likely to occur—for example, antecubital region, wrist, dorsal surface of the hand; areas with recent venipuncture sites, sclerosed veins; or areas of previous surgery such as skin grafts, side of mastectomy, lumpectomy, node dissection, or partial amputation.

O. Immediately prior to administration, verification of the order, drugs, or routes to be administered and the correct sequence of administration (Mancini & Modlin, 2011), dose calculations, volumes, expiration times and dates, drug appearance and physical integrity of the drugs, rate set on the infusion pump when required, and accuracy of two different patient identifiers
P. Monitoring central or peripheral IV administration
   1. Verify presence of blood return before, during, and after administration of therapy.
   2. Observe for signs and symptoms of infiltration.
Q. Administration of prechemotherapy hydration, antiemetics, and other medications, if ordered
R. Administration of chemotherapy drugs according to agency policy and procedures, following safe handling procedures and according to the five rights:
   1. Right medication
   2. Right time
   3. Right route
   4. Right dose
   5. Right patient
S. Assessment of the patient for signs of infiltration (burning, pain, swelling, redness)
T. Flushing the IV tubing with appropriate solution after administering each agent and at completion of the infusion
U. After drug administration, removal of intact administration setup; the spike from the IVF containers should not be removed or tubing reused.
V. Removal of the needle or IV catheter
   1. Apply an adhesive bandage to the peripheral IV site.
   2. Apply gentle pressure to the site to reduce local bleeding.
W. Washing potentially contaminated surfaces with water and detergent
X. Discarding contaminated materials in the appropriate hazardous waste container; Table 22-3 lists chemotherapies requiring PPE for longer than 48 hours.
Y. Documentation of medication administration, infusion site, patient education, and outcomes or response according to agency policy
II. Interventions to minimize risk of extravasation (Schulmeister, 2011)
   A. Prevention is the best approach for avoiding extravasation injury.
      1. Chemotherapy administration should be limited to knowledgeable and clinically competent individuals.
      2. Risk for extravasation should be assessed prior to treatment administration. Vigilance is always required during administration.
      3. Policies and procedures in the management of extravasations should be clearly delineated,

Table 22-3

Chemotherapies Needing Personal Protection for Greater Than 48 Hours

Chemotherapeutic Agent	Metabolites present in Urine	Metabolites in Feces or Bile
Carmustine	4 days+	
Cisplatin	5 days+	
Docetaxel	6% excretion	Up to 1 wk
Doxorubicin	5% excretion up to 5 days	Up to 1 wk
Etoposide	5 days+	
Gemcitabine	7 days+	
Methotrexate (oral)	Up to 5 days	Up to 5 days
Mitoxantrone	Up to 5 days	Up to 5 days
Teniposide	Up to 5 days	
Vincristine	Minimal	Up to 3 days
Vinorelbine	Minimal	3 days+

Data from Eisenberg, S. (2011). Drug administration. In Polovich, M. (Ed.). *Safe handling of hazardous drugs* (2nd ed., pp. 3–4). Pittsburgh: Oncology Nursing Society.

readily accessible in all sites where vesicants may be administered, and periodically reviewed.

B. If extravasation is suspected, appropriate materials and agents should be obtained for the management of extravasation.

1. Extravasation—infiltration or leakage of an IV antineoplastic agent into the local tissues
   a. Irritants—agents that cause a local inflammatory reaction but do not cause tissue necrosis
   b. Vesicants—agents that have the potential to cause cellular damage or tissue destruction if leakage into extravascular tissue occurs; see Table 22-4 for a list of agents associated with extravasation and tissue injury. ⚠
      (1) Observe for swelling, redness, lack of blood return, IV that slows or stops infusing, leaking around needle or catheter.
      (2) Instruct the patient to report pain, burning, or changes in sensations during chemotherapy administration.
      (3) Administer vesicants in larger veins of the arm, above the wrist and below the elbow. Avoid areas of flexion or areas with minimal overlying tissue.
      (4) Assess patency every 2 to 3 mL when administering IV push and every 5 minutes for piggyback infusion.
   c. If extravasation occurs or is suspected, do the following:
      (1) Immediately discontinue infusion, leaving needle or IV catheter in place.

Table 22-4

Agents Associated with Extravasation or Tissue Injury

Agent	Antidote	Type
Amsacrine (m-AMSA)	None	Vesicant
Bendamustine (Treanda)	None	Vesicant or irritant
Bleomycin (Blenoxane)	None	Vesicant or irritant
Carboplastin (Paraplatin)	Unknown	Irritant
Carmustine (BCNU, BiCNU)	Unknown	Vesicant
Cisplatin (Platinol)	Sodium thiosulfate	Vesicant if >20 mL of 0.5 mg/mL concentration extravasates
Dacarbazine (DTIC-Dome)	None	Irritant
Dactinomycin (Actinomycin D)	None	Vesicant
Daunorubicin (Cerubidine)	Dexrazoxane	Vesicant
Doxorubicin (Adriamycin)	Dexrazoxane	Vesicant
Liposomal doxorubicin (Doxil)	None	Irritant
Epirubicin (Ellence)	Dexrazoxane	Vesicant
Etoposide (VePesid, VP-16)	None	Vesicant or irritant
Idarubicin (Idamycin)	Dexrazoxane	Vesicant
Ifosfamide (Ifex)	Unknown	Irritant
Mechlorethamine (Mustargen)	Isotonic sodium thiosulfate	Vesicant
Melphalan (Alkeran)	None	Vesicant
Mitomycin (Mutamycin)	None	Vesicant
Mitoxantrone (Novantrone)	Unknown	Vesicant (ulceration rare unless infiltrated in concentrated dose)
Paclitaxel (Taxol)	None	Vesicant or irritant
Plicamycin (Mithracin)	None	Vesicant
Streptozocin (Zanosar)	None	Vesicant
Teniposide (VM 26)	None	Irritant
Vinblastine (Velban)	Hyaluronidase	Vesicant
Vincristine (Oncovin)	Hyaluronidase	Vesicant
Vindesine (Eldisine)	Hyaluronidase	Vesicant
Vinorelbine (Navelbine)	Hyaluronidase	Vesicant

Data from Schulmeister, L. (2009). Extravasation. In Whitford, J., Olsen, M., Polovich, M. (Eds.) *Chemotherapy and biotherapy guidelines and recommendations for practice* (3rd ed., pp. 105–111). Pittsburgh: Oncology Nursing Society; Schulmeister, L. (2011). Extravasation management: Clinical update. *Seminars in Oncology Nursing, 27*(1), 82–90.

Part 3

Table 22-5

Specific Toxicities and Nursing Interventions for Selected Chemotherapeutic Agents

Toxicity	Chemotherapeutic Agents	Nursing Interventions
Hypersensitivity	Asparaginase Paclitaxel Bleomycin Carboplatin Cisplatin Docetaxel Liposomal doxorubicin hydrochloride	Identify patients at risk—patients with previous allergic reactions to this or other medications; cycle of therapy. Assess for early signs of hypersensitivity—urticaria, pruritus, generalized uneasiness, hypertension, progressing to more severe reactions, including shortness of breath, chest pain, back pain, hypotension, bronchospasm, cyanosis, rigors, chills. Taxane reactions generally occur at onset of first and/or second infusion; platin reactions generally occur after fifth infusion and during the infusion. Assess for signs of anaphylaxis-type reactions. Provide supportive care, as indicated. Premedicate, as ordered. Administer bleomycin test dose to patients with lymphoma (may not be predictive of reaction before first dose).
Pulmonary injury (pulmonary toxicity presenting as pneumonitis that may progress to pulmonary fibrosis)	Bleomycin Mitomycin Cyclophosphamide Methotrexate Cytosine arabinoside Carmustine Procarbazine	Monitor cumulative dose of bleomycin, which should not exceed 400 units; doses above this limit significantly increase risk of pulmonary toxicity. Assess for signs of pulmonary toxicity—dry persistent cough, dyspnea, tachypnea, cyanosis, and basilar rales. Provide pulmonary toilet or adequate exercise. Higher levels of fraction of inspired oxygen (FiO_2) increase bleomycin toxicity potential.
Renal toxicity	Cisplatin High-dose methotrexate	Monitor creatinine, blood urea nitrogen (BUN), and urinary output. Avoid use of other nephrotoxic agents. Provide adequate hydration or diuresis. Premedicate with chemoprotective agent, if ordered, for cisplatin.
Ototoxicity	Cisplatin	Teach patient to report tinnitus. Monitor dose levels; risk increases with dosage $> 60\text{-}75 \text{ mg/m}^2$. Refer patient for audiography, if indicated.
Hemorrhagic cystitis	Cyclophosphamide Ifosfamide	Ensure adequate fluid intake $> 3000 \text{ mL/day}$ unless contraindicated. Have the patient void every 2-4 hr during day and every 4 hr at night. Assess for signs of cystitis. Administer mesna or continuous bladder irrigation (CBI), as ordered. Oral doses of cyclophosphamide should be given early in the day.
Cardiotoxicity manifested by electrocardiography (ECG) changes, congestive heart failure (CHF), cardio myopathy, angina, dysrhythmias, tachycardia, bradycardia	Doxorubicin Daunorubicin Epirubicin Idarubicin Cyclophosphamide (high dose) 5-Fluorouracil Capecitabine Mitoxantrone	Monitor cumulative doses of agents; maximal cumulative dose is 550 mg/m^2 for doxorubicin—doses above this significantly increase risk for cardiotoxicity; maximal cumulative dose for doxorubicin is 450 mg/m^2 if patient received or is concurrently receiving radiation to mediastinum or cyclophosphamide. Assess for signs of cardiotoxicity, including ECG changes; signs of CHF, including weight gain, pedal edema, shortness of breath, and jugular vein distention (JVD). Mitoxantrone—risk is not as great as with daunorubicin and doxorubicin; risk is increased with cumulative doses $> 125 \text{ mg/m}^2$.
Diarrhea	Irinotecan	Early and late diarrhea can be dose-limiting. Early diarrhea occurs within 24 hr of administration and is generally cholinergic; treatment may include atropine. Late diarrhea occurs >24 hr after dose and is managed with loperamide on schedule recommended by manufacturer.
Peripheral neuropathy	Paclitaxel Cisplatin Carboplatin Oxaliplatin	Monitor for sensory and motor nerve changes and stocking-glove distribution of dysesthesia. Peripheral neuropathy appears in the distal extremities of hands and feet and progresses proximally. Loss of sense includes loss of sense of proprioception, vibration, pain, temperature, and touch.
Hypotension	Etoposide	Rapid infusion may precipitate hypotension; administer over 30-60 min. Monitor blood pressure.

Continued

Table 22-5

Specific Toxicities and Nursing Interventions for Selected Chemotherapeutic Agents—cont'd

Toxicity	Chemotherapeutic Agents	Nursing Interventions
Neurotoxicity (central)	Ifosfamide Methotrexate Vincristine Cytarabine Intrathecal administration	Monitor creatinine, BUN, and albumin; risk of neurotoxicity increases with decreased renal function and low albumin level. Neurologic checks should be performed every 4 hr for patients at risk. Teach patients and families to report early signs of neurotoxicity.
Neurotoxicity (peripheral)	Paclitaxel Docetaxel Vincristine Vinorelbine Vinblastine Cisplatin	Assess for numbness of hands and feet, footdrop, slapping gait, tingling of fingertips and toes, decreased fine and gross motor abilities. Monitor for constipation as a potential early sign of neurotoxicity. Teach patient to report symptoms of neurotoxicity.

Data from DeVita, V., Lawrence, T., Rosenberg, S., et al., (2011). *DeVita, Hellman, and Rosenberg's cancer: Principles & practice of oncology* (9th ed., pp. 375-421). Philadelphia: Lippincott Williams & Wilkins; Chu, E. & DeVita, V. (2013). *Physicians' cancer chemotherapy drug manual 2013*. Burlington, MA: Jones & Bartlett Learning; Polovich M., (2009). *Chemotherapy and biotherapy guidelines and recommendations for practice* (3rd ed., pp. 25–34). Pittsburgh: Oncology Nursing Society.

(2) Aspirate residual medication and blood from the IV tubing.

(3) Remove the IV needle or device.

(4) Assess symptoms or suspected site of extravasation.

(5) For most medications, treatment of extravasation is nonpharmacologic.

    (a) Avoid applying pressure to the area to decrease spread of drug infiltrate.

    (b) Administer antidote, if appropriate. Apply a sterile dressing; use heat or cold compresses as indicated for the agent extravasated.

    (c) Elevate the affected extremity to decrease swelling.

(6) Notify the physician of extravasation; arrange follow-up.

(7) Document extravasation in the medical record to include date, time, needle size and type, site, method of administration, medications administered, sequence of antineoplastic agents, approximate amount of agent extravasated, subjective symptoms reported by patient, nursing assessment of site, interventions, notification of physician, instructions given to patient, measurements and photographs, follow-up measures, and signature.

III. Interventions to decrease the incidence and severity of complications of chemotherapy (Table 22-5)

EVALUATION

The oncology nurse systematically and regularly evaluates the patient's as well as the family's responses to interventions to determine progress toward the achievement of expected outcomes. Relevant data are collected, and actual findings are compared with expected findings. Nursing diagnoses, outcomes, and plans of care are reviewed and revised, as necessary.

References

Abu-Khalaf, M., & Harris, L. N. (2011). Antimicrotubule agents. In V. DeVita, T. S. Lawrence, & S. Rosenberg (Eds.), *DeVita, Hellman, and Rosenberg's cancer: Principles & practice of oncology* (9th ed., pp. 413–421). Philadelphia: Lippincott Williams & Wilkins.

Chu, E., & DeVita, V. T. (2013). *Physicians' cancer chemotherapy drug manual 2013*. Burlington, MA: Jones & Bartlett Learning.

Eisenberg, S. (2011). Drug administration. In M. Polovich (Ed.), *Safe handling of hazardous drugs* (2nd ed., pp. 35–47). Pittsburgh: Oncology Nursing Society.

Glynn-Tucker, E. M. (2011). Definition of hazardous drugs. In M. Polovich (Ed.), *Safe handling of hazardous drugs* (2nd ed., pp. 3–4). Pittsburgh: Oncology Nursing Society.

Mancini, R., & Modlin, J. (2011). Chemotherapy administration sequence: A review of the literature and creation of a sequencing chart. *Journal of Hematology Oncology Pharmacy, 1*(1), 17–25.

Neuss, M., Polovich, M., McNiff, K., Esper, P., Gilmore, T. R., LeFebvre, K., et al. (2013). 2013 Updated American Society of Clinical Oncology/Oncology Nursing Society chemotherapy administration safety standards including standards for the safe administration and management of oral chemotherapy. *Oncology Nursing Forum, 40*(3), 225–233.

Oncology Nursing Society (ONS). (2011). *ONS position statement on the education of the RN who administers and cares for the individual receiving chemotherapy and biotherapy. Position statements/education, certification, and role delineation.* ons.org/aboutONS/ONS.

Polovich, M. (2009). Safe handling. In M. Polovich, J. M. Whitford, & M. Olsen (Eds.), *Chemotherapy and biotherapy guidelines and recommendations for practice* (3rd ed., pp. 73–84). Pittsburgh: Oncology Nursing Society.

Power, L. (2011). Drug compounding. In M. Polovich (Ed.), *Safe handling of hazardous drugs* (2nd ed, pp. 27–35). Pittsburgh: Oncology Nursing Society.

Rasheed, Z. A., & Rubin, E. H. (2011). Topoisomerase-interacting agents. In V. DeVita, T. S. Lawrence, & S. Rosenberg (Eds.), *DeVita, Hellman, and Rosenberg's cancer: Principles & practice of oncology* (9th ed., pp. 402–412). Philadelphia: Lippincott Williams & Wilkins.

Reed, E. (2011a). Platinum analogs. In V. DeVita, T. S. Lawrence, & S. Rosenberg (Eds.), *DeVita, Hellman, and Rosenberg's Cancer: Principles & practice of oncology* (9th ed., pp. 386–392). Philadelphia: Lippincott Williams & Wilkins.

Reed, S. (2011b). Cell cycle. In V. DeVita, T. S. Lawrence, & S. Rosenberg (Eds.), *DeVita, Hellman, and Rosenberg's cancer:*

Principles & Practice of oncology (9th ed., pp. 68–81). Philadelphia: Lippincott Williams & Wilkins.

Schulmeister, L. (2009). Extravasation. In M. Polovich, J. M. Whitford, & M. Olsen (Eds.), *Chemotherapy and biotherapy guidelines and recommendations for practice* (3rd ed., pp. 105–111). Pittsburgh: Oncology Nursing Society.

Schulmeister, L. (2011). Extravasation management: Clinical update. *Seminars in Oncol Nurs, 27*(1), 82–90.

Shelburne, N. (2009). Principles of antineoplastic therapy. In M. Polovich, J. M. Whitford, & M. Olsen (Eds.), *Chemotherapy and biotherapy guidelines and recommendations for practice* (3rd ed., pp. 25–34). Pittsburgh: Oncology Nursing Society.

Tew, K. (2011). Alkylating agents. In V. DeVita, T. S. Lawrence, & S. Rosenberg (Eds.), *DeVita, Hellman, and Rosenberg's cancer: Principles & practice of oncology.* (9th ed, pp. 375–385). Philadelphia: Lippincott Williams & Wilkins.

CHAPTER 23

Nursing Implications of Targeted Therapies and Biotherapy

Brenda Keith and Kristine Deano Abueg

OVERVIEW

I. Definition

A. Terms *biotherapy* and *targeted therapy* —encompass a wide range of modalities, targets, and mechanisms

B. Targeted therapies—use of drugs to block growth and spread of cancer by interfering with specific molecules, referred to as *molecular targets*, involved in tumor growth and progression (National Cancer Institute [NCI], 2012)

1. Molecular targeted therapy (MTT) focuses on molecular and cellular changes that are specific to cancer and may be more effective than other types of treatment and less harmful to normal cells.

2. Many of these therapies focus on proteins that are involved in cell signaling pathways.

  a. Most signals are initiated by ligands outside of the cell that bind to receptors found on the cell membrane. Binding of a ligand to a receptor stimulates the activities of proteins necessary to continue transmission of the signal inside of the cell, resulting in biologic processes necessary for cell function.

  b. Disruption or alterations of signal transduction pathways can cause disease. For example, tumors may produce excessive ligands such as growth factors, resulting in continued growth of the tumor.

  c. Mutations in signaling pathways are found in many cancers (Cantley, Carpenter, Hahn, & Myerson, 2011).

3. Other targeted therapies can cause cancer cell death in the following ways:

  a. Directly, by specifically inducing apoptosis

  b. Indirectly, by stimulating the immune system to recognize and destroy cancer cells

  c. By delivering toxic substances directly to cancer cells (NCI, 2012)

4. The development of targeted therapies requires identification of appropriate targets that are known to play a role in cancer cell growth and survival.

C. Biotherapy—use of biologically derived substances to elicit biologic responses

1. Better understanding of the biology of cancer cells has led to the development of biologic agents that mimic some of the natural signals that the body uses to control cell function.

2. Clinical trials have shown that this cancer treatment, called *biologic response modifier (BRM) therapy*, *biologic therapy*, *biotherapy*, or *immunotherapy*, is effective for several cancers (American Cancer Society [ACS], 2012).

3. BRMs are compounds that are used to treat cancer by altering or augmenting naturally occurring processes within the body.

  a. BRMs use the body's immune system, either directly or indirectly, for the following purposes:

    (1) To enhance the activity of the immune system to increase the body's natural defense mechanisms against cancer (CancerQuest, 2011)

    (2) To lessen the side effects that may be caused by some cancer treatments

  b. BRMs include interferons, interleukins, colony-stimulating factors, monoclonal antibodies (MAbs), vaccines, gene therapy, and nonspecific immunomodulating agents.

    (1) BRMs such as interferons and interleukins provide nonspecific active immunity, whereas the monoclonal antibodies provide passive immunity.

    (2) Hematopoietic factors such as granulocyte colony-stimulating factor are used to increase general immunity and prevent opportunistic infection (Bisht, Bist, & Dhasmana, 2010).

(3) Other molecular targeted therapy approaches such as small molecule inhibitors (e.g., tyrosine kinase and proteasome inhibitors) are not considered biologic therapy.

D. Focus of this chapter—biotherapies and molecular targeted agents approved by the U.S. Food and Drug Administration (FDA) for the treatment of cancers

II. Goals and approaches

A. Cancer panomics—understanding the complex combination of genes, proteins, molecular pathways, and unique patient characteristics that together drive the disease of cancer, as well as understanding how to target these factors in combination to develop prevention strategies and curative therapies (American Society of Clinical Oncology [ASCO], 2012)

B. Diagnosis of cancer
1. MAbs used in the differential diagnosis of cancer
   a. Classification of leukemia or lymphoma (recognition of cell surface markers) with flow cytometric analysis
   b. Radiolabeled MAbs (low-dose radioisotopes tagged to MAbs) used as highly specific diagnostic tools to detect tumors using special scans
      (1) OncoScint for diagnosis of some colorectal cancers and other types of cancers
      (2) CEA-Scan for metastatic colon cancer diagnosis (Wagner & Kempken, 2013)

C. Treatment of cancer
1. Neoadjuvant treatment to achieve a pathologic complete response, downstage the tumor (e.g., pertuzumab in combination with trastuzumab and docetaxel for the neoadjuvant treatment of HER2-positive breast cancer), or both (Gianni et al., 2012)
2. Primary treatment
   a. Single agent (e.g., imatinib mesylate) for the treatment of newly diagnosed adult patients with Philadelphia chromosome–positive chronic myelogenous leukemia in the chronic phase (Hughes et al., 2010)
   b. Combination therapy—for example, CHOP (cyclophosphamide, doxorubicin, vincristine [Oncovin], prednisone) plus rituximab (Rituxan) for high-grade lymphoma (Coiffier et al., 2002)
3. Adjuvant therapy
   a. After surgery to maintain the disease-free interval (e.g., imatinib mesylate following complete gross resection of KIT (CD117)-positive gastrointestinal stromal tumor (GIST) (Scandinavian Sarcoma Group, 2009)
   b. Combination therapy—for example, TCH (docetaxel, carboplatin, trastuzumab) for human epidermal growth factor receptor-2 (HER2)–positive breast cancer (Slamon et al., 2011)
4. Treatment of metastatic disease
   a. Used as single agent or combined with other treatment modalities such as chemotherapy
   b. First-line treatment for metastatic disease
      (1) Sunitinib for first-line treatment of metastatic renal cell carcinoma (Motzer et al., 2009)
      (2) Bevacizumab in combination with chemotherapy for first-line treatment of metastatic nonsquamous non–small cell lung cancer (NSCLC) (Sandler et al., 2006)
   c. Second-line metastatic disease, refractory disease, palliative treatment
      (1) Cabozantinib for progressive medullary thyroid cancer (Elisei et al., 2013)
      (2) Ipilimumab for unresectable or metastatic melanoma (Hodi et al., 2010)
5. Maintenance therapy
   a. Ongoing treatment to lower the risk of recurrence following initial therapy
   b. Treatment to lower progression or metastases in advanced cancer (e.g., erlotinib as maintenance treatment of NSCLC if the disease has not progressed after first-line therapy)
6. Combination therapy
   a. With other biologic agents (e.g., hematopoietic growth factors used in stimulation of dendritic cells [DCs])
   b. Synergistic effects of MAbs with chemotherapy
   c. Dual targets
      (1) Two targeted agents used simultaneously to address multiple molecular mutations
      (2) Example—pertuzumab and trastuzumab in HER2-positive metastatic breast cancer that both target HER2 but at different regions of the receptor (Baselga et al., 2012)
   d. Conjugated MAb
      (1) Conjugated with radioisotopes to deliver radiotherapy to targeted cancer cells (e.g., tositumomab, ibritumomab tiuxetan)
      (2) Conjugated with chemotherapy to deliver cytotoxic chemotherapy to targeted cancer cells (e.g., ado-trastuzumab emtansine)
   e. Radiosensitization—for example, increased radiotherapy benefit for initial treatment of locally or regionally advanced squamous cell

cancer of the head and neck with concurrent cetuximab (Bonner et al., 2010)

D. Supportive therapy
   1. Hematopoietic growth factors after antineoplastic therapy to decrease the incidence and severity of neutropenia, anemia, and thrombocytopenia
   2. For the prevention of skeletal-related events in patients with bone metastases from solid tumors (e.g., denosumab)

E. Targeted therapy in many cancers and clinical situations still under investigation
   1. Many applications currently supported in the literature have not received regulatory (FDA) approval.

III. Targets
   A. Cell signaling pathways—effectively relay external signals (cell proliferation, apoptosis, responses to stimuli, and migration) to the cell nucleus, which is the communication network governing and mediated by the interaction between tyrosine kinases
      1. Tyrosine kinases—regulate cell signal transmission by catalyzing the transfer of an activating phosphate group between sequential proteins
      2. Cascade sequence
         a. Growth factors interact with the extracellular portion of a membrane-bound tyrosine kinase.
         b. The bound tyrosine kinase dimerizes, and this activates the receptor, allowing the transfer of its phosphate group (located on the intracellular portion) to the next protein in the sequence.
         c. Sequential proteins are activated (phosphorylated) in a specific sequence.
         d. Ultimately, the sequence of protein activation results in gene activation.
      3. Mutations in specific proteins—result in aberrant proliferation, migration, apoptotic control, and stimulus response dysregulation; several such mutations include the following:
         a. Overexpression of membrane-bound tyrosine kinases, as in the example of HER-2 tyrosine kinase receptor, or the epidermal growth factor receptor (EGFR) tyrosine kinase receptor
         b. Autophosphorylation of pathway proteins, resulting in overactivation of the cell signal in the absence of regulating growth factors
      4. Interaction of targeted therapies with selected mutant proteins or gene sequence along the cell signaling pathway (see modalities below)
         a. Monoclonal antibodies exert effects on targets by one or more of the following:
            (1) Prevents ligand binding to the membrane-bound receptor by interaction with extracellular membrane-bound receptors and extracellular serum growth factors
            (2) Blocks signals from the receptor to the nucleus of the cell
            (3) Mediates antibody-dependent cell-mediated cytotoxicity (ADCC) by recruiting immune system cells to activate a systemic immune response (Scott, Allison, & Wolchok, 2012)
            (4) Sensitizes cancer cells to chemotherapy
         b. Small molecules interact and inhibit tyrosine kinase domains of specific intracellular proteins. Table 23-1 compares MAbs and small-molecule kinase inhibitors.
   B. Targeted cancer therapies that have been approved for use in specific cancers—drugs that interfere with cell growth signaling or tumor blood vessel development promote the specific death of cancer cells, stimulate the immune system to destroy specific cancer cells, and deliver toxic drugs to cancer cells (NCI, 2012); several key pathways identified as carcinogenic drivers in specific cancers:
      1. Vascular endothelial growth factor (VEGF) plays a key role in tumor angiogenesis, thereby contributing to metastases, drug resistance, and tumor growth.
         a. Targeted therapy mechanisms
            (1) Inhibition of the intracellular tyrosine kinase domain of VEGF receptor (VEGF-R) and platelet-derived growth factor receptor (PDGF-R) using small-molecule inhibitors

Table 23-1

Comparison of Monoclonal Antibodies and Small-Molecule Kinase Inhibitors

	Monoclonal Antibodies	Small-Molecule Kinase Inhibitors
Size	Large molecule	Small molecule
Site(s) of action	Extracellular	Intracellular
Method of administration	Injected	Oral
Half-life	Days	Hours
Type of target	Single target	Single or multiple
Potential for immune system activation	Yes	No
Potential for drug-drug interactions	No	Yes

(2) Inhibition of the extracellular domain using monoclonal antibodies

b. Examples include bevacizumab, sunitinib malate, and sorafenib.

c. Key adverse events of antiangiogenesis agents—wound healing complications, bleeding, hypertension, and proteinuria

2. Human epidermal growth factor receptors (HER) are a family of four related cell surface–bound tyrosine kinases; HER1/EGFR, HER2, HER3, and HER4. Receptor activation occurs through ligand-independent and ligand-dependent processes (e.g., dimerization). Receptors may pair with like receptors, which is referred to as *homodimerization*. Pairing of different HER receptors is called *heterodimerization*. Activation of the receptor triggers a series of downstream cell-signaling cascades such as MAPK and PI3K, which regulate key cellular processes. Development of agents targeting this pathway has largely been focused on the membrane-bound tyrosine kinase molecules, particularly HER1/EGFR and HER2.

a. Dysregulation of the HER2 molecules expressed via overexpression of the HER proteins and gene amplification

b. HER1 also commonly referred to as *EGFR*

(1) The external domain of the HER1/EGFR tyrosine kinase is the target of anti-EGFR MAbs, including cetuximab and panitumumab.

(2) The internal domain of the HER1/EGFR tyrosine kinase is the target of small-molecule inhibitors, including erlotinib and gefitinib.

c. HER2

(1) Receptor overexpression can create excessive HER2 signaling, resulting in cell proliferation, DNA synthesis, and tumorigenesis.

(2) In vivo, HER2 is the preferred dimerization partner for all HER2 receptors and thus presents an important target in HER2-involved tumors.

(a) The external domain of the HER2 tyrosine kinase is the target of trastuzumab, pertuzumab, and ado-trastuzumab emtansine.

(b) The internal domain of the HER2 tyrosine kinase is the target of the small-molecule inhibitor lapatinib. Figure 23-1 depicts HER family receptors and targeted therapies.

3. PI3K/Akt—these molecules regulate signaling pathways involved in proliferation, survival, cell growth, and motility; overexpression of

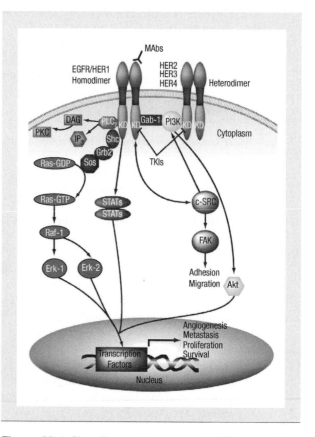

Figure 23-1 Signaling pathways and inhibitors of the HER family of receptors. *From Sachdev, J. & Jahanzeb, M. (2012). Blockade of the HER family of receptors in the treatment of HER2-positive metastatic breast cancer. Clinical Breast Cancer, 12(1), 19–29.*

PI3K (phosphoinositide 3-kinase inhibitor) and Akt inappropriately transforms normal into malignant cells; PI3K is also thought to induce angiogenesis, critical for continued tumor growth and metastasis.

4. Mammalian target of rapamycin (mTOR) pathway regulates cellular processes, including cell survival, proliferation, and growth.

a. mTOR regulates cell growth, proliferation, differentiation, tumor cell motility, and metastases (Zhou & Huang, 2011).

b. Agents include temsirolimus (for renal cell cancer) and everolimus (for renal cell cancer, subependymal giant cell astrocytoma, and renal angiomyolipoma).

c. PI3K activation activates Akt which activates mTOR (de Lartigue, 2011)

5. Phosphatase and tensin homolog (PTEN) is a tumor suppressor gene that negatively regulates PI3K and Akt; loss of this signaling molecule allows overexpression of the PI3K-Akt pathway.

6. The mitogen-activated protein kinase (MAPK) pathway communicates a signal from the surface

of the cell to the deoxyribonucleic acid (DNA) in the nucleus. A defect in this pathway leads to uncontrolled growth. It is also known as the *Ras-Raf-MEK* (mitogen-activated extracellular signal regulated kinase 1)-*ERK* (extracellular signal–regulated protein kinase) pathway.

a. The proteins produced by a family of three closely related genes, the *Ras* genes (KRas, NRas, HRas), regulate cell proliferation, adhesion, and migration. Increased activation in cancer caused by mutations in *Ras* genes allows for unregulated cell growth. The first drug approved to act on this pathway was sorafenib.

b. There are three isoforms of Raf (ARaf, BRaf, and CRaf).

c. MEK is a protein that is downstream from Ras in the MAPK pathway. Blocking the activity of the MEK protein may be an indirect method to attack tumors with mutated Ras proteins or other proteins that influence MAPK activity (NCI, 2013).

d. Ras-Raf-MEK-ERK signaling is especially important in melanoma, with several agents approved for treatment (Ascierto et al., 2012). Figure 23-2 depicts signaling pathways altered in melanoma, including the Ras-Raf-MEK-ERK pathway.

7. *BCR-ABL* (breakpoint cluster region-Abelson) is a fusion gene resulting from the mutated translocation of arms of chromosomes 9 and 22 (residing on the mutated Philadelphia

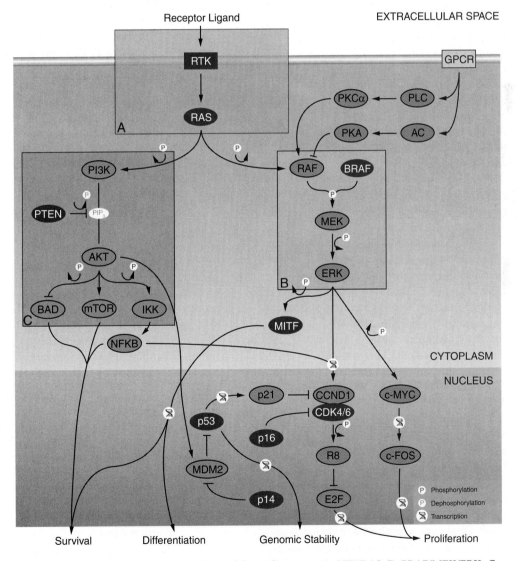

Figure 23-2 Signaling pathways altered in melanoma. A, RTK/RAS. **B,** BRAF/MEK/ERK. **C,** PI3K/PTEN/AKT. Mutated or genetically abnormal molecules are shown in gray. *From Haluska, F., Pemberton, T., Ibrahim, N., & Kalinsky, K. (2007). The RTK/RAS/BRAF/PI3K pathways in melanoma: Biology, small molecule inhibitors, and potential applications. Seminars in Oncology, 34(6), 546–554.*

chromosome). The gene encodes the BCR-ABL fusion protein associated with increased cell division and growth implicated in chronic myeloid leukemia, acute lymphoblastic leukemia, and chronic neutrophilic leukemia.

   a. Targeted therapy mechanisms—interferes with a critical binding site of the BCR-ABL, effectively stopping its ability to interact with enzymes and switching off the downstream pathways that promote leukemia cell growth (Patel, Suthar, Patel, & Singh, 2010)

   b. Examples—imatinib mesylate, dasatinib, nilotinib, ponatinib

8. MET is an integral plasma membrane protein that relays signals from the extracellular environment into the cytoplasm. MET is activated when its extracellular domain binds to hepatocyte growth factor (HGF) (Appleman, 2011). MET activates key oncogenic pathways and is involved in angiogenesis.

9. The Janus-associated kinase (JAK)/STAT pathway mediates the signaling of a number of cytokines and growth factors for hematopoiesis and immune and inflammatory responses in the body (Sawyer, 2011). Ruxolitinib is a JAK1 and JAK2 inhibitor used in the treatment of myelofibrosis.

10. The *ALK* fusion gene is an alteration in a normal gene called anaplastic lymphoma kinase (ALK) and is thought to play a critical role in the growth of some NSCLCs. Crizotinib is used in the treatment of ALK-positive NSCLC.

11. Hedgehog pathway mutations may result in cancer development. Vismodegib is used in the treatment of metastatic basal cell carcinoma. It binds to Smoothened, a transmembrane protein involved in Hedgehog signal transduction.

12. Programmed death 1 protein (PD-1) and its ligand (PD-L1) play a role in the ability of tumor cells to evade the host's immune system. PD-L1 on the tumor cell surface inhibits T cells that might otherwise attack the tumor cell. Anti–PD-1 and anti–PD-L1 antibodies potentiate an immune response by blocking the interaction between the PD-1 protein and one of its ligands, PD-L1 (Helwick, 2013). Nivolumab and lambrolizumab are being developed to target PD-1; MDPL3280A is a PD-L1 agent that is under investigation.

13. The poly (ADP-ribose) polymerase (PARP) family of enzymes is involved in many functions of the cell, including the repair of DNA damage and maintenance of DNA integrity. PARP1 overexpression has been associated with overall prognosis in cancer, especially in breast cancer. PARP1 and PARP2 inhibitors have demonstrated activity in breast and ovarian cancers caused by mutations in either *BRCA1* or *BRCA2* (Kummar et al., 2012). These agents are being studied in clinical trials.

14. Fms-like tyrosine kinase 3 (*FLT3*) gene mutations can be detected in approximately 30% of patients with acute myeloid leukemia (AML) and is associated with a poor clinical outcome. Long-term outcomes of patients with *FLT3* internal tandem duplication (ITD) may be improved with FLT3 inhibitors (Takahashi et al., 2013). These agents remain investigational.

15. Polo-like kinase 1 (Plk1) is an enzyme that regulates cell division (mitosis) and is considered a potential target for cancer therapy. High levels of Plk1 correlate with a poor prognosis. Volasertib is a potent inhibitor of Plk1. This inhibition results in cell cycle arrest and subsequent cell death (apoptosis). Studies are being conducted using volasertib in AML (The ASCO Post, 2013b).

IV. Types of targeted therapies

  A. Targeted therapies interact with selected proteins along the cell signaling pathway, thereby interrupting the transmission of the signal and activation of cancerous DNA.

  B. Targeted therapies may have direct cytotoxic action on tumor cells, indirect action to restore, augment, or modulate the immune system to facilitate the destruction of tumor cells, promote cell differentiation, interfere with neoplastic changes, or prevent metastases (Bisht et al., 2010).

    1. MAbs target the extracellular domain (i.e., the receptor) of the membrane-bound tyrosine kinase and extracellular serum growth factors. They are antibodies directed against molecules that are either overexpressed or mutated in cancer cells (Vapiwala & Geiger, 2010). Refer to Table 23-2 for a list of FDA-approved MAbs.

     a. Classified in two groups for cancer treatment

      (1) Unconjugated or naked MAbs, which work by themselves with no drug or radioactive material attached

      (2) Conjugated Mabs, which are attached to a chemotherapy drug, radioactive particle, or a toxin; sometime referred to as *antibody drug conjugates* (ADCs), *tagged, labeled,* or *loaded antibodies*

     b. MAb types depending on the portion of mouse antibody

      (1) Murine (suffix, -*momab*)—derived from mouse antibody

      (2) Chimeric (suffix, -*ximab*)—combination of mouse and human antibody

Table 23-2

Monoclonal Antibodies Currently FDA-Approved in Oncology

Antibody	Target	FDA-Approved Indications	Mechanism of Action
Rituximab (Rituxan) Chimeric IgG1	CD20	For treatment of CD20-positive B-cell NHL and CLL; for maintenance therapy for untreated follicular CD20-positive NHL; for treatment of granulomatosis with polyangiitis; for treatment of microscopic polyangiitis	Unconjugated; ADCC; direct induction of apoptosis, CDC
Trastuzumab (Herceptin) Humanized IgG1	HER2	For treatment of HER2-positive breast cancer, as a single agent or in combination with chemotherapy for (a) adjuvant or (b) metastatic disease; for treatment of HER2-positive metastatic gastric or gastroesophgeal junction carcinoma in combination with cisplatin and capecitabine/5-fluorouracil	Unconjugated; inhibition of HER2 signaling; ADCC
Bevacizumab (Avastin) Humanized IgG1	VEGF	For treatment of metastatic colorectal cancer, renal cell cancer, glioblastoma multiforme, and nonsquamous, non-small cell lung cancer	Unconjugated; inhibition of VEGF signaling
Cetuximab (Erbitux) Chimeric IgG1	HER1/EGFR	For first-line treatment of KRAS mutation-negative, EGFR-expressing metastatic colorectal cancer; for treatment of squamous cell cancer of the head and neck	Unconjugated; inhibition of EGFR signaling; ADCC
Panitumumab (Vectibix) Human IgG2	EGFR/HER1	As a single agent for treatment of pretreated EGFR-expressing metastatic colorectal carcinoma	Unconjugated; inhibition of EGFR signaling
Eculizumab (Soliris) Humanized IgG2	C5	For treatment of paroxysmal nocturnal hemoglobinuria and for treatment of atypical hemolytic uremic syndrome	Unconjugated; complement inhibitor
Ofatumumab (Arzerra) Human IgG1	CD20	For treatment of patients with CLL refractory to fludarabine and alemtuzumab	Unconjugated
Ipilimumab (Yervoy) Human IgG1	CTLA-4	For treatment of unresectable or metastatic melanoma	Unconjugated; inhibition of CTLA-4 signaling
Pertuzumab (Perjeta) Humanized	HER2	For first-line treatment of metastatic HER2-positive breast cancer; for neoadjuvant treatment of HER2-positive breast cancer	Unconjugated; HER2 dimerization inhibitor that blocks ligand-dependent heterodimerization of HER2
Denosumab (Xgeva) Human IgG2	RANKL	For prevention of skeletal-related events in patients with bone metastases from solid tumors; for treatment of giant cell tumor of the bone	Unconjugated; prevents RANKL from activating its receptor
Ibritumomab tiuxetan (Zevalin) Murine IgG1	CD20	For treatment of low-grade or follicular B-cell NHL	Immunoconjugate; delivery of the radioisotope yttrium-90
Brentuximab vedotin (Adcetris) Chimeric IgG1	CD30	For treatment of patients with relapsed or refractory Hodgkin lymphoma or systemic anaplastic lymphoma	Antibody drug conjugate; delivery of microtubule disrupting agent
Ado-trastuzumab emtansine (Kadcyla) Humanized IgG1	HER2	For treatment of HER2-positive metastatic breast cancer	Antibody drug conjugate; delivery of cytotoxic derivative of maytansine; ADCC; inhibits HER2 signaling; prevents HER2 shedding
Obinutuzumab (Gazyva) Humanized IgG1	CD20	For treatment of patients with previously untreated CLL	Unconjugated; CDC; ADCC; antibody-dependent cellular phagocytosis; direct activation of intracellular death signaling pathways

ADCC, Antibody-dependent cellular cytotoxicity; *CD,* clusters of differentiation; *CDC,* complement-dependent cytotoxicity; *CLL,* chronic lymphocytic leukemia; *CTLA-4,* cytotoxic T-lymphocyte protein 4; *EGFR,* epidermal growth factor receptor; FDA, U.S. Food and Drug Administration; *HER,* humanized epidermal growth factor receptor; *IgG,* immunoglobulin; *NHL,* non-Hodgkin lymphoma; *RANKL,* receptor activator of nuclear factor kappa-B ligand; *VEGF,* vascular endothelial growth factor.

Part 3

      (3) Humanized (suffix, -*zumab*)—small part mouse fused with human antibody

      (4) Human (suffix, -*umab*) —totally human antibody

  c. Characteristics of an ideal antigen for MAb-based targeted therapy

    (1) Overexpression on the tumor cell and therefore accessible to the MAb

    (2) Homogenous expression on tumor cells

    (3) Plays an important role in cancer progression and contributes to the hallmarks of cancer (Modjtahedi, Ali, & Essapen, 2012)

2. Small-molecule kinase inhibitors interact with domains of specific intracellular proteins. These agents may be receptor protein kinases (i.e., they have extracellular ligand-binding domains) or nonreceptor protein kinases (i.e., they are confined to the cytoplasm or nuclear compartment) (Weinberg, 2014). Many of the targets of small-molecule inhibitors are tyrosine kinases, which are enzymes found within cells that transfer phosphate groups and affect molecular signaling (Vapiwala & Geiger, 2010). Table 23-3 lists current FDA-approved small-molecule kinase inhibitors.

3. Proteasome inhibitors (Crawford, Walker, & Irvine, 2011; Hideshima, Richardson, & Anderson, 2011) disrupt regulated degradation of pro-growth cell cycle proteins, resulting in apoptosis. Examples include bortezomib and carfilzomib, which are used to treat multiple myeloma.

4. *Cytokine* is a generic term for proteins released by cells that affect the function of other cells. Many agents are pleotrophic—that is, possess multiple effects.

  a. Interferons (IFNs)—family of glycoprotein hormones with immunomodulatory, antiproliferative, and antiviral effects

  b. Interleukins (ILs)—"between leukocytes," protein molecules responsible for the signaling and communication among cells of the immune system

  c. Hematopoietic growth factors—family of glycoprotein molecules that regulate the reproduction, maturation, and functional activity of blood cells

  d. Tumor necrosis factor (TNF)—a proinflammatory cytokine produced by monocytes and macrophages that has antineoplastic effects but also causes inflammation (as in rheumatoid arthritis)

5. Vaccines condition the patient's own immune system to recognize and respond to specific antigens.

  a. Types—dendritic cell–based vaccines, virus-based vaccines, DNA vaccines, and cell-based vaccines (Drake, 2011)

  b. Clinical uses

  c. Preventive vaccines designed to target infectious agents that can cause cancer (e.g., human papilloma virus [HPV] to protect females against many but not all cases of cervical, vaginal, or vulvar cancer)

  d. Therapeutic vaccines (e.g., sipuleucel-T to treat advanced prostate cancer)

6. Differentiating agents—loss of differentiation is one of the hallmarks of malignancy. Retinoids, histone deacetylase inhibitors, vitamin A analogues, and inhibitors of DNA methylation have been shown to induce differentiation and arrest proliferation in tumor cell lines (Bisht et al., 2010).

  a. DNA and histone proteins that make up chromatin (condensed DNA in nondividing cells) can be modified by the attachment of chemical groups that can then determine which genes are expressed. These modifications are referred to as *epigenetic alterations*. The addition of acetyl groups (acetylation) or methyl groups (methylation) to histones is frequently dysregulated in cancer cells. Histone modifications are catalyzed by enzymes. Histone acetyltransferase (HAT) and histone deacetylases (HDACs) catalyze acetylation, and methylation is catalyzed by histone methyltransferase (HMTs) and histone demethylases (HDMs) (Lartigue, 2013). The tight coiling of DNA that results from the deacetylation of histones inhibits the transcription of tumor suppressor genes. HDAC inhibitors cause DNA relaxation, allowing tumor suppressor genes to be accessible for transcription (Kavanaugh, White, & Kolesar, 2010). Histone deacetylase HDAC inhibitors include vorinostat and romidepsin, both used in the treatment of cutaneous T-cell lymphoma (CTCL).

  b. Retinoids include bexarotene for CTCL, alitretinoin for the treatment of cutaneous lesions in AIDS-related Kaposi sarcoma, and tretinoin for inducing remission in acute promyelocytic leukemia. Major toxicities of retinoids include dry skin, bone tenderness, hyperlipidemia, reversible hepatic enzyme abnormalities, cheilitis, and retinoic acid syndrome (Aronson, 2010).

7. Fusion proteins direct cytocidal action or toxin to cells that express the targeted receptor or

Table 23-3

Small-Molecule Kinase Inhibitors Currently FDA-Approved for Oncology

Small-Molecule Kinase Inhibitors	Target	FDA-Approved Indications
Imatinib mesylate (Gleevec)	BCR-ABL, PDGF, SCF, c-Kit (CD117)	Newly diagnosed and refractory Ph+ CML; adjuvant and recurrent KIT (CD117)-positive GIST; newly diagnosed and refractory Ph+ ALL; myelodysplastic and myeloproliferative diseases; dermatofibrosarcoma protuberans; hypereosinophilic syndrome; aggressive systemic mastocytosis
Erlotinib (Tarceva)	HER1/EGFR	NSCLC as first-line treatment with EGFR mutation; maintenance treatment of NSCLC where disease has not progressed after first-line therapy; progressive NSCLC; first-line treatment of advanced pancreatic cancer
Lapatinib (Tykerb)	HER1/EGFR and HER2	Advanced or metastatic HER2+ breast cancer
Vandetanib (Caprelsa)	Multiple tyrosine kinases	Symptomatic or progressive medullary thyroid gland cancer
Sunitinib malate (Sutent)	Multiple tyrosine kinases	Advanced RCC; GIST after disease progression or intolerance to imatinib mesylate; PNET
Sorafenib (Nexavar)	Multiple intracellular and cell surface kinases	Advanced RCC; unresectable HCC
Dasatinib (SPRYCEL)	Multiple kinases	Newly diagnosed Ph+ CML in chronic phase; Ph+ CML in chronic, accelerated, or blast phase with resistance or intolerance to prior therapy, including imatinib; Ph+ ALL with resistance or intolerance to prior therapy
Nilotinib (Tasigna)	BCR-ABL	Newly diagnosed Ph+ CML in chronic phase; Ph+ CML in chronic or accelerated phase with resistance or intolerance to prior therapy, including imatinib
Pazopanib (Votrient)	Multiple tyrosine kinases	Advanced RCC; advanced soft tissue sarcoma after prior therapy
Crizotinib (Xalkori)	Multiple tyrosine kinases	Locally advanced or metastatic NSCLC that is ALK-positive
Axitinib (Inlyta)	Multiple VEGFR tyrosine kinases	Advanced RCC after failure of one prior systemic therapy
Bosutinib (Bosulif)	BCR-ABL; Src family	Ph+ CML in chronic, accelerated, or blast phase with resistance or intolerance to prior therapy
Vemurafenib (Zelboraf)	Serine-threonine kinase	Unresectable or metastatic malignant melanoma with BRAF V600E mutation
Regorafenib (Stivarga)	Multiple membrane-bound and intracellular kinases	Metastatic colorectal cancer previously treated with chemotherapy and anti-VEGF therapy; GIST tumors previously treated with imatinib mesylate and sunitinib malate
Cabozantinib (Cometriq)	Multiple tyrosine kinases	Progressive metastatic medullary thyroid cancer
Dabrafenib (Tafinlar)	BRAF kinases	Unresectable melanoma or for metastatic melanoma with BRAF V600E mutation
Trametinib (Mekinist)	MEK1	Unresectable or metastatic melanoma with BRAF V600E or V600K mutations
Ibrutinib (Imbruvica)	BTK	Mantle cell lymphoma treated with at least one prior therapy
Afatinib (Gilotrif)	EGFR, HER2, HER4	First-line treatment of metastatic NSCLC whose tumors have EGFR exon 19 deletions or exon 21 substitution mutations

ALK, Anaplastic lymphoma kinase; *ALL*, acute lymphoblastic leukemia; *BCR-ABL*, breakpoint cluster region-Abelson; *BTK*, Bruton tyrosine kinase; *CD*, clusters of differentiation; *CML*, chronic myelogenous leukemia; *GIST*, gastrointestinal stromal tumor; *HER1/EGFR*, human epidermal growth factor receptor 1/epidermal growth factor receptor; *HER2*, human epidermal growth factor receptor 2; *HCC*, hepatocellular carcinoma; *MEK1*, mitogen-activated extracellular signal regulated kinase 1; *NSCLC*, non–small cell lung cancer; *Ph+*, Philadelphia chromosome positive; *PDGF*, platelet-derived growth factor; *PNET*, pancreatic neuroendocrine tumor; *RCC*, renal cell cancer; *SCF*, stem cell factor; *VEGFR*, vascular endothelial growth factor receptor.

inhibit key processes needed for cell growth and survival. Antibody-enzyme fusion proteins have been used in two major ways for cancer therapy: (1) antibody-directed prodrug therapy (ADEPT), where the fusion protein is targeted to cancer and used to activate a subsequently administered prodrug, or (2) the fusion protein is directly toxic when internalized (Andrady, Sharma, & Chester, 2011).

a. Denileukin diftitox targets the CD25 component of the IL-2 receptor for the treatment of CTCL. It consists of IL-2 protein sequences fused to diphtheria toxin.

b. Ziv-aflibercept targets portions of two different VEGF receptors fused to a portion of the immunoglobulin G1 (IgG1) immune protein for the treatment of metastatic colorectal cancer. By binding to VEGF, ziv-aflibercept prevents it from interacting with receptors on endothelial cells, thereby blocking the growth and development of new blood vessels (NCI, 2012).

8. Nonspecific immunomodulating agents are substances that stimulate or indirectly augment the immune system. Bacillus Calmette-Guerin (BCG) is used in the treatment of superficial bladder cancer following surgery to prevent recurrence. BCG has a preference for entering bladder cancer cells where the proteins are broken down. The fragments are combined with histocompatibility antigens and displayed on the cell surface as a target for cell destruction via a cytokine or cytotoxicity response (Steinberg, Sachdeva, & Curti, 2012).

9. Heat shock proteins (Hsps) are sometimes referred to as *molecular chaperones*. Chaperones help newly formed proteins assume the proper shape needed to perform their specific biologic function. Hsp inhibitors have the potential to disable numerous proteins that contribute to the growth of cancer. They may also work in patients who develop mutations that result in resistance to traditional targeted drugs, because blocking the chaperone will inhibit the function of the mutated proteins as well (The ASCO Post, 2013a). In lung cancer, proteins such as EGFR and ALK depend on Hsp90 for activation (Broderick, 2013; Ramalingam et al., 2013).

10. Gene therapy remains investigational in cancer treatment. It includes three main strategies:
    a. The insertion of a normal gene into cancer cells to replace a mutated gene
    b. Genetic modification to silence a mutated gene
    c. Genetic approaches to directly kill cancer cells (U.S. Department of Energy Genome Programs, 2011)

C. Adverse events of targeted therapies
1. Drug-drug and drug-food interactions—must be monitored in any patient on oral agents, especially small-molecule targeted therapies⚠
   a. Most of the orally administered agents are metabolized in the liver by the cytochrome P450 enzyme family.
   b. Substances (drugs or foods) that affect enzyme activity will, in turn, increase or inhibit drug bioavailability.
      (1) P450 inhibitors will suppress enzyme activity and increase drug bioavailability.
      (2) P450 inducers will accelerate enzyme activity and reduce drug bioavailability.
2. Infusion reactions
   a. Allergic reactions to foreign proteins such as IgE–mediated reaction and classified as type 1 hypersensitivity responses (Vogel, 2010)
   b. Nonallergic infusion reactions—MAbs have a unique potential for a nonallergic infusion reaction caused by cytokine release (Vogel, 2010)
3. Cardiac toxicities of various types reported with targeted therapies (Lenihan & Kowey, 2013)
   a. Arterial hypertension is a common adverse event of the VEGF pathway and is reported in patients being treated with sorafenib, sunitinib, bevacizumab, and pazopanib.
   b. Decreases in left ventricular ejection fraction (LVEF) may occur with anti-HER2 therapies and may be asymptomatic or symptomatic.
   c. Arrhythmias related to QTc prolongation have been documented with numerous small-molecule inhibitors.
   d. VEGF-targeted agents should be used with caution in patients with clinically significant cardiovascular disease or pre-existing congestive heart failure (CHF).
4. Diarrhea associated with HER1/EGFR inhibitors
5. Metabolic dyscrasias
   a. Hypomagnesemia is a relatively common side effect of cetuximab and panitumumab therapy (Fakih & Vincent, 2010).
   b. mTOR inhibitors are most commonly associated with disorders of metabolism and nutrition (hypercholesterolemia and hyperglycemia). The insidious nature of these disorders means that symptoms are generally lacking until the condition becomes so severe that organ damage occurs (Eisen et al., 2012).
   c. Hypothyroidism is very common with sunitinib and also noted with other agents in the class.
6. Dermatologic reactions—associated with EGFR-directed therapies; examples of EGFR inhibitors include erlotinib, cetuximab, and panitumumab, which can result in

papulopustular eruption, xerosis, pruritus, paronychia, alopecia, and hypertrichosis of the face, with trichomegaly of the eyelashes (Lacouture, 2013); characteristic rash associated with EGFR inhibitors may have potential as a surrogate marker of efficacy in patients with KRAS wild-type tumors (Fakih & Vincent, 2010).
   7. mTOR inhibitors associated with treatment-related infections because of their immunosuppressive properties; noninfectious pneumonitis is a class effect of mTOR inhibitors (Eisen et al., 2012).
   8. Gastrointestinal perforation (GIP) —a rare but potentially fatal complication reported in association with bevacizumab and sorafenib
   9. Venous thromboembolism (VTE)—a common complication in cancer patients in general, but treatment-related VTE and arterial thromboembolism (ATE) reported with bevacizumab, sunitinib, and temsirolimus
   10. Bevacizumab and mTOR inhibitors shown to adversely affect the process of wound healing
   11. Capillary leak syndrome—movement of fluid from the vasculature into the tissues; seen with IL-2 and also with IL-11; end results are edema, weight gain, hypotension, and decreased urinary output
   12. Everolimus-associated stomatitis—one of the most frequent dose-limiting toxicities; has a rapid onset, usually within the first week of therapy (Barroso-Sousa et al., 2013)

ASSESSMENT

I. Pertinent personal history
   A. Disease status
      1. Site of cancer
      2. Stage of cancer
   B. Goals of therapy; line of treatment
   C. Biomarkers indicating targeted therapy sensitivity
      1. Immunohistochemistry used to stain receptors
      2. In situ hybridization testing fluorescence in situ hybridization (FISH) used to determine gene copy numbers
      3. FDA-approved companion diagnostic assays that measure levels of proteins, genes, or specific mutations and are used to provide a specific therapy (e.g., cobas 4800 BRAF V600E Mutation Test to aid in selecting melanoma patients whose tumors carry the BRAF V600E mutation for treatment with vemurafenib; therascreen KRAS RGQ PCR Kit to detect mutations in the *KRAS* gene to determine which patients are most likely to benefit from treatment with MAb EGFR inhibitors; therascreen EGFR RGQ PCR Kit to determine if a patient with lung cancer expresses EGFR mutations that may benefit from treatment with afatinib; cobas EGFR Mutation Test to detect lung cancer mutations that may benefit from treatment with erlotinib) (FDA, 2013).
   D. Assessment of current medications, especially those that may be contraindicated with targeted therapies and biotherapies
      1. CYP450 substrates
      2. Warfarin
      3. Aspirin
      4. Steroids—contraindicated with ILs
      5. Nonsteroidal anti-inflammatory drugs (NSAIDs)
      6. Medications that may alter mentation or coagulation
      7. Immunosuppressants
      8. Antihypertensive therapy
      9. Herbal preparations
   E. Assessment for chronic illnesses that may be exacerbated by side effects associated with targeted therapy and biotherapy, such as heart disease, diabetes, neurologic or psychiatric disorders, pulmonary disease, hypertension, psoriasis
   F. Assessment for history of, and response to, prior cancer therapies
   G. Allergies
II. Physical examination—thorough physical assessment by body system before initiation of therapy (to serve as a baseline for comparison) and at regular intervals during the course of therapy to evaluate tolerance to therapy
   A. Cardiovascular—heart rate and rhythm, abnormal heart sounds, blood pressure, and orthostatic blood pressure with agents known to cause hypotension or hypertension; identification of risk factors for the development of cardiotoxicity; baseline studies pertinent for specific agent
      1. Blood pressure changes must be monitored regularly for patients treated with anti-VEGF agents.
      2. LVEF and assessment for cardiomyopathy (peripheral edema, jugular vein distention, auscultation of heart sounds, auscultation of lung sounds) must be monitored regularly for patients treated with anti-HER2 agents (Anderson & Wimberly, 2013).
      3. Electrolyte concentrations (e.g. serum calcium, potassium, and magnesium) must be evaluated and imbalances corrected before initiating therapy with small-molecule kinase inhibitors (e.g., vandetanib, nilotinib, pazopanib, vemurafenib). Patients must be routinely monitored with continued therapy (Lenihan & Kowey, 2013). Serum electrolytes, including serum magnesium, potassium, and calcium, should be closely monitored during and after cetuximab (Bristol-Myers Squibb, 2013).

4. QT interval prolongation should be evaluated with electrocardiography (ECG) at baseline and periodically during treatment with small-molecule kinase inhibitors (e.g., lapatinib, sunitinib, pazopanib, vandetanib, nilotinib) (Lenihan & Kowey, 2013).

B. Pulmonary—respiratory rate, breath sounds, shortness of breath, cyanosis, and clubbing

C. Gastrointestinal (GI) and nutritional—weight, eating patterns, abdominal girth, mucositis, xerostomia, and bowel pattern

D. Musculoskeletal—range of motion, functional status, and presence and patterns of arthralgias

E. Neurologic—affect, orientation, memory, attention span, social engagement, sensory perception, and peripheral neuropathy

F. Integumentary—erythema, rash, lesions, injection site reactions, dryness, decreased turgor, and alopecia

G. General—presence of fever and flulike symptoms and fatigue

III. Psychosocial examination

A. Assessment of baseline mental status

B. Assessment of current social structure, including support systems, primary caretaker, housing and living arrangements, and work status

C. Assessment of type, number, and effectiveness of previous coping strategies used by client and family

D. Determination of response to illness and emotional state

E. Assessment for ability to perform self-care activities (especially important if therapy is to be administered in the ambulatory setting)

F. Assessment for patient adherence, especially regarding oral targeted therapies, to identify specific barriers

G. Consideration of financial status—need for referral to social worker or access to pharmaceutical company reimbursement assistance programs

H. Assessment for cultural factors and health-related beliefs

IV. Evaluation of laboratory data

A. Hematologic—white blood cell (WBC) count, differential, hemoglobin and hematocrit levels, and platelet count

B. Renal function—blood urea nitrogen (BUN) level, creatinine level, glomerular filtration rate (GFR), and proteinuria

C. Liver function—lactate dehydrogenase (LDH), alkaline phosphatase, aspartate aminotransferase (AST—formerly known as *serum glutamic oxaloacetic transaminase* or SGOT), alanine aminotransferase (ALT—formerly known as *serum glutamate pyruvic transaminase* or SGPT), and bilirubin levels

D. Nutritional parameters—electrolytes, protein, albumin levels, glucose, and cholesterol

E. Diagnostic and staging results

F. Thyroid function (especially before starting sunitinib therapy)

V. Client's and family's perceptions of treatment goals and demands

A. Treatment goals (e.g., diagnostic, therapeutic, supportive, or investigational)

B. Requirements of treatment such as length of hospitalization, follow-up clinic visits, laboratory and diagnostic test requirements, and financial obligations

C. Expected side effects of targeted therapies

D. Self-care skills required

PROBLEM STATEMENTS AND OUTCOME IDENTIFICATION

I. Risk for Decreased Cardiac Output (NANDA-I)

A. Expected outcome—patient maintains left ventricular ejection fraction above normal limits.

B. Expected outcome—patient demonstrates adequate cardiac output as evidenced by blood pressure and pulse rate and rhythm within normal parameters for client; strong peripheral pulses; adequate urine output; and an ability to tolerate activity without symptoms of dyspnea, syncope, or chest pain.

C. Expected outcome—patient maintains a QTc interval > 480 msec.

D. Expected outcome—patient participates in baseline and routine ECG and echocardiography monitoring.

E. Expected outcome—patient remains free of myocardial infarction.

II. Impaired Skin Integrity (NANDA-I)

A. Expected outcome—skin rash is effectively managed.

B. Expected outcome—overlying skin infection is prevented.

III. Risk for Bleeding (NANDA-I)

A. Expected outcome—morbidity and mortality from hemorrhage are prevented.

B. Expected outcome—toxicity is reduced (Oncology Nursing Society [ONS] Putting Evidence into Practice [PEP], 2009b).

IV. Fatigue (NANDA-I)

A. Expected outcome—cause of fatigue is managed to allow patients to remain on therapy.

V. Diarrhea (NANDA-I)

A. Expected outcome—morbidity and mortality from diarrhea are prevented.

B. Expected outcome—patient and family verbalize and use effective preventive and treatment techniques for diarrhea.

C. Expected outcome—patient maintains adequate hydration, fluid balance, and electrolyte and acid-base balance.

VI. Risk for Metabolic Imbalance

A. Expected outcome—concomitant metabolic changes (hypomagnesemia, hyperglycemia) are identified and corrected.

B. Expected outcome—morbidity and mortality from metabolic imbalance are prevented.

VII. Deficient Knowledge (NANDA-I), related to type of targeted therapy or biotherapy biologic agent and potential side effects

A. Expected outcome—patient correctly performs a desired or prescribed health behavior.

VIII. Risk for Drug-Drug and Drug-Food Interactions

A. Expected outcome—patient and family identify key potentially dangerous drug-drug and drug-food interactions.

B. Expected outcome—patient and family collaborate with interdisciplinary health care team to evaluate possible interactions among all prescription, over-the-counter, and herbal preparations.

IX. Risk for Imbalanced Body Temperature (NANDA-I)

A. Expected outcome—abnormal body temperatures are prevented.

X. Impaired Oral Mucous Membrane (NANDA-I)

A. Expected outcome—stomatitis is effectively managed.

B. Expected outcome—life-threatening consequences are prevented.

PLANNING AND IMPLEMENTATION

I. Interventions to minimize cardiac dysfunction

A. Routine monitoring of LVEF (via echocardiography [ECHO] or multigated acquisition scan [MUGA])

1. Obtaining baseline LVEF

2. When ejection fraction is less than 50% to 55% of institutional normal, dose reduction may be indicated or therapy may be held, depending on specific therapy

3. Assessment for signs and symptoms of congestive heart failure (dependent edema, lung sounds, dyspnea)

B. Routine monitoring of ECG

1. Obtaining baseline ECG

2. Referral to agent-specific package insert for recommended ECG monitoring schedule

3. Assessment of ECG for QTc interval changes, especially for prolongation greater than 480 msec

C. Routine monitoring for hypertension

1. Monitoring blood pressure (BP) before, during, and after treatment infusion

2. Controlling hypertension prior to administration of targeted therapy

3. Treatment for hypertension, as needed, with standard therapy (appropriate for the patient's individual situation)

4. Suspending targeted therapy or permanently discontinuing if hypertension is life-threatening

5. Identification and appropriate management of other factors contributing to hypertension (e.g., smoking, obesity, sedentary lifestyle)

D. Collaboration with cardiologist for appropriate diagnosis, management, and monitoring of cardiac effects

II. Interventions to maintain skin integrity (ONS PEP, 2010)

A. Teaching patient and family to report earliest signs of EGFR-related skin rash

B. Teaching patient and family expected trajectory of EGFR-related rash

C. Teaching pre-emptive proactive techniques to minimize discomfort associated with EGFR-related skin rash before rash becomes dose-limiting

D. Techniques to decrease severity of rash

1. Protecting skin from the sun with physical sunblocks (e.g., zinc oxide, titanium dioxide) with 30 SPF that block UVA and UVB

2. Tetracyclines—minocycline, doxycycline, tetracycline

3. Topical steroids

4. Skin moisturizer

E. Treatment of papulopustular skin rash

1. Use of low-strength topical steroids on face and medium-strength topical steroids on the body

2. Use of topical antibiotics (e.g., clindamycin, erythromycin) to treat papulopustular skin rash

3. Obtaining culture if bacterial infection suspected

F. Management of EGFR inhibitor–induced paronychia

1. Frequent application of petroleum jelly to the periungual soft tissue

2. Oral antibiotics for infections

3. Silver nitrate or ferric subsulfate solution

4. Clipping or removing nails

5. Daily white vinegar soaks (1:10 concentration)

6. Cushioning of fingers and toes to prevent injury

7. Topical corticosteroid cream

G. Management of EGFR inhibitor–induced itching

1. Emollients

2. Topical antipruritics (e.g., Aveeno Anti-Itch, Sarna Ultra)

3. Topical agents for scalp itching—fluocinonide 0.05%, clobetasol foam, steroid shampoo (e.g., fluocinolone acetonide)
4. Cold compresses
5. Antihistamines with sedative effects (e.g., diphenhydramine) in the evening and at bedtime
6. Pregabalin for intractable itch

III. Interventions to reduce risk of bleeding
   A. Control of hypertension
   B. Educating patients about management of minor bleeding (e.g., epistaxis with bevacizumab)
   C. Exercising caution before initiating anticoagulant therapy
   D. Platelet threshold maintenance

IV. Interventions to manage fatigue (ONS PEP, 2011)
   A. All patients with cancer screened for presence or absence of fatigue at regular intervals
   B. Focused evaluation of fatigue to include history and assessment of contributing factors (e.g., anemia, hypothyroidism, cardiomyopathy, dehydration)
   C. Education and counseling regarding known patterns of fatigue
   D. General management strategies, including self-monitoring, energy conservation, use of distraction
   E. Exercise as an effective strategy for fatigue

V. Interventions to treat and prevent diarrhea (ONS PEP, 2008)
   A. Complete thorough subjective and objective assessment to rule out other potential infectious, pharmaceutical, or dietary causes.
      1. Complete applicable laboratory assessments, including *Clostridium difficile* or other tests, to rule out or diagnose an infectious process.
      2. Complete chemistry panel to assess electrolyte imbalance.
      3. Complete blood cell count to rule out neutropenia.
      4. Assess stool consistency and number of stools per day.
   B. Recommendations for dietary modifications to treat diarrhea
      1. Avoidance of foods commonly associated with diarrhea such as greasy, spicy, or fried items
      2. Avoidance of foods that increase gas accumulation and cramping such as Brussels sprouts, broccoli, cabbage, and other cruciferous vegetables
      3. Initiating "BRAT" diet of bananas, rice, applesauce, and toast
      4. Maintaining or increasing intake to at least 3 to 4 liters of fluid daily with emphasis on liquids containing electrolytes

5. Restriction of milk products
6. Avoiding or limiting caffeine
7. Eating small, frequent meals
8. Reinforcement of education about prescribed pharmaceuticals
9. Adequate skin care

VI. Interventions related to metabolic imbalance
   A. Hyperglycemia (Eisen et al., 2012)
      1. For treatment with mTOR inhibitors, obtaining optimal glycemic control in diabetic patients before initiating treatment
      2. Advising patients to report excessive thirst or polyuria
      3. Monitoring fasting serum glucose level before treatment and periodically thereafter
   B. Hypomagnesemia (Fakih & Vincent, 2010)
      1. Monitoring for symptoms of hypomagnesemia, which may be cardiovascular, neuromuscular, or behavioral
      2. Monitoring electrolytes and magnesium during and for 8 weeks after the completion of anti-EGFR therapy
      3. Administering appropriate replacement, although oral supplementation is often ineffective and poorly tolerated because of diarrhea; intravenous replacement therapy important for patients with grade 3 or 4 hypomagnesemia

VII. Interventions related to deficient knowledge
   A. Assessing patient's barriers to learning
   B. Observing patient's ability and readiness to learn
   C. Explaining disease state
   D. Ensuring that patient recognizes the need for medications and understands treatments
      1. Explaining the difference among chemotherapy, radiation therapy, and molecular targeted treatment
      2. Describing potential side effects of molecular targeted treatment
      3. Incorporating strategies to improve adherence (e.g., Helping Your Patient Stay on Course Toolkit, ONS, 2009a).

VIII. Interventions to minimize deleterious drug-drug and drug-food interactions
   A. Educating client and family regarding potentially dangerous interactions and providing specific instructions about common foods
   B. Obtaining complete medication list and performing routine medication reconciliation, ensuring no drug-drug and drug-food interactions

IX. Interventions to manage imbalanced body temperature

A. Identification of treatments that result in fever associated with infusion reactions (e.g., first infusions of select monoclonal antibodies)

B. Identification of patients at risk for infusion reactions, hypersensitivities

C. Administration of premedications, as indicated

D. Closely monitoring patients at risk for infusion reactions

E. Administration of therapies for patients experiencing infusion reactions (Vogel, 2010)

X. Interventions to manage oral stomatitis (ONS PEP, 2009c)

A. Implementing an oral care protocol; use of nonalcoholic mouthwash

B. Assessment for pain and infections and implementing treatment accordingly

C. Instituting low-level laser therapy for severe stomatitis

EVALUATION

The oncology nurse recognizes that targeted therapies have a different mechanism of action compared with chemotherapy or radiation therapy. As a result, the side effect profile may be very different from that of more traditional types of therapies.

The oncology nurse systematically and regularly evaluates the responses of the client and family to interventions to determine progress toward the achievement of expected outcomes. Relevant data are collected, and actual findings are compared with expected findings. Nursing diagnoses, outcomes, and plans of care are reviewed and revised, as necessary.

References

American Cancer Society (ACS). (2012). *The history of cancer.* http://www.cancer.org/acs/groups/cid/documents/webcontent/002048-pdf.pdf.

American Society of Clinical Oncology (ASCO). (2012). *Shaping the future of oncology: Envisioning cancer care in 2030.* http://www.asco.org/sites/default/files/shapingfuture-lowres.pdf.

Anderson, S., & Wimberly, B. (2013). Anthracyclines, trastuzumab, and cardiomyopathy. In A. Fadol (Ed.), *Cardiac complications of cancer therapy.* Pittsburgh: Oncology Nursing Society.

Andrady, C., Sharma, S., & Chester, K. (2011). Antibody-enzyme fusion proteins for cancer therapy. *Immunotherapy, 3*(2), 193–211. http://dx.doi.org/10.2217/imt.10.90.

Appleman, L. (2011). MET signaling pathway: A rational target for cancer therapy. *Journal of Clinical Oncology, 29*(36), 4837–4838.

Aronson, J. (2010). Retinoids. In J. Aronson (Ed.), *Meyler's side effects of drugs used in cancer and immunology* (15th ed.). San Diego, CA: Elsevier.

Ascierto, P., Ascierto, M., Capone, M., Elaba, Z., Murphy, M., & Palmieri, G. (2012). Molecular pathogenesis of melanoma: Established and novel pathways. In M. Murphy (Ed.), *Diagnostic and prognostic biomarkers and therapeutic targets in melanoma.* New York: Humana Press.

Barroso-Sousa, R., Santana, I., Testa, L., de Melo Gagliato, D., & Mano, M. (2013). Biological therapies in breast cancer: Common toxicities and management strategies. *The Breast, 22*(6), 1009–1018.

Baselga, J., Cortes, J., Kim, S., Im, S., Hegg, R., Im, Y., et al. (2012). Pertuzumab plus trastuzumab plus docetaxel for metastatic breast cancer. *The New England Journal of Medicine, 366*(2), 109–119.

Bisht, M., Bist, S. S., & Dhasmana, D. C. (2010). Biological response modifiers: Current use and future prospects in cancer therapy. *Indian Journal of Cancer, 47,* 443–451.

Bonner, J., Harari, P., Giralt, J., Azarnia, N., Shin, D. M., Cohen, R. B., et al. (2010). Radiotherapy plus cetuximab for locoregionally advanced head and neck cancer: 5-year survival data from a phase 3 randomized trial, and relation between cetuximab-induced rash and survival. *Lancet Oncology, 11*(1), 21–28.

Bristol-Myers, Squibb. (2013). Erbitux [package insert]. Princeton, NJ: Author.

Broderick, J. (2013). *Novel Hsp inhibitor may offer NSCLC salvage option.* http://www.onclive.com/conference-coverage/asco-2013/Novel-Hsp-Inhibitor-May-Offer-NSCLC-Salvage-Option.

CancerQuest. (2011). *Biological response modifiers (BRM).* http://www.cancerquest.org/biological-response-modifiers.html.

Cantley, L., Carpenter, C., Hahn, W., & Meyerson, M. (2011). Cell signaling, growth factors and their receptors. In V. Devita Jr., T. Lawrence, & S. Rosenberg (Eds.), *Cancer: Primer of the molecular biology of cancer.* Philadelphia: Lippincott Williams & Wilkins.

Coiffier, B., LePage, E., Briere, J., Herbrecht, R., Tilly, H., Bouabdallah, R., et al. (2002). CHOP chemotherapy plus rituximab compared to CHOP alone in elderly patients with diffuse large B-cell lymphoma. *The New England Journal of Medicine, 346,* 235–242.

Crawford, L., Walker, B., & Irvine, A. (2011). Proteasome inhibitors in cancer therapy. *Journal of Cell Communication Signaling, 5*(2), 101–110.

de Lartigue, J. (2011). *Targeting Pi3K/Akt pathway: 20 years of progress.* http://www.onclive.com/publications/oncology-live/2011/october-2011/targeting-pi3kakt-pathway-20years-of-progress/2.

Drake, C. (2011). Update on prostate cancer vaccines. *Cancer Journal, 17*(5), 294–299.

Eisen, T., Sternberg, C., Robert, C., Mulders, P., Pyle, L., Zbinden, S., et al. (2012). Targeted therapies for renal cell carcinoma: Review of adverse event management strategies. *Journal of the National Cancer Institute, 104*(2), 93–113.

Elisei, R., Schlumberger, M., Muller, S., Schoffski, P., Brose, M. S., Shah, M. H., et al. (2013). Cabozantinib in progressive medullary thyroid cancer. *Journal of Clinical Oncology, 31*(29), 3639–3646.

Fakih, M., & Vincent, M. (2010). Adverse events associated with anti-EGFR therapies for the treatment of metastatic colorectal cancer. *Current Oncology, 17*(Suppl. 1), S18–S30.

Gianni, L., Pienkowski, T., Im, Y., Roman, L., Tseng, L. M., Liu, M. C., et al. (2012). Efficacy and safety of neoadjuvant pertuzumab and trastuzumab in women with locally advanced, inflammatory, or early HER2-positive breast cancer (NeoSphere): A randomized multicenter, open-label phase 2 trial. *The Lancet, 13*, 25–32.

Helwick, C. (2013). *Impressive results shown for immune checkpoint inhibitors: Anti-PD1 and anti-PD-L1 antibodies.* http://www.ascopost.com/issues/june-10,-2013/impressive-results-shown-for-immune-checkpoint-inhibitors-anti-pd1-and-anti-pd-l1-antibodies.aspx.

Hideshima, T., Richardson, P., & Anderson, K. (2011). Mechanism of action of proteasome inhibitors and deacetylase inhibotors and the biological basis of synergy in multiple myeloma. *Molecular Cancer Therapeutics, 10*, 2034–2042.

Hodi, F., O'Day, S., McDermott, D., Weber, R. W., Sosman, J. A., Haanen, J. B., et al. (2010). Improved survival with ipilimumab in patients with metastatic melanoma. *The New England Journal of Medicine, 363*(8), 711–723.

Hughes, T., Hochhaus, A., Branford, S., Muller, M. C., Kaeda, J. S., Foroni, L., et al. (2010). Long-term prognostic significance of early molecular response to imatinib in newly diagnosed chronic myeloid leukemia: An analysis from the International Randomized Study of Interferon and STI571 (IRIS). *Blood, 116* (19), 3758–3765.

Kavanaugh, S., White, L., & Kolesar, J. (2010). Vorinostat: A novel therapy for the treatment of cutaneous T-cell lymphoma. *American Journal of Health-System Pharmacy, 67*(10), 793–797.

Kummar, S., Chen, A., Parchment, R., Kinders, R., Ji, J., Tomaszewski, J., et al. (2012). Advances in using PARP inhibitors to treat cancer. *BMC Medicine, 25*(10), 25, http://dx.doi.org/10.1186/1741-7015-10-25.

Lacouture, M. (2013). *Dermatologic adverse events associated with targeted therapies.* http://www.cancernetwork.com/binary_content_servlet.

Lartigue, J. (2013). *Targeting epigenetics for cancer therapy: Scores of agents capture interest of researchers.* http://www.onclive.com/publications/Oncology-live/2013/October-2013/Targeting-Epigenetics-for-Cancer-Therapy-Scores-of-Agents-Capture-Interest-of-Researchers.

Lenihan, D., & Kowey, P. (2013). Overview and management of cardiac adverse events associated with tyrosine kinase inhibitors. *The Oncologist, 18*(8), 900–908.

Modjtahedi, H., Ali, S., & Essapen, S. (2012). Therapeutic application of monoclonal antibodies in cancer: Advances and challenges. *British Medical Bulletin, 104*(1), 41–59.

Motzer, R., Hutson, T., Tomczak, P., Michaelson, M., Bukowski, R., Oudard, S., et al. (2009). Overall survival and updated results for sunitinib compared with interferon alfa in patients with metastatic renal cell carcinoma. *Journal of Clinical Oncology, 27*(22), 3584–3590.

National Cancer Institute (NCI). (2012). *Targeted cancer therapies.* http://www.cancer.gov/cancertopics/factsheet/Therapy/targeted.

National Cancer Institute (NCI). (2013). *MEK: A single drug target shows promise in multiple cancers.* http://www.cancer.gov/cancertopics/research-updates/2013/MEK.

Oncology Nursing Society (ONS). (2008). *Diarrhea.* http://www.ons.org/Research/PEP/Diarrhea.

Oncology Nursing Society (ONS). (2009a). *Adherence to oral therapies for cancer: Helping your patients stay on course toolkit.* http://www.ons.org/ClinicalResources/OralTherapies/Toolkit.

Oncology Nursing Society (ONS). (2009b). *Prevention of bleeding.* http://www.ons.org/Research/PEP/Bleeding.

Oncology Nursing Society (ONS). (2009c). *Mucositis.* http://www.ons.org/Research/PEP/Mucositis.

Oncology Nursing Society (ONS). (2010). *Skin reactions.* http://www.ons.org/Research/PEP/Skin.

Oncology Nursing Society (ONS). (2011). *Fatigue.* http://www.ons.org/Research/PEP/Fatigue.

Patel, D., Suthar, M., Patel, V., & Singh, R. (2010). BCR ABL kinase inhibitors for cancer therapy, http://www.ijpsdr.com/pdf/vol2-issue2/1.pdf.

Ramalingam, S., Goss, G., Andric, Z., Bondarenko, I., Zaric, B., Ceric, T., et al. (2013). A randomized study of ganetespib, a heat shock protein 90 inhibitor, in combination with docetaxel versus docetaxel alone for second-line therapy of lung adenocarcinoma (GALAXY-1). *Journal of Clinical Oncology, 31* (Suppl. Abstract CRA8007).

Sachdev, J., & Jahanzeb, M. (2012). Blockade of the HER family of receptors in the treatment of HER2-positive metastatic breast cancer. *Clinical Breast Cancer, 12*(1), 19–29.

Sandler, A., Gray, R., Perry, M., Brahmer, J., Schiller, J., Dowlati, A., et al. (2006). Paclitaxel-carboplatin alone or with bevacizumab for non-small-cell lung cancer. *The New England Journal of Medicine, 355*(24), 2542–2550.

Sawyer, C. (2011). Targeted therapy with small molecule kinase inhibitors. In V. Devita Jr., T. Lawrence, & S. Rosenberg (Eds.), *Cancer: Primer of the molecular biology of cancer.* Philadelphia: Lippincott Williams & Wilkins.

Scandinavian Sarcoma Group and Sarcoma Group of the AIO, Germany. (2009). *Short (12 months) versus long (36 months) duration of adjuvant treatment with the tyrosine kinase inhibitor imatinib mesylate of operable GIST with a high risk for recurrence: a randomized phase III study.* http://www.ssg-org.net/wp-content/uploads/2011/05/SSG-XVIII-April20091.pdf.

Scott, A., Allison, J., & Wolchok, J. (2012). Monoclonal antibodies in cancer therapy. *Cancer Immunity, 12*, 14.

Slamon, D., Eiermann, M., Robert, N., Pienkowski, T., Martin, M., Press, M., et al. (2011). Adjuvant trastuzumab in HER2-positive breast cancer. *The New England Journal of Medicine, 365*(14), 1273–1283.

Steinberg, D., Sachdeva, K., & Curti, B. (2012, September 27). *Bacillus Calmette-Guerin immunotherapy for bladder cancer.* Medscape. http://emedicine.medscape.com/article/1950803-overview#aw2aab6b2.

Takahashi, K., Kantarjian, H., Pemmaraju, N., Andreeff, M., Borthakur, G., Faderl, S., et al. (2013). Salvage therapy using FLT3 inhibitors may improve long-term outcomes of relapsed or refractory AML with patients with FLT3-ITD. *British Journal of Haematology, 161*(5), 659–666.

The American Society of Clinical Oncology (ASCO) Post. (2013a). *Novel heat shock protein inhibitor effective in combination with docetaxel as second-line therapy for advanced lung cancer.* Retrieved from, http://www.ascopost.com/ViewNews.aspx?nid=4216.

The American Society of Clinical Oncology (ASCO) Post. (2013b). *FDA grants volasertib breakthrough designation in AML.* http://www.ascopost.com/issues/november-1,-2013/fda-grants-volasertib-breakthrough-therapy-designation-in-aml.aspx.

U.S. Department of Energy Genome Programs. (2011, August 11). *Gene therapy.* http://www.ornl.gov/sci/techresources/Human_Genome/medicine/genetherapy.shtml.

U.S. Food and Drug Administration (FDA). (2013). *Medical devices: Device approval and clearances.* http://www.fda.gov/MedicalDevices/ProductsandMedicalProcedures/DeviceApprovalsandClearances/default.htm.

Vapiwala, N., & Geiger, G. (2010). *Introduction to targeted therapy.* http://www.oncolink.org/treatment/article1.cfm?c=204&id=255.

Vogel, W. (2010). Infusion reactions: Diagnosis, assessment, and management. *Clinical Journal of Oncology Nursing, 14*(2), E10–E20.

Wagner, R., & Kempken, R. (2013). Past, present and future of monoclonal antibodies. *Monograph Monoclonal Antibodies.* www.actip.org/pages/library/MonoclonalAntibodies.html.

Weinberg, R. (2014). Growth factors, receptors, and cancer. In R. Weinberg (Ed.), *The biology of cancer* (2nd ed.). New York: Garland Science.

Zhou, H., & Huang, S. (2011). Role of mTOR signaling in tumor cell motility, invasion and metastasis. *Current Protein and Peptide Science, 12*(1), 30–42.

Part 3

CHAPTER 24

Nursing Implications of Support Therapies and Procedures

Dawn Camp-Sorrell

Blood Component Therapy

OVERVIEW

I. Use of blood component therapy in cancer care has increased because of the following reasons (National Comprehensive Cancer Network [NCCN], 2013; Schrijvers, 2011; Watson & Hearnshaw, 2010):
  A. Advancement of surgical oncology techniques
  B. Use of more aggressive single-modality and multimodality cancer therapy and the resulting bone marrow suppression
  C. Development of donor programs, hemapheresis technology, hematopoietic stem cell transplantation therapies, all of which serve to increase the available range of blood component therapies
II. Types of blood component therapy (see Table 24-1)
III. Sources of blood components
  A. Homologous blood component—blood collected from screened donors for transfusion to another individual
  B. Autologous blood—blood collected from the intended recipient
    1. Self-donation usually made before elective surgery
    2. Red blood cell (RBC) salvage during surgery by use of automated "cell saver" device or manual suction equipment
  C. Directly donated blood—blood component collected from a donor designated by the intended recipient

IV. Potential complications of blood component therapy (Bilgin, van de Watering, & Brand, 2011; DomBourian & Holland, 2012; Eisenberg, 2010; Federici, Vanelli, & Arrigoni, 2012; Ferreira, Zulli, Soares, de Castro, & Moraes-Souza, 2011; Gilliss, Looney, & Gropper, 2011; NCCN, 2013; Pandey & Vyas, 2012; Schrijvers, 2011; Watson & Hearnshaw, 2010)
  A. Acute reactions

  1. Hemolytic reactions
  2. Febrile nonhemolytic reactions
  3. Allergic reactions
  4. Anaphylaxis
  5. Volume overload
  6. Hypothermia
  7. Air emboli
  8. Bacteremia or sepsis
  9. Coagulation problems in massive transfusion such as dilution of clotting factors or hemorrhage
  10. Metabolic derangement
  11. Acute lung injury
  12. Urticaria reaction
  B. Delayed—develops days, months or years later
  1. Hemolytic reactions causing immune destruction of transfused RBCs, which are attacked by the recipient's antibodies
  2. Iron overload from frequent RBC transfusions
  3. Refractory to blood products
  4. Post-transfusion purpura
  5. Transfusion-associated graft-versus-host disease (GVHD)
  6. Alloimmunization, which may occur when patient develops alloantibodies against the donor's antigens
  7. Transmission of virus such as hepatitis virus, human immunodeficiency virus, herpesvirus
  C. Transfusion of the incorrect product to the incorrect patient

ASSESSMENT

I. Need for some form of blood component therapy for all patients with a diagnosis of cancer during the course of their illness (Federici et al., 2012; NCCN, 2013; Valent & Schiffer, 2011)
II. Need for factors that increase the likelihood for receipt of blood component therapy

Table 24-1

Types of Blood Component Therapy

Blood Component	Indication	Consideration
Whole blood	Replacement of blood volume Replacement of RBCs	Rarely used, except in extreme loss of volume
RBCs (packed)	Anemia, for replacement of RBCs	Volume overload
Leukocyte-poor packed RBCs	Prior febrile reactions to packed RBCs May delay alloimmunizations	May use a leukocyte filter to further reduce risk of reaction
Washed or plasma-poor RBCs	Prior urticarial reaction, IgA deficiency, need to avoid complete transfusion	Increased viscosity of blood; thin with normal saline before transfusion
Frozen packed RBCs	Rare blood types, autologous donations; a separate process removes plasma and leukocytes	Used for severe RBC reactions
Platelets, random	Control or prevent bleeding; platelet count < 10,000–20,000/mm^3 or patient is bleeding or preoperative	Few RBCs present; ABO compatibility not required
Single-donor platelets	May delay alloimmunization, lower risk of infection, exposure to one donor	Poor increase in platelet count
Leukocyte-poor platelets	Prior febrile reaction to platelets	Febrile reactions; poor increase in platelet count
HLA–matched platelets	Poor response to prior platelet transfusion because of alloimmunization	Only obtain increase in platelet count if HLA-matched platelets are used
Granulocytes	Documented infection from bacteria or fungi not responsive to therapy, with severe neutropenia, not expected to recover for several days to 1 wk	Long-term therapeutic effect questionable
Fresh-frozen plasma	Increase in the level of clotting factors in patient with documented deficiency	Plasma compatibility preferred; when thawed, must transfuse within 24 hr; watch for fluid overload
Cryoprecipitate	Increase in levels of factors VIII and XIII, fibrinogen, and von Willebrand factor	Plasma compatibility preferred; when thawed, must transfuse within 6 hr; if pooled, within 4 hr
Factor VIII	Hemophilia A or low AT III levels	In patients with volume overload problems, plasma cannot be used
Factor IX	Hemophilia B deficiency	Need replacement of factor
Colloid solutions	Expand blood volume	ABO compatibility not required
Plasma substitutes	Chiefly 5% and 25% albumin and PPF	Provide volume expansion and colloid replacement without risk of hepatitis or HIV
Serum immune globulins	To provide passive immunity protection (e.g., against cytomegalovirus) or treat hypogammaglobulinemia	Avoid transfusion for patient with allergic reactions to plasma

AT, Antithrombin; *HIV*, human immunodeficiency virus; *HLA*, human leukocyte antigen; *IgA*, immunoglobulin A; *PPF*, plasma protein fraction; *RBCs*, red blood cells.

A. Cancer treatment—surgery, radiation therapy, chemotherapy, targeted therapy, stem cell transplantation
B. Cancer that has invaded the bone marrow
C. Drugs that suppress bone marrow production
D. Chronic bacterial infection
E. Chronic or acute viral infection
F. Aging
G. Malnutrition including deficiencies in folate, vitamin B$_{12}$, and iron
H. Stress
I. Chronic immune deficiency
J. Comorbidities—heart disease, diabetes, renal failure, liver disease

K. Acute blood loss
III. Physical assessment (see Chapter 27)
IV. Evaluation of laboratory data (Apelseth, Hervig, & Bruserud, 2011; Carson et al., 2012; Drewniak & Kuijpers, 2009; Estcourt, Stanworth, & Murphy, 2011; NCCN, 2013; Novaretti & Dinardo, 2011; Sharma, Sharma, & Tyler, 2011; Valent & Schiffer, 2011)
A. ABO type
B. Hemoglobin—typically less than 8 g/dL
C. Platelet count
1. Less than 10,000/mm^3, with or without bleeding
2. Less than 20,000/mm^3, with active bleeding

3. Less than 50,000/mm^3 and scheduled for surgical procedure

D. Neutrophils—less than 500/mm^3, with an infection unresponsive to antibiotic therapy

E. International normalized ratio (INR) greater than 1.69 and partial thromboplastin time (PTT) and prothrombin time (PT) prolonged

F. Disseminated intravascular coagulation (DIC)— laboratory assessment, if indicated: fibrinogen less than 150 mg/dL, fibrin/fibrinogen degradation products (FDPs) greater than 40, D-dimer assay elevated

G. Immunoglobulin G (IgG) level decreased

PROBLEM STATEMENTS AND OUTCOME IDENTIFICATION

I. Deficient Knowledge (NANDA-I), related to need for and risks of blood component therapy

A. Expected outcome—patient discusses blood component therapy rationale.

B. Expected outcome—patient describes blood component therapy risk factors.

C. Expected outcome—patient describes blood component therapy benefit.

II. Risk for Injury (NANDA-I) ⚠

A. Expected outcome—patient receives blood component therapy without reaction.

B. Expected outcome—risk of blood component therapy reaction is reduced through accurate assessment and preventive intervention.

C. Expected outcome—patient lists potential signs and symptoms of reactions to blood component therapy that should be reported to the health care team.

PLANNING AND IMPLEMENTATION

(Carson et al., 2012; Federici et al., 2012; Pandey & Vyas, 2012; Watson & Hearnshaw, 2010)

I. Interventions to maximize patient safety ⚠

A. Obtaining, storing, and administering blood components according to institutional protocol

1. Review of institutional protocol to confirm need for filter and irradiation

2. Review of institutional protocol for specific tubing, priming solution, and flushing procedure

B. Checking blood component type with medical order

C. Checking blood component type and identification numbers with another registered nurse

D. Comparing blood component identification information with patient identification information before administration

E. Examining blood product for clots, bubbles, particulates, and discoloration

F. Ensuring that medications are never added to blood products

II. Interventions to monitor for complications of blood component therapy (NCCN, 2013; Sharma et al., 2011)

A. Assessment for general signs and symptoms—fever, chills, muscle aches and pain, back pain, chest pain, headache, and warmth or redness at site of infusion or along vessel

B. Assessment for respiratory signs and symptoms— shortness of breath, tachypnea, apnea, cough, wheezing, rales, and/or air embolism

C. Assessment for cardiovascular signs and symptoms—bradycardia or tachycardia, hypotension or hypertension, facial flushing, cyanosis of extremities, cool clammy skin, distended neck veins, and edema

D. Assessment for integumentary signs and symptoms—rash, hives, swelling, urticaria, post-transfusion purpura, diaphoresis

E. Assessment for gastrointestinal (GI) signs and symptoms—nausea, vomiting, abdominal cramping and pain, and diarrhea

F. Assessment for renal signs and symptoms—dark, concentrated, red- to brown-colored urine

G. Assessment for other delayed complications— delayed hemolytic transfusion reaction, graft-versus-host disease (from nonirradiated blood), iron overload, alloimmunization, infections—hepatitis, human immunodeficiency virus (HIV), cytomegalovirus (CMV), bacterial contamination

H. Assessment for changes in laboratory values such as hypocalcemia and hyperkalemia, resulting from anticoagulants in blood products

III. Interventions to decrease incidence and severity of side effects (Apelseth et al., 2011; DomBourian & Holland, 2012; Estcourt et al., 2011; Gilliss et al., 2011; Harris, 2009; NCCN, 2013; Pandey & Vyas, 2012; Rimajova, Sopko, Martinka, Kubalova, & Mistrik, 2012; Valent & Schiffer, 2011)

A. Premedicating patient with antipyretics and antihistamines, as ordered, usually acetaminophen and diphenhydramine

B. Attaching appropriate filter, blood component, or both to the blood product

1. Use of leukocyte reduction filter to reduce the number of leukocytes transfused to the patient in a unit of RBCs

2. Administering irradiated blood components to all allogeneic hematopoietic stem cell transplantation (HSCT) recipients, and others, as ordered, to prevent the transfusion of leukocytes

3. Administering single-donor platelet products, as ordered

4. Administering CMV-negative products, as ordered, to patients who do not have the virus to prevent infection

C. Use of 20-gauge or larger needle for infusion, preferably a needle-free system when transfusing RBCs and platelets

D. Infusion of component over time, according to institutional guidelines
1. Packed RBCs—infused slowly over initial 15 minutes, then remainder over 1 to 2 hours per unit; no longer than 4 hours per unit
2. Platelets—infused random donor or single-donor platelets over 30 to 60 minutes, or according to volume
3. Granulocytes—infused slowly over 2 to 4 hours
4. Fresh-frozen plasma—each unit administered slowly or as tolerated by fluid volume
5. Cryoprecipitate—infused rapidly over 15 minutes or less
6. Concentrated factor VIII or factor IX—infused rapidly over 15 minutes or less

E. Observing for signs and symptoms of transfusion reaction—fever, chills, shortness of breath, dyspnea, wheezing, hives, flank or back pain, blood in urine, hypotension, tachycardia, chest pain, and headache
1. If a reaction occurs, the following should be done:
   a. Stop infusion and keep intravenous (IV) line open with normal saline solution.
   b. Report reaction to the provider and the transfusion service or blood bank.
   c. Check identifying tags and numbers on the blood component at the bedside.
   d. Treat symptoms noted, as ordered.
      (1) Diphenhydramine—administer 25 to 50 mg intravenously.
      (2) Hydrocortisone—have 50 to 100 mg available.
      (3) Meperidine (Demerol)—administer 25 to 50 mg IV to treat uncontrolled rigors or shaking.
      (4) Acetaminophen—administer 650 to 1000 mg by mouth (PO).
      (5) Subsequently, the patient should be premedicated with acetaminophen and diphenhydramine.
      (6) Oxygen—administer if indicated.
      (7) Diurectic—administer for fluid overload.
      (8) Epinephrine or solumedrol—administer for allergic or anaphylactic reaction.
   e. Monitor vital signs every 15 minutes, or more frequently, if clinically indicated.
   f. Send blood bag and attached administration set and labels to the transfusion service or blood bank.
   g. Collect blood and urine samples, as ordered.
   h. Document transfusion reaction.
      (1) Date and time noted
      (2) Signs and symptoms observed
      (3) Actions taken
      (4) Patient monitored for approximately 2 hours after transfusion to ensure that a reaction does not occur

F. Benefits of transfusion (Novaretti & Dinardo, 2011; Shrijvers, 2011; Sharma et al., 2011)
1. RBCs—correction of anemia
   a. Need to observe for increase of hemoglobin of 1 g/dL or hematocrit by 3% with 1 unit
   b. Improvement of symptoms (e.g., fatigue, pallor, weakness, shortness of breath)
2. Platelets—correction of thrombocytopenia
   a. Need to observe for increase of 30 to 60×10^3/mL with 1 unit of apheresis platelets
   b. Decrease in signs of bleeding
3. Plasma—to restore clotting factor, expand blood volume, and provide osmotic diuresis
4. White blood cells (WBCs)—need to observe increase of WBCs and decrease of infection risk
5. Cryoprecipitate—corrects dilution of clotting factors secondary to massive hemorrhage, extensive transfusion, liver failure or consumption coagulopathy secondary to DIC by raising fibrinogen level by 5 to 10 mg/dL
6. IgG—to maintain antibody levels, prevent infection, confer passive immunity

IV. Interventions to incorporate patient and family into care
A. Educating about the purpose of the transfusion or blood component therapy
B. Review of procedure for administration of blood component therapy
C. Teaching about the signs and symptoms of transfusion reaction that should be reported to the health care team

V. Interventions to monitor for response to blood component therapy
A. Monitoring changes in laboratory values
B. Assessment for changes in subjective responses of patients to blood component therapy (e.g., reduction in fatigue or shortness of breath)
C. Monitoring for signs and symptoms and bleeding

VI. Interventions for pharmacologic management (see also Chapter 25) (Aapro, 2012; Pirker, 2009; Valent & Schiffer, 2011)
A. Recombinant factor VIIa for patients with existing coagulopathy
1. Activates factor X to factor Xa; activated factor Xa converts prothrombin to thrombin, which then acts to convert fibrinogen to fibrin, forming a hemostatic plug
2. Approved by the U.S. Food and Drug Administration (FDA) for the treatment of bleeding episodes in hemophilia A or B patients with inhibitors to factor VIII or factor IX

3. Potential use in those with DIC, liver disease, and thrombocytopenia refractory to human leukocyte antigen (HLA)–matched platelets
B. Vitamin K—essential for activating factors II, VII, IX, and X because its deficiency impairs the function of clotting factors
C. Warfarin (Coumadin)—acts by inhibiting vitamin K–dependent coagulation factors
D. Heparin
   1. In combination with antithrombin III (heparin cofactor), inhibits thrombosis by inactivating activated factor X and inhibiting the conversion of prothrombin to thrombin
   2. Inactivates thrombin and prevents conversion of fibrinogen to fibrin
   3. Prevents the formation of a stable fibrin clot by inhibiting the activation of the fibrin
E. Artificial plasma indicated for treatment of shock, acute liver failure, acute respiratory distress syndrome (ARDS), severe hyponatremia, renal dialysis

VII. Interventions for patients who refuse blood component therapy (NCCN, 2013)
A. Discussion about reasons for refusal, such as religious beliefs that prohibit the use of blood products or personal preference
B. Techniques for minimization of blood loss
   1. Minimization of routine blood testing
   2. Use of pediatric blood collection tubes
   3. Providing aggressive mucositis treatment
   4. Suppressing menstrual cycles in patients with thrombocytopenia
   5. Minimizing GI bleeding with proton pump inhibitors and bowel management
   6. Iron component therapy for iron deficiency
   7. Growth factor therapy

EVALUATION

The oncology nurse systematically and regularly evaluates the patient's and the family's responses to blood component therapy to determine progress toward the achievement of normal blood counts, normalized coagulation profile, and repleted IgG levels. Relevant data are collected, and actual findings are compared with expected findings. Problem statements and outcome identification, outcomes, and plans of care are reviewed and revised, as necessary.

Access Devices—Venous, Arterial, Peritoneal, Intraventricular, and Epidural or Intrathecal

OVERVIEW

I. Access devices essential in the care of patients with cancer because of the following (Baskin et al., 2012; Camp-Sorrell, 2011; Camp-Sorrell, 2010; Chopra,

Anand, Krein, Chenoweth, & Saint, 2012; Jan et al., 2012; Schiffer et al., 2013; Zaghal et al., 2012) (Table 24-2):
A. Increased use of combination intravenous (IV) therapy in the treatment of cancer
B. Increased use of supportive therapy (nutritional support, antibiotics, blood component therapy) in cancer care
C. Increased laboratory monitoring required with aggressive therapy
D. Increased use of arterial, peritoneal, epidural, intrathecal, and intraventricular therapy in the treatment of cancer
E. Increased diversity of access devices and the technology of the devices

II. Types of venous access devices (Camp-Sorrell, 2011; Camp-Sorrell, 2010; Chung & Behestiti, 2011; Schiffer et al., 2013)
A. Short-term or intermediate-term peripheral catheters—defined as those devices that are in place less than 14 days and used to infuse fluids, medications, blood products, and total parenteral nutrition (TPN) and to obtain blood specimens
   1. Description—single-lumen or multilumen catheters
      a. Insertion—peripherally in forearm or antecubital fossa into the cephalic, basilic, or median cubital vein
      b. Material—silicone elastomer, polyurethane, or elastomeric hydrogel
   2. Types
      a. Catheter—14 to 28 gauge with single lumen from ⅝ to 2 inches; inserted into a peripheral vein
      b. Midline catheters—3 to 8 inches long; 18 to 23 gauge; used for therapy for 1 to 4 weeks or longer
B. Nontunneled venous short-term catheters
   1. Description—catheters placed directly into jugular, femoral, or subclavain veins
   2. Material
      a. Short-term catheters made of silastic or polyurethane material in sizes of 14 to 24 gauge
      b. Single or multilumen
   3. Insertion of nontunneled catheters centrally in jugular vein, subclavian vein, superior vena cava (SVC), or inferior vena cava
C. Long-term venous catheters—maintained for months to years
   1. Overview—distal tip lies in the lower third of the superior vena cava (SVC)
      a. Made of silicone, polyurethane, or a combination
      b. Radiopaque available
      c. Power catheters available for delivery of power injection flow rates required for contrast-enhanced injections; can withstand high infusion pressures

Table 24-2

Criteria and Indications for Access Devices

Type of Device	Clinical Indications	Patient Selection Criteria
Short-term venous catheters	Infusion of chemotherapy, antibiotics, TPN, PPN, blood components, and analgesics Infusion of vesicant or irritating agents that may damage peripheral veins Urgent venous access needed	Limited venous access available Frequent venous access required Peripheral lines and midlines: need to consider osmolality of solution infused through vein (dextrose ≤ 12.5%)
Long-term venous catheters	Infusion of chemotherapy, antibiotics, TPN, blood components, analgesics Collection of blood samples	Limited venous access available; frequent venous access needed for prolonged period of time Long-term catheterization desired by the patient; ability to take care of device is necessary
Implanted ports	Infusion of all of the above agents Collection of blood samples	Limited venous access available for continuous or intermittent therapy anticipated; patient or family unable to take care of external device
PICCs	All above therapies Blood collection samples	Patient does not desire device in chest or is unable to undergo surgical procedure
Arterial catheters and implanted ports	Delivery of high concentration of chemotherapy directly into tumor	Tumor with direct arterial access Tumor sensitive to antineoplastic agents
Intraperitoneal catheters or implanted ports	Delivery of high concentration of chemotherapy to disease in peritoneal cavity	Metastatic cancer into the abdomen and peritoneum; diagnosis of cancer of the ovary or colon, mesothelioma, or malignant ascites
Intraventricular device	Delivery of high concentration of chemotherapy or antibiotic to the CSF	Malignant CSF leukemia or lymphoma, meningeal carcinomatosis, or CSF infections
Intraventricular or epidural devices	Delivery of high concentration of opioid analgesics, anesthetic medications, chemotherapy, and antispasmodic agents	Chronic intractable pain; postsurgical pain Patients with spasticity, intrathecal chemotherapy for neurologic cancers, or neoplastic meningitis

CSF, Cerebrospinal fluid; *PICCs*, peripherally inserted central catheters; *PPN*, peripheral parenteral nutrition; *TPN*, total parenteral nutrition.

d. Available with pressure-activated safety valve (PASV) located in the catheter hub; designed to permit fluid infusion and decrease risk of blood reflux
e. Insertion performed under maximal sterile barriers
2. Tunneled (Heberlein, 2011)
   a. Description—single-lumen or multilumen catheters
      (1) Tip of catheter open or closed in sizes of 2.7 to 12.5 French (Fr)
      (2) Dacron cuff attached to the catheter becoming embedded into the subcutaneous tissue after tunneling
         (a) Stabilizes the catheter
         (b) Minimizes the risk of ascending infections up the tunnel
      (3) Antimicrobial cuff available, in a biodegradable collagen matrix, at the exit site to prevent ascending microbes; releases antimicrobial activity for approximately 4 to 6 weeks
   b. Insertion—percutaneous insertion using the subclavian or internal jugular in the interventional radiology (IR) or surgery

(1) Once vein is cannulated, the guidewire is advanced into the vein.
(2) An introducer is threaded over the guidewire.
(3) Guidewire is removed and catheter is advanced into the vein.
(4) Catheter is tunneled through the subcutaneous (SC) tissue to exit on the anterior chest, typically above the nipple line midway between the sternum and clavicle.
3. Implanted port (Bassi, Giri, Pattanayak, Abraham, & Pandey, 2012; Gonda & Li, 2011; Teichgraber, Pfitzmann, & Hofmann, 2011; Zaghal et al., 2012)
   a. Description—single- or double-port device
      (1) Port body with reservoir inside covered with self-sealing septum
      (2) Port body size 16.5 to 40 mm with an attached or nonattached catheter in sizes of 4 to 12 Fr
      (3) Port is accessed with a straight or angled noncoring needle or noncoring over-the-needle catheter (needle removed and catheter left in port)

(4) Port body is made of plastic, titanium, polysulfone, or combination of materials

b. Types
(1) Anterior chest placement
(2) Peripheral ports—placed in basilic, cephalic, or median cubital veins with port above or below antecubital fossa
(3) Open or closed catheter tip

c. Insertion in IR or surgery
(1) Catheter insertion procedure similar to tunnel catheter
(2) Port sutured into a subcutaneous pocket near the vessel in which the catheter is inserted

4. Peripherally inserted central catheters (PICCs) (Chopra et al., 2012)
a. Description
(1) Size, 16 to 28 gauge, 15 to 27 inches long
(2) Securement or stabilization device used to stabilize external portion at the antecubital fossa

b. Insertion at the bedside or IR
(1) Inserted peripherally into the cephalic, accessory cephalic, basilic, or median cubital
(2) Several techniques used to advance PICC into correct position with or without ultrasound guidance

c. Types—open or closed catheter tips, single- or double-lumen (staggered distal lumens)

III. Types of nonvenous access devices
A. Arterial catheters (Bertino, 2008; Ganeshan, 2008)
1. Descriptions—for short- or long-term chemotherapy administration
a. Smaller internal diameters and thicker walls because of higher vascular arterial pressure
b. Size ranges from 2 to 5 Fr
c. One-way valve to prevent retrograde blood flow

2. Material
a. Silicone, radiopaque-beaded, branded catheter
b. Pump with collapsible reservoir that can be filled with medication and a catheter attached
(1) Programmable—variable delivery rates adjusted through radiofrequency control
(2) Nonprogrammable—predetermined constant rate

3. Insertion in IR or surgery
a. Catheter inserted into in the artery for perfusion, usually hepatic artery, similar to venous placement; subclavian, hypogastric, femoral, and brachial arteries used

b. Port or pump surgically placed in subcutaneous pocket over a bony prominence

4. Types
a. Nontunneled percutaneous catheter—short-term access; catheter removed immediately when therapy completed
b. Implanted arterial port—similar to venous port with a beaded or branded catheter to place within the artery
c. Implanted arterial pump—a flexible medication delivery pump with a reservoir that contains medication

B. Peritoneal catheters—for administration of chemotherapy into the peritoneal cavity or for the treatment of ascites (Abdel-Aal, Gaddikeri, & Saddekni, 2011; Helm, 2012)
1. Descriptions
a. A single lumen in catheter; may have multiple side holes to permit increased distribution of solution
b. Temporarily or permanently implanted into the peritoneal cavity

2. Material—silicone or polyurethane with radiopaque markings
a. Tunneled catheters may have one or two cuffs to secure the catheter within the peritoneal cavity.
b. Titanium ports or plastic port body with self-sealing septum with attached catheter

3. Insertion
a. Catheter placed through the anterior abdominal wall at the level of the umbilicus with tip directed toward cul-de-sac of the pelvis
b. Tunnel—catheter tunneled in the SC tissue to the side of the midline or abdomen
c. Port—placed in SC pocket over a bony prominence, usually a lower rib

4. Types
a. Temporary catheter remaining in place for procedure, then removed
b. Tunneled catheter similar to venous
c. Implanted port similar to venous

C. Intraventricular catheter (Ommaya reservoir) —for access to the ventricular system as an alternative to repeated lumbar punctures; provides direct access to cerebral spinal fluid (CSF) (Zairi, LeRhun, Tetard, Kotecki, & Assaker, 2011)
1. Description—dome-shaped with catheter attached
2. Material
a. Self-sealing silicone reservoir with catheter
b. Reservoir volume 1.5 to 2.5 mL
c. Radiopaque reservoir

3. Insertion—reservoir surgically placed under the scalp and the catheter threaded into the lateral ventricle

D. Epidural and intrathecal catheters—for administration of opioid analgesics and anesthetic mediations, chemotherapy, CSF sampling and antispasmodic agents intrathecally (Heran, Smith, & Legiehn, 2008)

1. Description
   a. Epidural—catheter placed in the epidural space
   b. Intrathecal—catheter inserted below the dura where CSF circulates
2. Material
   a. Temporary—radiopaque, polyurethane, or nylon catheters with open or closed tips with three-eyed multiport configuration
   b. Tunnel—silicone polyurethane material with radiopaque material with attached cuff
   c. Pump—similar to arterial, as described above
3. Insertion
   a. Catheter inserted into the epidural space approximately 4 cm, usually at L2-3; L3-4; or L4-5
   b. Catheter inserted into the intrathecal space approximately 4 cm, usually at L2-3; L3-4; or L4-5
   c. Catheter tunneled subcutaneously in the SC tissue; exits the waist or side of the abdomen
   d. Pump implanted into a created SC pocket and placed over a bony prominence
4. Types
   a. Temporary catheter for short-term use
   b. Tunneled catheter similar to venous
   c. Implanted pump with catheter attached similar to arterial pumps
   d. Ports—similar to venous ports with portal body attached to a catheter, except epidural and intrathecal ports have a 60-micron filter within the reservoir and the low profile systems have a 20-micron filter, preventing large particulate matter from entering the catheter and CSF

IV. Potential complications associated with access devices (Baskin et al., 2012; Bhutta & Culp, 2011; Chopra et al., 2012; Debourdeau et al., 2013; Camp-Sorrell, 2011; Jan et al., 2012; Meek, 2011; Narducci et al., 2011; O'Grady et al., 2011; Petree, Wright, Sanders, & Killion, 2012; Schiffer, et al., 2013; Teichgraber et al., 2011; Zairi et al., 2011)

A. Infection—presence of redness, pain, swelling, warmth, or drainage at exit site or along tunnel, or pocket
   1. Preventive measures
      a. Most infections occur from contamination of insertion or access site, hub of catheter, or both.
      b. Catheters coated with chlorhexidine, silver sulfadiazine, or antibiotics are recommended to decrease infection in short-term venous catheters.
      c. Hubs can be coated with anti-infective agents such as chlorhexidine.
      d. Removal of catheter should be based on clinical judgment and the need for the device.
   2. Dressing changes (Macklin, 2010; O'Grady et al., 2011; Schiffer et al., 2013; Webster, Gillies, O'Riordan, Sherriff, & Rickard, 2011)
      a. Gauze—changed every other day or prn (as needed) if soiled or nonocclusive
      b. Transparent—changed every 5 to 7 damages or prn if soiled or nonocclusive
      c. Exit site cleansed with chlorhexidine solution
      d. Use of needleless connectors and positive-pressure values to minimize risk of infections recommended
   3. Strict aseptic technique for all procedures; sterile technique for nonvenous procedures such as peritoneal, epidural, intraventricular.
   4. Bundle care to include the following:
      a. Frequent hand washing before and after use
      b. Maximal barrier precautions on insertion of device
      c. Alcohol hub decontamination before each access

B. Occlusion—inability to infuse fluid, or difficulty infusing, or inability to withdraw blood or body cavity fluid—that is, peritoneal fluid (Baskin et al., 2012; Marnejon, Angelo, Abu, & Gemmel, 2012)
   1. Occlusion—occurs in 14% to 36% of patients within 1 to 2 years of device placement
      a. Thrombosis—occurs in up to 66% in long-term venous devices
      b. Fibrin sheath—may form at the catheter tip, causing a one-way valve effect, allowing infusion of IV fluids into the patient but causing withdrawal occlusion, which most commonly occurs within 24 hours and up to 2 weeks after placement
      c. Intraluminal blood clot—may cause complete obstruction
      d. Mural thrombus—a clot that adheres to the vessel wall and occludes the tip of the catheter
      e. Deep vein thrombosis—occludes the vein
   2. From medications, total parenteral nutrition, or lipids
   3. Mechanical withdrawal occlusions
      a. Pinch-off syndrome—catheter becomes pinched between the clavicle and the first rib, with possible catheter fracture (Sugimoto, Nagata, Hayashi, & Kano, 2012).

b. Secondary collapse of catheter lumen caused by negative pressure

c. Catheter abutted against a vein wall so that attempts to aspirate will cause an occlusion

4. Preventive measures with flushing (Macklin, 2010; O'Grady et al., 2011; Schiffer et al., 2013)

  a. Venous (10 units/mL versus 100 units/mL heparin flush; normal saline only)

    (1) Short term—3 to 5 mL normal saline

    (2) Tunnel—3 mL/day; 3 mL every other day; 5 mL three times a week; 5 mL weekly

    (3) Port—5 mL every 4 to 8 weeks

    (4) PICC—3 mL/day; 3 mL every other day

    (5) Closed-end catheters—5 to 10 mL normal saline weekly

    (6) Normal saline 5 to 20 mL flush after use, such as blood withdrawal, medications, blood products

  b. Arterial

    (1) Catheters—3 to 5 mL of 1000 to 5000 units/mL daily

    (2) Ports—2000 to 5000 units/mL of 5 mL weekly

    (3) Pumps—no flush

  c. Peritoneal

    (1) Catheters—20 mL sterile normal saline

    (2) Port—20 mL sterile normal saline followed by heparinized saline

  d. Intraventricular—flush after using with reserved CSF or preservative-free saline

  e. Epidural or intrathecal

    (1) Catheter—1 to 2 mL with preservative-free normal saline before and after use

    (2) Port—3 mL preservative-free normal saline before and after use

    (3) Pump—no flush; refill as needed.

5. Preventive for radiographic imaging after placement to ensure correct placement

C. Catheter tip migration—regional discomfort, pain, swelling, or difficulty in using device, or catheter fracture or tear (Gibson, & Bodenham, 2013)

1. Preventive measure—self-adhesive anchoring devices to secure device

2. Monitoring of length of catheter (tunnel, midline, PICC) to ensure placement intact; radiography ordered for long-term catheters to confirm placement

D. Air embolism—presence of sudden-onset pallor or cyanosis, shortness of breath, cough, or tachycardia; catheter closely monitored after placement

E. Pneumothorax—presence of shortness of breath, chest pain, or tachycardia (Teichgraber et al., 2011)

1. Preventive measures—follow-up imaging after placement

2. Close monitoring of patient; chest radiography to assess for pneumothorax

F. Arterial injury—bleeding at exit or entrance site caused by puncture of artery near access site; close monitoring of patient after placement

G. Phlebitis—mechanical or chemical irritation that may cause injury to vein; close monitoring of exit site

H. Extravasation—infiltration of vesicant agent outside vein causing tissue damage

1. Preventive measures—placement checked prior to administering medications for blood return and ensuing catheter tip in correct placement

2. Monitoring of patient for signs of extravasation such as complaints of burning, difficulty in administering the medication

3. Frequent checks of exit sites of ventricular assist devices (VADs)

4. Stabilize needle within port.

I. Arrhythmia—caused by line placement in right atrium or ventricle; close monitoring of patient

J. Dislodgement—increase in the length of the external catheter, pain during infusion of fluids, swelling along the catheter tract or insertion site, or catheter embolization if shears off or fractures

K. Skin erosion—port or tunnel catheter breaks through underlying skin and becomes a source of infection (Bassi et al., 2012); exit site assessed at each patient contact

ASSESSMENT

(Camp-Sorrell, 2011)

I. Identification of potential candidates for access devices (Table 24-2)

II. Physical examination

A. Evaluation of site of potential device insertion

B. Evaluation of condition of skin over potential insertion site

C. Assessment of patency of access device

D. Evaluation of patient for potential infection, because most devices would not be placed in the presence of a bloodstream infection

E. Assessment for coagulopathies, low platelet numbers, as ordered, to assess for bleeding potential

F. Assessment of current medications, especially for anticoagulants and aspirin

III. Psychosocial examination

A. Ability of patient or family to care for the access device

B. Knowledge of procedures for use of access device for therapy

C. Concerns expressed about implications of insertion of device

D. Anxiety related to the procedure

PROBLEM STATEMENTS AND OUTCOME IDENTIFICATION

I. Risk for Infection (NANDA-I) ⚠
  A. Expected outcome—patient remains free of infection, or infection is recognized early and promptly treated.
II. Deficient Knowledge (NANDA-I), related to care of access devices
  A. Expected outcome—patient and family demonstrate appropriate care of access devices.
  B. Expected outcome—patient and family describe the rationale, benefits, and risks of access device.
  C. Expected outcome—patient and family list the signs and symptoms of complications of access device to report to a member of the health care team.

PLANNING AND IMPLEMENTATION

(Gibson & Bodenham, 2013; Petree et al., 2012).
I. Interventions to maximize patient safety ⚠

  A. Maintaining aseptic technique when entering or manipulating the system
  B. Teaching patient and family emergency procedures if the device is damaged
  C. Obtaining radiographic confirmation of catheter or port placement before using device (radiographic examination not necessary for peripheral and midlines)
  D. Teaching family and patient how to care for and maintain access device according to agency policy and procedure
    1. Evaluation of understanding of care, including return demonstration
    2. Providing visual aids in the teaching process
II. Interventions to minimize risks for complications of venous, arterial, or peritoneal devices (Bassi et al., 2012; Baskin et al., 2012; Bhutta & Culp, 2011; Chopra et al., 2012; Debourdeau et al., 2013; Gibson & Bodenham, 2013; Marnejon et al., 2012; Meek, 2011; Nakazawa, 2010; O'Grady et al., 2011; Schulmeister, 2010; Zairi et al, 2011) (Table 24-3)

Part 3

Table 24-3

Interventions for Complications of Access Devices

Complication	Prevention	Restoration
Loss of blood return	Maintain flushing routine, flush with push-stop method to cause swirling action in device.	Change patient position, roll on to right or left side, sit up, lie flat. Change intrathoracic pressures: have patient inhale fully and hold breath or exhale fully and hold breath. Attempt push-pull method using normal saline-filled syringe (avoid using high force or high pressure) or a thrombolytic agent.
Occlusion	Maintain flushing routines, flush with push-stop method to cause swirling, prevent clotting. Always flush with normal saline before and after drug administration, blood withdrawal, and administration of blood products. Avoid incompatible drugs.	If occlusion the result of clotted blood, tPA may be instilled with a physician order. If drug precipitate, determine type of drug, check with pharmacist for drug to dissolve precipitate such as the following: • Lipids dissolve with ethyl alcohol 70% via 22-mcg filter. • Drugs dissolve with sodium bicarbonate (1 mEq/mL) or hydrochloric acid (0.1 N).
Pinch-off syndrome	Proper placement by surgeon	Surgical removal is performed, as indicated, to avoid fracture.
Infection	Wash hands thoroughly. Follow strict aseptic techniques when using device.	Culture blood, body fluids, and exit site. Administer antibiotic, as ordered, by the physician. Remove device, as indicated.
Dislodgement	Avoid pulling on the catheter. Tape device securely. Teach patient to avoid manipulation of catheter or port and prevent trauma to catheter.	Refer to physician for resuturing if tip of the catheter remains in the vessel. Remove device, as indicated
Catheter migration	Protect device from trauma. Anchor device appropriately with sutures.	Refer to physician for repositioning catheter using fluoroscopy. Remove device, as indicated
Catheter pinholes, tracks, cuts	Avoid use of scissors or sharp objects near the catheter. Clamp properly, over reinforced area on catheter.	Repair using appropriate repair kit.

Continued

Table 24-3

Interventions for Complications of Access Devices—cont'd

Complication	Prevention	Restoration
Erosion of port through subcutaneous tissue	Avoid placing port at sites of actual or potential tissue damage (in radiation field). Avoid trauma or pressure over port.	Refer to physician to remove device.
Port-catheter separation	Avoid trauma and high-pressure infusions, or flushing with 1- or 3-mL syringes when clogged.	Refer to physician for removal of device.
Dislodgement of port access needle	Tape needle securely in place. Avoid tension on the needle or tubing.	Remove needle, and reaccess port using a sterile noncoring needle.

A. Obtaining cultures, as indicated
  1. Blood cultures drawn peripherally and through device
  2. Culture exit or entrance site
  3. Culture body fluid such as peritoneal or spinal fluid
B. Administering antibiotics, as indicated
  1. Vancomycin recommended for empiric therapy
  2. Adjustment of antibiotics on the basis of culture results
  3. Antibiotic lock therapy in conjunction with systemic therapy indicated for long-term devices when device salvage is the goal
C. Removal of access device, as indicated
  1. Complicated infection
  2. Endocarditis, osteomyelitis, or septic thrombosis
  3. Tunnel or port pocket infection
  4. Totally occluded catheter from thrombosis or precipitation
  5. Therapy completed
D. Obtaining radiographic confirmation prior to accessing the device initially to ensure correct placement; radiographic imaging ordered if the device needs to be reassessed because of lack of blood draw or inability to infuse
E. Instituting care bundles to reduce potential infection (Schiffer, et al., 2013)
  1. Maximum sterile barriers prior to insertion
  2. Hand hygiene
  3. Chlorhexidine cleansing agent
  4. Optimal catheter site insertion
  5. Assessment of device necessity
F. Administering anticoagulant or fibrinolytic, as indicated
  1. Symptomatic venous catheter–related thrombosis—anticoagulation therapy for 3 months
  2. Tissue plasminogen activator (tPA) administered, as indicated, to restore patency

EVALUATION

The oncology nurse systematically and regularly evaluates the patient's and family's responses to access devices to facilitate therapy in a safe manner. Relevant data are collected, and actual findings are compared with expected findings. Problem statements and outcome identification, outcomes, and plans of care are reviewed and revised, as necessary.

Infusion Systems

OVERVIEW

(Camp-Sorrell, 2011; Health Devices, 2010; Wang, Moeller, & Ding, 2012).
  I. Infusion systems critical in the care of patients with cancer because of the following:
    A. Increased emphasis on timing and use of antineoplastic therapy
    B. Increased number of IV therapies
    C. Need to minimize entry into the infusion system to minimize infection
    D. Increased alternative approaches to administration of opioids
    E. Increased use of antibiotic and antifungal therapy in the patient's home
    F. Increased use of nutritional therapy in the patient's home
  II. Uses for infusion systems
    A. Controlling the rate of infusions
    B. Providing positive pressure for infusions
    C. Providing alarms for early identification of a problem
    D. Designed for small volumes, such as an antibiotic, or large volumes, such as TPN
  III. Types of infusion systems (Camp-Sorrell, 2011; Manrique-Rodriguez et al., 2012)
    A. Peristaltic pumps
      1. Smart pump technology or dose error reduction system—available with downloaded drug

libraries; checks programmed doses against preset limits stored in the drug libraries; alert given if programmed doses exceed preset limits

2. Used to administer RBCs, antibiotics, parenteral nutrition, and IV fluids (including chemotherapy)
3. Intermittent or continuous infusion
4. Wide range of infusion rates and volumes
5. Linear and peristaltic or rotary peristaltic—propels fluid forward using appendages that move in wavelike motion

B. Syringe pumps—typically used to administer highly concentrated drugs or antibiotics
1. Lightweight, portable, and easy for patients to use
2. Smart pump technology with a disposable syringe
3. Motor-driven gear mechanism propels fluid by forcing plunger or piston on syringe barrel

C. Elastomeric pumps
1. Lightweight, portable, and easy to use
2. Used to administer small volumes of medications such as antibiotics and chemotherapy
3. Elastomeric membrane—generates infusion pressure when filled with fluid as gravity or positive pressure causes membrane to deflate and fluid is forced out
4. Disposable unit

IV. Potential complications associated with infusion systems
A. Occlusion
1. Empty reservoir—increased risk for clot formation
2. Kinked tubing
3. IV catheter infiltration
4. Pump malfunction
B. Severed or leaking infusion tubing
C. Mechanical errors—power failure, error in programming, insufficient fluid volume, error in setting up the system

ASSESSMENT

I. Identification of potential candidates to receive therapy using infusion systems
A. Requires long-term or short-term, controlled-rate IV therapy
B. Has peripheral or access device established such as venous, arterial, peritoneal, or epidural

II. Physical examination
A. Site of venous, arterial, peritoneal, or epidural access—color, temperature, and contour, drainage of entry site, exit site, or tunnel of catheter
B. Patency of access device

III. Psychological examination
A. Ability of patient and family to care for infusion device if used at home
B. Concerns expressed about infusion device use

PROBLEM STATEMENTS AND OUTCOME IDENTIFICATION

I. Risk for Injury (NANDA-I) ⚠
A. Expected outcome—patient remains free of complications from infusion system and complications are recognized early and promptly treated.
B. Expected outcome—fluids, medications, or blood components are infused safely and accurately.

II. Deficient Knowledge (NANDA-I), related to management of infusion systems
A. Expected outcome—patient and family demonstrate proper technique in managing infusion systems.
B. Expected outcome—patient and family monitor infusion systems for proper function.
C. Expected outcome—patient and family promptly report signs of potential complications to appropriate health care provider.

PLANNING AND IMPLEMENTATION

I. Interventions to maximize safety for the patient ⚠
A. Maintaining aseptic technique when entering or manipulating the system
B. Teaching patient and family emergency procedures to use if the system's tubing is disengaged
C. Maintaining electrical safety—checking wiring, plugs, and accessory power packs; keeping electrical equipment away from water hazards; not overloading electrical outlets
D. Giving patient and caregiver information on who to call or contact if problems arise

II. Interventions to minimize risks of complications from infusion system
A. Checking patency of system with each system component change
B. Assessment of intactness of system, rate of infusion, remaining volume to be infused, and site of infusion at regular intervals
C. Use of accessory components designed for the specific system
D. Operating infusion systems only for their intended use
E. Replacing equipment and accessory components at intervals recommended by the manufacturer or institutional policy

III. Interventions to monitor for complications of infusion system
A. Assessment for redness, pain, swelling, and purulent exudate at infusion site

B. Assessment of patient response to fluids or medications being infused

C. Assessment of the system when any alarm sounds

EVALUATION

The oncology nurse systematically and regularly evaluates the patient's and family's responses to infusion systems to determine progress toward the achievement of expected outcomes. Relevant data are collected, and actual findings are compared with expected findings. Problem statements and outcome identification, outcomes, and plans of care are reviewed and revised, as necessary.

References

Aapro, M. (2012). Emerging topics in anaemia and cancer. *Annals of Oncology, 23*(Suppl. 10), 289–293.

Abdel-Aal, A. K., Gaddikeri, S., & Saddekni, S. (2011). Technique for peritoneal catheter placement under fluoroscopic guidance. *Radiology, Research and Practice,* 1–4. http://dx.doi.org/10.1155/2011/141707.

Apelseth, T. O., Hervig, T., & Bruserud, O. (2011). Current practice and future directions for optimization of platelet transfusions in patients with severe therapy-induced cytopenia. *Blood Reviews, 25*(3), 113–122. http://dx.doi.org/10.1016/j.blre.2011.01.006.

Baskin, J. L., Reiss, U., Wilimas, J. A., Metzger, M. L., Ribeiro, R. C., Pui, C. H., et al. (2012). Thrombolytic therapy for central venous catheter occlusion. *Haematologica, 97,* 641–650. http://dx.doi.org/10.3324/haematol.2011.050492.

Bassi, K. K., Giri, A. K., Pattanayak, M., Abraham, S. W., & Pandey, K. K. (2012). Totally implantable venous access ports: Retrospective review of long-term complications. *Indian Journal of Cancer, 49*(1), 114–118. http://dx.doi.org/10.4103/0019-509x.98934.

Bertino, J. R. (2008). Implantable pump for long-term chemotherapy administration via the hepatic artery: Has it fulfilled its promise? *Journal of Clinical Oncology, 26,* 4528–4529. http://dx.doi.org/10.1200/JCO.2008.18.0117.

Bhutta, S. T., & Culp, W. C. (2011). Evaluation and management of central venous access complications. *Techniques in Vascular and Interventional Radiology, 14*(4), 217–224. http://dx.doi.org/10.1053/j.tvir.2011.05.003.

Bilgin, Y. M., van de Watering, L. M. G., & Brand, A. (2011). Clinical effects of leucoreduction of blood transfusions. *The Netherlands Journal of Medicine, 69,* 441–450.

Camp-Sorrell, D. (2010). State of the science of oncology vascular access devices. *Seminars in Oncology Nursing, 26,* 80–87. http://dx.doi.org/10.1016/j.soncn.2010.02.001.

Camp-Sorrell, D. (Ed.). (2011). *Access device guidelines: Recommendations for nursing practice and education* (3rd ed.). Pittsburgh: Oncology Nursing Society.

Carson, J. L., Grossman, B. J., Kleinman, S., Tinmouth, A. T., Marques, M. B., Fung, M. K., et al. (2012). Red blood cell transfusion: A clinical practice guidelines from the AABB. *Annals of Internal Medicine, 157*(1), 49–58. http://dx.doi.org/10.7326/0003-4819-157-1-201206190-00429.

Chopra, V., Anand, S., Krein, S. L., Chenoweth, C., & Saint, S. (2012). Bloodstream infection, venous thrombosis, and peripherally inserted central catheters: Reappraising the evidence. *American Journal of Medicine, 125,* 733–741. http://dx.doi.org/10.1016/j.amjmed.2012.04.010.

Chung, H. Y., & Beheshti, M. V. (2011). Principles of non-tunneled central venous access. *Techniques in Vascular and Interventional Radiology, 14*(4), 186–191. http://dx.doi.org/10.1053/j.tvir.2011.05.005.

Debourdeau, P., Farge, D., Beckers, M., Baglin, C., Bauersachs, R. M., Brenner, B., et al. (2013). International clinical practice guidelines for the treatment and prophylaxis of thrombosis associated with central venous catheters in patients with cancer. *Journal of Thrombosis and Haemostasis, 11,* 71–80. http://dx.doi.org/10.1111/jth.12071.

DomBourian, M., & Holland, L. (2012). Optimal use of fresh frozen plasma. *Journal of Infusion Nursing, 35*(1), 28–32. http://dx.doi.org/10.1097/NAN.0b013e31823b9a2b.

Drewniak, A., & Kuijpers, T. W. (2009). Granulocyte transfusion therapy: Randomization after all? *Haematologica, 94,* 1644–1648. http://dx.doi.org/10.3324/haematol.2009.013680.

Eisenberg, S. (2010). Refractory response to platelet transfusion therapy. *Journal of Infusion Nursing, 33*(2), 89–97. http://dx.doi.org/10.1097/NAN.0b013e318cfd392.

Estcourt, L. J., Stanworth, S. J., & Murphy, M. F. (2011). Platelet transfusions for patients with haematological malignancies: Who needs them? *British Journal of Haematology, 154,* 425–440. http://dx.doi.org/10.1111/j1365-2141.2010.8483x.

Federici, A. B., Vanelli, C., & Arrigoni, L. (2012). Transfusion issues in cancer patients. *Thrombosis Research, 129*(Suppl. 1), S60–S65. http://dx.doi.org/10.1016/S0049-3848(12)70018-X.

Ferreira, A. A., Zulli, R., Soares, S., de Castro, V., & Moraes-Souza, H. (2011). Identification of platelet refractoriness in oncohematologic patients. *Clinics (São Paulo, Brazil), 66*(1), 35–40. http://dx.doi.org/10.1590/S1807-59322011000100007.

Ganeshan, A., Upponi, S., Hon, L., Warakaulle, D., & Uberoi, R. (2008). Hepatic arterial infusion of chemotherapy: The role of diagnostic and interventional radiology. *Annals of Oncology, 19,* 847–851. http://dx.doi.org/10.1093/annonc/mdm528.

Gibson, F., & Bodenham, A. (2013). Misplaced central venous catheters: Applied anatomy and practical management. *British Journal of Anaesthesia, 110,* 333–346. http://dx.doi.org/10.1093/bja/aes497.

Gilliss, B. M., Looney, M. R., & Gropper, M. A. (2011). Reducing non-infectious risks of blood transfusion. *Anesthesiology, 115,* 635–649. http://dx.doi.org/10.1097/ALN.0b013e31822a22d9.

Gonda, S. J., & Li, R. (2011). Principles of subcutaneous port placement. *Techniques in Vascular and Interventional Radiology, 14*(4), 198–203. http://dx.doi.org/10.1053/j.tvir.2011.05.007.

Harris, D. J. (2009). The resurgence of granulocyte transfusions. *Journal of Infusion Nursing, 32,* 323–329. http://dx.doi.org/10.1097?NAN.0b013e3181bd519e.

Health Devices. (2010). Elastomeric pain pumps. *Health Devices, 39,* 366–375.

Heberlein, W. (2011). Principles of tunneled cuffed catheter placement. *Techniques in Vascular and Interventional Radiology, 14,* 192–197. http://dx.doi.org/10.1053/j.tvir.2011.05.008.

Helm, C. W. (2012). Ports and complications for intraperitoneal chemotherapy delivery. *British Journal of Gynecology, 119,* 150–159. http://dx.doi.org/10.1111/j.1471-0528.2011.03179.x.

Heran, M. K. S., Smith, A. D., & Legiehn, G. M. (2008). Spinal injection procedures: A review of concepts, controversies, and complications. *Radiologic Clinics of North America, 46,* 487–514. http://dx.doi.org/10.1016/j.rel.2008.02.005.

Jan, H. C., Chou, S. J., Chen, T. H., Lee, C. I., Chen, T. K., & Lou, M. A. (2012). Management and prevention of complications of subcutaneous intravenous infusion port. *Surgical Oncology, 21*(1), 7–13. http://dx.doi.org/10.1016/j.suronc.2010.07.001.

Macklin, D. (2010). Catheter management. *Seminars in Oncology Nursing, 26,* 113–120. http://dx.doi.org/10.1016/j.soncn.2010.02.002.

Manrique-Rodriguez, S., Sanchez-Galindo, A., Fernandez-Llamazares, C. M., Lopez-Herce, J., Echarri-Martinez, L., Escudero-Vilaplana, V., et al. (2012). Smart pump alerts: All that glitters is not gold. *International Journal of Medical Informatics, 81,* 344–350. http://dx.doi.org/10.1016/j.ijmedinf.2011.10.010.

Marnejon, T., Angelo, D., Abu, A. A., & Gemmel, D. (2012). Risk factors for upper extremity venous thrombosis associated with peripherally inserted central venous catheters. *The Journal of Vascular Access, 13,* 231–238. http://dx.doi.org/10.5301/jva.5000039.

Meek, M. E. (2011). Diagnosis and treatment of central venous access-associated infections. *Techniques in Vascular and Interventional Radiology, 14*(4), 212–216. http://dx.doi.org/10.1053/j.tvir.2011.05.009.

Nakazawa, N. (2010). Infectious and thrombotic complications of central venous catheters. *Seminars in Oncology Nursing, 26,* 121–131. http://dx.doi.org/10106/j.soncn.2010.02.007.

Narducci, F., Jean-Laurent, M., Boulanger, L., El Bedoui, S., Mallet, Y., Houpeau, J. L., et al. (2011). Totally implantable venous access port systems and risk factors for complications: A one-year prospective study in a cancer centre. *European Journal of Surgical Oncology, 37,* 913–918. http://dx.doi.org/10.1016/j.ejso.2011.06.016.

National Comprehensive Cancer Network (NCCN). (2013). *Cancer and chemotherapy-induced anemia guidelines, version 1.* http://www.nccn.org/professionals/physician_gls/pdf/anemia.pdf

Novaretti, M. C. Z., & Dinardo, C. L. (2011). Clinical applications of immunoglobulin: Update. *Revista Braserlia de Hematolgia Hemoterapia, 33,* 221–230. http://dx.doi.org/10.5581/1516-8484.20110058.

O'Grady, N. P., Alexander, M., Burns, L. A., Dellinger, P., Garland, J., Heard, S. O., et al. (2011). *Guidelines for the prevention of intravascular catheter-related infections.* 1–83. www.cdc.gov/hicpac/bsi/bsi-guidelines-2011.html

Pandey, S., & Vyas, G. N. (2012). Adverse effects of plasma transfusion. *Transfusion, 52*(Suppl. 1), 65S–79S. http://dx.doi.org/10.1111/j1537-2995.2012.03663.x.

Petree, C., Wright, D. L., Sanders, V., & Killion, J. B. (2012). Reducing blood stream infections during catheter insertion. *Radiology Technology, 83,* 532.540.

Pirker, R. (2009). Erythropoiesis-stimulating agents in patients with cancer: Update on safety issues. *Expert Opinion on Drug Safety, 8,* 515–522. http://dx.doi.org/10.1517/14740330903158929.

Rimajova, V., Sopko, L., Martinka, J., Kubalova, S., & Mistrik, M. (2012). Granulocyte transfusions. *Bratislavske Leerske Listy, 113*(3), 175–181.

Schiffer, C. A., Mangu, P. B., Wade, J. C., Camp-Sorrell, D., Dope, D. G., El-Rayes, B. F., et al. (2013). Central venous catheter care for the patient with cancer: American Society of Clinical Oncology clinical practice guideline. *Journal of Clinical Oncology,* 1–15. http://dx.doi.org/10.1200/JOP.2012.000780, e-pub.

Schrijvers, D. (2011). Management of anemia in cancer patients: Transfusions. *The Oncologist, 16*(suppl 3), 12–18.

Schulmeister, L. (2010). Management of non-infectious central venous access device complications. *Seminars in Oncology Nursing, 26,* 132–141. http://dx.doi.org/10106/j.soncn.2010.02.003.

Sharma, S., Sharma, P., & Tyler, L. N. (2011). Transfusion of blood and blood products: Indications and complications. *American Family Physician, 83,* 719–724.

Sugimoto, T., Nagata, H., Hayashi, K., & Kano, N. (2012). Pinch-off syndrome: Transection of implantable central venous access device. *BMJ Case Reports,* November 30, *2012.* http://dx.doi.org/10.1136/bcr-2012-006584.

Teichgraber, U. K., Pfitzmann, R., & Hofmann, H. A. F. (2011). Central venous port systems as an integral part of chemotherapy. *Deutsches Ärzteblatt International, 108*(9), 147–154. http://dx.doi.org/10.3238/arztebl.2011.0147.

Valent, J., & Schiffer, C. A. (2011). Thrombocytopenia and platelet transfusions in patients with cancer. *Cancer Treatment and Research, 157,* 251–265. http://dx.doi.org/10.1007/978-1-4419-7073-2_15.

Wang, J., Moeller, A., & Ding, Y. S. (2012). Effects of atmospheric pressure conditions on flow rate of an elastomeric infusion pumps. *American Journal of Health-System Pharmacy, 69,* 587–591. http://dx.doi.org/10.2146/ajhp110296.

Watson, D., & Hearnshaw, K. (2010). Understanding blood groups and transfusion in nursing practice. *Nursing Standards, 24*(30), 41–48.

Webster, J., Gillies, D., O'Riordan, E., Sherriff, K. L., & Rickard, C. M. (2011). Gauze and tape and transparent polyurethane dressings for central venous catheters. *Cochrane Database System Review, 9*(11), CD003827. http://dx.doi.org/10.1002/14651858.CD003827.pub2.

Zaghal, A., Khalife, M., Mukherji, D., El Majzoub, N., Shamseddine, A., Hoballah, J., et al. (2012). Update on totally implantable venous access devices. *Surgical Oncology, 21,* 207–215. http://dx.doi.org/10.1016/j.suronc.2012.02.003.

Zairi, F. Le, Rhun, E., Tetard, M. C., Kotecki, N., & Assaker, R. (2011). Complications related to the placement of an intraventricular chemotherapy device. *Journal of Neuro-Oncology, 104,* 247–252. http://dx.doi.org/10.1007/s11060-010-0474-4.

Part 3

CHAPTER 25

Pharmacologic Interventions

Kenneth Utz and Carol Viele

Antimicrobials

OVERVIEW

I. Rationale and indications (Gea-Banacloche & Segal, 2011)
   A. For use in the treatment of infections
      1. Infections are a major complication of cancer and cancer therapy.
      2. Individuals with cancer have suppressed immune function and increased risk of infection because of their disease, its treatment, or both.
      3. Infections are the most common cause of death in persons with cancer.
      4. As a result of changes in immune functions, many of the usual signs and symptoms of infection are absent in the patient diagnosed with cancer or receiving cancer treatment.
II. Types of antimicrobial drugs (Table 25-1)
   A. Principles of medical management (Freifeld et al., 2011; Gea-Banacloche & Segal, 2011)
      1. At the first sign of temperature greater than 101° F (38.3° C) or a sustained temperature of greater than 100.4° F (38° C) for 1 hour, a fever workup is indicated.
         a. Temperature—should not be taken from the axilla because it is unreliable or from the rectum because of the risk of colonizing bacteria entering the surrounding area
         b. History and physical examination
         c. Blood cultures—two sets of blood cultures
            (1) One should be peripheral and one central if patient has an indwelling central venous catheter or port.
            (2) Two peripheral cultures should be drawn if no central catheter is in place.
            (3) If patient has poor access, one culture may suffice, depending on organizational procedures.
         d. Urine culture in all patients if suspicion of a urinary tract infection

         e. Sputum culture if symptoms or high risk
         f. Chest radiography if symptoms are present or in high-risk patients
            (1) Anticipated neutropenia of longer than 7 days
            (2) Multiple comorbidities
            (3) Progenitor cell transplantation patients
            (4) Patients with a hematologic malignancy
         g. Other cultures from wounds and drainage, if applicable
   B. Initiation of empiric antimicrobial therapy (Freifeld et al., 2011; Irwin et al., 2013; National Comprehensive Cancer Network [NCCN], 2013f)
      1. Selection of antibiotics is based on the following:
         a. Broad-spectrum coverage of antibiotic regimen vital
         b. Coverage for common infectious organisms in persons with cancer
         c. Most antibiotic regimens developed using the most current information regarding prevalence rates for microorganisms and the patterns of resistance in the institution
      2. Intravenous (IV) doses and schedules are designed to provide bactericidal serum levels for as long as possible between each dose interval.
      3. Duration of treatment is sufficient for the resolution of the fever without exposure to unnecessary antimicrobial side effects.
         a. Negative culture results—if no organisms were isolated, treatment continues for a minimum of 7 days.
         b. Afebrile for 3 days
         c. Neutrophil count greater than 500 cells/mm^3
      4. If fever is unresponsive to initial antibiotic therapy, the risk of a nonbacterial cause, infectious organisms resistant to antimicrobial therapy (e.g., methicillin-resistant *Staphylococcus aureus*, vancomycin-resistant *Enterococcus*), inadequate serum and tissue levels of antimicrobials, or drug fever should be considered.

Table 25-1

Antimicrobials Used for Neutropenic Fever

	Coverage	Dose	Comments
Antibacterials			
Penicillins			
Piperacillin-tazobactam (Zosyn)	Gram-positive bacteria Gram-negative bacteria Anaerobic bacteria	4.5 h IV every 6 hr	• First-line therapy for neutropenic fever • May produce false-positive galactomannan • Should not be used for meningitis • Dose adjustment required for renal dysfunction
Carbapenems			
Imipenem-cilastatin (Primaxin)	Gram-positive bacteria Gram-negative bacteria Anaerobic bacteria	500 mg IV every 6 hr	• Increasing resistance • Lowers seizure threshold • Dose adjustment required for renal dysfunction
Meropenem (Merrem)	Gram-positive bacteria Gram-negative bacteria Anaerobic bacteria	1 g IV every 8 hours (2 g for meningitis)	• First-line therapy for neutropenic fever • Effective for meningitis, nosocomial pneumonia, and intra-abdominal infections • Carbapenemase-producing bacteria have been documented. • Dose adjustment required for renal dysfunction
Cephlasporins			
Ceftazidime (Fortaz)	Streptococcus Gram-negative bacteria	2 g IV every 8 hr	• Limited activity against gram-positive bacteria • Strongly consider additional gram-positive coverage if used • Increased resistance reported • Second-line therapy for neutropenic fever • Dose adjustment needed for renal dysfunction
Cefepime (Maxipime)	Gram-positive bacteria Gram-negative bacteria	2 g IV every 8 hr	• First-line therapy for neutropenic fever • Not ideal for intra-abdominal infections • Dose adjustments needed for renal dysfunction
Ceftaroline (Teflaro)	Gram-positive bacteria MRSA Gram-negative bacteria	600 mg IV every 12 hr	• Indicated for community-acquired pneumonia and cutaneous infections • False-positive direct Coombs test • Dose adjustments needed for renal dysfunction
Fluoroquinolones			
Ciprofloxacin (Cipro)	Gram-negative bacteria Atypical bacteria Limited gram-positive bacteria	500 mg PO every 12 hr (with amoxicillin or clavulanic acid for low-risk febrile neutropenia) 400 mg IV every 8 hr	• Often used as double coverage for *Pseudomonas* infections • Not as effective as others in the class for respiratory infections • Dose adjustments needed for renal dysfunction • Should be used with caution in pediatric patients (tendon rupture)
Levofloxacin (Levaquin)	Gram-positive bacteria Gram-negative bacteria Atypical bacteria Limited anaerobic bacteria	500 mg PO every 24 hr (prophylaxis of neutropenic fever) 500-750 mg IV every 24 hr	• Use as prophylaxis may increase gram-negative resistance • Do not use for febrile neutropenia if used as prophylaxis. • Limited date as empiric therapy for febrile neutropenia • Dose adjusted for renal dysfunction
Moxifloxacin (Avelox)	Gram-positive bacteria Limited gram-negative bacteria Atypical bacteria Anaerobic bacteria	400 mg PO every 24 hr 400 mg IV every 24 hr	• As effective as ciprofloxacin or amoxicillin-clavulanic acid for low-risk febrile neutropenia • Not effective for gram-negative double coverage
Aminoglycosides			
Tobramycin	Gram-negative bacteria	Weight-based dosing variable	• Good activity against *Pseudomonas* • Used for double coverage of gram-negative infections • Often adjusted based on pharmacokinetic parameters • Nephrotoxicity and ototoxicity limit use

Continued

Table 25-1

Antimicrobials Used for Neutropenic Fever—cont'd

	Coverage	Dose	Comments
Gentamicin	Gram-positive bacteria (synergy with beta-lactams) Gram-negative bacteria	Weight-based dosing variable	• Not as active against *Pseudomonas* as tobramycin • Nephrotoxicity and ototoxicity limit use
Miscellaneous Antibiotics			
Vancomycin	Gram-positive bacteria	Weight-based dosing	• Often added to cover gram-positive infection in patients with febrile neutropenia • Only indicated as empiric therapy for some patients • Doses adjusted based on trough concentrations
Linezolid (Zyvox)	Gram-positive bacteria	600 mg IV/PO every 12 hr	• Hematologic toxicity limits use • Active against vancomycin-resistant enterococci
Daptomycin (Cubicin)	Gram-positive bacteria	Weight-based dosing variable	• Active against vancomycin-resistant enterococci • May cause rhabdomyolysis; monitor creatine phosphokinase (CPK) weekly • Not active against pulmonary infections • Dose adjusted for renal function
Sulfamethoxazole-trimethoprim (Bactrim, Septra)	*Pneumocystis jiroveci*	Single-strength tablet once daily Double-strength tablet Monday, Wednesday, and Friday	• Used as prophylaxis and treatment of *P. jiroveci*
Antifungals **Azoles**			
Fluconazole (Diflucan)	*Candida* (except *C. glabrata* and *C. krusei*)	100-0 mg IV/PO daily	• No activity with molds • Used as prophylaxis in high-risk patient populations (e.g., transplantation, acute leukemia) • Dose adjusted for renal function
Voriconazole (Vfend)	*Candida* *Aspergillus* Dimorphic fungi	6 mg/kg IV twice daily × two doses; then 4 mg/kg IV twice daily	• First-line therapy for aspergillosis • Used as empiric therapy in febrile neutropenia • Dose adjustment for renal function in IV formulation only • Evidence suggests dose adjustments by weekly troughs increases efficacy. • Target concentration for TDM=1-5.5 mg/L
Posaconazole (Noxafil)	*Candida* *Aspergillus* *Zygomycetes* Dimorphic fungi	200 mg PO three times daily (prophylaxis) 200 mg PO four times daily (salvage therapy)	• Absorption related to stomach pH; avoid acid suppressants. • Take with fatty food, nutritional substitute, or acidic beverage to increase absorption. • Effective as prophylaxis in patients with acute myeloid leukemia and chronic graft-versus-host disease
Amphotericin B Formulations			
Amphotericin B deoxycholate	*Candida* *Aspergillus* (not *Aspergillus terrus*) *Zygomycetes* *Cryptococcus* Dimorphic fungi	0.5-1.5 mg/kg IV once daily	• Nephrotoxicity, electrolyte wasting, and infusion reaction limit use • Alternative formulations have replaced this in clinical practice. • Prehydration with normal saline and premedication with acetaminophen and diphenhydramine are necessary.
Liposomal amphotericin B (Ambisome)	*Candida* *Aspergillus* (not *Aspergillus terrus*) *Zygomycetes* *Cryptococcus* Dimorphic fungi	3-5 mg/kg IV once daily	• Significantly less toxicity than deoxycholate • Prophylaxis is not necessary • 3 mg/kg is as effective as 10 mg/kg for invasive mold infections.

Continued

Part 4

Table 25-1

Antimicrobials Used for Neutropenic Fever—cont'd

	Coverage	Dose	Comments
Amphotericin B lipid complex (Abelcet)	*Candida* *Aspergillus* (not *Aspergillus terrus*) *Zygomycetes* *Cryptococcus* Dimorphic fungi	5 mg/kg IV once daily	• Significantly less toxicity than deoxycholate • Prophylaxis not needed • Possibly more nephrotoxicity than with liposomal formulation
Echinocandins Caspofungin (Cancidas)	*Candida* *Aspergillus*	70 mg IV once daily × 1 dose; then 50 mg IV once daily	• First-line therapy for candidiasis • Empiric therapy for febrile neutropenia • Salvage therapy for aspergillosis
Micafungin (Mycamine)	*Candida* *Aspergillus*	50 mg IV once daily (prophylaxis) 100-150 mg IV once daily	• As effective as fluconazole for prophylaxis in stem cell transplantation patients • Similar uses as caspofungin
Antivirals Acyclovir	HSV VZV	400 mg PO twice daily (prophylaxis) or 200 mg three to five times daily 5-10 mg/kg IV three times daily	• Effective as prophylaxis for patients who are HSV-positive • Fluid hydration is necessary if therapeutic IV doses are used. • Doses based on ideal body weight
Valacyclovir	HSV VZV	500 mg PO once daily (prophylaxis)	• Metabolized to acyclovir • Improved bioavailability as compared with acyclovir
Ganciclovir	HSV VZV CMV HHV-6	5 mg/kg IV twice daily	• Effective preemptive therapy for CMV in high-risk patients • Hematologic toxicity
Valganciclovir	HSV VZV Cytomegalovirus HHV-6	900 mg PO once daily (prophylaxis) 900 mg PO twice daily × two wk minimum; then taper dose	• Metabolized to ganciclovir • Hematologic toxicity • Prophylaxis used for patients with previous CMV reactivation
Cidofovir	HSV VZV CMV Adenovirus	5 mg/kg IV every week × two doses; then every two doses	• Significant renal toxicity requires aggressive pre- and post hydration • Ocular toxicity • Myelosuppression • Give probenecid to prevent renal reabsorption. • Second-line therapy for CMV • First-line therapy for adenovirus

CMV, Cytomegalovirus; *HHV-6*, human herpes virus 6; *HSV*, herpes simplex virus; *IV*, intravenous; *PO*, by mouth; *TDM*, therapeutic drug monitoring *VZV*, varicella zoster virus.

Adapted from National Comprehensive Cancer Network. (2013f). *Prevention and treatment of cancer-related infections (v1.2013).* http://www.nccn.org/professionals/physician_gls/pdf/infections.pdf.

a. Continue current antimicrobials if clinical condition is unchanged and evaluation reveals no new information.
b. Change antimicrobial program if evidence of progressive infection is present.
c. Add an antifungal agent to the antimicrobial program.
  (1) One third of febrile neutropenic patients who do not respond to 1 week of antimicrobial therapy have a systemic fungal infection.
  (2) Most common organisms include *Candida* and *Aspergillus*.

5. Antiviral therapy should be considered if patient has a past history of positive titers or positive history of an outbreak during chemotherapy (e.g., herpes simplex, herpes zoster).
6. Consider consultation with infectious disease specialist.
III. Potential adverse effects of antimicrobial therapy (see Table 25-1)
  A. Suprainfection
  B. Renal toxicity—acute renal tubular necrosis, nephritis, electrolyte imbalances
  C. Hematologic—thrombocytopenia, neutropenia, anemia

D. Hepatotoxicity—elevated liver function tests

E. Cardiovascular—phlebitis, hypotension, arrhythmias, prolonged QT interval

F. Gastrointestinal (GI)—nausea, vomiting, anorexia, diarrhea, colitis

G. Neurotoxicity—seizures, dizziness, ototoxicity

H. Dermatologic—rash, Stevens-Johnson syndrome, thrush, esophagitis, vaginitis

I. Fluid and electrolyte imbalances—hypokalemia, hypernatremia, hypomagnesemia, dehydration, fluid volume overload

J. Hypersensitivity reactions

ASSESSMENT

I. Assessment for presence of risk factors (see Chapter 4) (Freifeld et al., 2011; Gea-Banacloche & Segal, 2011; NCCN, 2013f)

A. Disruption of primary barriers to organisms
   1. Surgical disruption of skin
   2. Invasive procedures (e.g., insertion of central vascular access catheters, indwelling urinary catheters)
   3. Extravasation of vesicant antineoplastic agents
   4. Stomatitis or mucositis
   5. Rectal fissures
   6. Burns

B. Alteration in immune function
   1. Neutropenia with granulocyte count less than 1000/mm^3
   2. Length of time patient has been neutropenic
   3. Steroid use
   4. Calcineurin inhibitors
   5. Cyclosporine
   6. Tacrolimus
   7. Previous antibiotic therapy
   8. Functional asplenia
   9. Graft-versus-host disease
   10. Hematologic malignancy
   11. Stem cell transplantation

C. Concurrent disease states
   1. Diabetes
   2. Cardiovascular disease
   3. Renal disease
   4. Liver disease
   5. GI disease
   6. Fistula, abscesses
   7. Stress
   8. Pulmonary disease (e.g., chronic obstructive pulmonary disease [COPD])

D. Tumor necrosis and invasion

E. Previous cancer treatment that causes significant alteration in B- and T-cell function (chemotherapy, biotherapy or radiotherapy)
   1. Fludarabine
   2. Alemtuzumab
   3. Rituximab
   4. Antithymocyte globulin

II. History of drug allergies or drug reaction or intolerance

III. Physical examination (see Chapter 27)

IV. Current medications

V. Evaluation of diagnostic and laboratory data
   A. Culture and sensitivity—blood, urine, sputum
   B. Complete blood cell count with differential
   C. Complete metabolic panel (CMP)
   D. Imaging with or without biopsy
      1. Chest radiography
      2. Computed tomography (CT)
      3. Magnetic resonance imaging (MRI)
      4. Esophagogastroduodenoscopy (EGD)
      5. Bronchoscopy

VI. Assessment of patient's and family's cultural and ethnic background, particularly health care practices and values and beliefs related to pharmacotherapy
   A. Assessment of understanding and adherence to Western medicine
   B. Determining if patient and family are also consulting traditional healers and practitioners of Eastern medicine or homeopathy, and taking herbal preparations and megavitamins (potential drug interactions)
   C. Determining patient's racial group because biologic variations among racial groups may affect drug metabolism rates, clinical drug responses, and side effects of drugs

NURSING DIAGNOSES AND OUTCOME IDENTIFICATION

I. Risk for Infection (NANDA-I)
   A. Expected outcome—patient remains free of infection, or infection is recognized early and treated promptly.
   B. Expected outcome—current sepsis initiatives and antibiotics will be initiated within 1 hour of fever spike in neutropenic patients.

II. Risk for Imbalanced Body Temperature (NANDA-I)
   A. Expected outcome—patient maintains body temperature within normal range.

III. Deficient Knowledge (NANDA-I), related to infection
   A. Expected outcome—patient and family describe personal risk factors for infection.
   B. Expected outcome—patient and family discuss the rationale for immediate evaluation of fever.
   C. Expected outcome—patient lists signs and symptoms of adverse effects of antimicrobial drug therapy to report to the health care team.
   D. Expected outcome—patient and family describe rationale for adhering to and completing prescribed medication regimen.

PLANNING AND IMPLEMENTATION

I. Interventions to manage elevated body temperature and prevent infection (see Chapter 27)⚠

II. Interventions to educate the patient and family
   A. Education about risk factors for infection (see Assessment)
   B. Discussion regarding signs and symptoms of infection
   C. Providing the rationale for the use of antimicrobial drug therapy and for taking antimicrobials as scheduled
   D. Providing information about potential adverse effects to report to the health care team and strategies to manage adverse effects
   E. Discussion about the importance of adherence and strategies to promote adherence, such as medication boxes and electronic reminders

III. Interventions to decrease the incidence and monitor for adverse effects of antimicrobial therapy (Table 25-1)

IV. Interventions to monitor for therapeutic response to antimicrobial therapy
   A. Monitoring temperature, pulse, respirations, and blood pressure
   B. Discussion about rationale for immediate evaluation of fever⚠
   C. Assessment of changes in laboratory values or fluid volume status

EVALUATION

The oncology nurse systematically and regularly evaluates the patient's risk of infection and the patient's and family's responses to interventions that prevent and manage infection. Relevant data are collected, and actual findings are compared with expected findings. Nursing diagnoses, outcomes, and plans of care are reviewed and revised, as necessary.

Anti-Inflammatory Agents

OVERVIEW

I. Rationale and indications (Grossman & Nesbit, 2008)
   A. To reduce inflammation and pain
      1. Although the inflammatory process is a protective mechanism, in certain situations it may cause harm and pain to the patient.
         a. The inflammatory process involves the production of prostaglandins by the action of the enzyme cyclo-oxygenase (also known as *prostaglandin synthetase*).
         b. Prostaglandins mediate nociceptive pain caused by inflammation.
         c. Inhibition of cyclo-oxygenase by anti-inflammatory agents will inhibit production of prostaglandins, which decreases pain signaling and the inflammatory response.

II. Types of anti-inflammatory agents
   A. Nonsteroidal anti-inflammatory drugs (NSAIDs) (Table 25-2)
   B. Corticosteroids (Table 25-3)

III. Principles of medical management
   A. Pain management (see Chapter 34)
      1. Treatment of mild to moderate pain
         a. Step 1 on the World Health Organization ladder (see Chapter 34)
         b. Few patients with cancer have adequate pain control with anti-inflammatory agents alone.
      2. Adjuvant pharmacologic pain management with opiates
         a. Addition of NSAIDs can reduce opioid dose requirements.
   B. Symptom management
      1. Tumor lysis fever
      2. Bony metastases

IV. Potential adverse effects (Table 25-4)⚠
   A. Gastrointestinal bleeding
   B. Renal toxicity
   C. Bleeding
   D. Cardiac toxicity
   E. Confusion, especially in older adults

ASSESSMENT

I. Identification of patients at risk (Grossman & Nesbit, 2008)
   A. For pain (see Chapter 34)—patients with cancers that commonly metastasize to bone (e.g., prostate, breast, lung)
   B. Patients with fever from tumor lysis (see Chapter 40)
   C. Patients at risk for toxicities with NSAIDs⚠
      1. Age older than 60 years
      2. History of GI bleed or ulcers
      3. Thrombocytopenia
      4. Renal insufficiency
      5. Comorbid disease
         a. Diabetes
         b. Multiple myeloma

II. Goals of therapy
   A. Level of pain relief consistent with the patient's goal

III. Physical examination
   A. Vital signs
   B. Pain assessment (see Chapter 34)
      1. Patient reported pain using a pain rating scale
      2. Impairment of physical and psychological activities because of pain
      3. Impairment in performing activities of daily living
   C. Assess for effects of tumor lysis (see Chapter 40)

IV. Current medications
   A. NSAIDs should be used with caution with any medications that increase the risk of bleeding (e.g., warfarin, heparins).⚠

Table 25-2

Commonly Used Nonsteroidal Anti-Inflammatory Drugs in Cancer

NSAIDs	Usual Adult Oral Dosages (Max. Dosage per 24 hr)	Notable Drug Information
Propionic Acids		
Fenoprofen (Nalfon, various generics)	300-600 mg q4-6h (max. 3000 mg)	Prescription required; dizziness, GI side effects
Ibuprofen (various generics [OTC])	400-800 mg q4-6h (max. 3200 mg)	200 mg available OTC; GI side effects
Ketoprofen (Orudis)	25-60 mg q6-8h (max. 300 mg)	GI side effects, headache, dizziness
Naproxen (Naprosyn, Aleve [OTC])	250-275 mg q6-8h (max. 1250 mg)	Weight gain; do *not* crush tablets.
Acetic Acids		
Diclofenac (Voltaren)	50-75 mg q8-12h (max. 200 mg)	GI side effects; take with food.
Etodolac (Lodine, Lodine XL)	200-400 mg q6-8h (max. 1200 mg)	GI side effects, fluid retention
Indomethacin (Indocin)	25 mg q8-12h (max. 200 mg)	Renal toxicity, GI side effects
Ketorolac (Toradol)	10 mg q4-6h (max. 40 mg)	Use lower doses in older adults.
Sulindac (Clinoril)	200 mg q12h (max. 400 mg)	Less renal toxicity
Tolmetin (Tolectin)	200-600 mg q8h (max. 1800 mg)	Fewer GI side effects; take on empty stomach
Oxicam		
Piroxicam (Feldene)	20 mg daily (max. 40 mg)	Long half-life allows for once daily dosing; use with caution in older patients; causes fluid retention
Salicylates		
Acetylsalicylic acid, aspirin	325-650 mg q3-4h (max. 6000 mg)	Do not combine with NSAIDs; potent antiplatelet effects
Choline magnesium trisalicylate (Trilisate)	1500 mg q12h (max. 3000 mg)	Has no antiplatelet effect
Salsalate (Disalcid; various generics)	750 mg q8-12h (max. 3000 mg)	Has no antiplatelet effect
Cyclo-oxygenase-2 Selective Inhibitor		
Celecoxib (Celebrex)	100-200 mg q12h (max. 400 mg)	GI safety advantages yet to be demonstrated with chronic use. Fewer GI and platelet side effects; renal elimination 27%; mostly hepatic metabolism by CYP-2C9; fluconazole may increase concentrations of celecoxib. Give antacids 1 hr apart from celecoxib to avoid decreased absorption; interacts with warfarin, lithium, and methotrexate to increase levels and toxicity

GI, Gastrointestinal; *NSAIDs*, nonsteroidal anti-inflammatory drugs; *OTC*, over-the-counter.

Table 25-3

Corticosteroids Used in the Treatment of Cancer

Corticosteroids	Equivalent Dose	Notable Drug Information
Short-Acting (8-12 hr)		
Cortisone (various trade names)	30 mg	Sodium and water retention
Hydrocortisone (various trade names)	20 mg	Sodium and water retention
Intermediate-Acting (12-36 hr)		
Methylprednisone (Medrol)	4 mg	Minimal sodium-retaining activity
Prednisolone (various trade names)	5 mg	Minimal sodium-retaining activity
Prednisone (various trade names)	5 mg	Metabolized to prednisolone
Long-Acting		
Dexamethasone (Decadron)	0.75 mg	No sodium-retaining activities with lower dose

Table 25-4

Adverse Effects of Nonsteroidal Anti-inflammatory Drugs (NSAIDs) and Corticosteroids

Adverse Effects	Nursing Implications
NSAIDs	
Gastrointestinal	
Ulceration, bleeding, gastritis, dyspepsia, abdominal pain, constipation, PUD	Administer with food or milk.
	Note guaiac stool.
Risks increase with age, chronic use, concomitant corticosteroid use and history of PUD; misoprostal (Cytotec) can be used to prevent NSAID-induced ulcers.	Assess for signs and symptoms of GI bleeding.
Pancreas	
Pancreatitis reported with sulindac	Monitor serum amylase and lipase levels and urinary amylase level results.
	Monitor for signs and symptoms of pancreatitis (e.g., sudden and intense epigastric pain, nausea and vomiting, low-grade fever, jaundice).
Hepatic	
Increased ALT, AST, bilirubin levels; risks for hepatotoxicity include alcoholism, chronic active hepatitis, history of hepatitis, cirrhosis, and CHF	Monitor liver enzymes, bilirubin laboratory results.
	Assess health history for risk factors.
Central Nervous System	
Dizziness, drowsiness, light-headedness or vertigo, somnolence, mental confusion	Neurologic examination for alertness and orientation
	Advise clients and families to avoid driving or other hazardous activities that require mental alertness until CNS effects can be determined.
	Implement measures for client safety, as needed (e.g., assist with ambulation, fall precautions).
Malaise, fatigue	Avoid alcohol and other CNS depressants.
	Assess level of fatigue.
	Provide for rest periods.
Headache	Monitor CBC laboratory test results.
	Assess level of headache, and administer pain medications, as needed.
Cardiovascular	
CHF, peripheral edema, fluid retention, hypertension	Monitor fluid status, lung sounds, pitting edema, vital signs, and daily weights.
Renal	
Acute renal failure, elevated BUN and serum creatinine levels and proteinuria; risks include age, chronic renal disease, CHF	Monitor intake and output.
	Monitor BUN, creatinine, urinalysis laboratory test results, and blood pressure.
	Assess for edema.
	Assess health history for risk factors.
Hematologic	
Neutropenia, leukopenia, thrombocytopenia, decreased hemoglobin and hematocrit levels; *exception:* choline magnesium trisalicylate (Trilisate)	Monitor CBC results with differential.
	Assess and implement measures to manage infection, bleeding, and fatigue (see Chapters 27 and 34).
Platelet Aggression	
Prolonged bleeding time	Monitor platelet levels.
	No IM shots
	Implement bleeding precautions per institution protocol.
Special Senses	
Visual disturbance, blurred vision, photophobia, ocular cataracts, glaucoma, ear pain, tinnitus	Stress the importance of regular eye examinations and hearing tests.
	Educate client about reporting blurred vision, eye pain, ear pain, and tinnitus to health care provider and about darkening room or wearing sunglasses if photophobic.
Hypersensitivity	
Asthma and anaphylaxis	Monitor for hypersensitivity reactions—changes in respiratory status, itching, hives, fever, pain, changes in pulse rate, decrease in blood pressure, decrease in urinary output. Assess breath sounds; elevate HOB to ease breathing.
	Administer oxygen, as needed.
	Administer bronchodilators, antihistamines, agents, as needed.

Continued

Table 25-4

Adverse Effects of Nonsteroidal Anti-inflammatory Drugs (NSAIDs) and Corticosteroids—cont'd

Adverse Effects	Nursing Implications
Respiratory Dyspnea, hemoptysis, bronchospasm, shortness of breath	NSAIDs are contraindicated in clients with ASA allergy, nasal polyps, bronchospastic disease. Perform respiratory assessment; monitor breath sounds. Examine sputum for color and consistency. Elevate HOB to ease breathing. Administer bronchodilators and oxygen, as needed.
Dermatologic and Skeletal Rash, erythema, urticarial, photosensitivity, osteoporosis, poor wound healing, skin thinning, growth arrest	Observe for rash and monitor wounds for prolonged healing time or changes in wound bed. Advice clients to use sunblock, wear protective clothing, protect skin, avoid prolonged exposure to sunlight. Monitor height.
Pituitary Adrenal insufficiency caused by prolonged use and rapid withdrawal	Monitor blood glucose and electrolyte laboratory test results. Monitor vital signs and presence of peripheral edema.
Infectious Disease Immunosuppressive with increased risk of infections—bacterial, fungal, viral; activation of tuberculosis and spread of herpes conjunctivitis	Observe for signs of cortisol insufficiency, such as fever, orthostatic hypotension, syncopal episodes, disorientation, myalgia, and arthralgia. Cultures, dermatologic examination. Administer antimicrobial drugs and antipyretics as needed. Be aware that signs and symptoms of infection may be masked by NSAIDs.
Corticosteroids Cushing Syndrome with Long-Term Use Central obesity, moon face, buffalo hump, easy bruising, acne, hirsutism, striae, skin atrophy	Assess patient's body image concerns. Provide opportunity for client to share concerns and discuss coping strategies. Educate regarding care of skin and safety precautions
Electrolyte and Metabolic Imbalances Hyperglycemia, hypernatremia, hypokalemia, and hypocalcemia, leading to edema, hypertension, diabetes, osteoporosis	Monitor laboratory results (blood glucose, electrolytes, calcium), vital signs, body weight. Assess for edema.
Neuromuscular and Skeletal Arthralgia, myalgia, fatigue, muscle weakness, myopathy, osteoporosis, muscle wasting, fractures	Monitor muscle strength. Administer pain medication, as needed. Encourage regular exercise to promote bone development. Implement safety measures to prevent falls and injuries.
Ocular Effects Cataracts and glaucoma	Regular eye examinations Educate client to report any eye pain or blurred vision, to health care provider. Those with open-angle glaucoma should avoid corticosteroids.
Suppression of Pituitary-Adrenal Function With long-term use, sudden withdrawal may cause acute adrenal insufficiency and dependence, fever, myalgia, arthralgia, malaise; unable to respond to stress	Monitor blood pressure for hypotension. Monitor electrolytes for hyponatremia. Assess for dehydration, fatigue, diarrhea, anorexia. Monitor vital signs and muscle and joint pain; administer pain medication. Educate regarding stressful situations, both physiologic and emotional, and when to contact a health care professional for assistance.
Psychiatric Disturbances Paranoia, psychosis, hallucinations	Observe for and report any mental status changes. Suicide precautions, if needed Refer to mental health professional, as needed.
Gastrointestinal Peptic ulcers, GI bleeding	Assess for epigastric pain 1-3 hr after meals. Assess for nausea or vomiting, and observe for hematemesis. Monitor CBC and guaiac stools or emesis.
Miscellaneous Poor wound healing, immunosuppression, menstrual irregularities, arrest of growth	Assess any wounds for prolonged healing. Monitor CBC with differential; assess and manage effects of low white blood cell, red blood cell, and platelet counts (see Chapter 27). Monitor height.

ALT, Alanine aminotransferase; *ASA*, acetylsalicylic acid; *AST*, aspartate aminotransferase; *BUN*, blood urea nitrogen; *CBC*, complete blood cell count; *CHF*, congestive heart failure; *CNS*, central nervous system; *GI*, gastrointestinal; *HOB*, head of bed; *IM*, intramuscular; *NSAIDs*, nonsteroidal anti-inflammatory drugs; *PUD*, peptic ulcer disease.

V. Evaluation of diagnostic and laboratory data
   A. Complete blood cell count
   B. Renal function
VI. Assessment of patient's and family's cultural and ethnic background, particularly health care practices and values and beliefs related to pharmacotherapy (see Antimicrobials, Assessment sections)

NURSING DIAGNOSES AND EXPECTED OUTCOMES

I. Acute Pain or Chronic Pain (NANDA-I)
   A. Expected outcome—patient states that the pain is reduced or relieved to his or her satisfaction.
II. Risk for Imbalanced Body Temperature (NANDA-I)
   A. Expected outcome—patient maintains body temperature within normal range.
III. Deficient Knowledge (NANDA-I), related to anti-inflammatory drug therapy
   A. Expected outcome—patient describes potential adverse effects of anti-inflammatory drug therapy.
   B. Expected outcome—patient describes measures to manage adverse effects of anti-inflammatory drug therapy.
   C. Expected outcome—patient lists signs and symptoms of adverse effects of anti-inflammatory agents to report to the health care team.
   D. Expected outcome—patient describes rationale for prescribed anti-inflammatory drug therapy.

PLANNING AND IMPLEMENTATION

I. Interventions to manage pain (see Chapter 34) and fever from tumor lysis (see Chapter 40)
II. Interventions to educate patient
   A. Rationale for use of anti-inflammatory drug therapy and for taking anti-inflammatory drugs as scheduled
   B. Adverse effects and strategies to prevent and manage adverse effects
   C. Adverse effects to report to health care team⚠
III. Interventions to monitor for adverse effects of anti-inflammatory drug therapy (see Table 25-4)
IV. Interventions to decrease the incidence and manage the adverse effects of anti-inflammatory drug therapy (see Table 25-4)⚠
   A. Establishing patient's allergies before administering NSAIDs
      1. NSAIDs are contraindicated in patients with aspirin allergy or hypersensitivity to acetylsalicylic acid (ASA), nasal polyps, and bronchospastic disease.
   B. Review of patient's current medications for potential drug interactions
      1. For example, NSAIDs may increase the effects of phenytoin (Dilantin), sulfonamide, and warfarin (Coumadin).

2. NSAIDs should be withheld if a patient is taking intravenous methotrexate because NSAIDs decrease renal clearance of methotrexate.
   C. Review of the use of complementary therapy that may alter the metabolism of NSAIDs
V. Interventions to monitor for therapeutic response to anti-inflammatory drug therapy
   A. Assessment of patient for adequate symptom relief (e.g., pain)
   B. Assessment of patient for infection because the antipyretic and anti-inflammatory actions of NSAIDs may mask signs and symptoms of infection⚠

EVALUATION

The oncology nurse systematically and regularly evaluates the patient's pain or fever and responses to NSAIDs to determine progress toward alleviation of pain or fever. Relevant data are collected, and actual findings are compared with expected findings. Nursing diagnoses, outcomes, and plans of care are reviewed and revised, as necessary.

Antiemetic Therapy

OVERVIEW

I. Rationale and indications (Hainsworth, 2008; Hesketh, 2008)
   A. For prevention and treatment of nausea and vomiting
   B. Causes of nausea and vomiting
      1. Chemotherapy (Table 25-5)
         a. One of the most feared side effects of chemotherapy by patients
         b. Estimated incidence of 70% to 80% without prophylaxis
      2. Radiation therapy
      3. Surgery
      4. Direct effect of tumor (e.g., bowel obstruction)
      5. Concomitant pharmacologic therapy (e.g., opiates, antibiotics)
      6. Concomitant medical complications
         a. Fluid and electrolyte disturbances
            (1) Volume depletion
            (2) Hypercalcemia
            (3) Hypo- or hypernatremia
            (4) Hypo- or hyperglycemia
         b. Infection (e.g., septicemia, meningitis)
         c. Constipation and bowel obstruction
   C. Complications of treatment-induced nausea and vomiting
      1. Malnutrition
         a. Increased weight loss
         b. Immune suppression
         c. Fluid and electrolyte imbalance

Part 4

Table 25-5

Emetogenic Potential, Onset, and Duration of Action of Select Chemotherapeutic Agents

Incidence[+]	Agent
High (>90%)	Carmustine > 250 mg/m^2*
	Cisplatin
	Cyclophosphamide > 1500 mg/m^2
	Dacarbazine
	Mechlorethamine
	Streptozocin
	Doxorubicin > 60 mg/m^2*
	Epirubicin > 90 mg/m^2*
	Ifosfamide > 2 g/m^2*
	AC (doxorubicin/ cyclophosphamide)
Moderate (30%-90%)	Aldesleukin (IL-2)
	Amifostine ≥ 300 mg/m^2
	Arsenic trioxide
	Azacitidine
	Bendamustine
	Busulfan
	Carboplatin*
	Carmustine < 250 mg/m^2*
	Clofarabine
	Cyclophosphamide < 1500 mg/m^{2†}
	Cytarabine > 200 mg/m^2*
	Daunorubicin
	Dactinomycin
	Doxorubicin ≤ 60 mg/m^2*
	Epirubicin ≤ 90 mg/m^2*
	Etoposide[†]
	Idarubicin
	Ifosfamide ≤ 2 g/m^2*
	Irinotecan
	Melphalan[†]
	Methotrexate > 250 mg/m^2*
	Oxaliplatin
	Temazolomide
Low (10%–30%)	Amifostine < 300 mg/m^2*
	Altretamine
	Brentuximab vedotin
	Cabazitaxol
	Carfilzomib
	Cytarabine ≤ 200 mg/m^2
	Docetaxel
	Doxorubicin (liposomal)
	Erubilin
	Etoposide[†]
	Fluorouracil
	Floxuridine
	Gemcitabine
	Ixabepilone
	Lomustine*
	Mercaptopurine
	Methotrexate < 250 mg/m^2*
	Mitomycin-C*
	Mitoxantrone
	Paclitaxel
	Paclitaxel (albumin-bound)
	Pemetrexed
	Pentostatin
	Pralatrexate
	Romidepsin

Continued

Table 25-5

Emetogenic Potential, Onset, and Duration of Action of Select Chemotherapeutic Agents—cont'd

Incidence	Agent
	Thiotepa
	Topotecan
Very low (<10%)	Alemtuzumab
	Asparaginase
	Bevicizumab
	Bleomycin
	Bortezomib
	Bacillus Calmette-Guerin (BCG)
	Cetuximab
	Chlorambucil
	Cladribine
	Decitabine
	Denileukin diftitox
	Fludarabine
	Ipilimumab
	Nelarabine
	Ofatumumab
	Panitumumab
	Pegaspargase
	Rituximab
	Pertuzumab
	Trastuzumab
	Temsirolimus
	Tretinoin
	Vinblastine
	Vincristine
	Vincristine (lipsomal)
	Vinorelbine

*Dose-related; potential increases with higher doses.

[†]Route and dose-related.

[+]Incidence estimate if prophylaxis is not used.

Adapted from National Comprehensive Cancer Network. (2013). *Antiemesis (v 1.2013).* http://www.nccn.org/professionals/physician_gls/pdf/antiemesis.pdf; and Hesketh, P.J. (2008). Chemotherapy-inducing nausea and vomiting. *New England Journal of Medicine, 358,* 2482–2494.

2. Mallory-Weiss tear—esophageal tear caused by vomiting
3. Decreased compliance
4. Decreased quality of life
5. Fatigue
D. Classifications of nausea and vomiting
    1. Acute
        a. Occurs within 24 hours of chemotherapy administration
            (1) Chemotherapy-mediated release of serotonin from enterochromaffin cells; substance P and other mediators also released
            (2) Neurotransmission through vagal afferent neurons to chemotherapy trigger zone
            (3) Vomiting center then activated

2. Late or delayed
  a. Occurs 24 to 120 hours after chemotherapy administration
    (1) Mechanism not well understood
    (2) Biggest risk factor development of acute nausea or vomiting
    (3) Could continue after 120 hours if severe
3. Anticipatory
  a. Arises from the cortex and limbic region of the brain
  b. Classic Pavlovian conditioned response in patients with prior episodes of poorly controlled nausea and vomiting
  c. Nonthreatening cues (auditory, visual, or sensory) may trigger reaction
  d. Provoked by anxiety
4. Breakthrough
  a. Nausea or vomiting occurring despite medical prophylaxis
5. Refractory
  a. Breakthrough nausea or vomiting not responsive to standard therapy
II. Risk factors (Hainsworth, 2008; Hesketh, 2008; NCCN, 2013b).
  A. Divided into treatment-specific and patient-specific
    1. Treatment-specific
      a. Chemotherapeutic agents in specific regimen
      b. Dose of chemotherapeutic agents
      c. Route of administration
      d. Rate of administration
      e. Cycle of therapy
    2. Patient-specific
      a. History of chemotherapy-induced nausea and vomiting (CINV)
      b. History of other forms of nausea and vomiting
      c. Pregnancy
      d. Motion sickness
      e. Female gender
      f. Age (<50 years)
      g. Anxiety
      h. Alcohol use or abuse (less alcohol use increases risk)
III. Types of antiemetic drugs (Table 25-6) (Feyer & Jordan, 2011; Hainsworth, 2008; Hesketh, 2008; NCCN, 2013b).
  A. Mechanism of most antiemetics—interference of neurotransmission of nausea to the vomiting center via trough disruption of signaling pathways
    1. Major neurotransmitter targets
      a. Serotonin (5-HT3 antagonists; e.g., ondanstron)
      b. Neurokinin (NK1 antagonists; e.g., aprepitant)
      c. Dopamine (D2 antagonists; e.g., prochlorperazine)

d. Histamine (H1 antagonists; e.g., promethazine)
e. Acetylcholine (muscarinics; e.g., scopolamine)
f. Cannabinoid (cannabinoid agonists; e.g., dronabinol)
IV. Principles of medical management (Basch et al., 2011; Feyer & Jordan, 2011; Hainsworth, 2008; Hesketh, 2008; Irwin, Brant, & Eaton, 2012; NCCN, 2013b)
  A. Goal—prevention of nausea and vomiting
  B. Lowest effective antiemetic dose used before chemotherapy
  C. Selection of appropriate antiemetics (see Table 25-6) based on the emetogenic potential of the chemotherapy as well as patient risk factors
  D. Antiemetics administered prophylactically to cover onset, peak, and duration period of each chemotherapeutic agent
  E. Assessment of the patient for risk of delayed emesis and prophylactic therapy, if indicated
  F. Follow-up assessment of outcomes 48 to 72 hours after chemotherapy and guidance, if indicated
V. Prophylaxis of nausea and vomiting (Basch et al., 2011; Feyer & Jordan, 2011; Hainsworth, 2008; Hesketh, 2008; NCCN, 2013b)
  A. Highly emetogenic agents
    1. Neurokinin 1 inhibitor + 5-HT3 antagonist + dexamethasone
    2. Dexamethasone days 2 to 4
    3. Lorazepam
    4. Proton pump inhibitor or H2 blocker
  B. Moderately emetogenic agents
    1. 5-HT3 antagonist + dexamethasone
    2. Dexamethasone days 2 and 3
    3. Lorazepam
    4. Proton pump inhibitor or H2 blocker
  C. Low emetogenic agents
    1. Dexamethasone before chemotherapy on day 1 or metoclopramide or prochlorperazine
    2. Proton pump inhibitor or H2 blocker
  D. No emetogenic risk
    1. No current therapy
VI. Agents for breakthrough nausea and vomiting (Basch et al., 2011; Feyer & Jordan, 2011; Hainsworth, 2008; Hesketh, 2008; NCCN, 2013b)
  A. Prochlorperazine
  B. Droperidol
  C. Promethazine
  D. Dexamethasone
  E. Dronabinol
  F. Lorazepam
  G. Ondansetron
  H. Metoclopramide
VII. Potential adverse effects (Hesketh, 2008)
  A. Adverse effects of drug therapy (see Table 25-6)

ASSESSMENT

I. Identification of patients at risk for nausea and vomiting (see Chapter 28)
   A. Current treatments and medical history
      1. Chemotherapy agent, dose, and schedule
      2. Radiation therapy, location, and dosage
      3. Other medical problems
      4. Current medications
   B. Patient-related factors
      1. Age younger than 50 years—may have more anticipatory vomiting
      2. Heavy ethanol intake—may have lower incidence
      3. Women more than men
      4. Positive history of pregnancy-related nausea and vomiting
      5. Positive history of motion sickness
II. Physical examination (see Chapter 28)
   A. Number and volume of emetic episodes
   B. Retching
   C. Lack of oral intake; intake and output
   D. Fluid balance, signs and symptoms of dehydration—poor skin turgor, weight loss, concentrated urine, low urine output, orthostatic hypotension
   E. Presence of blood in vomitus
   F. Vital signs—orthostatic hypotension
   G. History of present health problems (e.g., patients with glaucoma should avoid many of the antiemetics, patients with QT interval prolongation)
III. Evaluation of diagnostic and laboratory data
   A. Serum electrolyte values
   B. Electrocardiography (ECG) to determine any arrhythmias, heart block, QT interval
IV. Assessment of patient's and family's cultural and ethnic background, particularly health care practices and values and beliefs related to pharmacotherapy (see Antimicrobials, Assessment sections)

NURSING DIAGNOSES AND EXPECTED OUTCOMES

I. Nausea (NANDA-I)
   A. Expected outcome—patient states absence of nausea and has no vomiting episodes.
II. Risk for Deficient Fluid Volume (NANDA-I)
   A. Expected outcome—patient maintains fluid volume and electrolyte balance.
III. Deficient Knowledge (NANDA-I), related to antiemetic drug therapy
   A. Expected outcome—patient discusses the rationale for the use of antiemetic drug therapy and the schedule of administration.
   B. Expected outcome—patient describes potential adverse effects of antiemetic drug therapy.
   C. Expected outcome—patient describes measures to manage adverse effects of antiemetic drug therapy.
   D. Expected outcome—patient lists signs and symptoms of adverse effects of antiemetic drug therapy to report to the health care team.

PLANNING AND IMPLEMENTATION

I. Interventions to manage nausea and vomiting (see Chapter 28)
   A. Following recommended schedules for administration (e.g., administration of oral antiemetics 30 to 40 minutes before treatment, intravenous [IV] bolus approximately 10 to 30 minutes before treatment)
   B. Assessment of patient's nausea and vomiting status during and after chemotherapy administration; follow-up in outpatient setting 24 hours after dosing
   C. Ensuring patient has access to medication for breakthrough nausea
II. Interventions to manage fluid deficit
   A. Encouraging hydration as patient is able when nausea and vomiting subsides
   B. Providing IV hydration when patient is unable to maintain adequate oral intake
III. Interventions to educate patient
   A. Rationale for use of antiemetic drug therapy and for receiving antiemetics as scheduled
   B. Adverse effects and strategies to manage adverse effects
   C. Adverse effects to report to health care team
IV. Interventions to decrease the incidence, monitor response, and manage antiemetic drug therapy adverse effects (see Table 25-6)
   A. Implementing strategies to maximize patient safety⚠
      1. Assessment for mental status changes, dizziness, sedation; implementing safety measures (e.g., fall precautions), as needed
   B. Monitoring for response to antiemetic therapy following chemotherapy and prior to each consecutive treatment

EVALUATION

The oncology nurse systematically and regularly evaluates the patient's nausea and vomiting and responses to antiemetic therapy to effectively prevent and manage nausea and vomiting. Relevant data are collected, and actual findings are compared with expected findings. Nursing diagnoses, outcomes, and plans of care are reviewed and revised, as necessary.

Table 25-6

Antiemetic Therapy: Select Pharmacologic Agents for the Control of Chemotherapy-Induced Nausea and Vomiting

Name	Route	Dose/Schedule (Adult)	Adverse Effects of Class	Nursing Implications
Serotonin Antagonists				
Ondansetron	IV	8-16 mg before chemotherapy or 0.15 mg/kg q8h for three doses	Headache	Assess for headache, and consider acetaminophen for headache. Reduced incidence of headache with granisetron compared with the rest
			Constipation	Assess for number and consistency of stools. Administer stool softeners (docusate) and stimulants (senna) to prevent constipation. Increase fluids and roughage in diet.
	PO	8-32 mg before chemotherapy		
Granisetron	IV	1 (0.01 mg/kg) before chemotherapy	Transient increases in serum AST, GPT	Monitor liver function test results. Administration: Give higher doses over at least 30 minutes to prevent dizziness, headache, hypotension
	PO	2 mg before chemotherapy		
Dolasetron	PO	100 mg before chemotherapy		Consider ECG for tachycardia or new onset of shortness of breath.
Palonosetron	IV	0.25 mg before chemotherapy	ECG changes	
Neurokinin Antagonists				
Aprepitant	PO	125 mg on day 1 prior to chemotherapy; then 80 mg daily on days 2 and 3	Constipation	Assess for number and consistency of stools. Administer stool softeners (docusate) and stimulants (senna) to prevent constipation. Increase fluids and roughage in diet.
Fosaprepitant	IV	150 mg before chemotherapy	Diarrhea	Monitor for stool number and consistency.
			Hiccups	Monitor for hiccups. If persistent, then consider chlorpromazine (Thorazine), or a muscle relaxer may be considered. Possibly related to dexamethasone
			Fatigue	Likely from chemotherapy administration and not the drug itself
Substituted Benzamide				
Metoclopramide	IV	10 mg as needed very 4-6 hr	Sedation	Assess level of sedation. Have patients avoid tasks that require alertness until drug response is established. Have patients avoid alcohol and other CNS depressants.
	PO	2 mg/kg q2h × 4 0.5-2.0 mg/kg q3-4h 20-40 mg q4-6h	Extrapyramidal symptoms (EPSs) (e.g., akathisia, acute dystonic reactions); increased incidence in patients <40 years	Assess for EPS reactions. Prophylactic diphenhydramine to prevent EPSs for high doses; may be used with lower doses if EPSs occur
			Diarrhea (high doses)	Assess number and consistency of stools. Administration: Do not administer to patients with prior hypersensitivity to procaine or procainamide, epilepsy or pheochromocytoma, or if stimulation of GI motility is contraindicated (e.g., mechanical obstruction, GI bleeding).

Continued

Table 25-6

Antiemetic Therapy: Select Pharmacologic Agents for the Control of Chemotherapy-Induced Nausea and Vomiting—cont'd

Name	Route	Dose/Schedule (Adult)	Adverse Effects of Class	Nursing Implications
Phenothiazines				
Prochlorperazine	IV	10 mg every 4-6 hr scheduled or as needed	Sedation	Have patients avoid tasks that require alertness until drug response is established. Have patients avoid alcohol and other CNS depressants.
	PO	10 mg every 4-6 hr as scheduled or needed	Blurred vision	Assess vision and impact on safety.
	PR	25 mg every 12 hr as needed	EPSs (e.g., akathisia)	Monitor for and be prepared to treat EPSs with diphenhydramine 25 mg IV or PO.
Promethazine	IV	12.5-25 mg every 4 hr as scheduled or needed	Dry mouth	Have patient suck on ice chips or sugar-free hard candy.
	PO	12.5-25 mg every 4 hr as scheduled or needed	Orthostatic hypotension	Frequent intake of fluids. Monitor VS and BP lying and sitting or standing for orthostatic changes. Educate patient to rise slowly from lying or sitting position.
			Anticholinergic crisis with overuse	Give benztropine (Cogentin) or diphenhydramine for treatment for anticholinergic crisis. See Prochlorperazine.
			Rash (promethazine)	Monitor for new rash with therapy.
			Photosensitivity (promethazine)	Patients should avoid sun exposure.
			Respiratory depression (promethazine)	Particular caution for patients taking concomitant opioids
Corticosteroids				
Dexamethasone	IV	10-20 mg before chemotherapy	Dyspepsia	Take with food or milk.
	PO	4-8 mg twice daily for four to six doses on days 2 through 4	Increased appetite.	Monitor weight.
			Hiccups	Assess for prolonged hiccups.
			Euphoria and insomnia	Assess emotional status and ability to sleep.
			Fluid retention	Monitor intake and output and weight. Assess for edema.
			Hyperglycemia	Monitor blood sugar and electrolyte results.
			Hypokalemia	Assess for effects of low potassium.
Methylprednisolone	IV	125 mg before chemotherapy	Burning with infusion	Slow IV infusion to prevent perineal itching/burning (see Table 10-4)
Dopamine (D2) Antagonists				
Haloperidol	IV	0.5-2.0 mg every 4-6 hr as needed	Sedation	Assess level of sedation. Avoid tasks that require alertness until drug response is established.
	PO	0.5-2 mg every 4-6 hr as needed	EPSs (e.g., akathisia)	Avoid alcohol and other CNS depressants. Monitor for and be prepared to treat EPSs with diphenhydramine 25 mg IV or PO.
			Orthostatic hypotension	Monitor VS and BP lying and sitting or standing for orthostatic changes. Educate patient to rise slowly from lying or sitting position.

Continued

Table 25-6

Antiemetic Therapy: Select Pharmacologic Agents for the Control of Chemotherapy-Induced Nausea and Vomiting—cont'd

Name	Route	Dose/Schedule (Adult)	Adverse Effects of Class	Nursing Implications
Droperidol	IV	0.625 mg every 6 hr as needed	Sedation	Assess level of sedation. Patient should avoid tasks that require alertness until drug response is established. Patient should avoid alcohol and other CNS depressants.
			EPSs (e.g., akathisia)	Monitor for and be prepared to treat EPSs with diphenhydramine 25 mg IV or PO.
			Hypotension	Monitor VS.
			Prolongation of QT interval	Monitor ECG and check for the QTc level each time. Do not administer if 500 msec or over. If patient complains of shortness of breath or skipped heartbeats, notify health care provider. Black box warning or sudden depth due to prolonged QT interval.
Cannabinoid				
Dronabinol	PO	5-10 mg every 3 or 6 hr	Sedation and dizziness	Assess level of sedation. Patient should avoid tasks that require alertness until drug response is established. Patient should avoid alcohol and other CNS depressants.
			Dry mouth	Patient should suck on ice chips or hard candy. Encourage frequent intake of fluids.
			Euphoria or dysphoria	Assess emotional status (more common in older adult patients).
			Orthostatic hypotension	Monitor VS and BP lying and sitting or standing for orthostatic changes. Educate patient to rise slowly from lying or sitting position.
Benzodiazepine				
Lorazepam	IV PO	0.5-2.0 mg every 4-6 hr 0.5-2.0 mg every 4–6 hr	CNS side effects (sedation, disorientation, dizziness, weakness)	Assess patient's level of consciousness and risk for oversedation. Patient should avoid tasks that require alertness until drug response is established. Patient should avoid alcohol and other CNS depressants. Implement measures for patient safety, such as fall precautions.
			Autograde amnesia	Assess memory. Refer to mental health professional, as needed.
			Hypotension	Monitor VS.

AST, Aspartate transaminase; *bid*, twice daily; *BP*, blood pressure; *CNS*, central nervous system; *ECG*, electrocardiography; *GI*, gastrointestinal; *GPT*, glutamic-pyruvic transaminase; *IM*, intramuscular; *IV*, intravenous; *PO*, by mouth; *PR*, per rectum; *prn*, as needed; *SL*, sublingual; *tid*, three times daily; *VS*, vital signs.

Adapted from National Comprehensive Cancer Network. (2013b). *Antiemesis (v 1.2013).* http://www.nccn.org/professionals/physician_gls/pdf/antiemesis.pdf.

Analgesics

OVERVIEW

I. Definition, rationale, and indications (DeSandre & Quest, 2010; Grossman & Nesbit, 2008; Induru & Lagman, 2011; NCCN, 2013a)

A. Pain is defined as an unpleasant, multidimensional sensory and emotional experience associated with actual or potential tissue damage or described in relation to such damage.

B. It is estimated that 90% of cancer pain can be controlled with currently available medications.

C. Pain is caused by the tumor itself 70% of the time, diagnostic (e.g., biopsy) or therapeutic (e.g., surgery, chemotherapy) approaches 20% of the time, paraneoplastic syndromes less than 10% of the time, and unrelated to the malignancy less than 10% of time.

D. Goals of therapy
1. To reduce the effect of noxious stimuli caused by thermal, chemical, or mechanical injury that elicits pain
2. To improve quality of life

E. Analgesics work by interfering with the pain transduction, transmission, or modulation in the primary afferent neuronal fibers, spinothalamic tract, collateral fibers, and higher brain centers.

F. Analgesics are used to manage both nociceptive (somatic and visceral) and neuropathic pain (see Chapter 34).

II. Types of analgesics
A. Opioids (Table 25-7)

B. Nonopioid analgesics (see Anti-inflammatory Agents section)

C. Co-analgesics (see Psychotropic Drugs: Sedative or Hypnotic and Antianxiety Agents and Anti-inflammatory Agents sections)

III. Principles of medical management (DeSandre & Quest, 2010; Grossman & Nesbit, 2008; Induru & Lagman, 2011; Irwin, Lee, Rodgers, Starr, & Webberm, 2012; NCCN, 2013a)

A. Selection of appropriate analgesia is based on pharmacokinetic factors (see Table 25-7) and the patient's physical needs, age, history of analgesia usage, and organ function.

B. The most appropriate dose is the one that controls pain through a 24-hour period.

C. If opioids are used, patients should have long-acting and breakthrough options available when pain is constant.

D. As doses are titrated to effective levels, both long-acting and breakthrough doses should be

Table 25-7

Pharmacokinetic Features of Opioids

Drug	Equivalent Potency	Onset of Effect (min)	Peak Effect (min)	Duration of Effect (hr)
Morphine				
IV	10 mg	5-10	10-15	3-5
Oral	30 mg	30	60	4-6
Codeine	200 mg	30	45-90	4-6
Fentanyl				
IV	0.1 mg (100 mcg)	6	6-10	30-60
Patch	Variable	18-24 hours	6 days	Prolonged
Buccal	400 mcg	5-15	30-60	4-5
Hydromorphone				
IV	1.5 mg	5-10	10-15	3-5
Oral	7.5 mg	30-60	30-60	4-6
Levorphanol				
IV	2 mg	—	—	6-8
Oral	4 mg	30	60-90	6-8
Meperidine				
IV	75 mg	15	30-60	2-3
Oral	300 mg	—	—	3-6
Methadone	10 mg (depends on total morphine dose)	—	—	6-8
Oxycodone				
Immediate release	20 mg	15	45-60	3-6
Delayed release	—	30	60	12
Oxymorphone				
IV	1 mg	10	30-90	3-6
Oral	10 mg	—	—	—

IV, Intravenous; *PO*, by mouth; *PR*, per rectum.

Adapted from National Comprehensive Cancer Network. (). *NCCN guidelines for supportive care: Adult cancer pain (v1.2013).* http://www.nccn.org/professionals/physician_gls/pdf/pain.pdf.

increased; the breakthrough dose should be 10% to 20% of the 24-hour long-acting dose.

E. Prophylaxis for constipation with a stool softener and bowel stimulant should be considered for all patients started on opioid analgesics.

F. The effectiveness and the side effect profile should be reassessed (see Chapter 34).

G. Tolerance occurs in patients who take opioids regularly; that is, they require higher doses to achieve the same amount of analgesia.

H. Physical dependence occurs in all patients who take opioids regularly; a withdrawal syndrome will occur if the opioid is abruptly stopped.

I. Psychological dependence is addiction that occurs when patients crave the opioid, use the drug compulsively, and continue use despite harm.

IV. Routes of administration
  A. Oral
    1. Most convenient
    2. Preferred
    3. Immediate- and extended-release dosing available
  B. Transdermal
  C. Parenteral
    1. Intravenous
    2. Intrathecal
    3. Subcutaneous
  D. Topical
  E. Buccal, transmucosal, or nasal for rapid-onset opioids
  F. Rectal

V. Potential adverse effects
  A. Adverse effect profile of opioid analgesics (Table 25-8)
  B. Dependence
    1. Physical dependence is universal.
      a. Doses of opioids should not be abruptly withdrawn to avoid opioid withdrawal.
    2. Opioid withdrawal
      a. Not a sign of psychological addiction
      b. Symptoms
        (1) Nausea and vomiting
        (2) Diarrhea
        (3) Perspiration
        (4) Tachycardia
        (5) Chills
        (6) Restless legs syndrome
        (7) Dysphoria
        (8) Anxiety or paranoia
        (9) Insomnia
  C. Drug interactions with multidrug regimens (Table 25-9)
    1. Other sedative or hypnotic drugs—potentiate sedative properties of opioids and combination opiate substances ⚠

    2. Drugs that lower seizure threshold ⚠
      a. Increased risk of seizures with concomitant administration
      b. Concomitant drugs that alter mental status equilibrium
      c. Other drugs that alter hepatic metabolism, renal excretion
      d. Other drugs that alter bioavailability, absorption, or pharmacokinetics of the administered drug
  D. Causes of abnormalities in drug absorption
    1. Gastrointestinal
      a. Surgical resections, including gastrectomy, jejunectomy, and duodenectomy, may increase transit time, decrease absorption, or both.
      b. Feeding tubes inserted at various points in the GI tract may not be the appropriate point of absorption of an individual drug.
        (1) Tube feedings or fluids administered through tubes may increase transit time and decrease absorption.
      c. Pharmacologically induced changes in gut motility
        (1) Laxatives
        (2) Muscarinics (e.g., atropine)
        (3) Prokinetic agents (e.g., metoclopramide)
    2. Topical or transdermal absorption
      a. Skin integrity
        (1) Moisture content
        (2) Ulcerations
        (3) Fat-to-lean body ratio
      b. Occlusive dressings increase absorption.
      c. Heat
  E. Potential adverse effects caused by compromised organ systems
    1. Renal insufficiency—may slow rate of elimination of drug, metabolites, or both, leading to increased potential for toxicities
      a. Morphine
      b. Codeine
      c. Meperidine
      d. Hydromorphone (metabolites exist but clinical significance is unknown)
      e. Tramadol
    2. Hepatic insufficiency—may increase amount of drug available to body because of decreased first-pass effect, altered enzyme pathways, other metabolic pathways
      a. Fentanyl
      b. Morphine (caution with extended-release formulations)
      c. Tramadol
      d. Oxycodone (caution with extended-release formulations).

Part 4

Table 25-8

Side Effect Profile of Opioid Analgesics

Side Effects	Nursing Implications
Gastrointestinal	
Nausea, vomiting	Monitor nausea and number of vomiting episodes and effect on comfort and fluid balance; administer antiemetic drug therapy as needed.
Constipation	Assess bowel elimination patterns and compare with patient's normal pattern; administer stool softeners and/or stimulant cathartics.
Narcotized bowel	Increase fluid and dietary fiber intake; abdominal assessment; report decreased or absent bowel sounds and increased abdominal pain.
Cardiovascular	
Arteriolar vasodilation and reduced peripheral resistance; decrease in blood pressure; tachycardia, bradycardia	Monitor vital signs, blood pressure for orthostatic hypotension. Provide for patient safety if blood pressure is low.
Respiratory	
Depressant effect on brainstem reduces respiratory rate, minute volume, tidal exchange; irregular and periodic breathing; respiratory arrest	Monitor level of sedation; respiratory rate and depth; arterial blood gases; vital signs, O_2 saturations; have available narcotic antagonist and measures for respiratory assistance.
Decreased cough reflex	Monitor coughing ability postoperatively; use aspiration precautions.
Central Nervous System	
Drowsiness, alteration in mood and mental clouding; visual and auditory hallucinations, euphoria, dizziness, disorientation, paranoia; lethargy, inability to concentrate, apathy; seizures, uncontrollable twitching, myoclonus	Neurologic assessment Provide for patient safety. Institute fall precautions, as needed. Monitor for preseizure activity, especially in patients taking meperidine; monitor for twitching. Level of sedation may indicate degree of respiratory depression. Methylphenidate (Ritalin), 5-10 mg, PO bid or tid, may be helpful for somnolence or mental clouding from opioids.
Pupil	
Miosis	Monitor pupil size and response to light (contraction).
Smooth Muscle	
Contraction of gallbladder, bile duct, sphincter of Oddi	Monitor for signs of gastric upset; if present, evaluate liver and pancreatic function tests.
Genitourinary	
Urinary retention	Monitor urine output, palpate bladder, catheterize (straight or indwelling), as needed.
Dermatologic	
Skin rash, cutaneous vasodilation	Monitor skin integrity. Administer antihistamines for allergic reactions. Educate patient to avoid scratching. Provide cool environment.

bid, Twice daily; *PO*, by mouth; *tid*, three times daily.

3. Central nervous system (CNS)—brain metastases, underlying seizure disorders may predispose to CNS toxicity
4. Urinary—benign prostatic hypertrophy may contribute to urinary retention.
5. Respiratory—underlying restrictive or obstructive disease may potentiate respiratory compromise from opioids. ⚠
   a. Chronic obstructive pulmonary disease (COPD)
   b. Emphysema
   c. Obstructive sleep apnea
6. Cardiovascular—coronary artery disease, congestive heart failure

ASSESSMENT

I. Identification of patients at risk for pain (see Chapter 34)
   A. Assessment of type of pain—description, cause, classification, degree of pain
   B. History of past and current analgesia regimens and their effectiveness
      1. Time to onset of pain relief
      2. Duration of time of pain relief
      3. Quality or rating of decrease of pain

Table 25-9

Common Drug Interactions of Analgesics

Drug	Effect
Methadone	
Barbiturates, carbamazepine (Tegretol), phenytoin, rifampin (Rifadin)	Reduced methadone plasma levels by enhancing CYP2D6 metabolism
Fluconazole (Diflucan), itraconazole (Sporanox), ketoconazole (Nizoral)	Increased methadone plasma levels by inhibiting CYP3A4 metabolism; enhanced sedation may be observed.
Opioid Analgesics	
Barbiturates	Enhanced CNS depressant effects
Cimetidine (Tagamet)	Enhanced respiratory and CNS depressant effects
Chlorpromazine (Thorazine)	Enhanced CNS depression and hypotension
Monoamine oxidase inhibitors	Enhanced CNS depressant effects. Increased adverse reactions (excitation, sweating, rigidity, hypertension)
Meperidine	
Isoniazid (INH)	Potentiates isoniazid
Phenytoin	Reduced meperidine plasma levels
NSAIDs	
ACE inhibitors	Reduced antihypertensive effect
Alpha-adrenergic receptor blockers	Reduced antihypertensive effect
Corticosteroids	Increased incidence of GI ulceration
Hydralazine (Apresoline)	Reduced antihypertensive effect
Prazosin (Minipress)	Reduced antihypertensive effect
Potassium-sparing diuretics	Decreased renal function
Salicylates	
Warfarin (Coumadin)	Increased risk of bleeding
Acetazolamide (Diamox)	May enhance renal salicylate excretion and increase salicylate penetration into the brain, causing CNS salicylate toxicity
Alcohol (ETOH)	Increased risk of GI blood loss
Heparin (Liquaemin)	Increased risk of bleeding
Methotrexate (Folex, Mexate)	Increased risk of methotrexate toxicity
Probenecid (Benemid)	Inhibits uricosuric effects of probenecid
Sulfinpyrazine (Anturane)	Inhibits uricosuric effects of sulfinpyrazone
Antacids	Reduced salicylate levels; increased renal elimination of salicylates
Antidiabetic agents	Increased response of sulfonylureas; chlorpropamide most likely affected

ACE, Angiotensin-converting enzyme; *CNS*, central nervous system; *CYP2D6*, cytochrome P450 enzyme 2D6; *CYP3A4*, cytochrome P450 enzyme 3A4; *GI*, gastrointestinal; *NSAIDs*, nonsteroidal anti-inflammatory drugs.

C. Assessment of side effects from previous regimens
  1. Description of side effects
  2. Onset and duration of side effects
  3. Pharmacologic and other interventions to control or alleviate side effects
  4. Severity of side effects
II. Physical examination
  A. Review of systems
  B. Examination of the area of pain, originating site of pain, or both—redness, temperature changes, atrophy, tenderness (see Chapter 34)
III. Current medications
IV. Evaluation of diagnostic and laboratory data
  A. Renal indices—serum creatinine and blood urea nitrogen (BUN) levels, intake and output
  B. Hepatic indices—aspartate aminotransferase (AST), alanine aminotransferase (ALT), bilirubin, alkaline phosphatase
  C. Electrocardiography (ECG), electroencephalography (EEG), if indicated
  D. QT interval prolongation—may occur in patients taking methadone
  E. Radiographic examination, bone scan, CT, MRI, positron emission tomography (PET), ultrasonography
V. Assessment of patient's and family's cultural and ethnic background, pain beliefs, health care practices, and values and beliefs related to pharmacotherapy (see Antimicrobials, Assessment sections)

NURSING DIAGNOSES AND EXPECTED OUTCOMES

I. Acute Pain or Chronic Pain (NANDA-I)
   A. Expected outcome—patient states pain is relieved or reduced to his or her satisfaction.
II. Deficient Knowledge (NANDA-I), related to pharmacologic management of pain
   A. Expected outcome—patient discusses the rationale for the use of analgesics, including the schedule of administration.
   B. Expected outcome—patient describes adverse effects of use of analgesics and measures to manage adverse effects.
   C. Expected outcome—patient understands the importance of adherence to attain comfort goals.
   D. Expected outcome—patient lists signs and symptoms of adverse effects of analgesics to report to the health care team.
   E. Expected outcome—patient and family discuss that the risk of addiction is rare.

PLANNING AND IMPLEMENTATION

I. Interventions to manage pain (see Chapter 34)
II. Interventions to educate patient
   A. Rationale for taking analgesic medications, including schedule of administration—long-acting and breakthrough agents
   B. Adverse effects and strategies to manage adverse effects
   C. Adverse effects to report to health care team
III. Interventions to decrease the incidence and manage adverse effects of analgesics (see Table 25-8)
   A. Assessment of baseline data (e.g., vital signs, CNS—orientation, alertness, affect; respiratory effort, oxygen saturation, rate, depth, sedation score)
   B. Review of patient's medical history for existing or previous conditions, such as acute alcoholism, impaired hepatic or renal function, advanced age, increased intracranial pressure
   C. Assessment of normal bowel patterns
   D. Review of patient's medications for possible drug interactions
IV. Interventions to monitor for response to analgesia
   A. Assessment of patient's pain experience and response to treatment
   B. Assessment for adverse effects, toxicity, and drug interactions

EVALUATION

The oncology nurse systematically and regularly evaluates the patient's pain and responses to analgesics to determine progress toward optimal comfort. Relevant data are collected, and actual findings are compared with expected findings. Nursing diagnoses, outcomes, and plans of care are reviewed and revised, as necessary.

Psychotropic Drugs: Anxiolytics and Sedative-Hypnotics

OVERVIEW

I. Rationale and indications (Dy & Apostol, 2010; Traeger, Greer, Fernandez-Robles, Temel, & Pirl, 2012)
   A. Definition of anxiety
      1. An unpleasant, multifactorial experience of a psychosocial, emotional, or spiritual nature that interferes with the ability to cope with cancer, its physical symptoms, or its treatments
      2. Commonly referred to as *distress*, because this is a more socially acceptable term
      3. Incidence
         a. Anxiety present in an estimated one third or more of all patients with cancer
         b. Could occur at any time during the cancer trajectory
         c. Most common times of high risk for anxiety
            (1) Cancer diagnosis
            (2) During treatment
            (3) Disease status change (e.g., remission, progression)
            (4) End of life
      4. Risk factors for anxiety
         a. Previous diagnosis of an anxiety disorder
         b. History of psychiatric disorder
         c. Cancer-related fears
            (1) Situational anxiety (e.g., diagnosis, treatment)
            (2) Existential (e.g., death, failure)
         d. Comorbidity (e.g., pain, fatigue)
      5. Common uses of anxiolytics in patients with cancer
         a. To reduce anxiety associated with cancer and its management
         b. To manage comorbid anxiety, depression, or seizures
         c. To reduce pain associated with anxiety
         d. To manage alcohol or narcotic withdrawal
         e. To prevent anticipatory nausea or vomiting or treat chemotherapy-induced nausea and vomiting
   B. Insomnia
      1. Definition
         a. Difficulty falling asleep at night or waking up during the night
         b. Different from waking up with confusion (delirium), sleep apnea, depression or anxiety
      2. Factors that increase insomnia
         a. Excessive sleeping during the day
         b. Other unrelieved cancer symptoms (e.g., pain, dyspnea)
         c. Substance use
            (1) Caffeine
            (2) Alcohol

d. Anxiety
e. Medications (e.g., corticosteroids)
3. Common uses of sedative or hypnotic medications
   a. Induction of sleep
   b. Maintenance of sleep
   c. Amnesia (reduced recall) of medical procedure
II. Types of anxiolytics, sedative-hypnotic medications (Dy & Apostol, 2010; Traeger et al., 2012)
   A. Benzodiazepines (Table 25-10 and Table 25-11)
   B. Nonbenzodiazepines (see Table 25-10)

C. Barbiturates
D. Used infrequently for treating anxiety or insomnia
E. Other medications (see Table 25-10)
   1. Buspirone
   2. Melatonin agonist
      a. Ramelteon
      b. Melatonin
F. Selective serotonin reuptake inhibitors (SSRIs) (see Table 25-11)
G. Serotonin norepinephrine reuptake inhibitors (see Table 25-11)

Table 25-10

Common Sedative, Hypnotic, or Anxiolytic Drugs

Drug	Dose	Adverse Effects (Class effect unless noted)	Comments (Class)
Benzodiazepines*			
Chlorazepate (rapid acting)	7.5-15 mg by mouth every 6 to 12 hr		Intermediate-acting agents are better tolerated in cancer patients.
Diazepam (rapid acting)	2-10 mg intravenously or by mouth every 6-12 hr	Sedation Cognitive impairment	Lorazepam, oxazepam, alprazolam, and temazepam are preferred over triazolam, flurazepam, and chlordiazepoxide.
Alprazolam (intermediate acting)	0.25-0.5 mg by mouth every 8 hr (usual max daily dose 4 mg)		CNS side effects are increased with when given to elderly patients.
Chlordiazepoxide (intermediate acting)	5-100 mg by mouth	Dizziness Lightheadedness	These medications increase the risk of falls. Fall precautions should be used for any patient receiving these medications.
Clonazepam (intermediate acting)	0.5 mg by mouth every 8 hr (usual max daily dose of 20 mg)		
Lorazepam (intermediate acting, hypnotic)	0.5-2 mg intravenously or by mouth every 4-6 hr (usual max daily dose of 6 mg)	Information recall	Midazolam is the most frequently used benzodiazepine to use this side effect clinically.
Oxazepam (intermediate acting, hypnotic)	10-30 mg by mouth every 6-8 hr	Morning somnolence	Carryover effect from medication is worse with agents with a long half-life (see Table 10-11)
Triazalom (rapid acting, used for insomnia)	0.125-0.25 mg by mouth at bedtime		Withdrawal symptoms are more common and more severe with short-acting agents.
Estazolam (intermediate acting, used for insomnia)	1-2 mg by mouth at bedtime	Withdrawal	Symptoms of withdrawal include psychosis, seizures and coma.
Temazepam (intermediate acting, used for insomnia)	15-30 mg by mouth at bedtime	Respiratory Depression	Use with caution patients with respiratory comorbidities.
		Rebound insomnia (dependence)	Occurs after extended use.
Nonbenzodiazepine†			
Buspirone	7.5 mg by mouth twice daily Increase dose every 3 days Max dose is 60 mg	Side effects are similar, but occur in a reduced incidence and severity.	Similar to above.

GABA, Gamma-aminobutyric acid.

*These agents bind to GABA receptors, inhibiting CNS excitation and resulting in CNS depression.

†Mechanism of action is similar to that of benzodiazepines, but with a different structure.

Part 4

Table 25-11

Pharmacokinetic Comparison of Selected Benzodiazepines

Drug	Equivalent Potency (mg)	Metabolic Pathway	Half-Life (Hours)
Alprazolam	0.5	CYP3A4	12–15
Chlordiazepoxide	10	CYP3A4	30–100
Clonazepam	0.25-0.5	CYP3A4	18–50
Diazepam	5	CYP2C19 and CYP3A4	50–100
Lorazepam	1	Glucuronidation	10–14
Temazepam	5	Glucuronidation, CYP2C19, and CYP3A4	10–40
Triazolam	0.1	CYP3A4	2–5

CYP pathway: Knowledge of the particular CYP enzymes involved in the metabolism of medications is important to predict drug-drug interactions. If a medication that is metabolized by one or multiple CYP enzymes is given concomitantly with a medication that inhibits those enzymes, resulting in a drug-drug interaction, an adverse medication event could occur because of accumulation of the inhibited drug. If you have questions or concerns about the potential for drug-drug interactions while caring for a patient, consider a pharmacy consult.

From Lexi-Comp Online: *Lexi-drugs online.*

III. Principles of medical management (Dy & Apostol, 2010; NCCN, 2013d; Traeger et al., 2012)
   A. Selection of therapy
      1. Psychotherapy
      2. Pharmacologic (see Tables 25-10)
         a. Half-life
         b. Sedative properties
         c. Psychomotor and memory impairment
         d. Dose-response profiles
         e. Cost
         f. Duration of therapy
         g. Dosage conversion
         h. Routes of administration
         i. Compromised organ function
         j. Age-related alterations
IV. Potential adverse effects (see Tables 25-10)
   A. CNS effects
      1. Sedation
      2. Dizziness
      3. Lightheadedness
      4. Cognitive impairment
   B. Rebound insomnia for short-acting agents
   C. Complex sleep-related behaviors (e.g., sleep walking)
   D. Motor incoordination
   E. Behavioral changes
   F. Delirium
      1. Particularly in older adults
   G. Respiratory suppression
      1. Caution should be used in patients with pulmonary disease (e.g., COPD)
V. Drug interactions ⚠
   A. Alcohol
      1. Concomitant consumption of alcohol and these medications should be avoided.
   B. Inhibitors or inducers of hepatic enzyme CYP3A4 (e.g., clarithromycin, ketoconazole, ritonavir, rifampin, carbamazepine)

ASSESSMENT

I. Identification of patients at risk for anxiety disorders (see Chapter 38), sleep disorders (see Chapter 34)
   A. Assessment for signs and symptoms of anxiety and sleep disorders
II. Physical examination (see Chapters 34 and 38)
III. Current medications
IV. Evaluation of diagnostic and laboratory data
   A. Screening tools for distress (NCCN, 2013d; Traeger et al., 2012)
   B. Electrolyte abnormalities and blood glucose levels
   C. Drug levels
V. Assessment of patient's and family's cultural and ethnic background, particularly health care practices and values and beliefs related to pharmacotherapy (see Antimicrobials, Assessment sections)
   A. Determination of patient's racial group because biologic variations among racial groups may affect drug metabolism rates, clinical drug responses, and drug-related side effects

NURSING DIAGNOSES AND EXPECTED OUTCOMES

I. Anxiety (NANDA-I)
   A. Expected outcome— patient describes a reduction in anxiety.
II. Disturbed Sleep Pattern (NANDA-I)
   A. Expected outcome—patient achieves adequate amount of sleep.
   B. Expected outcome—patient discusses the rationale for the use of sedative-hypnotic or anxiolytic drugs, including schedule of administration.
   C. Expected outcome—patient describes adverse effects of use of sedative-hypnotic or anxiolytic drugs.

D. Expected outcome—patient describes measures to manage adverse effects of sedative-hypnotic or anxiolytic drugs.

E. Expected outcome—patient lists signs and symptoms of adverse effects of sedative-hypnotic or anxiolytic drugs to report to the health care team.

F. Expected outcome—patient aware of what medications to avoid because of drug-drug interactions.

III. Acute Pain or Chronic Pain (NANDA-I)

A. Expected outcome—patient takes anxiolytics and sedatives or hypnotics to maintain comfort.

PLANNING AND IMPLEMENTATION

I. Interventions to manage sleep disorders and pain (see Chapter 34) and anxiety (see Chapter 38)

II. Interventions to educate patient

A. Rationale for use of sedative-hypnotic or anxiolytic drug therapy and taking them as scheduled

B. Adverse effects and strategies to manage adverse effects

C. Adverse effects to report to health care team

III. Interventions to monitor for adverse effects of sedative-hypnotic or anxiolytic drugs (see Table 25-10)

IV. Interventions to decrease the incidence and manage the adverse effects of sedative-hypnotic or anxiolytic drugs (see Table 25-10)

A. Assessment of baseline data (e.g., vital signs, CNS—orientation, alertness, affect; respiratory effort, rate, depth)

B. Review of patient's medical history for existing or previous conditions

C. Review of patient's medications for potential drug interactions ⚠️

V. Interventions to monitor for response to psychotropic drugs

A. Psychiatry or psychology consultation, as needed

B. Assessment for level of anxiety and amount of restful sleep

EVALUATION

The oncology nurse systematically and regularly evaluates the patient's and family's responses to anxiolytics and sedatives-hypnotics to determine progress toward alleviation of anxiety and promotion of sleep. Relevant data are collected, and actual findings are compared with expected findings. Nursing diagnoses, outcomes, and plans of care are reviewed and revised, as necessary.

Antidepressants

OVERVIEW

I. Rationale and indications (Li, Fitzgerald, & Rodin, 2012; McMenamin, 2011)

A. For treatment of depression

1. Depression—may range from minor mood changes to major emotional responses of suicidal ideation

2. Symptoms of depression (one of the first two, with four additional)

3. Depressed mood
   a. Anhedonia (inability to experience pleasure)
   b. Appetite disturbance
   c. Sleep disturbance
   d. Psychomotor agitation or retardation
   e. Fatigue
   f. Feelings of worthlessness
   g. Difficulty concentrating
   h. Suicidal ideation ⚠️

4. Risk factors for depression
   a. Younger age
   b. History of depression
   c. Less social support
   d. Attachment anxiety
   e. Poor communication with health care providers
   f. Maladaptive coping
   g. Increasing physical burden of cancer
      (1) Metastatic disease
      (2) Disability from disease or treatment
      (3) Number or severity of physical symptoms present
      (4) Uncontrolled pain

5. Types of depression
   a. Bipolar—with manic phase
   b. Major depression—unipolar only
   c. Situational depression
   d. Drug- or food-induced depression

B. Purposes of antidepressants

1. To treat clinical unipolar or bipolar depression or anxiety

2. To treat depression associated with chronic pain

3. As adjuvant pharmacologic pain management in pain conditions, including postherpetic neuralgia, migraine and chronic tension headaches, sundowner syndrome

4. To treat insomnia

II. Types of antidepressants (Table 25-12)

A. SSRIs

B. Mixed action

III. Principles of medical management (Li et al., 2012)

A. Selection of therapy

1. Depression
   a. Psychotherapy types
   b. Pharmacologic therapy (see Table 25-12)

IV. Potential adverse effects (see Table 25-12)

A. Drug-drug interactions

B. Dietary restrictions

Table 25-12

Common Antidepressants

Drug	Initial Dose	Anticholinergic	Sedation	Orthostatic Hypotension	Conduction Abnormalities	GI Distress	Weight Gain	Comments
Tricyclic Antidepressants								
Amitriptyline	25-75 mg q HS	4+	4+	3+	3+	1+	4+	Also used for chronic pain
Desipramine	25-75 mg q HS	1+	2+	2+	2+	-	1+	—
Imipramine	25-75 mg q HS	3+	3+	4+	3+	1+	4+	—
Nortriptyline	25-50 mg q HS	2+	2+	1+	2+	0	2+	—
Serotonin Reuptake Inhibitors								
Citalopram	20 mg q AM	0	0	0	0	3+	1+	Significant sexual dysfunction
Escitalopram	10 mg q AM	0	0	0	0	3+	1+	Significant sexual dysfunction
Fluoxetine	10-20 mg q AM	0	0	0	0	3+	1+	CYP2B6 and 2D6 inhibitor (do not use with tamoxifen); significant sexual dysfunction
Paroxetine	10-20 mg q AM	1+	1+	0	0	3+	2+	CYP2B6 and 2D6 inhibitor (do not use with tamoxifen); significant sexual dysfunction
Sertraline	20-50 mg once daily	0	0	0	0	3+	1+	CYP2B6 and 2D6 inhibitor (do not use with tamoxifen); significant sexual dysfunction
Mixed-Action Agents								
Bupropion	150 mg q AM; bid (SR tab)	0	0	0	1+	1+	0	Contraindicated with seizures, bulimia, or anorexia; low incidence of sexual dysfunction
Duloxetine	40-60 mg once daily	1+	1+	0	1+	3+	0	Also used for neuropathy
Venlafaxine	37.5 mg once daily (XR tab)	1+	1+	0	1+	3+	0	Frequency of hypertension increases with dose; often used for hot flashes from tamoxifen
Desvenlafaxine	50 mg once daily	0	1+	1+	0	3+	0	—
Mirtazapine	15 mg q HS	1+	3+	1+	1+	0	3+	Doses > 15 mg/day less sedating low; incidence of sexual dysfunction; reported to increase appetite
Trazodone	50 mg tid	0	4+	3+	1+	1+	2+	Often used for insomnia (50-150 mg q HS)

AM, Morning; *bid*, twice daily; *HS*, at bedtime; *q*, every; *SR*, sustained-release; *tid*, three times a day; *XR*, extended-release.

Adapted from Lacy CF, Armstrong LL, Goldman MP, Lance LL. (2011). *Drug information handbook* (20th ed.; pp. 1143–1147). Hudson, OH: Lexi-Comp.

ASSESSMENT

I. Identification of patients at risk for depression
   (see Chapter 38)
   A. Age—younger more than older persons
   B. Health conditions (e.g., advanced stage of disease),
      negative body image
   C. Mental health history—family or individual
      history of depression or substance abuse
   D. Disease recurrence, treatment failure
   E. Unrelieved symptoms, especially pain
   F. Interactions with other medications
      1. Antihypertensive and cardiovascular drugs—
         guanethidine (Ismelin), methyldopa (Aldomet),
         reserpine (Serpalan, Serpasil), propranolol
         (Inderal), metoprolol (Lopressor), prazosin
         (Minipress), clonidine (Catapres), digitalis
      2. Sedative-hypnotic agents—alcohol, chloral
         hydrate (Noctec), benzodiazepines,
         barbiturates, meprobamate (Equanil)
      3. Anti-inflammatory agents and analgesics—
         indomethacin (Indocin), phenylbutazone,
         opioids, pentazocine (Talwin)
      4. Steroids—corticosteroids, oral contraceptives,
         estrogen withdrawal
      5. Miscellaneous—antiparkinsonian drugs,
         antineoplastic agents (interferon, Aldesleukin
         [interleukin-2]), ethambutol (Myambutol),
         neuroleptics, stimulant withdrawal
   G. Concomitant medical diseases
      1. Endocrine disorders—hypothyroidism,
         hyperthyroidism, diabetes mellitus,
         hyperparathyroidism, Cushing disease,
         Addison disease
      2. CNS disorders—brain tumors, Parkinson
         disease, multiple sclerosis, Alzheimer disease,
         Huntington disease
      3. Cardiovascular disorders—myocardial
         infarction (MI), cerebral vascular accident
         (CVA), congestive heart failure (CHF)
      4. Miscellaneous disorders—rheumatoid arthritis,
         pancreatic disease, cancer, systemic lupus
         erythematosus, infectious disease, metabolic
         abnormalities, pernicious anemia, malnutrition
II. Identification of patients at risk for pain (see Chapter 34)
III. Assessment for signs and symptoms (see Chapters 34
    and 38)
IV. Physical examination (see Chapters 34 and 38)
V. Evaluation of diagnostic and laboratory data
   A. Electrolyte disorders
   B. Fluid imbalances
VI. Assessment of patient's and family's cultural
    and ethnic background, particularly health care
    practices and values and beliefs related to
    pharmacotherapy (see Antimicrobials, Assessment
    sections)

NURSING DIAGNOSES AND EXPECTED OUTCOMES

I. Ineffective Coping (NANDA-I)
   A. Expected outcome—patient experiences adequate
      management of his or her depression with minimal
      adverse effects from medications.
II. Risk for Self-Directed Violence (NANDA-I)⚠
   A. Expected outcome—patient verbalizes suicidal
      ideations and agrees to contract not to act on
      impulse.⚠
III. Acute Pain or Chronic Pain (NANDA-I)
   A. Expected outcome—patient states that the pain is
      reduced or relieved to his or her satisfaction.
IV. Deficient Knowledge (NANDA-I), related to
    antidepressant therapy
   A. Expected outcome—patient discusses rationale for
      use of antidepressant drug therapy, including
      schedule of administration.
   B. Expected outcome—patient describes potential
      adverse effects of antidepressants.
   C. Expected outcome—patient describes measures to
      manage adverse effects of antidepressants.
   D. Expected outcome—patient lists signs and
      symptoms of adverse effects of antidepressants to
      report to the health care team.

PLANNING AND IMPLEMENTATION

I. Interventions to manage effects of depression
   (see Chapter 38) and pain (see Chapter 34)
II. Interventions to educate patient
   A. Rationale for use of antidepressant drug
      therapy and taking antidepressants as scheduled
   B. Adverse effects and strategies to manage adverse
      effects
   C. Adverse effects to report to health care team
III. Interventions to monitor for adverse effects of
    antidepressants (see Table 25-12)
IV. Interventions to decrease the incidence and
    manage the adverse effects of antidepressants
    (see Table 25-12)
V. Interventions to monitor for therapeutic response to
   antidepressants
   A. Monitoring patient for emotional changes, suicidal
      ideation⚠
   B. Obtaining psychiatric or psychological
      consultation, as needed
   C. Monitoring patient for response to pain
      management interventions
   D. Assessment for adverse effects, toxicity, and drug-
      drug interactions

EVALUATION

The oncology nurse systematically and regularly evaluates
the patient's and family's responses to interventions for
depression to determine progress toward the achievement

of improved mood and quality of life. Relevant data are collected, and actual findings are compared with expected findings. Nursing diagnoses, outcomes, and plans of care are reviewed and revised, as necessary.

Anticonvulsants

OVERVIEW

I. Rationale and indications (Weller, Stupp, & Wick, 2012)
   A. For prophylaxis and treatment of seizure activity
      1. Incidence of seizure more common in patients with cancer than patients without cancer
      2. Tumors possible in patients with cancer with primary brain tumor, metastatic cancer to the brain or leptomeninges, or localized tumors outside of the CNS
      3. Seizures—may be the first symptoms of primary or metastatic disease
      4. Seizures more common in primary brain tumors because of CNS infiltrative characteristics that are typically not part of metastatic solid tumors
      5. Causes of tumors in cancer patients
         a. Tumor infiltration (e.g., glioblastoma)
         b. Tissue damage and edema (e.g., solid tumors)
         c. Chemotherapy
            (1) Ifosfamide
            (2) High-dose methotrexate
            (3) Busulfan
         d. Stroke (hemorrhagic or ischemic)
         e. Infection (e.g. meningitis)
         f. Metabolic abnormalities (e.g., sodium imbalance, syndrome of inappropriate diuretic hormone [SIADH])
   B. As adjuvant pharmacologic therapy for pain with neurologic cause (e.g., trigeminal neuralgia, phantom limb pain, peripheral neuropathy)
II. Types of anticonvulsants (Table 25-13)
   A. Enzyme-inducing (e.g., phenobarbital, carbamazepine, phenytoin)
      1. Not commonly used
      2. Drug-drug interactions problematic
   B. Non-enzyme-inducing medications (e.g., valproic acid, levatriacetam, lamotrigine)
      1. More commonly used
      2. Well tolerated, with limited drug-drug interactions
III. Principles of medical management (Weller et al., 2012)
   A. Diagnosis of appropriate seizure activity
      1. Understanding the cause of the seizure is important.
      2. Neurology consultation should be considered.
      3. Seizure should not be presumed to be from tumor.
      4. Evaluation of other causes should be undertaken.
      5. No anticonvulsant has been shown to be more effective than another.
      6. No evidence suggests that dual therapy is more effective than monotherapy.
      7. Therapeutic selection is based on drug interactions and tolerance.

Table 25-13

Common Anticonvulsants and Adjunct Therapy

Drug	Dose Range	Target Concentration	Side Effects	Drug Interactions
Phenobarbital	50-300	10-40	Sedation, cognitive decline, allergy	Enzyme induction
Phenytoin	200-350	10-20	Dizziness, allergy, hepatotoxicity, gingival hyperplasia, cerebellar atrophy, rash	Enzyme induction
Carbamazepine	600-2000	4-8	Dizziness, nausea, ataxia, hyponatremia, leukopenia, hepatotoxicity, rash	Enzyme induction
Oxcarbazepine	900-2400	4-8	Hyponatremia, leucopenia, rash	Enzyme induction
Valproic acid	1200-2400	10-35	Tremor, weight gain, coagulation disorders, thrombocytopenia, teratogenicity	Enzyme inhibition
Lamotrigine	100-300	2-15	Rash, tremor, sedation	Enzyme substrate
Gabapentin	900-3000	2-20	Sedation, weight gain	—
Levetiracetam	1000-3000	3-30	Sedation, psychiatric effects	—
Lacosamide	100-400	10-20	Dizziness, nausea, headache, cognition decline, rash	—
Zonisamide	300-500	20-30	Dizziness, ataxia, anorexia	—
Tiagabine	15-70	0.02-0.08	Dizziness, fatigue	Enzyme substrate
Vigabatrin	200-300	0.8-36	Visual field defects, fatigue, sedation	Decreases phenytoin concentrations

Adapted from Weller, M., Stupp, R., & Wick, W. (2012). Epilepsy meets cancer: When, why and what to do about it? *Lancet Oncology, 13,* 375–382.

8. Resistant disease is defined as using two or more anticonvulsants at appropriate dosing with breakthrough epileptic activity.
   A. Diagnosis of appropriate pain syndrome
   B. Selection of appropriate pharmacologic therapy (see Table 25-13)
IV. Potential adverse effects (see Table 25-13)

ASSESSMENT

I. Identification of patients at risk for seizure activity
   A. Underlying seizure disorder
      1. Previous seizure history
   B. Drugs that lower seizure threshold (e.g., bupropion, isoniazid, tricyclic antidepressants, meperidine, propoxyphene, phenothiazines)—see www.professionals.epilepsy.com.
   C. Medical conditions that lower seizure threshold
      1. Trauma
      2. Febrile episodes
      3. Tumor pressure in brain
II. Identification of patients at risk for neurologic pain
   A. Chemotherapy (e.g., paclitaxel, vincristine, bortezomib, thalidomide, oxaliplatin)
   B. Diabetes
   C. Amyloidosis
III. Physical examination
   A. Neurologic examination
      1. Mental status—general appearance, level of consciousness, mood and affect, thought content and intellectual capacity
      2. Cranial nerve assessment
      3. Sensory function
      4. Motor function
      5. Assessment of reflexes
IV. Evaluation of diagnostic and laboratory data
   A. Anticonvulsant serum levels
   B. Serum electrolyte values
   C. Analysis of cerebrospinal fluid (CSF)
   D. EEG, CT, MRI, PET
V. Assessment of patient's and family's cultural and ethnic background, particularly health care practices and values and beliefs related to pharmacotherapy (see Antimicrobials, Assessment sections)

NURSING DIAGNOSES

I. Risk for Injury (NANDA-I)⚠️
   A. Expected outcome—patient remains safe during a seizure.
   B. Expected outcome—patient experiences adequate seizure control with minimal side effects.
II. Acute Pain or Chronic Pain (NANDA-I)
   A. Expected outcome—patient states pain is relieved or reduced to his or her satisfaction.
III. Deficient Knowledge (NANDA-I), related to use of anticonvulsant drug therapy

A. Expected outcome—patient discusses the rationale for the use of anticonvulsants, including schedule of administration.
B. Expected outcome—patient describes potential adverse effects of anticonvulsants.
C. Expected outcome—patient describes measures to manage adverse effects of anticonvulsants.
D. Expected outcome—patient and family list the signs and symptoms of adverse effects of anticonvulsants to report to the health care team.

PLANNING AND IMPLEMENTATION

I. Interventions to ensure patient safety in the event of a seizure⚠️
   A. Instituting seizure precautions.
   B. Providing a safe environment, free of physical hazards
   C. Assessment for injuries after completion of the seizure activity
      1. Vital signs
      2. Neurologic examination
II. Interventions to manage pain (see Chapter 34)
III. Interventions to educate the patient
   A. Rationale for use of anticonvulsant drug therapy and taking anticonvulsants as scheduled
   B. Adverse effects and strategies to manage adverse effects
   C. Adverse effects to report to health care team
IV. Interventions to monitor for adverse effects of anticonvulsants (see Table 25-13)
V. Interventions to decrease the incidence and manage the adverse effects of anticonvulsants (see Table 25-13)
   A. Assessment of baseline data (e.g., neurologic status)
   B. Review of patient's medical history for existing or previous conditions
   C. Review of patient's medications for potential drug-drug interactions
   D. Conducting patient and family teaching (e.g., good oral hygiene, avoiding driving or other potentially hazardous activity that requires mental alertness)
VI. Interventions to monitor for a therapeutic response to anticonvulsant drug therapy
   A. Assessment of neurologic status and pain level
   B. Assessment for adverse effects, toxicity, and drug interactions

EVALUATION

The oncology nurse systematically and regularly evaluates the patient's seizures or pain and responses to anticonvulsants to determine progress toward the achievement of safety and comfort. Relevant data are collected, and actual findings are compared with expected findings. Nursing diagnoses, outcomes, and plans of care are reviewed and revised, as necessary.

Hematopoietic Growth Factors

OVERVIEW

I. Rationale and indications (Metcalf, 2010; Wilkes & Barton-Burke, 2010).

   A. Hematopoietic growth factors (HGFs)—glycoproteins that stimulate the proliferation of bone marrow progenitor cells and their maturation into fully differentiated circulating blood cells

      1. Growth factors—target either one or multiple cell cells

      2. Functions of growth factors

         a. Promote cellular proliferation

         b. Induce cellular maturation

         c. Prevent apoptosis

      3. Immune enhancement

         a. White blood cell (WBC) growth factors (e.g., filgrastim, pegfilgrastim, sargramostim) increase the activity of multiple immune cells, including neutrophils and macrophages.

   B. Cancer-related indications

      1. Granulocyte colony-stimulating factor (G-CSF) and granulocyte-macrophage colony-stimulating factor (GM-CSF)

         a. Prevention of febrile neutropenia after chemotherapy

         b. Shorten duration of neutropenia after hematopoietic transplantation or treatment for acute myeloid leukemia

         c. Mobilize hematopoietic stem cells prior to stem cell transplantation

      2. Erythropoietin (epoetin alfa and darbepoetin alfa)

         a. Anemia caused by chemotherapy in patients with an incurable malignancy

II. Types of growth factors in clinical use (Metcalf, 2010)

   A. Single-lineage factors

      1. G-CSF (filgrastim and pegfilgrastim)

         a. Produced by macrophages, fibroblasts, and endothelial cells

         b. Stimulate target cells that include a late precursor committed to the neutrophil lineage and the mature neutrophil

         c. Increase phagocytic activity

         d. Increase antimicrobial killing

         e. Enhance antibody-dependent cell-mediated cytotoxicity

      2. Erythropoietin (epoetin alfa and darbepoetin alfa)

         a. Naturally produced by the kidneys

         b. Production regulated by a feedback mechanism involving the perception of decreased oxygen tension in tissue

         c. Interacts with specific receptors on erythroid burst-forming units and erythroid colony-forming units

         d. Binding of the stimulating factor and these units, leading to erythropoiesis and subsequent production and differentiation of erythrocytes, or red blood cells (RBCs)

      3. Oprelvekin (interleukin-11)

         a. Stimulates hematopoietic stem cells and megakaryocytes

         b. Increases differentiation and production of platelets

   B. Multilineage factors

      1. GM-CSF (sargramostim)

         a. Receptors exist on myeloid cell lines.

         b. Major effect stimulates the proliferation and differentiation of the cells destined for the neutrophil and macrophage lines.

         c. GM-CSF enhances functional activities of neutrophils and monocytes or macrophages, leading to enhanced activity in clearing bacterial and fungal organisms.

         d. GM-CSF stimulates production of secondary cytokines such as tumor necrosis factor (TNF), IL-1, and macrophage colony-stimulating factor (M-CSF).

III. Principles of medical management (Cooper, Madan, Whyte, Stevenson, & Akehurst, 2011; NCCN, 2013c; NCCN, 2013e; Rizzo, Brouwers, & Hurley, 2010)

   A. G-CSF and GM-CSF

      1. Prevention of febrile neutropenia with G-CSF or GM-CSF is more effective than treatment of febrile neutropenia with G-CSF or GM-CSF.

      2. Prevention of neutropenia by using G-CSF or GM-CSF is indicated in patients with 20% or more risk of febrile neutropenia.

      3. The risk of neutropenia is determined primarily by chemotherapeutic regimen (review NCCN guidelines for an extensive list of regimens with ≥20% risk of febrile neutropenia).

      4. Risk is increased in select patients.

         a. Increased age (>65 years)

         b. Extensive previous treatments (chemotherapy and radiation therapy)

         c. Hematologic malignancy

         d. Multiple comorbidities (e.g., diabetes, COPD)

      5. G-CSF has been shown to decrease days on antibiotics and hospital stay by 1 day, but it does not decrease mortality.

      6. Pegfilgrastim is at least as effective as filgrastim in the prevention of febrile neutropenia.

         a. Some data suggest it may be a more effective agent, but this has not been shown in randomized controlled trials.

      7. Filgrastim is used to mobilize stem cells from the bone marrow to be collected peripherally prior to allogeneic or autologous stem cell transplantation.

      8. Pegfilgrastim has limited use in stem cell mobilization at this time.

B. Erythropoietin (EPO)
1. EPO causes an increase in hemoglobin (>2 g/dL) more effectively than placebo in patients with anemia caused by chemotherapy.
   a. EPO also decreases the number of RBC transfusions required to treat anemia.
2. Concern has been raised by multiple clinical trials suggesting a decrease in progression-free and overall survival in patients receiving EPO during chemotherapy, radiotherapy, or no active treatment.⚠
   a. The U.S. Food and Drug Administration (FDA) requires a risk evaluation and migration strategy (REMS).
   b. REMS for EPO requires providers to submit documentation that the risks of using EPO have been discussed with the patient when used for chemotherapy-induced anemia.
   c. EPO is not recommended in select patient populations.
      (1) Cancer patients not receiving active treatment
      (2) Cancer patients receiving chemotherapy with a curative intent
   d. EPO has been shown to increase the risk of venous thromboembolism as well.⚠
3. EPO should not be given in patients with hemoglobin greater than 10 g/dL.
4. Treatment goals
   a. To prevent RBC transfusions
   b. To ensure that the starting dose and maintenance dose are lowest to prevent RBC transfusion.
5. It is important to evaluate iron stores prior to use.
   a. Iron is an important component of RBCs.
   b. Patients who are iron-deficient will not respond to EPO.

C. Oprelvekin
1. The FDA has approved this drug to reduce platelet transfusions caused by low platelet nadirs from myelotoxic chemotherapy.
2. Oprelvekin has not been shown to decrease mortality.
3. High cost and significant toxicity (fluid retention) limit its use.
4. This is rarely used; thrombocytopenia is typically managed with platelet transfusion.

IV. Potential adverse effects
A. Side effects (Table 25-14)

ASSESSMENT

I. Identification of patients at risk for the following:
A. Neutropenia—absolute neutrophil count less than $500/mm^3$ (see Chapter 27)
B. Anemia—hemoglobin level less than 10 g/dL (see Chapter 27)
C. Thrombocytopenia—platelet count less than 75,000 cells/mm^3 (see Chapter 27)

Table 25-14

Growth Factors

Drug	Indications	Side Effects	Nursing Implications
GM-CSF or sargramostim (Leukine)	Myeloid recovery after autologous BMT BMT graft failure or engraftment delay Following induction chemotherapy for acute myelogenous leukemia; use if bone marrow hypoplastic with <5% blasts on day 10.	*Low dose:* Bone pain, local skin reaction, fever, flulike symptoms, headache, arthralgias, myalgias *High dose:* Pericardial effusions, capillary leak syndrome, third spacing Phlebitis with peripheral IV administration	*Low dose:* Monitor level of pain; acetaminophen for bone, joint, muscle pain, headache, fever; monitor VS, especially temperature; encourage fluids and rest *High dose:* cardiovascular assessment, VS, monitor fluid balance and edema, intake and output, breath sounds; monitor electrolyte and CBC laboratory test results Monitor IV site for pain and redness; discontinue IV if present. Monitor CBC laboratory test results for return of granulocytes and monocytes. *Administration:* Subcutaneous administration standard; IV administration may require albumin in IV carrier.
Pegfilgrastim (pegylated G-CSF, Neulasta)	Antineoplastic, chemotherapy-induced neutropenia	Bone pain Adult respiratory distress syndrome (rare)	Monitor level of pain; administer acetaminophen for bone pain. Assess respiratory status (breath sounds, rate, pattern and depth of respirations, oxygen saturation); notify physician of worsening symptoms.

Continued

Table 25-14

Growth Factors—cont'd

Drug	Indications	Side Effects	Nursing Implications
		Splenic rupture (rare)	Abdominal assessment and pain; notify physician Monitor CBC laboratory test results for return of neutrophils *Precautions:* Contraindicated in patients with known hypersensitivity to *Escherichia coli*–derived proteins; do not administer sooner than 24 hours after chemotherapy and in the case of pegfilgrastim must be no sooner than 14 days before chemotherapy.
G-CSF or filgrastim (Neupogen)	Antineoplastic, chemotherapy-induced neutropenia	Bone pain	Monitor level of pain; administer acetaminophen for bone pain. Monitor CBC for increase in neutrophils. *Precautions:* Contraindicated in patients with known hypersensitivity to *E. coli*–derived products; do not shake vial vigorously if giving subcutaneous injection.
Erythropoietin (Epogen, Procrit)	Cancer patients receiving chemotherapy Anemia of chronic cancer Zidovudine-treated HIV-infected patients Chronic renal failure	Hypertension Thrombotic events Seizures Headaches Skin rashes, urticaria; transient rash at injection site	Monitor blood pressure. Assess for possible emboli in lower extremities or lungs. Assess for seizure activity; implement seizure precautions as needed. Assess level of headache; administer pain medication as needed. Assess skin before the start of treatment and during treatment; rotate injection sites. Monitor CBC laboratory test results for increase in red blood cell count.
Darbepoetin, NESP (Aranesp)	Renal failure Chemotherapy-induced anemia in patients with nonmyeloid malignancies, chronic renal failure not on dialysis	Hypertension Fatigue Edema Vascular access thrombosis and thrombotic events Fever, pneumonia, dyspnea, sepsis Seizures Nausea, vomiting, diarrhea, dehydration	Contraindicated in patients with uncontrolled hypertension; closely monitor blood pressure of all patients; rotate injection sites; monitor blood counts. Assess level of fatigue; provide for periods of rest between activities; educate about energy-conserving strategies. Assess skin for edema; elevate lower extremities; protect skin from damage; intake and output; assess breath sounds. Assess for possible emboli in lower extremities or lungs and in vascular access devices; report positive evidence to physician. Monitor VS; monitor respiratory status e.g., (breath sounds; rate, depth, ease, and pattern of respirations; dyspnea, shortness of breath; oxygen saturation); administer antipyretics and antimicrobials as needed. Assess for seizure activity; implement seizure precautions as needed. GI assessment and effect of nausea, vomiting, and diarrhea on comfort, fluid balance, perineal skin; intake and output; administer antiemetic and antidiarrheal drugs as needed; encourage fluids if tolerated; monitor signs of dehydration (dry skin and mucous membranes, concentrated urine, thirst, fever). Monitor CBC laboratory test results for increase in red blood cell count.

BMT, Bone marrow transplantation; *CBC,* complete blood cell count; *G-CSF,* granulocyte colony-stimulating factor; *GI,* gastrointestinal; *GM-CSF,* granulocyte-macrophage colony-stimulating factor; *HIV,* human immunodeficiency virus; *IV,* intravenous; *VS,* vital signs.

II. Physical examination (see Chapter 27)

III. Current medications

IV. Evaluation of diagnostic and laboratory data (see Chapter 27)

V. Assessment of patient's and family's cultural and ethnic background, particularly health care practices and values and beliefs related to pharmacotherapy (see Antimicrobials, Assessment sections)

NURSING DIAGNOSES AND EXPECTED OUTCOMES

I. Risk for Infection (NANDA-I)

A. Expected outcome—patient remains free of infection, or infection is recognized early and treated promptly.

B. Expected outcome—patient and family describe personal risk factors for infection.

II. Risk for Anemia

A. Expected outcome—patient maintains adequate hemoglobin level balanced with the potential risk of disease progression when using EPO.

III. Deficient Knowledge (NANDA-I), related to HGF drug therapy

A. Expected outcome—patient and family demonstrate self-care skills required to administer HGF, as applicable (e.g., subcutaneous injections).

B. Expected outcome—patient identifies the type of and describes the rationale for treatment with HGFs, including schedule of administration.

C. Expected outcome—patient describes potential adverse effects of HGF therapy.

D. Expected outcome: patient describes measures to manage adverse effects of HGF therapy.

E. Expected outcome—patient lists signs and symptoms of adverse effects of HGF therapy to report to the health care team.

PLANNING AND IMPLEMENTATION

I. Interventions to manage neutropenia or infection, thrombocytopenia or bleeding, and anemia or fatigue (see Chapters 27 and 34)

II. Interventions to educate patient

A. Rationale for need of medications and taking as scheduled

B. Administration of HGF (e.g., subcutaneous injection)

C. Adverse effects and strategies to manage adverse effects

D. Adverse effects to report to health care team

III. Interventions to monitor for adverse effects of HGFs (see Table 25-14)

IV. Interventions to decrease the incidence and manage the adverse effects of HGFs (see Table 25-14).

A. Assessment of baseline data (e.g., vital signs, neurologic status)

B. Review of patient's medical history for existing or previous conditions

C. Review of patient's medications for potential drug interactions

D. Conducting patient and family teaching (e.g., on side effects and self-management; medication administration)

V. Interventions to monitor for response to HGFs.

A. Monitoring laboratory results (e.g., complete blood cell count)

B. Assessment of activity level, presence of infection and bleeding, as applicable

C. Assessment for adverse effects, toxicity, and drug interactions

EVALUATION

The oncology nurse systematically and regularly evaluates the patient's responses to HGFs to determine progress toward prevention or treatment of neutropenia and correction of anemia. Relevant data are collected, and actual findings are compared with expected findings. Nursing diagnoses, outcomes, and plans of care are reviewed and revised, as necessary.

References

Basch, E., Prestrud, A. A., Hesketh, P. J., Kris, M. G., Feyer, P. C., Somerfield, M. R., et al. (2011). Antiemetics: American Society of Clinical Oncology clinical practice guideline update. *Journal of Clinical Oncology, 2,* 4189–4198.

Cooper, K. L., Madan, J., Whyte, S., Stevenson, M. D., & Akehurst, R. L. (2011). Granulocyte colony-stimulating factors for febrile neutropenia prophylaxis following chemotherapy: Systematic review and meta-analysis. *BMC Cancer, 23,* 404.

DeSandre, P. L., & Quest, T. E. (2010). Management of cancer-related pain. *Hematology Oncology Clinics of North America, 24,* 643–658.

Dy, S. M., & Apostol, C. C. (2010). Evidence-based approaches to other symptoms in advanced cancer. *Cancer Journal, 16,* 507–513.

Feyer, P., & Jordan, K. (2011). Update and new trends in antiemetic therapy: The continuing need for novel therapies. *Annals of Oncology, 22,* 30–38.

Freifeld, A. G., Bow, E. J., Sepkowitz, K. A., Boeckh, M. J., Ito, J. I., Mullen, C. A., et al. (2011). Clinical practice guideline for the use of antimicrobial agents in neutropenic patients with cancer: 2010 update by the Infectious Diseases Society of America. *Clinical Infectious Diseases, 52,* e56.

Gea-Banacloche, J., & Segal, B. H. (2011). Infections in the cancer patient. In V. T. DeVita, T. S. Lawrence, & S. A. Rosenberg (Eds.), *Cancer: Principles and practice of oncology* (pp. 2262–2299). Philadelphia: Lippincott Williams & Wilkins.

Grossman, S., & Nesbit, S. (2008). Cancer pain. In M. D. Abeloff, J. O. Armitage, J. E. Niederhuber, M. B. Kastan, & W. G. McKenna (Eds.), *Abeloff's clinical oncology* (pp. 565–577). Philadelphia: Churchill Livingstone.

Hainsworth, J. (2008). Nausea and vomiting. In M. D. Abeloff, J. O. Armitage, J. E. Niederhuber, M. B. Kastan, & W. G. McKenna (Eds.), *Abeloff's clinical oncology* (pp. 565–577). Philadelphia: Churchill Livingstone.

Hesketh, P. J. (2008). Chemotherapy-induced nausea and vomiting. *New England Journal of Medicine, 358,* 2482–2494.

Induru, R. R., & Lagman, R. L. (2011). Managing cancer pain: Frequently asked questions. *Cleveland Clinic Journal of Medicine, 78*, 449–464.

Irwin, M., Brant, J., & Eaton, L. (2012). Putting evidence into practice: Improving oncology patient outcomes pharmacologic and nonpharmacologic interventions for pain oncology nursing society. *Oncology Nursing Society*, 1–33.

Irwin, M., Erb, C., Williams, C., Wilson, B., Zitella, L., Irwin, M., et al. (2013). Putting evidence into practice: Improving oncology patient outcomes prevention of infection, oncology nursing society. *Oncology Nursing Society*, 6–8.

Irwin, M., Lee, J., Rodgers, C., Starr, P., & Webberm, J. (2012). Putting evidence into practice: Improving oncology patient outcomes chemotherapy-induced nausea and vomiting. *Oncology Nursing Society*, 1–9.

Lacy, C. F., Armstrong, L. L., Goldman, M. P., & Lance, L. L. (2011). *Drug information handbook* (20th ed., pp. 1143–1147). Hudson, OH: Lexi-Comp.

Lexi-Comp Online. (2013). *Lexi-drugs online.* Hudson.

Li, M., Fitzgerald, P., & Rodin, G. (2012). Evidence-based treatment of depression in patients with cancer. *Journal of Clinical Oncology, 30*, 1187–1196.

McMenamin, E. (2011). Cancer pain management. In C. Yarbro, D. Wucjik, & B. Gobe (Eds.), *Cancer nursing principles and practice* (pp. 685–712). Sudbury, MA: Jones and Bartlett.

Metcalf, D. (2010). The CSFs and cancer. *Nature Reviews Cancer, 10*, 425.

National Comprehensive Cancer Network. (2013a). *Adult cancer pain (v 1.2013).* http://www.nccn.org/professionals/physician_gls/pdf/pain.pdf.

National Comprehensive Cancer Network. (2013b). *Antiemesis (v 1.2013).* http://www.nccn.org/professionals/physician_gls/pdf/antiemesis.pdf.

National Comprehensive Cancer Network. (2013c). *Cancer- and chemotherapy-induced anemia (v 1.2013).* http://www.nccn.org/professionals/physician_gls/pdf/anemia.pdf.

National Comprehensive Cancer Network. (2013d). *Distress management (v 2.2013).* http://www.nccn.org/professionals/physician_gls/pdf/distress.pdf.

National Comprehensive Cancer Network. (2013e). *Myeloid growth factors (v 12013).* http://www.nccn.org/professionals/physician_gls/pdf/myeloid_growth.pdf.

National Comprehensive Cancer Network. (2013f). *Prevention and treatment of cancer-related infections (v1.2013).* http://www.nccn.org/professionals/physician_gls/pdf/infections.pdf.

Rizzo, J. D., Brouwers, M., Hurley, P., Seidenfeld, J., Somerfield, M. R., & Temin, S. (2010). American Society of Clinical Oncology/American Society of Hematology clinical practice guideline update on the use of epoetin and darbepoetin in adult patients with cancer. *Journal of Clinical Oncology, 28*, 4996–5010.

Traeger, L., Greer, J. A., Fernandez-Robles, C., Temel, J. S., & Pirl, W. F. (2012). Evidence-based treatment of anxiety in patients with cancer. *Journal of Clinical Oncology, 30*, 1197–1205.

Weller, M., Stupp, R., & Wick, W. (2012). Epilepsy meets cancer: When, why and what to do about it? *Lancet Oncology, 13*, e375–e382.

Wilkes, G., & Barton-Burke, M. (2010). *Oncology Nursing Drug Handbook* (pp. 391–394). Burlington, MA: Jones & Bartlett Learning.

CHAPTER 26

Complementary and Integrative Modalities

Lori Johnson and Roberta Bourgon

OVERVIEW

I. Definitions—therapies that may be used to enhance the efficacy of conventional (allopathic, biologic, scientific, orthodox, Western) medicine therapy, alleviate side effects of conventional treatment, and improve the patient's sense of well-being and quality of life, or both
  A. Complementary therapies are often used in conjunction with conventional medicine.
    1. Complementary therapies have been scientifically tested, but currently a large body of evidence does not exist to support many complementary therapies. Current evidence may be equivocal for many complementary therapies.
    2. Many complementary therapies may be referred to as supportive care (e.g., massage, acupuncture).
  B. Alternative therapies are used in place of conventional treatments.
    1. This refers to unproven, non–evidence-based interventions often advertised by proponents to be able to cure cancer.
    2. Patients pursue alternative therapies for various reasons such as fear of side effects from conventional treatment, traditional or cultural practice, and cost-effectiveness.
  C. *Complementary and alternative medicine* (CAM) is the term used to describe the entire domain of therapies that fall outside of conventional medicine.
  D. *Integrative medicine, integrative health care*, and *integrative oncology* are some terms that refer to combining complementary therapies with conventional treatment regimens.
    1. A personalized and holistic approach that takes into account each patient's unique circumstances (e.g., diagnosis, patient values and preferences, expected toxicities related to standard treatment regimen) to customize treatment programs (Lawenda, 2012)
  E. *Holism* or *holistic health care* refers to modalities that integrate the body-mind-emotion-spirit-environment of a person (Dossey & Keegan, 2013).

II. Current trends in the United States
  A. Growing trend in the use of CAM across the United States (U.S.)
    1. Nearly 40% of Americans report using CAM therapies outside of conventional medicine (National Center for Complementary and Alternative Medicine [NCCAM], 2013).
  B. Most commonly used CAM therapies by adults in the U.S. include a range of products (e.g., nutritional supplements), whole-medicine systems (e.g., chiropractic and osteopathic), and mind-body approaches (e.g., meditation and yoga) (Barnes, Bloom, & Nahin, 2008) (Figure 26-1).
  C. Continued increase in the use of dietary supplements (Gahche et al., 2011)
    1. Over 40% of American adults used supplements in 1994, increasing to more than 50% in 2006.
    2. Approximately 40% of adults report taking multivitamins and multiminerals, making these the most commonly used dietary supplements.
    3. In 2006, 61% of women older than 60 years reported using supplemental calcium, up from 28% in 1994.
    4. The use of supplements containing vitamin D has increased in both men and women between the ages of 40 and 59 from 26% in 1994 to 45% in 2006. For adults older than 60, the increase was from 23.7% in 1994 to 56.3% in 2006.
    5. Reasons for using CAM include health maintenance or disease prevention (77%), pain management (73%), treatment of specific acute or chronic health conditions (59%), and as supplements to conventional medicine (53%) (Dossey & Keegan, 2013).
    6. A growing number of conventional medicine providers are offering complementary therapies, which has resulted in the increasing utilization of integrative oncology approaches.
      a. In palliative care and hospice settings, 41.8% of providers offered complementary and

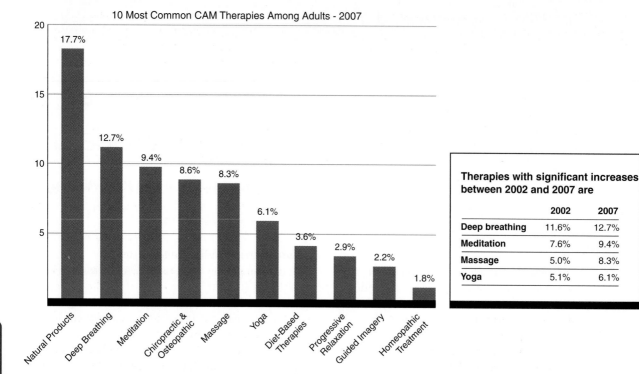

Figure 26-1 Ten Most Common Complementary and Alternative Therapies among Adults.
From Barnes, P. M., Bloom, B., & Nahin, R. (2008). Complementary and alternative medicine use 387 among adults and children: United States, 2007 (DHHS Publication No. 2009-1240). *Hyattsville, MD: National Center for Health Statistics.*

alternative therapies (Bercovitz, Sengupta, Jones, & Harris-Kojetin, 2011).

    (1) Among hospice care providers, 71.7% offered massage, supportive group therapy (69%), music therapy (62.2%), pet therapy (58.6%), and guided imagery or other relaxation techniques (53.7%).

  b. Many academic and private cancer treatment centers are offering a range of complementary services.

III. Major categories of CAM—no single standard for categorizing CAM; the National Center for Complementary and Alternative Medicine (NCCAM) distinguishes two broad categories of health care practices that fall outside of conventional medical treatments:

  A. Natural products

  B. Mind and body practices (NCCAM, 2013).

  C. The National Care Institute (NCI) Office of Cancer Complementary and Alternative Medicine (NCI OCCAM, 2013) lists eight major categories of CAM therapy:

    1. Alternative medical systems

    2. Energy therapies

    3. Exercise therapies

    4. Manipulative and body-based methods

    5. Mind-body interventions

    6. Nutritional therapeutics

    7. Pharmacologic and biologic treatments

    8. Spiritual therapies

IV. Whole medical systems

  A. Ayurveda—taken from Sanskrit, *ayus,* which means "life or lifespan," and *veda,* which means "knowledge"

    1. Ayurveda—based on the principle that maintaining balance in the body, mind, and consciousness is used to preserve health and treat illness

    2. Specific interventions—driven by the individual's *prakriti* (nature), which is determined by the three *gunas* (ways of being: *tamas, rajas, sattva*); human physiology believed to be the result of the combination of the three *doshas* (*pitta, kapha,* and *vatta*) in each individual; energy (or *prana*) flows through the body through channels or *nadis*; disruption in the flow of energy results in disease.

    3. Interventions—aimed at rebalancing the *doshas* and restoring the flow of energy; may include proper diet, hydration, and lifestyle (e.g., following a set sleep-wake routine, detoxification or cleansing techniques, specific massage techniques [*marma* therapy], specific movements or spoken words [*mantras*])

B. Chiropractic medicine—emphasizes structural alignment of the spine
  1. Adjustments are made through manipulation of the spine and joints to re-establish normal central nervous system (CNS) functioning.
  2. Interventions may include massage, nutrition, and specialized kinesiology.
  3. Chiropractic medicine is contraindicated in patients with bone metastasis, spinal cord compression, thrombocytopenia, or venous thrombosis.
C. Homeopathy—based on the precept of healing through the administration of specific substances
  1. Substances are chosen according to the following beliefs:
    a. Like cures like.
    b. The more a remedy is diluted, the greater is the potency.
    c. Illness is specific to the individual.
  2. This form of medicine is based on the belief that symptoms are an indication that the body is attempting to rid itself of disease.
  3. Treatment is based on the person as a whole being, as opposed to focusing on the symptoms.
D. Osteopathic medicine—focuses on the relationship between the structure and function of the body; osteopaths are fully licensed to diagnose, treat, and prescribe in conventional medicine
  1. Recognizes that structure and function are subject to a range of disorders
  2. Uses physical manipulation to facilitate self-healing in the individual, as well as conventional medical therapies
E. Traditional Chinese medicine (TCM)—originated in China and evolved over thousands of years
  1. Includes key concepts:
    a. Yin-yang—concept of two opposing complementary forces that are brought into balance to maintain healthy body and mind
    b. Meridians—pathways or channels that run throughout the body through which *qi* (energy, pronounced "chee") or energy flows; disruption in the flow of qi results in disease; acupuncture and other techniques used to direct, redirect, or unblock the flow of qi
    c. Five elements—fire, earth, metal, water, and wood, which correspond to various organs and tissues in the body
    d. Eight principles—used in TCM to analyze symptoms; principles include cold-heat, interior-exterior, excess-deficiency, and yin-yang
  2. Interventions—include use of herbs, acupuncture, and other methods

[e.g., moxibustion, cupping, mind-body therapy] to enhance health and treat illness
V. Manipulative and body-based practices
  A. Acupuncture—an ancient Oriental technique, associated with TCM, used to restore or promote health and well-being through the use of fine-gauge needles inserted into specific points on the body to stimulate or disperse the flow of energy
    1. Used in conjunction with methods such as massage, herbal remedies, and nutritional counseling
    2. May be a safe and effective treatment for chronic lymphedema related to breast cancer treatment (Cassileth et al., 2013)
    3. Contraindicated in patients who are neutropenic or severely thrombocytopenic
  B. Acupressure—the use of finger or hand pressure over specific points on the body to relieve symptoms or to influence specific organ function
    1. May be used to release tension, reestablish the natural flow of energy, or both
    2. Contraindicated in patients with bleeding disorders or thrombocytopenia and in those taking anticoagulant medications such as warfarin (Coumadin)
    3. Should not be done over body areas with tumor, lymphadenopathy, or both
  C. Alexander technique—uses movement and touch to restore balance in the body and neuromuscular function, thus allowing the body to regain a relaxed, healthy posture
  D. Aromatherapy—uses essential oils extracted from herbs and other plants
    1. Treats physical imbalances and restores psychological and spiritual well-being
    2. Essential oils are inhaled, applied topically, or ingested
    3. Currently no standardization of practice; a wide range of quality in essential oils, because processing is not regulated
    4. Topical application of essential oils to be avoided unless they are prepared by a trained specialist
  E. Cranial osteopathy—uses gentle manipulation of the skull to re-establish natural configuration and movement
    1. Disorders manifested throughout the body can be improved by realigning the skull.
  F. Dance therapy—dance and music combined to facilitate uplifting of the mind, body, and spirit through natural body movement
  G. Feldenkrais method—a somatic education system that teaches movement and gentle manipulation to increase body awareness and improve body function
    1. Used to improve posture and promote flexibility and freedom of movement

H. Lymphatic therapy—the use of vigorous massage to stimulate flow of lymphatic fluid
   1. Intended to move lymph fluid and release toxins stored in the lymphatic system
   2. Refreshes the immune system
   3. Manual, gentle lymphatic drainage used to prevent and treat lymphedema following breast cancer surgery (Zimmermann, Wozniewski, Szklarska, Lipowicz, & Szuba, 2012)

I. Massage—the use of manual pressure and strokes on muscle tissue
   1. Used to reduce emotional and physical tension, increase circulation, and relieve muscular pain
   2. Can provide comfort and increased body awareness

J. Neuromuscular therapy—a type of massage therapy that uses moderate pressure on muscles, nerves, and trigger points to decrease pain and tension

K. Physical therapy—used to correct mechanical body ailments and restore normal musculoskeletal functioning
   1. Procedures designed to relieve pain, reduce swelling, strengthen muscles, and restore range of motion
   2. Can include a combination of massage, electrostimulation, ultrasonography, and prescribed exercises

L. Qigong—a Chinese meditative practice that combines physical postures with focused intention and breathing techniques to release, cleanse, strengthen, and circulate energy
   1. Used for stress reduction and to enhance the body's natural healing abilities
   2. May increase vitality and awareness of internal energy that furthers the mind-body connection
   3. Can be performed with patient in either standing or sitting position

M. Shiatsu—a Japanese form of body work similar to acupressure
   1. Uses finger and palm pressure to manipulate energetic pathways to improve the flow of energy
   2. Pressure applied to specific points in a continuous rhythmic sequence
   3. Used to calm an overactive sympathetic nervous system, improve circulation, relieve muscle tension, and alleviate stress
   4. The patient is fully clothed during the treatment, unlike other massage techniques, and no oil is applied to the body.
   5. May not be safe in cancer patients, who are at increased risk of blood clots, because the type of manipulations may dislodge a blood clot

N. Trigger point therapy—a method of compression of specific points in muscle tissue to relieve pain and tension

   1. May be used together with therapeutic massage and passive stretching
   2. Treatment goals aimed at decreasing swelling and stiffness and increasing range of motion
   3. Like physical therapy, exercises assigned to be performed at home between treatment sessions

VI. Mind-body modalities
A. Art therapy—uses a variety of art techniques using different mediums (drawing, coloring, painting, sculpting, and multimedia) to assist the patient in restoring, maintaining, or improving physical, mental, emotional, and spiritual well-being
   1. Based on the concept that the creative process helps people resolve inner conflict and process issues, reduce stress, increase self-esteem and self-awareness, and achieve insight
   2. Requires a master's degree in art therapy and may require licensure, credentials, or both, depending on the state

B. Color therapy (chromotherapy)—uses electronic instrumentation and color receptivity to integrate the nervous system and body-mind
   1. Based on premise that color conveys energy at different frequencies and the human body responds to these vibrational frequencies
   2. May be used to increase well-being and is used to treat acute and chronic ailments

C. Eye movement desensitization and reprocessing (EMDR)—a psychotherapy technique based on the concept that distressing events are associated with specific rapid eye movements
   1. The therapist helps the patient recall distressing events, eliciting the associated rapid eye movements, and then redirects the eye movements through stimulation or distraction, thereby breaking the connection that is causing distressing thoughts and feelings to persist (Triscari, Faraci, D'Angelo, Urso, & Catalisano, 2011).

D. Guided imagery—a structured process that uses live or recorded scripts describing different scenarios or detailed images to guide the patient through a process
   1. May lead the patient through progressive muscle relaxation or through a visualization of a treatment process (e.g., visualization of chemotherapy entering the body and seeking out cancer cells to remove them from the body)
   2. Techniques—use of a coach who narrates the imagery, an audio recording, or a video recording

E. Meditation—a method of quieting the mind to facilitate inner peace; numerous forms of meditation, ranging from simple focused breathing to transcendental meditation; practices share characteristics, and often involve focused breathing and a relaxed yet alert state that promotes control over thoughts and feelings

  1. Studies have shown that achieving a relaxed state of mind may decrease perceived levels of stress, relieve muscle tension, enhance sense of well-being, and boost the immune response (Pritchard, Elison-Bowers, & Birdsall, 2010).
  2. Mindfulness-based stress reduction (MBSR) is a technique whereby patients are trained to development awareness of experiences moment by moment and in the context of all senses (Davidson, Kabat-Zinn, Schumacher et al., 2003).
  3. Yoga Nidra meditation teaches patients to explore sensations, emotions, and thoughts and then to dissociate from them.
  4. Transcendental meditation uses a *mantra* (a word, sound, or phrase) to direct focus and to prevent distraction.

  F. Music therapy—an applied psychotherapy that uses making or listening to music to explore behavioral, emotional, or spiritual disruption, and to assist the patient in resolving these issues
   1. Some states require therapists to have a master's degree, certification, or both.
  G. Neurolinguistic programming (NLP)—a systematic approach to changing thought patterns, thereby changing feelings or perceptions
   1. One example is the use of a "gratitude journal." The patient is instructed to record daily entries in a journal, specifically recalling positive aspects of his or her life, to promote a positive outlook over time. The concept is that one gets more of whatever one focuses on.
  H. T'ai chi—an ancient Chinese practice of movements coordinated with breathing techniques
   1. Derived from martial art form
   2. Enhances coordination and balance and promotes physical, emotional, and spiritual well-being
  I. Yoga—strength and flexibility achieved through the use of specific postures and controlled breathing
   1. Has evolved into mainstream practice with multiple variations, ranging from restorative (gentle) yoga to promote well-being in frail patients to power yoga, which uses a vigorous, fitness-based approach and is often taught in gyms
   2. Has a meditative component that brings harmony to body, mind, and spirit

VII. Biologically based practices
  A. Biofeedback—a technique for teaching the patient to recognize, observe, and learn to control biologic responses to stress
   1. Monitors are used to give feedback to the patient about vital signs (blood pressure, heart rate, and respiratory rate), and the patient is taught to relax through visualization and focused breathing, among other methods.
   2. By conscious effort, patients learn to bring about change in vital functions.
  B. Herbal therapy—the use of herbs and their chemical properties to treat specific conditions or to improve general health and well-being
   1. Herbal preparations are used in alcohol extractions, liquid extractions, salves, teas, capsules, oils, liquids, or in their raw forms and are taken internally, inhaled, or applied directly to the body. Therapeutic aims are restoration of health and providing support to the body's mechanisms of immunity, elimination, detoxification, and homeostasis.
   2. The use of herbal medicines should be monitored by a knowledgeable provider, members of the health care team, or both.
   3. Caution should be used with herbs that are known to affect the CYP3A4267 pathway because of the potential for herb–drug interactions (e.g., St. John's wort).
  C. Hydrotherapy—the application of water to the body in its various forms (ice, water, steam) and at an extreme temperature (hot or cold) to restore and maintain health
   1. Treatments include water baths, steam baths, saunas, and the application of hot or cold compresses.
  D. Nutritional counseling—the use of diet, nutritional supplements, or both to prevent and manage illness or to enhance and maintain health
  E. Energy work, energy therapy, biofield therapy—a broad category of work aimed at influencing the major energy centers (*chakras*) of the body and the flow of a patient's internal and external energy; energy work can be used to treat physical symptoms and emotional or spiritual distress, or enhance well-being.
   1. Reiki—an energy healing modality whereby the practitioner uses his or her hands to direct the flow of energy to various parts of the body to facilitate healing and relaxation; hands are placed on the body in specific patterns without deep pressure to redirect or restore energy flow.
   2. Therapeutic touch—a technique for balancing the flow of energy in the body through the transfer of human energy
     a. Based on the concept that disruption in energy flow leads to disease and restoring that flow can lead to health, growth, order, and wholeness
   3. Healing touch—an energy healing technique that uses the nursing process (Hart, Freel, Haylock, & Lutgendorf, 2011)

a. Developed by Janet Mentgen, a registered nurse, in the 1980s

b. Includes specific protocols, all of which include assessment, intervention, and evaluation of the patient's response

c. Standardized training

4. Magnetic therapy—the use of magnets to influence magnetic fields to positively affect the nervous system, organs, and tissues to stimulate healing

ASSESSMENT

I. Use of CAM—may negatively interfere or interact with conventional cancer treatment; nursing assessment to include questions directed at determining patient use of CAM and discussion regarding the risks and benefits, as needed ⚠

II. Relevant patient demographics and clinical information

A. Demographics—should include age, gender, education, residence, economic status, ethnic and cultural identity

B. Clinical information—should include comorbidities, allergies, medications (including CAM), and cancer disease information: type, stage, cancer treatments

III. Initial and ongoing assessment of the patient with regard to CAM—should include a comprehensive assessment

A. Disturbances or imbalances in the following areas:

1. Physical well-being
2. Nutritional status
3. Functional performance status
4. Psychosocial status
5. Emotional and mental well-being
6. Sexual functioning
7. Age-related developmental issues
8. Spiritual well-being
9. Energy field disturbances

B. Identification of risk in the areas of the following:

1. Environmental factors
2. Cultural practices
3. Family dynamics
4. Socioeconomic status
5. Health behaviors

C. Patient values and preferences:

1. Meaning of health and well-being
2. Religious and spiritual practices
3. Cultural practices
4. Lifestyle patterns

PROBLEM STATEMENTS AND OUTCOME IDENTIFICATION

I. Deficient Knowledge, related to cancer treatment and its effects and CAM practices (NANDA)

A. Expected outcomes

1. The patient will verbalize understanding of prescribed conventional treatment and CAM.

2. The patient will be able to identify risks and benefits of CAM practices in relation to CAM use with conventional medicine.

3. The health care team will demonstrate increased knowledge regarding CAM and provide CAM resources available in the institution, community, and Internet.

PLANNING AND IMPLEMENTATION

I. Interventions to increase patient knowledge about CAM and its effects on conventional therapy.

A. Encouraging open communication about conventional therapy options and CAM

1. Support of informal dialogue initiated by nurses, patients, and their families

a. Success depends on building rapport, ensuring a culturally sensitive and nonjudgmental social and professional environment.

b. Nurses must recognize that quick dismissals of CAM may shut down further communication.

c. All CAM therapies used by patient and who is guiding the use of the therapies, if known, should be documented.

d. Disclosure of CAM use is an ongoing process that is shaped by patient's health concerns and rapport with the health care team.

2. Explaining conventional therapies in a way that patients can understand them

3. Making an effort to comprehend why conventional medicine may not satisfy patient (e.g., lack of psychosocial support, poor symptom control, inconvenience, lack of understanding)

4. Exploring patient rationales for using CAM or contemplating CAM use (e.g., accessibility, fear of side effects, social pressure, agency and empowerment)

5. Emphasizing and supporting the patient's right to choose among therapeutic options

a. Therapeutic objectives for patient may not be the same as those of the health care team.

B. Ability to differentiate CAM practices that interfere with conventional medicine from those that complement it

1. Validating the appropriate use of CAM and explaining how some CAM practices may interfere with conventional medicine (e.g., cause antagonistic or other undesirable biophysical results, delay in or termination of conventional treatment).

2. Incorporation of compatible CAM practices into conventional medicine

II. Interventions to increase health care provider's knowledge about CAM, its effects on conventional therapy, and resources

A. Supporting the need for a well-informed health care team

1. Familiarity with CAM resources available in the institution, community, and Internet
2. Knowledge about CAM sources (including health food vendors)
3. Recognition that patients are important sources of information about CAM
4. Awareness that CAM may reflect cultural preferences and is an integral component of a patient's family and social identity
5. Ability to effectively discuss CAM from a scientific, evidence-based perspective
   a. Recognition that failure to offer objective information about safety and efficacy compromises patient-initiated dialogue about CAM
   b. Offering appropriate referrals to trusted trained professionals, as indicated

EVALUATION

The oncology nurse systematically and regularly evaluates the responses of the patient and those of the family or significant other to interventions to determine progress toward the achievement of expected outcomes. Relevant data are collected, and actual findings are compared with expected findings. Nursing diagnoses, outcomes, and plans of care are reviewed and revised, as necessary.

References

Barnes, P. M., Bloom, B., & Nahin, R. (2008). *Complementary and alternative medicine use among adults and children: United States, 2007 (DHHS Publication No. 2009-1240)*. Hyattsville, MD: National Center for Health Statistics.

Bercovitz, A., Sengupta, M., Jones, A., & Harris-Kojetin, L. D. (2011). *Complementary and alternative therapies in hospice: The National Home and Hospice Care Survey: United States, 2007 (DHHS Publication No. 2011-1250)*. Hyattsville, MD: National Center for Health Statistics.

Cassileth, B. R., Van Zee, K. J., Yeung, K. S., Coleton, M. I., Cohen, S., Chan, Y. H., et al. (2013). Acupuncture in the treatment of upper-limb lymphedema. *Cancer, 119*(13), 2455–2461.

Davidson, R. J., Kabat-Zinn, J., Schumacher, J., Rosenkranz, M., Muller, D., Santorelli, S. F., et al. (2003). Alterations in brain and immune function produced by mindfulness meditation. *Psychosomatic Medicine, 65*(4), 564–570.

Dossey, B. M., & Keegan, L. (2013). *Holistic nursing: A handbook for practice* (6th ed.). Burlington, MA: Jones & Bartlett.

Gahche, J., Bailey, R., Burt, V., Hughes, J., Yetley, E., Dwyer, J., et al. (2011). Dietary supplement use among U.S. adults has increased since NHANES III (1988-1994). *National Center for Health Statistics Data Brief, 61*, 1–8.

Hart, L. K., Freel, M. I., Haylock, P. J., & Lutgendorf, S. K. (2011). The use of healing touch in integrative oncology. *Clinical Journal of Oncology Nursing, 15*(5), 519–525.

Lawenda, B. D. (2012). *Integrative oncology essentials: A patients' guide to cancer care and prevention (Version 1.09.12)*. www.integrativeoncology-essentials.com.

National Cancer Institute, Office of Cancer Complementary and Alternative Medicine (NCI OCCAM). (2013). *Annual report on complementary and alternative fiscal year 2011*. Washington, DC: Author.

National Center for Complementary and Alternative Medicine (NCCAM). (2013). *What is CAM? All about complementary and alternative medicine*. nccam.nih.gov/health/whatiscam.

Pritchard, M., Elison-Bowers, P., & Birdsall, B. (2010). Impact on integrative restoration (irest) meditation on perceived stress levels in multiple sclerosis and cancer outpatients. *Stress and Health, 26*, 233–237.

Triscari, M. T., Faraci, P., D'Angelo, V., Urso, V., & Catalisano, D. (2011). Two treatments for fear of flying compared: Cognitive behavioral therapy combined with systematic desensitization or eye movement desensitization and reprocessing. *Aviation Psychology and Applied Human Factors, 1*(1), 9–14. http://dx.doi.org/10.1027/2192-0923/a00003, 419.

Zimmermann, A., Wozniewski, M., Szklarska, A., Lipowicz, A., & Szuba, A. (2012). Efficacy of manual lymphatic drainage in preventing secondary lymphedema after breast cancer surgery. *Lymphology, 45*(3), 103–112.

Part 4

CHAPTER 27

Alterations in Hematologic and Immune Function

Sandra Kurtin

OVERVIEW

I. Definition—*myelosuppression*, a reduction in bone marrow function that results in a reduced production of red blood cells (RBCs), white blood cells (WBCs), and platelets (Plt) into the peripheral circulation

II. Physiology (Kurtin, 2012; Metcalf, 2010; Undevia, Gomez & Ratain, 2005)

A. The bone marrow is the primary source for development of the components of blood (hematopoiesis), including myeloid and lymphoid progenitor cells.
   1. Myeloid cells include granulocytes (neutrophils, eosinophils, basophils, monocytes), RBC, and platelets.
   2. Lymphoid cells include B and T lymphocytes.

B. Risk factors for myelotoxicity are broadly categorized into three types: disease-related, patient-related, and treatment-related.

C. Chemotherapy-induced myelosuppression is the most common dose-limiting adverse event in cancer treatment.
   1. Each anti-neoplastic agent varies with respect to the onset and duration of cytopenias, depending on pharmacokinetic variables: dose, frequency, route of administration, absorption, distribution, metabolism, and excretion.

D. Treatment-related myeloid cytopenias, neutropenia and thrombocytopenia, are most common.
   1. Neutropenia—absolute neutrophil count (ANC) below 1500/mm^3 places the patient at increased risk of infection and sepsis.
   2. Thrombocytopenia—platelet count below the normal range; places the patient at increased risk of bleeding
   3. Anemia—hemoglobin below 10 g/dL places the patient at increased risk of fatigue and tissue hypoxia.

E. The severity of myeloid cytopenias is based on common grading criteria (Table 27-1).

F. Treatment-related lymphopenia is less common.
   1. Lymphopenia, a reduction in the number of B or T lymphocytes, places the patient at risk for opportunistic infections.

Neutropenia

OVERVIEW

I. Definition—a decrease in number of circulating neutrophils in the blood evidenced by ANC less than the lower limit of normal (LLN) (see Table 27-1)

A. Normal WBC—4.5 to 13.0 1000/μL

B. Neutrophils comprise 44% to 76% of the total WBC
   1. First line of defense against infection
   2. Life span—1 to 3 days (as little as 6 hours in stress situations)

C. ANC = % neutrophils (segs and bands) × WBC
   1. Grade 1—ANC < lower limit of normal to 1500/mm^3
   2. Grade 2—ANC <1500 to 1000/mm^3
   3. Grade 3—ANC <1000 to 500/mm^3
   4. Grade 4—ANC <500/mm^3
   5. Febrile neutropenia (FN)—ANC <1000/mm^3 and a single temperature of >38.3 ° C (101 ° F) or a sustained temperature of ≥38 ° C (100.4 ° F) for more than 1 hour (Freifeld, Bow, & Sepkowitz, 2010)
   6. Sample calculation of ANC
      a. WBC = 3.1 1000/μL
      b. Neutrophils (25%) + bands (10%) = 35%
      c. ANC = 3100 × 0.35 = 1085/mm^3 = grade 2 neutropenia

II. Physiology (Carlesso & Cardoso, 2010; Metcalf, 2010)

A. Chemotherapy-induced neutropenia (CIN) is one of the most common dose-limiting toxicities associated with systemic treatment for cancer.

Table 27-1

National Cancer Institute Common Criteria for Adverse Events, Version 4: Myelotoxicity (NCI-CTCAEv4)

Myelotoxicity	Definition	Grading
Anemia	A disorder characterized by an reduction in the amount of hemoglobin in 100 mL of blood	Grade 1: Hgb <LLN—10.0 g/dL Grade 2: Hgb <10.0-8.0 g/dL Grade 3: Hgb <8.0 g/dL, transfusion indicated Grade 4: Hgb <6.2-4.9 g/dL, Life-threatening consequences; urgent intervention indicated
Neutropenia	A finding based on laboratory test results that indicates a decrease in number of neutrophils in a blood specimen	Grade 1: ANC <LLN—1500/mm^3 Grade 2: ANC <1500-1000/mm^3 Grade 3: ANC <1000-500/mm^3 Grade 4: ANC <500/mm^3
Febrile neutropenia	A disorder characterized by an ANC < 1000/mm^3 and a single temperature of >38.3° C (101° F) or a sustained temperature of ≥38° C (100.4° F) for more than one hour	Grade 3: ANC < 1000/mm^3 with a single temperature of >38.3° C (101° F) or a sustained temperature of ≥38° C (100.4° F) for more than 1 hour Grade 4: Life-threatening consequences; urgent intervention indicated
Thrombocytopenia	A finding based on laboratory test results that indicate a decrease in number of platelets in a blood specimen	Grade 1: Plt < LLN–75,000/mm^3 Grade 2: Plt < 75,000-50,000/mm^3 Grade 3: Plt < 50,000-25,000/mm^3 Grade 4: Plt < 25,000/mm^3

ANC, Absolute neutrophil count; *Hgb*, hemoglobin; *LLN*, lower limit of normal; *Plt*, platelet.

Adapted from National Cancer Institute. (2013). *Common terminology criteria for adverse events (CTCAE) version 4.0.* ctep.cancer.gov/protocolDevelopment/electronic_applications/ctc.htm#ctc_40.

B. Neutrophils divide rapidly and are susceptible to the cytotoxic effects of chemotherapy.

C. Chemotherapy and radiation therapy may also damage the bone marrow microenvironment, including the stroma and cytokine milieu.

 1. Radiation to bone marrow–producing regions—pelvis, ribs, sternum, skull, metaphyses of the long bones—may cause prolonged cytopenias.

III. Risk factors (Aapro, Crawford, & Kamioner, 2010; Ahn & Lee, 2012; Daniel & Crawford, 2006; Kurtin 2010; Kurtin, 2012; Park et al., 2010; Schwenkglenks, et al., 2011) (Table 27-2)

A. Host-related factors

 1. Age greater than 65 years; more fat and less cellular marrow than in younger counterparts

 2. Female gender

 3. Eastern Cooperative Oncology Group (ECOG) performance scale (PS) >1

Table 27-2

Factors Associated with High Risk for Chemotherapy-Induced Myelotoxicity

Host-Related Factors	Disease- and Treatment-Related Factors
Age >65 yr	High tumor burden or extensive disease
Female gender	Previous history of chemotherapy or radiation
Eastern Cooperative Oncology Group (ECOG) performance scale (PS) >1	Preexisting cytopenias
Malnutrition	Bone marrow involvement with tumor
Immunosuppression	Type of chemotherapy
Comorbidities: chronic obstructive pulmonary disease, diabetes, renal impairment, liver disease	Dose intensity of chemotherapy
Open wounds or recent surgery	Elevated lactate dehydrogenase (LDH) level
Active infection or preexisting fungal infections	Hypoalbuminemia
Drug-drug interactions	Hyperbilirubinemia
	Hematologic malignancy
	Hospitalization

From Kurtin, S. (2012). Myeloid toxicity of cancer treatment. *Journal of the Advanced Practitioner in Oncology, 3,* 209–224.

4. Malnutrition
5. Immunosuppression
6. Comorbidities—chronic obstructive pulmonary disease (COPD), diabetes, renal impairment, liver disease
7. Open wounds or recent surgery
8. Active infection or pre-existing fungal infections
9. Drug-drug interactions
10. Tumor cell invasion into bone marrow
11. Hematologic malignancies
12. High tumor burden or extensive disease
13. Neutropenia lasting more than 4 days after an episode of FN
14. Concurrent mucositis, colitis, or typhlitis
15. Intensive care unit (ICU) admission
16. Disseminated intravascular coagulation (DIC)
17. Cross-reactive protein level greater than 100 mg/L at day 5 of treatment for FN
18. Confusion or altered mental status
19. Bleeding that is severe enough to require transfusion
20. Arrhythmia or electrocardiographic changes requiring treatment

  B. Treatment-related factors
1. Previous history of chemotherapy or radiation
2. Pre-existing cytopenias
3. Bone marrow involvement with tumor
4. Type of chemotherapy (Table 27-3)
5. Dose intensity of chemotherapy
6. Elevated lactate dehydrogenase (LDH)
7. Hypoalbuminemia
8. Hyperbilirubinemia
9. Hematologic malignancy
10. Hospitalization

  C. Biotherapy and steroids—may place the patient at risk due to immunosuppression and lymphopenia

IV. Principles of medical management (Aapro et al., 2010; Crawford et al., 2011; Klastersky, Awada, Paesmans, & Aoun, 2011; Kurtin, 2012; Talcott et al., 2011; Wingard & Elmongy, 2009) (Table 27-4)

  A. Prevention
1. Identification of patients at high risk
2. Patient and caregiver education for infection prevention that is appropriate to the level of risk
3. Prophylactic use of colony-stimulating factors (CSFs) recommended for the following reasons:
    a. Risk of CTC-AE grade 3/4 CIN or FN greater than 20% in the setting of potentially curable disease or where dose intensity is necessary for optimal clinical outcomes (see Table 27-1)
    b. Risk of CTC-AE grade 3/4 CIN of FN is 10% to 20% in patients with high-risk profile (see Table 27-1)

4. U.S. Food and Drug Administration (FDA)–approved agents for stimulation of neutrophils (Crea, Giovannetto. Zinzani, & Danesi, 2009; National Comprehensive Cancer Network [NCCN], 2013a)
    a. Filgrastim (Neupogen) 5 mcg/kg daily (rounding to the nearest vial size by institution-defined weight limits)
      (1) 24 hours or up to 4 days after treatment until post-nadir ANC recovers to normal or near-normal levels by laboratory standards
    b. Pegfilgrastim (Neulasta)
      (1) A single dose of 6 mg per cycle of treatment
      (2) Most often given the day after treatment; limited data support administration on the final day of chemotherapy
    c. Sargramostin (Leukine)
      (1) Used in clinical trials at a dose of 250 μg/m^2/day
      (2) 24 hours or up to 4 days after treatment, until post-nadir ANC recovery to normal or near normal levels by laboratory standards
    d. Prophylactic use of CSFs with concurrent chemotherapy or radiation not recommended
    e. Most common adverse events (AEs) associated with granulocyte CSF (G-CSF) agents—include bone pain, myalgia, arthralgia, and fever
    f. Bone pain managed with naproxyn 225 mg and loratadine 10 mg every 12 hours at the onset of bone pain and continued until resolved (generally 48-72 hours)

5. Prophylactic antibiotics considered only for patients with hematologic malignancies or at very high risk for FN—fluoroquinolone with or without glycopeptide, antifungal and antiviral agents; institution- or region-specific regimen based on common infectious agents

  B. Neutropenia without fever or active infection
1. Implementation of primary prevention, as above
2. Establishment of a plan for close monitoring of blood counts in initial phase of treatment when risk is greatest
3. Review of reportable signs and symptoms with patient and caregivers, including who to contact and how ⚠
4. Subsequent treatment requiring dose modification, dose delay, or administration of G-CSF agents as secondary prophylaxis
5. Low-risk patients with anticipated early recovery managed in an outpatient setting

Table 27-3

Common Chemotherapeutic Regimens for Selected Tumor Types with Intermediate to High Risk for Myelotoxicity

Bladder Cancer

MVAC (methotrexate, vinblastine, doxorubicin, cisplatin) (H)

Breast Cancer

AC→T→with trastuzumab (I)	AT (doxorubicin, paclitaxel (H)
CMF (cyclophosphamide, methotrexate, 5-fluorouracil) (I)	Dose-dense AC→T (doxorubicin, cyclophosphamide, paclitaxel) (H)
Docetaxel every 21 days (I)	Docetaxel+trastuzumab (H)
Epirubicin as a single agent or in sequential regimens with cyclophosphamide, 5-fluorouracil, methotrexate (I)	TAC (docetaxel, doxorubicin, cyclophosphamide) (H)
FEC→T (fluorouracil, epirubicin, cyclophosphamide, and sequential docetaxel) (I)	Paclitaxel+lapatinib (I)
Paclitaxel every 21 days (I)	Vinblastine (I)

Cervical Cancer

Cisplatin+topotecan (I)	Topotecan (I)	Irinotecan (I)

Colorectal Cancer

FOLFOX (fluorouracil, leucovorin, oxaliplatin) (I)

Esophageal and Gastric Cancer

DCF (docetaxel, cisplatin, fluorouracil) (H)	
Irinotecan, cisplatin (I)	ECF (epirubicin, cisplatin, 5-fluorouracil) (I)

Hodgkin Lymphoma

ABVD (doxorubicin, bleomycin, vinblastine, dacarbazine) (I)

BEACOPP (bleomycin, etoposide, doxorubicin, cyclophosphamide, vincristine, procarbazine, prednisone) (H)

Stanford V (mechlorethamine, doxorubicin, vinblastine, bleomycin, etoposide, prednisone) (I)

Kidney Cancer

Doxorubicin, gemcitabine (H)

Melanoma

Dacarbazine-based combinations with or without IL2 (H)

Non-Hodgkin Lymphoma (variation by subtype of NHL)

ICE (ifosfamide, carboplatin, etoposide) (H)	MINE (mesna, ifosfamide, novantrone, etoposide) (H)
CHOP-R -14 (cyclophosphamide, vincristine, doxorubicin, prednisone) (H)	Hyper-CVAD (rituximab, cyclophosphamide, vincristine, doxorubicin, methotrexate, cytarabine–alternating regimens) (H)
DHAP (dexamethasone, cisplatin, cytarabine) (H)	FC/FCR (fludarabine, Cytoxan, rituximab) (I)
ESHAP (etoposide, methyprednisolone, cisplatin, cytarabine) (H)	R-GEMP (rituximab, gemcitabine, methylprednisolone) (H)
CHOP-R (cyclophosphamide, doxorubicin, vincristine, prednisone) (I)	GDP (gemcitabine, dexamethasone, cisplatin)(I)

Non–Small Cell Lung Cancer

Docetaxel/carboplatin (H)	Etoposide/cisplatin (H)
Cisplatin/vinorelbine/cetuximab (H)	Paclitaxel/cisplatin (I)
Docetaxel/cisplatin (I)	Vinorelbine/cisplatin (I)

Ovarian Cancer

Docetaxel (H)	Paclitaxel (H)
Topotecan (H)	Carboplatin/docetaxel (I)

Sarcoma

MAID (mesna, doxorubicin, ifosfamide, dacarbazine) (H)

Small Cell Lung Cancer

ACE (doxorubicin, cyclophosphamide, etoposide) (H) Topotecan (H)	ICE (ifosfamide, carboplatin, etoposide) (H)
Topotecan/cisplatin (I)	Etoposide/carboplatin (I)

Testicular Cancer

VeIP (vinblastine, ifosfamide, cisplatin) (H)	VIP (etoposide, ifosfamide, cisplatin) (H)
BEP (bleomycin, etoposide, cisplatin) (H)	TIP (paclitaxel, ifosfamide, cisplatin) (H)
Etoposide/cisplatin (I)	

Uterine Cancer

Docetaxel (I)

Intermediate risk (I) is defined as 10% to 20%, and high risk (H) is defined as >20%. This excludes myeloid malignancies and multiple myeloma.

From Kurtin, S. (2012). Myeloid toxicity of cancer treatment. *Journal of the Advanced Practitioner in Oncology, 3,* 209–224.

Table 27-4

Recommendations for Prevention and Management of Chemotherapy-Induced Neutropenia (CIN) and Febrile Neutropenia (FN)

Assessment of risk	• See Table 27-2 and Table 27-3 for consideration for description of risk factors for CIN caused by disease-related, host-related, and treatment-related factors.

Prevention	• Patient and caregiver education for infection prevention appropriate to the level of risk
	• Prophylactic use of colony-stimulating factors (CSFs) is recommended when:
	  • Risk of CTC-AE grade 3/4 CIN or FN is >20% in the setting of potentially curable disease or where dose intensity is necessary for optimal clinical outcomes
	  • Risk of CTC-AE grade 3/4 CIN or FN is 10% to 20% in patients with high-risk profile
	• FDA-approved agents:
	  • Filgrastim (Neupogen) dosing guidelines (www.neupogen.com)
	  • Pegfilgrastim (Neulasta) dosing guidelines (www.neulasta.com)
	• Consider prophylactic antibiotics for patients with hematologic malignancies at very high risk for FN—fluoroquinolone with or without glycopeptide, antifungal, antiviral agents.

Management of CIN	• Implement primary prevention, as above. • Establish a plan for close monitoring of blood counts in initial phase of treatment when risk is greatest. • Review reportable signs and symptoms with patient and caregivers, including who to contact and how. • Subsequent treatment may require dose modification, dose delay, or administration of granulocyte CSF (G-CSF) agents as secondary prophylaxis. • Low-risk patients with anticipated early recovery can be managed in an outpatient setting. • Most common adverse events (AEs) associated with G-CSF agents include bone pain, myalgia, arthralgia, and fever. • Bone pain can be effectively managed with naproxyn 225 mg and loratadine 10 mg every 12 hr at the onset of bone pain and continued until resolved (generally 48-72 hr).
Management of FN	• FN is considered a medical emergency. • Prompt intervention is critical to avoid morbidity and mortality. • Rapid assessment should be performed for risk of clinical deterioration. • Implement institutional standard of care for FN, including obtaining cultures (blood and urine), chest radiography (posteroanterior and lateral), viral and vancomycin-resistant enterococci (VRE) swabs, if indicated, and prompt administration of intravenous antibiotics (cefepime most common first-line agent). • Unstable patients should be transported by emergency medical services equipped with Advanced Cardiac Life Support (ACLS) capabilities. • Patients at very high risk for poor prognosis may require ICU admission.

From Kurtin, S. (2012). Myeloid toxicity of cancer treatment. *Journal of the Advanced Practitioner in Oncology, 3*, 209–224.

C. Febrile neutropenia ⚠

1. Considered a medical emergency
2. Prompt intervention critical to avoid morbidity and mortality
3. Rapid assessment for risk of clinical deterioration
   a. Hypotension—systolic blood pressure (SBP) less than 90 mm Hg
   b. Tachypnea—respiratory rate (RR) greater than 24 breaths/min
   c. Serum albumin— less than 3.3 g/dL
   d. Serum bicarbonate level—less than 21 mmol/L
   e. Cross-reactive protein level—greater than 20 mg/L at baseline
   f. High procalcitonin level—greater than 2.0 ng/mL
   g. Circulating soluble triggering receptor (sTREM-1) —greater than100 pg/mL
   h. High pentraxin 3 (PTX3) levels at the onset of FN
4. Implementation of institutional standard of care for FN—obtaining cultures (blood and urine), chest radiography (posteroanterior and lateral), viral and VRE (vancomycin-resistant enterococci) swabs, if indicated, and prompt administration of intravenous antibiotics (cefepime most common first-line agent)
5. Rapid deterioration in patients with FN; prompt management of these patients essential to avoid more severe AEs such as cardiovascular collapse or death
6. Unstable patients to be transported by emergency medical services equipped with Advanced Cardiac Life Support (ACLS) capabilities
7. Intensive care unit (ICU) admission for patients with FN at high risk for poor prognosis

V. Potential sequelae of prolonged neutropenia
  A. Delay in administering treatment on time or dose delays; dose reductions
  B. Circulatory collapse
  C. Acute respiratory failure
  D. Sepsis and septic shock
  E. Death

ASSESSMENT

I. History (Flores & Ershler, 2009; Kurtin, 2012)
  A. Review of current and previous cancer therapy
  B. Chemotherapy, radiation therapy, biotherapy, or multimodal therapy
  C. Previous incidence of neutropenia or neutropenic fevers
  D. Hematopoietic growth factor use
  E. Review of bone marrow biopsy report, if available, to determine bone marrow involvement or hypocellularity
  F. Review of comorbid conditions and current medications placing the patient at increased risk (see Risk Factors)
  G. Review of infection history, including bacterial, fungal, and viral infections
  H. Review of current antibiotic regimen such as trimethoprim-sulfamethoxazole (Bactrim) or amphotericin B, which can decrease the neutrophil count
II. Physical examination (Flores & Ershler, 2009; Klastersky et al., 2007; Kurtin, 2012)
  A. Assessment of vital signs—fever the most common manifestation of infection
    1. Rigors should be treated emergently in a patient with neutropenia.
    2. Hypotension (SBP < 90 mm Hg) or tachypnea (RR > 24) are indicative of high risk for clinical deterioration.
  B. Characteristic signs of infection (erythema, induration, drainage, and cough)—may not be apparent because of suppression of the phagocytic response
    1. Commonly infected sites—include the respiratory tract, gastrointestinal (GI) tract, genitourinary tract, perineum, anus, and skin
    2. Assessment of all indwelling catheter sites
    3. Assessment of for abnormal breath sounds
    4. Assessment of the oral cavity for thrush, plaque, redness, infected ulcerations
    5. Assessment for abdominal tenderness, stiffness, and guarding
    6. Assessment for change in mental status
    7. Assessment of nutritional status—protein-calorie malnutrition causes lymphopenia, diminished levels of the complement system, and a decrease of certain immunoglobulins

C. Laboratory data
  1. Complete blood cell count (CBC) with differential
  2. Calculation of ANC
  3. Culture and sensitivity testing of urine, blood, stool, sputum, cerebrospinal fluid (CSF), wound, and drainage tubes or bags
D. Radiology
  1. Chest radiography (PA and lateral)

PROBLEM STATEMENTS AND OUTCOME IDENTIFICATION

I. Risk for Imbalanced Body Temperature (NANDA-I)
  A. Expected outcome—patient maintains a normal body temperature.
II. Risk for Infection (NANDA-I)
  A. Expected outcome—patient does not develop major infectious complications as a result of neutropenia.
  B. Expected outcome—patient's ANC is greater than 1000/mm^3.
III. Deficient Knowledge (NANDA-I), related to infection precautions
  A. Expected outcome—patient accurately describes appropriate infection precautions.

PLANNING AND IMPLEMENTATION

I. Pharmacologic—see Section IV of Overview.
II. Nonpharmacologic (Flores & Ershler, 2009; Kurtin, 2012) ⚠
  A. Interventions to minimize the occurrence of infection
    1. Using strict hand washing technique
    2. Encouraging patient to bathe daily, taking care to maintain meticulous personal hygiene, including oral and perineal care
    3. Restricting presence of vases with fresh flowers or other sources of stagnant water
    4. Limiting visitors to those without communicable illness, especially children
    5. Changing water in pitchers, denture cups, and nebulizers daily
  B. Use of aseptic technique for all nursing interventions, including all indwelling catheters (e.g., venous access devices, urinary, biliary or feeding tubes), wounds, or invasive procedures; specific institutional guidelines to be referred to for management of central catheters
III. Interventions to monitor for complications
  A. Establishing a plan for monitoring blood counts based on the patients individual risk profile (see risk factors and Table 27-2)
  B. Monitoring for nadir (the lowest point of the blood cell levels after cancer treatment)
    1. Nadir becomes apparent as immature cells in the marrow are destroyed and become absent in the bloodstream.

2. Usually 7 to 14 days after chemotherapy, with variability for combined modality treatments, nitrosourea agents, and radiation to the pelvis
3. Occasional occurrence after biotherapy
4. Usually after multimodal treatment; nadir occurring sooner and more severely than from single-modality therapy

C. Cancer treatment usually held for an ANC less than 1000 to 1500/mm^3.

D. Monitoring for signs and symptoms of infection

IV. Interventions to incorporate patient and family in care

A. Teaching about personal hygiene measures to minimize the occurrence of infection—examples: wiping the perineal area from front to back after voiding and after a stool; daily bathing ⚠

B. Teaching about infection precautions and how to minimize the risk of infection—example: strict hand washing ⚠

C. Teaching about subcutaneous administration of hematopoietic growth factors

D. Teaching about the symptoms for which to call the physician or nurse, such as temperature higher than 100.5° F (38.1° C), productive cough, painful urination, or sore throat ⚠

EVALUATION

The oncology nurse systematically and regularly evaluates the patient's and family's responses to neutropenia to prevent infection. Relevant data are collected, and actual findings are compared with expected findings. Nursing diagnoses, outcomes, and plans of care are reviewed and revised, as necessary.

Anemia

OVERVIEW

I. Definition— a disorder characterized by a reduction in the amount of hemoglobin in 100 mL of blood (CTC-AE version 4)

A. Normal values—gender-specific
1. Female—hemoglobin (Hgb): 11.5 to 15.5 g/dL; hematocrit (Hct): 35% to 46%
2. Male—Hgb: 13.5 to 17.5 g/dL; Hct: 40% to 51%

B. RBC life span—120 days

C. Patients at increased risk of fatigue, tachycardia, tachypnea, chest pain, dyspnea, and syncope

D. Risk related to severity of anemia
1. Grade 1—(Hgb) less than LLN to 10.0 g/dL; less than LLN to 6.2 mmol/L; less than LLN to 100 g/L
2. Grade 2—Hgb less than 10.0 to 8.0 g/dL; less than 6.2 to 4.9 mmol/L; less than 100 to 80 g/L
3. Grade 3—Hgb less than 8.0 g/dL; less than 4.9 mmol/L; less than 80 g/L; transfusion indicated
4. Grade 4—life-threatening consequences; urgent intervention

II. Physiology (Carlesso & Cardoso, 2010; Metcalf, 2010)

A. Erythrocytes are developed from the myeloid stem cells in bone marrow.

B. Function of RBCs is to carry oxygen to all cells in the body.

C. Anemia is a common finding in patients with cancer, with an incidence ranging from 30% to 90% (Rodgers et al., 2012).

III. Risk factors (Daniel & Crawford, 2006; Kurtin, 2012; Slichter, 2007; Slichter et al., 2010)

A. Patient-related factors
1. Risk factors for neutropenia or myelosuppression
2. Any disorder with occult blood loss

B. Disease-related factors
1. Risk factors for neutropenia or myelosuppression
2. Autoimmune hemolytic anemia
3. Chronic GI blood loss
4. Malnutrition with deficiencies of folic acid, vitamin B$_{12}$
5. Iron deficiencies—gastric bypass surgery, inability to absorb oral iron
6. Chronic renal insufficiency
7. Invasion of tumor cells in the bone marrow or cancers involving the bone marrow such as multiple myeloma, lymphoma, leukemia, or myelodysplastic syndromes
8. Erythroid leukemia
9. Myelodysplastic syndromes
10. Rare genetic disorders that affect RBC production—thalassemia

C. Treatment-related factors
1. Most chemotherapeutic agents affect granulocytes and platelets before measurable effects on the RBCs seen; some agents known to cause treatment-related anemia such as cisplatin
2. Drug-induced red blood cell aplasia (rare)
3. Evaluation of anemia in relation to other cytopenias

IV. Principles of medical management (Kurtin, 2010; Kurtin, 2011; Slichter, 2007; Slichter et al., 2010; Triulzi et al., 2012) (Box 27-1)

A. Prevention of anemia
1. Identification of patients at high risk for anemia and the secondary effects
   a. Evaluation of symptoms and underlying disease
   b. Determination of chronicity
2. Consideration of individual characteristics of the patients such as underlying comorbidities affected by anemia, cardiovascular and pulmonary diseases
3. Patient and caregiver education for conservation of energy, planning of activities, and reportable sign and symptoms

---

Box 27-1

Recommendations for Management of Chemotherapy-Induced Anemia (CIA)

Assessment of Risk

- High risk factors for more serious complications of anemia include:
  - Cardiopulmonary disease, progressive or rapid decline in hemoglobin (Hgb) with or without recent chemotherapy or radiation, sustained symptoms such as tachycardia, tachypnea, chest pain, dyspnea, syncope, debilitating fatigue

Treatment

General Principles of Treatment

- Establishment of the underlying cause(s)—bleeding, nutritional, inherited, renal insufficiency, treatment, chronic disease, hemolysis
- Treatment of the underlying cause(s)
- Evaluation of symptoms of anemia with consideration of individual patient characteristics
- Weighing of the risks and benefits of each treatment approach (packed red blood cell [PRBC] transfusion, erythropoiesis-stimulating agent [ESA] administration)

Transfusion of PRBCs

- Requires informed consent
- Asymptomatic patients—transfuse to maintain Hgb 7 to 9 g/dL
- Symptomatic with hemorrhage—transfuse to maintain hemodynamic stability
- Symptomatic with Hgb < 10 g/dL—transfuse to maintain Hgb 8 to 10 g/dL
- Acute coronary syndromes with anemia—transfuse to maintain Hgb > 10 g/dL

Benefits

- Rapid increase in Hgb may improve fatigue in some patients

Risks

- Viral transmission—HIV: 3.1/100,000; hepatitis C: 5.1/100,000; hepatitis B: 3.41-3.43/100,000
- Transfusion-related acute lung injury (TRALI)—0.81/100,000

- Transfusion-associated circulatory overload (TACO)—1% to 6% to higher in ICU and postoperative settings
- Fatal hemolysis—1.3 to 1.7 per 1 million transfused units
- Febrile nonhemolytic reactions—1.1% to 2.15%

ESA Administration

- FDA-approved agents: Aranesp (darbepoetin alfa), Procrit (epoetin alfa), Epogen (epoetin alfa)
- Not indicated in patients receiving chemotherapy with curative intent
- Requires REMS compliance and training for providers (ESA APPRISE Oncology Program) (https://www.esa-apprise.com/ESAAppriseUI/ESAAppriseUI/default.jsp)
- Requires informed consent from patients
- Goal—to administer the lowest dose necessary to avoid PRBC transfusion not to exceed Hgb of 10 g/dL
- If Hgb rises >1 g/dL in any 2-week period, dose reductions are required; see prescribing information at https://www.esa-apprise.com/ESAAppriseUI/ESAAppriseUI/default.jsp

Benefits

- Avoidance of transfusions

Risks

- Inferior survival and decreased time to progression, most notably with target Hgb > 12 g/dL
- www.fda.gov/cder/drug/infopage/RHE/default.htm
- Thrombosis—increased with risk with history of coagulopathy, obesity, coronary artery disease, thrombocytosis, hypertension, immobilization, hospitalization, selected hormonel therapies, immunomodulatory agents (www.nccn.org/professionals/physician_gls/f_guidelines.asp#supportive)
- Hypertension or seizures
- Pure red blood cell aplasia (rare)

From Kurtin, S. (2012). Myeloid toxicity of cancer treatment. *Journal of the Advanced Practitioner in Oncology, 3,* 209–224.

Part 4

---

4. Establishing a plan of care for monitoring blood counts and follow-up
5. Maintaining a current type and screen for patients requiring frequent transfusions

B. Packed RBC transfusions
  1. Benefits—improvement in symptoms of anemia
  2. Risks
     a. Viral transmission—human immunodeficiency virus (HIV): 3.1/100,000;

hepatitis C: 5.1/100,000; hepatitis B: 3.41 to 3.43/100,000
     b. Transfusion-related acute lung injury (TRALI)—0.81/100,000
     c. Transfusion-associated circulatory overload (TACO)—1% to 6% to higher in ICU and postoperative settings
     d. Fatal hemolysis—1.3 to 1.7 per million transfused units

e. Febrile nonhemolytic reactions—1.1% to 2.15%

f. Exacerbation of underlying cardiopulmonary disease, including congestive heart failure

g. Iron overload and secondary organ toxicity

3. Administration

a. Requires informed consent

b. Asymptomatic patients—transfuse to maintain Hgb at 7 to 9 g/dL

c. Symptomatic with hemorrhage—transfuse to maintain hemodynamic stability

d. Symptomatic with Hgb less than 10 g/dL— transfuse to maintain Hgb at 8 to 10 g/dL

e. Acute coronary syndromes with anemia— transfuse to maintain Hgb at greater than 10 g/dL

C. Erythropoietin-stimulating proteins (ESAs) (see Box 27-1)

1. Benefits—avoidance of transfusions

2. Risks

a. Inferior survival and decreased time to progression—most notably with target Hgb greater than 12 g/dL

b. Thrombosis—increased risk with history of coagulopathy, obesity, coronary artery disease, thrombocytosis, hypertension, immobilization, hospitalization, selected hormonel therapies, immunomodulatory agents

c. Hypertension or seizures

d. Pure RBC aplasia (rare)

3. Administration

a. FDA-approved agents

(1) Darbepoetin alfa (Aranesp), epoetin alfa (Procrit or Epogen)

(2) Not indicated in patients receiving chemotherapy with curative intent

(3) Requires Risk Evaluation and Mitigation Strategy (REMS) compliance and training for providers (ESA APPRISE Oncology Program) www.esa-apprise. com/ESAAppriseUI/ESAAppriseUI/ default.jsp

(4) Requires informed consent from patients

b. Goal—to administer the lowest dose necessary to avoid packed RBC (PRBC) transfusion not to exceed Hgb of 10 g/dL

c. If Hgb rises greater than 1 g/dL in any 2-week period, dose reductions required—see prescribing information (www.esa-apprise. com/ESAAppriseUI/ESAAppriseUI/ default.jsp).

ASSESSMENT

See Kurtin, 2012; Slichter, 2007.

I. History

A. Previous cancer treatment such as chemotherapy, radiation therapy, or multimodal therapy

B. Current medications that could alter RBC function

C. Social history of alcohol intake and illicit drug use

II. Physical examination (Kurtin, 2012)

A. Assessment for bleeding such as from rectum, nose, ears, oral cavity

B. Assessment of all stool, urine, and vomitus for blood

C. Assessment of the skin for pallor

D. Assessment for menstrual bleeding and the number of sanitary napkins or tampons used

E. Assessment for changes that indicate intracranial bleeding—changes in level of consciousness, restlessness, headache, seizures, pupil changes, ataxia

III. Laboratory data

A. CBC with platelets and differential

B. Evaluation of contributing factors for anemia

1. Iron deficiency

2. Folate deficiency

3. Vitamin B_{12} deficiency

4. Gastrointestinal blood loss

5. Hemolysis screening

6. Thyroid function

7. Testosterone level

C. Serum erythropoietin level

PROBLEM STATEMENTS AND OUTCOME IDENTIFICATION

I. Deficient Knowledge (NANDA-I), related to energy conservation

A. Expected outcome—Patient accurately describes appropriate energy conservation strategies.

II. Risk for Injury (NANDA-I)

A. Expected outcome—patient can describe reportable signs and symptoms that require emergent medical care. ⚠

B. Expected outcome—patient has resolution of anemia.

C. Expected outcome—patient does not develop any complications as a result of anemia.

D. Expected outcome—patient will not fall or sustain any injuries.

PLANNING AND IMPLEMENTATION

I. Pharmacologic—see Section IV of Overview.

II. Nonpharmacologic (Kurtin, 2012; Kurtin et al., 2012) ⚠

A. Interventions to minimize secondary effects of anemia

B. Cancer treatment generally held for Hgb less than 7.5 g/dL with the exception of known bone marrow disorders

C. PRBC transfusions based on World Health Organization (WHO) guidelines for transfusion

III. Implementation of strategies to incorporate patient and family in care ⚠
   A. Teaching the family and patient about energy conservation and reportable signs and symptoms
   B. Teaching the family and patient about signs of transfusion reactions
   C. Teaching about safety measures to decrease the potential for injury caused by syncope or dyspnea during periods of anemia

EVALUATION

The oncology nurse systematically and regularly evaluates the patient's responses to anemia and its treatment to prevent secondary organ effects or injury. Relevant data are collected, and actual findings are compared with expected findings. Nursing diagnoses, outcomes, and plans of care are reviewed and revised, as necessary.

Thrombocytopenia

OVERVIEW

I. Definition—decrease in the circulating platelets below the LLN based on institutional laboratory measures—(CTC-AE version 4)
   A. Normal count—150,000 to 400,000/mm^3
   B. Life span—10 to 12 days (as little as 24 hours in stressful situations)
   C. Patients with thrombocytopenia at an increased risk of bleeding
   D. Risk related to the severity of thrombocytopenia
      1. Grade 1—platelets (Plt) less than LLN to 75,000/mm^3
      2. Grade 2—Plt less than 75,000 to 50,000/mm^3
      3. Grade 3—Plt less than 50,000 to 25,000/mm^3
      4. Grade 4—Plt less than 25,000/mm^3
II. Physiology (Carlesso & Cardoso, 2010; Metcalf, 2010)
   A. Megakaryocytes develop and form the myeloid stem cells in bone marrow.
   B. Each megakaryocyte produces millions of platelets each day and can be measured in peripheral blood.
   C. The function of platelets is to maintain vascular hemostasis, prevent blood loss through platelet adhesion to block small breaks in blood vessels, and initiate clotting mechanisms.
III. Risk factors (Daniel & Crawford, 2006; Kurtin, 2012; Slichter, 2007; Slichter et al., 2010).
   A. Patient-related factors
      1. Risk factors for neutropenia
      2. Concurrent administration of anti-platelet agents
   B. Disease-related factors
      1. Risk factors for neutropenia or myelosuppression
      2. Underlying platelet disorders—idiopathic thrombocytopenic purpura or thrombotic thrombocytopenic purpura causing accelerated platelet destruction

3. Coagulation abnormalities
   a. Hypocoagulation—vitamin K deficiency from malnutrition or liver disease alters the development of prothrombin and several clotting factors.
   b. Hypocoagulation—paraneoplastic syndromes, DIC, and thrombosis, increase the use of platelets
4. Splenomegaly—platelet sequestration in the spleen
5. Invasion of tumor cells into bone marrow or cancers involving bone marrow such as multiple myeloma, lymphoma, leukemia, or myelodysplastic syndromes
6. Megakaryocytic leukemia
   C. Treatment-related factors
      1. Risk factors for neutropenia or myelosuppression, including chemotherapy and radiation
         a. Platelet count—usually decreases in 7 to 14 days after administration or sooner with multimodal treatment
         b. Usually decrease in platelet count after the drop in WBCs
         c. Recovery usually occurs within 2 to 6 weeks
      2. Endotoxins released from bacteria during an infection—can damage platelets and alter platelet aggregation
      3. Some medications can alter platelet development; such as aspirin, clopidogrel (Plavix), digoxin (Lanoxin), furosemide (Lasix), heparin, phenytoin (Dilantin), quinidine, sulfonamides (Bactrim), and tetracycline.
IV. Principles of medical management (Kurtin, 2010; Kurtin, 2012; Slichter, 2007; Slichter et al., 2010; Triulzi et al., 2012) (Box 27-2)
   A. Prevention of thrombocytopenia
      1. Identification of patients at high risk for thrombocytopenia and bleeding
         a. WHO bleeding grades
            (1) Grade 1—petechiae, ecchymosis, occult blood in body secretions, mild vaginal spotting
            (2) Grade 2—evidence of gross hemorrhage not requiring RBC transfusion over routine needs: epistaxis, hematuria, hematemesis
            (3) Grade 3—hemorrhage of one or more units of PRBCs per day
            (4) Grade 4—life-threatening hemorrhage, defined as either massive bleeding causing hemodynamic compromise or bleeding into a vital organ (e.g. intracranial, pericardial, or pulmonary hemorrhage).

Box 27-2

Recommendation for Management of Chemotherapy-Induced Thrombocytopenia

Assessment of Risk

- CTC-AE risk (see Table 27-4) and WHO bleeding grades
  - Petechiae, ecchymosis, occult blood in body secretions, mild vaginal spotting
  - Evidence of gross hemorrhage not requiring red blood cell (RBC) transfusion over routine needs: epistaxis, hematuria, hematemesis
  - Hemorrhage of one or more units of packed RBCs (PRBCs) per day
  - Life-threatening hemorrhage, defined as either massive bleeding causing hemodynamic compromise or bleeding into a vital organ (e.g., intracranial, pericardial, or pulmonary hemorrhage)
- Evaluation of symptoms and underlying disease
- Determination of chronicity
- Consideration of individual characteristics of the patient, including proximity to treatment center, concomitant anticoagulation therapy or antiplatelet drugs, prior response to platelets, concurrent inflammatory process or infection, CNS disease

Prevention of Risk

- Evaluation of bleeding risk, as above
- Establishing a plan of care for monitoring blood counts and follow-up
- Maintaining a current type and screen for patients requiring frequent transfusions
- Withholding anticoagulation therapy for platelet count less than 50,000/μL
- Educate the patient and caregivers about bleeding precautions and reportable sign and symptoms.

Platelet Products
Random Donor Platelets (RDPs)

- Centrifuged from whole blood
- Common dose administered, 4 to 6 random donor units (pooled from multiple units of whole blood)
- Larger volume—1 unit = 60 mL, 6 units = 360 mL
- Exposure to more donors

Single-Donor Platelets (SDPs)

- Single donor undergoes apheresis—process requires 1.5 to 2.5 hr
- Approximately 200 mL
- Process is costly—more than twice the cost of RDPs
- Leuko reduced product from more recent procedures

Platelet (Plt) Transfusions Based on Platelet Levels and Patient Characteristics

- Plt $\leq$ 10,000/μL—threshold for therapeutic platelet transfusions
- Patients with a history of bleeding or an active infectious process—may require higher threshold for transfusion
- Surgical or invasive procedure—platelets to be maintained at >50,000 μL; for more aggressive procedures and for patients with complicating factors, higher platelet count may be required
- Neurosurgical procedures—platelets to be maintained at >100,000 μL/L
- Premedication for platelets required in patients with history of urticaria
- Evaluation of response to platelets performed by obtaining post-platelet count 30 to 60 min after infusion

From Kurtin, S. (2012). Myeloid toxicity of cancer treatment. *Journal of the Advanced Practitioner in Oncology, 3*, 209–224.

---

b. Evaluation of symptoms and underlying disease
c. Determination of chronicity

2. Consideration of individual characteristics of the patients, including proximity to treatment center, concomitant anticoagulation therapy or antiplatelet drugs, prior response to platelets, concurrent inflammatory process or infection, central nervous system (CNS) disease
3. Patient and caregiver education for bleeding precautions or risks and reportable sign and symptoms ⚠
4. Establishing a plan of care for monitoring blood counts and follow-up
5. Maintaining a current type and screen for patients requiring frequent transfusions
6. Withholding anticoagulation therapy for platelet count less than 50,000/μL ⚠

B. Platelet transfusions
  1. Random donor platelets (RDP)
     a. Centrifuged from whole blood
     b. Common dose administered is 4 to 6 random donor units (pooled from multiple units of whole blood)
     c. Larger volume—1 unit = 60 mL; 6 units = 360 mL
     d. Results in patient exposure to more donors

2. Single-donor platelets (SDP)
   a. Single donor undergoes apheresis—process requires 1.5 to 2.5 hours
   b. Approximately 200 mL
   c. Process costly—more than twice the cost of RDP transfusion
   d. Leuko reduced product from more recent procedures
3. Platelet less than 10,000/μL—threshold for therapeutic platelet transfusion
4. Patients with a history of bleeding or an active infectious process—may require higher threshold for transfusion
5. Surgical or invasive procedure—maintain platelets greater than 50,000 μL; more aggressive procedures and for patients with complicating factors may require higher platelet count. ⚠
6. Neurosurgical procedures—platelets maintained at greater than 100,000 μL/L ⚠
7. Premedication for platelets required in patients with history of urticarial reactions
8. Evaluation of response to platelets by obtaining post–platelet count 30 to 60 minutes after infusion

C. Administration of plasma to replenish clotting factors when patient is actively bleeding and becomes refractory to platelets
D. Progestational agents prescribed to decrease menstrual bleeding
E. Drug-induced or disease-related bleeding treated with steroids

V. Potential sequelae of prolonged thrombocytopenia
   A. Delay in administering treatment on time or dose delays; dose reductions
   B. Refractory to platelet transfusions (alloimmunization)
   C. Internal bleeding such as intracranial, GI, or respiratory tract bleeding
   D. Transfusion reaction or transmitted disease
   E. Death

ASSESSMENT

See Kurtin, 2012; Slichter, 2007.
I. History
   A. Previous cancer treatment such as chemotherapy, radiation therapy, or multimodal therapy
   B. Current medications that could alter platelet production
   C. Social history of alcohol intake and illicit drug use
II. Physical examination (Kurtin, 2012)
   A. Assessment for bleeding such as from rectum, nose, ears, oral cavity
   B. Assessment for petechiae, which usually appear initially on the upper and lower extremities, then on pressure points, elbows, and the oral palate
   C. Assessment of all stool, urine, and vomitus for blood
   D. Assessment of the skin for ecchymosis, purpura, or oozing of puncture sites
   E. Assessment for conjunctiva hemorrhage and sclera injection
   F. Assessment for menstrual bleeding and the number of sanitary napkins or tampons used
   G. Assessment for changes that indicate intracranial bleeding, such as changes in level of consciousness, restlessness, headache, seizures, pupil changes, ataxia
III. Laboratory data
   A. Platelet count
   B. Coagulation values—fibrinogen, prothrombin time, partial thromboplastin time
   C. Antiplatelet antibodies

PROBLEM STATEMENTS AND OUTCOME IDENTIFICATION

I. Deficient Knowledge (NANDA-I), related to bleeding precautions
   A. Expected outcome—patient accurately describes appropriate bleeding precautions.
II. Risk for Injury (NANDA-I)
   A. Expected outcome—patient has resolution of thrombocytopenia.
   B. Expected outcome—patient does not develop any complications as a result of thrombocytopenia.
   C. Expected outcome—patient will not fall or sustain any injuries.

PLANNING AND IMPLEMENTATION

I. Pharmacologic—see Section IV of Overview.
II. Nonpharmacologic (Kurtin, 2012) ⚠
   A. Interventions to minimize the occurrence of bleeding
      1. Avoiding the use or overinflation of a blood pressure cuff or use of a tourniquet when the platelet count is less than 20,000/mm^3
      2. Avoiding invasive procedures such as enema, taking rectal temperature, administering suppositories, bladder catheterization, venipuncture, finger stick, use of nasogastric tubes, administering subcutaneous or intramuscular injection
      3. Preparation of the environment to avoid trauma (e.g., padding side rails, arranging furniture to eliminate sharp corners, clearing walkways)
      4. Applying firm direct pressure to venipuncture site for 5 minutes
   B. Encouraging patient to wear shoes during ambulation to maintain skin integrity
   C. Encouraging patient to avoid sharp objects such as a straight-edge razor

D. If bleeding not controlled, applying absorbable gelatin sponges or liquid thrombin
E. For nosebleeds, placing the patient in high Fowler position and applying pressure to the nose
F. Applying ice packs to decrease the bleeding
G. Implementing a bowel elimination regimen to prevent constipation
H. Use of soft toothbrushes by patient to avoid gingival trauma
I. Instructing patient to avoid physical activity that may lead to trauma
J. Monitoring platelet levels
K. Cancer treatment usually withheld for platelet count less than 50,000 to 100,000/mm^3
L. Platelet transfusion based on WHO guidelines for transfusion

III. Implementation of strategies to incorporate patient and family in care ⚠
A. Teaching the family and patient bleeding precautions
B. Teaching the family and patient signs of bleeding that should be called to the attention of the physician or nurse
C. Teaching about safety measures to decrease the occurrence of bleeding when performing activities of daily living, including fall prevention

EVALUATION

The oncology nurse systematically and regularly evaluates the patient's responses to thrombocytopenia and its treatment to prevent bleeding. Relevant data are collected, and actual findings are compared with expected findings. Nursing diagnoses, outcomes, and plans of care are reviewed and revised, as necessary.

Infection

OVERVIEW

See NCCN, 2013b; Wood & Payne, 2011.
I. Definition—when the body or a part of the body is invaded by a microorganism or virus and an infection develops, depending on three factors
A. Infectious diseases an important factor in morbidity and mortality in cancer patients
II. Physiology (Wood & Payne, 2011).
A. Susceptibility to cancer-related infections results from the nature of the malignancy and cancer treatments.
1. Impairment of host defense mechanisms—skin and mucosal barriers (mucositis, dermatologic reactions, invasive procedures), neutropenia, immunosuppression
2. Increased susceptibility to infections with variable risk throughout the cancer diagnosis
3. Prolonged immunosuppression, which increases the risk of opportunistic infections (viruses,

fungi, mycobacteria, rare bacterial strains) and more severe consequences of common pathogens
B. Most important physical barrier against invasion of organism—the skin and mucosal barriers
C. WBCs, particularly neutrophils, an important defense against infection
III. Risk factors (NCCN, 2013b; Wood & Payne, 2011)
A. Patient-related factors
1. Immunodeficiency associated with primary malignancy
2. Neutropenia
3. Disruption of mucosal barriers
4. Splenectomy and functional asplenia
5. Corticosteroids and other lymphotoxic agents
6. Comorbid conditions
7. Malnutrition; hypoalbuminemia
8. Hypogammaglobulinemia
9. Chronic obstructive pulmonary disease (COPD)
10. Renal or hepatic insufficiency
11. Poor performance status
12. Age greater than 65 years
B. Disease- and treatment-related factors
1. Hematologic or lymphoid malignancy
2. Hematopoietic stem cell transplantation; graft-versus-host disease (GVHD)
3. High tumor burden
4. Remission status
5. Prior exposure to chemotherapy and intensity of immunosuppressive therapy
6. Solid organ transplantation
7. Cytotoxic chemotherapy—depth and duration of neutropenia (see Neutropenia)
8. T- and B-cell suppressants, steroids, purine analogs, alemtuzumab
9. Barriers breached—vascular access device (VAD), mucositis, surgery
10. Radiation therapy
11. Stem cell transplantation or GVHD (see Chapter 20)
12. HIV
13. Chronic neutropenic conditions
IV. Principles of medical management
A. Identification of patients at risk
B. Instituting preventive antimicrobial treatments for patients at high risk for viral, fungal, or opportunistic bacterial infections
C. Isolation of the source, if possible
D. Administration of antibiotics, according to organism isolated
E. Using meticulous skin, mucosal, and wound care
F. Administration of WBC line growth factors, as appropriate (see Neutropenia)

V. Potential sequelae of prolonged infection
  A. Delay in treatment or ineligibility for selected treatment because of infection history
  B. Pneumonia and acute respiratory distress
  C. Cardiovascular collapse
  D. Septic shock
  E. Resistance to antibiotics or superinfection
  F. Death

ASSESSMENT

I. History (NCCN, 2013b; Wood & Payne, 2011)
  A. Review of previous cancer therapy such as chemotherapy, radiation therapy, biotherapy, or multimodal therapy
  B. Review of infection history
  C. Review of known allergies to medications, especially antibiotics
  D. Review of immunosuppressive therapy
II. Physical examination (NCCN 2013b; Wood & Payne, 2011).
  A. Complete physical examination to isolate potential source: skin, mucosa, lungs, sinus, perirectal, abdomen, wounds, indwelling catheters
  B. Assessment of mental status for orientation, confusion, memory recall, alertness
  C. Assessment of rapidity of onset of symptoms
  D. Vital signs
    1. Fever—pattern, severity, associated symptoms
    2. Blood pressure and respirations—hypotension (SBP < 90 mm Hg) or tachypnea (RR >24) indicative of high risk for clinical deterioration
    3. Heart rate—tachycardia may be present
    4. Assessment of vital signs every 4 to 8 hours or more often as indicated for trends or deviations from the normal
  E. Assessment of urine or stool for color, consistency or clarity, odor, presence of blood
III. Laboratory data
  A. CBC with differential
  B. Culture and sensitivity testing of the urine, stool, blood, sputum, wounds, drainage bags or tubes
  C. Rectal swabs for VRE
  D. Oral swabs for viruses
  E. Stool for *Clostridium difficile*
  F. Skin or wound swabs for bacterial, viral, fungal infections
  G. Skin punch biopsy to isolate fungal infections
IV. Radiology
  A. Chest radiography (PA and lateral)
  B. Additional radiology testing based on suspected source

PROBLEM STATEMENTS AND OUTCOME IDENTIFICATION

I. Risk for Infection (NANDA-I)
  A. Expected outcome—patient accurately describes appropriate infection precautions.

II. Risk for Injury (NANDA-I)⚠
  A. Expected outcome—patient does not develop major complications from the infectious process.

PLANNING AND IMPLEMENTATION

I. Pharmacologic—see Section IV of Overview.
II. Nonpharmacologic (NCCN, 2013b; Wood & Payne, 2011)
  A. Interventions to minimize infections ⚠
    1. Using strict hand washing before and after all contact with patient
    2. Promoting and encouraging meticulous personal and oral hygiene, perineal care
    3. Avoiding unnecessary invasive procedures such as giving enemas, taking rectal temperatures, bladder catheterization, and venipuncture
    4. Administering vaccinations such as flu vaccine, Pneumovax, to prevent communicable infections
    5. Use of aseptic technique when performing nursing interventions
    6. Ensuring adequate hydration and a high-calorie, high-protein diet
  B. Interventions to locate source of infection
    1. Obtaining appropriate cultures such as blood, sputum, stool, urine, and wounds, as indicated
    2. Educating the patient and family about signs and symptoms of infection and when to call the physician or nurse ⚠
    3. Having chest radiography performed, as ordered
    4. Reporting critical changes in patient assessment parameters to physician ⚠

EVALUATION

The oncology nurse systematically and regularly evaluates the patient's responses to infection and its treatment to determine progress toward the achievement of safety and lack of untoward outcomes. Relevant data are collected, and actual findings are compared with expected findings. Nursing diagnoses, outcomes, and plans of care are reviewed and revised, as necessary.

Hemorrhage

OVERVIEW

I. Definition—the occurrence of abnormal internal or external discharge of blood
II. Physiology
  A. Hemostasis is the process of a solid clot forming in the blood from a fluid component.
  B. Coagulation is the mechanism of forming a stable fibrin clot.
  C. Hemorrhage occurs in cancer patients from alterations in hemostasis or coagulation mechanisms.
III. Risk factors (Kurtin, 2012; NCCN, 2013b; Wood & Payne, 2011).

Part 4

A. Disease-related
  1. Cerebral hemorrhage may occur with severe thrombocytopenia or with brain metastases.
  2. Myeloproliferative disorders such as polycythemia vera, myelofibrosis, and thrombocythemia may cause hemorrhage phenomena.
  3. DIC may result from prostate cancer or acute promyelocytic leukemia.
  4. Paraneoplastic syndromes may stimulate bleeding.
  5. Splenomegaly may cause bleeding.
B. Treatment related
  1. Bone marrow or hematopoietic stem cell transplantation may cause a diffuse alveolar hemorrhage characterized by cough, dyspnea, and hypoxemia.
  2. DIC may occur as a result of cancer treatment.
  3. High-dose chemotherapy such as with cyclophosphamide (Cytoxan) may cause hemorrhagic cystitis or myocardial hemorrhage.
  4. All types of surgical procedures pose a risk for hemorrhage, especially if the tumor is embedded within arteries or veins.
IV. Principles of medical management (NCCN, 2013b)
  A. Administration of appropriate blood products
  B. Administration of oxygen
  C. Vasopressor drugs—may control severe bleeding
  D. Lavage with iced saline through a nasogastric tube—may control gastric bleeding
V. Potential sequelae of prolonged hemorrhage
  A. Viral disease from numerous blood transfusions
  B. Shock
  C. Transfusion reaction
  D. Death

ASSESSMENT

I. History (NCCN, 2013b; Wood & Payne, 2011)
  A. Review of previous cancer therapy such as chemotherapy, radiation therapy, or multimodal treatment
  B. Ascertaining recent traumatic events
  C. Review of the cancer
  D. Evidence of metastasis to the brain or bone marrow
  E. Leukemia, especially nonlymphocytic leukemia, which may cause hemorrhage as a result of a paraneoplastic process
  F. Review of past medical history for the occurrence of peptic or gastric ulcer disease or esophageal varices
II. Physical examination
  A. Assessment for signs of hemorrhage complications such as weak pulse, irregular pulse, pale skin, cold and moist skin
  B. Assessment of all urine, stool, vomitus, and sputum for blood
  C. Assessment of vital signs
  D. Assessment for neurologic deficits such as reduced level of alertness or orientation

III. Laboratory data
  A. CBC
  B. Coagulation factors
  C. Occult stool test
  D. Bleeding time

PROBLEM STATEMENTS AND OUTCOME IDENTIFICATION

I. Risk for Deficient Fluid Volume (NANDA-I)
  A. Expected outcome—patient does not develop complications as a result of hemorrhage.
  B. Expected outcome—patient has resolution of hemorrhage.
II. Ineffective Peripheral Tissue Perfusion (NANDA-I)
  A. Expected outcome—patient does not have tissue compromise as a result of hemorrhage.

PLANNING AND IMPLEMENTATION

I. Pharmacologic—see Section IV of Overview.
II. Nonpharmacologic (Kurtin, 2012; NCCN, 2013b).
  A. Interventions to minimize the bleeding
    1. Applying occlusive dressings to bleeding wounds after cleansing the area
    2. If applicable, elevating the body part above the heart level and applying firm pressure over the area
    3. Administering plasma and other blood components
  B. Interventions to monitor for complications ⚠
    1. Hemodynamic measurements—decrease in cardiac output and decrease in blood pressure
    2. Strict intake and output records to detect negative fluid balance
    3. Reporting critical changes in the patient's assessment parameters to the physician, such as change in mental status, decrease in blood pressure, increase in bleeding

EVALUATION

The oncology nurse systematically and regularly evaluates the patient's responses to hemorrhage interventions to determine progress toward hemodynamic stability. Relevant data are collected, and actual findings are compared with expected findings. Nursing diagnoses, outcomes, and plans of care are reviewed and revised, as necessary.

Fever and Chills

OVERVIEW

I. Definition—elevation of body temperature above 100.4° F (38° C) to 101.3° F (38.5° C) orally (CTC-AE version 4)
  A. Chills (shivering) occur as a body's response to heat loss when the body's temperature abruptly increases, as with fever or a drug reaction.

B. Involuntary contractions of the skeletal muscles occur with shivering.

C. The internal body temperature is maintained by shivering, which is a thermoregulatory mechanism.

D. Shivering is a subjective feeling of cold.

E. Fever is initiated by the release of endogenous pyrogens from phagocytic WBCs.

F. Vasodilation and sweating are physiologic mechanisms used to increase heat loss.

G. Vasoconstriction and shivering are the body's mechanisms for conserving or producing heat.

H. Production of fever occurs as a response to the elevation of the set point in the temperature-regulating center in the hypothalamus.

I. Shivering results in an increase in metabolic activity and oxygen consumption brought about by an increase in muscle tone.

J. Skin temperature drops because of vasoconstriction, which decreases heat loss.

K. Each degree of temperature Fahrenheit results in a 7% increase in metabolic rate and increases the demands on the heart.

II. Physiology

  A. The thermoregulatory center in the hypothalamus controls body temperature.

  B. Various heat loss mechanisms help return the temperature to normal levels during fevers.

III. Risk factors

  A. Disease related

    1. See Neutropenia and Infection sections.

    2. Tumor involving the hypothalamus, where the temperature control for the body is located

    3. Paraneoplastic syndromes

    4. Pyrogens released by the tumor cells, which produce a fever, especially in the presence of uncontrolled tumor growth

    5. Most common tumors associated with tumor-induced fever—include Hodgkin disease, osteogenic sarcoma, lymphoma, liver metastasis

  B. Treatment related

    1. See Neutropenia and Infection sections.

    2. Chemotherapy side effects from agents that can cause a drug fever or flulike syndrome (e.g., bleomycin [Blenoxane], daunorubicin [Cerubidine], thiotepa [Thioplex], methotrexate [Mexate], dacarbazine (DTIC-Dome), plicamycin [Mithracin])

    3. Blood transfusion reaction

    4. Biotherapy side effect from interferon, monoclonal antibody, or interleukin

    5. Steroid-induced adrenal insufficiency

    6. Drug-induced, as with vancomycin or amphotericin B

    7. Invasive procedure

IV. Principles of medical management (NCCN, 2013b)

  A. Assessment of patient for possible causes, clinical manifestations

  B. Administering acetaminophen alternated with ibuprofen every 2 hours to decrease fever and drug toxicity; caution with use in patients with thrombocytopenia

  C. Administering nonsteroidal anti-inflammatory drugs (NSAIDs) for tumor-induced fever; caution with use in patients with thrombocytopenia or renal insufficiency

  D. Treating the underlying cause

V. Potential sequelae of prolonged fever and chills

  A. Increase in fatigue, muscle weakness, myalgia; reduced quality of life

  B. Dyspnea

  C. Cardiopulmonary compromise

  D. Death

ASSESSMENT

I. History (NCCN, 2013b)

  A. Previous cancer treatments and any reactions

  B. Previous exposure to infections

  C. Type of cancer and extent of disease

  D. Previous blood transfusions

  E. Current medications

  F. History of hypersensitivity reactions

II. Physical examination (NCCN, 2013b; Wood & Payne, 2011)

  A. Frequent assessment of vital signs

  B. Complete physical examination to ascertain the source of fever

  C. Review of laboratory data, additional laboratory analysis based on suspected cause (e.g., neutropenia-related fevers, drug reactions, cholangitis)

PROBLEM STATEMENTS AND OUTCOME IDENTIFICATION

I. Risk for Imbalanced Body Temperature (NANDA-I)

  A. Expected outcome—patient's fever and chills resolve.

II. Ineffective Thermoregulation (NANDA-I)

  A. Expected outcome—patient does not develop complications as a result of fever and chills.

  B. Expected outcome—patient participates in strategies to maximize comfort.

PLANNING AND IMPLEMENTATION

I. Pharmacologic—see section IV of Overview.

II. Interventions to locate the source of infection

  A. Obtaining cultures from the blood, throat, urine, stool, sputum, and wounds when an infection is suspected, including cultures from all access devices

III. Interventions to provide comfort

A. Promoting slow cooling of the skin and mucous membranes
B. Tepid sponge baths
C. Reduced amount of patient clothing
D. Mechanical cooling blankets
E. Reduction of the environmental temperature
F. Avoiding rapid reduction in body temperature that can cause chilling by providing warm blankets or heating pads at the first sign of chilling
G. Changing damp clothing immediately to prevent chilling
H. Administering acetaminophen, aspirin or ibuprofen to reduce fever ⚠
   1. Acetaminophen—not to exceed 4000 mg in a 24-hour period; to be used with caution in patients with liver disease
   2. Aspirin—to be used with caution in patients with platelet disorders
   3. Ibuprofen—to be used with caution in patients with renal impairment
I. Increasing fluid intake to prevent dehydration
J. Educating patient as to self-care measures for fever or chills, including medication management

IV. Interventions to minimize the occurrence of infection in common sites
A. Encouraging patient to cough and take deep breaths every 4 to 8 hours while awake
B. Encouraging patient to perform oral hygiene every 4 hours while awake
C. Encouraging patient to void frequently
D. Instructing the patient to avoid the use of douches or tampons
E. Encouraging the patient to eat well-balanced meals and increase fluid intake

EVALUATION

The oncology nurse systematically and regularly evaluates the patient's responses to interventions for fever and chills to determine progress toward the achievement of expected outcomes. Relevant data are collected, and actual findings are compared with expected findings. Nursing diagnoses, outcomes, and plans of care are reviewed and revised, as necessary.

References

Aapro, M., Crawford, J., & Kamioner, D. (2010). Prophylaxis of chemotherapy-induced febrile neutropenia with granulocyte-stimulating factors: Where are we now? *Supportive Care in Cancer, 18,* 529–541.

Ahn, S., & Lee, Y. S. (2012). Predictive factors for poor prognosis febrile neutropenia. *Current Opinion in Hematology, 24,* 376–380.

Carlesso, N., & Cardoso, A. (2010). Stem cell regulatory niches and their role in normal and malignant hematopoiesis. *Current Opinion Hematology, 17,* 281–286.

Crawford, J., Allen, J., Armitage, J., Blayney, D. W., Cataland, S. R., Heanwey, M. L., et al. (2011). Myeloid growth factors. *Journal of the National Comprehensive Cancer Network, 9,* 914–932.

Crea, F., Giovannetti, E., Zinzani, P. L., & Danesi, R. (2009). Pharmacological rationale for early G-CSF prophylaxis in cancer patients and role of pharmacogenetics in treatment optimization. *Critical Reviews in Oncology Hematology, 72,* 21–44.

Daniel, D., & Crawford, J. (2006). Myelotoxicity from chemotherapy. *Seminars in Oncology, 33,* 74–85.

Flores, I. Q., & Ershler, W. (2009). Managing neutropenia in older patients with cancer receiving chemotherapy in a community setting. *Clinical Journal of Oncology Nursing, 14,* 81–86.

Freifeld, A., Bow, E., & Sepkowitz, K. (2010). Clinical practice guideline for the use of antimicrobial agents in neutropenic patients with cancer: 2010 update by the Infectious Diseases Society of America. *Clinical Infectious Diseases, 52,* e56–e93, 2011.

Klastersky, J., Ameye, L., Maertens, J., Georgala, A., Muanza, F., Aoun, M., et al. (2007). Bacteraemia in febrile neutropenic cancer patients. *International Journal of Antimicrobial Agents, 30* (Suppl. 1), S51–S59.

Klastersky, J., Awada, A., Paesmans, M., & Aoun, M. (2011). Febrile neutropenia: A critical review of the initial management. *Critical Reviews in Oncology Hematology, 78,* 185–194.

Kurtin, S. (2010). Risk analysis in the treatment of hematologic malignancies in the elderly. *Journal of the Advanced Practitioner in Oncology, 1,* 119–129.

Kurtin, S. (2011). Leukemia and myelodysplastic syndromes. In C. H. Yarbro, D. Wujcik, & B. H. Gobel (Eds.), *Cancer nursing: Principles and practice.* (7th ed., pp. 1369–1398). Sudbury, MA: Jones and Bartlett.

Kurtin, S. (2012). Myeloid toxicity of cancer treatment. *Journal of the Advanced Practitioner in Oncology, 3,* 209–224.

Metcalf, D. (2010). The colony-stimulating factors and cancer. *Nature Reviews Cancer, 10,* 425–434.

National Comprehensive Cancer Network. (2013a). *NCCN clinical practice guidelines in oncology. Myeloid growth factors, version 1.2013.* www.nccn.org.

National Comprehensive Cancer Network. (2013b). *NCCN clinical practice guidelines in oncology. Prevention and treatment of cancer-related infections, version 1.2013.* www.nccn.org.

Park, Y., Kim, D. S., Park, S. J., Seo, H. Y., Lee, S. R., Sung, H. J., et al. (2010). The suggestion of a risk stratification system for febrile neutropenia with hematologic disease. *Leukemia Research, 34,* 294–300.

Rodgers, G. M., Becker, P. S., Blinder, M., Cella, D., Chanan-Khan, A., Cleeland, C., et al. (2012). Cancer and chemotherapy-induced anemia. *Journal of the National Comprehensive Cancer Network, 10,* 628–653.

Schwenkglenks, M., Pettengell, R., Jackisch, C., Paridaens, R., Constenal, M., Bosly, A., et al. (2011). Risk factors for chemotherapy-induced neutropenia occurrence in breast cancer patients: Data from the INC-EU Prospective. Observational European Neutropenia Study. *Supportive Care in Cancer, 19*(4), 483–490.

Slichter, S. J. (2007). Evidence-based platelet transfusion guidelines. *Hematology, 2007*(1), 172–178.

Slichter, S., Kaufman, R. M., Assmann, S. F., McCullough, J., Triulzi, D. J., Strauss, R. G., et al. (2010). Dose of prophylactic platelet transfusions and prevention of hemorrhage. *New England Journal of Medicine, 362,* 600–613.

Talcott, J. A., Yeap, B. Y., Clark, J. A., Siegel, R. D., Loggers, E. T., Lu, C., & Godley, P. A. (2011). Safety of early discharge for low-risk patients with febrile neutropenia: A multicenter randomized controlled trial. *Journal of Clinical Oncology, 29,* 3977–3983.

Triulzi, D. J., Assmann, S. F., Strauss, R. G., Ness, P. M., Hess, J. R., Kaufman, R. M., et al. (2012). The impact of platelet transfusion characteristics on post-transfusion platelet increments and clinical bleeding in patients with hypoproliferative thrombocytopenia. *Blood, 119,* 5553–5562.

Undevia, S. D., Gomez-Abuin, G., & Ratain, M. (2005). Pharmacokinetic variability of anticancer agents. *Nature Reviews Cancer, 5,* 447–458. http://dx.doi.org/dx.doi.org/10.1038/nrc1629.

Wingard, J. R., & Elmongy, M. (2009). Strategies for minimizing complications of neutropenia: Prophylactic myeloid growth factors or antibiotics. *Critical Reviews in Oncology Hematology, 72,* 144–154.

Wood, S., & Payne, J. (2011). Cancer-related infections. *Journal of the Advanced Practitioner in Oncology, 2,* 356–371.

Part 4

CHAPTER 28

Alterations in Gastrointestinal Function

Leslie Nelson

Xerostomia

OVERVIEW

I. Definition—a subjective sensation of dryness in the mouth caused by a reduction in the quantity of saliva produced or a change in its composition (Visvanathan & Nix, 2010)

II. Pathophysiology—causes include medications with antimuscarinic properties, radiotherapy (RT) to the head and neck area, uncontrolled diabetes, and specific diseases of the salivary gland (Visvanathan & Nix, 2010)

III. Risk factors and causes (Box 28-1)
   A. Disease-related
      1. Primary tumor involving the salivary or parotid glands
      2. Metastatic tumor involving the salivary glands
      3. Other diseases or conditions—diabetes, infection, candidiasis, Sjögren syndrome, obsessive-compulsive disorder, and anxiety states
   B. Treatment-related
      1. Surgical removal of salivary glands
      2. Pharmacologic therapy for symptom management and other comorbid conditions: antihistamines, decongestants, anticholinergics, diuretics, antidepressants, opioids, phenothiazines, anorexic agents, antihypertensives, antipsychotics, antiparkinsonian agents, diuretics, hypnotics, anxiolytics
      3. RT effects (Jensen et al., 2010)
         a. Can be transient or prolonged
         b. Increases risk of oral infections and carious destruction of teeth, oral mucosal discomfort and pain, hampered oral functioning, and a worsened nutritional state
         c. Most frequent and permanent complaint after conventional RT to the head and neck related to the cumulative RT dose and the volume of salivary gland tissue included in the treatment portals
         d. Timing—decreased salivary flow rates within first week of treatment; second phase may be noted after RT
   C. Lifestyle-related—alcohol, caffeine, nicotine, and ingestion of drugs that decrease the flow of saliva (Visvanathan & Nix, 2010)
   D. Age—younger people more likely to recover salivary flow compared with older adults

IV. Principles of medical management (Visvanathan & Nix, 2010)
   A. General or supportive measures—avoidance of drugs that cause xerostomia; taking frequent sips of water; and obtaining counseling for recognized anxiety states, treatment for underlying oral candidiasis if present, and early referral for dental care
   B. Salivary stimulation—has a greater benefit over salivary substitutes in patients who have residual salivary function
      1. Salivary stimulants
         a. Chewing gum
         b. Vitamin C (ascorbic acid)—less effective than other stimulants
         c. Malic acid—found in fruits such as apples and pears
         d. Pilocarpine—available in 5-mg tablets; recommended dose up to 30 mg/day; up to 12 weeks to reach maximum effectiveness; cholinergic effects contraindicate agent in patients with asthma, chronic obstructive pulmonary disease (COPD), heart disease, epilepsy, Parkinson disease, or hyperthyroidism
   C. Salivary substitutes—contain electrolytes that correspond to normal saliva, mucin, or methylcellulose-based preparations; mucin-based products better tolerated and have a longer duration of action
   D. Surgical interventions—salivary reservoirs, reconstruction of mandibular dentition

Box 28-1

Causes of Xerostomia

....

Drugs Causing Xerostomia
Bronchodilators
Antiparkinsonian drugs
Tricyclic antidepressants
Antipsychotics
Decongestants
Antihistamines
Mydriatic eye drops
Drugs for urinary incontinence
Antihypertensives
Diuretics
Drugs used for irritable bowel and diverticular disease

Diseases Causing Xerostomia
Primary Sjögren syndrome
Secondary Sjögren syndrome
Rheumatoid arthritis
Systemic lupus erythematosus
Diabetes mellitus
Sarcoidosis
Human immunodeficiency infection
Primary biliary cirrhosis
Scleroderma

Other Causes of Xerostomia
Anxiety or depression
Amyloidosis
Wegener granulomatosis
Radiotherapy to the head and neck
Bone marrow transplantation
Chronic graft-versus-host disease

Adapted from Visvanathan, V. & Nix, P. (2010). Managing the patient presenting with xerostomia: A review. *International Journal of Clinical Practice*, 64(3), 404–407.

E. Dental prophylaxis with frequent cleaning and fluoride treatments before, during, and after RT
F. Prophylactic oral antimicrobial therapy

ASSESSMENT

I. History
   A. Previous therapy for cancer
   B. Prescription and nonprescription medications and supplements (e.g., vitamins and mineral supplements)
   C. Pattern of xerostomia—incidence, frequency, alleviating and aggravating factors
   D. Impact of xerostomia on food taste, intake, swallowing, digestion, and communication, as well as psychosocial response to condition
II. Physical examination
   A. Dry, shiny mucous membranes of oral cavity; thin, pale-looking mucosa

B. Thick, ropy, and scant saliva; may result in cracked lips, dry tongue, mouth sores, and periodontal disease
   C. Difficulty swallowing, chewing, and communicating
   D. Salivary gland examination—parotid and submandibular often enlarged (Visvanathan & Nix, 2010)
      1. Sialometry—normal saliva flow variable, less than 0.12 to 0.16 mL/min considered abnormal
      2. Histology of minor salivary gland biopsy
III. Laboratory findings—to rule out autoimmune or other disease process
   A. Complete blood cell (CBC) count—abnormal in some autoimmune diseases
   B. Biochemistry—signs of dehydration
   C. Liver function tests—elevated in cirrhosis patients
   D. Immunology—rule out rheumatoid arthritis (RA), human immunodeficiency virus (HIV), Sjögren syndrome
IV. Psychosocial examination—presence of fear, anxiety, or both

PROBLEM STATEMENTS AND OUTCOME IDENTIFICATION

I. Risk for Impaired Oral Mucous Membrane (NANDA-I)
   A. Expected outcome—patient describes risk factors for development of xerostomia.
II. Risk for Infection (NANDA-I)
   A. Expected outcome—patient states signs, symptoms, and complications of infection and participates in interventions that may prevent infection.
III. Disturbed Sensory Perception: gustatory ⚠
   A. Expected outcome—patient verbalizes appropriate diet to protect oral cavity.

PLANNING AND IMPLEMENTATION

I. Interventions to minimize the risk of occurrence and severity of xerostomia
   A. Measures to increase salivary flow by stimulating residual parenchyma
      1. Offering salivary stimulants (agents that affect salivary glands)
         a. Chewing gum, vitamin C, malic acid (e.g., apples and pears)
         b. Salivary enzyme products (e.g., Biotene, sugarless gum, toothpaste, mouthwash containing xylitol)
         c. Pilocarpine (Salagen) to stimulate remaining salivary function
   B. Interventions to provide moisture to the oral mucosa
      1. Moistening of foods with liquids, milk, or gravies
      2. Sipping liquids with and between meals at frequent intervals
      3. Increasing intake to eight glasses of liquid per day unless contraindicated

4. Using artificial saliva such as oxygenated glycerol triester spray or aqueous electrolyte spray (Furness, Worthington, Bryan, Birchenough, & McMillan, 2011)
5. Use of ice chips, popsicles, effervescent vitamin C (except when receiving RT), malic acid, pilocarpine (Visvanathan & Nix, 2010)
6. Use of room humidifier, humidified face mask, or both at night; use of hyperthermic humidification, which has shown some promise
7. Use of protective enzymes present in some foods
   a. Papain, which is found in papaya juice
   b. Amylase, present in pineapples (use frozen to minimize stinging)
   c. Meat tenderizer, which helps dissolve and break up thick saliva (mouth to be swabbed before meals)
8. Lubricating the mucosa with ⅛ teaspoon of butter or vegetable or corn oil before meals, starting 2 to 3 weeks after RT has been completed
9. Use of lip balm
10. Nonpharmacologic measures (Cho, 2013)
    a. Acupressure—application of physical techniques such as neck massage, pressure on the sternal notch, or both, tailored to patient preference
    b. Psychotherapy to aid in pain relief
    c. Hypnosis
    d. Relaxation techniques
    e. Imagery training

C. Interventions to decrease risk of complications of xerostomia
1. Frequent assessments for early detection
2. Encouraging patient to maintain meticulous oral hygiene with mechanical and chemical debridement of accumulated plaque and microorganisms at regular intervals at least before and after each meal; every 2 hours ideal
3. Having patient avoid physical, chemical, and thermal irritants such as poorly fitting dental prosthetics, hydrogen peroxide, alcohol, tobacco, commercial mouthwashes, and food items such as dry, bulky, spicy, and acidic foods

II. Interventions to monitor for complications related to xerostomia
A. Examination of oral cavity daily; observation of lips, tongue, buccal area membranes, throat, swallow, roof and floor of mouth, saliva, and voice quality
B. Encouraging periodic dental examinations
C. Advising patient to seek prompt and appropriate medical treatment if infection develops

EVALUATION

The oncology nurse systematically and regularly evaluates the patient's and family's responses to xerostomia interventions to determine progress toward oral cavity protection and restoration. Relevant data are collected, and actual findings are compared with expected findings. Problem statements, outcomes, and plans of care are reviewed and revised, as necessary.

Dysphagia

OVERVIEW

I. Definition—any disruption in the swallowing process during bolus transport from the oral cavity to the stomach (Gaziano, 2013)
II. Pathophysiology, cause, and risk factors
A. Neurologic impairment
1. Loss of innervation (i.e., of cranial nerves V, VII, IX, X, XI, and/or XII; thus loss of swallow reflex)
2. Loss of vocal cord control
B. Tumor infiltration and impingement of the esophagus and mouth by tumor, treatment-related effects, or both (Gaziano, 2013)
1. Major surgery that impairs the ability to hold food in mouth, lateralize, masticate, form a bolus, and move a bolus through the oropharynx and esophagus
2. RT to the site causing fibrosis or stenosis
3. Mucositis, aphthous ulceration, candidiasis
4. Chemotherapy effects on the oral cavity and esophagus
5. Changes in character of oral secretions from RT and chemotherapy
C. Iatrogenic factors
1. Psychotropic medications that impair gag reflex and swallowing
2. Anticholinergic drugs
D. Lifestyle-related effects (e.g., emotional responses to disease and treatment)
III. Progression of dysphagia
A. Usually insidious and slowly progressive
B. Usually manifested as difficulty swallowing solids, progressing to difficulty swallowing liquids, including saliva, increasing the risk for aspiration, pneumonia, or both
C. Usually associated with weight loss, anorexia, nausea, dehydration, protein-calorie malnutrition, cachexia, muscle wasting, and negative nitrogen wasting
D. Older adults at increased risk, as well as patients with certain cancer types—head and neck cancer, esophageal and lung carcinomas with lymph node involvement

IV. Principles of medical management (Raber-Durlacher et al., 2012)
   A. Treatment for underlying disease—nodal RT, laser surgery, antifungal and antibiotic medications
   B. Endoscopic laser therapy
   C. Alternative method for feedings; may require short- or long-term interventions
   D. Use of thickening agents (e.g., Thick-It, Nutra-Thik, Thick'N Easy) to lessen the risk for flow of liquids into the airway causing choking and aspiration
   E. Medications—steroids, expectorants, bronchodilators, pain and anxiety medications to relieve symptoms related to dysphagia
   F. Swallowing therapy, direct swallowing exercise, or both

ASSESSMENT

I. History
   A. Previous treatments for cancer
   B. Presence of underlying systemic disease—infection, cardiac disease, or stroke
   C. Patterns of dysphagia—incidence; pattern; alleviating, aggravating, and precipitating factors
   D. Impact on lifestyle, comfort, activities of daily living, and quality of life (QOL)
II. Physical examination
   A. Observation for presence of facial droop, drooling, oral retention, choking, coughing after swallowing, and gurgling voice quality
   B. Determining patient's ability to masticate, hold food in mouth, and propel food to oropharynx using tongue
   C. Eliciting patient's subjective report of pain or discomfort; weakness of lips, tongue, or jaw; "lump in the throat"
   D. Assessment of lungs because of potential for aspiration

PROBLEM STATEMENTS AND OUTCOME IDENTIFICATION

I. Impaired Swallowing (NANDA-I)
   A. Expected outcome—patient participates in measures to minimize the complications of impaired swallowing.
II. Risk for Aspiration (NANDA-I) ⚠
   A. Expected outcome—patient participates in measures to minimize aspiration.
   B. Expected outcome—patient and family demonstrate competence in emergency techniques related to aspiration, regurgitation, and airway obstruction.
III. Risk for Injury (NANDA-I) ⚠
   A. Expected outcome—patient and family list symptoms or changes that require professional assistance and management, including aspiration,

airway obstruction, weight loss greater than 5% of body weight, and dehydration.
   B. Expected outcome—patient and family identify resources in the community to assist with coping.

PLANNING AND IMPLEMENTATION

I. Nonpharmacologic interventions that minimize the risk of occurrence or complications of dysphagia (Gaziano, 2013)
   A. Management of the underlying cause of dysphagia
   B. Consultation with speech or occupational therapist to perform a swallow test to determine extent of problem
   C. Educating patient and family about methods to facilitate the effectiveness and ease of swallowing (Gaziano, 2013)
      1. Head posture
         a. Chin tuck
         b. Turning head to weaker side
         c. Tilting head to stronger side or backward
      2. Body posture
         a. Upright at 90 degrees
         b. Lying on one side
      3. General swallowing tips
         a. Decreasing rate of intake
         b. Multiple swallows per bolus
         c. Alternating solids with liquids
         d. Decreasing bolus size
         e. Liquids by spoon or puree by syringe
   D. Providing appropriate assist devices—straws, plunger spoon, Asepto syringe, and/or pastry tube.
   E. Ensuring adequate food and calorie intake with high-calorie, high-protein foods, providing enteral feedings, or both throughout the day (e.g., eight small feedings)
   F. Educating patient and family about decreasing pain with swallowing—ice chips, soft or pureed foods, semisolid foods, avoidance of hot and spicy foods, use of local anesthetics
   G. Nutrition consult
   H. Occupational therapy consultation for evaluation of swallowing
II. Interventions to maximize safety (Kaspar & Ekberg, 2012) ⚠
   A. Prevention of aspiration by using mechanical techniques
      1. Elevating head of bed 45 to 90 degrees, with head slightly forward while patient is eating and having the patient maintain position for 45 to 60 minutes after oral intake
      2. Assisting with moving food from front of tongue to posterior area using a long-handled spoon or a syringe, as needed
   B. Minimizing swallowing difficulty by having the patient avoid milk products and alternate solids with liquids and encouraging chewing thoroughly on the strongest side of the mouth

C. Explaining all procedures before occurrence to decrease fear or anxiety associated with attempts to swallow and staying with patient during feedings

D. Having patient avoid small pieces of solids that can become lost in the mouth

E. Consultation with dietitian to provide thickening agents to minimize aspiration

F. Use of a variety of foods served in an appetizing way, in a progressive manner—pureed to ground to soft-textured to all textures, based on serial swallow tests

III. Interventions to monitor complications related to dysphagia (Kaspar & Ekberg, 2012)

A. Maintaining a daily food record

B. Weighing the patient daily, or at least every other day if daily weighing upsets the patient

C. Assessment for signs and symptoms—dehydration, aspiration, increased or decreased secretions

D. Exploring the need for alternative methods for providing nutrition, for example, total parenteral nutrition (TPN); enteral feedings via percutaneous endoscopic gastrostomy (PEG); nasogastric (NG), low-profile gastrostomy; or percutaneous endoscopic jejunal access device if oral intake is not possible via oral route

E. Eliciting patient's subjective reports of changes in patterns of dysphagia and measures that enhance or aggravate swallowing—room temperature foods versus cold or hot foods, consistency

IV. Interventions to involve patient and family in care (Gaziano, 2013)

A. Determining the willingness of significant other to assist with care

B. Teaching patient and family about all aspects of care, including emergency measures, pulmonary hygiene, oral hygiene, and appropriate time to report complications to a member of the health care team

V. Interventions to enhance adaptation (Gaziano, 2013)

A. Providing ongoing support to patient in a situation that may potentially cause fear, anxiety, and inability to cope

B. Providing detailed written and audiovisual materials

C. Initiating early referral to speech therapist and dietitian for nutritional advice

VI. Interventions that are complementary

A. Exploring awareness and use of complementary and alternative medicine (CAM) such as mind-body interventions, homeopathy, acupuncture, vitamins, or herbal products

B. Identification of the methods that are practiced, if they were used before cancer diagnosis or after diagnosis, and patient's feelings about effectiveness

EVALUATION

The oncology nurse systematically and regularly evaluates the patient's and family's responses to interventions for dysphagia to determine progress toward adequate nutrition and safety. Relevant data are collected, and actual findings are compared with expected findings. Problem statements, outcomes, and plans of care are reviewed and revised, as necessary.

Mucositis or Esophagitis

OVERVIEW

I. Definition—inflammatory lesions of the oral and gastrointestinal (GI) tracts caused by high-dose cancer therapies; *alimentary tract mucositis* refers to mucosal injury across the oral and GI mucosa, from the mouth to the anus (Farrington, Cullen, & Dawson, 2010)

A. Stomatitis—mucositis or inflammation and ulcerative reaction of the oral cavity

B. Esophagitis—mucositis in the esophagus

C. Mucositis—can involve all mucous membranes, including the intestine (Zur, 2012)

II. Pathophysiology

A. Drugs interfere with deoxyribonucleic acid (DNA), ribonucleic acid (RNA), or protein synthesis and cause destruction of rapidly proliferating cells. Cellular proliferation rates differ throughout the GI tract, which explains the difference in onset of symptoms related to toxicity (Zur, 2012).

1. Small intestine proliferation rate is approximately 4 days.

2. Dermal proliferation is approximately 34 days.

3. Oral or esophageal tissue is somewhere between these two.

B. As the host's marrow function becomes more suppressed, the damage is greater.

C. Incidence is multifactorial—for example, diagnosis and treatment regimens for cancer.

1. Oral mucositis occurs in approximately 40% of patients receiving standard-dose chemotherapy.

2. Up to 70% in patients receiving chemotherapy higher doses seen with bone marrow transplantation (Zur, 2012).

III. Risk factors (Barasch & Epstein, 2011)

A. Disease- or host-related

1. Infiltration of mucosal membranes of the GI tract by primary or metastatic tumor, contributing to the mucositis

2. Age of the patient; those younger than 20 years old have a higher risk.

3. Type and location of tumor—oral problem frequency two to three times higher in hematologic malignancies than solid tumors

B. Treatment-related
1. Damage directly related to the dose; may be dose-limiting toxicity
2. May be acute; manifests as mucosal inflammation, ulceration, infection, and mucosal hemorrhage; small intestine will show damage within a few days of cytotoxic exposure and large intestine a short while later (Zur, 2012).
3. May be chronic; manifests as changes in healthy tissues from xerostomia, taste alterations, trismus (spasms and muscular fibrosis), soft tissue or bone necrosis
4. Drug administration—antineoplastic therapies exert both direct and indirect effects on the GI mucosal tissue (Zur, 2012).
   a. Chemotherapy—attacks the stratified squamous nonkeratinizing epithelium of the oral mucosa because of the following:
      (1) Direct effect of treatment on the oral mucosa; interference with proliferation of mucosal cells—direct somatotoxicity
      (2) Indirect effect on salivary glands, which causes damage to the permeable barrier that helps protect the mucosa from invasion of organisms—indirect somatotoxicity (Barasch & Epstein, 2011)
   b. Drugs—antimetabolites, antitumor antibiotics, miscellaneous drugs such as methotrexate, 5-fluorouracil (5-FU), cisplatin (Platinol), cytarabine (ara-C, cytosine arabinoside, Cytosar-U), etoposide (VP-16, Etopophos, VePesid), cyclophosphamide (Cytoxan), mechlorethamine (nitrogen mustard, Mustargen) vinblastine (Velban), vincristine (Oncovin), hydroxyurea (Hydrea, Mylocel), procarbazine (Matulane), capcitabine (Xeloda), liposomal doxorubicin (Doxil), irinotecan (Camptosar), and the mTOR inhibitors (Afinitor, Torisel) and tyrosine kinase inhibitor (Sutent), in which effects are dose-related and cumulative
   c. Depends on the method of infusion; for example, continuous infusion schedules have greater negative effect than short infusions
   d. Correlates directly with the white blood cell (WBC) nadir
   e. RT—radiation-induced damage different from chemotherapy-induced damage in that the tissues from RT remain in jeopardy throughout the life of the patient (Farrington et al., 2010).

5. RT
   a. Effects greater when chest, abdomen, head and neck, and intestines are in the field
   b. Higher doses of RT given to larger volumes over shorter periods increase the severity of mucositis.
   c. Severity of mucositis related to the daily RT dose, total cumulative dose, and volume of irradiated tissue (Farrington et al., 2010)
      (1) Medications such as antimicrobials and steroids
      (2) Oral graft-versus-host disease (GVHD)
      (3) Immunosuppression—cancer and cancer treatments decrease the body's immune system and alter protective barriers.

C. Lifestyle-related
1. Inadequate oral hygiene; periodontal disease
2. Exposure to irritants—chemical (citrus, spicy, mouthwashes, tobacco, alcohol) or physical (temperature extremes, poor-fitting prosthesis)
3. Dehydration
4. Malnutrition
5. Age—frequency greater in younger than older age
6. Renal and hepatic dysfunction both alter drug metabolism.
7. Quality of life—how well the patient is functioning

IV. Principles of medical management (Oncology Nursing Society [ONS], 2013; Worthington et al., 2010)
   A. Antimicrobial agents, growth factors, cytokines, coating agents, and anti-inflammatory agents the main treatments for radiation-induced oral mucositis; effectiveness not established (Harris et al., 2008); however, may be a soothing agent to patients; antifungal and antiviral agents controversial (ONS, 2014)
   B. Increasing oral protein intake—may enhance oral tissue healing
   C. Treatment based on the following factors:
      1. Presence of a working GI tract
      2. Cancer treatment modalities
         a. Surgery—location and extent of surgery
         b. Chemotherapy—type and dose
         c. RT—location and dose of radiation
         d. Targeted therapy
      3. QOL and the expected outcome of the cancer
   D. Systemic therapy such as acetaminophen, nonsteroidal anti-inflammatory drugs (NSAIDS), antacids, and opioids
   E. Topical analgesics (e.g., lidocaine solution)
   F. Topical protective and coating agents such as benzocaine (Orabase, Oratect Gel, Hurricane), and lidocaine (Zilactin)

G. Cryotherapy (ice) before and during administration of 5-FU—serves as a preventive method to decrease drug exposure to the oral mucosa (ONS, 2014)

H. Low-level laser therapy

I. Dietary and vitamin supplements such as oral liquid supplements that contain whey proteins have been found to improve total energy or protein consumption.

J. Biologic response modifiers—prostaglandin E2, interleukin, fibronectin, immunoglobulin, beta-carotene, and epidermal growth factors

K. Antidiarrheal medications

L. Problem-specific approaches—xerostomia, taste changes, anorexia, hemorrhage (thrombin-soaked collagen gauzes with ice and/or vasoconstricting agents)

V. Potential sequelae of prolonged mucositis or esophagitis

A. Impaired integrity of the mucous membranes

B. Infection, pain, ulceration, bleeding

C. Difficulty swallowing and speaking

D. Inadequate nutritional intake, absorption, or both leading to nutritional deficits, weight loss, and potential malnutrition and wasting; complications related to nutritional replacement may also occur (van Vilet, Harmsen, deBont, & Tissing, 2010).

E. Diarrhea

F. Bleeding or hemorrhage

ASSESSMENT

I. History

A. Previous therapy for cancer

B. Chemical exposure, physical exposure, or both

C. Routine oral hygiene practices

D. Weight history

1. Measurement of the percentage (%) of weight change from usual body weight (the current measured weight is divided by the usual weight and multiplied by 100)

a. This percentage should be evaluated for differences from pre-illness, pre-diagnosis, and after-diagnosis weights; weight loss of 2% to 5% is considered severe (Zur, 2012).

E. Changes in eating and drinking and how long changes have lasted

F. Symptoms affecting eating and drinking—nausea and vomiting, diarrhea, constipation, sores in the mouth, dry mouth, taste and smell changes, food likes and dislikes

G. Other illness that may affect nutrition

H. Patterns of mucositis—incidence; frequency; precipitating, alleviating, and aggravating factors; overall pattern of mucositis along the entire GI tract

I. Impact of stomatitis or mucositis on lifestyle, comfort, nutrition, activities of daily living, and QOL

J. Assessment for prolonged neutropenia because metabolic needs may increase 25% with a body temperature of 102° F (38.9° C)

II. Physical examination

A. An oral assessment tool and grading scale are used on an ongoing basis so that changes can be consistently qualified as they occur and compared with the baseline assessment.

1. Multiple tools to assess the oral cavity exist in the literature.

2. Institutions should choose one and use it exclusively and consistently.

3. The National Cancer Institute Common Toxicity Criteria scale (NCI, 2010) is as follows:

a. Grade 1: Mild symptoms

b. Grade 2: Moderate pain, not interfering with oral intake

c. Grade 3: Severe pain, interfering with oral intake

d. Grade 4: Life-threatening; urgent intervention needed; hospitalization

e. Grade 5: Death

B. Timing of complications in relation to the chemotherapy, RT, or both should be immediately recognized.

1. Complaints of mucous membrane burning within 3 to 10 days of chemotherapy frequently precede objective signs; erythema may develop and progress to erosion or ulceration over the next 3 to 5 days.

2. Neutropenic patients frequently found to have mucosal ulcerations infected by *Candida* throughout the GI tract but often asymptomatic (Zur, 2012)

C. The oral cavity and throat should be examined and palpated for redness, swelling, presence of white patches, shiny appearance, pain or burning, decreased or increased salivation, and presence of sensation changes. Dental appliances should be removed and the area underneath assessed.

D. Mucosal inflammation—in the anorectal area, stomal, vaginal—should be observed.

E. Weight loss, loss of fat under skin, muscle wasting, fluid collection in the legs, and the presence of ascites should be assessed.

PROBLEM STATEMENTS AND OUTCOME IDENTIFICATION

I. Deficient Fluid Volume (NANDA-I)

A. Expected outcome—patient maintains hydration status and describes strategies to maintain hydration with mucositis.

II. Diarrhea (NANDA-I)

A. Expected outcome—diarrhea is controlled within 48 hours.

III. Acute Pain (NANDA-I)

A. Expected outcome—pain is well controlled according to patient goal.

IV. Deficient Knowledge (NANDA-I), related to mucositis
  A. Expected outcome—patient discusses measures to minimize risk of occurrence, severity, and complications of mucositis.
  B. Expected outcome—patient and family list situations that require professional assistance and interventions, including temperature elevations greater than 101° F (38.3° C), significant decrease in oral intake, and poorly controlled pain or diarrhea, such as more than five stools per day.

PLANNING AND IMPLEMENTATION

I. Interventions to prevent oral complications during cancer treatment (ONS, 2014; Worthington et al., 2010)
  A. Providing information before cancer treatments and encouraging early intervention
    1. Regular dental care; dental examination may be necessary prior to treatment
    2. Consistent oral assessments
    3. Initiation of a standardized oral hygiene program

II. Interventions to minimize the risk of occurrence and severity of mucositis (ONS, 2014)
  A. Use of palifermin (Kepevance) for prevention of severe mucositis in transplantation settings; administered intravenously before stem cell or bone marrow infusion
  B. Nonpharmacologic measures to decrease inflammation of mucous membranes
    1. Encouraging oral and perineal hygiene measures
    2. Encouraging fluid intake of greater than 3000 mL/day, if tolerated
    3. Ensuring avoidance of exposures to chemical and physical irritants
  C. Measures to increase comfort (ONS, 2014)
    1. Use of topical protective agents (e.g., benzocaine magnesium hydroxide)
    2. Increasing frequency of oral hygiene
    3. Use of normal saline or salt and baking soda rinses (half a teaspoon each in one cup of warm water)
    4. Administering systemic (e.g., opioids, NSAIDs) or topical analgesics (e.g., viscous lidocaine)
    5. Encouraging sitz baths
  D. Measures to decrease risk of complications of mucositis or esophagitis
    1. Modifying intake to bland, soft, liquid, high-calorie, high-protein foods
    2. Use of amifostine (Ethyol) (acts as a radioprotector), as appropriate, when RT is used (Eisbruch, 2011)
    3. Encouraging oral assessment daily and a systematic oral care regimen consisting of cleansing, lubricating, and coating, because

systematic performance (compliance) is of more value than the actual agents used
    4. Discouraging sexual intercourse and douching during the inflammatory stage of mucositis and encouraging meticulous perineal care

III. Interventions to monitor patient response to symptom management
  A. Monitoring changes in level of comfort
  B. Monitoring changes in integrity of the mucous membranes
  C. Monitoring adherence with measures to decrease severity of mucositis and to reduce the incidence of complications

IV. Interventions to incorporate patient and family in care
  A. Teaching about oral and perineal hygiene measures
  B. Teaching about signs and symptoms of infection, impaired skin integrity, and complications to report to the health care team
  C. Exploring ways to enhance QOL issues that affect patient comfort, appetite, communication, and general well-being

EVALUATION

The oncology nurse systematically and regularly evaluates the patient's and family's responses to interventions for mucositis to determine progress toward the achievement of comfort and adequate nutrition and hydration. Relevant data are collected, and actual findings are compared with expected findings. Problem statements, outcomes, and plans of care are reviewed and revised, as necessary.

Nausea and Vomiting

OVERVIEW

I. Definitions
  A. Nausea is characterized by a queasy sensation, the urge to vomit, or both (Rangwala, Zafar, & Abernathy, 2012).
  B. Vomiting is a reflex involving motor and autonomic responses that result in the forceful expulsion of gastric contents through the mouth, activated by humoral or neuronal stimuli (Getto, Zesterson, & Breyer, 2011).

II. Pathophysiology (Figure 28-1) (Hesketh, 2008)
  A. The vomiting center (VC) is located in the brainstem and is directly activated by the visceral and vagal afferent pathways from the GI tract, the chemotherapy trigger zone vestibular apparatus, and the cerebral cortex.
  B. Chemotherapy, RT, and other toxins cause cellular damage to the GI mucosa. The damaged mucosa causes enterochromaffin cells in the GI tract to release serotonin, activating 5-HT3 receptors on the visceral afferent fibers in the vagus nerve,

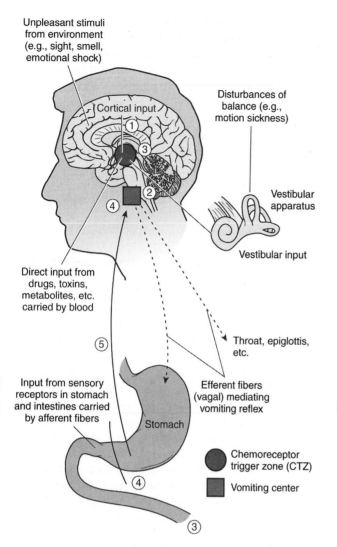

Unpleasant stimuli from environment (e.g., sight, smell, emotional shock)

Cortical input

Disturbances of balance (e.g., motion sickness)

Vestibular apparatus

Vestibular input

Direct input from drugs, toxins, metabolites, etc. carried by blood

Throat, epiglottis, etc.

Input from sensory receptors in stomach and intestines carried by afferent fibers

Stomach

Efferent fibers (vagal) mediating vomiting reflex

Chemoreceptor trigger zone (CTZ)

Vomiting center

Figure 28-1 Mechanisms of nausea and vomiting. *From Clayton, B.D., & Willihnganz, M.J. (2013). Basic pharmacology for nurses (16th ed.). St. Louis: Mosby.*

which, in turn, induces impulses to areas in the medulla responsible for vomiting (Wickham, 2012).

C. Other neurotransmitters, including dopamine and gamma-aminobutyric acid (GABA), are involved.

III. Risk factors

A. Disease-related
1. Primary or metastatic tumor of the central nervous system (CNS) that includes the VC or increased intracranial pressure (Getto et al., 2011)
2. Delayed gastric emptying
3. Obstruction of a portion of the GI tract
4. Food toxins, infection, or motion sickness
5. Metabolic abnormalities such as hyperglycemia, hyponatremia, hypercalcemia, renal or hepatic dysfunction, or a combination of all these factors.

B. Treatment-related
1. Stimulation of the receptors of the labyrinth in the inner ear
2. Obstruction, irritation, inflammation, and delayed gastric emptying stimulating the GI tract through vagal visceral afferent pathways
3. Stimulation of the VC by chemotherapy (Wickham, 2012)
4. Stimulation of the VC through afferent pathways from RT of the GI tract
5. Type of chemotherapy
6. Medication side effects
7. Side effects of concentrated nutritional supplements

C. Situational
1. Increased incidence in those younger than 50 years old
2. Increased incidence in females
3. Increased levels of stress, emotions, and anxiety
4. Increase in noxious odors or visual stimuli
5. Conditioned (anticipatory) responses to previous cancer treatment and other stressful experiences; occurs in up to 75% of chemotherapy patients (Wickham, 2012)

IV. Principles of medical management (National Comprehensive Cancer Network [NCCN], 2014)

A. Treatment of underlying disease

B. Antiemetic therapy
1. Serotonin antagonists (e.g., ondansetron [Zofran], granisetron [Kytril] granisetron transdermal system [Sancuso], dolasetron [Anzemet], palonosetron [Aloxi]) (Grunberg, Clark-Snow, & Koeller, 2010)
2. Neurokinin-1 receptor antagonist (aprepitant [Emend]/fosaprepitant) (dos Santos, Souza, Brunetto, Sasse, & Lima, 2012)
3. Dopamine receptor antagonists such as metoclopramide (Reglan), haloperidol (Haldol), droperidol (Inapsine)
4. Phenothiazines such as prochlorperazine (Compazine), chlorpromazine (Thorazine)
5. Corticosteroids such as dexamethasone (Decadron); most effective when paired with serotonin antagonists
6. Benzodiazepines such as lorazepam (Ativan); most effective when combined with other agents
7. Cannabinoids such as dronabinol (Marinol) and nabilone (Cesamet)
8. Miscellaneous—megestrol acetate (likely to be effective), olanzapine, mirtazapine, ginger (effectiveness not yet established but some evidence exists)

C. Nonpharmacologic interventions
1. Relaxation and distraction techniques, including guided imagery and music therapy, progressive muscle relaxation for anticipatory nausea

2. Acupressure—may decrease intensity of nausea (Wickham, 2012)
3. Acupuncture
4. Ginger

D. Management of concurrent symptoms such as fatigue and pain (Wickham, 2012)

V. Potential sequelae of prolonged nausea
   A. Vomiting
   B. Taste changes, development of food aversions
   C. Anorexia with weight loss, fluid and electrolyte imbalances, dehydration
   D. Noncompliance or refusal to complete treatment plan
   E. Altered QOL (Glare, Miller, Nikolova, & Tickoo, 2011)

ASSESSMENT

I. History
   A. Presence of risk factors for nausea, including a history of motion sickness or pregnancy-induced nausea, prior history of chemotherapy (Thompson, 2012)
   B. Current symptoms
   C. Patient's perception of possible correlation between occurrence of nausea and distress (anticipatory chemotherapy-induced nausea and vomiting [CINV]; anxiety)
   D. Perceived meaning of nausea on work, role, responsibilities, and mood
   E. Patterns of nausea—onset, frequency, associated symptoms to rule out other causes: mental status changes, confusion, brain tumor or metastasis; bowel obstruction, precipitating factors, aggravating factors, and alleviating factors; anticipatory, acute, delayed CINV; treatment differences—that is, benzodiazepines for anticipatory, 5-HT3 antagonist for acute, dopamine receptor antagonist for delayed

II. Physical examination
   A. Signs of sweating, tachycardia, dizziness, pallor, excessive salivation, weakness
   B. Laboratory reports to assess for other causes—serum electrolytes, liver and renal function tests, intake and output
   C. Weight
   D. Signs of dehydration

III. Grading (NCI, 2010)
   A. Nausea
      1. Grade 1: Loss of appetite
      2. Grade 2: Oral intake decreased, no significant weight loss or dehydration
      3. Grade 3: Inadequate oral caloric or fluid intake, TPN, hospitalization
   B. Vomiting
      1. Grade 1: 1 to 2 episodes in 24 hours
      2. Grade 2: 3 to 5 episodes in 24 hours

      3. Grade 3: More than 6 episodes in 24 hours, total parenteral nutrition (TPN), feeding tube, hospitalization may be indicated

IV. Psychosocial assessment
   A. Exploration of anxiety-producing events and coping abilities
   B. Identification of strengths of patient and family

PROBLEM STATEMENTS AND OUTCOME IDENTIFICATION

I. Nausea (NANDA-I)
   A. Expected outcome—patient describes personal risk for nausea.
   B. Expected outcome—patient participates in measures to minimize the risk of occurrence of nausea.

II. Imbalanced Nutrition: Less than Body Requirements (NANDA-I)
   A. Expected outcome—nutritional status will be maintained without weight loss.

III. Risk for Imbalanced Fluid Volume (NANDA-I)
   A. Expected outcome—patient and family list changes in the condition suggestive of dehydration and describe strategies to maintain fluid status.

PLANNING AND IMPLEMENTATION

I. Interventions to minimize the risk of occurrence, severity, or complications of nausea
   A. Individualizing treatment according to emetic potential of chemotherapy, expected duration of nausea and vomiting, and current pattern of symptoms (Shoemaker, Estfan, Induru, & Declan Walsh, 2011)
   B. Modification of the environment—cool, well ventilated, lowered lighting and noise levels, absence of noxious sights and smells
   C. Modification of diet to include bland, chilled foods, with liquids served separately
   D. Having patient avoid movement and recline for the first 30 minutes after eating
   E. Replacement of fluids with popsicles, sports drinks (e.g., Gatorade), intravenous hydration
   F. Administering antiemetics around the clock until the nausea cycle is broken; switching to agent with different mechanism if emesis persists
   G. Encouraging nonpharmacologic treatments (see Treatment section) (Thompson, 2012)

II. Interventions to maximize safety ⚠
   A. Positioning during vomiting episodes to reduce risk of aspiration (Glare et al., 2011)
   B. Anticipating needs arising as a result of weakness, sedative effects of antiemetics, or both
   C. Providing assistance with ambulation by using raised side rails and placing the call bell and emesis basin within patient's reach

Part 4

III. Interventions to monitor for complications of nausea
   A. Observing for signs of dehydration, electrolyte imbalance, and profound loss of weight in a short time frame
   B. Observing for side effects that may be associated with antiemetic therapy
IV. Interventions to incorporate patient and family in care
   A. Teaching home management techniques to avoid or minimize emetic events, including use of medications around the clock, avoidance of strong scents (food, perfume, air fresheners)
   B. Encouraging the use of self-care diaries and logs to record frequency and severity of nausea and response to therapies; referral to dietician or nutritionist
   C. Teaching the importance of reporting critical changes in patient condition to the health care team, including presence of vomiting; signs and symptoms of aspiration, dehydration, or other pathologic condition
   D. Instructing patient and family on use of nonpharmacologic interventions
   E. Instructing patient and family to recognize concurrent symptoms such as pain or fatigue that may increase the experience of nausea

EVALUATION

The oncology nurse systematically and regularly evaluates the patient's and family's responses to nausea and vomiting interventions to determine progress toward the achievement of optimal comfort and fluid and nutritional maintenance. Relevant data are collected, and actual findings are compared with expected findings. Problem statements and outcome identification, outcomes, and plans of care are reviewed and revised, as necessary.

Ascites

OVERVIEW

See Kipps, Tan, & Kaye, 2013.
   I. Definition—pathologic accumulation of fluid in the abdominal cavity
   II. Pathophysiology
   A. Cancer cells attach to peritoneal lining, proliferate and invade; suggestion that transcoelomic metastasis is associated with ascites production
   B. Impaired drainage from peritoneal cavity—lymphatic obstruction
   C. Increased filtration into the abdominal cavity from portal vein hypertension or vascular endothelial growth factor (VEGF) involvement
   III. Risk factors
   A. Disease-related risk factors

1. Associated with various tumors, mainly intra-abdominal malignancies: ovarian (accounts for 38%), endometrial, uterine
2. Breast, lung, and lymphatic tumors most common, extra-abdominal sites
3. Colon, gastric, pancreatic, mesothelial, testicular, and sarcomatous tumors
4. Liver metastasis
   B. Treatment-related risk factors—previous radiation to the abdomen, surgical modification of venous or lymphatic channels, or both
IV. Principles of medical management
   A. Treatment of underlying cause; need to rule out non-neoplastic causes
   B. Diet (salt and water restrictions) and diuresis—with cirrhosis
   C. Repeated therapeutic removal of fluid by paracentesis—leads to protein depletion
   D. Intraperitoneal—chemotherapy or biotherapy instilled into the peritoneal cavity
   E. Systemic chemotherapy or monoclonal antibody therapy (e.g., bevacizumab [Avastin], VEGF inhibitor)
   F. Peritoneovenous shunting (LeVeen or Denver shunt)—diverts fluid from the abdomen into the blood circulation)
   G. External drains (Tenchoff, PleurX)—PleurX drainage system recommended for malignant ascites
   H. Ultrasound-guided insertion of a peritoneogastric shunt (from peritoneal cavity to gastrostomy tube)
V. Potential sequelae of progressive ascites
   A. Discomfort, anorexia, early satiety, decreased bladder capacity, bowel obstruction, electrolyte imbalance, nausea and vomiting, infection, shortness of breath, respiratory compromise, lower extremity edema, impaired skin integrity, abdominal distention, fatigue, weight gain
   B. Appearance of ascites in advanced disease indicative of a poor prognosis

ASSESSMENT

I. History
   A. Presence of risk factors associated with malignant ascites
   B. Pattern of ascites
   1. Subjective indicators—indigestion, early satiety, swollen ankles, easy fatigability, shortness of breath, constipation, reduced bladder capacity
   2. Increasing abdominal girth
   3. Review of previous treatment strategies for ascites and current or recent treatment for cancer and anticipated side effects

C. Presence of self-care strategies
1. Ability to perform interventions to relieve or minimize effects of ascites
2. Willingness to self-monitor weight, girth; record keeping

II. Physical examination
   A. Presence of weight gain, distended abdomen, fluid wave, shifting dullness, bulging flanks, everted umbilicus, stretched skin, increased abdominal girth
   B. Presence of lower extremity edema
   C. Laboratory tests—high carcinoembryonic antigen (CEA) (>12 mg/mL), total protein, lactate dehydrogenase (LDH), differential albumin, fibronectin, and cholesterol level; cytologic confirmation of the presence of malignant cells in ascitic fluid, immunohistochemical staining, cytology examination result, and character of transudate (usually bloody or serosanguineous)
   D. Radiology—ultrasonography (can detect as little as 100 mL of fluid), computed tomography (CT) of abdomen (radiography shows a ground-glass appearance with loss of detail) (Gordon, 2012)

PROBLEM STATEMENTS AND OUTCOME IDENTIFICATION

I. Excess Fluid Volume (NANDA-I)
   A. Expected outcome—peritoneal fluid is minimized with appropriate interventions.
   B. Expected outcome—patient states the personal risk for potential recurrence of ascites and early symptoms that need to be reported to lessen the extent of fluid accumulation and discomfort from urinary retention.

II. Deficient Knowledge (NANDA-I), related to ascites
   A. Expected outcome—patient and family state the changes in condition that require professional assistance and intervention, such as weight gain of more than 2 pounds per day and increased abdominal girth, acute respiratory distress, fever, changes in level of pain, and edema noted in other body parts such as the lower legs and feet.

PLANNING AND IMPLEMENTATION

I. Nonpharmacologic interventions to minimize the risk of occurrence, severity, or complications of ascites (Kipps et al., 2013)
   A. Maximizing measures to promote comfort
      1. Teaching patient and family about need to maintain high Fowler position
      2. Having patient avoid restrictive clothing
      3. Reminding patient about the need to use nonpharmacologic techniques for pain relief (e.g., relaxation, imagery, music, distraction, healing touch)
      4. Use of methods to assist with activities, as needed

II. Interventions to incorporate patient and family in care
   A. Encouraging family to provide foods within dietary restrictions
   B. Teaching patient and family about dietary restrictions to help control fluid development
   C. Educating about signs and symptoms of dehydration, infection, respiratory distress, and malnutrition, which may be associated with ascites
   D. Teaching family how to measure abdominal girth and weight daily and to assess changes such as fullness, bloating, and abdominal pressure

III. Medical and pharmacologic interventions to reduce ascites (Reshamwala, 2010)
   A. Routine paracentesis to drain fluid
   B. Chemotherapy or targeted therapy to reduce ascites
   C. PleurX drain placement for chronic reaccumulation of ascites
   D. Palliative care consultation if no relief from chemotherapy

EVALUATION

The oncology nurse systematically and regularly evaluates the patient's and family's responses to interventions for ascites to determine progress toward achievement of comfort and fluid management. Relevant data are collected, and actual findings are compared with expected findings. Problem statements, outcomes, and plans of care are reviewed and revised, as needed.

Constipation

OVERVIEW

I. Definition—decreased frequency in defecation (typically less than three bowel movements in a week); often accompanied by discomfort (Rangwala et al., 2012)
II. Physiology—slowing of intestinal mobility by one of the following mechanisms:
   A. Primary—results from extrinsic factors that slow peristalsis: decreased physical activity, lack of time or privacy for defecation, low-fiber diet
   B. Secondary—results from pathologic processes such as bowel obstruction, spinal cord compression, hypercalcemia, hypokalemia, and hypothyroidism
   C. Iatrogenic—from use of pharmacologic agents such as opioids, chemotherapy, anticonvulsants, and psychotropic medications (Rangwala et al., 2012)
III. Risk factors
   A. Disease-related
      1. Internal or external obstruction of bowel by tumor
      2. Fluid and electrolyte imbalances—dehydration, hypercalcemia, hypokalemia

3. Decreased physical activity, immobility, or both
4. Spinal cord compression at T8-L3 (levels that control bowel innervation)
5. Anorexia causing decreased food and fluid intake
6. Pressure from ascites
7. Neurologic disorders such as multiple sclerosis, Parkinson disease, chronic idiopathic intestinal pseudo-obstruction, or stroke
8. Metabolic and endocrine disorders such as diabetes, hypothyroidism or hyperthyroidism, or uremia
9. Systemic disorders such as amyloidosis, lupus, or scleroderma
B. Treatment related
1. Manipulation of intestines during surgery
2. Surgical trauma to neurogenic pathways to intestines, rectum, or both
3. Neurotoxic effects of cancer chemotherapeutic agents such as vincristine (Oncovin, Vincasar PFS) and vinblastine (Velban)
4. Nutritional deficiencies, decreased fiber, roughage, and fluid intake
5. Side effects of pharmacologic agents such as opioids, analgesics, cholinergics, antacids
C. Situational
1. Lack of privacy (Shoemaker et al., 2011)
2. Interference with usual bowel movement routine
3. Failure to respond to defecation reflex because of pain, fatigue, social activities, or inability to reach the toilet
4. Depression, decreased physical activity
IV. Principles of medical management (Shoemaker et al., 2011)
A. Surgical correction of obstructive disease
B. Correction of fluid and electrolyte imbalances
C. Enemas or irrigations
D. Medications such as laxatives, stool softeners, fiber supplements
E. Increased fiber in diet
V. Potential sequelae of constipation
A. Fecal impaction (also called *dyschezia* or *terminal reservoir syndrome*)
B. Paralytic ileus
C. Intestinal obstruction
D. Laxative dependence

ASSESSMENT

I. History
A. Presence of risk factors
B. History of defining characteristics of constipation
1. Change in usual patterns of bowel elimination such as decreased frequency, hard stool, abdominal cramping, increased use of laxatives

2. Date of last bowel movement
3. Change in factors contributing to bowel elimination such as activity level, fluid intake, dietary fiber intake, and laxative use
4. History of constipation, chronic laxative use, or both
5. Anxiety regarding bowel movement patterns
6. Perception of incomplete evacuation following defecation
7. Rectal pain associated with inability to defecate
8. Sudden onset of diarrhea (may be a symptom of severe impaction)
C. GI symptoms—nausea, vomiting, anorexia
D. Pattern of occurrence of constipation—onset; frequency; severity-associated symptoms; precipitating, aggravating, and alleviating factors
E. Perceived effectiveness of self-care measures to relieve constipation
F. Perceived impact of constipation on comfort, activities of daily living, mood
G. History of rectal fissures or abscesses
II. Physical findings
A. Inspection of abdomen
1. Symmetry
2. Contour
3. Distention
4. Bulges
5. Peristaltic waves
B. Auscultation of character, frequency, and presence or absence of bowel sounds in the four quadrants of the abdomen
C. Palpation of abdomen
1. Masses or stool in the colon
2. Areas of increased resistance or tenderness
D. Rectal examination to check for fecal impaction, hemorrhoids, or fissures

PROBLEM STATEMENTS AND OUTCOME IDENTIFICATION

I. Constipation (NANDA-I)
A. Expected outcome—patient reports normal pattern of bowel functioning.
B. Expected outcome—patient manages constipation through self-care measures.
II. Risk for Constipation (NANDA-I)
A. Expected outcome—patient and family identify and manage factors that may affect constipation such as diet, stress, physical activity, and neurogenic conditions.
B. Expected outcome—patient manages constipation through titration of laxatives.
C. Expected outcome—patient and family contact an appropriate health team member when unable to relieve constipation through self-care measures.

PLANNING AND IMPLEMENTATION

I. Interventions to minimize risk and severity of constipation
  A. Nonpharmacologic interventions (Shoemaker et al., 2011)
    1. Encouraging intake of at least 3000 mL of fluid per day unless contraindicated
    2. Modifying diet, as tolerated, to include high-fiber foods and roughage, fresh fruits, vegetables, whole grains, and dried beans to 20 to 35 g of fiber per day
    3. Having the patient maintain or increase physical activity level
    4. Establishing a daily bowel movement routine
  B. Effective interventions usually used by patient to alleviate constipation that are not contraindicated by health status
    1. Prune juice
    2. Dietary modification
  C. Pharmacologic interventions
    1. Stimulant laxatives—chemically stimulate the smooth muscles of the bowel to increase contractions (Shoemaker et al., 2011)
      a. Bisacodyl (Dulcolax)
      b. Cascara (various generics)
      c. Senna (Senokot)
    2. Osmotic laxatives—increase the bulk of the stools by retaining water
      a. Magnesium salts
      b. Sodium phosphate
      c. Polyethylene glycol (MiraLax)
    3. Bulk-forming laxatives—nondigestible substances that pass through the stomach and increase the bulk of the stools
      a. Methylcellulose
      b. Psyllium
    4. Emollient and lubricant laxatives—agents that soften hardened feces and facilitate the passage through the lower intestine
      a. Docusate
      b. Mineral oil
    5. Miscellaneous laxatives
      a. Glycerin suppositories
      b. Lactulose
    6. Methylnaltrexone (Relistor)—for opioid-induced constipation (Shoemaker et al., 2011)
  D. Initiate a prophylactic bowel regimen with opioid or vinca alkaloid therapy.
II. Interventions to maximize patient safety ⚠
  A. Checking for impaction if symptoms such as decreased or absent bowel sounds, abdominal distention, loss of appetite are present
  B. Avoidance of digital rectal examinations if patient is neutropenic, thrombocytopenic, or both
III. Interventions to monitor for complications from constipation (Calixto-Lima, Martins de Andrade, Gomes, Geller, & Siqueira-Batista, 2012)
  A. Assessment for interference with deep breathing related to abdominal distention
  B. Monitoring signs of social withdrawal related to flatulence and focus on elimination
  C. Monitoring untoward responses to symptom management
    1. Abdominal cramping or diarrhea with laxatives
    2. Rectal emptying and aggravation of constipation with enemas
    3. Dehydration or decreased fluid intake, which reduces effectiveness of stool softeners
  E. Reporting critical changes to the physician
    1. Abdominal distention
    2. Fecal impaction
    3. Bleeding
    4. Absence of bowel sounds
    5. Nausea and vomiting (bowel obstruction must be ruled out)
IV. Implementation of strategies to enhance adaptation and rehabilitation (Calixto-Lima et al., 2012)
  A. Educating patient about laxative dependence and independence with a combination of laxatives and stool softeners
  B. Emphasizing dietary control of constipation with foods high in fiber such as celery, bran, whole wheat bread
  C. Encouraging adoption of a daily fluid intake of 3000 mL, unless contraindicated
  D. Recommending adoption of a daily bowel movement routine
    1. Daily schedule for evacuation (e.g., after meals when gastrocolic reflexes are active)
    2. Privacy
    3. Medications such as stool softeners or expanders, natural laxative mixtures; avoidance of pharmaceutical laxatives, if possible
    4. Enemas or irrigation procedures, if necessary (ONS, 2014)
V. Interventions to incorporate patient and family in care
  A. Teaching about controlling constipation through fluid intake, dietary control, activity level
  B. Providing information about hazards of laxative dependence ⚠

EVALUATION

The oncology nurse systematically and regularly evaluates the patient's and family's responses to interventions for constipation to determine progress toward achievement of regular bowel movements. Relevant data are collected, and actual findings are compared with expected findings. Problem statements, outcomes, and plans of care are reviewed and revised, as necessary.

Diarrhea

OVERVIEW

I. Definition—passage of more than three unformed stools in 24 hours (Rangwala et al., 2012)
  A. Classification
    1. By volume
      a. Large volume—results from a larger than usual amount of water, intestinal secretion, or both in the intestine
      b. Small volume—results from excessive intestinal mobility
    2. By acuity—acute or chronic, depends on underlying pathologic condition
  B. Physiology
    1. Osmotic—unabsorbable substances in intestine draw water into intestinal lumen by osmosis, increasing the weight and volume of stool
      a. Lactose intolerance
      b. Enteral tube feedings
      c. Intestinal hemorrhage
    2. Secretory—intestinal mucosa secretes excessive fluid and electrolytes
      a. Bacteria such as *Escherichia coli* and *Clostridium difficile*
      b. Laxatives
      c. Neuroendocrine tumors
    3. Hypermotility—limited absorption because of increased motility of intestines
      a. Inflammatory bowel disease
      b. Radiation proctitis
      c. Chemotherapy drugs
      d. GVHD (Getto et al., 2011)
II. Risk factors
  A. Disease-related (Rangwala et al., 2012)
    1. Obstruction of bowel from intrinsic or extrinsic tumor
    2. Intestinal bacteria or viruses
    3. GVHD, in which immunocompetent cells of the allogeneic donor marrow recognize the normal GI cells as foreign and initiate an immune reaction that leads to cell destruction of target tissues in the gut
    4. Intestinal neuroendocrine tumors with liver metastases
    5. Food intolerance or allergies
  B. Treatment related
    1. Surgical resection of significant portions of bowel—may cause fluid malabsorption syndrome
    2. RT to abdominal area—causes increased cellular destruction in bowel lumen and increased intestinal motility
    3. Chemotherapeutic agents such as ironotecan, fluorouracil, cetuximab, erlotinib, sorafenib, and sunitinib—may cause increased cellular destruction in bowel lumen and heighten intestinal motility (Getto et al., 2011)
    4. Medications such as antibiotics, antacids, or laxatives
    5. Nutritional therapies such as tube feedings and dietary supplements
    6. Fecal impaction—may create paradoxical diarrhea
  C. Lifestyle-related
    1. Increased stress and anxiety because of inadequate coping strategies
    2. Changes in usual dietary habits, for example, increases in dietary fiber or other foods containing natural laxative properties
III. Principles of medical management (Table 28-1)
  A. Pharmacologic management of symptoms (Rangwala et al., 2012)
  B. Modification of associated therapy such as radiation, chemotherapy, nutritional supplements, or antibiotics
  C. Treatment of associated conditions such as *C. difficile* infection or GVHD
  D. Decompression or surgery for bowel obstruction
  E. Hormone inhibition therapy such as with octreotide (Shaw & Taylor, 2012)
IV. Potential sequelae of prolonged diarrhea
  A. Dehydration
  B. Electrolyte imbalances such as hypokalemia or hyponatremia
  C. Impaired skin integrity of perineal area
  D. Decreased social interaction
  E. Fatigue

ASSESSMENT

I. History
  A. Review of previous and current therapy for cancer
  B. Review of prescription and nonprescription medications
  C. Usual bowel movement pattern—frequency, color, amount, odor, consistency of stool
  D. Recent changes in factors contributing to usual fecal elimination patterns
    1. Increased levels of stress
    2. Dietary changes such as addition of fiber and roughage, fruit juices, coffee, alcohol, fried foods, or fatty foods, which increase bowel motility.
    3. Recent course of antibiotic therapy
  E. Known food or medication intolerance or allergies
  F. Presence of flatus, cramping, abdominal pain, urgency to defecate, recent weight loss, decreased urinary output of 500 mL less than intake, complaints of bloating
  G. Fluid intake
  H. Weight loss greater than 1% to 2% in 1 week
II. NCI grading criteria (NCI, 2010)
  A. Grade 1: Increase of more than 4 stools per day over baseline
  B. Grade 2: Increase of 4 to 6 stools per day
  C. Grade 3: Increase of more than 7 stools per day, hospitalization indicated

Table 28-1

Comparison of ASCO and ONS Evidence-Based Guidelines

Topic	American Society of Clinical Oncology (ASCO)	Oncology Nursing Society (ONS)
First-line treatment	Dietary modifications Loperamide 4 mg followed by 2 mg every 4 hr	Dietary modifications Loperamide 4 mg followed by 2 mg every 4 hr
Diarrhea refractory to loperamide: mild to moderate diarrhea (ASCO) or grade 2 or 3 (ONS)*	CID: Octreotide 100-500 mcg with dose escalation as needed or tincture of opium or budesonide RID: Continue loperamide 2 mg every 2 hr; replace fluid and electrolytes.	Likely to be effective for CRID: 150 mcg octreotide, SC tid, for 5 days Likely to be effective for RID: Octreotide 100 mcg, SC tid
Complicated (ASCO) or severe (ONS) diarrhea	Complicated CID: IV octreotide 100-150 mcg, SC or IV tid, with dose escalation until controlled, and an antibiotic (fluoroquinolone); hospitalization may be necessary; stool workup; laboratory tests. Complicated RID: Hospitalization may not be necessary; continue loperamide; may not need octreotide, and antibiotics may worsen.	Recommended for severe CID: Octreotide 100 mcg, SC tid, for 3 days, then 50 mcg SC tid for 3 days Likely to be effective for severe CID: 30 mg long-acting repeatable octreotide intramuscularly 7-14 days prior to day 1 of chemotherapy, then every 28 days up to six doses Likely to be effective for RID grade 2 or 3†: Octreotide 100 mcg, SC tid
Prevention	The ASCO states that no definitive data exist, but the future is promising.	Effectiveness not established: Budesonide, oral alkalization, charcoal, and levofloxacin for irinotecan-induced diarrhea; probiotics and glutamine for CID prevention
Important facts	Assessment recommendations: Increase monitoring (weekly assessment of gastrointestinal toxicity); blood tests no more than 48 hr prior to chemotherapy; increased management such as antibiotic treatment if diarrhea lasts more than 24 hr; discontinue chemotherapy if severe CID, may lead to death	Benefits balanced with risks: Amifostine infusion; neomycin for irinotecan-induced diarrhea Effectiveness not established: Antioxidants (vitamins E and C) for treatment of RID Effectiveness unlikely: Sulfasalazine and selenium supplementation for prevention of RID; pentosan polysulfate for treatment of RID Not recommended for practice: Sucralfate for prevention of RID

CID, Chemotherapy-induced diarrhea; *CRID*, chemotherapy- and radiation-induced diarrhea; *RID*, radiation-induced diarrhea; *SC*, subcutaneously; *tid*, three times daily.

*According to the Oncology Nursing Society, budesonide's effectiveness has not been established; however, the American Society of Clinical Oncology recommends it.

†ONS does not offer recommendations for RID higher than grade 3.

From Shaw, C., & Taylor, L. (2012). Treatment-related diarrhea in patients with cancer. *Clinical Journal of Oncology Nursing, 16*(4), 413–417. doi: 10.1188/12.CJON.413-417.

D. Grade 4: Life-threatening, urgent intervention needed

E. Grade 5: Death

III. Physical examination

A. Hypotension

B. Tachycardia

C. Hyperactive bowel sounds

D. Hard stool in rectum

E. Perineal skin irritation

F. Poor skin turgor

G. Dry mucous membranes

H. Abdominal tenderness with palpation

I. Abdominal distention

IV. Psychosocial examination

A. Presence of fear

B. Presence of anxiety

C. Complaints of isolation

V. Diagnostic studies

A. Stool culture for *C. difficile*, ova and parasites, WBC count

B. Serum electrolytes

C. Daily weights

PROBLEM STATEMENTS AND OUTCOME IDENTIFICATION

I. Diarrhea (NANDA-I)

A. Expected outcome—patient reestablishes and maintains a normal pattern of bowel function.

II. Impaired Skin Integrity (NANDA-I)

A. Expected outcome—patient and family identify and manage factors that impair skin integrity caused by diarrhea.

III. Deficient Fluid Volume (NANDA-I)

A. Expected outcome—patient experiences adequate fluid volume and electrolyte balance.

B. Expected outcome—patient and family contact an appropriate health care team member when diarrhea is severe, prolonged (12 to 24 hours), uncontrollable with self-care measures, interferes with quality of life, or is accompanied by fever, nausea, vomiting, or reduced urine output.

PLANNING AND IMPLEMENTATION

I. Interventions to minimize diarrhea occurrence and severity (Calixto-Lima et al., 2012)
   A. Pharmacologic interventions
      1. Antidiarrheals
         a. Loperamide (Imodium A-D)
         b. Diphenoxylate (Lomotil)
      2. Antispasmodic: Atropine
      3. Anti-inflammatory: Mesalamine
      4. Antibiotics
         a. Metronidazole (Flagyl)
         b. Neomycin (Shaw & Taylor, 2012)
   B. Nonpharmacologic interventions
      1. Modification of dietary plan to avoid foods the patient cannot tolerate
      2. Decreasing fiber and roughage
      3. Encouraging smaller, more frequent meals (Calixto-Lima et al., 2012)
II. Implementation of strategies to decrease bowel motility
   A. Pharmacologic interventions
      1. Opioids: Tincture of opium
      2. Octreotide (Sandostatin)
      3. Bulk-forming—Methylcellulose (Citrucel), psyllium (Metamucil)
      4. Loperamide (Imodium)
   B. Nonpharmacologic
      1. Serving foods and liquids at room temperature
      2. Encouraging avoidance of coffee and alcohol
      3. Encouraging avoidance of spicy, fried, or fatty foods and food additives
      4. Teaching strategies such as relaxation, distraction, or imagery to modify stress response
      5. Recommending low-residue diet for patients with bowel irritation
      6. Recommending low-lactose diet for patients with known or temporary lactose intolerance
         a. Diet is maintained for 2 weeks after diarrhea subsides.
         b. Dairy products may be reintroduced slowly (Calixto-Lima et al., 2012).
III. Interventions to maximize patient safety ⚠
   A. Monitoring level of weakness and fatigue
   B. Providing assistance with ambulation and activities of daily living, as indicated
IV. Interventions to monitor for complications related to diarrhea
   A. Assessment of the character of bowel movement at each stool

B. Assessment of the perineal area every 8 hours or with a change in symptoms
C. Monitoring intake and output ratio; electrolyte, creatinine, blood urea nitrogen (BUN) levels
D. Monitoring for subtle changes in patient affect, neuromuscular responses, activity level, and cognitive status as cues for potential electrolyte imbalances
E. Weighing the patient daily
F. Reporting significant changes in condition to the physician
G. Implementing rectal skin care regimen
H. Monitoring changes in skin turgor and mucous membranes
V. Interventions to improve social interactions
   A. Determining impact of diarrhea on social interactions and activities
   B. Teaching the patient about the interventions to minimize impact of diarrhea in daily living
VI. Interventions to incorporate the patient and family in care (Calixto-Lima et al., 2012)
   A. Teaching patient about a perineal hygiene program that includes cleansing perineal area with mild soap, rinsing thoroughly, patting area dry, and applying a skin barrier after each bowel movement; assessment of any skin breakdown around stoma if this applies
   B. Teaching about dietary modifications to minimize diarrhea and replace electrolytes
   C. Teaching about signs and symptoms to report to a member of the health care team
   D. Instructing patient to limit use of gas-producing foods such as cabbage, beans, green peppers, and onions while planning meals

EVALUATION

The oncology nurse systematically and regularly evaluates the patient's and family's responses to interventions for diarrhea to determine progress toward the achievement of normal bowel movements and fluid and electrolyte balance. Relevant data are collected, and actual findings are compared with expected findings. Problem statements, outcomes, and plans of care are reviewed and revised, as necessary.

Bowel Obstruction

OVERVIEW

I. Definition—any process preventing forward movement of bowel contents (O'Connor & Creedon, 2011).
II. Pathophysiology
   A. Mechanical obstruction—most common in end-stage cancer, may be partial or complete (Soriano & Mellar, 2011)

B. Functional obstructions—caused by changes to peristalsis (Badari, Farolino, Nasser, Mehboob, & Crossland, 2012)
   1. Causes
      a. Adhesions resulting from surgery or RT
      b. Pseudo-obstruction from paraneoplastic destruction of enteric neurons in rare cases
      c. Severe ileus from anticholinergic drugs
      d. Intraluminal tumors that may occlude the lumen or act as a point of intussusception
      e. Intramural tumors that may extend to the mucosa and obstruct the lumen or impair peristalsis
      f. Mesenteric and omental masses or malignant adhesions that may kink or angulate the bowel, creating an extramural obstruction
      g. Tumors that infiltrate into the mesentery bowel muscle or the enteric or celiac plexus and cause dysmotility
      h. Objects blocking the intestinal lumen—for example, foreign bodies and fecal or barium impaction
C. Location
   1. Small intestine obstructions
      a. Postoperative intra-abdominal adhesions—entrap a loop of intestine and contract, causing an obstruction and possibly strangulation; may develop a few days following surgery or many years later
      b. Nonsurgical adhesions following an infection such as peritonitis or following RT; may occur at any time following the infection or completion of RT
      c. Hernias
      d. Miscellaneous conditions such as inflammatory bowel disease
   2. Large bowel obstructions, most often in the sigmoid colon, caused by the following:
      a. Cancer
      b. Volvulus
      c. Diverticulitis
III. Risk factors
   A. Disease-related (O'Connor & Creedon, 2011)
      1. Obstruction of bowel by tumor
      2. Cholangiocarcinoma and pancreatic and gallbladder carcinoma the most common tumors causing duodenal obstruction
      3. Ovarian and colon cancers, which cause distal obstructions
      4. Hernia
      5. Inflammatory bowel disease
      6. Gallstones
      7. Peptic ulcers
      8. Pancreatitis
      9. Diverticular disease

B. Treatment-related
   1. Manipulation of intestines during surgery
   2. Surgical trauma to neurogenic pathways to intestines, rectum, or both
   3. Previous intestinal obstruction
   4. RT to abdominal area
IV. Principles of medical management (Rangwala et al., 2012)
   A. Surgical options
      1. Resection and reanastomosis
      2. Decompression with a colostomy or ileostomy
      3. Bypass of an obstructing lesion
      4. Lysis of adhesions
   B. Nothing by mouth (NPO)
   C. Abdominal decompression
      1. Nasogastric suction
      2. Percutaneous gastrostomy
      3. Enema
      4. Rectal tube
      5. Intestinal stenting—a large-caliber stent placed using fluoroscopic and endoscopic guidance (Dolan, 2011)
   D. Correction of fluid and electrolyte imbalances
   E. Parenteral nutrition
   F. Pharmacologic management (O'Connor & Creedon, 2011)
V. Potential sequelae of bowel obstruction
   A. Dehydration
   B. Peritonitis
   C. Bowel perforation
   D. Hypotension
   E. Hypovolemic or septic shock

ASSESSMENT

I. History
   A. Presence of risk factors
   B. Symptoms
      1. Abdominal pain and intestinal colic from intestinal stretching and pressure of peristalsis as the bowel tries to push its contents past the obstruction; may help identify the obstruction's type and severity
         a. Small intestine obstructions—associated with greater symptoms but fewer signs; severe nausea and greater number of emesis episodes, but fairly normal radiographic plain films of the abdomen
         b. Large intestine obstructions—radiographic plain abdominal films show air in bowels; pain is severe (Soriano & Mellar, 2011)
         c. Mechanical obstructions—cramping and spasmodic
         d. Nonmechanical obstructions—diffuse, constant, and less intense pain, which can be described as pressure or fullness

e. Partial obstructions—cramping pain after eating, along with mild to moderate hypomotility

f. Complete bowel obstruction—pain intensifies and comes in waves or spasms as the bowel tries to push intestinal contents past the obstruction; peristalsis may stop when bowel becomes exhausted.

g. Strangulation—constant, intense pain intensified with movement

2. Nausea and vomiting

a. Gastric outlet obstruction—sour emesis that is not bile-colored and often contains undigested food

b. Proximal small intestine obstruction—rapid-onset, bitter, bile-stained emesis that may be projectile

c. Distal small intestine obstruction or colonic obstruction with an incompetent ileocecal valve—orange-brown, malodorous feculent emesis

3. Anorexia

4. Constipation

a. May experience lack of bowel movements and flatus or may have paradoxical diarrhea (if partial blockage exists)

b. Bowel may evacuate below an obstruction; obstipation may develop.

C. Past and present patterns of elimination

1. Any recent changes in stool consistency or bowel habits

2. Date and time of last bowel movement

3. Use of antacids, laxatives, or enemas

D. Other

1. Current medications

2. Endocrine history

3. Immunologic history

4. Diet

II. Physical findings

A. Abdominal distention

1. The lower the obstruction, the longer it lasts.

a. The more complete it is, the more severe the distention will be.

2. Baseline measurement of abdominal girth should be obtained and section of measurement marked.

3. Board like abdomen may indicate peritonitis.

B. Abnormal bowel sounds

1. Intermittent borborygmi (loud prolonged gurgles of hyperperistalsis)

2. Mechanical obstruction

a. Proximal to obstruction—high-pitched, tinkling, or hyperactive bowel sounds that may be heard in clusters or rushes

b. Distal to the obstruction—bowel sounds hypoactive or absent

3. Nonmechanical

a. Hypoactive, low-pitched gurgles or weak tinkles

b. Absent bowel sounds indicating a paralytic ileus (Dolan, 2011)

III. Diagnostic tests

A. Abdominal radiography

B. CT of the abdomen (Viswanathan et al., 2012)

C. Contrast medium studies

1. Oral barium is not used if bowel perforation is suspected or until colonic obstruction is ruled out.

2. Barium enema is used to evaluate colonic obstruction.

D. Endoscopy

E. Magnetic resonance imaging (MRI)

PROBLEM STATEMENTS AND OUTCOME IDENTIFICATION

I. Acute Pain (NANDA-I)

A. Expected outcome—patient reports adequate pain relief.

II. Risk for Deficient Fluid Volume (NANDA-I)

A. Expected outcome—patient has adequate fluid volume and electrolyte balance.

III. Imbalanced Nutrition: Less than Body Requirements (NANDA-I)

A. Expected outcome—patient receives adequate nutrition when bowel is obstructed, according to patient goals.

B. Expected outcome—patient and family contact an appropriate health care team member when symptoms of bowel obstruction occur.

PLANNING AND IMPLEMENTATION

I. Interventions to minimize risk and severity of bowel obstruction

A. Promoting comfort

1. Pharmacologic interventions

a. Opiate analgesics

b. Analgesic adjuncts

c. Smooth muscle relaxants

d. Antiemetics

e. Corticosteroids (O'Connor & Creedon, 2011)

f. Antisecretory agents—octreotide

2. Nonpharmacologic interventions

a. Ensuring a relaxing environment

b. Providing back rubs or massage

c. Positioning patient on side and support with pillows

d. Providing frequent oral care; use of moistened sponge sticks; avoidance of lemon or glycerin swabs

B. Administering fluid and electrolyte replacement therapy

C. Helping patient ambulate early, according to the patient's tolerance

D. Encouraging deep-breathing exercises

II. Interventions to maximize patient safety

A. Elevating head of bed to 45 degrees to improve ventilation and prevent aspiration

B. Providing care of nasogastric tube

1. Assessment of pressure around nostrils every shift

2. Applying a water-soluble lubricant to nasal mucosa

3. Irrigating the tube with normal saline

C. Reporting critical changes to the provider ⚠

1. Fever and chills

2. Local, intense, constant pain

3. Absence of bowel sounds after full 5 minutes of auscultation

4. Muscle guarding, rigidity, rebound tenderness

5. Sudden worsening of patient's condition

III. Interventions to monitor for complications related to bowel obstruction

A. Assessment for signs and symptoms of dehydration—dry mouth and lips, poor skin turgor, decreased urinary output

B. Assessment for interference with deep breathing related to abdominal distention

C. Assessment for signs and symptoms of peritonitis—boardlike abdomen, increased pain on movement, shallow respirations, tachycardia

D. Measurement of abdominal girth during every shift

E. Monitoring intake and output ratio, including gastric output

F. Monitoring key laboratory values

1. Electrolytes—sodium, potassium, chloride levels

2. Renal function tests—BUN, creatinine levels

3. CBC—hemoglobin, hematocrit levels

4. Arterial blood gas (ABG)—bicarbonate level, arterial blood pH

5. Serum enzymes—amylase, alkaline phosphatase, creatine kinase, LDH levels

IV. Interventions to incorporate the patient and family in care

A. Explaining all treatments and the rationales for them

B. Instructing the patient on deep-breathing exercises

C. Instructing the patient on interventions that reduce anxiety and provide comfort—for example, relaxation techniques, mental imagery, and music

D. Instructing the patient to breathe through the nose to decrease the amount of air swallowed

E. Teaching about signs and symptoms of bowel obstruction to report to the health care team

F. Teaching about signs and symptoms of infection to report to the health care team

EVALUATION

The oncology nurse systematically and regularly evaluates the patient's and family's responses to interventions for bowel obstruction to determine progress comfort and alleviation of bowel obstruction. Relevant data are collected, and actual findings are compared with expected findings. Problem statements, outcomes, and plans of care are reviewed and revised, as necessary.

Bowel Ostomies

OVERVIEW

I. Definition—a surgical creation of an opening between the colon and the abdominal wall

A. Surgical considerations (Gainant, 2011)

1. Ostomies created for muscle-invasive cancer and locally advanced cancer in the pelvis (e.g., gynecologic and rectal malignancies)

2. Extent of colonic resection determined by blood supply and distribution of lymph nodes

3. Distal sigmoid, rectosigmoid, rectum, and anus are removed through an abdominal and perineal approach, resulting in a permanent colostomy.

4. Wide excision done in cancer of the low rectum to remove lymph nodes, remove bulky tumor in the pelvis, and obtain adequate margins

5. Potency and continence are preserved; nerves are spared because of dissection around hypogastric and pelvic plexus.

B. Types (Gainant, 2011)

1. Temporary—indicated for bowel decompression in the presence of an obstructing tumor or fistulas involving the colon or rectum or to allow for bowel to heal following surgery

2. Permanent—indicated when the distal bowel, rectum, and anus are removed because of rectal cancer

C. Location of colostomy—determines consistency and volume of output

1. Cecostomy or ascending type—produces semifluid to mushy stool that contains residual enzymes and occurs throughout the day

2. Transverse ostomy—drains mushy stool at irregular intervals, usually after meals, and contains no enzymes

3. Descending or sigmoid type—produces soft to formed stool and can be regulated by irrigation

D. Stomas—may be identified by the type of surgical construction: end, loop, or double-barrel (Gainant, 2011)

1. End stoma—constructed by dividing the bowel and bringing the proximal end of the bowel through an opening in the abdominal wall

a. Distal bowel segment removed in abdominal perineal resection

b. Distal bowel segment sutured closed and left in place, called *Hartmann's pouch*, and continues to produce mucus from the rectum

2. Loop stoma—constructed by bringing a loop of bowel out through an incision and stabilizing it on the abdomen

   a. Usually created in the transverse loop

   b. Temporary procedure to relieve an obstruction or as palliation

3. Double-barrel stoma—indicates two stomas side by side or apart from one another

   a. Distal stoma—often referred to as a *mucous fistula*

   b. Proximal stoma—produces stool

II. Risk factors

A. Low rectal cancers

B. Ulcerative colitis or Crohn disease

C. Pelvic radiation

D. Chemotherapy

E. Diverticulitis

III. Effects of treatment (Soriano & Davis, 2011)

A. Pelvic exenteration may result in a urinary diversion, fecal diversion, or both.

B. Pelvic and abdominal radiation causes damage to the mucosa.

C. Mucosal damage may occur when the stoma is located in the radiation field.

D. Antineoplastic agents such as 5-FU, mitomycin C, and vincristine (Oncovin) may cause stomatitis, diarrhea, and constipation (Dolan, 2011).

ASSESSMENT

I. Pertinent personal history

A. Type of surgery and stoma

B. Previous pelvic or abdominal radiation or chemotherapy treatments

C. Changes in patterns of elimination

D. Difficulty in catheterizing a continent diversion

E. Diet habits and fluid consumption

F. History of chronic ulcerative colitis

II. Physical findings

A. Characteristics of stoma and peristomal skin

B. Effectiveness of pouching system

C. Characteristics of effluent (e.g., volume, consistency, color)

PROBLEM STATEMENTS AND OUTCOME IDENTIFICATION

I. Impaired Skin Integrity (NANDA-I)

A. Expected outcome—patient's stoma remains red and moist.

B. Expected outcome—skin surrounding stoma is intact.

II. Deficient Knowledge (NANDA-I), related to management of fecal diversions

A. Expected outcome—patient contacts the wound/ostomy/continence nurse for ongoing evaluations and maintaining up-to-date equipment.

B. Expected outcome—patient manages care of ostomy/urinary diversion.

III. Disturbed Body Image (NANDA-I)

A. Expected outcome—patient verbalizes feelings about the ostomy diversion and effect on body image.

B. Expected outcome—patient and significant other demonstrate confidence in their ability to resume previous sexual activities.

C. Expected outcome—patient is aware of available support groups.

PLANNING AND IMPLEMENTATION

I. Interventions to minimize incidence and severity of complications associated with fecal diversions

A. Stoma care (Haugen & Ratliff, 2013)

1. Stoma placement

   a. Scars, bony prominences, skin creases, or belt line avoided

   b. Site marked while patient is lying, standing, and sitting

   c. Site location within borders of rectus muscle

2. Appliance selection based on type of effluent, abdominal contour, manual dexterity, patient preference, cost

3. Changing appliance every 5 days and as needed for leakage or complaint of peristomal skin discomfort

4. Cutting pouch opening so barrier clears stoma by ⅛ inch and protecting exposed skin with skin barrier paste, if needed

5. Gently removing pouch by pushing down on skin while lifting up on pouch

6. Cleansing peristomal skin with water, and patting dry

7. Assessment of stoma and skin around stoma for erythema, dermatitis, bleeding, infection, stomal protrusion, retraction, mucoseparation, prolapse, herniation, and stenosis with each appliance change

8. Emptying pouch when one-third to one-half full

9. Protecting stoma from injury

10. Using silver nitrate sticks to stop bleeding of stoma

B. Management of diversion

1. Monitoring volume, color, and consistency of effluent

2. Monitoring function of new colostomies, which usually commences 3 to 5 days after surgery

3. Catheterizing new continent diversions beginning 3 to 4 weeks after surgery

4. Stopping irrigation of colostomy until RT or chemotherapy is completed

II. Interventions to address knowledge deficit and enhance adaptation and rehabilitation

   A. Teaching the patient how to irrigate the colostomy as a management option for regulating function of a descending and sigmoid colostomy

   B. Teaching the patient about measures to control gas and odor

   C. Teaching about ways to manage constipation and diarrhea

   D. Teaching about the importance of adequate intake of dietary fiber and fluid

   E. Discussing the signs and symptoms of urinary tract infections and when to seek medical attention

   F. Providing information about support resources available, for example, the United Ostomy Association

   G. Referral to the wound, ostomy, continence nurse for stoma marking and follow-up

   H. Assessment for presence of sexual dysfunction

   I. Referring patient and partner to appropriate resources for sexual counseling and treatment (D'Orazio & Goldberg, 2011)

EVALUATION

The oncology nurse systematically and regularly evaluates the patient's and family's responses to bowel ostomies to determine progress toward normal bowel function and ostomy adjustment. Relevant data are collected, and actual findings are compared with expected findings. Problem statements and outcome identification, outcomes, and plans of care are reviewed and revised, as necessary.

References

Badari, A., Farolino, D., Nasser, E., Mehboob, S., & Crossland, D. (2012). A novel approach to paraneoplastic intestinal pseudo-obstruction. *Supportive Care in Cancer, 20*, 425–428.

Barasch, A., & Epstein, J. B. (2011). Management of cancer therapy-induced oral mucositis. *Dermatologic Therapy, 24*(4), 424–431.

Calixto-Lima, L., Martins de Andrade, E., Gomes, A. P., Geller, M., & Siqueira-Batista, R. (2012). Dietetic management in gastrointestinal complications from antimalignant chemotherapy. *Nutrition Hospital, 27*(1), 65–75.

Cho, W. C. S. (Ed.). (2013). *Evidence-based non-pharmalogical therapies for palliative cancer care: Evidence-based anticancer complementary and alternative medicine.* (pp. 253–274). Berlin: New York.

Dolan, E. (2011). Malignant bowel obstruction: A review of current treatment strategies. *American Journal of Hospice and Palliative Medicine, 28*(8), 576–582.

D'Orazio, M., & Goldberg, M. (2011). Ostomy management and quality of life. *Journal of Wound, Ostomy, and Continence Nursing, 38*(5), 493–494.

dos Santos, L., Souza, F., Brunetto, A., Sasse, A., & Lima, J. (2012). Neurokinin-1 receptor antagonists for chemotherapy -induced nausea and vomiting: A systematic review. *Journal of the National Cancer Institute, 104*(17), 1280–1292.

Eisbruch, A. (2011). Amifostine in the treatment of head and neck cancer: Intravenous administration, subcutaneous administration, or none of the above. *Journal of Clinical Oncology, 29*(2), 119–121.

Farrington, M., Cullen, L., & Dawson, C. (2010). Assessment of oral mucositis in adult and pediatric oncology. *Otorhinolaryngology and Head-Neck Nursing, 28*(3), 8–15.

Furness, S., Worthington, H. V., Bryan, G., Birchenough, S., & McMillan, R. (2011). Interventions for the management of dry mouth: Topical therapies. *Cochrane Database of Systematic Reviews,* (12), CD008934.

Gainant, A. (2011). Emergency management of acute colonic cancer obstruction. *Journal of Visceral Surgery, 149*, e3–e10.

Gaziano, J. M. (2013). *Eating and swallowing issues—dysphagia.* oralcancerfoundation.org/dental/e_s_issues.html.

Getto, L., Zesterson, E., & Breyer, M. (2011). Vomiting, diarrhea, constipation and gastroeneteritis. *Emergency Medicine Clinics of North America, 29*(1), 211–237. http://dx.doi.org/10.1016/j.emc.2011.01.005.

Glare, P., Miller, J., Nikolova, T., & Tickoo, R. (2011). Treating nausea and vomiting in palliative care: A review. *Clinical Interventions in Aging, 6*, 243–259.

Gordon, F. (2012). Ascites. *Clinical Liver Disorders, 16*, 285–289.

Grunberg, S., Clark-Snow, R. A., & Koeller, J. (2010). Chemotherapy-induced nausea and vomiting: Contemporary approaches to optimal management: Proceedings from a symposium at the 2008 Multinational Association of Supportive Care in Cancer (MASCC) Annual Meeting. *Supportive Care in Cancer, 8* (Suppl. 1), S1–S10.

Harris, D. J., Eilers, J., Harriman, A., Cashavelly, B. J., & Maxwell, C. (2008). Putting evidence into practice: Evidence-based interventions for the management of oral mucositis. *Clinical Journal of Oncology Nursing, 12*(1), 141–152. http://dx.doi.org/10.1188/08.CJON.141-152.

Haugen, V., & Ratliff, C. (2013). Tools for assessing peristomal skin complications. *Journal of Wound, Ostomy, and Continence Nursing, 40*(2), 131–134.

Hesketh, P. J. (2008). Chemotherapy-induced nausea and vomiting. *New England Journal of Medicine, 358*(23), 2482–2494.

Jensen, S. B., Pedersen, A. M., Vissink, A., Andersen, E., Brown, C. G., Davies, A. N., et al. (2010). A systematic review of salivary gland hypofunction and xerostomia induced by cancer therapies: Prevalence, severity and impact on quality of life. *Supportive Care in Cancer, 18*(8), 1039–1060.

Kaspar, K., & Ekberg, O. (2012). Identifying vulnerable patients: Role of the EAT-10 and the multidisciplinary team for early intervention and comprehensive dysphagia care. *Nestle Nutrition International Workshop Series, 72*, 19–31.

Kipps, E., Tan, D., & Kaye, S. (2013). Meeting the challenge of ascites in ovarian cancer: New avenues for therapy and research. *Nature Reviews/Cancer,* 1-11.

National Cancer Institute. (2010). *Common terminology criteria for adverse events v 4.03.* evs.nci.nih.gov/ftp1/CTCAE/CTCAE_4.03_2010-06-14_QuickReference_5x7.pdf.

National Comprehensive Cancer Network. (2014). *Antiemesis, 2014.* www.nccn.org/professionals/physician_gls/pdf/antiemesis.pdf.

O'Connor, B., & Creedon, B. (2011). Pharmacological treatment of bowel obstruction in cancer patients. *Expert Opinion on Pharmacotherapy, 12*(14), 2205–2214.

Oncology Nursing Society (ONS). (2014). Putting evidence into practice. *Mucositis.* https://www.ons.org/practice-resources/pep/mucositis.

Raber-Durlacher, J. E., Brennan, M., Verdonk-de Leeuw, I., Gibson, R., Eilers, J., Waltimo, T., et al. (2012). Swallowing dysfunction in cancer patients. *Supportive Care in Cancer, 20*(3), 433–443.

Rangwala, R., Zafar, Y., & Abernathy, A. (2012). Gastrointestinal symptoms in cancer patients with advanced disease: New methodologies, insights and a proposed approach. *Journal of Supportive and Palliative Care, 6*(1), 69–75.

Reshamwala, P. A. (2010). Management of ascites. *Critical Care Nursing Clinics of North America, 22*(3), 309–314. http://dx.doi.org/10.1016/j.ccell.2010.04.003.

Shaw, C., & Taylor, L. (2012). Treatment-related diarrhea in patients with cancer. *Clinical Journal of Oncology Nursing, 16*(4), 413–417.

Shoemaker, L., Estfan, B., Induru, I., & Declan Walsh, T. (2011). Symptom management: An important part of cancer care. *Cleveland Clinic Journal of Medicine, 78*(1), 25–33.

Soriano, A., & Mellar, D. (2011). Malignant bowel obstruction: Individualized treatment near the end of life. *Cleveland Clinic Journal of Medicine, 78*(3), 197–206.

Thompson, N. (2012). Optimizing treatment outcomes in patients at risk for chemotherapy-induced nausea and vomiting. *Clinical Journal of Oncology Nursing, 16*(3), 309–313.

van Vilet, M., Harmsen, H., deBont, E., & Tissing, W. (2010). The role of intestinal microbiota in the development and severity of chemotherapy-induced mucositis. *Plos Pathogens, 6*(5), 1–7.

Visvanathan, V., & Nix, P. (2010). Managing the patient presenting with xerostomia: A review. *International Journal of Clinical Practice, 64*(3), 404–407.

Viswanathan, C., Bhosale, P., Ganeshan, D., Truong, M., Silverman, P., & Balachandran, A. (2012). Imaging of complications of oncological therapy in the gastrointestinal system. *Cancer Imaging, 12,* 163–172.

Wickham, R. (2012). Evolving treatment paradigms for chemotherapy-induced nausea and vomiting. *Cancer Control, 19*(2), 3–9.

Worthington, H. V., Clarkson, J. E., Bryan, G., Furness, S., Glenny, A. M., Littlewood, A., et al. (2010). Interventions for preventing oral mucositis for patients with cancer receiving treatment. *Cochrane Database of Systematic Reviews,* (12), CD000978.

Zur, E. (2012). Gastrointestinal mucositis: Focus on the treatment of the effects of chemotherapy and radiotherapy on the rectum. *International Journal of Pharmaceutical Compounding, 16*(2), 117–123.

CHAPTER 29
Alterations in Genitourinary Function

Sally L. Maliski

Urinary Incontinence

OVERVIEW

I. Physiology
  A. Definition
    1. Urinary incontinence—involuntary loss of urine to the extent that it becomes a problem
      a. Stress—involuntary loss of urine during laughing, coughing, sneezing, or other physical activities that increase abdominal pressure
      b. Urge—involuntary loss of urine associated with an abrupt and strong desire to void
      c. Reflex—involuntary loss of urine with no sensation of urge voiding or bladder fullness
      d. Functional—state in which an individual experiences incontinence because of difficulty in reaching or inability to reach the toilet before urination
      e. Total—continuous loss of urine without distention or awareness of bladder fullness
      f. Urinary retention—chronic inability to void followed by involuntary voiding (overflow incontinence) caused by overdistention of the bladder (Doughty, 2005)
  B. Mechanisms
    1. Urinary incontinence—a voiding dysfunction that can be classified as storage (stress, urge, total, functional), emptying (urinary retention), and combination of storage and emptying (reflex) problems (Doughty, 2005)
    2. Storage problems
      a. Involuntary contracting of bladder during filling
      b. Reduced compliance of bladder wall
      c. Sensory urgency
      d. Loss of bladder neck and proximal urethra support
      e. Intrinsic sphincter dysfunction
    3. Emptying problems
      a. Loss of or impaired contractility
      b. Urethral or prostatic obstruction

4. Storage and emptying problems
  a. Loss of voluntary control of voiding
  b. Loss of bladder-sphincter coordination (Doughty, 2005)
5. Postprostatectomy incontinence
  a. Sphincter competence depends primarily on integrity of the rhabdosphincter (Bauer et al., 2011; Campbell, Glazener, Hunter, Cody, & Moore, 2012).
  b. Incompetence of the rhabdosphincter is the primary cause and may result from reduced sphincter mobility from scarred or atrophied tissue, tissue injury caused by ischemia during surgery, pudendal nerve injury, or shortening of the urethra.
  c. Urge is caused by bladder muscle (detrusor) instability, low bladder wall compliance, or both.
  d. Combination of stress and urge incontinence results from damage to the rhabdosphincter along with detrusor instability.
  e. Atrophy of the rhabdosphincter and neural degeneration are evident with advancing age (Campbell et al., 2012).
6. Female
  a. Loss of estrogen during menopause may cause urethral epithelium thinning.
  b. Obstruction may be caused by severe pelvic organ prolapse (Banakhar, Al-Shaiji, & Hassouna, 2012; Dillon, Lee, & Lemack, 2012; Jung, Jeon, & Bai, 2008).
7. Risk factors
  a. Disease related
    (1) Loss of ability to inhibit bladder or rectal contractions in clients with lesions in the brain cortex as a result of a cerebrovascular accident, multiple sclerosis, Parkinson disease, or primary or metastatic tumor (Doughty, 2005; Krogh & Christenson, 2009)

(2) Loss of bladder and bowel reflex contractions, which may occur in clients with suprasacral lesions of the spinal cord, spinal cord tumors, compression following radical pelvic surgery, or diabetic neuropathy (Doughty, 2005; Krogh & Christenson, 2009)

(3) Loss of sphincter competency, which affects the bladder's ability to store urine; may be acquired after radical prostatectomy, radiation treatment, trauma, or sacral cord lesions (Doughty, 2005; Iyengar, Levy, Choi, Lee, & Kuban, 2011; Krogh & Christenson, 2009)

(4) Impaired or lost sensation of the bladder caused by inflammation, chronic infection, or prolonged bladder distention

(5) Obstruction of the bladder caused by tumor, prostatic hyperplasia, or fecal impaction

(6) Immobility commonly associated with chronic degenerative disease

(7) Endocrine conditions such as hyperglycemia and diabetes insipidus, which cloud the sensorium and induce diuresis

(8) Loss of functional ability, which often accompanies cognitive impairment in patients with central nervous system (CNS) metastases, Alzheimer disease, and delirium

(9) Previous transurethral resection of the prostate, anastomotic stricture, stage of disease, surgical technique, experience of the surgeon (Doughty, 2005)

b. Treatment related

(1) Surgical intervention that disrupts neural pathways, which may occur with abdominal perineal resection or radical prostatectomy

(2) Inflammatory reaction from the effects of radiation therapy (RT) on bladder and bowel, which may result in fibrosis or stenosis

(3) Chemotherapy agents such as vincristine (Oncovin), oxaliplatin (Eloxatin), and ifosfamide (Ifex), which cause neurotoxic side effects

(4) Fistula formation as a complication of disease, surgery, or RT

(5) Cryosurgery, which may cause urinary incontinence, urethral sloughing, bladder neck obstruction (Kimura et al., 2010)

(6) Medications, including anticholinergics, diuretics, narcotics, sedatives, hypnotics, tranquilizers, and laxatives

(7) Complications associated with indwelling catheters, including urinary tract infections, urinary stones, epididymitis, scrotal abscess, urethritis, urethral erosion, fistula formation, bladder cancer (Doughty, 2005; Jahn, Beutner, & Langer, 2012)

II. Principles of medical management

A. Treatment of underlying condition affecting incontinence

B. Surgical treatment considered for postprostatectomy incontinence, if incontinence persists 6 to 12 months following radical prostatectomy

C. Surgical treatment such as bladder neck suspension, pubovaginal sling, artificial urinary or rectal sphincter, rectal sphincter repair, augmentation cystoplasty, or fecal or urinary diversion

D. Drug therapy

E. Dietary modifications

1. Limiting alcohol intake and beverages containing caffeine

2. Limiting fluid intake several hours prior to bedtime

F. Bladder training programs (Doughty, 2005; Nazarko, 2013)

III. Potential sequelae of prolonged incontinence

A. Perianal skin irritation and excoriation

B. Changes in role relationship and lifestyle

C. Embarrassment that may prevent seeking needed health care

ASSESSMENT

I. History

A. Personal history

1. Cognitive ability

2. Neurologic disease or symptoms

3. Motivation to self-care in toileting

4. Manual dexterity and mobility

5. Living arrangements

6. Identification of caregiver and degree of caregiver involvement

7. Prescription and nonprescription medications

8. Impact of incontinence on self-esteem and interpersonal relationships

B. Past and present patterns of elimination

1. Precipitants of incontinence—caffeine and alcohol consumption, physical activity, surgery, trauma, recent illnesses

2. Daily fluid intake

3. Urinary tract symptoms—nocturia, dysuria, hesitancy, enuresis, straining, poor stream

4. Duration of incontinence

5. Frequency and amount of continence and incontinence

6. Previous treatments and its effects

7. Bladder diary for 3 days (Doughty, 2005)

II. Physical findings
  A. Presence of abdominal masses
  B. Palpation of full bladder
  C. Pelvic organ prolapse
  D. Fecal impaction to be ruled out
  E. Neurologic assessment, including balance, gait, deep tendon reflexes, sphincter tone, external anal sphincter contraction, perineal sensation
  F. Presence of incontinence, odor, perineal skin irritation or breakdown
III. Diagnostic testing
  A. Urinalysis and culture and sensitivity to assess for hematuria, bacteriuria, and glucosuria
  B. Cough stress test
  C. Presence and amount of postvoiding residual urine (Doughty, 2005)
  D. Urodynamic and imaging studies (e.g., cystometrography; voiding cystourethrography; electromyography to evaluate micturition, bladder filling, and storing function)
  E. Cystoscopy to identify site of obstruction (Doughty, 2005)

PROBLEM STATEMENTS AND OUTCOME IDENTIFICATION

I. Impaired Urinary Elimination (NANDA-I)
  A. Expected outcome—patient will achieve or experience improvement urinary continence.

PLANNING AND IMPLEMENTATION

I. Interventions to promote urinary continence
  A. Determining cause of or contributing factors of incontinence
  B. Reducing environmental barriers to using toileting facilities
  C. Nonpharmacologic interventions
    1. Supportive techniques
      a. Daily assessment of perianal skin
      b. Cleaning area after every voiding or bowel movement with soft washcloth and perianal cleanser, rinsing thoroughly, and patting dry
      c. Applying moisture barrier ointment or skin barrier after each incontinent episode
      d. Use of absorbent pads or briefs (Fader, Cottenden, & Getliffe, 2008)
      e. Use of penile compression devices for males and pessaries for females (Bauer et al., 2011)
      f. Use of external (condom) and internal catheters as a final method to manage incontinence (Jahn et al., 2012)
    2. Implementation of appropriate behavioral techniques
      a. Establishing a routine schedule for voiding, such as every 2 to 3 hours (habit training)
      b. Asking the patient on a regular basis about voiding (prompt voiding)
      c. Teaching the patient to suppress the urge to void to rebuild bladder capacity (bladder retraining).
      d. Teaching the patient how to perform Kegel exercises to strengthen pelvic floor muscles
      e. Having the patient do Kegel exercises, at least three sets of 10 repetitions per day
      f. Having the patient decrease fluid intake in the evening to decrease possibility of nighttime incontinence or nocturia
      g. Having the patient reduce intake of caffeine-containing beverages such as coffee, tea, and colas and reduce intake of alcohol and other bladder irritants
    3. Electrostimulation, which is delivered by means of electrodes attached to a portable stimulator to stimulate muscle contractions for 30 minutes daily (Bendaña et al., 2009)
    4. Urology consultation for evaluation of voiding problems, appropriate treatment, and behavioral modification or bladder retraining
  D. Pharmacologic interventions
    1. Anticholinergics (e.g., oxybutynin [Ditropan], tolterodine [Detrol], darifenacin [Enablex], fesoterodine [Toviaz], propiverine)
    2. Tricyclic antidepressants (e.g., imipramine [Tofranil], duloxetine [Cymbalta])
    3. Potassium channel openers (Doughty, 2005)
  E. Adherence to incontinence management program
    1. Monitoring subjective reports of the patient and family of changes in the pattern of incontinence
    2. Monitoring the client's compliance to the incontinence management program
    3. Monitoring effectiveness of measures implemented to manage incontinence
  F. Incorporating patient and family in care
    1. Teaching pelvic muscle exercises
    2. Teaching proper use of devices to control incontinence
    3. Teaching toileting programs (e.g., prompted voiding, bladder retraining)
    4. Instructing on critical factors that need to be reported to the physician
      a. Signs and symptoms of urinary tract infections and retention
      b. Worsening pattern of elimination

EVALUATION

The oncology nurse systematically and regularly evaluates the patient's and family's responses to nonpharmacologic and pharmacologic interventions to determine progress toward achieving urinary continence. Relevant data are collected, and actual findings are compared with expected findings. Nursing diagnoses, outcomes, and plans of care are reviewed and revised, as needed.

Part 4

Ostomies and Urinary Diversions

OVERVIEW

I. Urinary diversions
   A. Surgically created to divert the urine stream away from the original lower urinary tract
      1. Performed in situations in which the bladder is removed—that is, radical cystectomy or radical cystoprostatectomy for cancer of the bladder
      2. Involves removal of the bladder, pelvic lymph nodes, prostate (in men) and uterus, fallopian tubes, ovaries, and anterior vaginal wall, possibly urethra (in women)
      3. Sexual dysfunction common because of neural damage from surgery (Colwell, Goldberg, & Carmel, 2004; Yarbro, Wujik, & Holmes, 2010)
   B. Types of urinary diversions
      1. Ileal conduit
         a. Created from segment of small bowel; as the proximal end is sutured closed, the distal end is brought out through the abdominal wall; a stoma is created, and the ureters are implanted into the small bowel segment.
         b. Urine produced almost continuously
         c. Requires an external collection device
         d. As a freely refluxing system, high risk for chronic urinary tract infections, which increases the risk of stone formation (Colwell et al., 2004)
   C. Continent diversions
      1. Reservoir constructed from ileum or large intestine, which stores up to 800 mL of urine
      2. Continence maintained by the construction of the reservoir via a one-way flap valve (Colwell et al., 2004)
      3. External collection device not needed
         a. Patient will need to catheterize through the stoma to drain urine from the reservoir every 4 to 6 hours (Lester, 2012).
   D. Orthoptic neobladder
      1. Newer urinary reconstructive procedure in which a surgically constructed bladder is created from the intestine and attached to the urethra
      2. Intermittent catheterization needed for urinary retention
      3. Voiding accomplished by relaxation of the urinary sphincters and simultaneously practicing a Valsalva maneuver
      4. Factors that would exclude creation of neobladder—cancer extending into urethra, past history of inflammatory bowel disease, radiation, or short gut syndrome from previous bowel resection (Colwell et al., 2004)

II. Risk factors
   A. Pelvic radiation
   B. Chemotherapy
   C. Bladder cancer with muscle invasion (Colwell et al., 2004)
III. Effects of treatment
   A. Pelvic exenteration may result in a urinary diversion, fecal diversion, or both.
   B. Pelvic and abdominal radiation cause damage to the mucosa, resulting in diarrhea and cystitis.
   C. Mucosal damage may occur when the stoma is located in the field of radiation treatment (Colwell et al., 2004).

ASSESSMENT

I. Pertinent personal history
   A. Type of surgery and stoma
   B. Previous pelvic or abdominal radiation or chemotherapy treatments
   C. Changes in patterns of urinary elimination
   D. Recurrent or chronic urinary tract infections
   E. Difficulty in catheterizing a continent diversion
   F. Diet habits and fluid consumption
II. Physical findings
   A. Characteristics of stoma and peristomal skin
   B. Presence of leakage of urine from a continent diversion

PROBLEM STATEMENTS AND OUTCOME IDENTIFICATION

I. Deficient Knowledge (NANDA-I), related to management of urinary diversions
   A. Expected outcome—patient independently manages his or her urinary diversion; urinary diversion is patent and functioning properly.
II. Disturbed Body Image (NANDA-I), related to urinary diversion
   A. Expected outcome—patient demonstrates enhanced body image and self-esteem as evidenced by ability to look at, touch, talk about, and care for urinary diversion.

PLANNING AND IMPLEMENTATION

I. Interventions regarding care of urinary diversion to ensure proper functioning and to prevent or minimize complications
   A. Teaching patient how to care for urinary diversion
      1. Stoma placement
         a. Scars, bony prominences, skin creases, belt line, or site of hernia to be avoided
      2. Appliance selection based on type of effluent, abdominal contour, manual dexterity, patient preference, cost

3. Change of appliance every 5 days and as needed for leakage or complaint of peristomal skin discomfort

4. Cutting pouch opening so that barrier clears stoma by ⅛ inch and protecting exposed skin with skin barrier paste, if needed

5. Gently removing pouch by pushing down on the skin while lifting up on the pouch

6. Cleansing peristomal skin with water and patting dry

7. Assessment of stoma and skin around stoma for erythema, dermatitis, bleeding, infection, stomal protrusion, retraction, mucoseparation, prolapse, herniation, and stenosis with each appliance change

8. Emptying pouch when one-third to one-half full and before chemotherapy treatment

9. Protecting stoma from injury (Colwell et al., 2004)

10. Monitoring volume, color, and consistency of effluent

11. Monitoring functioning of new urinary diversion, which usually commences 3 to 5 days after surgery
    a. Patient may have several tubes in place postoperatively.
       (1) Jackson Pratt drain—to collect bodily fluids from surgical site
       (2) Two ureteral stents—one for each kidney
           (a) Allows healing of uretero-enteric anastamoses
           (b) Collects majority of urine output on the first 5 to 7 postoperative days

12. Catheterizing new continent diversions beginning about 3 to 4 weeks after surgery (Colwell et al., 2004)
    a. Ureteral stents are irrigated with 10 to 20 mL of normal saline every 6 to 8 hours for several weeks postoperatively.
    b. When urinary output from the new continent diversion increases, urine output from ureteral stents decreases.
       (1) Ureteral stents are removed.
       (2) Patient will need to catheterize through the stoma to drain urine from the reservoir every 4 to 6 hours (Lester, 2012).

13. Referral to the wound, ostomy, continence nurse for follow-up care (Colwell et al., 2004)

II. Interventions to promote body image and self-esteem
   A. Acknowledgment of normalcy of emotional response to change in urinary function and use of urinary diversion
   B. Encouraging patient to verbalize positive or negative feelings about having urinary diversion device

   C. Assisting patient in incorporating actual changes into activities of daily living (ADLs), social life, interpersonal relationships, and occupational activities
   D. Helping patient identify ways to cope that have been useful in the past
   E. Referring patient and caregivers to support groups and provide resources (e.g., United Ostomy Association), as needed

EVALUATION

The oncology nurse systematically and regularly evaluates the patient's and family's responses to interventions to determine progress toward the achievement of expected outcomes. Relevant data are collected, and actual findings are compared with expected findings. Nursing diagnoses, outcomes, and plans of care are reviewed and revised, as necessary.

Renal Dysfunction

OVERVIEW

I. Pathophysiology
   A. Kidneys regulate fluid and electrolyte balance by filtering essential substances from the blood, selectively reabsorbing needed fluid and electrolytes, and excreting those not needed in the urine (Thomas, 2008).
   B. Mechanism of chemotherapy-induced renal dysfunction generally includes damage to vasculature or structures of the kidneys, intrarenal damage, hemolytic-uremic syndrome (consists of anemia, thrombocytopenia, and acute renal failure), prerenal perfusion deficits, postrenal obstruction from tumor lysis syndrome, and development of obstructive stones.
   C. Severe and prolonged renal hypoperfusion may promote intrinsic renal damage.
   D. Damage to the renal tubules, renal blood vessels, or interstitium or glomerulus of the kidney leads to kidney dysfunction.
   E. Injury to the renal tubules causes electrolyte loss, renal tubular acidosis, loss of urine-concentrating ability, and reduction of glomerular filtration rate (Thomas, 2008).
II. Risk factors
   A. Effects of disease
      1. Compression of ureters by metastatic tumor of the surrounding lymph nodes may cause obstruction, resulting in hydronephrosis (Givens & Wethern, 2009).
      2. Compression of blood vessels by mass or tumor may cause venous occlusion of the kidney, arterial occlusion of the kidney, or both.
         a. Reduction of blood flow may impair kidney function.

3. Loss of ability by the kidneys to concentrate urine occurs in hypercalcemia of malignancy.
   a. Kidneys are attempting to excrete all of the calcium in blood, which leads to diuresis and accompanying electrolyte disturbances such as hypophosphatemia.
   b. Hypercalcemia of malignancy occurs more commonly in cancers such as breast cancer with metastases; multiple myeloma; squamous cell cancer of the lung and head and neck; renal cell cancer; lymphomas; and leukemia (Thomas, 2008; Yarbro et al., 2010).
4. Advanced prostate or cervical cancer renal problems are related to postrenal obstructive uropathy (Yarbro et al., 2010).
B. Treatment-related
   1. Radiation to renal structures may lead to permanent fibrosis and atrophy.
   2. Precipitation of uric acid or calcium phosphate crystallization from lysis of tumor cells may result in obstruction or formation of stones.
   3. Fluid and electrolyte imbalances caused by chemotherapy agents may have an indirect effect on kidney function and may lead to renal failure.
   4. Nephrotoxic agents such as antineoplastic agents cisplatin (Platinol), carboplatin (Paraplatin), ifosfamide (Ifex), gemcitabine (Gemzar), high-dose methotrexate (MTX), carmustine (BiCNU), semustine (Lomustine), pentostatin (Nipent), diaziquone (AZQ), interferon-α (Alferon-N), mitomycin-C (Mutamycin), streptozocin (Zanosar), aminoglycoside antibiotics, and amphotericin B (Fungizone) cause a direct effect.

ASSESSMENT

I. Pertinent personal history to identify risk factors
   A. Advanced age
   B. Diuretics, cardiac and nephrotoxic medications
   C. Type of malignancy
   D. Comorbidities such as hypertension, diabetes insipidus, diabetes mellitus
   E. Previous pelvic or abdominal radiation or chemotherapy treatments
   F. Renal stones
   G. Pre-existing renal impairment
II. Physical findings
   A. Cardiovascular—arrhythmias, rapid thready pulse, orthostatic hypotension
   B. Neurologic—lethargy, confusion
   C. Poor skin turgor, dry mucous membranes
   D. Gastrointestinal (GI)—nausea, vomiting, polydipsia, splenomegaly
   E. Genitourinary—nocturia, polyuria, oliguria, flank pain, dysuria

III. Laboratory data
   A. Serum creatinine and blood urea nitrogen (BUN) levels reflect renal function.
   B. Creatinine clearance study is often done before implementing chemotherapy to assess renal function.
   C. Elevation of serum uric acid and calcium levels and a decrease in potassium and magnesium levels may suggest renal impairment (Thomas, 2008; Yarbro et al., 2010).

PROBLEM STATEMENTS AND OUTCOME IDENTIFICATION

I. Excess Fluid Volume (NANDA-I)
   A. Expected outcome—patient maintains adequate fluid volume and electrolyte balance; patient identifies and manages factors that may affect renal function, for example, diet, medications, and physical activity.

PLANNING AND IMPLEMENTATION

I. Interventions to maintain adequate fluid volume and electrolyte balance
   A. Monitoring for signs and symptoms of renal toxicity
      1. Verifying baseline renal function
      2. Nonpharmacologic interventions
         a. Monitoring intake and output closely
            (1) Urine output—less than 30 mL/hr may indicate renal impairment
            (2) Maintaining adequate fluid intake.
            (3) Maintaining a greater intake than output, unless contraindicated, if patient is receiving diuretics.
            (4) Ensuring aggressive hydration before, during, and after cisplatin (Platinol-AQ) administration
            (5) Maintaining adequate fluid intake
            (6) Monitoring for obstructive diuresis (urine output of more than 2000 mL in 8 hours) following the removal of obstruction
            (7) Straining urine for stones, if indicated
         b. Monitoring vital signs and postural blood pressure
         c. Monitoring laboratory data— serum creatinine, BUN, phosphorus, potassium, magnesium, sodium, uric acid, calcium, glucose, and creatinine clearance levels
         d. Recording daily weights
         e. Maximizing mobility
            (1) Changing patient position every 2 hours
            (2) Performing passive range of motion exercises for patients on bed rest
            (3) Encouraging weight bearing and ambulation if patient is able (Yarbro et al., 2010)

B. Pharmacologic interventions
   1. Saline hydration with appropriate diuretic to maintain fluid balance (Thomas, 2008)
   2. Oral sodium bicarbonate to maintain alkaline urine
   3. Amifostine and sodium thiosulfate for cisplatin nephrotoxicity (Thomas, 2008)
   4. Replacing electrolytes, as needed
   5. Administering diuretics, as needed

II. Interventions to incorporate patient and family in care
   A. Teaching the patient about importance of maintaining adequate hydration and safe weight-bearing activity
   B. Teaching the patient and family about the signs and symptoms of electrolyte imbalance (e.g., hyper- and hypocalcemia, hyper- and hypokalemia, hyponatremia), and fluid volume excess and the appropriate time to seek medical attention
   C. Explaining properties of medications prescribed

EVALUATION

The oncology nurse systematically and regularly evaluates the patient's and family's responses to interventions to determine progress toward the achievement of fluid and electrolyte balance. Relevant data are collected, and actual findings are compared with expected findings. Nursing diagnoses, outcomes, and plans of care are reviewed and revised, as necessary.

References

Banakhar, M. A., Al-Shaiji, T. F., & Hassouna, M. M. (2012). Pathophysiology of overactive bladder. *International Urogynecology Journal, 23*(8), 975–982.

Bauer, R. M., Gozzi, C., Hübner, W., Nitti, V. W., Novara, G., Peterson, A., et al. (2011). Contemporary management of postprostatectomy incontinence. *European Urology, 59*(6), 985–996.

Bendaña, E. E., Belarmino, J. M., Dinh, J. H., Cook, C. L., Murray, B. P., Feustel, P. J., et al. (2009). Efficacy of transvaginal biofeedback and electrical stimulation in women with urinary urgency and frequency and associated pelvic floor muscle spasm. *Urologic Nursing, 29*(3), 171.

Campbell, S. E., Glazener, C. M., Hunter, K. F., Cody, J. D., & Moore, K. N. (2012). Conservative management for postprostatectomy urinary incontinence. *Cochrane Database Systematic Reviews, 1*, CD001843, http://dx.doi.org/10.1002/14651858.CD01843.pub4.

Colwell, J. C., Goldberg, M. T., & Carmel, J. E. (2004). *Fecal & urinary diversions.* St. Louis: Mosby.

Dillon, B. E., Lee, D., & Lemack, G. E. (2012). Urodynamics: Role in incontinence and prolapse: A urology perspective. *Urologic Clinics of North America, 39*(3), 265–272. http://dx.doi.org/10.1016/j.ucl.2012.05.001.

Doughty, D. B. (2005). *Urinary and fecal incontinence: Current management concepts* (3rd ed.). St Louis: Mosby Elsevier.

Fader, M., Cottenden, A. M., & Getliffe, K. (2008). Absorbent products for moderate-heavy urinary and/or fecal incontinence in men and women. *Cochrane Database Systematic Reviews. 4*, CD007408, http://dx.doi.org/10.1002/14651858.CD007408.

Givens, M. L., & Wethern, J. (2009). Renal complications in oncologic patients. *Emergency Medicine Clinics of North America, 27*(2), 283–291.

Iyengar, P., Levy, L. B., Choi, S., Lee, A. K., & Kuban, D. A. (2011). Toxicity associated with postoperative radiation therapy for prostate cancer. *American Journal of Clinical Oncology, 34*(6), 611–618. http://dx.doi.org/10.1097/coc.06013e3181f946dc.

Jahn, P., Beutner, K., & Langer, G. (2012). Types of indwelling urinary catheters for long-term bladder drainage in adults. *Cochrane Database Systematic Reviews. 10*, CD004997, http://dx.doi.org/10.1002/14651858.CD004997.pub3.

Jung, B. H., Jeon, M. J., & Bai, S. W. (2008). Hormone-dependent aging problems in women. *Yonsei Medicine Journal, 49*(3), 345–351. http://dx.doi.org/10.3349/ymj.2008.49.3.345.

Kimura, M., Mouraviev, V., Tsivian, M., Moreira, D. M., Mayes, J. M., & Palasike, T. J. (2010). Analysis of urinary function using validated instruments and uroflowmetry after primary and salvage prostate cryoablation. *Urology, 76*(5), 1258–1265. http://dx.doi.org/10.1016/j.urology.2009.09.062.

Krogh, K., & Christenson, P. (2009). Neurogenic colorectal and pelvic floor dysfunction. *Best Practice and Research in Clinical Gastroenterology, 23*(4), 531–543. http://dx.doi.org/10.1016/j.bpg.2009.04.012.

Lester, J. (2012, August). Restoring and maintaining urinary function. *Seminars in Oncology Nursing, 28*(3), 163–169.

Nazarko, L. (2013). Urinary incontinence: Providing respectful, dignified care. *British Journal of Community Nursing, 18*(2), 58, 60, 62-4.

Thomas, N. (Ed.). (2007). *Renal nursing* (3rd ed.). Edinburgh: Elsevier.

Yarbro, C. H., Wujik, D., & Holmes, G. (2010). *Cancer nursing: Principles and practice* (7th ed.). Sudbury, MA: Jones & Bartlett.

Part 4

CHAPTER 30

Alterations in Musculoskeletal, Integumentary, and Neurologic Functions

Kathryn Renee Waitman

Alterations in Musculoskeletal Functions

OVERVIEW

I. Definitions
   A. Musculoskeletal alterations—affecting the body's joints, ligaments, muscles, nerves, tendons, and structures that support limbs, neck, and back
   B. Impaired physical mobility (immobility)—a state in which the patient experiences or is at risk for a limitation in independent, purposeful physical movement of the body or one or more extremities (North American Nursing Diagnosis Association [NANDA], 2003)

II. Physiology
   A. Quantitative decline in muscle mass (sarcopenia) (Reid & Fielding, 2012)
   B. Inactivity and limited use or disuse of muscle groups may decrease the muscles' ability to contract and may lead to decreased muscle size, muscle atrophy, and weakness.
   C. Motor impairment (spasticity, muscle weakness, paralysis, hemiparesis, ataxia) may occur in primary cancer (brain tumors, multiple myeloma) or as a secondary effect in metastatic disease (spinal cord compression), infections, and cancer therapy or in nonmalignant conditions.

III. Risk factors
   A. Disease related (Martin, 2014; Oncology Nursing Society [ONS], 2009)
      1. Skeletal system tumor
      2. Tumors of the brain and spinal cord
      3. Obstruction in lymphatic or systemic circulation
      4. Bone pain
      5. Pain, stiffness, fatigue
      6. Spinal cord compression
      7. Sensory-perceptual alterations
      8. Nonmalignant conditions—herniated disks, vertebral fractures secondary to osteoporosis, ear infections
      9. Complications of bed rest
      10. Complications of cardiopulmonary disorders
      11. Dehydration
   B. Treatment related
      1. Side effects of corticosteroid therapy
      2. Side effects of radiation therapy
      3. Side effects of chemotherapy
      4. Nerve and muscle damage from surgical intervention
   C. Lifestyle related
      1. Changes in physical activity level
      2. High or low stress level
      3. Independent versus dependent personality
   D. Psychological and social issues
      1. Presence or absence of social support
      2. Depression

ASSESSMENT

I. History
   A. Presence of risk factors
   B. Recent treatment and anticipated side effects
   C. Decreased activity level
   D. Functional status
   E. Presence of pain, muscle weakness, and fatigue
   F. Presence of dyspnea, activity intolerance
   G. Presence of vertigo, ringing in ears, or blurred vision
   H. Evaluation of fall risk
   I. History of alcohol or drug use
   J. Current exercise practice
   K. Current therapy

II. Physical examination
   A. Changes in muscle tone, strength, and muscle mass
   B. Unintentional weight loss
   C. Strength and motor function
   D. Mobility and sensory function
   E. Changes in sexual function

F. Changes in bowel and bladder function

G. Incontinence and loss of sphincter control

H. Range of joint motion

I. Positive Babinski sign and reflexes

J. Alignment, balance, gait, and joint structure

K. Muscle mass, tone, and strength

L. Difficulty changing position from sitting to standing

M. Difficulty writing name

III. Psychosocial examination

A. Depression

B. Anxiety

C. Lack of motivation

IV. Laboratory data

A. Hypercalcemia

B. Electrolyte abnormalities

C. Lumbar puncture results

PROBLEM STATEMENTS AND OUTCOME IDENTIFICATION

I. Impaired Physical Mobility (NANDA-I)

A. Expected outcome—patient will actively participate in measures to maintain optimal physical function and prevent complications of immobility.

II. Activity Intolerance (NANDA-I)

A. Expected outcome—patient maintains activity level within capabilities.

III. Risk for Injury (NANDA-I)

A. Expected outcome—patient and family will verbalize and use safety measures to minimize risk for injury. ⚠

IV. Risk for Impaired Skin Integrity (NANDA-I)

A. Expected outcome—patient's skin remains intact.

PLANNING AND IMPLEMENTATION

I. Interventions to increase physical functioning (Albrecht & Taylor, 2012; Martin, 2014; ONS, 2009)

A. Having the patient perform active range of motion (AROM) exercises on unaffected limbs at least three or four times per day and passive range of motion (PROM) on affected limbs

B. Monitoring progress from AROM to functional activities

C. Maintaining body alignment while the patient is in bed

D. Changing the patient's position every 2 hours

E. Observing the patient before, during, and after activity or exercise

F. Obtaining appropriate assistive devices (e.g., splints, walker, cane, overhead trapeze)

G. Consulting with rehabilitation services for physical and occupational therapy

II. Interventions to decrease risk of further complications of immobility

A. Establishing a routine for activities of daily living (ADLs)

B. Providing assistance and supervision, as needed

C. Placing the call light within reach when the patient is left alone

III. Interventions to maximize safety for the patient ⚠

A. Protecting areas of decreased sensation from extreme heat and cold

B. Teaching the patient with decreased perception of extremities to check where the limb is placed when changing positions

C. Placing the bed in low position and the two side rails at the head of bed (HOB) up

D. Clearing pathways in room and hallways

IV. Interventions to enhance adaptation and rehabilitation

A. Positive reinforcement for behaviors that contribute to positive outcomes

B. Having the patient and family responsible for aspects of care according to their capabilities

C. Initiating and following up with referrals to rehabilitation services

V. Interventions to incorporate patient and family in care

A. Instructing patient and family about signs and symptoms to report

B. Discussing risk factors for impaired mobility

EVALUATION

The oncology nurse systematically and regularly evaluates the patient's mobility status and responses to interventions to optimize physical functioning and mobility. Relevant data specific to function are collected, and actual findings are compared with expected findings. Nursing diagnoses, outcomes, and plans of care are reviewed and revised, according to the patient's overall goals.

Alterations in Integumentary Function

OVERVIEW

I. Physiology

A. The skin is composed of three layers—the epidermis, the dermis, and the subcutaneous tissue (Figure 30-1).

1. The epidermis is the avascular outer layer, which serves as a barrier to prevent water loss and renews itself continuously through cell division.

2. The dermis, the inner connective tissue layer, is highly vascular, with afferent sensory nerve receptors, which provides nutritional support to the avascular epidermal layer.

3. The subcutaneous tissue is composed of adipose tissue, which serves as a cushion to trauma, an insulator to temperature changes, and an energy reservoir.

B. Intact skin protects the body from bacteria, temperature changes, physical trauma, and radiation.

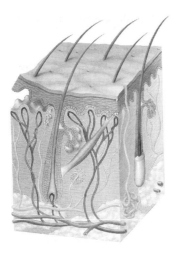

Figure 30-1 Normal skin. *From Herlihy, B. (2007). The human body in health and illness (3rd ed.). St. Louis: Saunders.*

C. Skin is the first line of defense by regulating thermal processes, protecting underlying structures, and excreting waste (Bergstrom, 2011).

II. Risk factors
  A. Disease related (Morse, 2014; O'Leary & Catania, 2014; Rodriguez, 2014; Vogel, 2014; Zitella, 2014)
    1. Thrombocytopenia
    2. Cutaneous metastases (late manifestation in the course of the illness for solid tumors of the breast and lung, squamous cell carcinoma of the head and neck, malignant melanoma, lymphoma, Kaposi sarcoma)
    3. Cutaneous paraneoplastic syndromes—acanthosis nigricans, acquired ichthyosis, Paget disease, telangiectasia, hypertrichosis, lanuginosa acquisita, erythroderma
    4. Primary malignant skin cancer (melanoma, basal cell carcinoma, squamous cell carcinoma, Kaposi sarcoma)
    5. Mycosis fungoides (slow, progressive, cutaneous T-cell lymphoma)
    6. Premalignant lesions (actinic keratosis, leukoplakia, dysplastic nevus syndrome)
  B. Treatment related (McCann, Akilov, & Geskin, 2012; Morse, 2014; O'Leary & Catania, 2014; Ridner, 2014; Vogel, 2014) (Table 30-1)
    1. Desquamative skin reaction (radiation enhancement, radiation recall, combined modality therapy) as a result of chemotherapy in association with radiation therapy
    2. Fragile skin from steroid therapy
    3. Erythema multiforme (widespread, scattered, cutaneous vesicles) associated with multiple drugs
    4. Erythema nodosum (tender, subcutaneous, anterior leg nodules)—hypersensitivity reaction to penicillin or sulfonamides
    5. Graft-versus-host disease (skin reaction related to bone marrow transplantation)
    6. Side effects of biologic response modifiers and epidermal growth factor receptor (EGFR) inhibitors
    7. Side effects of chemotherapy—mucositis, compromised nutritional status
    8. Side effects of radiation therapy—immunosuppression, compromised nutritional status, diarrhea
    9. Extravasation of chemotherapy (anthracyclines, taxanes, antimetabolites)
    10. Adhesive dressings (central and peripheral intravenous [IV] access)
    11. Tubes
      a. Chest tubes, Foley catheter, biliary catheters
      b. Feeding tubes—gastrostomy, jejunostomy
      c. Tubes for decompression and drains
    12. Malnutrition—decreased protein stores
    13. Other effects—alopecia, pressure ulcers, (lymph) edema, pruritus, jaundice, incontinence, infection

ASSESSMENT

I. History
  A. Presence of risk factors
  B. Patient's age
  C. General health status
  D. Exposure to infection
  E. Recent treatment and anticipated side effects
  F. Current drug therapy
  G. Past and current skin conditions
  H. Review of personal hygiene practices
  I. Nutritional status
  J. Smoking habits
  K. Incontinence of bowel or bladder
II. Physical examination (Figure 30-2)
  A. Skin—color, integrity, temperature, texture, turgor, presence of sloughing, rash
  B. Presence of redness, petechiae, purpura, ecchymosis, jaundice
  C. Presence of erythema, dry desquamation, moist desquamation
  D. Presence and grade of rash
  E. Local inflammation at injection site (erythema, induration, blisters)
  F. Ulcerations of mouth; dry, cracked mucous membranes and lips
  G. Presence of alopecia
  H. Presence of pruritus
  I. Integrity of tube sites, perirectal tissue, perineal tissue
  J. Presence of pressure ulcers
  K. Presence of pain

Table 30-1

Etiologic Factors of Skin Reactions

Skin Reaction	General Class of Reaction	Drug Class or Mechanism
Skin Reactions Found with Radiation Therapy Alone		
Acute radiation dermatitis	Immediate dermatitis occurring in radiated areas with erythema, pain, dermal swelling, itching, necrosis	May occur with all radiation therapy Mechanism is free radical damage to tissue
Chronic radiation dermatitis	Long-term effects of radiation therapy in port area with thinning of skin, scarring and contractures, telanglectasias, long-term skin sensitivity to irritants and environmental agents	May occur with all radiation therapy Mechanism is free radical damage to tissue Severity depends on port size and total dose
Skin Reactions Found with Chemotherapy and Radiation Therapy in Combination		
Radiation recall dermatitis	Occurs in previously irradiated skin within 1-2 wk following chemotherapy; erythema, edema, superficial ulcerations, superficial skin sloughing	Many drugs
Skin Reactions Found with Chemotherapy alone		
Allergic or Immune Complex Reactions		
Activation of already existing immune complex reaction in collagen vascular diseases of systemic lupus erythematosus and progressive systemic sclerosis (scleroderma)	Chemotherapy drug activates immune complexes already circulating due to underlying collagen vascular disease process, causing circular red scaly rash	Many drugs
Contact allergy (activated T cells)	Allergic response where drug touches skin (erythema, local swelling, desquamation, blistering, necrosis possible)	Nitrogen mustard (mechlorethamine)
Erythema multiforme (antigen-antibody complexes)	Rash with typical target lesions involving extremities, including palms and soles, can progress to generalized	Many drugs
Immunoglobulin E (IgE)–mediated	Itching, redness, swelling, within 1 hour after infusion begun; if life-threatening, termed *anaphylaxis* and includes decreased blood pressure, decreased level of consciousness, airway and breathing compromise	Platinum derivatives (cisplatin, carboplatin)
Serum sickness (antigen-antibody complexes)	Flulike symptoms, which may progress to life-threatening	Rituximab
Vasculitis (from antigen-antibody complexes	Generalized vascular inflammation with end-organ damage	Methotrexate
Extravasation injury (drug leaks from IV site into surrounding tissue)	Varying severity depending on specific drug (swelling, redness, irritation, local tissue loss, necrosis)	Many drugs
Light-Related Reactions		
Photo enhancement	Drug given several days after sunburn causes sunburn to reappear in that area.	Many drugs
Photosensitivity	Patient more sensitive to sun in solar-exposed areas and may develop severe sunburn.	Antitumor antibiotics; many drugs
Phototoxicity	Allergic response on solar-exposed areas may be severe with edema, erythema, severe path, blistering; if very severe, may result in permanent hyperpigmentation	Many drugs
Nail Changes		
Beah lines	Transverse lines in nails, bands corresponding to when drug was given or time when critical illness occurred	Any chemotherapy agent or critical illness

Continued

Table 30-1

Etiologic Factors of Skin Reactions—cont'd

Skin Reaction	General Class of Reaction	Drug Class or Mechanism
Oncholysis	Nail lifts up from base	Paclitaxel, docetaxel, cyclophosphamide, doxorubicin, 5-fluorouracil (5-FU), hydroxyurea, combination of vinblastine + bleomycin
Nail inflammation	Inflammatory changes around nail, including paronychia	EGFR (epidermal growth factor receptor) inhibitors (cetuximab, gefitinib), taxanes (docetaxel)
Pigment Changes of Skin, Mucous Membranes, Nails, Hair		
Drug secreted in sweat may induce pigmentation. Flag sign	Under areas where adhesive tape applied and skin sweats	Docetaxel, thiotepa, ifosfamide
Generalized hyperpigmentation of all skin	Pigment loss of hair during time drug is given; all skin involved	Many drugs Busulfan (termed *busulfan tan*), pegylated liposomal doxorubicin, hydroxyurea, methotrexate Cyclophosphamide
Gums	Permanent hyperpigmentation of gums	Cisplatin, hydroxyurea, bleomycin
Hyperpigmentation in areas of pressure or injury	Injured skin only, although inciting injury may be mild	Tegafur (5-FU derivative)
Hyperpigmentation of palms, soles, nails	Circular areas of hyperpigmentation in these locations	Daunorubicin
Hyperpigmentation of solar-exposed skin	Sun-exposed areas only	Daunorubicin
Scalp hyperpigmentation Variety of pigmentary changes of skin and appendages	Circular hyperpigmented areas in scalp General types of pigmentary changes especially common with drugs listed to right	Various cytotoxic drugs (alkylating agents, tumor-directed antibiotics)
Various types of hyperpigmentation—serpentine, generalized, other	Generalized hyperpigmentation (all skin), of sun-exposed areas only, serpentine (follows underlying vein where drug infused), mucosa of tongue, nails, conjunctiva of eyes	5-FU
Rashes		
Generalized rash of hands and feet	Usually localized, but can become more generalized	Tyrosine kinase signal transduction inhibitors (occurs with 50% of patients on higher doses of imatinib)
Acneiform rash	Papules and pustules similar to acne although this rash contains *no* comedones; commonly involves face and also back, upper chest	EGFR inhibitors (cetuximab, gefitinib)
Hand-foot syndrome, or acral erythema	Erythema of hands and feet, dysesthesias	Various chemotherapy drugs
Toxicity to rapidly dividing cells	Alopecia, mouth ulcers, gastrointestinal (GI) tract ulcers, GI yeast overgrowth and other infections from decreased mucous production (mucous is protective), bone marrow effects of anemia, decreased platelets, decreased white blood cells (WBCs), decreased production of sperm and ova	Most chemotherapy drugs; probability of occurrence depends on how much the drug affects rapidly dividing cell groups

From DeHaven C, Chemotherapy and radiotherapy effects on the skin, 2007, http://www.spsscs.org/feature-articles/chemotherapy-and-radiotherapy-effects-on-the-skin. Used with permission.

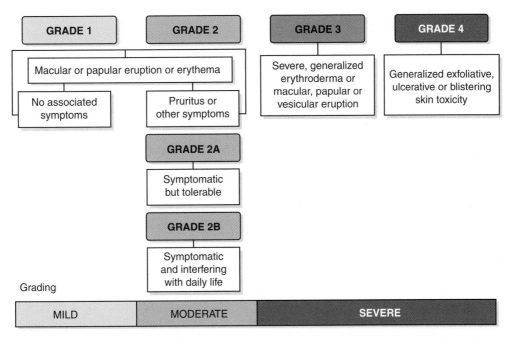

Figure 30-2 Modified grading system for skin rash mediated by epidermal growth factor receptor (EGFR) inhibition. *Data from Pérez–Soler, R., et al. (2005). Her1/EGFR inhibitor–associated rash: future directions for management and investigation outcomes from the her1/EGFR inhibitor rash management forum. Oncologist, 10, 345–356.*

III. Psychosocial examination
 A. Social isolation
 B. Anxiety
 C. Depression
IV. Laboratory data
 A. Complete blood cell (CBC) count
 B. Blood chemistries
 C. Platelet count
 D. Serum albumin—total protein

PROBLEM STATEMENTS AND OUTCOME IDENTIFICATION

 I. Impaired Skin Integrity (NANDA-I)
 A. Expected outcome—patient and family verbalize strategies and actively participate in routine and preventive skin management.
 II. Impaired Oral Mucous Membranes (NANDA-I)
 A. Expected outcome—patient verbalizes strategies to minimize the risk of and to manage mucositis.
 III. Situational Low Self-Esteem (NANDA-I)
 A. Expected outcome—patient and family discuss effects of skin alterations on self-concept and body image.
 B. Expected outcome—patient engages in strategies to be more involved with others.
 IV. Imbalanced Nutrition: Less than Body Requirements (NANDA-I)
 A. Expected outcome—patient increases and/or maintains adequate dietary and fluid intake.

 V. Risk for Infection (NANDA-I)
 A. Expected outcome—patient does not develop an infection.
 B. Expected outcome—patient identifies the risk factors and initial signs and symptoms of infection to report to a member of the health care team.

PLANNING AND IMPLEMENTATION

 I. Assessment of knowledge of risk factors and side effects of therapy
 II. Interventions to increase or maintain dietary and fluid intake
 A. Offering small frequent meals with increased protein and calories
 B. Moistening foods with liquids, sauces, and gravy
 C. Having the patient increase fluid intake to 3 L/day if not medically contraindicated (e.g., water and calorie-dense fluids such as protein drinks, milk, juice)
 D. Having the patient rinse the oral cavity with normal saline or a nonalcoholic mouthwash
 III. Interventions to decrease inflammation of mucous membranes (see Chapter 28)
 IV. Interventions to teach self-care techniques and prevent complications
 A. Teaching the patient and family to assess the skin every 4 hours
 B. Teaching patient and family tube and drain management

C. Assisting with turning and positioning every 2 hours

D. Massaging uninjured areas gently

E. Use of an air mattress, specialty bed, or water mattress for high-risk persons

F. Instructing on gentle skin cleansing with mild pH-balanced skin cleanser

G. Rinsing soap thoroughly off skin and patting skin dry

H. Moisturizing and lubricating skin

I. Use of dry, clean, wrinkle-free linens and devices such as an egg crate mattress

J. Use of specialty beds

V. Interventions to protect skin integrity

A. Teaching about the effects of treatments on skin

B. Teaching about the use of protective film, skin barriers, or collection devices around drains and tubes with copious drainage

C. Teaching about the use of sterile technique for invasive procedures such as insertion of tubes

D. Teaching about hand washing

E. Keeping patient's fingernails smooth and short

F. Teaching about reportable signs and symptoms of infection

G. Recommending about the use of cotton clothing and avoidance of restrictive clothing

H. Reporting changes in skin color, integrity, pain, increased pruritus, drainage (amount, odor, color, consistency) to health care provider

VI. Interventions for oral, perineal, and general hygiene

A. Use of soft toothbrush or oral sponges

B. Applying moisturizers to oral mucosa

C. Cleansing the perineal area with mild soap, rinsing thoroughly, patting the area dry, and applying a skin barrier after each bowel movement

D. Applying adhesive perineum pad or panty liner without deodorant to the undergarment

E. Gently cleansing skin with mild soap and tepid water and patting dry with soft cloth

VII. Nonpharmacologic interventions

A. Adding emollients to bath water, skin lubricants to skin other than to irradiated sites

B. Oatmeal baths

C. Application of cool or warm compresses

D. Avoiding alcohol-based skin lotions

VIII. Pharmacologic interventions

A. Prophylactic medications

B. Medications to manage rash (Figure 30-3)

IX. Interventions to adapt and cope with hair loss (see Chapter 36)

X. Interventions for radiation-induced acute and chronic skin reactions (see Chapter 21)

EVALUATION

The oncology nurse systematically and regularly evaluates the patient's skin integrity and performs interventions to promote optimal health and to prevent infections. Relevant data are collected, and actual findings are compared with expected findings. Nursing diagnoses, outcomes, and plans of care are reviewed and revised, as necessary.

Neuropathies

OVERVIEW

I. Physiology (Brant, 2014; Fields, 2014; Matthews & Berger, 2014; Wilkes, 2014)

A. Neuropathies—any functional disturbances, pathologic changes, or both in the peripheral nervous system (PNS): cranial, sensory, and motor nerves and portions of the autonomic nervous system

B. Neuropathies of the central nervous system (CNS)—seizures, encephalopathy, cerebellar dysfunction, ophthalmologic toxicities and ototoxicities, mental status changes, and peripheral neuropathies with sensory and motor dysfunction

C. Incidence and severity of neuropathies—may vary, depending on administration of immunosuppressive therapy

D. Toxicities—may be dose related and reversible on discontinuation of therapy

II. Risk factors

A. Disease related

1. Effects of cancer

2. Postherpetic neuralgia (PHN)

3. Presence of infiltrative emergencies (e.g., spinal cord compression)

4. Other diseases (e.g., history of hepatic or neurologic dysfunction)

5. Pre-existing neuropathies as a result of diabetes mellitus, human immunodeficiency virus (HIV) infection, preexisting vitamin B complex deficiency (Tofthagen, Visovsky, & Hopgood, 2013)

B. Treatment related

1. Side effects of high-dose chemotherapy (e.g., cerebellar dysfunction, strokelike reaction, generalized weakness, gait disturbance, numbness of feet, loss of proprioception, vibratory sensation)

2. Peripheral neuropathies—tingling of fingers and toes, jaw pain, footdrop, muscular atrophy (Tofthagen, 2010; Tofthagen et al., 2013; Wilkes, 2014)

3. Side effects of radiation therapy (e.g., ataxia, dysarthria, nystagmus, radicular pain)

4. Age—older than 60 years

5. Pre-existing neuropathy related to radiation therapy

C. Situation related

1. Psychological issues

2. Social issues

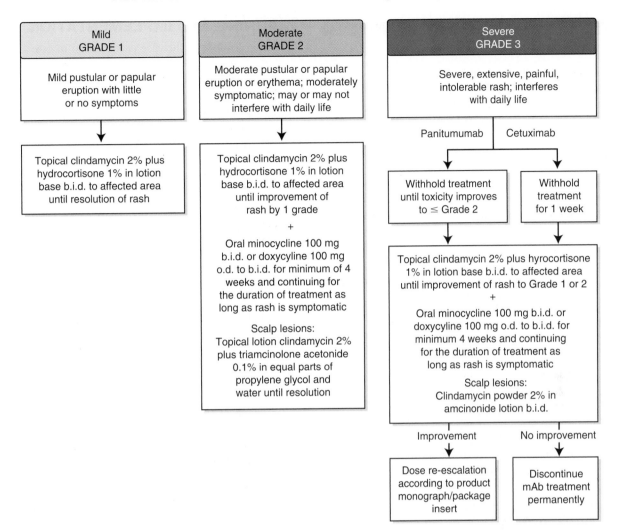

Figure 30-3 Treatment recommendations for rash mediated by monoclonal antibody (mAb) targeting of epidermal growth factor receptor, by severity. *b.i.d.,* Twice daily; *o.d.,* once daily. *Data from Pérez–Soler, R., Delord J.P., Halpern, A., et al. (2005). Her1/EGFR inhibitor-associated rash: future directions for management and investigation outcomes from the her1/EGFR inhibitor rash management forum. Oncologist, 10, 345–356.*

ASSESSMENT

I. History
  A. Presence of risk factors or other comorbidities such as diabetes, idiopathic neuropathy prior to chemotherapy
  B. Psychiatric and current life problems
  C. Acute herpes zoster
  D. Recent chemotherapy treatment and anticipated side effects
  E. Presence of weakness
  F. Presence of burning, numbness, tingling in feet and hands, perioral numbness, paresthesias—stocking-glove distribution (Tofthagen, 2010; Tofthagen et al., 2013; Wilkes, 2014)
  G. Presence of paresthesia of hands and feet, constipation, loss of deep tendon reflex
  H. Presence of cerebellar involvement (e.g., tremors, loss of balance)
  I. Inability to perform ADLs
  J. Performance of occupational and recreational activities
  K. Current medication therapy
  L. Presence of anxiety, low self-esteem
II. Physical examination (Table 30-2)
  A. Vital signs
  B. Baseline sensory, mobility, and motor function
  C. Baseline autonomic function
  D. Baseline cranial nerve assessment
  E. Baseline cerebellar function
  F. Speech or language ability
  G. Sight-related changes (e.g., blurred vision, impaired color perception)

Part 4

Table 30-2

Assessment of Neuropathy

Function	Procedure
Cerebellar and proprioception	• Evaluate rapid alternating movement of hands. • Observe for accurate movement of extremities. • Evaluate balance using Romberg test: Have patient stand with feet together, arms at side with eyes closed. A slight sway is normal. • Observe gait for stride and stance.
Sensory function	• Test for response to touch and pain. • Check vibration sense using a tuning fork. • Evaluate position sense: Move a finger or great toe up and down while patient's eyes are closed; have patient identify position of the digit. • Assess for discrimination between sharp and dull sensations. • Evaluate the ability to distinguish the body part being touched. • Evaluate for stereognosis, the ability to distinguish a common object, such as a coin. • Evaluate for graphesthesia, the ability to identify a common letter or number drawn on the hand.
Deep tendon reflexes	• Test deep tendon reflexes (biceps, brachioradial, triceps, patellar, Achilles). • Check for clonus.

From Marrs, J., Newton, S. (2003). Updating your peripheral neuropathy "know how." *Clinical Journal of Oncology Nursing, 7*(3), 299–303.

III. Psychological examination
    A. Anxiety management strategies
    B. Coping style and ability
IV. Laboratory data
    A. Nerve conduction studies (e.g., electromyography [EMG])
    B. Muscle or nerve biopsy

PROBLEM STATEMENTS AND OUTCOME IDENTIFICATION

I. Risk for Injury (NANDA-I) ⚠
    A. Expected outcome—patient verbalizes measures to maximize safety and manage self-care.
II. Impaired Physical Mobility (NANDA-I)
    A. Expected outcome—patient maintains or increases mobility.
III. Acute Pain or Chronic Pain (NANDA-I)
    A. Expected outcome—patient verbalizes a satisfactory relief of pain.
IV. Constipation (NANDA-I)
    A. Expected outcome—patient maintains regular bowel function.

PLANNING AND IMPLEMENTATION

I. Interventions to increase participation in care
    A. Assessment of knowledge of early signs and symptoms of neuropathies
    B. Teaching about side effects of chemotherapy
    C. Teaching about hand and foot care (use of massage and lotions)
    D. Referral to occupational and rehabilitation services
    E. Before start of chemotherapy, instructing patient about potential neurologic side effects
    F. Instructing patient on how to maintain a safe environment both at home and at work
    G. Giving positive feedback and honest reassurance
    H. Empowering patient to communicate with physician and nurse about symptoms
II. Interventions to maximize safety for the patient (see Alterations in Mobility, Planning, and Implementation sections) ⚠
III. Interventions to promote stool softening
    A. Monitoring and recording characteristics of stools
    B. Use of stool softeners or laxatives, as needed, for bowel movement regimen
    C. Having patient increase fluid intake to 3000 mL/day unless medically contraindicated
    D. Modifying diet to include gradual increase of high-fiber foods
IV. Interventions to minimize diminished sensations ⚠
    A. Having patient protect hands and feet from cold through use of gloves and socks
    B. Having patient avoid excess stimulation of skin and avoid tight clothing
    C. Having patient wear gloves for gardening activities
    D. Teaching about inspection of affected areas for burns, cuts, abrasions
    E. Infusion rates of paclitaxel—can be infused over longer duration to decrease incidence of peripheral neuropathy
V. Pharmacologic interventions for pain reduction (Brant, 2014; Donovan, 2009; Tofthagen et al., 2013; Smith et al., 2013; Wilkes, 2014;)
    A. Mild analgesics—acetaminophen (Tylenol) and nonsteroidal anti-inflammatory drugs
    B. Antidepressants—amitriptyline (Elavil), imipramine (Tofranil), nortriptyline (Pamelor, duloxetine [Cymbalta])
    C. Anticonvulsants (e.g., gabapentin [Neurontin], pregabalin [Lyrica], valproic acid [Depakote])
    D. Opioids
    E. Lidocaine 5% patch
    F. Glutamine
    G. Use of creams (e.g., application of capsaicin cream three or four times daily)
VI. Interventions to promote self-care and decrease mobility impairment

Part 4

A. Collaborating with physical and occupational rehabilitation services
B. Developing an exercise and muscle-strengthening program
C. Use of assistive devices
D. Assisting in performance of ADLs, as needed

VII. Nonpharmacologic interventions to manage pain, anxiety, depression (Brant, 2014; Marrs & Newton, 2003; Tofthagen et al., 2013; Wilkes, 2014)
A. Exercise
B. Transcutaneous electrical nerve stimulation (TENS)
C. Acupuncture and acupressure
D. Relaxation techniques—yoga, meditation, guided imagery
E. Biofeedback
F. Art and music therapy

EVALUATION

The oncology nurse systematically and regularly evaluates the patient for evidence of nerve dysfunction and implements interventions to promote ability to carry out ADLs, decrease pain, and improve quality of life. Relevant data are collected, and actual findings are compared with expected findings. Nursing diagnoses, outcomes, and plans of care are reviewed and revised, as necessary.

Alterations in Mental Status

OVERVIEW

I. Physiology
A. With alterations in mental status, changes may occur in general appearance, cognition (process that involves perception, memory, and thinking; changes in behavior/personality), and self-care skills (Fields, 2014; Matthews & Berger, 2014).
B. Components of behavior or personality involve a person's presence or consciousness noted in thoughts, emotions, and actions.
C. An alteration in mental status may also result in loss of the ability to carry out ADLs and meet self-care needs.

II. Risk factors
A. Disease related
   1. CNS neoplasm, primary or metastatic disease
   2. Metabolic emergencies (e.g., hypercalcemia, hyperuricemia, sodium or potassium imbalances)
   3. Uncontrolled pain
   4. Head injury
   5. Pre-existing depression
   6. HIV-related dementia
   7. Opportunistic infections (e.g., toxoplasmosis, encephalitis, cryptococcal meningitis)
   8. Liver disease

B. Treatment related
   1. Side effects of chemotherapy (e.g., sleep disturbance, headache, hyperkinesis)
   2. Side effect of biologic response modifier therapy (e.g., lethargy, somnolence, disturbance in recent memory)
   3. Side effect of steroid therapy (e.g., depression, psychotic reactions)
   4. Side effects of specific agents such as ifosfamide and interleukin-2 (IL-2) (encephalopathy and psychosis)
   5. Side effects of analgesics
   6. Dehydration
   7. Electrolyte imbalance (e.g., hyperuricemia, hyponatremia, hypokalemia)
C. Situation related
   1. Emotionally traumatic situations
   2. Significant loss
   3. Depression with melancholia, anxiety, anger
   4. Rejection and abandonment
   5. Hopelessness
   6. Powerlessness

ASSESSMENT

I. History
A. Presence of risk factors
B. Analgesics
C. Recent head injury, trauma, falls
D. Medication history, steroid use
E. Opioid use
F. Alcohol abuse
G. Reported confusion at night
H. Uncontrolled pain

II. Physical examination
A. Neurologic examination
B. Cognitive mental status screening
C. Impaired memory, recent and remote
D. Impaired problem solving
E. Impaired communication and language

III. Psychosocial examination
A. Changes in emotional and behavioral affect
B. Mood swings
C. Anxiety
D. Hallucinations, illusions
E. Impaired judgment
F. Decreased level of consciousness
G. Agitation, restlessness, seizures, shakiness
H. Tremors, confusion, grand mal seizures, coma, death
I. Influence of culture
J. Information on baseline status to be obtained from family members or caregivers

IV. Laboratory data
A. CBC
B. Serum electrolyte levels
C. Thyroid and liver function

PROBLEM STATEMENTS AND OUTCOME IDENTIFICATION

I. Disturbed Thought Processes
   A. Expected outcome—patient demonstrates improvement or adjustment to altered orientation, behavioral patterns, or mood states.

II. Bathing Self-Care Deficit, Dressing Self-Care Deficit, Feeding Self-Care Deficit, Toileting Self-Care Deficit (NANDA-I)
   A. Expected outcome—patient participates in ADLs and self-care activities to the limits of his or her ability.

III. Risk for Injury (NANDA-I) ⚠
   A. Expected outcome—patient remains free from injury related to cognitive impairment.

IV. Anxiety (NANDA-I)
   A. Expected outcome—patient demonstrates a reduction in anxiety experienced.

PLANNING AND IMPLEMENTATION

I. Interventions to maintain or regain patient's cognitive functions
   A. Assessment of degrees of altered attention and concentration
   B. Reorienting the patient to time, place, and reason for hospitalization
   C. Providing clear, concise information, using simple terms, with face-to-face interaction with patient
   D. Providing a structured, organized environment
   E. Providing cues for orientation—clock, calendar, personal items
   F. Maintaining a quiet environment; approaching the patient in a slow, unhurried manner
   G. Providing structure in routine activities—specific time for breakfast, hygiene, medications, lunch, visitors
   H. Proving explanation for distortion in patient's feelings and thoughts
   I. Allowing time for response to questions and decisions
   J. Discussion with primary care provider about medications to manage psychosis

II. Psychoeducational interventions (Fields, 2014; Matthews & Berger, 2014)
   A. Use of counseling and psychotherapy
   B. Use of behavior therapy
   C. Providing education about disease process, self-care management
   D. Encouraging patient attendance at a support group

III. Interventions to involve patient and family in care
   A. Assessment of the family's understanding and educating family members about potential cognitive dysfunction
   B. Engaging patient and family in discussion of illness from their perspective, including influence of culture
   C. Discussing appropriate cultural interventions that may complement the medical regimen
   D. Providing opportunities for family members to ask questions and obtain information
   E. Teaching family to monitor changes in cognitive status
   F. Instructing patient and family about signs and symptoms to report to the health care team
   G. Reinforcing information that the health care provider discussed during visits
   H. Teaching about avoidance of alcohol and nonessential medications

IV. Interventions to ensure a safe environment in the inpatient and outpatient settings (Fields, 2014; Matthews & Berger, 2014) ⚠
   A. Maintaining the bed in the lowest position with wheels locked; ensuring that the call light is within patient's reach
   B. Providing sufficient light so that patient can see surroundings, especially if in a new, strange environment
   C. Use of a chair as a barrier to inhibit patient from wandering out of room or area
   D. Use of an alarm system to alert nurse or nurses' station when patient is attempting to get out of bed or chair
   E. Requesting a sitter if patient is considered unsafe
   F. Use of side rails as a last resort
      1. If patient has a tendency to climb out of bed, side rails may increase the risk of injury.
      2. If any form of restraint is used, the relevant Joint Commission on Accreditation of Healthcare Organizations (JCAHO) regulations should be considered.
   G. Providing a rocking chair during the day to help patient use up some energy
   H. Assessment of limitations in, and assisting with, ADLs, as needed
   I. Assessment for the presence of pharmacologic agents that may alter cognitive function
   J. Assessment of the person's thoughts and feelings toward staff and the need for hospitalization
   K. Discussing the patient's fears and concerns

V. Nonpharmacologic interventions to manage anxiety and depression
   A. Cognitive distraction—imagery, music therapy
   B. Psychoeducation
   C. Art therapy
   D. Massage therapy
   E. Pet therapy

EVALUATION

The oncology nurse systematically and regularly evaluates the patient mental status and responses to interventions to optimize cognitive abilities and safety. Relevant data are collected, and actual findings are compared with expected findings. Nursing diagnoses, outcomes, and plans of care are reviewed and revised, as necessary.

References

Albrecht, T. A., & Taylor, A. G. (2012). Physical activity in patients with advanced-stage cancer: A systematic review of the literature. *Clinical Journal of Oncology Nursing, 16*(3), 293–300.

Bergstrom, K. (2011). Development of a radiation skin care protocol and algorithm using the Iowa model of evidence-based practice. *Clinical Journal of Oncology Nursing, 15*(6), 593–595.

Brant, J. M. (2014). Pain. In C. H. Yarbro, D. Wujcik, & B. H. Gobel (Eds.), *Cancer symptom management* (4th ed., pp. 69–89). Burlington, VT: Jones and Bartlett.

DeHaven, C. (2007). *Chemotherapy and radiotherapy effects on the skin.* http://www.spsscs.org/feature-articles/chemotherapy-and-radiotherapy-effects-on-the-skin.

Donovan, D. (2009). Management of peripheral neuropathy caused by microtubule inhibitors. *Clinical Journal of Oncology Nursing, 13*(6), 686–694.

Fields, M. M. (2014). Increased intracranial pressure. In C. H. Yarbro, D. Wujcik, & B. H. Gobel (Eds.), *Cancer symptom management* (4th ed., pp. 439–453). Burlington, VT: Jones and Bartlett.

Marrs, J., & Newton, S. (2003). Updating your peripheral neuropathy "know how." *Clinical Journal of Oncology Nursing, 7*(3), 299–303.

Martin, V. R. (2014). Arthralgias and myalgias. In C. H. Yarbro, D. Wujcik, & B. H. Gobel (Eds.), *Cancer symptom management* (4th ed., pp. 13–23). Burlington, VT: Jones and Bartlett.

Matthews, E. E., & Berger, A. M. (2014). Sleep disturbances. In C. H. Yarbro, D. Wujcik, & B. H. Gobel (Eds.), *Cancer symptom management.* (4th ed., pp. 93–109). Burlington, VT: Jones and Bartlett.

McCann, S., Akilov, O. E., & Geskin, L. (2012). Adverse effects of denileukin difitox and their management in patients with cutaneous T-cell leukemia. *Clinical Journal of Oncology Nursing, 16*(5), E164–E172.

Morse, L. (2014). Skin and nail bed changes. In C. H. Yarbro, D. Wujcik, & B. H. Gobel (Eds.), *Cancer symptom management.* (4th ed., pp. 587–608). Burlington, VT: Jones and Bartlett.

North American Nursing Diagnosis Association (NANDA). (2003). *Nursing diagnoses: Definitions and classification 2003–2004.* Philadelphia: NANDA.

O'Leary, C., & Catania, K. (2014). Extravasation. In C. H. Yarbro, D. Wujcik, & B. H. Gobel (Eds.), *Cancer symptom management* (4th ed., pp. 541–552). Burlington: Jones and Bartlett.

Oncology Nursing Society (2009). *Fatigue.* www.ons.org/Research/PEP/Fatigue.

Reid, K. F., & Fielding, R. A. (2012). Skeletal muscle power: A critical determinate of physical functioning in older adults. *Exercise and Sports Sciences Review, 40*(1), 1–12.

Ridner, S. H. (2014). Lymphedema. In C. H. Yarbro, D. Wujcik, & B. H. Gobel (Eds.), *Cancer symptom management* (4th ed., pp. 555–564). Burlington, VT: Jones and Bartlett.

Rodriguez, A. L. (2014). Bleeding and thrombotic complications. In C. H. Yarbro, D. Wujcik, & B. H. Gobel (Eds.), *Cancer symptom management* (4th ed., pp. 287–313). Burlington, VT: Jones and Bartlett.

Smith, E., Pang, H., Cirrincione, C., et al. (2013). Effect of duloxetine on pain, function, and quality of life among patients with chemotherapy-induced painful peripheral neuropathy: A randomized clinical trial. *JAMA, 309*(13), 1359–1367.

Tofthagen, C. (2010). Patient perceptions associated with chemotherapy-induced peripheral neuropathy. *Clinical Journal of Oncology Nursing, 14*(3), E22–E28.

Tofthagen, C., Visovsky, C. M., & Hopgood, R. (2013). Chemotherapy-induced peripheral neuropathy: An algorithm to guide nursing management. *Clinical Journal of Oncology Nursing, 17*(2), 138–144.

Vogel, W. H. (2014). Hypersensitivity reactions to antineoplastic drugs. In C. H. Yarbro, D. Wujcik, & B. H. Gobel (Eds.), *Cancer symptom management* (4th ed., pp. 115–130). Burlington, VT: Jones and Bartlett.

Wilkes, G. M. (2014). Peripheral neuropathy. In C. H. Yarbro, D. Wujcik, & B. H. Gobel (Eds.), *Cancer symptom management.* (4th ed., pp. 457–489). Burlington, VT: Jones and Bartlett.

Zitella, L. J. (2014). Infection. In C. H. Yarbro, D. Wujcik, & B. H. Gobel (Eds.), *Cancer symptom management* (4th ed., pp. 131–151). Burlington, VT: Jones and Bartlett.

CHAPTER 31
Alterations in Respiratory Function

Leslie V. Matthews

Anatomic or Surgical Alterations

OVERVIEW

I. Definition—inadequate ventilation or oxygenation resulting from anatomic or surgical alterations (Hong et al., 2010; Shannon et al., 2010)
  A. Anatomic alterations
    1. Space-occupying lesions within the lung itself or in the pleural space (e.g., from primary or metastatic cancer to the lung)
    2. Airway obstruction of tracheobronchial tree from direct extension of primary or metastatic tumors or enlarged lymph nodes
    3. Abnormal accumulation of fluid within lung or pleural space (Shannon et al., 2010)
      a. Pneumothorax—abnormal accumulation of air within the pleural space
      b. Hemothorax—abnormal accumulation of blood within the pleural space
      c. Hydrothorax (effusion)—abnormal accumulation of fluid within the pleural space
      d. Empyema—abnormal accumulation of infected fluid or pus in the pleural space caused by recent chest surgery, immunocompromise, or lung infection
    4. Compression of tracheobronchial tree from bronchospasm, laryngeal swelling from hypersensitivity reactions related to chemotherapy and/or biotherapy treatments, or superior vena cava syndrome (SVCS) (see Chapter 41)
  B. Surgical alterations
    1. Thoracic surgery for removal of primary or metastatic cancer of the lung (Hong et al., 2010)
      a. Pneumonectomy—surgical removal of an entire lung
      b. Lobectomy—removal of a lobe of the lung
      c. Segmental resection—removal of one or more segments of a lung lobe
      d. Wedge resection—removal of a small wedge-shaped localized area near the lung surface
    2. Tracheostomy following head and neck surgery, laryngectomy
II. Risk factors (DeVita, Lawrence, & Rosenberg, 2011; Jarvis, 2012)
  A. Primary or metastatic cancer of the lung
  B. Recent surgery (especially thoracic or abdominal), immobility, or situations in which hypoventilation is likely
  C. Cancers associated with SVCS (see Chapter 41)
  D. Thoracic or head and neck surgery
  E. Primary or adjuvant tracheobronchial surgeries
  F. Surgery for palliation, tumor debulking
  G. History of obstructive or restrictive pulmonary disease
  H. History of cardiovascular disease
  I. Smoking history or environmental exposure to irritants such as pollution, pesticides, chemicals, or other irritants

ASSESSMENT

I. History (Hong et al., 2010; Jarvis, 2012; Yarbro, Wujcik, & Gobel, 2011)
  A. Cough
    1. Acute—less than 2 to 3 weeks; chronic—longer than 2 months
    2. Sputum production, hemoptysis
  B. Dyspnea—shortness of breath; tachypnea—rapid breathing; orthopnea—difficulty breathing when supine; paroxysmal nocturnal dyspnea—awakening from sleep with shortness of breath
  C. Wheeze, stridor, chest pain, hoarseness
  D. Ability to carry out activities of daily living (ADLs)
  E. Tobacco use—pack history
  F. Exercise or activity tolerance
  G. Number of pillows used for sleep and comfort
  H. Anxiety and apprehension
II. Presence of risk factors
III. Diagnostic tests (Hong et al., 2010)

A. Chest radiography, computed tomography (CT), magnetic resonance imaging (MRI), and positron emission tomography (PET) to delineate anatomic extent of involvement

B. Pulmonary function tests (PFTs) to quantify air flow limitation

C. Arterial blood gases (ABGs)

D. Ventilation-perfusion scans

E. Bronchoscopy for direct visualization

F. Endobronchial thoracentesis

IV. Physical examination (Cash & Glass, 2011)

A. Abnormal or altered breathing patterns
1. Tachypnea
2. Pursed-lip breathing or use of accessory muscles of respiration

B. Abnormal breath sounds—wheezes, decreased or absent breath sounds

C. Sputum—amount, color, presence of blood

D. Cyanosis
1. Hypoxemia
2. Chronic obstructive pulmonary disease (COPD)

E. Vital signs and pulse oximetry

F. Evaluate airway swelling, oropharyngeal swelling

G. Presence of enlarged lymph nodes or masses in the head and neck area

PROBLEM STATEMENTS AND OUTCOME IDENTIFICATION

I. Impaired Gas Exchange (NANDA-I)
A. Expected outcome—patient maintains optimal gas exchange.

II. Ineffective Breathing Pattern (NANDA-I)
A. Expected outcome—patient's breathing pattern and rate are regular.
B. Patient and family verbalize correct understanding of medication regimen for managing respiratory symptoms.

III. Activity Intolerance (NANDA-I)
A. Expected outcome—patient maintains activity level within capabilities.
B. Expected outcome—patient uses measures to conserve energy expenditure.

IV. Deficient Knowledge (NANDA-I), related to respiratory complications and management
A. Expected outcome—patient and family identify correct procedures and precautions for oxygen use.
B. Expected outcome—patient and family identify critical symptoms or changes in current status to report to health care providers.

PLANNING AND IMPLEMENTATION

See Cash & Glass, 2011; Yarbro et al., 2011.

I. Interventions to minimize the risk of occurrence, severity, or complications of respiratory distress

A. Treatment aimed at the underlying disease process
1. Radiation therapy (RT), chemotherapy, biotherapy, and targeted agents for primary or metastatic cancer of the lung or to reduce obstruction of the tracheobronchial tree
2. Thoracentesis to remove abnormal accumulated contents in pleural space
3. Systemic antibiotic treatment for empyema

B. Using measures to ease and increase the effectiveness of breathing and to promote physical comfort
1. Supplemental oxygen administration
2. Proper positioning, use of pillows
3. Incorporating measures to minimize pain, which may contribute to ineffective breathing (see Chapter 31)

C. Prioritizing patient activity and exercise and use of energy conservation strategies

II. Interventions to maximize safety ⚠
A. Encouraging patient to use supplemental oxygen, as needed, with ambulation to prevent hypoxia and potential falls
B. Encouraging the use of assistive devices (e.g., cane, walker, wheelchair), as needed, for ambulation, ADLs

III. Interventions to monitor for complications
A. Assessment of level of consciousness, mental status
B. Assessment of heart rate and rhythm, respiratory effort, vascular perfusion, and pulse oximetry readings
C. Reporting critical changes to the oncology provider

IV. Interventions to monitor response to management
A. Assessment of respiratory rate, rhythm, effort
B. Assessment for signs of respiratory impairment
1. Dyspnea and or tachypnea
2. Dry persistent cough
3. Basilar rales
C. Monitoring for adequate relief of symptoms
1. Subjective reports from patient and family of the following:
a. Changes in the respiratory pattern
b. Psychological responses to respiratory distress
c. Comfort, relief of dyspnea and cough

V. Interventions to educate patient and family regarding the following:
A. Activity prioritization and energy conservation strategies
1. Frequent rest periods
2. Easy-to-prepare meals
3. Often-used items within reach
B. Emergency care, available community resources, and medication management
C. Signs and symptoms to report to the health care team

Part 4

EVALUATION

The oncology nurse systematically and regularly evaluates the patient's and family's responses to interventions that alleviate respiratory distress related to anatomic or surgical alterations. Relevant data are collected and synthesized. Nursing diagnoses, outcomes, and plans of care are reviewed and revised, as necessary.

Pulmonary Toxicity Related to Cancer Therapy

OVERVIEW

I. Definition—parenchymal pulmonary disease caused by antineoplastic therapy, radiation, chemotherapy, biologic agents, targeted therapies (Polovich, Whitford, & Olsen, 2009)
II. Classification
   A. Radiation-induced pneumonitis (Rovirosa & Valduvieco, 2010; Zhang et al., 2012)
      1. Subacute inflammatory response to radiation exposure to the lung; occurs in 1% to 20% of patients receiving thoracic radiation
      2. Toxic effects are proportionate to the following:
         a. Total radiation dose and volume of lung tissue irradiated
         b. Fractionation schedule; hyperfractionation schedules may cause less RT pneumonitis
         c. Concomitant administration of chemotherapy (Table 31-1)
   B. Chemotherapy, biotherapy, or target therapy–induced pulmonary toxicity (Perry, 2012) (Table 31-2)
      1. Targets rapidly proliferating cells and may impart direct injury to parenchymal endothelial cell membranes of lung, causing bilateral interstitial infiltrates or fibrosis
      2. Systemic release of cytokines, hypersensitivity reaction, or immune complex–related reaction
III. Risk factors (Barber & Ganti, 2011; Guntur & Dhand, 2012; Yarbro et al., 2011)
   A. RT (Rovirosa & Valduvieco, 2010)
      1. Occurs in 5% to 15% of all patients receiving RT
      2. Concurrent chemotherapy or RT
      3. Pre-existing pulmonary disease, interstitial lung disease
      4. Smoking history
      5. Poor performance status
      6. More severe in older adults and in females
   B. Chemotherapy induced (Ryu, 2010)
      1. Age—older than 60 years
      2. Cumulative dose of administered drug
      3. Pre-existing pulmonary disease, interstitial lung disease (e.g., COPD), renal dysfunction
      4. Smoking history
      5. Concomitant or sequential RT to lungs
      6. Oxygen therapy at high concentration (>35%)
   C. Targeted therapy–induced (Peerzada, Spiro, & Daw, 2010)
      1. Pre-existing lung disease or cardiovascular disease

ASSESSMENT

I. History (Barber & Ganti, 2011; Rovirosa & Valduvieco, 2010)
   A. RT-induced pulmonary toxicity
      1. Early nonspecific symptoms include nonproductive cough, mild dyspnea, low-grade temperature, pleuritic chest pain
      2. May occur 6 to 12 weeks after completion of RT, although symptoms can range from 1 to 6 months after RT
      3. Exclude other causes of pulmonary infiltrates—infection, recurrent tumors, thromboembolic disease, lymphangitic carcinomatosis
   B. Chemotherapy-induced pulmonary toxicity
      1. Dyspnea the cardinal symptom; also nonproductive cough, malaise, fatigue, fever.
      2. Generally develops over weeks to months, but can also develop quickly (within hours) and may occur years following drug exposure
   C. Targeted therapy–induced
      1. Dyspnea
      2. Acute cough
II. Physical examination (Guntur & Dhand, 2012; Ryu, 2010)
   A. RT induced
      1. Physical examination—may be unreliable
         a. Moist rales, pleural friction rub
         b. Evidence of pleural fluid heard over the area of irradiation
         c. Tachypnea, cyanosis (late)

Table 31-1

Chemotherapy and Biologic Agents Predisposing to Radiation Pneumonitis

Chemotherapy Agents	Targeted Therapies
Bleomycin	Alemtuzumab
Busulfan	Bevacizumab
Chlorambucil	Cetuximab
Cyclophosphamide	Rituximab
Doxorubicin	Trastuzumab
Ifosfamide	
Methotrexate	
Mitomycin	
Vinblastine	
Vincristine	

Data from Rovirosa, A. & Valduvieco, I. (2010). Radiation pneumonitis. *Clinical Pulmonary Medicine, 17*(5), 218–222.

Table 31-2

Chemotherapy and Targeted Therapy–Related Pulmonary Abnormalities

Pattern of Lung Involvement	Specific Agents	Radiologic Abnormality
Acute pneumonitis	Bortezomib, cetuximab, dasatinib, erlotinib, everolimus, gefitinib, gemcitabine, imatinib, irinotecan, pemetrexed, piritrexim, procarbazine, rituximab, sorafenib, sunitinib, temozolomide, temsirolimus, thalidomide, trastuzumab	Diffuse patchy ground-glass opacities, diffuse reticular pattern
Bronchiolitis	Bortezomib, busulfan, cetuximab, panitumumab, topotecan	Hyperinflation, air trapping
Hemoptysis	Bevacizumab	Bilateral ground-glass opacities, consolidation
Hypersensitivity reactions	Alpha-interferon, cetuximab, etoposide, gemcitabine, L-asparaginase, panitumumab, rituximab, taxanes, vinca alkaloids	Air flow obstruction, airway hyperreactivity, hyperinflation
Interstitial pneumonitis	Erlotinib, everolimus, gefitinib, ofatumumab, rituximab, sorafinib, sinitinib, temsirolimus, thalidomide, trastuzumab	Diffuse, patchy, ground-glass opacities
Isolated acute chest pain	Bleomycin, doxorubicin, etoposide, methotrexate	Nonspecific
Isolated cough	Alpha-interferon, IL-2, methotrexate	Nonspecific
Isolated diminished diffusion capacity of lungs for carbon monoxide (DLCO)	Bischloroethylnitrosourea (BCNU; carmustine), gemcitabine, paclitaxel	Nonspecific
Mediastinal lymphadenopathy	Bleomycin, interferon, methotrexate	Hilar, mediastinal lymphadenopathy
Pleural effusion	Bleomycin, bortezomib, busulfan, dasatinib, etoposide, fludarabine, gemcitabine, imatinib, IL-2, methotrexate, procarbazine, taxanes, thalidomide	Pleural effusion
Pneumothorax	Carmustine	Pneumothorax
Pulmonary edema	Ara-C, alpha-interferon, azathioprine, decitabine, granulocyte colony-stimulating factor (G-CSF), gemcitabine, imatinib, nitrogen mustard, paclitaxel, vinorelbine	Diffuse alveolar infiltrates, without cardiomegaly or pleural effusion
Pulmonary embolus (PE)	Bevacizumab, lenalidomide, thalidomide	Acute PE

Adapted from Guntur, V.P. & Dhand, R. (2012). Pulmonary toxicity of chemotherapeutic agents. In Perry, M.C. (Ed.). (2012). *Perry's chemotherapy source book* (5th ed., pp. 206–213). Philadelphia: Lippincott Williams & Wilkins; Barber, N.A., Ganti, A.K. (2011). Pulmonary toxicities from targeted therapies: A review. *Targeted Oncology*, 6(4), 235–243.

2. Radiographic changes
   a. Early—diffuse haziness, ground-glass opacification
   b. Late—infiltrates or dense consolidation corresponding to the region of radiation exposure
B. Chemotherapy induced (Torrisi et al., 2011)
   1. Physical examination
      a. Results may be normal, early onset, as late as 2 months, or years after therapy
      b. End-inspiratory basilar rales
      c. Tachypnea
   2. Radiographic changes
      a. Classic diffuse reticular pattern, ground-glass opacities, usually bilateral
      b. Results—may also be normal
C. Targeted therapy–induced
   1. Physical examination

   a. Asymptomatic or present with dyspnea and dry cough
   b. Low-grade fever, congestion
   2. Radiographic changes
      a. Diffuse bilateral lung infiltrates
      b. Results—may also be normal
III. Diagnostic tests and findings.
   A. PFTs—may reveal restrictive defect or obstructive pattern
      1. Decreased lung volume
      2. Decreased restrictive ventilatory pattern, diminished diffusion capacity of the lungs for carbon monoxide (DLCO); DLCO measures the ability of the lungs to transfer gas from inhaled air to the RBCs in pulmonary capillaries
   B. High-resolution CT
      1. Detection of radiation fibrosis
      2. Abnormality is generally nonspecific

C. ABGs
   1. Hypoxia
   2. Hypocapnia, respiratory alkalosis

PROBLEM STATEMENTS AND OUTCOME IDENTIFICATION

I. Impaired Gas Exchange (NANDA-I)
   A. Expected outcome—patient maintains optimal gas exchange.
II. Ineffective Breathing Pattern (NANDA-I)
   A. Expected outcome—patient's breathing pattern and rate are regular.
   B. Expected outcome—patient and family identify critical symptoms or changes in current status to report to health care providers.
III. Activity Intolerance (NANDA-I)
   A. Expected outcome—patient maintains activity level within capabilities and uses measures to reduce or conserve energy expenditure.

PLANNING AND IMPLEMENTATION

I. Interventions to medically manage treatment-related pulmonary toxicity
   A. RT induced (Graves, Siddiqui, Anscher, & Movsas, 2010; Iwamoto, Haas, & Gosselin, 2012).
      1. Mild symptoms—cough suppressants, antipyretics, rest
      2. Severe symptoms and impaired gas exchange—glucocorticoid therapy until symptoms improve, then taper slowly; pneumonitis may flare if taper is too rapid; about 50% respond to glucocorticoid therapy
   B. Chemotherapy induced (Guntur & Dhand, 2012; Ryu, 2010)
      1. Monitoring baseline PFTs and limiting cumulative dose
      2. Concurrent or prior use of oral or intravenous corticosteroids
      3. Discontinuation of suspected agent
   C. Targeted therapy induced (Barber & Ganti, 2011; Hadjinicolaou, Nisar, Parfrey, Chilvers, & Ostor, 2011)
      1. Rare, but may be life threatening
      2. Prompt resolution with dose reduction or discontinuation
II. Interventions to monitor patient (Graves et al., 2010; Joyce, 2010; Polovich et al., 2009)
   A. Ensuring that PFTs are performed routinely
   B. Assessment of respiratory rate, rhythm, effort
   C. Assessment for signs of pulmonary toxicity—dyspnea, dry persistent cough, basilar rales, tachypnea, pleuritic pain
III. Encouraging balanced activity training to decrease or prevent adverse effects of therapy (Decker & Lee, 2010; Lakoski, Eves, Douglas, & Jones, 2012)
   A. Evaluation of cardiorespiratory fitness

B. Monitoring activities to minimize energy expenditure
C. Monitoring for adequate relief of symptoms

EVALUATION

The oncology nurse systematically and regularly evaluates the patient's pulmonary responses to chemotherapy, biotherapy, and targeted therapy to determine goal attainment of optimal gas exchange. Relevant data are collected, and actual findings are compared with expected findings. Nursing diagnoses, outcomes, and plans of care are reviewed and revised, as necessary.

Dyspnea

OVERVIEW

I. Definition—a subjective sensation of difficulty breathing, the feeling of inability to get enough air, and the reaction to the sensation (Campbell, 2011; Disalvo, Joyce, Tyson, & Mackay, 2008; Gaguski, Brandsema, Gernalin, & Martinez, 2010)
II. Risk factors
   A. Disease related
      1. Tumors that impinge on respiratory structures and decrease air flow
      2. Conditions that increase metabolic demands (e.g., fever, infection)
      3. Cerebral metastasis, which affects the respiratory center or stimulates the central and peripheral chemoreceptors
      4. Metastatic effusions in the pleural or cardiac space or abdominal cavity, which compromise lung expansion, gas exchange, or blood flow to the lungs
      5. Coexisting pulmonary, cardiac or neuromuscular disease, which compromises lung expansion or blood flow to the lungs
      6. Advanced disease or terminal illness
   B. Treatment related (Joyce, 2010; Polovich et al., 2009)
      1. Incisional pain that may compromise lung expansion
      2. Immediate and long-term effects of RT to the lung fields
      3. Antineoplastic agents that may cause pulmonary toxicity
         a. May be acute or delayed (up to 10 years after treatment)
         b. May be dose related, reversible, or chronic
      4. Anaphylactic reactions to antineoplastic agents, biologic response modifiers, or targeted therapy agents
      5. Pneumothorax related to placement of vascular access catheters, fine-needle aspiration, or thoracentesis

C. Lifestyle related
1. Strong emotional responses, particularly anxiety or anger, contribute to the sensation of dyspnea.
2. Tobacco use or exposure to environmental toxic substances—asbestos, chromium, coal products, ionizing radiation, vinyl chloride, chloromethyl ethers
3. Obesity

ASSESSMENT

See Campbell, 2011.
I. History
   A. Presence of risk factors such as smoking, chemical exposure
   B. Subjective reports of shortness of breath, "can't catch breath," "smothering," "air hunger," uncomfortable breathing, anxiety, or panic
   C. Pattern of dyspnea—onset, frequency, severity, associated symptoms, aggravating or alleviating factors
   D. Impact of dyspnea on ADLs, lifestyle, relationships, role responsibilities, emotional well-being, sexuality, and body image
II. Physical findings
   A. Tachypnea, hypercapnea, increased respiratory excursion
   B. Use of accessory muscles, retraction of intercostal spaces, nostril flaring
   C. Clubbing of digits caused by chronic hypoxemia; cyanosis, pallor, jugular vein distention, upper extremity swelling, venous congestion in thorax or chest region
III. Psychological signs and symptoms
   A. Concentration difficulties, memory difficulties, or both; confusion
   B. Restlessness
IV. Diagnostic tests and findings (DeVita et al., 2011; Foster, Mistry, Peddi, & Sharma, 2010; Jarvis, 2012).
   A. Dyspnea-like pain, subjective; abnormal findings may be lacking
   B. Complete blood cell (CBC) count—hemoglobin deficiencies
   C. Pulse oximetry—severity of hypoxia
   D. Chest radiography and CT—structural abnormalities, PFTs
   E. Bronchoscopic examination
   F. Sputum or bronchial cultures
   G. ABGs
V. Assessment scales such as a numeric rating scale to measure degree of patient's dyspnea (Gaguski et al., 2010)

PROBLEM STATEMENTS AND OUTCOME IDENTIFICATION

I. Activity Intolerance (NANDA-I)
   A. Expected outcome—patient uses measures to conserve energy.
   B. Expected outcome—patient maintains activity level within capabilities.
II. Anxiety (NANDA-I)
   A. Expected outcome—patient describes a decrease in anxiety.
III. Deficient Knowledge (NANDA-I), related to management of dyspnea
   A. Expected outcome—patient and family understand the use of medications, including opioids, to manage dyspnea.
   B. Expected outcome—patient and family identify critical symptoms or changes in current status to report to health care providers.

PLANNING AND IMPLEMENTATION

I. Interventions to manage treatment-related dyspnea (Gaguski et al., 2010; Joyce, 2010)
   A. Treatment of underlying disease with thoracentesis, RT, chemotherapy, antimicrobial medications
   B. Pharmacologic agents
      1. Glucocorticoids—decrease local inflammation
      2. Opioids and anxiolytics—decrease pain and anxiety
      3. Bronchodilators—increase air flow to the lungs
      4. Diuretics—decrease fluid overload
   C. Supplemental oxygen, as indicated
II. Interventions to manage discomfort of dyspnea (Cheung & Zimmerman, 2011; Disalvo et al., 2008; Qaseem et al., 2008)
   A. Recommended for practice
      1. Immediate-release oral and parenteral opioids, which decrease central respiratory drive by reducing ventilatory demand
      2. Oxygen for short-term relief of hypoxia
   B. May alleviate dyspnea in some patients
      1. Oxygen therapy in hypoxia
      2. Benzodiazepines for anxiety
      3. Increased ambient air flow directed at face or nose
      4. Cooler temperatures.
      5. Promotion of relaxation and stress reduction techniques
      6. Providing educational, emotional, and psychosocial support to patient and caregiver; referral to other disciplines, as appropriate
   C. Effectiveness not established—more studies needed
      1. Oxygen therapy in nonhypoxia
      2. Pharmacologic agents—extended-release morphine, midazolam plus morphine, nebulized opioids, furosemide, lidocaine
      3. Further evaluation needed for use of acupuncture and cognitive behavioral approaches

Part 4

D. Expert opinion—low-risk interventions
   1. Avoidance of volume overload
   2. Encouraging positioning to facilitate breathing—upright position; forward position with elbows on knees, table, or pillows
   3. Instruction to patient about diaphragmatic breathing techniques with slow exhalation; may not be effective and may be harmful in patients with pulmonary restrictive disease
   4. Recommendation for assistive devices such as wheelchair, walker, and portable oxygen, as needed
   5. Exercise rehabilitation (Decker & Lee, 2010; Lakoski et al., 2012)

III. Interventions to maximize safety ⚠
   A. Encouraging use of assistive devices such as cane, walker, or wheelchair, as needed, for ambulation and ADLs
   B. Using activity limitation, conservation of energy strategies
      1. Frequent rest periods
      2. Use of ready-made meals
      3. Often-used items within reach

IV. Interventions to monitor for complications
   A. Assessment of level of consciousness and mental status
   B. Monitoring intake and output
   C. Assessment of heart rate and rhythm, respiratory effort, vascular perfusion
   D. Reporting to the oncology provider critical changes such as unresponsiveness, tachypnea, tachycardia, chest pressure, or acute pain, consistent with patient goals

V. Interventions to monitor response to management
   A. Observing and reporting physical symptoms such as decreased shortness of breath, increased energy, ease of breathing
   B. Monitoring subjective reports of the changes in the pattern of dyspnea or psychological responses to dyspnea such as anxiety or distress

VI. Interventions to educate patient and family
   A. Teaching about activity limitation, energy conservation strategies
   B. Providing information about accessing emergency care, available community resources

VII. Behavioral interventions to decrease the sense of dyspnea and enhance psychosocial well-being
   A. Encouraging use of relaxation techniques, prayer and meditation, aromatherapy
   B. Use of language that is easy to understand (e.g., shortness of breath instead of dyspnea)
   C. Use of complementary and alternative therapies such as relaxation techniques and stress reduction strategies

EVALUATION

The oncology nurse systematically and regularly evaluates the patient's and family's response to interventions to alleviate dyspnea and achieve patient comfort and optimal air exchange. Relevant data are collected, and actual findings are compared with expected findings. Nursing diagnoses, outcomes, and plans of care are reviewed and revised, as necessary.

Pleural Effusions

OVERVIEW

I. Definition—presence of excess fluid in the pleural space

II. Classification (Davidson, Firat, & Michael, 2012; Light, 2011)
   A. Benign pleural effusion—may be caused by the following:
      1. Increased hydrostatic pressure (congestive heart failure [CHF])
      2. Increased permeability in microvascular circulation (infection, trauma)
      3. Increased negative pressure in the pleural space (atelectasis)
      4. Decreased oncotic pressure in the microvasculature (nephrotic syndrome, cirrhosis, hypoalbuminemia)
   B. Malignant pleural effusion, the presence of malignant cells in the pleura, signifies distant spread of disease; may be caused by the following:
      1. Direct extension of primary tumor to the pleura or mediastinum or mesothelioma involving the pleura
      2. Impaired lymphatic drainage from the pleural space resulting from obstruction caused by tumor
      3. Increased permeability caused by inflammation or disruption of the capillary endothelium
      4. Altered mucosal lung or mediastinal tissue resulting from RT

III. Risk factors (Quinn, Alam, Aminazad, Marshall, & Choong, 2013)
   A. Primary tumors of lung, breast, hematopoietic system
   B. Prior pleural effusion
   C. Radiation to the chest, thorax, or abdomen
   D. Surgical modification of venous or lymphatic vessels

ASSESSMENT

I. History (Hong et al., 2010; Maskell, 2012)
   A. Presence of risk factors
      1. Breast or lung cancer
      2. Previous treatment modalities

B. Symptoms—severity related to the speed of accumulation, not amount; usually caused by pulmonary compression
  1. Dyspnea, progressive, exertional
  2. Cough usually dry and nonproductive
  3. Chest pain
II. Physical examination (Walker & Bryden, 2010)
  A. Tachypnea
  B. Restricted chest wall expansion
  C. Dullness to percussion
  D. Auscultation—diminished or absent breath sounds, egophony (an increased resonance of voice sounds heard when auscultating the lungs, often caused by lung consolidation and fibrosis), pleural friction rub
  E. Fever
  F. General manifestations—compression atelectasis or mediastinal shift if pleural effusion severe
III. Diagnostic tests (Light, 2011; Quinn et al., 2013).
  A. Chest radiography—effusion size, position of mediastinum and diaphragm; blunting of costophrenic angle
  B. Chest CT—to identify loculated effusion or alternative diagnosis
  C. Ultrasonography—to identify optimal site for thoracentesis
  D. Thoracentesis—pleural fluid withdrawal for cytology, chemical analysis, and culture (rule out infection); diagnostic and therapeutic
  E. Pleural fluid evaluation (lactate dehydrogenase [LDH], glucose, protein)—to determine transudative or exudative fluid
    1. Transudative—systemic factors causing effusion, such as CHF, cirrhosis, nephrotic syndrome, hypoalbuminemia
    2. Exudative—local factors causing effusion
      a. Neoplastic—metastatic or primary tumor
      b. Infectious—bacterial, fungal, viral, parasitic
      c. Pulmonary embolus
      d. Gastrointestinal (GI) disease—GI abscess, pancreatic disease, post-abdominal surgery
      e. Pleural biopsy—increases diagnostic yield when combined with cytologic studies

PROBLEM STATEMENTS AND OUTCOME IDENTIFICATION

I. Impaired Gas Exchange (NANDA-I)
  A. Expected outcome—patient maintains optimal gas exchange.
II. Ineffective Breathing Pattern (NANDA-I)
  A. Expected outcome—patient's breathing pattern and rate are regular.
III. Activity Intolerance (NANDA-I)
  A. Expected outcome—patient maintains activity level within capabilities.
  B. Expected outcome—patient uses measures to conserve energy.

IV. Readiness for Enhanced Self-Care (NANDA-I)
  A. Expected outcome—patient and family identify correct procedures and precautions for oxygen use and/or indwelling pleural catheter (IPC) management.
  B. Expected outcome—patient and family identify critical symptoms or changes in current status to report to health care providers.

PLANNING AND IMPLEMENTATION

See Walker & Bryden, 2010; Yarbro et al., 2011.
I. Interventions to manage pleural effusions (Davis, 2012; Kastelik, 2013; Maskell, 2012) (Figure 31-1)
  A. Therapeutic aspiration using intrapleural chemical agent; talc most efficacious, evidence-based
    1. Obliterates the pleural space to prevent fluid reaccumulation
    2. May improve patient comfort, relieve dyspnea for palliation
    3. Reaccumulation of fluid is common
    4. Potential for hypoproteinemia, pneumothorax, empyema, fluid loculation
  B. Thorascopic drainage and talc poudrage
  C. Video-assisted thoracoscopic surgery (VATS)
    1. Hydrodissection with irrigation device into the pleural space
    2. Talc pleurodesis if large effusion or recurrent
  D. IPC—for palliative relief
  E. Chemotherapy and mediastinal radiation—may be effective in responsive tumors (lymphoma, small cell lung cancer [SCLC])
II. Interventions to decrease symptom severity associated with pleural effusion
  A. Teaching about measures to increase the ease and effectiveness of breathing
  B. Incorporating measures to minimize discomfort (e.g., opioid analgesia before chest tube insertion and as needed)
  C. Recommending the use of relaxation techniques, as indicated, for coping with anxiety
III. Interventions to maximize safety ⚠
  A. Encouraging use of assistive devices, as needed, for ADLs
  B. Using activity limitation and conservation of energy strategies
  C. Instructing family in use of and precautions related to oxygen therapy
  D. Instructing family or caregivers in the appropriate use of medications to manage disease
IV. Interventions to monitor the consequences of therapy
  A. Assessment of respiratory rate, rhythm, effort, adventitious breath sounds
  B. Assessment of characteristics of pain and relief measures
  C. Monitoring subjective response to drainage and rate of fluid reaccumulation

Part 4

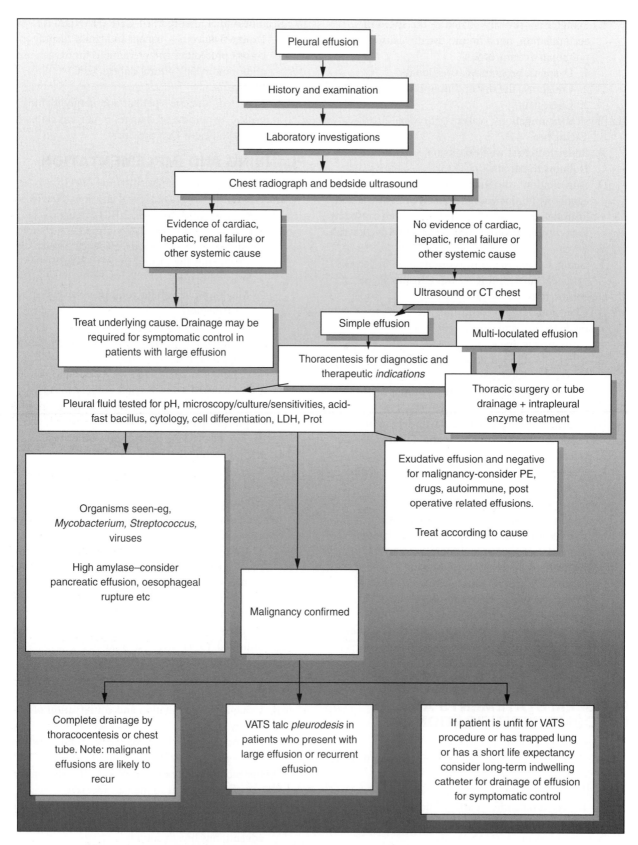

Figure 31-1 Decision Making and Management of Pleural Effusion. *From Quinn, T., Alam, N., Aminazad, A., Marshall, M. B., & Choong, C. K. C. (2013). Decision making and algorithm for the management of pleural effusions.* Thoracic Surgery Clinics, 23(1), 11–16.

D. Reporting critical changes to the oncology provider
  1. Chest pain
  2. Fever
  3. Change in character of respiration
V. Interventions to educate patient and family regarding the following:
  A. Activity limitation, conservation of energy strategies
  B. Emergency care, available community resources
  C. Signs and symptoms to report to the health care team
  D. Procedures that may be required to alleviate pleural effusions
VI. Interventions to enhance adaptation or rehabilitation
  A. Assisting the patient to maintain independence within the limitation of symptoms
  B. Encouraging the patient and family to express concerns

EVALUATION

The oncology nurse systematically and regularly evaluates patient and family responses to interventions to determine progress toward the achievement of expected outcomes. Relevant data are collected, and actual findings are compared with expected findings. Nursing diagnoses, outcomes, and plans of care are reviewed and revised, as necessary.

References

Barber, N. A., & Ganti, A. K. (2011). Pulmonary toxicities from targeted therapies: A review. *Targeted Oncology, 6*(4), 235–243.

Campbell, M. L. (2011). Dyspnea. *AACN Advanced Critical Care, 22*(3), 257–264.

Cash, J. C., & Glass, C. A. (2011). *Family practice guidelines* (2nd ed.). New York: Springer.

Cheung, W. Y., & Zimmerman, C. (2011). Pharmacologic management of cancer-related pain, dyspnea, and nausea. *Seminars in Oncology, 38*(3), 450–459.

Davidson, B., Firat, P., & Michael, C. W. (2012). *Serous effusions.* London: Springer-Verlag.

Davis, H. E., Mishra, E. K., Kahan, B. C., Wrightson, J. M., Stanton, A. E., Guhan, A., et al. (2012). Effect of an indwelling pleural catheter vs chest tube and talc pleurodesis for relieving dyspnea in patients with malignant pleural effusion: The TIME2 randomized controlled trial. *JAMA, 307*(22), 2383–2389.

Decker, G. M., & Lee, C. O. (2010). *Handbook of integrative oncology nursing: Evidence-based practice.* Pittsburgh: Oncology Nursing Society.

DeVita, V. T., Lawrence, T. S., & Rosenberg, S. A. (2011). *DeVita, Hellman, and Rosenberg's cancer: Principles and practice of oncology* (9th ed.). Philadelphia: Lippincott Williams & Wilkins.

Disalvo, W. M., Joyce, M. M., Tyson, L. B., & Mackay, K. (2008). Putting evidence into practice: Evidence-based interventions for cancer-related dyspnea. *Clinical Journal of Oncology Nursing, 12*(2), 341–352.

Foster, C., Mistry, N., Peddi, P. F., & Sharma, S. (2010). *The Washington manual of medical therapeutics* (33rd ed.). Philadelphia: Lippincott Williams & Wilkins.

Gaguski, M. E., Brandsema, M., Gernalin, L., & Martinez, E. (2010). Assessing dyspnea in patients with non-small cell lung cancer in the acute care setting. *Clinical Journal of Oncology Nursing, 14*(4), 509–513.

Graves, P. R., Siddiqui, F., Anscher, M. S., & Movsas, B. (2010). Radiation pulmonary toxicity: From mechanisms to management. *Seminars in Radiation Oncology, 20*(3), 201–207.

Guntur, V. P., & Dhand, R. (2012). Pulmonary toxicity of chemotherapeutic agents. In M. C. Perry (Ed.), *Perry's the chemotherapy source book* (5th ed., pp. 206–213). Philadelphia: Lippincott Williams & Wilkins.

Hadjinicolaou, A. V., Nisar, M. K., Parfrey, H., Chilvers, E. R., & Ostor, A. J. (2011). Non-infectious pulmonary toxicity of rituximab: A systematic review. *Rheumatology, 51*(4), 653–662.

Hong, W. K., Bast, R. C., Hait, W. N., Pollock, R. E., Weichselbaum, R. R., Holland, J. F. et al. (Eds.). (2010). *Holland-Frei cancer medicine* (8th ed.). Shelton, CT: Peoples Medical Publishing House-USA.

Iwamoto, R. R., Haas, M. L., & Gosselin, T. K. (2012). *Manual for radiation oncology nursing practice and education* (4th ed.). Pittsburgh: Oncology Nursing Society.

Jarvis, C. (2012). *Physical examination and health assessment* (6th ed.). St. Louis: Elsevier Saunders.

Joyce, M. M. (2010). Dyspnea. In C. G. Brown (Ed.), *A guide to oncology symptom management* (pp. 199–220). Pittsburgh: Oncology Nursing Society.

Kastelik, J. A. (2013). Management of malignant pleural effusion. *Lung, 191*(2), 165–175.

Lakoski, S. G., Eves, N. D., Douglas, P. S., & Jones, L. W. (2012). Exercise rehabilitation in patients with cancer. *Nature Reviews Clinical Oncology, 9,* 288–296.

Light, R. W. (2011). Pleural effusions. *The Medical Clinics of North America, 95*(6), 1055–1070.

Maskell, N. A. (2012). Treatment options for malignant pleural effusions: Patient preference does matter. *JAMA, 307*(22), 2432–2433.

Peerzada, M. M., Spiro, T. P., & Daw, H. A. (2010). Pulmonary toxicities of biologics: A review. *Anti-Cancer Drugs, 21*(2), 131–139.

Perry, M. C. (2012). *Perry's the chemotherapy source book* (5th ed.). Philadelphia: Lippincott Williams & Wilkins.

Polovich, M., Whitford, J. M., & Olsen, M. (2009). *Chemotherapy and biotherapy guidelines and recommendations for practice* (3rd ed.). Pittsburgh: Oncology Nursing Society.

Qaseem, A., Snow, V., Shekelle, P., Casey, D. E., Jr., Cross, J. T., Jr., Owens, D. K., et al. (2008). Evidence-based interventions to improve the palliative care of pain, dyspnea, and depression at the end of life: A clinical practice guideline from the American College of Physicians. *Annals of Internal Medicine, 148*(2), 141–146.

Quinn, T., Alam, N., Aminazad, A., Marshall, M. B., & Choong, C. K. C. (2013). Decision making and algorithm for the management of pleural effusions. *Thoracic Surgery Clinics, 23*(1), 11–16.

Rovirosa, A., & Valduvieco, I. (2010). Radiation pneumonitis. *Clinical Pulmonary Medicine, 17*(5), 218–222.

Ryu, J. H. (2010). Chemotherapy-induced pulmonary toxicity in lung cancer patients. *Journal of Thoracic Oncology, 5*(9), 1313–1314.

Shannon, V. R., Jiminez, C. A., Travis, E. L., Safdar, A., Adachi, R., Balachandran, D. D., et al. (2010). In W. K. Hong, R. C. Bast, D. W. Kufe, R. E. Pollock, R. R. Weichselbaum, & J. F. Holland (Eds.), *Cancer Medicine* (pp. 1849–1870). Shelton, CT: People's Medical Publishing House-USA.

Torrisi, J. M., Schwartz, L. H., Gollub, M. J., Ginsberg, M. S., Bosl, G. J., & Hricak, H. (2011). CT findings of chemotherapy-induced toxicity: What radiologists need to know about the clinical and radiologic manifestations of chemotherapy toxicity. *Radiology, 258,* 41–56.

Walker, S. J., & Bryden, G. (2010). Managing pleural effusions: Nursing care of patients with a Tenckhoff catheter. *Clinical Journal of Oncology Nursing, 14*(1), 1092–1095.

Yarbro, C. H., Wujcik, D., Gobel, B. H. (Eds.). (2011). *Cancer nursing: Principles and practice* (7th ed.). Sudbury, MA: Jones and Bartlett.

Zhang, X., Sun, J., Sun, J., Ming, H., Wang, X., Wu, L., et al. (2012). Prediction of radiation pneumonitis in lung cancer patients: A systematic review. *Journal of Cancer Research and Clinical Oncology, 138*(12), 2103.

Part 4

CHAPTER 32

Alterations in Cardiovascular Function

Deborah Kirk Walker

Lymphedema

OVERVIEW

I. Definition—obstruction of the lymphatic system that causes accumulation of lymph fluid in interstitial spaces

II. Pathophysiology—occlusion or damage to the venous side of capillaries or the lymphatic system, which decreases reabsorption of lymphatic fluid made up of protein, water, fats, and wastes from cells, thereby causing swelling or lymphedema (Ridner, 2013)

  A. Primary lymphedema—genetic or familial abnormalities that can be present at birth and many years later

  B. Secondary lymphedema caused by damage or destruction of the lymphatic system

III. Incidence

  A. Varies per cancer diagnosis; increases with lymph node dissection and disease involvement of the lymph system

  B. May occur within days of a traumatic event to lymphatic system and last a lifetime if the event is permanent (e.g., lymph node dissection)

IV. Risk factors (Lasinski, 2013)

  A. Surgical—lymph node dissection, number of lymph nodes removed, type of surgery

  B. Infection—affected extremity, concurrent illness

  C. Seroma formation following surgery (Fu et al., 2011)

  D. Obesity or elevated body mass index (BMI) (Helyer, Varnic, Le, Leong, & McCready, 2010; Ridner, Dietrich, Stewart, & Armer, 2011)

  E. Air travel with suboptimal cabin pressure, long distance travel, prolonged immobilization

  F. Traumatic injury to affected extremity

  G. Excessive physical use of affected extremity; prolonged standing (lower extremity)

  H. Poor nutrition

  I. Genetics (Ridner, 2013)

  J. Thrombophlebitis

  K. Taxane therapy (Fontaine et al., 2010).

  L. Skin inflammation or chronic disorders of the skin

  M. Radiation therapy—location and formation of scars or fibrosis

  N. Tumor invasion, advanced disease, or both

ASSESSMENT

I. Physical findings (Wanchai, Beck, Stewart, & Armer, 2013a)

  A. Tightness of clothing, shoes, wrist watch, jewelry

  B. Visible puffiness

  C. Pain, stiffness, weakness, numbness, paresthesia of affected extremity

  D. Redness, warmth of affected extremity

  E. Tends to occur distal to proximal

  F. Thickening, pitting, and erythema of skin; peau d'orange changes

  G. Increased pigmentation or superficial veins, stasis dermatitis

  H. Induration with nonpitting edema

  I. Secondary cellulitis

  J. Decreased range of motion, feeling of heaviness of affected extremity

II. Assessment tools (Bernas, 2013; Ridner, 2013)

  A. Extremity measurements

    1. Arm measured 5 and 10 cm above and below the olecranon process and compared with the other extremity

    2. Leg measured at the level of the calf

  B. Water displacement—measuring limb volume

  C. Radiofrequency devices to measure fluid content

III. Clinical staging and grading

  A. Staging of lymphedema by examination—evaluates the progression of the disease (International Society of Lymphology [ISL], 2009; National Cancer Institute [NCI], 2013)

    1. Stage 1—mild, spontaneously reversible

      a. Heaviness of extremity

      b. Skin smooth-textured, with pitting edema

      c. May have pain and erythema

    2. Stage 2—moderate, irreversible

      a. May have tissue fibrosis

      b. Skin stretched, shiny, with nonpitting edema

3. Stage 3—severe, lymphostatic elephantiasis, irreversible
   a. Skin discolored, stretched, firm; nonpitting edema
   b. Rare in patients with breast cancer
B. Grading—evaluates severity of signs and symptoms (NCI, 2013)
   1. Grade 1—swelling, pitting edema; 5% to 10% difference in size at greatest point or mass of limbs
   2. Grade 2—obvious obstruction, taut skin; 10% to 30% difference in size at greatest point or mass of limbs
   3. Grade 3—limb starts to look disfigured; interferes with activities of daily living (ADLs); more than 30% difference in size at greatest point or mass of limbs
   4. Grade 4—often progresses to malignancy; disabling and may need removal of affected extremity; 5% to 10% difference in size or mass of limbs
IV. Laboratory and diagnostic tests (Bernas, 2013)
   A. Lymphoscintigraphy—radioactive mapping of lymphatic vessels
   B. Ultrasonography for evaluation of tissue and fluid
   C. Computed tomography (CT), magnetic resonance imaging (MRI), or positron emission tomography (PET) not approved for evaluation of lymphedema but can be used to evaluate soft tissue or a possible mass

PROBLEM STATEMENTS AND OUTCOME IDENTIFICATION

I. Acute Pain or Chronic Pain (NANDA-I)
   A. Expected outcome—patient reports acceptable level of pain control.
II. Impaired Physical Mobility (NANDA-I)
   A. Expected outcome—patient will use resources to help maintain level of functioning of affected lymphedema area
III. Disturbed Body Image (NANDA-I)
   A. Expected outcome—patient will communicate feelings about body image changes.
   B. Expected outcome—patient will talk with someone who has experienced lymphedema to discuss feelings of body image changes
IV. Risk for Impaired Skin Integrity (NANDA-I) ⚠
   A. Expected outcome—patient or caregiver will implement strategies to prevent skin breakdown and infection and will carry out a skin care regimen.
   B. Expected outcome—patient will protect affected extremity from trauma.

PLANNING AND IMPLEMENTATION

See Figure 32-1.
I. Interventions to treat symptoms associated with lymphedema (Chang & Cormier, 2013; Lasinski, 2013; Ridner, 2013; Wanchai et al., 2013b)
   A. Nonpharmacologic interventions—should be used in conjunction with other modalities to reduce symptoms associated with lymphedema (Wanchai, Armer, & Stewart, 2013a)
      1. Complete decongestive therapy—standard of care
         a. Compression bandaging, compression garment
         b. Manual lymphatic drainage
         c. Exercise of extremity with strength training
         d. Skin care program with proper bathing, drying, lubrication
      2. Other needed measures:
         a. Avoiding prolonged standing
         b. Elevating affected extremity
         c. Avoiding extreme heat—may worsen the swelling (e.g., hot tubs)
   B. Pharmacologic interventions to treat symptoms associated with lymphedema

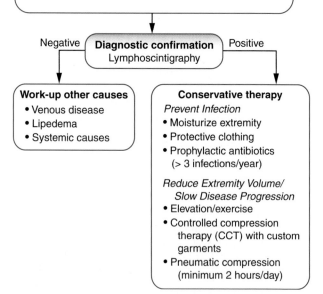

Figure 32-1 Treatment algorithm for lymphedema.
Modified from Slavin, S. A., Schook, C. C., Greene, A. K. (2011). Lymphedema management (pp. 211–220). In M. P. Davis, P. Feyer, P. Ortner, & C. Zimmermann (Eds.). Supportive oncology (pp. 211–220). Philadelphia: Saunders.

1. Early antibiotic treatment for suspected infections
2. Pain management for acute or chronic pain

II. Interventions for patient education (National Lymphedema Network, 2011)
   A. Measures to prevent lymphedema
   B. Signs and symptoms to report (e.g., high risk for infection)
   C. Need for lifelong follow-up
   D. A low-sodium, high-fiber, weight-controlling diet
   E. Importance of skin care to maintain skin integrity
   F. Education to eliminate safety hazards to prevent injury ⚠

EVALUATION

The oncology nurse systematically and regularly evaluates the client's and family's responses to interventions for lymphedema to determine progress toward the achievement of comfort and optimal mobility. Relevant data are collected, and actual findings are compared with expected findings. Nursing diagnoses, outcomes, and plans of care are reviewed and revised, as necessary.

Edema

OVERVIEW

I. Definition—fluid accumulation in interstitial spaces
II. Pathophysiology (Kalra & Aggarwal, 2012)—movement of fluid from the vascular space into the interstitial space by an alteration in one or more of the following:
   A. Increased capillary pressure—when volume of blood is expanded or with obstruction (e.g., heart disease, renal disease, cirrhosis, deep venous thrombosis)
   B. Increased capillary permeability—from vascular injury (e.g., burns, radiation, drug reactions, infection); treatment with interleukin-2 (IL-2) or vascular endothelial growth factors (VEGFs)
   C. Obstruction of lymph system—see Lymphedema
   D. Decreased plasma oncotic pressure—results in increased fluid in the tissues (e.g., proteinuria, hepatic failure, protein malnutrition)
   E. Raised hydrostatic pressure—fluid driven from the capillaries into the interstitial spaces (e.g., venous obstruction, fluid retention, prolonged standing)
III. May be associated with the following (Bonita & Pradhan, 2013; ISL, 2009; Kalra & Aggarwal, 2012; Ryberg, 2013):
   A. Lymphatic obstruction by tumor or deep vein thrombosis
   B. Cancer—common in kidney, liver, ovarian tumors
   C. Systemic conditions—heart failure, nephrotic syndrome, liver failure

   D. Medications—may include hormones, nonsteroidal anti-inflammatory drugs (NSAIDs), calcium channel blockers, tricyclic antidepressants, steroids, IL-2 therapy, corticosteroids, beta-blockers
   E. Chemotherapy—cisplatin, docetaxel, gemcitabine; targeted therapies—imatinib mesylate; anti-angiogenesis agents—thalidomide; monoclonal antibodies
   F. Allergic response or septic shock, which leads to histamine release
   G. Poor nutrition, hypoproteinemia, hypoalbuminemia
   H. Iatrogenic causes—plasma expanders, intravenous (IV) fluid overload, blood component therapy
   I. Hypothyroidism
   J. Burns, trauma, sepsis
   K. Allergic reactions
   L. Malignant ascites
IV. Incidence
   A. Unknown because the problem is underreported
   B. May be increasing because of longer survival rates

ASSESSMENT

See Bonita & Pradhan, 2013; ISL, 2009; Kalra & Aggarwal, 2012; Ryberg, 2013.
I. Risk factors
   A. Pre-existing cardiac, renal, or liver disease
   B. Cancer and treatment for cancer
   C. Decreased mobility
   D. Long distance travel
   E. Prior history of edema
   F. Certain medications
   G. Deep venous thrombosis
   H. Hypertension
II. Physical findings
   A. Tightness of clothing, shoes, jewelry, watch
   B. Pain or stiffness
   C. Weight gain
   D. Shortness of breath, dyspnea on exertion, orthopnea, paroxysmal nocturnal dyspnea, rales
   E. Frequent or decreased urination
   F. Presence of S3 or S4 heart sound
   G. Increased jugular venous pressure
   H. Increased blood pressure and tachycardia
   I. Ascites, hepatomegaly
   J. Dependent edema (extremities, sacrum)
   K. Skin thickening or skin tightness
   L. Decreased peripheral pulses
III. Laboratory and diagnostic tests
   A. Serum albumin and protein—may be decreased
   B. Creatinine, blood urea nitrogen (BUN)—may be increased with kidney disease
   C. Liver function—may be increased with cirrhosis
   D. Thyroid studies—to rule out thyroid disease

E. Brain natriuretic peptide (BNP)—will be elevated with edema that may be caused by heart failure

F. Chest radiography (CXR)—evidence of fluid overload, increased size of heart shadow

G. Echocardiography—decreased ejection fraction (EF) in heart failure

H. Ultrasonography—to rule out deep venous thrombosis or thrombophlebitis if edema is unilateral

PROBLEM STATEMENTS AND OUTCOME IDENTIFICATION

I. Risk for Impaired Skin Integrity (NANDA-I)
   A. Expected outcome—patient will maintain intact skin.
   B. Expected outcome—patient or caregiver will implement strategies to prevent skin breakdown.
II. Excess Fluid Volume (NANDA-I)
   A. Expected outcome—patient weight returns to baseline and remains stable.
   B. Expected outcome—patient's skin turgor remains normal.
III. Ineffective Peripheral Tissue Perfusion (NANDA-I)
   A. Expected outcome—patient maintains moderate activity level to promote circulation.
   B. Expected outcome—patient acknowledges the importance of protecting involved extremity from injury. ⚠
IV. Impaired Physical Mobility and Activity Intolerance (NANDA-I)
   A. Expected outcome—patient will maintain function of affected lymphedema area.
   B. Expected outcome—patient maintains muscle strength and joint range of motion. ⚠

PLANNING AND IMPLEMENTATION

I. Interventions to manage edema and possible side effects from treatment
   A. Nonpharmacologic
      1. Elevate extremities above level of heart.
      2. Compression stockings
      3. Maintain lubrication of skin
      4. Bed rest to promote diuresis; reposition every 2 hours
      5. Fluid restriction
      6. Treatment of underlying cause
      7. Monitor intake and output, electrolytes, serum albumin
      8. Protect extremity from injury ⚠
      9. Walk or other exercise
      10. Protect from extreme temperatures ⚠
   B. Pharmacologic (Kalra & Aggarwal, 2012)
      1. Diuretics
      2. Angiotensin-converting enzyme inhibitors (ACEIs) or, if not tolerated, angiotensin receptor blockers (ARBs)

      3. Beta-blockers
      4. Analgesics, as needed
II. Interventions for patient education
   A. Low-sodium, well-balanced diet
   B. Use of appropriate skin care strategies
   C. Avoidance of prolonged standing or sitting with legs crossed
   D. Avoidance of hepatotoxic drugs and alcohol
   E. Fluid restriction may be warranted
   F. Walking or other exercise to maintain muscle strength and joint range of motion
   G. Daily weigh-ins by patient and reporting greater than a 3- to 4-pound gain
   H. Educating patient and family regarding the risks for electrolyte disturbance and possible interventions if symptoms occur

EVALUATION

The oncology nurse systematically and regularly evaluates the client's and family's responses to interventions for edema to determine progress toward the achievement of weight maintenance and fluid balance. Relevant data are collected, and actual findings are compared with expected findings. Nursing diagnoses, outcomes, and plans of care are reviewed and revised, as necessary.

Malignant Pericardial Effusion

OVERVIEW

I. Definition—accumulation of fluid in the pericardial sac that affects cardiac function, resulting in decreased cardiac output
II. Pathophysiology (Burazor, Imazio, Markel, & Adler, 2013)
   A. Malignant pericardial effusions may develop from the following:
      1. Metastatic disease that has moved into the cardiac space through local advancement, spread by blood or lymph systems, or obstruction from adenopathy
      2. Treatment complications from radiation causing damage to structure; chemotherapy causing damage to endothelial cells or cardiomyocytes
      3. Infection in an immunocompromised patient
III. May be associated with the following (Burazor et al., 2013; Maisch, Ristic, & Pankuweit, 2010):
   A. Primary tumors of the pericardium; mesothelioma most common
   B. Direct tumor invasion of the myocardium; more common with lung tumors, thymoma, esophageal tumors, lymphoma
   C. Obstruction of mediastinal lymph nodes by tumor
   D. Infection (bacterial, viral, fungal)

E. Fibrosis secondary to radiation therapy (RT)

F. Drug-induced

G. Autoimmune disease

IV. Incidence (Kim et al., 2010)

A. Poor prognosis once diagnosed

B. Death within first year in 86% of cases

ASSESSMENT

I. Risk factors (Burazor et al., 2013)

A. Coexisting cardiac disease, systemic lupus erythematosus, bacterial endocarditis

B. RT of 3000 cGy to more than 33% of heart; fractions more than 300 cGy/day

C. High-dose chemotherapy or biotherapy agents that cause capillary permeability

1. Chemotherapy—cytosine arabinoside, cyclophosphamide, busulfan

2. Biologic agents—interferon, IL-2, IL-11, granulocyte-macrophage colony-stimulating factor (G-CSF)

3. Targeted agents—imatinib

4. Arsenic trioxide

5. All-trans retinoic acid

D. Rare causes include hemorrhagic tamponade from direct injury or infection.

II. Physical findings (Burazor et al., 2013)

A. Symptoms—reflect chronicity

1. Slowly developing effusions—may have little or no symptoms

2. Rapidly developing effusions—may be symptomatic at 50 to 80 mL (normal pericardial fluid volume = 15 to 50 mL)

B. Fatigue, malaise, weakness

C. Dyspnea at rest and with exertion

D. Dull, nonpositional chest pain; distant, muffled heart sounds late findings

E. Nonproductive cough

F. Tachycardia, hypotension, jugular vein distention, decreased peripheral pulses

G. Anxiousness, restlessness

H. Nausea and vomiting

I. Pericardial friction rub more likely to occur with radiation-induced or nonmalignant effusions

J. Point of maximal impulse shifted to left

K. Moderately increased central venous pressure (15-18 cm H_2O or 8-12 mm Hg)

L. 2+ to 3+ pedal edema with slowly developing effusions; may be absent with rapid development of effusion

M. Narrowing pulse pressure, pulsus paradoxus greater than 13 mm Hg

N. Cool, clammy extremities

O. Hepatomegaly or splenomegaly

III. Laboratory and diagnostic tests (Burazor et al., 2013)

A. CXR indicating cardiac enlargement, widened mediastinum, "water bottle" shape of heart, pulmonary infiltrates

B. Electrocardiography (ECG) changes, including low-voltage QRS, tachycardia, nonspecific ST-T changes; electrical alternans a rare finding

C. Echocardiography—a definitive test for effusion and cardiac function

D. CT of chest especially helpful with large tumor burden

E. May evaluate pericardial fluid for lactate dehydrogenase, protein, and tumor markers

F. Cardiac catheterization—may be indicated if the diagnosis is uncertain

G. Troponins—may be elevated

H. White blood cell (WBC) count—will be elevated with infection

I. Cross-reactive protein elevated with inflammation

J. BNP elevated with fluid overload

PROBLEM STATEMENTS AND OUTCOME IDENTIFICATION

I. Acute Pain (NANDA-I)

A. Expected outcome—patient reports acceptable level of pain control.

II. Decreased Cardiac Output and Risk for Ineffective Peripheral Tissue Perfusion (NANDA-I)

A. Expected outcome—skin will remain warm and dry.

B. Expected outcome—patient will exhibit no pedal edema.

C. Expected outcome—patient will maintain ejection fraction (EF) within 5% of baseline.

D. Expected outcome—patient will demonstrate normal vital signs and oxygenation.

III. Risk for Activity Intolerance (NANDA-I)

A. Expected outcome—patient will modify activities to adjust to decreased activity tolerance.

B. Expected outcome—patient will seek necessary help in performing activities.

IV. Ineffective Breathing Pattern (NANDA-I)

A. Expected outcome—patient will report feeling comfortable when breathing.

PLANNING AND IMPLEMENTATION

(See Burazor et al., 2013.)

I. Interventions to relieve symptoms and improve quality of life

A. Nonpharmacologic interventions

1. Drainage of pericardial fluid (e.g., percutaneous pericardiocentesis)

2. Radiation—may be indicated, but not common

3. Elevation of head of bed to relieve dyspnea

4. Minimizing patient activities to conserve energy

5. No treatment may be elected, with close follow-up if asymptomatic
6. Consultation with palliative care specialist
   B. Pharmacologic interventions
      1. Chemotherapy—may be indicated if tumor responsive (e.g., lymphoma, leukemia, breast cancer)
      2. Administration of sclerosing agents into pericardial space
      3. Oxygen therapy
      4. Diuretics probably not beneficial
      5. Pain management
II. Interventions for patient education
   A. Preparation for pericardial drainage
   B. Energy conservation methods
   C. Relaxation techniques
   D. Activity modification to conserve energy

EVALUATION

The oncology nurse systematically and regularly evaluates the client's and family's responses to malignant pericardial effusion to determine progress toward the achievement of expected outcomes. Relevant data are collected, and actual findings are compared with expected findings. Nursing diagnoses, outcomes, and plans of care are reviewed and revised, as necessary.

Cardiovascular Toxicity Related to Cancer Therapy

OVERVIEW

I. Definition—damage to the cardiac muscle related to cancer therapies that may cause alterations in cardiac function (Davis & Witteles, 2013)
II. Pathophysiology (Bonita & Pradhan, 2013; Ryberg, 2013)
   A. Cardiotoxicity
      1. Alkylating agents—associated with acute myopericarditis, pericardial effusions, and heart failure (e.g., cyclophosphamide, ifosfamide)
      2. Anthracyclines—may cause toxicity from injury of free radicals that result in myocardial cell loss, fibrosis, and loss of contractility (e.g., doxorubicin, epirubicin, idarubicin, mitoxantrone)
      3. Taxanes—may cause early heart failure and left ventricular dysfunction (LVD); shown to be more toxic if administered with doxorubicin (e.g., paclitaxel, docetaxel); cremophor EL in paclitaxel contributes to the process (Minotti, Menna, Salvatorelli, Cairo, & Gianni, 2004)
      4. Monoclonal antibodies—inhibit certain pathways critical to cardiac function, which may increase the risk for cardiac toxicity (e.g., VEGF).

a. Bevacizumab—increases blood pressure, may cause arterial thromboembolic events (ATE); toxicity usually reversible
b. Trastuzumab—may cause acute heart failure and cardiomyopathy when used with or following anthracyclines; reversible
c. Pertuzumab—LVD and symptoms of heart failure have been observed (Lenihan et al., 2012)
d. Rituximab—arrhythmias and angina have been reported; can be life-threatening
e. Aflibercept—ATE; congestive heart failure has been observed
      5. Tyrosine kinase inhibitors (TKIs)—although the incidence is small, TKIs (e.g., dasatinib, lapatinib, imatinib, sunitinib) may cause cardiotoxicities through inhibition of the various targeted pathways (e.g., EGFR, VEGFR, BRAF)
      6. Proteasome inhibitors—may cause cardiotoxicity from stress to the cell endoplasmic reticulum (e.g., bortezomib) (Hawkes, Okines, Plummer, & Cunningham, 2011)
      7. Antimetabolites—may cause coronary artery spasm, resulting in angina, arrhythmia, myocardial infarction, cardiac arrest, and sudden death; coronary artery thrombosis and apoptosis of myocardial cells (e.g., 5-fluorouracil [5-FU], capecitabine)
      8. Radiation to areas near the heart may cause fibrosis of cardiac structures, resulting in injury and dysfunction leading to pericardial effusions, tamponade, valvular insufficiency, constrictive pericarditis, and myocardial infarction (Martinou & Gaya, 2013)
   B. Hypertension (Bonita & Pradhan, 2013; Ryberg, 2013)
      1. Drugs that may cause hypertension— bevacizumab, sorafenib, sunitinib, pazopanib, vandetanib, axitinib, afibercept, imatinib
   C. QT prolongation—may occur from targeted therapies and drug-drug interactions and cause lethal arrhythmias (Bonita & Pradhan, 2013; Ryberg, 2013)
      1. Arsenic trioxide, pazopanib, sunitinib, vandetanib, lapatinib, dasatinib, nilotinib
   D. Venous thromboembolism (VTE), with or without ATE (Bonita & Pradhan, 2013; Ryberg, 2013)
      1. ATE—bevacizumab, aflibercept, dasatinib
      2. Both ATE and VTE—sunitinib, sorafenib, pazopanib
III. Incidence (Bonita & Pradham, 2013)
   A. Acute reactions—infrequent, reversible
      1. Occur within 24 hours of drug administration
      2. Usually self-limiting and cease when the drug is stopped

3. May not require discontinuation of the drug

B. Early onset within 1 year after treatment —infrequent

C. Late onset after 1 year of completing therapy
   1. Occurs with cumulative doses of drugs
   2. Dilated cardiomyopathy may occur

ASSESSMENT

(See Carver, Szalda, & Ky, 2013.)

I. Risk factors
   A. Pre-existing heart disease, hypertension, hyperlipidemia
   B. History of smoking
   C. Age younger than 15 years or advanced age, older than 65
   D. Certain cardiotoxic drugs
      1. Doses that place patient at risk:
         a. Doxorubicin greater than 550 mg/m^2
         b. Liposomal doxorubicin greater than 900 mg/m^2
         c. Epirubicin greater than 720 mg/m^2
         d. Mitoxantrone greater than 120 mg/m^2
         e. Idarubicin greater than 90 mg/m^2
   E. Exceeding recommended total doses of chemotherapy or high dose in short period
   F. Radiation to the chest
   G. Acute cardiac event during treatment
   H. Combination of chest radiation with anthracycline
   I. Other—female gender, obesity, comorbid disease

II. Physical findings
   A. Palpitations, chest pain, orthostatic symptoms, arrhythmias, jugular vein distention, bilateral pedal edema, presence of S3 or S4, murmurs with valvular abnormalities, decreased cardiac EF
      1. Tachycardia—early sign in anthracycline toxicity
   B. Shortness of breath, dyspnea, orthopnea, nonproductive cough
   C. Exercise intolerance, fatigue
   D. Weight gain
   E. Syncope

III. Laboratory and diagnostic tests to monitor (Bonita & Pradhan, 2013; Cardinale, Bacchiani, Beggiato, Colobo, & Cipolla, 2013; Carver et al., 2013)
   A. ECG changes
      1. Premature atrial contractions, premature ventricular contractions
      2. Nonspecific ST-T wave changes
   B. Echocardiography or multigated acquisition (MUGA) scan
      1. Left ventricular function—usually decreased EF
         a. Decreased EF to less than 45% or decrease of more than 5% over baseline requiring drug discontinuation
      2. Pericardial effusion
      3. Left ventricular hypertrophy
   C. MRI—gold standard for evaluation of left ventricular volumes, mass and function; however, it is cost prohibitive
   D. BMI or waist circumference
   E. Laboratory changes that may affect cardiac function—potassium, magnesium, calcium, renal function, cardiac biomarkers (e.g., troponins, BNP), thyroid, lipid levels; electrolytes should be monitored, especially with drugs that may prolong the Q-T interval

PROBLEM STATEMENTS AND OUTCOME IDENTIFICATION

I. Decreased Cardiac Output and Risk for Ineffective Peripheral Tissue Perfusion (NANDA-I)
   A. Expected outcome—patient will perform activity within limitations of prescribed heart rate.
   B. Expected outcome—patient will exhibit no pedal edema.
   C. Expected outcome—patient maintains EF within 5% of baseline.
   D. Expected outcome—patient demonstrates normal vital signs and oxygenation level.

II. Risk for Activity Intolerance (NANDA-I)
   A. Expected outcome—patient will seek help in performing activities as needed.
   B. Expected outcome—patient will verbalize acceptance of decreased activity level.

III. Risk for Imbalanced Fluid Volume (NANDA-I)
   A. Expected outcome—patient will remain hemodynamically stable.
   B. Expected outcome—patient will maintain adequate fluid balance consistent with underlying disease restriction.

IV. Anxiety (NANDA-I)
   A. Expected outcome—patient will identify factors that cause anxious behavior.
   B. Expected outcome—patient will discuss activities to decrease anxious behavior.

PLANNING AND IMPLEMENTATION

See Bonita & Pradhan, 2013; Cardinale et al., 2013; Carver et al., 2013.

I. Interventions for cardiotoxicity—prevention important
   A. Documentation of total cumulative dose of drug; discontinuation when maximum dose is achieved
      1. Doxorubicin—550 mg/m^2
      2. Daunorubicin (Cerubidine, DaunoXome)—600 mg/m^2
      3. Mitoxantrone (Novantrone)—160 mg/m^2
      4. High-dose cyclophosphamide—144 mg/kg for 4 days
   B. Monitoring baseline and interval ECG or MUGA scan

C. Monitoring vital signs and weight

D. Use of liposomal doxorubicin decreases cardiotoxicity

E. Monitoring exposure of RT

II. Interventions to treat cardiotoxicity with nonpharmacologic methods (Curigliano et al., 2012)

A. Cardiovascular risk assessment before treatment starts

B. Screening of cardiovascular function at appropriate intervals

C. Valvular surgery—may be indicated with radiation-induced valvular disease

D. Management of underlying disease—both cancer and cardiac disease

E. Radiation management to reduce exposure to cardiac structure

III. Interventions to treat cardiotoxicity with pharmacologic methods based on underlying event (Curigliano et al., 2012)

A. Lipid-lowering agents if indicated for hyperlipidemia

B. Beta-blockers and ACE inhibitors

1. Can be used for LVD

2. Trastuzumab cardiotoxicity—currently evidence-based guidelines lacking; withdrawal of treatment and management of cardiac dysfunction with beta-blockers and ACEIs recommended

C. ARBs concurrent with anthracyclines—helps prevent cardiac damage (Nakamae et al., 2005)

D. ACEIs and calcium channel blockers to treat hypertension from angiogenesis inhibitors

E. Q-T prolongation

1. Avoidance of drug-drug interactions

2. Monitoring electrolytes and treating imbalance

F. Administration of cardioprotective iron chelating agents such as dexrazoxane (Zinecard), to prevent doxorubicin-induced cardiotoxicity in patients with metastatic breast cancer who require more than 300 mg/m^2 of drug (Huh, Jaffe, Durand, Munsell, & Herzog, 2010; Van Dalen, Caron, Dickinson, & Kremer, 2011)

IV. Interventions for patient education

A. Signs and symptoms to report

B. Well-balanced diet, with a focus on any restrictions

C. Importance for medically approved exercise program (Scott et al., 2013)

EVALUATION

The oncology nurse systematically and regularly evaluates the client's and family's responses to cancer therapies that cause cardiac toxicity to determine progress toward the achievement of normal cardiac function. Data are collected, and actual findings are compared with expected findings. Nursing diagnoses, outcomes, and plans of care are reviewed and revised, as necessary.

Thrombotic Events

OVERVIEW

I. Definition—venous thrombus or arterial embolus interfering with venous drainage or obstructing arterial blood flow

II. Pathophysiology (Young et al., 2012)

A. A thrombus may form in the setting of stasis, endothelial injury, or a hypercoagulable state (Virchow triad).

1. The thrombus is composed of red blood cells (RBCs), fibrin, and platelets; it fills the vessel lumen, causing partial or complete obstruction of blood flow, or may shed emboli, causing a pulmonary embolus or cerebrovascular accident.

2. The thrombus may float freely in the blood vessel, leading to embolization, where it lodges in a blood vessel, causing partial or complete obstruction of blood flow.

B. Tumor cells may be associated with procoagulant activities.

1. Tumor cells deposit fibrin in tissues and act late in the clotting cascade, providing a surface for prothrombinase assembly.

2. Microvasculature becomes hyperpermeable, allowing clotting proteins to leak into extravascular space.

3. Procoagulants released from cancer cells initiate the clotting cascade.

III. May be associated with the following (Connolly & Khorana, 2010; Conti et al., 2013; Kearon et al., 2012; Mandala et al., 2010; Schmidt, Horvath-Puho, Thomsen, Smeeth, & Sorensen, 2012):

A. Thrombocytosis (platelet count > 400,000/mm^3)

B. Metastatic cancer

C. Presence of venous access device

D. Disseminated intravascular coagulation

E. Cancer treatments

1. Cytotoxic agents

2. Hormonal therapy

3. Antiangiogenic agents—thalidomide, lenalidomide

F. Sepsis

G. Cardiac disease, pulmonary disease, renal disease

H. Clotting abnormalities (e.g., factor V Leiden, protein C and protein S deficiency, antiphospholipid antibodies)—less likely in persons with cancer

I. Microangiopathic hemolytic anemia (MAHA) associated with thrombotic thrombocytopenic purpura (TTP)

J. Smoking, obesity (BMI >35 kg/m^2), immobility
K. Heparin-induced thrombocytopenia
L. History of venous thromboembolism
M. Hospitalization (Centers for Disease Control and Prevention [CDC], 2012)
N. Erythropoietic stimulating agents, blood transfusions, major surgery (Bennett et al., 2008; Rogers et al., 2012)
O. Advanced age
P. Lymphadenopathy

IV. Incidence rates—vary in persons with cancer by disease; more common with the following (DeMartino et al., 2012; Young et al., 2012):
A. High risk—cancers of the lung, gastrointestinal tract, pancreatic, prostate, ovary
B. Leukemias, multiple myeloma, Hodgkin and non-Hodgkin lymphoma
C. Advanced disease or metastatic disease

ASSESSMENT

See Conti et al., 2013; Mandala et al., 2010; National Comprehensive Cancer Network [NCCN], 2013.

I. Risk factors
A. Estrogen, tamoxifen use
B. Smoking
C. Recent surgery
D. Bed rest or decreased activity status
E. Recent long distance plane or car travel.
F. Obesity—BMI >35 kg/m^2.
G. Advanced age
H. Prior venous thromboembolism (VTE)
I. Cancer diagnosis
J. Lymphadenopathy
K. Familial hypercoagulability
L. Comorbidities—such as infection, heart failure, ATE, diabetes

II. Physical findings
A. Venous occlusion
1. Dull ache, tight feeling, or pain in the calf, especially with walking
2. Tenderness over involved vein, palpable venous cord
3. Unilateral edema of involved extremity
4. Distention of superficial collateral veins
B. Arterial embolus
1. Severe pain in the involved extremity
2. Extremity coolness, pallor
3. Absent or decreased pulse
C. Pulmonary embolus
1. Chest pain
2. Dyspnea, shallow respirations, tachypnea
3. Sudden onset of anxiety
4. Cardiopulmonary arrest
5. Decreased pulse oximetry
6. Decreased breath sounds with pleural friction rub

D. Clotting abnormalities
1. Easy bruising
2. Bleeding from mucous membranes, in urine or stool

III. Laboratory and diagnostic tests (Farge et al., 2013; NCCN, 2013)
A. Complete blood cell (CBC) count and platelet count—thrombocytosis; platelets more than 400,000/mm^3
B. Abnormal venous duplex scan or venography with VTE
C. Liver function tests, BUN, creatinine
D. Abnormal arteriography with arterial embolus
E. Abnormal spiral CT or ventilation-perfusion (V-Q) scan with pulmonary embolism
F. Prothrombin time (PT), partial thrombin time (PTT), international normalized ratio (INR), abnormal clotting factors
G. Magnetic resonance venography for pelvic and iliac veins and vena cava—can be cost-prohibitive

PROBLEM STATEMENTS AND OUTCOME IDENTIFICATION

I. Risk for Decreased Cardiac Tissue Perfusion (NANDA-I)
A. Expected outcome—patient's extremities are of normal warmth and color.

II. Impaired Gas Exchange (NANDA-I), related to pulmonary emboli
A. Expected outcome—patient maintains normal respiratory rate.
B. Expected outcome—patient will carry out activities of daily living (ADLs) without weakness or fatigue.

III. Activity Intolerance (NANDA-I)
A. Expected outcome—patient demonstrates tolerance of physical activity.
B. Expected outcome—patient will identify factors that cause fatigue.

IV. Acute Pain (NANDA-I)
A. Expected outcome—patient reports acceptable level of pain control.
B. Expected outcome—patient will rate pain less than 3 on a scale of 1 to 10.

PLANNING AND IMPLEMENTATION

See Farge et al., 2013; Kearon et al., 2012.

I. Interventions to promote prevention in high-risk patients
A. Nonpharmacologic
1. Frequent ambulation, leg exercises if bedridden
2. Elevation of foot with knee flexed
3. Use of elastic stockings, pneumatic compression device
4. Referral to physical therapy, occupational therapy, or both

B. Pharmacologic (Siegal & Garcia, 2012)
 1. Prophylaxis is not recommended in patients receiving standard chemotherapy.
 2. Prophylaxis should be considered in patients with pancreatic or lung cancer.
  a. Acetylsalicylic acid (aspirin, ASA), 81 mg
  b. Low-molecular–weight heparin (LMWH)

II. Interventions to treat existing embolus
 A. Nonpharmacologic
  1. Placement of inferior vena cava filter if pharmacologic management is contraindicated
  2. Arterial embolectomy
  3. Thrombolysis consider on case by case basis
  4. Monitor laboratory parameters—PT, PTT, INR
 B. Pharmacologic
  1. LMWH
  2. Heparin infusion
  3. Warfarin (adjusted to INR of 2-3)
  4. Oxygen for pulmonary embolism
  5. Pain management

III. Interventions for patient education
 A. Medication administration
 B. Preventive measures
 C. Bleeding precautions if patient taking anticoagulant
 D. Dietary restrictions—avoid foods high in vitamin K
 E. Smoking cessation
 F. Activity restrictions

EVALUATION

The oncology nurse systematically and regularly evaluates the client's and family's responses to interventions to prevent and manage thromboembolism. Relevant data are collected, and actual findings are compared with expected findings. Nursing diagnoses, outcomes, and plans of care are reviewed and revised, as necessary.

References

Bennett, C. L., Silver, S. M., Djulbegovic, B., Samaras, A. T., Blau, C. A., Gleason, K. J., et al. (2008). Venous thromboembolism and mortality associated with recombinant erythropoietin and darbepoetin administration for the treatment of cancer-associated anemia. *JAMA, 299*(8), 914–924. http://dx.doi.org/10.1001/jama.299.8.914.

Bernas, M. (2013). Assessment and risk reduction in lymphedema. *Seminars in Oncology Nursing, 29*(1), 12–19. http://dx.doi.org/10.1016/j.soncn.2012.11.003.

Bonita, R., & Pradhan, R. (2013). Cardiovascular toxicities of cancer chemotherapy. *Seminars in Oncology, 40*(2), 186–198. http://dx.doi.org/10.1053/j.seminoncol.2013.01.004.

Burazor, I., Imazio, M., Markel, G., & Adler, Y. (2013). Malignant pericardial effusion. *Cardiology, 124*(4), 224–232. http://dx.doi.org/10.1159/000348559.

Cardinale, D., Bacchiani, G., Beggiato, M., Alessndro, C., & Cipolla, C. M. (2013). Strategies to prevent and treat cardiovascular risk in cancer patients. *Seminars in Oncology, 40*(2), 186–198. http://dx.doi.org/10.1053/j.seminoncol.2013.01.008.

Carver, J. R., Szalda, D., & Ky, B. (2013). Asymptomatic cardiac toxicity in long-term cancer survivors: Defining the population and recommendations for surveillance. *Seminars in Oncology, 40*(2), 229–238. http://dx.doi.org/10.1053/j.seminoncol.2013.01.005.

Centers for Disease Control and Prevention. (2012). Venous thromboembolism in adult hospitalizations—United States, 2007-2009. *MMWR. Morbidity and Mortality Weekly Report, 61*(22), 401–404.

Chang, C. J., & Cormier, J. N. (2013). Lymphedema interventions: Exercise, surgery, and compression devices. *Seminars in Oncology Nursing, 29*(1), 28–40. http://dx.doi.org/10.1016/j.soncn.2012.11.005.

Connolly, G. C., & Khorana, A. A. (2010). Emerging risk stratification approaches to cancer associated thrombosis: Risk factors, biomarkers and a risk score. *Thrombosis Research, 125*(Suppl. 2), S1–S7. http://dx.doi.org/10.1016/S0049-3848(10)00227-6.

Conti, E., Romiti, A., Musumeci, B., Passerini, J., Zezza, L., Mastromarino, V., et al. (2013). Arterial thrombotic events and acute coronary syndromes with cancer drugs: Are growth factors the missed link? What both cardiologist and oncologist should know about novel angiogenesis inhibitors. *International Journal of Cardiology.* http://dx.doi.org/10.1016/j.ilcard.2013.01.052.

Curigliano, G., Cardinale, D., Suter, T., Plataniotis, G., de Azambuja, E., Sandri, M. T., et al. (2012). Cardiovascular toxicity induced by chemotherapy, targeted agents and radiotherapy: ESMO Clinical Practice Guidelines. *Annals of Oncology, 23*(Suppl. 7), vii155–vii166. http://dx.doi.org/10.1093/annonc/mds293.

Davis, M., & Witteles, R. M. (2013). Cardiac testing to manage cardiovascular risk in cancer patients. *Seminars in Oncology, 40*(2), 147–155. http://dx.doi.org/10.1053/j.seminoncol.2013.01.003.

DeMartino, R. R., Goodney, P. P., Spangler, E. L., Wallaert, J. B., Corriere, M. A., Rzucidio, E. M., et al. (2012). Variation in thromboembolic complications among patients undergoing commonly performed cancer operations. *Journal of Vascular Surgery, 55*(4), 1035–1040.

Farge, D., Debourdeau, P., Beckers, M., Baglin, C., Bauersachs, R. M., Brenner, B., et al. (2013). International clinical practice guidelines for the treatment and prophylaxis of venous thromboembolism in patients with cancer. *Journal of Thrombosis and Haemostasis, 11*(1), 56–70. http://dx.doi.org/10.1111/jth.12070.

Fontaine, C., Van Parijs, H., Decoster, L., Adriaenssens, N., Schallier, D. C., Vanhoey, M., et al. (2010). A prospective analysis of the incidence of postoperative lymphedema 1-2 years after surgery and axillary dissection in early breast cancer patients treated with concomitant irradiation and anthracyclines followed by paclitaxel. *Journal of Clinical Oncology, 28*(15), e11059.

Fu, M. R., Guth, A. A., Cleland, C. M., Lima, E. D., Kaval, M., Haber, J., et al. (2011). The effects of symptomatic seroma on lymphedema symptoms following breast cancer treatment. *Lymphology, 44*(3), 134–143.

Hawkes, E. A., Okines, A. F., Plummer, C., & Cunningham, D. (2011). Cardiotoxicity in patients treated with bevacizumab is potentially reversible. *Journal of Clinical Oncology, 29*(18), e560–e562. http://dx.doi.org/10.1200/JCO.2011.35.5008.

Helyer, L. K., Varnic, M., Le, L. W., Leong, W., & McCready, D. (2010). Obesity is a risk factor for developing postoperative lymphedema in breast cancer patients. *Breast Journal, 16*(1), 48–54. http://dx.doi.org/10.1111/j.1524-4741.2009.00855.

Huh, W. W., Jaffe, N., Durand, J. B., Munsell, M. F., & Herzog, C. E. (2010). Comparison of doxorubicin cardiotoxicity in pediatric sarcoma patients when given with dexrazoxane versus as continuous infusion. *Pediatric Hematology and Oncology, 27*(7), 546–557. http://dx.doi.org/10.3109/08880018.2010.503335.

International Society of Lymphology (ISL). (2009). The diagnosis and treatment of peripheral lymphedema. 2009 Consensus document of the International Society of Lymphology. *Lymphology, 42*, 51–60.

Kalra, O. P., & Aggarwal, A. (2012). Rational use of diuretics and pathophysiology of edema. *Medicine Update, 22*, 601–610.

Kearon, C., Akl, E. A., Comerota, A. J., Prandoni, P., Bounameaux, H., Goldhaber, S. Z., et al. (2012). Antithrombotic therapy for VTE disease: Antithrombotic therapy and prevention of thrombosis, 9th ed: American College of Chest Physicians Evidence-Based Clinical Practice Guidelines. *Chest, 141*(Suppl.), e419S–e494S. http://dx.doi.org/10.1378/chest.11-2301.

Kim, S. H., Kwak, M. H., Park, S., Kim, H. J., Lee, H. S., Kim, M. S., et al. (2010). Clinical characteristics of malignant pericardial effusion associated with recurrence and survival. *Cancer Research and Treatment, 42*(4), 201–216. http://dx.doi.org/10.4143/crt.2010.42.4.210.

Lasinski, B. B. (2013). Complete decongestive therapy for treatment of lymphedema. *Seminars in Oncology Nursing, 29*(1), 20–27. http://dx.doi.org/10.1016/j.soncn.2012.004.

Lenihan, D., Suter, T., Brammer, M., Neate, C., Ross, G., & Baselga, J. (2012). Pooled analysis of cardiac safety in patients with cancer treated with pertuzumab. *Annals of Oncology, 23*(3), 791–800. http://dx.doi.org/10.1093/annonc/mdr294.

Maisch, B., Ristic, A., & Pankuweit, S. (2010). Evaluation and management of pericardial effusion in patients with neoplastic disease. *Progress in Cardiovascular Disease, 53*(2), 157–163. http://dx.doi.org/10.1016/j.pcad.2010.06.003.

Mandala, M., Barni, S., Prins, M., Labianca, R., Tondini, C., Russo, L., et al. (2010). Acquired and inherited risk factors for developing venous thromboembolism in cancer patients receiving adjuvant chemotherapy: A prospective trial. *Annals of Oncology, 21*(4), 871–876. http://dx.doi.org/10.1093/annonc/mdp354.

Martinou, M., & Gaya, A. (2013). Cardiac complications after radical radiotherapy. *Seminars in Oncology, 40*(2), 178–185. http://dx.doi.org/10.1053/j.seminoncol.2013.01.007.

Minotti, G., Menna, P., Salvatorelli, E., Cairo, G., & Gianni, L. (2004). Anthracyclines: Molecular advances and pharmacologic developments in antitumor activity and cardiotoxicity. *Pharmacology Review, 56*, 185–229.

Nakamae, H., Tsumura, K., Terada, Y., Nakane, T., Nakamae, M., Ohta, K., et al. (2005). Notable effects of angiotensin II receptor blocker, valsartan, on acute cardiotoxic changes after standard chemotherapy with cyclophosphamide, doxorubicin, vincristine, and prednisolone. *Cancer, 104*(11), 2492–2498.

National Cancer Institute (NCI). (2013). *Lymphedema.* http://www.cancer.gov/cancertopics/pdq/supportivecare/lymphedema/healthprofessional/page.

National Comprehensive Cancer Network (NCCN). (2013). *Guidelines venous thromboembolic disease [v 1.2013].* http://www.nccn.org/professionals/physician_gls/f_guidelines.asp#site.

National Lymphedema Network. (2011). *Summary of risk reduction practices.* http://www.lymphnet.org/lymphedemaFAQs/riskReduction/riskReduction_summary.htm.

Ridner, S. H. (2013). Pathophysiology of lymphedema. *Seminars in Oncology Nursing, 29*(1), 4–11. http://dx.doi.org/10.1016/j.soncn.2012.002.

Ridner, S., Dietrich, M., Stewart, B., & Armer, J. (2011). Body mass index and breast cancer treatment-related lymphedema. *Supportive Care in Cancer, 19*, 853–857.

Rogers, M. A., Levine, D. A., Blumberg, N., Flanders, S. A., Chopra, V., & Langa, K. M. (2012). Triggers of hospitalization for venous thromboembolism. *Circulation, 125*(17), 2092–2099. http://dx.doi.org/10.1161/CIRCULATIONAHA.111.084467.

Ryberg, M. (2013). Cardiovascular toxicities of biological therapies. *Seminars in Oncology, 40*(2), 168–177. http://dx.doi.org/10.1053/j.seminoncol.2013.01.002.

Schmidt, M., Horvath-Puho, E., Thomsen, R. W., Smeeth, L., & Sorensen, H. T. (2012). Acute infections and venous thromboembolism. *Journal of Internal Medicine, 271*(6), 608–618. http://dx.doi.org/10.111/j.1365-2796.2011.02473.x.

Scott, J. M., Koelwyn, G. J., Hornsby, W. E., Khouri, M., Peppercorn, J., Douglas, P. S., & Jones, L. W. (2013). Exercise therapy as treatment for cardiovascular and oncologic disease after a diagnosis of early-stage breast cancer. *Seminars in Oncology, 40*(2), 218–228. http://dx.doi.org/10.1053/j.seminoncol.2013.01.001.

Siegal, D. M., & Garcia, D. (2012). Anticoagulants in cancer. *Journal of Thrombosis and Haemostasis.* http://dx.doi.org/10.1111/j.1538-7836.2012.04913.x, Sept 3.

Van Dalen, E. C., Caron, H. N., Dickinson, H. O., & Kremer, L. C. (2011). Cardioprotective interventions for cancer patients receiving anthracyclines. *Cochrane Database Systematic Review, 6*, CD003917. http://dx.doi.org/10.1002/14651858.CD003917.

Wanchai, A., Armer, J. M., & Stewart, B. R. (2013a). Complementary and alternative medicine and lymphedema. *Seminars in Oncology Nursing, 29*(1), 41–49. http://dx.doi.org/10.1016/j.soncn.2012.006.

Wanchai, A., Beck, M., Stewart, B. R., & Armer, J. M. (2013b). Management of lymphedema for cancer patients with complex needs. *Seminars in Oncology Nursing, 29*(1), 61–65. http://dx.doi.org/10.1016/j.soncn.2012.001.

Young, A., Chapman, O., Connor, C., Poole, C., Rose, P., & Kakkar, A. K. (2012). Thrombosis and cancer. *Nature Reviews. Clinical Oncology, 9*(8), 437–449. http://dx.doi.org/10.1038/nrclinonc.2012.106.

Part 4

CHAPTER 33
Alterations in Nutritional Status

Diane G. Cope

Weight Changes and Body Composition

OVERVIEW

(See Cunningham & Huhmann, 2011.)

I. Effects of cancer and cancer treatments—may cause overnutrition and undernutrition (weight gain, weight loss, and body composition), which may negatively affect cancer recurrence, survival, morbidity, and quality of life (QOL)

II. Causes of weight gain
   A. Disease related
      1. Weight gain experienced by patients with breast cancer as a result of multiagent chemotherapy regimens, regimens containing steroids, or both
      2. Effusions—pleural, pericardial, abdominal
      3. Edema
      4. Obstruction
      5. Inactivity
      6. Electrolyte imbalances
   B. Treatment related
      1. Hormonal drugs
      2. Steroids
      3. Electrolyte imbalances
      4. Metabolic complications
      5. Adjuvant chemotherapy for breast cancer
      6. Biologic medications such as interleukin-2 (IL-2)

III. Causes of weight loss
   A. Disease related
      1. Protein-calorie malnutrition caused by the metabolic effects of the tumor
      2. Location of the tumor—increased weight loss associated with upper respiratory and gastric tumors
   B. Surgery related, especially with head and neck cancers and esophageal, gastric, pancreatic, or colorectal surgeries
      1. May cause alterations in ability to eat
      2. May cause disrupted absorption of nutrients

   3. Postprandial dumping syndrome associated with gastric resections
   4. Frequent tests usually needed in surgical oncology patients; may limit intake, include dietary restrictions, or both
   5. Increased calories expended and energy needs increased during the perioperative period
   C. Treatment related
      1. Weight loss resulting from vomiting associated with chemotherapy and radiation
      2. Weight loss resulting from acute or chronic diarrhea caused by drugs (e.g., antibiotics, chemotherapy), dietary alterations, infectious processes (e.g., *Clostridium difficile*), intestinal ischemia, fecal impaction, irritable bowel disease, laxative abuse, endocrine disorders, malabsorption, surgery, and radiation colitis
      3. Post–stem cell transplantation acute and chronic graft-versus-host disease (GVHD)
      4. Presence of concurrent symptoms related to cancer treatment, including anorexia, taste alterations, mucositis, pain, anxiety, depression, fatigue
      5. Side effects of medications, including antibiotics, opioids, biologic and targeted therapies
   D. Insensible losses such as perspiration, gastric suction, surgical drains, fistulas, wounds

ASSESSMENT

I. History
   A. Previous dietary patterns, food preferences, cultural preferences, food allergies, eating habits, and history of weight changes
   B. Patterns of weight changes, including type, onset, duration, severity; early satiety; associated symptoms—nausea, food intolerances, taste abnormalities, mouth and throat pain, dysphagia, vomiting, diarrhea; other factors—precipitating, aggravating, alleviating factors

C. Previous self-care strategies
   1. Ability to carry out interventions to maintain weight
   2. Use of food, nutritional supplements, and other remedies
D. Current or recent treatment for cancer and experienced side effects
E. Assessment of patient for associated cultural, socioeconomic, emotional, and motivational factors that may affect weight loss or gain

II. Physical examination
   A. Determination of present weight and amount of total weight loss or gain
   B. Assessment for presence of dehydration, electrolyte imbalances, or both

PROBLEM STATEMENTS AND OUTCOME IDENTIFICATION

I. Imbalanced Nutrition: Less than Body Requirements (NANDA-I)
   A. Expected outcome—patient states the goals of interventions related to weight loss or gain.
   B. Expected outcome—patient states the personal risk for complications related to weight loss or gain and ways in which various cancer therapies may adversely affect nutritional reserves.
   C. Expected outcome—patient's nutritional intake is sufficient to maintain weight.

II. Disturbed Body Image (NANDA-I)
   A. Expected outcome—patient states the goals of interventions related to weight change.
   B. Expected outcome—patient states the personal risk for complications related to weight loss or gain and ways in which various cancer therapies may affect nutrition.
   C. Expected outcome—patient participates in measures to minimize risk of occurrence, severity, and complications of weight changes.
   D. Expected outcome—patient and family state awareness of resources in the community to assist with nutrition.

III. Diarrhea (NANDA-I)
   A. Expected outcome—patient states the changes in condition that require notification of health care provider; intervention, including number of stools, amount of diarrhea per day, or both

IV. Nausea (NANDA-I)
   A. Expected outcome notification patient states the changes in condition that require professional assistance, intervention, or both.
      1. Weight loss of greater than 5% of body weight
      2. Dehydration, increased insensible losses, edema
      3. Changes in skin integrity, wound healing, respiratory or cardiovascular status, presence of infection
      4. Inability to eat or drink
      5. Any area of concern for patient's well-being related to intake or lack of intake

PLANNING AND IMPLEMENTATION

I. Interventions to increase calorie and nutritional value of oral intake
   A. Teaching patient or family to do the following:
      1. Consume nutritionally dense and high-protein foods such as cottage cheese, puddings, and oatmeal.
      2. Eat frequently, in small portions throughout the day.
      3. Maximize food intake during periods of greatest strength and appetite, usually early in the day.
      4. Increase the kilocalorie (kcal) protein content of foods by adding protein powders, instant nonfat dry milk powder or instant breakfast powders to gravies, puddings, and other foods.
      5. Maximize food preferences and access to favorite foods within dietary restrictions.
      6. Choose high-protein, high-calorie, healthy snacks between meals.
      7. Try cold, room-temperature, and soft foods to improve intake.
   B. Administering oral supplements to increase protein-calorie intake between meals and at bedtime
   C. Limiting liquids at mealtime because they may cause early satiety and nausea
   D. Discussing taste changes and reviewing liquids and foods that patient may be able to tolerate

II. Interventions to promote maximal comfort and ease while eating
   A. Administering pain medications, if needed, 30 to 60 minutes before meals
   B. Assisting with oral care, as needed, before and after meals

III. Interventions to involve patient and family in care
   A. Assisting patient and family with calculating individualized calorie and protein requirements so that realistic goals can be set for weight changes; may need to consult with a nutritionist
   B. Using proper quantities of foods from the food groups that provide a balanced, nutritious diet for weight control
   C. Having the patient engage in regular exercise, if able
   D. Encouraging consultation with a dietitian

EVALUATION

The oncology nurse systematically and regularly evaluates the patient's and family's responses to interventions to determine progress toward the achievement of expected outcomes related to weight changes. Relevant data are collected, and actual findings are compared with expected findings. Nursing diagnoses, outcomes, and plans of care are reviewed and revised, as necessary.

Part 4

Taste Alterations

OVERVIEW

I. Definition—an actual or perceived change in taste sensation or loss of taste (Cunningham & Huhmann, 2011)
   A. Hypogeusesthesia—a decrease in the acuity of the taste sensation
   B. Dysgeusia—an unusual taste perception, perceived as unpleasant
   C. Ageusia—an absence of the taste sensation, "mouth blindness"
II. Pathophysiology, cause, and risk factors
   A. Disease related
      1. Excretion of amino acid–like substances from the tumor cells, which changes taste bud sensations (sweet, sour, bitter, salty)
      2. Invasion of tumor into the oral cavity or salivary glands
      3. Oral infections—for example, candidiasis
   B. Treatment related
      1. Specific surgical sites—oral cavity, tongue, salivary glands, pathway of the olfactory nerve, tracheostomy
      2. Radiation induced—changes in salivation production and consistency may precede mucositis or xerostomia
         a. Destruction of the taste buds occurs at minimum doses of 200 to 400 cGy; peaks 3 to 5 weeks after irradiation; may be nonexistent by the third or fourth week, return to baseline 6 to 12 months after treatment, or never return to normal (Haas, 2011; Hong et al., 2009)
         b. Saliva may become thick or tenacious early, and membranes may become dry at about day 10 to 14 during radiation treatment; condition may continue for 2 to 4 months following completion of radiation therapy (RT); beverages or foods, which are slightly tart or carbonated, may help thin secretions
      3. Chemotherapy induced
         a. Certain drugs have greater effect on taste sensation than others—for example, cisplatin (Platinol), ironotecan (Camptosar), cyclophosphamide (Cytoxan), dacarbazine (DTIC-Dome), dactinomycin (actinomycin D, Cosmegen), mechlorethamine (nitrogen mustard, Mustargen), methotrexate (Mexate), vincristine (Oncovin), and fluorouracil (5-FU, 5-fluorouracil) (Camp-Sorrell, 2011)
         b. Taste alterations
            (1) Constant or intermittent metallic and bitter taste
            (2) Increased or decreased threshold for the sweetness sensation, increased threshold for salty and sour tastes, usually decreased threshold for bitter taste
            (3) Aversion to meats, coffee, chocolate
   C. Lifestyle related
      1. Poor oral hygiene
      2. Nutritional deficiencies—zinc, copper, nickel, niacin, vitamin A
   D. Developmental
      1. Age-induced degeneration of the taste buds
      2. Learned aversions
         a. Taste changes or aversions that develop when a food is associated with unpleasant symptoms such as nausea and vomiting and pain
         b. Seem to develop most rapidly to new or novel foods
III. Principles of medical management
   A. Nutritional replacement liquid supplements
   B. Experimentation with different combinations of foods to mask or improve taste
IV. Potential consequences to taste alterations
   A. Anorexia—mainly caused by decreased intake, decreased quality of foods consumed, decreased volume of saliva and gastric secretions, which are necessary for effective digestion to take place
   B. Decreased intake because of food aversion that may persist up to 1 year after therapy
   C. Altered sense of taste, causing many patients to refuse meats, fish, poultry, eggs, tomatoes, and fried foods, which can lead to protein-calorie malnutrition and weight loss

ASSESSMENT

I. History
   A. Presence of hypogeusesthesia, ageusia, or dysgeusia
   B. History of risk factors, including degree and duration of taste alterations
   C. Subjective description of changes in taste and impact of taste alterations on nutritional status and usual lifestyle patterns
II. Physical examination
   A. Oral assessment
      1. Evaluation of oral cavity and throat for presence of erythema, desquamation, dryness or excess saliva, and ulceration
      2. Observing for signs and symptoms of secondary oral infection
   B. Weight
   C. Presence of other physical problems associated with altered intake
III. Laboratory findings associated with compromised nutritional status

A. Decreased levels of albumin, transferrin, and total lymphocytes
B. Decreased levels of zinc, copper, and nickel
C. Decreased levels of niacin and vitamin A

PROBLEM STATEMENTS AND OUTCOME IDENTIFICATION

I. Imbalanced Nutrition: Less than Body Requirements (NANDA-I)
   A. Expected outcome—patient states the goal of interventions related to taste alterations.
   B. Expected outcome—patient describes the personal risk for taste changes.
   C. Expected outcome—patient reports signs and symptoms related to taste alterations to health care team.
   D. Expected outcome—patient uses the appropriate interventions to achieve and maintain optimal nutrition.
   E. Expected outcome—patient uses interventions to minimize the degree, duration, and impact of taste alterations.
II. Impaired Oral Mucous Membranes (NANDA-I)
   A. Expected outcome—patient states the goal of interventions related to taste alterations.
   B. Expected outcome—patient describes the personal risk for changes in taste sensations.
   C. Expected outcome—patient reports signs and symptoms related to alterations in oral mucous membranes to health care team.
   D. Expected outcome—patient uses the appropriate interventions to achieve and maintain optimal nutrition.
   E. Expected outcome—patient uses interventions to minimize the degree and duration of taste alterations.

PLANNING AND IMPLEMENTATION

I. Interventions to minimize risk of occurrence and severity of taste alterations
   A. Instituting measures to increase sensitivity of taste buds
      1. Experimenting with spices and flavorings to enhance taste
      2. Use of the aroma of foods to stimulate taste
      3. Increasing fluid intake with meals
      4. Encouraging oral hygiene before and after meals
      5. Use of amifostine (Ethyol) with RT, as appropriate, to possibly prevent tissue damage and subsequent taste loss caused by RT (Tortorice, 2011)
   B. Instituting nonpharmacologic measures to decrease food aversion
      1. Adding increased sweeteners to foods and marinate meats in sweet juices

2. Substituting other sources of protein for poorly tolerated protein sources such as meats
3. Having patient avoid the sight and smell of foods causing unpleasantness
4. Having patient consume candies such as lemon drops or chew gum to change taste before meals and before chemotherapy treatment to reduce metallic taste and stimulate saliva
   C. Instituting nonpharmacologic measures to increase salivation and compensate for oral dryness
      1. Increasing water or juices at frequent intervals—for example, several times per hour
      2. Spraying water, saline, or artificial saliva on the mucous membranes
      3. Having patient suck on smooth, flat, tart candies or lozenges to stimulate saliva
      4. Having patient avoid alcohol, commercial mouthwashes, and smoking
      5. Humidifying the environmental air
      6. Offering foods that are moist or have gravy or sauces and discouraging intake of dry foods such as toast or crackers
II. Interventions to monitor for complications related to taste alterations
   A. Weighing patient at regular intervals
   B. Maintaining a daily diet record
   C. Teaching patients the importance of diligent oral care and inspection and ensuring that they are aware of conditions for which they should contact the health care team
III. Interventions to incorporate patient and family in care (see Anorexia, Planning and Implementation sections)
IV. Interventions patients may use in addition to or instead of conventional treatments (see Dysphagia, Planning and Implementation sections)

EVALUATION

The oncology nurse systematically and regularly evaluates the patient's and family's responses to taste changes to determine progress toward the achievement of expected outcomes such as improved appetite and improved oral intake. Relevant data are collected, and actual findings are compared with expected findings. Nursing diagnoses, outcomes, and plans of care are reviewed and revised, as necessary.

Anorexia

OVERVIEW

I. Definition—loss of appetite accompanied by decreased oral intake; may be insidious, with progressive weight loss and no other manifestations of disease prompting medical evaluation (Adams et al., 2008)
II. Causes of anorexia

Part 4

A. Physiologic factors (Adams et al 2008; Hopkinson, Wright, & Foster, 2008)
   1. Presence of concurrent symptoms, including nausea or vomiting, early satiety, diarrhea, constipation, pain, dysphagia, mucositis, ascites, alterations in taste or smell
   2. Structural problems such as esophageal of abdominal tumor, structural changes caused by surgery and/or dental involvement
   3. Metabolic disturbances such as hypercalcemia, hypokalemia, uremia, hyponatremia
   4. Medication side effects associated with opioids, antibiotics, and iron
   5. Treatment-related effects from chemotherapy, RT, surgery, and biotherapy
   6. A proinflammatory cytokine environment produced by cancer and its treatment, which contributes to anorexia (Gupta et al., 2011)
B. Psychological factors
   1. Anxiety, depression, fear, distress (Hopkinson et al., 2008)
   2. Loss of pleasure previously associated with food
C. Social factors (Walz, 2010)
   1. Changes in eating environment
   2. Changes in companionship during eating
III. Principles of medical and nursing management
   A. Early detection and ongoing evaluation of nutritional alterations (Adams et al., 2008; Granda-Cameron et al., 2010; Walz, 2010)
   B. Correcting the underlying cause such as uncontrolled pain, mucositis, nausea or vomiting, gastroesophageal reflux
   C. Providing support with nutritional supplementation or replacement
   D. Using nursing interventions to minimize occurrence, severity, and impact on nutritional status
IV. Sequelae of prolonged anorexia
   A. Contributes to decreased calorie and protein intake with subsequent loss of fat and muscle mass, weight loss, weakness, fatigue (Hopkinson et al., 2008)
   B. May lead to cachexia, which may affect prognosis by making patient less tolerant of therapy, causing dose or schedule changes that may diminish treatment effectiveness (Marian & Roberts, 2010; Sauer & Voss, 2012)
   C. Results in abnormalities of carbohydrate, protein, and fat metabolism
   D. Visceral and lean body mass depletion—muscle atrophy, visceral organ atrophy, hypoalbuminemia, anemia (Walz, 2010)
   E. Leads to compromised humoral and cellular immune function—impaired neutrophil function (chemotaxis, fungicidal, bactericidal) and delayed bone marrow production (Walz, 2010)

F. Protein-calorie malnutrition interferes with the delivery of oncologic therapy and increases the severity of side effects of treatment

ASSESSMENT

I. History
   A. Previous dietary patterns, food preferences, eating habits, bowel patterns, and history of anorexia with patient and family
   B. Patterns of anorexia—onset, frequency, severity; associated symptoms—food intolerances, early satiety, nausea, taste abnormalities, mouth or throat pain, dysphagia; other factors—precipitating, aggravating, alleviating factors
   C. Previous self-care strategies
      1. Ability to implement interventions to relieve anorexia
      2. Use of food and nutritional supplements
      3. Use of alternative or complementary nutritional products
   D. Current or recent treatment for cancer and side effects
II. Physical examination
   A. Determination of present weight and amount of total weight loss
   B. Assessment for presence of dehydration, electrolyte imbalances, or both—dry mouth, poor skin turgor, decreased urinary output
   C. Assessment of patient for associated ethnic, socioeconomic, emotional, and motivational factors that may affect the loss of weight or decreased oral intake
   D. Assessment of psychosocial responses to fear, anxiety, stress, depression, and noxious stimuli in the environment

PROBLEM STATEMENTS AND OUTCOME IDENTIFICATION

I. Imbalanced Nutrition: Less than Body Requirements (NANDA-I)
   A. Expected outcome—patient states the personal risk for complications related to loss of appetite and ways in which various cancer therapies may adversely affect nutritional intake.
   B. Expected outcome—patient and family participate in measures to minimize risk of occurrence, severity, and complications of anorexia.
   C. Expected outcome—patient's nutritional intake increases to appropriate calories needed to maintain weight.
   D. Expected outcome—patient demonstrates stable weight or progressive weight gain toward goal with normalization of laboratory values and is free of signs of malnutrition.

E. Expected outcome—patient participates in specific interventions to stimulate appetite or increase dietary intake.

F. Expected outcome—patient states the changes in condition that require professional assistance, intervention, or both.

1. Weight loss of greater than 5% of body weight
2. Dehydration, inability to eat or drink, or both
3. Changes in skin integrity and wound healing
4. Fever over 98.6 ° F (37 ° C), which increases the need for additional calories
5. Development or worsening of symptoms such as fatigue, early satiety, constipation, or nausea

II. Deficient Fluid Volume (NANDA-I)

A. Expected outcome—patient's fluid intake increases to maintain adequate hydration requirements.

B. Expected outcome—patient displays adequate fluid balance, as evidenced by stable vital signs, moist mucous membranes, good skin turgor, prompt capillary refill, and adequate urinary output.

III. Risk for Impaired Skin Integrity (NANDA-I)

A. Expected outcome—patient states the changes in condition that require professional assistance, intervention, or both.

1. Changes in skin integrity or wound healing
2. Fever over 100.5° F (38° C)

IV. Deficient Knowledge, related to personal risk for complications caused by loss of appetite and adverse effects of cancer therapies on nutritional reserves (NANDA-I)

A. Expected outcome—patient will verbalize understanding of condition or disease process and potential complications of anorexia.

B. Expected outcome—patient will identify relationship of signs and symptoms to the disease process and correlate symptoms with causative factors.

C. Expected outcome—patient will initiate necessary lifestyle changes and participate in treatment regimen.

V. Risk for Caregiver Role Strain (NANDA-I)

A. Expected outcome—patient and family state awareness of resources in the community to assist with nutrition.

PLANNING AND IMPLEMENTATION

See Weight Change: Planning and Implementation section.

I. Interventions to monitor complications related to anorexia

A. Maintaining a daily dietary intake record and weighing regularly

B. Assessment for signs and symptoms of electrolyte imbalances and dehydration

C. Assessment of overall skin and nail condition for adverse effects of poor nutrition or intake—skin breakdown, dehiscence, or poor wound healing

II. Interventions to include patient and family in care

A. Encouraging family to provide foods within dietary restrictions and to explore necessity of dietary restrictions when caloric or nutritional requirements are not being met as a result of restrictions (Hopkinson et al., 2008)

B. Teaching family methods to enhance protein-calorie content of foods and methods to enhance food intake

1. Providing a list of high-calorie, high-protein foods
2. Offering suggestions for supplementing nutritional value by adding protein or milk powders and supplements
3. Use of medications, as ordered by licensed provider—pain medications, vitamin supplements, medications that may stimulate appetite (e.g., corticosteroids or megestrol acetate [Megace]) (Adams et al., 2008)
4. Planning mealtimes that are relaxed, unhurried, and pleasant
5. Encouraging a positive eating environment by setting table attractively, listening to music, and avoiding eating from cartons or cans
6. Using a variety of foods to avoid taste fatigue
7. Avoiding fixating on intake to the point that it may become counterproductive

C. Teaching patient and family about the signs and symptoms of dehydration (dry skin and mucous membranes, poor skin turgor, decreased urinary output), delayed wound healing, malnutrition (wasting of skeletal mass, body fat decrease, weight loss, sepsis, reduced energy) and when to report critical symptoms to the treatment team

D. Developing a nurse-patient contract for increasing protein-calorie intake each day

III. Interventions to enhance adaptation and rehabilitation

A. Providing written and audiovisual materials on nutrition at the patient's level of education and understanding

B. Initiating early referral to a dietitian for nutritional assessment or intervention

EVALUATION

The oncology nurse systematically and regularly evaluates the patient's and family's responses to interventions to determine progress toward the achievement of expected outcomes related to anorexia such as weight gain, increase in fluid intake, improvement of fatigue, and understanding of potential complications of anorexia. Relevant data are collected, and actual findings are compared with expected findings. Nursing diagnoses, outcomes, and plans of care are reviewed and revised, as necessary, to minimize anorexia and associated symptoms.

Part 4

Cachexia

OVERVIEW

I. Definition—refers to progressive deterioration with muscle wasting that occurs when protein and calorie requirements are not met; characterized by anorexia, weight loss, skeletal muscle atrophy, and asthenia (Cunningham & Huhmann, 2011; Fearon et al., 2011)

II. Pathophysiology—may be primary or secondary (Harman, 2009)
  A. Primary cachexia—also known as the *anorexia-cachexia syndrome*
    1. Complex process involving anorexia, metabolic alterations, release of cytokines, and other catabolic factors that lead to skeletal muscle wasting (Cunningham & Huhmann, 2011; Harman, 2009)
    2. Appears to be mediated by proinflammatory cytokines, including tumor necrosis factor (TNF), interleukin (IL)-1, IL-6, interferon (IFN)-alpha, and IFN-beta, which may be produced by the tumor itself or by the immune system in response to the tumor (Laviano, Meguid, & Fanelli, 2006)
    3. Metabolic alterations—include decreased gluconeogenesis; alterations in glucose metabolism; increased metabolic rate; and changed lipid, protein, and carbohydrate metabolism
  B. Secondary cachexia—defined as involuntary weight loss and lethargy based on mechanical factors such as obstruction, malabsorption, or treatment-induced toxicities such as nausea and vomiting or alterations in taste (Cunningham & Huhmann, 2011; Suzuki, Asakawa, Amitani, Nakamura, & Inui, 2013)

III. Risk factors
  A. Disease related—cancer, especially lung and pancreatic cancers and gastric carcinomas, acquired immunodeficiency syndrome (AIDS), infections, septic states, inflammatory diseases
  B. Treatment related—chemotherapy; biotherapy; RT; surgery of the head, neck, stomach, pancreas, and bowel
  C. Situation related
    1. Psychological aspects of nutritional intake—cancer cachexia viewed by some to be the hallmark of terminal illness; thus, patients frequently "give up"
    2. Depression, inactivity, absence of an appetite, and functional losses affect the patient's QOL

IV. Principles of medical management
  A. Treatment of the underlying disease
  B. Pharmacologic interventions (Granda-Cameron, et al., 2010; Walz, 2010)
    1. Megestrol acetate (Megace)—has a dose-response effect
    2. Medroxyprogesterone—increases appetite
    3. Corticosteroids—dexamethasone (Decadron) methylprednisolone (Medrol) and prednisolone (Prednisone) are effective in improving appetite
    4. Metoclopramide (Reglan)—at low doses may stimulate gastrointestinal (GI) motility and decrease early satiety and nausea
    5. Metabolic inhibitors—to induce anabolism
    6. Other drugs currently being studied with uncertain efficacy—testosterone, nandrolone decanoate, and oxandrolone (Suzuki et al., 2013)
  C. Total parenteral nutrition (TPN) to replace nutritional deficiencies during cancer treatment and according to patient goals
    1. Enteral feedings—oral or tube feedings will help maintain normal GI flora and prevent atrophy of GI mucosa (Sauer & Voss, 2012)

V. Potential sequelae of cachexia
  A. Increased morbidity and mortality, present in 80% at death (Cunningham & Huhmann, 2011)
  B. Alterations in carbohydrate, protein, and lipid metabolism
  C. Decreased tissue sensitivity to insulin and decreased insulin response to glucose
  D. Impairment of immunocompetence—humoral, cellular, secretory, and mucosal immunity
  E. Poor wound healing and increased infection rates
  F. Protein-calorie malnutrition with resultant weight loss; visceral and somatic protein depletion that compromises enzymatic, structural, and mechanical functions
  G. Constipation caused by lack of food and fluid intake and the effects of cancer treatments

ASSESSMENT

I. History
  A. Previous dietary patterns, food preferences, eating habits, type and quantity of food consumed, history of anorexia discussed with patient and family
  B. Patterns of anorexia and presence of fatigue and malaise—assessment for onset, frequency, severity; associated symptoms—food intolerances, taste abnormalities, pain, dysphagia; other factors—precipitating, aggravating, alleviating factors
  C. Previous self-care strategies—ability to provide for own interventions to relieve anorexia; use of food, nutritional supplements, and other remedies
  D. Current or recent treatment for cancer and side effects experienced

E. Associated cultural, socioeconomic, emotional, and motivational factors that may affect the loss of weight

II. Physical examination

A. Determination of present weight and amount of total and recent weight loss

B. Assessment for presence of dehydration, electrolyte imbalances, or both

C. Assessment for muscle atrophy, loss of fat deposits, and presence of edema

D. Anthropometric measurements or consultation with a nutritionist

1. Triceps skinfolds and mid-arm muscle circumference

2. Height and weight (weight loss >5% in previous 3 months significant for diagnosis of protein-calorie malnutrition)

E. Review of biochemical measurements

1. Visceral protein stores—serum albumin, prealbumin, total iron-binding capacity, transferrin, electrolytes, nitrogen balance (Cunningham & Huhmann, 2011)

2. Lean body mass—computed tomography (CT) or dual energy x-ray absorptiometry (DEXA) (Di Sebastiano & Mourtzakis, 2012)

3. Degree of anemia

4. Deficiencies in trace metals and vitamins, and glucose intolerance

PROBLEM STATEMENTS AND OUTCOME IDENTIFICATION

(See Anorexia, Problem Statement and Outcome Identification section. Problem statements related to cachexia in addition to those listed in Anorexia section are given below.)

I. Adult Failure to Thrive (global decline with weight loss and functional decline)

A. Expected outcome—patient consumes frequent small feedings throughout the day by mouth or by alternative route as tolerated, according to goals.

B. Expected outcome—patient states the personal risk for complications related to cachexia and ways in which various cancer therapies may adversely affect nutritional reserves.

C. Expected outcome—family or significant other participates in measures to minimize risk of occurrence, severity, and complications of cachexia.

D. Expected outcome—patient states the changes in condition that require professional assistance, intervention, or both.

1. Weight loss of greater than 5% of body weight

2. Dehydration

3. Changes in skin integrity and wound healing, and infection

4. Inability to eat or drink

5. Any other area of concern for patient's sense of well-being related to food intake

E. Expected outcome—patient and family state awareness of resources in the community to assist with nutrition and caregiving support.

PLANNING AND IMPLEMENTATION

See Anorexia, Planning and Implementation sections.

EVALUATION

The oncology nurse systematically and regularly evaluates the patient's and family's responses to interventions to determine progress toward the achievement of expected outcomes to minimize risk of cachexia and associated complications. Relevant data are collected, and actual findings are compared with expected findings. Nursing diagnoses, outcomes, and plans of care are reviewed and revised, as necessary.

Nutrition Support Therapy

OVERVIEW

See Bosaeus, 2008; Cunningham & Huhmann, 2011; Fuhrman, 2010; Marian & Roberts, 2010.

I. Nutritional complications

A. Poor nutrition—a common consequence of cancer and its treatments; those with poor nutrition are:

1. Less able to tolerate therapy and receive optimal benefits from treatment

2. More susceptible to infection, debilitation, poor wound healing, skin breakdown, weakness, fatigue, depression, and apathy; poor nutrition affects quality of life

B. Effects of malignant tumors

1. Cancer cells compete with normal cells for nutrients needed for cellular division and growth.

2. Exact demands of the tumor on the host are unknown; the following metabolic changes are proposed:

a. Altered carbohydrate metabolism—glucose is mobilized for energy and results in glucose intolerance in selected patients, causing the following:

(1) Anaerobic glycolysis—produces two adenosine triphosphate (ATP) molecules where complete oxidation of glucose yields 36 ATP molecules; thus anaerobic glycolysis is less efficient; tumors use anaerobic glycolysis

(2) Increased rate of gluconeogenesis—an estimated 10% increase in energy expenditure for an individual with cancer

(3) Glucose intolerance—evidenced by a delayed clearing of intravenous (IV) or oral glucose, which could be caused by lack of tissue response to insulin or a defect of insulin response to hyperglycemia

b. Altered protein metabolism—muscle tissue mobilized to meet increased metabolic demands and results in muscle wasting, especially in those patients with cachexia, a severe syndrome of malnutrition (Marin Caro, Laviano, & Pichard, 2007; Sauer & Voss, 2012)
   (1) Prealbumin and serum albumin levels often used to measure protein status
   (2) Hypoalbuminemia common in patients with cancer—normal albumin level = 4 g/dL; average albumin level in patient with cancer = 2.9 g/dL
   (3) Increased uptake of amino acids by tumor
   (4) Decreased protein synthesis
   (5) Increased protein degradation; muscle protein breakdown is accelerated
   (6) Protein loss by abnormal leakage or exertion, leading to depletion of protein stores and decreased muscle mass
   (7) Use of protein for energy needs (Suzuki et al., 2013)
   (8) In cancer cachexia, protein wasted despite intake of protein, resulting in the following:
      (a) Weight loss that is often difficult to counteract, despite aggressive feeding
         (i) Results in negative nitrogen balance
         (ii) May affect survival and tolerance to treatment
      (b) Decrease in food intake, with partial starvation caused by conserving lean body mass and host depleting own muscle mass to provide amino acids needed
      (c) Loss of appetite, alteration in taste and smell, loss of appealing foods
      (d) Weakness, reduction of strength, decreased functional capacity
c. Fluid and electrolyte disturbances (Cunningham & Huhmann, 2011; Wujcik, 2011)
   (1) Hypercalcemia—high calcium levels in blood caused by certain tumors
   (2) Hyperuricemia—along with hyperphosphatemia and hyperkalemia, this is a result of chemotherapy breakdown of cells in some leukemias and lymphomas, leading to tumor lysis syndrome
   (3) Hyponatremia—common presentation with bronchogenic and small cell carcinoma causing syndrome of inappropriate antidiuretic hormone (SIADH) secretion and causing persistent loss of sodium and excessive retention of water by the kidneys
   (4) Hypokalemia may be caused by treatment with chemotherapy or antifungal therapy.
3. Cancer cells also produce biochemical substances that affect the desire for food, altering taste, causing anorexia (by central mechanisms or neurotransmitters) (Adams et al., 2008).
4. Malignant tumors may invade or compress structures and organs vital to the ingestion, digestion, and elimination of food and fluids or may increase metabolic demands.
   a. Fistula formation
   b. Obstruction
   c. Decubitus
   d. Ulcerations
C. Effects of cancer treatment
1. Structural changes in the GI system may result from surgery and result in the following (Cunningham & Huhmann, 2011):
   a. Inability to feed oneself
   b. Inability to masticate or swallow
   c. Inability to move food through the stomach and bowel
   d. Bowel diversion
   e. Nausea and vomiting
2. Functional changes from surgery, RT, or chemotherapy may result in the following (Cunningham & Huhmann, 2011):
   a. Malabsorption of fat
   b. Gastric hypersecretion of acid
   c. Water and electrolyte loss
   d. Dumping syndrome and changes in gastric motility
   e. Xerostomia
   f. Mucositis
   g. Constipation
   h. Changes in taste and smell
3. Metabolic changes may occur as a result of treatment or side effects of treatment such as increased energy demands that result from fever, stress, diarrhea, vomiting, and cell division or destruction.
II. Nutritional assessment
A. Nutritional screening—should be performed before therapy and at intervals during therapy (Charney & Cranganu, 2010)
1. Extensive nutrition history and dietary habits gathered
2. Anthropometric measurements—height, weight, mid-arm circumference, skinfold thickness, calculation of ideal body weight, body mass index (BMI)
3. Biochemical measurements of protein status— serum albumin (half-life, 20 days), transferrin (half-life, 8 days), prealbumin (half-life, 2 days);

assessing long-term, intermediate-term, and short-term protein status

III. Principles of medical management (Cunningham & Huhmann, 2011; Mattox & Goetz, 2010)

A. Controversies in nutritional support for long-term management in patients with cancer because of the following:

1. Nourishing a patient with cancer may enhance tumor growth by improving its nutrient supply
2. Beneficial effects of nutritional support are temporary

B. Goals of nutritional therapy

1. Determination of calorie and protein needs
2. Increase in weight
3. Maintaining of weight
4. Maintaining fluid and electrolyte balance
5. Improving sense of well-being
6. Prolonging life

C. Selection of type of nutritional therapy (enteral or parenteral) depends on the following:

1. Function of GI tract
2. Severity of nutritional problem
3. Ability of patient to masticate and swallow
4. Length of proposed oncologic therapy and prognosis
5. Community resources for management at home
6. Cost

D. Type of nutritional support (Baldwin, Spiro, Roger, & Emery, 2012; Fuhrman, 2010; Walz, 2010)

1. Increasing normal intake of food or liquids
   a. Five or six small meals per day
   b. High-protein snacks
   c. High-calorie, low-fat snacks
   d. Liquids that have calories, such as nutritional shakes, smoothies, or supplements
   e. Activities to increase appetite—for example, light exercise
   f. Avoiding empty-calorie food that does not offer nutrition
   g. Enteral or parenteral therapy used only if adequate oral intake cannot be maintained

2. Enteral therapy—provision of nutritional replacement through the GI tract through an entry other than the mouth—for example, gastrostomy (button), jejunostomy, or nasogastric (temporary) feeding tube or combination gastrostomy and jejunostomy tube
   a. Indicated if the need for nutritional support is anticipated for more than 1 month and attempts at oral intake have been unsuccessful; at least 30 cm of functioning small bowel required
   b. May require percutaneous endoscopic feeding tube placement

c. Potential complications of enteral tube placement and feedings included in Table 33-1

d. Selection of appropriate formula essential; different ones may need to be tried

   (1) Choice of formula is based on current nutritional requirements, any abnormalities of GI absorption, motility, or diarrhea loss and other coexisting diseases; also considered are laboratory data, amount of protein needed, nitrogen balance and metabolic rate of patient; lactose tolerance or intolerance.

   (2) Polymeric formulas contain nitrogen as a whole protein, carbohydrate is partially hydrolyzed starch, and fat contains long-chain triglycerides; most contain fiber.
      (a) Requires the gut to have some degree of digestive and absorptive capacity

   (3) Predigested formulas contain nitrogen as short peptides or, if elemental formula, proteins are free amino acids; carbohydrates provide much of the energy content and both long-chain and medium-chain triglycerides are present.
      (a) Indicated in presence of significant malabsorption

   (4) Disease-specific formulas are as follows:
      (a) Respiratory failure formulas contain low carbohydrate-to-fat ratio to minimize carbon dioxide production.
      (b) Renal failure formulas contain modified protein, electrolytes, and volume.

3. Maintenance of gut and maintenance of gut ability (including acid balance and luminal microflora) are the first line of defense against invaders into gut

4. Parenteral therapy provides feeding through an IV route when the GI tract cannot be used for nutritional replacement (Bosaeus, 2008; Marin Caro et al., 2007; Fuhrman, 2010)

   a. Parenteral therapy requires placement of a central venous line (CVL) or peripherally inserted central catheter (PICC) line, although peripheral parenteral nutrition (PPN) can be given with a lower glucose concentration.

   b. Infusion is a mixture of amino acids, glucose, fluid, vitamins, minerals, electrolytes, and trace elements. Lipid emulsions can be added to increase calories with smaller volume.

   c. Potential complications of parenteral therapy are presented in Table 33-2.

Part 4

Table 33-1

Potential Complications of Enteral Tube Placement and Feedings

Complication	Nursing Intervention
Nasogastric	
Malpositioned tube	Verify proper placement via chest radiography.
	Check placement each time before using tube.
	Aspirate gastric contents.
	Observe for air bubbles by placing distal end of tube in water.
	Inject air and listen with stethoscope over stomach.
	Tape tube securely to nose.
Aspiration	Give bolus feeding rather than continuous feeding.
	Administer no more than 350-400 mL over 20 minutes every 3 to 4 hr while patient is awake.
	Administer initial volume of 240 mL.
	Keep head of bed elevated by 30 degrees during and 1 hr after infusion.
Contaminated equipment, clogged tube	Change feeding bag and tube daily.
	Flush nasogastric tube with 30 mL of water after each feeding.
	If tube is clogged, flush with hot water or pulsating motions.
Abdominal distention, vomiting, cramping, diarrhea	Regulate infusion accurately over 20 min.
	Give formula at room temperature; you may need to decrease volume of formula given.
	Diarrhea may be caused by formula, lactose intolerance, bacterial contamination, osmolality, antibiotics, or *Clostridium difficile*.
Nasoduodenal	
Aspiration	Risk of occurrence is less because tube is in the small bowel.
	Give continuous rather than bolus feeding.
	Small bowel is sensitive to osmolarity; therefore administer at initial rate of 30-50 mL/hr for isotonic formula and increase by 25 mL/hr every 12 hr until desired volume is reached.
Contaminated equipment	Do not allow amount of formula in bag to exceed that which can be administered in 4 hr.
	Change entire administration set every 24 hr, and rinse with hot water every 8 hr.

Table 33-2

Potential Complications of Parenteral or Nutritional Therapy

Complications	Nursing Intervention
Technical or Mechanical	
Pneumothorax	May occur during insertion of subclavian catheter.
	Observe patient during insertion for chest pain, dyspnea, and cyanosis.
	Perform chest radiography after insertion to verify placement.
	Verify blood return before connecting IV tubing to catheter.
	Pneumothorax may occur during insertion.
Arterial puncture	Observe for bright red blood pulsating from catheter.
	Patient may complain of pain at site.
	Apply pressure to site for 15 min; you may need to apply a sandbag after this.
Malpositioned catheter	Monitor the catheter for migration from the superior vena cava to another vein. Note patient complaint of neck and shoulder pain and swelling in the surrounding area.
	NOTE: If unable to infuse solution through catheter and unable to obtain blood return, treat catheter occlusion according to institutional policy (see Section III of Overview under Vascular Access).
Clotted catheter	Infuse 10% dextrose in water solution peripherally or through other lumen of catheter at the same rate as with total parenteral nutrition (TPN) to prevent hypoglycemia.
Fluid overload	Regulate infusion on a volumetric pump for accuracy.
	Place a time tape on infusion, checking volume infused over each hour.
	Obtain daily weights, monitor input and output.
Air emboli	Secure all IV tubing connections with tape to prevent disconnection.
	If air emboli are suspected, clamp tubing immediately and place patient on left side in the Trendelenburg position.

Continued

Table 33-2

Potential Complications of Parenteral or Nutritional Therapy—cont'd

Complications	Nursing Intervention
Metabolic	
Hyperglycemia	Increase rate of infusion gradually. Check urine for sugar, ketones, and acetone every 6 hr. Monitor serum glucose levels daily.
Hypoglycemia	Administer insulin in TPN, as ordered. Monitor capillary blood glucose, as ordered. Observe for signs and symptoms of hypoglycemia. Monitor serum glucose levels. If sudden cessation of TPN occurs, infuse 10% dextrose in water solution peripherally at same rate as TPN. Per physician's order, administer 50 mL of 50% dextrose intravenously.
Infections	
Contaminated solution	Do not leave solution unrefrigerated for longer than 4 hr. Check each bottle or bag before and during infusion for color and clarity of solution.
Contaminated equipment	Change all IV tubing per institutional or agency procedure, using aseptic technique. Avoid interrupting TPN for other infusions or blood collecting.
Local site infection	Change dressing, using aseptic technique and following institutional procedure. Observe site for redness, tenderness, swelling, and exudates.
Fever	Monitor vital signs every 4 hr. Obtain both peripheral and central line blood cultures to identify source of infection.

ASSESSMENT

I. Nutritional assessment—includes an evaluation of the desire and ability of the patient to ingest and process nutritional products (Charney & Cranganu, 2010; Hopkinson et al., 2008; Walz, 2010)
   A. Ingestion
      1. Desire to eat
      2. Patterns of dietary intake
      3. Ability of patient to prepare food and feed self
      4. Food allergies and preferences
      5. Dentition
      6. Ability of patient to moisten, chew, and swallow nutrients
   B. Digestion
      1. Ability to digest food in stomach and small intestine
      2. Ability to move digested stomach contents through bowel
   C. Metabolism
      1. Presence of abnormal carbohydrate, fat, or protein metabolism
      2. Presence of vitamin and mineral deficiencies
   D. Excretion
      1. Fecal elimination patterns
      2. Urinary elimination patterns
      3. Characteristics of urine and stool
II. Nutritional assessment, including evaluation of the effects of dietary intake on the patient
   A. Physical assessment (Charney & Cranganu, 2010)
      1. Skin turgor
      2. Weight in comparison with ideal body weight
      3. Muscle mass as measured by the mid-arm circumference
      4. Fat stores as measured by triceps skinfold thickness
   B. Evaluation of laboratory data
      1. Serum prealbumin, total protein, and serum transferrin to assess protein stores
      2. Nitrogen balance to assess energy balance
      3. Hemoglobin and hematocrit index
      4. Electrolyte levels

PROBLEM STATEMENTS AND OUTCOME IDENTIFICATION

I. Imbalanced Nutrition: Less than Body Requirements (NANDA-I)
   A. Expected outcome—patient achieves adequate nutritional status according to individual goals.
   B. Expected outcome—patient demonstrates stable weight or progressive weight gain and is free of signs of malnutrition.
   C. Expected outcome—patient verbalizes individual interferences to adequate intake.
   D. Expected outcome—patient participates in specific interventions to stimulate appetite and increase dietary intake.
II. Risk for Infection (NANDA-I)
   A. Expected outcome—patient remains free of infection or infection is recognized early and promptly treated.

B. Expected outcome—patient will identify and participate in interventions to prevent and/or reduce risk of infection.

III. Diarrhea (NANDA-I)

A. Expected outcome—patient does not experience diarrhea during enteral feedings.

B. Expected outcome—patient will maintain usual bowel movement consistency or pattern.

IV. Risk for Aspiration (NANDA-I)

A. Expected outcome—patient maintains patent airway and does not aspirate tube feedings.

B. Expected outcome—patient is free of gastric contents in lung secretions.

V. Deficient Knowledge (NANDA-I), related to nutritional support therapy

A. Expected outcome—patient and family discuss rationale for nutritional support therapy.

B. Expected outcome—patient and family demonstrate necessary skills to manage nutritional support therapy.

C. Expected outcome—patient and family list signs and symptoms of complications of nutritional support therapy to report to the health care team.

PLANNING AND IMPLEMENTATION

I. Interventions to maximize patient safety ⚠

A. Administration of nutritional therapy, according to institutional protocol

B. Examination of nutritional supplement for abnormalities in color

C. Checking expiration date on nutritional supplement

D. Confirming placement of feeding tube or catheter before administering nutritional supplement.

II. Interventions to monitor for complications of nutritional therapy

A. Infection—fever and redness; swelling, pus, pain along feeding tube, catheter tract, or exit site

B. Respiratory complications—chest pain, dyspnea, cough, cyanosis

C. Fluid overload—weight gain, edema, shortness of breath, distended neck veins

D. Hyperglycemia—blood glucose monitoring every 6 hours, pattern of urinary elimination

E. GI—character of stool, bloating, pattern of fecal elimination

F. Electrolyte abnormalities—changes in mental status, weakness, fatigue, changes in neurologic examination (restlessness, agitation)

III. Interventions to decrease the incidence and severity of complications of nutritional support therapy (see Tables 33-1 and 33-2)

IV. Interventions to include patient and family in care

A. Teaching patient and family procedures needed to manage the feeding tube or catheter

B. Teaching patient and family about signs and symptoms of complications of nutritional support therapy

C. Encouraging participation of patient and family in decision making about nutritional therapy

EVALUATION

The oncology nurse systematically and regularly evaluates the patient's and family's responses to interventions to determine progress toward maintenance of adequate nutrition and weight. Relevant data are collected, and actual findings are compared with expected findings. Nursing diagnoses, outcomes, and plans of care are reviewed and revised, as necessary.

References

Adams, L., Shepard, N., Caruso, R., Norlling, M., Belansky, H., & Cunningham, R. (2008). Putting evidence into practice: Evidence-based interventions to prevent and manage anorexia. *Clinical Journal of Oncology Nursing, 13*(1), 95–102.

Baldwin, C., Spiro, A., Roger, A., & Emery, P. W. (2012). Oral nutritional interventions in malnourished patients with cancer: A systematic review and meta-analysis. *Journal of the National Cancer Institute, 104*, 1–15. http://dx.doi.org/10.1093/jnci/djr556.

Bosaeus, I. (2008). Nutritional support in multimodal therapy in cancer cachexia. *Supportive Care in Cancer, 16*, 447–451. http://dx.doi.org/10.107/s00520-007-0388-7.

Camp-Sorrell, D. (2011). Chemotherapy toxicities and management. In C. H. Yarbro, D. Wujcik, & B. H. Gobel (Eds.), *Cancer nursing: Principles and practice* (pp. 458–503). Sudbury, MA: Jones and Bartlett.

Charney, P., & Cranganu, A. (2010). Nutrition screening and assessment in oncology. In M. Marian & S. Roberts (Eds.), *Clinical nutrition for oncology patients* (pp. 21–44). Sudbury, MA: Jones and Bartlett.

Cunningham, R. S., & Huhmann, M. B. (2011). Nutritional disturbances. In C. H. Yarbro, D. Wujcik, & B. H. Gobel (Eds.), *Cancer nursing: Principles and practice* (pp. 818–844). Sudbury, MA: Jones and Bartlett.

Di Sebastiano, K. M., & Mourtzakis, M. (2012). A critical evaluation of body composition modalities used to assess adipose and skeletal muscle tissue in cancer. *Applied Physiology Nutrition and Metabolism, 37*(5), 811–821.

Fearon, K., Strasser, F., Anker, S. D., Bosaeus, I., Bruera, E., Fainsinger, R. L., et al. (2011). Definition and classification of cancer cachexia: An international consensus. *Lancet Oncology, 12*, 489–495. http://dx.doi.org/10.1016/51470-2045 (10)70218-7.

Fuhrman, M. P. (2010). Nutrition support for oncology patients. In M. Marian, & S. Roberts (Eds.), *Clinical nutrition for oncology patients* (pp. 45–63). Sudbury, MA: Jones and Bartlett.

Granda-Cameron, C., DeMille, D., Lynch, M. P., Huntzinger, C., Alcorn, T., Levicoff, J., et al. (2010). An interdisciplinary approach to manage cancer cachexia. *Clinical Journal of Oncology Nursing, 14*(1), 72–81. http://dx.doi.org/10.1188/10.CJON.72-80.

Gupta, S. C., Kim, J. H., Kannappan, R., Reuter, S., Doughert, P., & Aggarwal, B. (2011). Role of nuclear factor kB-mediated inflammatory pathways in cancer-related symptoms and their regulation by nutritional agents. *Experimental Biology and Medicine, 236*(6), 658–671.

Haas, M. L. (2011). Radiation therapy: Toxicities and management. In C. H. Yarbro, D. Wujcik, & B. H. Gobel (Eds.), *Cancer nursing: Principles and practice* (pp. 312–351). Sudbury, MA: Jones and Bartlett.

Harman, S. M. (2009). *Primary anorexia-cachexia syndrome in cancer patients.* http://www.healio.com/.

Hong, J. H., Omur-Ozbek, P., Stanek, B. T., Dietrich, A. M., Duncan, S. E., Lee, Y. W., et al. (2009). Taste and odor abnormalities in cancer patients. *Journal of Supportive Oncology, 7*(2), 58–65.

Hopkinson, J. B., Wright, D. N. M., & Foster, C. (2008). Management of weight loss and anorexia. *Annals of Oncology, 19*(Suppl. 7), vii289–vii293. http://dx.doi.org/10.1093/annonc/mdn452.

Laviano, A., Meguid, M. M., & Fanelli, F. R. (2006). Anorexia. In G. Montovani, S. D. Anker, & A. Inui (Eds.), *Cachexia and wasting: A modern approach* (pp. 139–148). Milan, Italy: Springer-Verlag Italia.

Marian, M., & Roberts, S. (2010). Introduction to the nutritional management of oncology patients. In M. Marian, & S. Roberts (Eds.), *Clinical nutrition for oncology patients* (pp. 1–20). Sudbury, MA: Jones and Bartlett.

Marin Caro, M. M., Laviano, A., & Pichard, C. (2007). Nutritional intervention and quality of life in adult oncology patients. *Journal of Clinical Nutrition, 26,* 289–301. http://dx.doi.org/10.1016/j.clnu.2007.01.005.

Mattox, T. W., & Goetz, D. E. (2010). Pharmacologic management of cancer cachexia-anorexia and other gastrointestinal toxicities associated with cancer treatments. In M. Marian, & S. Roberts (Eds.), *Clinical nutrition for oncology patients* (pp. 379–408). Sudbury, MA: Jones and Bartlett.

Sauer, A. C., & Voss, A. C. (2012). *Improving outcomes with nutrition in patients with cancer.* www.onsedge.com.

Suzuki, H., Asakawa, A., Amitani, H., Nakamura, N., & Inui, A. (2013). Cancer cachexia-pathophysiology and management. *Journal of Gastroenterology.* http://dx.doi.org/10.1007/s00535-013-0787-0, Epub.

Tortorice, P. V. (2011). Cytotoxic chemotherapy: Principles of therapy. In C. H. Yarbro, D. Wujcik, & B. H. Gobel (Eds.), *Cancer nursing: Principles and practice* (pp. 352–389). Sudbury, MA: Jones and Bartlett.

Walz, D. A. (2010). Cancer-related anorexia-cachexia syndrome. *Clinical Journal of Oncology Nursing, 14*(3), 283–287. http://dx.doi.org/10.1188/10.CJON.283-287.

Wujcik, D. (2011). Targeted therapy. In C. H. Yarbro, D. Wujcik, & B. H. Gobel (Eds.), *Cancer nursing: Principles and practice* (pp. 561–583). Sudbury, MA: Jones and Bartlett.

Part 4

CHAPTER 34

Comfort

Jeannine M. Brant, Amy Walton, and Lisa Dyk

Pain

OVERVIEW

I. Definition
   A. A sensory and emotional experience associated with actual or potential tissue damage or described in terms of such damage (International Association for the Study of Pain [IASP], 2012)
   B. Pain—defined as whatever the person says it is, existing whenever he or she says it does (McCaffery & Pasero, 1999)

II. Characteristics of pain (Brant, 2014)
   A. Acute pain—typically lasts less than 6 months; cause often known; pain behaviors more frequently exhibited
   B. Chronic pain—typically lasts longer than 3 months; cause of the pain often unknown with nonmalignant chronic pain; fatigue and depression common
   C. Cancer pain—includes acute and chronic cancer-related pain associated with direct tumor involvement, diagnostic or therapeutic procedures, or cancer treatment
      1. Pain may trigger fear of cancer progression or recurrence.
      2. Pain worsens anxiety, hopelessness, and depression.

III. Types of pain (Brant, 2014)
   A. Nociceptive pain—results from activation of nociceptors (pain fibers) in deep and cutaneous tissues
      1. Somatic pain—arises from the bone, joint, or connective tissue; described as sharp, throbbing, or pressure; well localized
      2. Visceral pain—results from nociceptor activation secondary to distention, compression, or infiltration of the thoracic or abdominal tissue (e.g., pancreas, liver, gastrointestinal [GI] tract); characterized by a diffuse, aching or cramping sensation; poorly localized

   B. Neuropathic pain—results from compression, inflammation, infiltration, ischemia, or injury to the peripheral, sympathetic, or central nervous system (CNS) (Bennett et al., 2012; IASP, 2012; Lema, Foley, & Hausheer, 2010)
      1. Peripheral neuropathic pain—caused by peripheral nerve injury, often characterized by a numbness and tingling sensation
      2. Centrally mediated pain—characterized by radiating and shooting sensations with a background of burning and aching
      3. Sympathetically maintained pain—centrally generated, caused by autonomic dysregulation; complex regional pain syndrome (CRPS)

IV. Physiology (Figure 34-1) (Brant, 2014)
   A. Transduction
      1. Initiated by a mechanical, thermal, or chemical noxious stimulus that sensitizes nociceptors (receptors sensitive to noxious stimuli)
      2. Neurotransmitters released at the time of injury include prostaglandins (PGs), bradykinin (BK), serotonin (5-HT), substance P (SP), and histamine (H), which initiate an inflammatory response
      3. An action potential or depolarization is generated along the neuron; sodium moves into the cell, potassium out of the cell; pain message begins its way to the CNS
   B. Transmission
      1. Action potential continues to the dorsal horn, where nociceptors terminate.
      2. Neurotransmitters and excitatory substances that inhibit presynaptic and postsynaptic nociceptive transmission are released in the spinal cord.
      3. Neurons continue to relay the message to the thalamus and other centers in the brain.
      4. The thalamus transmits the message to the cerebral cortex.
   C. Perception—the cerebral cortex processes the experience of pain and responds to the noxious

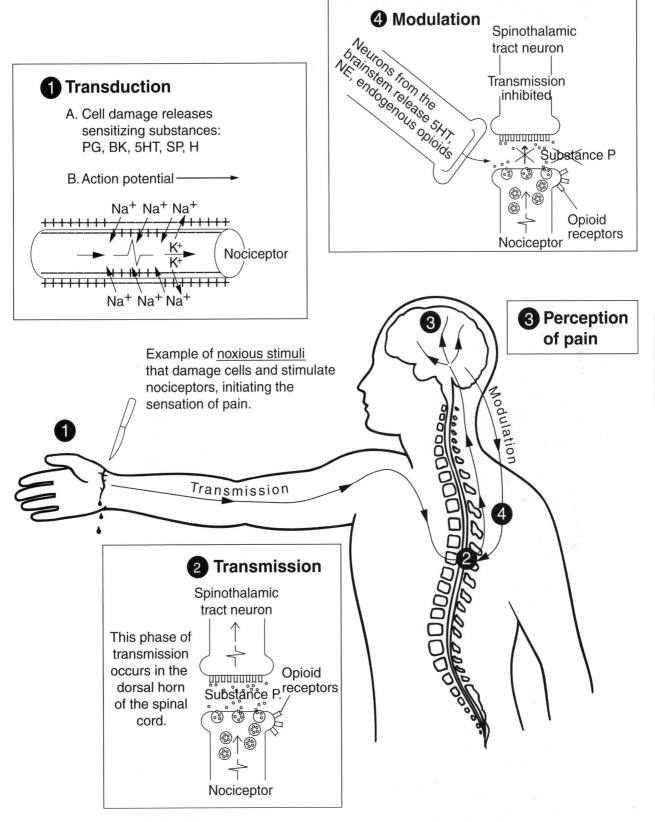

Figure 34-1 Physiology of pain. *5-HT*, Serotonin; *BK*, bradykinin; *H*, histamine; *NE*, norepinephrine; *PG*, prostaglandin; *SP*, substance P. *From McCaffery, M., & Pasero, C. (1999). Pain: Clinical manual (2nd ed.). St. Louis, MO: Mosby.*

stimuli to reduce pain perception via descending modulating mechanisms

D. Modulation
  1. Neurons in the brainstem (pons and medulla) descend to the dorsal horn and release neuromediators—endogenous opioids, norepinephrine, serotonin.
  2. Neuromediators inhibit the transmission of pain impulses at the dorsal horn.
  3. Opioids work at the dorsal horn by binding to receptors and preventing transmission of the pain signal to the higher brain centers.
V. Risk factors
  A. Disease-related factors
    1. Type of cancer (Brant, 2014)
      a. Head and neck cancer most common (70%)
      b. Gynecologic malignancies (60%)
      c. GI malignancy (59%)
    2. Bone metastases—most common source of cancer pain (Maccauro et al., 2011)
      a. Greatest incidence of bone metastases in breast, prostate, and lung cancers and multiple myeloma
      b. Bone destruction or compression of the bone on nerves and soft tissue
    3. Visceral pain—caused by tumor obstruction of the bowel, liver metastasis, blood flow occlusion to visceral organs, malignant ascites, and other causes
    4. Nerve compression or injury to peripheral, sympathetic, and central nervous systems (Maccauro et al., 2011).
      a. Spinal cord compression
      b. Plexopathies—pain is often a first sign followed by extremity weakness and sensory loss; characterized by shooting pain
      c. Peripheral neuropathies—characterized by painful numbness, tingling, weakness, sensory loss
  B. Treatment-related factors
    1. Chemotherapy-related pain
      a. Mucositis—antimetabolites, alkylating agents, anthracyclines, platinum-based chemotherapy, taxanes, and some targeted therapies (epidermal growth factor receptor [EGFR]) known to cause severe mucositis, as well as combination chemotherapy and high-dose regimens (Epstein et al., 2012)
      b. Peripheral neuropathies
        (1) Platinum compounds, vinca alkaloids, taxanes, thalidomide, and bortezomib—have the highest incidence of peripheral neuropathy (Beijers, Jongen, & Vreugdenhil, 2012)
        (2) Characterized by burning, numbness, tingling of hands and feet
      c. Herpetic neuralgia
        (1) Characterized by burning, aching, and shock like pain in the area of the lesions
        (2) Often results from immunosuppression from chemotherapy; topical agents such as lidocaine patch or gel and long-acting gabapentin are indicated for postherpetic neuralgia (Brant, 2010)
    2. Radiation therapy–related pain
      a. Mucositis—often occurs with radiation therapy to the head and neck but may occur anywhere along the GI tract
        (1) Usually manifests 2 to 3 weeks after the initiation of treatment (Epstein et al., 2012)
      b. Radiation skin changes—radiation dermatitis and radiation recall (Burris & Hurtig, 2010; Ryan, 2012)
    3. Chronic pain related to cancer surgery (Brant, 2011)
      a. Postmastectomy
        (1) Characterized by tightness in axilla, upper arm, chest
        (2) Often exacerbated with movement, extending, reaching, lifting, pulling, pushing; believed to be caused by intercostobrachial nerve damage
      b. Post-thoracotomy
        (1) Characterized by aching, numbness, and burning in the incisional area
        (2) Believed to be caused by intercostal nerve damage (occurs in up to 80% of patients in the first few months after surgery)
      c. Postsurgical head and neck cancer pain
        (1) Characterized by tightness, burning, shocklike pain
        (2) Thought to be caused by injury to the accessory and superficial cervical plexus, followed by denervation and atrophy of the trapezius muscle, subsequent downward and lateral scapula displacement, and thus shoulder dysfunction and pain
      d. Postnephrectomy—characterized by flank, groin, or abdominal heaviness or numbness
      e. Post–limb amputation—characterized by phantom or stump pain; may be neuropathic in nature
      f. Lymphedema—characterized as arm and shoulder fullness, heaviness, or tightness
        (1) May result from any cancer surgery that affects the lymphatic system (most commonly associated with breast cancer)
  C. Personal and psychosocial factors (Brant, 2014)
    1. Patient-related factors
      a. Reluctance to take opioid drugs for fear and misunderstanding of the terms *analgesic tolerance* and *addiction*

b. Fear that pain may be a sign of progressive disease; denial prevents patient from taking adequate analgesia

c. Desire to be a "good patient"

2. Provider-related factors

a. Misunderstanding of addiction, analgesic tolerance, physical dependence

b. Reluctance to prescribe—fear of recrimination by regulatory agencies

c. Suboptimal training in pain assessment and management

3. Age—older adults at higher risk for chronic pain and inadequate management

4. Culture—influences the perceptions and expression of pain

ASSESSMENT

See Brant, 2014; National Comprehensive Cancer Network [NCCN], 2013.

I. Special populations

A. Older adult population (Curtiss, 2010)

1. A comprehensive history of pharmacologic and supplemental medications

a. Many older adult patients taking numerous medications

b. Higher risk for polypharmacy interaction in populations older than 70 years taking five or more medications

2. Increased sensitivity to analgesics in many older adults

a. It is necessary to start with lower doses and titrate slowly.

b. Advanced age causes prolonged half-life and metabolism of the drug.

3. Appropriateness of pain screening scale

a. May need to use a nonverbal pain assessment tool if the patient cannot verbally report pain

4. Assessment for the presence of confusion and poor vision

5. Availability of home supervision

6. Cost to be considered when planning analgesics for older adults

B. Pediatric population (Chauhan, Weiss, & Warrier, 2010)

1. Assessment of pediatric population according to developmental age

2. Developmentally appropriate pain scale to be chosen

a. Pain faces are usually used in children ages 7 years and younger.

b. The 0 to 10 scale may be used for school-age and older children.

c. The Face, Legs, Activity, Cry, Consolability scale (FLACC) is used for children who cannot verbalize pain

(Merkel, Voepel-Lewis, Shayevitz & Malviya, 1997).

3. Starting dosage should be calculated according to weight.

II. Clinical pain assessment (Brant, 2012, 2014; Irwin, Brant, & Eaton, 2011) (Table 34-1)

A. Physical dimension

B. Psychological dimension

C. Social dimension

D. Spiritual or existential dimension

Table 34-1	
Pain: Assessment Parameters	
Domain	**Pain Assessment Components**

Physical	• **Onset:** When did the pain begin?
	• **Location:** Where is the pain located?
	• **Duration:** How long does the pain last? Is the pain constant or intermittent?
	• **Characteristics:** How would you describe the pain? (assists in diagnosis of the pain syndrome)
	  • Somatic pain—well-localized, constant, dull, aching, gnawing
	  • Visceral pain—poorly localized or referred, may come in waves, cramping, stretching
	  • Neuropathic pain—emanating from peripheral or central nervous system, burning, numb, radiating, shocklike
	• **Aggravating factors:** What makes the pain worse?
	  • Movement
	  • Activity
	  • Positioning
	• **Relieving factors:** What makes the pain better?
	  • Analgesics
	  • Positioning
	• **Treatment:** What treatments have you tried to control the pain?

Psychological	• History of anxiety, depression, or other psychological illness • Cognition, including confusion or delirium • Usual coping strategies • Psychological responses to pain and illness such as depression, anxiety, and fear
Social	• Interference of pain with activities of daily living, including physical or social withdrawal from activity • Family communication and response to illness • Support system
Spiritual, existential	• Presence of a spiritual community and its role related to pain and illness • Spiritual beliefs related to pain and illness • Influence of religion or spirituality on coping with pain

From Brant, J. M. (2012). Strategies to manage pain in palliative care. In M. O'Connor, S. Lee & S. Aranda. (Eds.). *Palliative care nursing: A guide to practice* (3rd ed., pp. 93-113). Victoria, Australia: Ausmed.

III. History and physical examination (NCCN, 2013)
   A. Medical history (current and prior oncologic treatment [chemotherapy, radiation therapy [RT], surgery], other significant comorbidities, pre-existing chronic pain)
   B. Evaluation of imaging studies (e.g., computed tomography [CT], magnetic resonance imaging [MRI], bone scan) and laboratory values (tumor markers)
   C. Physical and neurologic examination—assessment of pain behaviors (physical limitations, guarding), changes in muscle tone, loss of deep tendon reflexes
   D. Assessment for alterations in the following systems:
      1. Respiratory status—decreased rate and volume, increased carbon dioxide levels
      2. CNS changes—sedation or lethargy, euphoria, coordination, mood
      3. Cardiovascular system—hypotension
      4. GI system—constipation, bowel obstruction, inability to evacuate stool, nausea
      5. Genitourinary system—urinary retention, difficult urination
      6. Dermatologic system—diaphoresis, facial flushing, pruritus

IV. Evaluation and reassessment of pain (NCCN, 2013)
   A. Assessment or screening of each patient for pain at each contact (on admission to the hospital, during each home visit, or at outpatient clinic visits)
   B. Comprehensive pain assessment with each new report of pain
   C. Pain reassessed after appropriate intervals following pain interventions (e.g., evaluation of an oral medication should be approximately 1 hour after administration)
   D. Assessment of pain as the fifth vital sign

PROBLEM STATEMENTS AND OUTCOME IDENTIFICATION

I. Acute Pain or Chronic Pain (NANDA-I)
   A. Expected outcome—patient recognizes importance of preventing and controlling pain and reports pain intensity or temporality using standardized measures.
   B. Expected outcome—patient states that the pain is satisfactorily reduced or relieved.

II. Deficient Knowledge (NANDA-I), related to self-care and use of effective pain management strategies
   A. Expected outcome—patient verbalizes and uses appropriate pharmacologic and complementary interventions to control pain.

III. Social Isolation (NANDA-I)
   A. Expected outcome—patient participates in activities of daily living (ADLs) and collaborates with support network (family, friends, and spiritual leaders) to limit social isolation.

IV. Risk for Constipation (NANDA-I)
   A. Expected outcome—patient verbalizes need for or demonstrates use of stool softener and bowel stimulant while concurrently taking opioids to maintain normal GI motility.

PLANNING AND IMPLEMENTATION

I. Pharmacologic and nonpharmacologic management (NCCN, 2013)
   A. Treating the underlying cause of pain
   B. Tailoring pain management care according to the patient's individualized pain assessment
      1. Administering long-acting analgesics around the clock when pain is constant
      2. Distinguishing and managing breakthrough pain (Mercadante, 2011)
         a. Breakthrough pain (BTP)—a flare in the pain pattern that occurs in conjunction with persistent pain
            (1) Oral opioids—10% to 20% of the 24-hour dose
            (2) Parenteral opioids—25% to 50% of the hourly infusion rate; may be higher for incident pain that is predominant
         b. Incident pain—transient pain precipitated by any movement or activity
            (1) Analgesics at appropriate intervals to allow analgesics to work before anticipated pain-inducing activities
            (2) Use of BTP analgesics with a rapid onset; consider transmucosal fentanyl, immediate-release opioids, or subcutaneous or intravenous (IV) patient-controlled analgesia
         c. End-of-dose pain—pain that increases before the next scheduled dose, may be managed by increasing the opioid dose or frequency
      3. Use of equianalgesic conversion tables to guide opioid conversion
      4. Starting with least invasive route of administration (oral preferred, transdermal); change of routes or rotation of opioids if intolerable side effects or intractable pain occurs despite escalating doses
      5. Implementing strategies to minimize side effects of analgesic therapy: bowel regimen that includes stool softener and stimulant, antiemetics, H_2 antagonists, CNS stimulants to counteract sedation
   C. Pharmacologic pain management—use of the World Health Organization (WHO) analgesic ladder to manage pain (Figure 34-2) (Brant, 2012; NCCN, 2013; World Health Organization [WHO], 2012) (see Chapter 25)

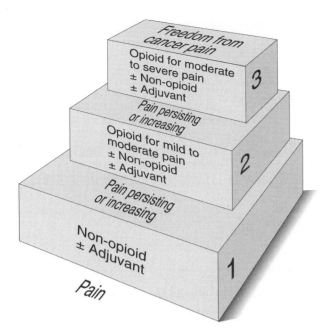

Figure 34-2 The World Health Organization (WHO) three-step analgesic ladder. *From World Health Organization. (1996). Cancer pain relief (2nd ed.). Geneva: WHO.*

1. Step 1—non opioid analgesics
   a. Used for mild pain or as adjuvants with opioid medications
   b. Examples—acetaminophen (Tylenol), acetylsalicylic acid (aspirin and ASA), nonsteroidal anti-inflammatory drugs (NSAIDs)
2. Step 2—opioid analgesics
   a. Use of opioids for mild to moderate pain or if pain persists or increases from step 1 of the WHO ladder
   b. Examples—hydrocodone and oxycodone in fixed combinations with acetaminophen or aspirin
   c. Opioids with acetaminophen combinations—have a ceiling dose; acetaminophen should not exceed 4000 mg in 24 hours and patients should not take more than 3000 mg in 24 hours unless recommended by a health care provider
   d. Use of mixed agonist-antagonists drugs (e.g., butorphanol [Stadol], pentazocin [Talwin]) to be avoided; converting from an opioid agonist to an agonist-antagonist could trigger a withdrawal crisis when given to a patient who has developed physical dependence on a pure opioid agonist
3. Step 3—opioid analgesics (Brant, 2010)
   a. For severe pain or if pain persists or increases from step 2 of the ladder
   b. Used most frequently in managing cancer related pain (e.g., morphine, oxycodone, hydromorphone, fentanyl)
      (1) To be avoided or used with caution in patients with renal impairment because of potential M3G and M6G metabolite accumulation, which may cause oversedation, respiratory depression, myoclonus
      (2) Meperidine to be avoided because the metabolite normeperidine may accumulate and cause CNS toxicity or cardiac arrhythmias
4. Analgesic adjuvant—used on each step of the WHO ladder to enhance analgesia, relieve concurrent symptoms that exacerbate pain, and relieve side effects associated with opioids (Table 34-2)
5. Miscellaneous interventions
   a. Pharmaceuticals for bone metastases
      (1) Radionuclides such as strontium-89 and samarium-153 for pain relief in disseminated metastatic bone cancer (Roqué I Figuls, Martinez-Zapata, Scott Brown, & Alonso-Coello, 2011)
      (2) Bisphosphonates (e.g., pamidronate, zoledronic acid) for relief of pain of osteolytic bone metastases (Loftus, Edwards-Bennett, & Sokol, 2012)
6. Intraspinal analgesia (Deer et al., 2011; Hayek, Deer, Pope, Panchal, & Patel, 2011; Lawson & Wallace, 2010)—can provide pain relief using lower doses of analgesics, thus limiting severity and toxicity of side effects; first-line agents include morphine, hydromorphone, bupivacaine
   a. Epidural
      (1) Approximately 10% of IV dose
      (2) Recommended for postsurgical pain following gynecologic surgery and other surgeries that cause pain at the waist level or below (Irwin et al., 2011)
      (3) Tunneled epidural analgesia—used to manage pain at the end of life when life expectancy is limited and an implantable pump is not feasible; catheter is tunneled from the spinal area around the waist and is attached to a pump that can deliver continuous infusion and optional bolus dose
   b. Intrathecal implantable pump
      (1) Approximately 10% of epidural dose
      (2) Used to manage intractable cancer pain, often toward the end of life
      (3) Patient selection

Part 4

Table 34-2

Adjuvant Analgesics

Drug Classifications	Indications	Side Effects
Acetaminophen (Tylenol)	Mild to moderate pain, fever	Hepatotoxicity, increased risk with alcohol consumption, liver failure Maximum recommended dose: 3000 mg/day or less or 4000 mg/day as recommended by a health care provider
Alpha$_2$-adrenergic agonist—clonidine hydrochloride (Catapres)	Epidural analgesia for neuropathic pain, postsurgical pain	Hypotension, bradycardia, central nervous system, depression, dry mouth
CNS Stimulants Caffeine Dextroamphetamine (Dexedrine) Methylphenidate (Ritalin) Modafinil (Provigil) Atomoxetine (Strattera)	Counteract psychomotor retardation; reduce sedation side effects of opioids	Nervousness, sleep disorder hypertension, palpitations, anxiety
Anticonvulsants Gabapentin (Neurontin) Pregabalin (Lyrica) Phenytoin (Dilantin) Carbamazepine (Tegretol) Lamotrigine (Lamictal) Topiramate (Topamax) Divalproex sodium (Depakote) Levetiracetam (Keppra) Zonisamide (Zonergran)	Neuropathic pain, trigeminal neuralgia, postherpetic neuralgia, brachial and lumbosacral plexopathies, chemoimmunotherapy-related neuropathies	Sedation, dizziness, ataxia, fatigue, bone marrow depression, nausea, rash, impaired concentration, edema
Tricyclic Antidepressants (TCAs) Amitriptyline (Elavil) Desipramine (Norpramin) Nortriptyline (Pamelor) **Selective Norepinephrine Reuptake Inhibitors** Venlafaxine (Effexor) Duloxetine (Cymbalta)	Neuropathic pain, postherpetic neuralgia, postsurgical neuropathies, chemoimmunotherapy-related neuropathies	Dry mouth, sedation, constipation, agitation, delirium, tachycardia, orthostatic hypotension, worsening of cardiac conduction abnormalities; more side effects with TCAs
Antispasmodic Baclofen (Lioresal)	Spastic pain, centrally mediated pain from spinal lesions	Drowsiness, slurred speech, hypotension, constipation, urinary retention
Benzodiazepines Alprazolam (Xanax) Clonazepam (Klonopin) Diazepam (Valium) Lorazepam (Ativan)	Anxiety associated with pain, panic attack, muscle spasm, procedure-related pain	Sedation, dementia, delirium, motor incoordination, hypotension, dizziness, respiratory depression
Corticosteroids Dexamethasone (Decadron) Methylprednisolone (Solu-Medrol)	Nerve compression (brachial and lumbosacral plexopathies), lymphedema and visceral distention, increased intracranial pressure	Euphoria, increased appetite, hyperglycemia, weight gain, Cushing syndrome, osteoporosis, psychosis, gastrointestinal (GI) bleeding, gastritis
Local Anesthetics Lidocaine, intravenous (IV) Lidocaine patch (Lidoderm) Mexiletine (Mexitil) Capsaicin cream (Zostrix) EMLA (eutectic mixture of local anesthetics) cream	Lidocaine for postherpetic neuralgia, peripheral neuropathy, postsurgical neuropathies EMLA cream for topical dermal anesthesia	Lidocaine patch may cause a mild rash at the application site
Muscle Relaxants Cyclobenzaprine (Flexeril) Carisoprodol (Soma)	Should be used short term for musculoskeletal pain, tetanus	Sedation, light-headedness, blurred vision, hypotension, akathisia

Continued

Table 34-2

Adjuvant Analgesics—cont'd

Drug Classifications	Indications	Side Effects
Metaxalone (Skelaxin) Methocarbamol (Robaxin) Tizanidine (Zanaflex)	Tizanidine may be used for longer periods of time; used for headache or neuropathic pain	
N-Methyl-D-Aspartate (NMDA) Antagonists		
Dextromethorphan with morphine (Morphidex) Ketamine Amantadine (Symmetrel) Memantine (Namenda)	Neuropathic pain, synergistic with opioids; may be helpful in preventing tolerance to opioids *Note:* Methadone also has NMDA activity	Psychotomimetic side effects, hallucinations, drowsiness
Nonsteroidal Anti-inflammatory Drugs (NSAIDs) **Selective Cyclooxygenase 2 (COX-2)** **Inhibitors** Celecoxib (Celebrex) **Nonselective COX Inhibitors** Ibuprofen (Advil, Motrin, Nuprin) Indomethacin (Indocin) Ketorolac (Toradol) Flurbiprofen (Ansaid) Diflunisal (Dolobid) Naproxen (Naprosyn, Aleve, Anaprox) Fenoprofen (Nalfon) Ketoprofen (Orudis, Actron) Choline magnesium trisalicylate (Trilisate) Sulindac (Clinoril)	Bone metastases, soft tissue infiltration, tumor, fever, inflammation	COX-1 inhibitors—may cause inhibition of platelet aggregation, gastric ulceration, renal toxicity, confusion in older adults COX-2 NSAIDs—more selective and cause fewer GI side effects

Adapted from American Pain Society. (2008). *Principles of analgesic use in the treatment of acute pain and cancer pain* (6th ed.). Glenview, IL: APS Press.

(a) Pain unrelieved by less invasive measures

(b) Successful intrathecal trial prior to pump implantation

(c) Patient factors such as proximity to medical care for pump care, home health or hospice with expertise in intrathecal delivery, and patient support systems

(d) Availability of an expert pain management team to implant pump, refill, and reprogram the device as needed

(e) Economic factors such as health insurance coverage of implantation and care; life expectancy of at least 3 to 6 months for cost of implantation to outweigh costs for alternative option of tunneled epidural catheter

7. RT—may alleviate painful bone metastases and reduce large localized bulky tumors (Yu, Tsai, & Hoffe, 2012)

8. Interventional or surgical strategies (NCCN, 2013)

a. Nerve blocks for well-localized pain syndromes

(1) Head and neck—peripheral nerve block

(2) Upper extremity—brachial plexus neurolysis

(3) Thoracic wall—epidural, intrathecal, intercostal, dorsal root ganglion neurolysis

(4) Abdominal—celiac plexus block, thoracic splanchnicectomy

(5) Pelvic—superior hypogastric plexus block

(6) Rectal—intrathecal neurolysis, midline myelotomy, superior hypogastric plexus block, ganglion impar block

(7) Unilateral pain—cordotomy

b. Neurostimulation for complex regional pain syndrome, neuralgias, peripheral neuropathy

c. Minimally invasive surgical procedures

(1) Percutaneous kyphoplasty or vertebroplasty—for treatment of osteoclastic lesions (spinal metastasis or compression fractures) to restore spinal stability

(2) Optimal debulking of tumor to limit pain or improve or maintain functional capabilities

D. Nonpharmacologic interventions (Irwin et al., 2011; NCCN, 2013)

1. Occupational and physical therapy, cancer rehabilitation

2. Acupuncture, acupressure, heat or cold therapy
3. Complementary therapies—distraction, music, guided imagery, hypnosis, massage, counseling and support groups

II. Interventions to increase comfort and patient and family knowledge
   A. Educating patients and families about strategies to prevent and manage pain
      1. Discussing the importance of adequate pain management in attaining optimal quality of life and the impact of pain on depression, sleep disturbance, and fatigue
      2. Informing patients about the potential for discomfort associated with treatments or procedures (e.g., bone marrow biopsy, lumbar puncture, IV or central line placement) to reduce anxiety of the unknown
      3. Educating patients and families about the use of pain rating scales to communicate pain and the responsiveness to interventions
      4. Encouraging the patient to take analgesics early in the pain experience to avoid severe pain and to take long-acting analgesics around the clock for constant pain
      5. Starting a bowel movement regimen on initiation of opioid analgesics; including a stool softener and bowel stimulant
      6. Educating the patient and family about multiple modalities available to control pain: non opioids, opioids, adjuvant analgesics, interventional procedures, complementary techniques
      7. Incorporating patient's social network (family leaders, minister, spiritual leader, healer) as appropriate.
   B. Differentiating among analgesic tolerance, physical dependence, addiction, and other pain terms (Brant, 2014; IASP, 2012)
      1. Analgesic tolerance—physiologic state of adaptation whereby the repeated exposure to a drug results in diminished effect of the drug over time and a possible need to increase the drug dose to achieve the same level of effect
      2. Physical dependence—physiologic state of adaptation manifested by the emergence of a withdrawal syndrome if drug use is abruptly stopped, rapidly decreased, or an antagonist is administered
      3. Addiction—neurobiologic disease with genetic, psychosocial, and environmental influences that results in psychological dependence on the use of substances for their psychic effects; characterized by cravings and compulsive use despite harm
   C. Monitoring the patient for safety
      1. Monitoring for side effects of opioid therapy, including respiratory depression

2. Educating patients who are at high risk for spinal cord compression to notify the health care team if early signs of impending compression occur

III. Interventions to facilitate coping
   A. Prevention of post-traumatic stress disorder related to uncontrolled pain with a judicious pain management plan
   B. Managing psychological distress, anxiety, and fear, which can aggravate cancer pain
   C. Use of complementary therapies to augment optimal pain management
      1. Use of adjunct therapies such as bubbles, pop-up books, magic gloves, and puppets to decrease pain perception in the pediatric population
      2. Providing information about additional complementary therapies, including relaxation, massage, hypnosis, guided imagery, and deep breathing, as appropriate
   D. Incorporating cultural and spiritual preferences into the plan of care

EVALUATION

The oncology nurse systematically and regularly evaluates the patient's and family's responses to pain interventions to achieve patient's individual comfort goal. Pain assessment data are collected, and the pain management plan is continuously modified to meet the patient's pain goal.

Pruritus

OVERVIEW

I. Definition—itching
II. Physiology (Cunha & Delfini Filho, 2012; Tey & Yosipovitch, 2011)
   A. Mediators
      1. Histamine released from mast cells and acts on H_1 receptors and C fibers
      2. Prostaglandins E_2 and H_2
      3. Substance P synthesized in C fibers
      4. Cytokines, serotonin, neuropeptides, and proteases
      5. Opioids along the afferent pathway
      6. Physical stimuli (electricity, pressure, temperature)
   B. Neural pathways
      1. The physiology of pruritus is closely linked to the physiology of pain.
      2. Polymodal C nociceptors are the neurons responsible for itch; they include 20% of the C fiber population.
      3. C fibers are sensitive to histamine.
      4. Impulse travels from the C fibers to the ipsilateral dorsal root ganglia to the opposite anterolateral spinothalamic tract to the

Table 34-3

Risk Factors for Pruritus

Patient- or Disease-Related Factors	Treatment-Related Factors	Lifestyle-Related Factors
Cancer Related Hematologic malignancies: Hodgkin lymphoma (30%), non-Hodgkin lymphoma, leukemia, multiple myeloma Solid tumors: lung, colon, breast, stomach Melanoma Anal and vulvar tumors (local itch) Prostate cancer (perineal and scrotal itch) Gliomas (face or nostril itch) Age: itch is experienced by 50%–70% of patients >70 years Infection	**Chemotherapy** L-asparaginase, cisplatin, cytarabine, taxanes *Allergic reaction and related pruritus—may occur with any agent* **Radiation Therapy** Skin reactions and pruritus—most common when the radiation dosage is >20 Gy **Immunotherapy or Targeted Therapy** Epidermal growth factor receptor (EGFR) inhibitors, mTOR (mammalian target of rapamycin) inhibitors, interferon, interleukin-2 Surgery Postsurgical wound healing	**Psychological** Stress, anxiety, depression, boredom, psychoses **Environmental** Dry atmospheric conditions Dehydration Clothing and laundering practices (chemical allergy) Overheating
Other Diseases Iron deficiency Cholestasis Polycythemia vera (30%–50%) Renal and hepatic disease Mycosis fungoides Thyroid dysfunction (Graves' disease or hypothyroidism) Diabetes (peripheral neuropathy)	**Medications** Opioids, aspirin, erythromycin, hormonal therapy, phenothiazines	

posterolateral ventral thalamic nucleus and ends at the cortex.
    5. The stimuli can originate anywhere along the afferent pathway.
  C. Risk factors (Table 34-3)

ASSESSMENT

I. Clinical assessment (Squiers et al., 2011)
  A. Review of medication history and potential allergies
  B. Presence of underlying disease
  C. Temporal patterns
    1. Patterns of pruritus, including circadian occurrence (pruritus typically increases at night), timing, onset, duration
    2. Aggravating and alleviating factors
    3. Impact of pruritus on daily activities
    4. Methods of assessment
      a. Patient's self-report
      b. Adjective lists describing pruritus—constant, intermittent, transient, burning, numbness
II. History and physical examination (Weisshaar et al., 2012)
  A. Potential laboratory findings
    1. Complete blood cell (CBC) count—elevated white blood cell (WBC) count, anemia, eosinophilia, polycythemia
    2. Blood chemistries—hyperglycemia, hyperuricemia, elevated blood urea nitrogen (BUN) or creatinine, abnormal liver function tests, bilirubin, alkaline phosphatase

    3. Thyroid function tests—hypoactive or hyperactive thyroid
    4. Other—low ferritin level, increased sedimentation rate, human immunodeficiency virus (HIV) antibody assay (if immunosuppression or lymphoma is a possibility)
    5. Urinalysis—glycosuria
  B. Physical and psychosocial findings
    1. New diagnosis of a malignancy—pruritus may be the presenting symptom
    2. Skin assessment—scratch marks, erythema, excoriation, thickening, dryness
    3. Vaginal discharge and erythema
    4. Presence of urea or bilirubin on the skin
    5. Presence of stress and anxiety

NURSING DIAGNOSES

I. Impaired Skin Integrity/Risk for Impaired Skin Integrity (NANDA-I)
  A. Expected outcome—patient's skin remains intact.
II. Ineffective Coping/Readiness for Enhanced Coping (NANDA-I)
  A. Expected outcome—patient and the family contact an appropriate health care team member when pruritus interrupts protective mechanisms and psychological well-being.
III. Deficient Knowledge (NANDA-I), related to readiness for enhanced knowledge of effective management strategies for pruritus

Part 4

A. Expected outcome—patient states the potential for pruritus with specific cancers, cancer therapies, and other related disease entities.

IV. Impaired Comfort (NANDA-I)
   A. Expected outcome—patient reports alleviation of pruritus and increased comfort.
   B. Expected outcome—patient and family describe interventions to manage pruritus, maximize comfort.

PLANNING AND IMPLEMENTATION

I. Interventions to manage pruritus
   A. Treating or removing the underlying cause
   B. Pharmacologic management (Table 34-4) (Tey & Yosipovitch, 2011)
   C. Nonpharmacologic management
      1. Medicated baths with antipruritics
      2. Application of creams and emollient lotions for comfort

II. Interventions to increase the patient and family knowledge base
   A. Educating patient and family about therapies that may cause pruritus
   B. Providing information about the signs and symptoms of infection related to pruritus: fever, erythema, edema, pain, purulent drainage
   C. Educating patient and family about self-care interventions to decrease the severity of pruritus

III. Interventions to maximize comfort (Seccareccia & Gebara, 2011; Weisshaar et al., 2012)
   A. Modifying the environment to prevent and minimize pruritus
      1. Keeping the room humidity at 40% or higher
      2. Keeping the room temperature cool to prevent vasodilation and limit sweating that may exacerbate itch; use of fans to circulate the air
      3. Use of cotton clothing and sheets; avoiding wool or fabrics that may irritate skin
      4. Use of mild, unscented, or hypoallergenic soaps; avoiding use of detergents
   B. Minimizing vasodilation
      1. Encouraging brief cool baths, showers, and environmental conditions; application of a mild moisturizing cream after bathing or showering; having the patient avoid fragrant topical agents
      2. Having the patient avoid alcohol, caffeine intake, and spicy foods
      3. Measures to reduce stress and anxiety
   C. Promoting skin integrity
      1. Encouraging fluid intake of 3000 mL/day
      2. Encouraging a diet high in iron, zinc, and protein
      3. Having the patient wear loose-fitting, nonirritating clothing
      4. Having the patient avoid scratching; education about wearing cotton gloves at night to avoid skin trauma

IV. Interventions to protect patient from potential sequelae
   A. Use of massage, pressure, and rubbing as alternatives to scratching
   B. Cutting patient's fingernails short and filing them smooth
   C. Instructing family about the importance of good hand hygiene
   D. Assessment of the pruritic areas for signs of infection

Table 34-4

Pharmacologic Management of Pruritus

Pharmacologic Agent	Type of Pruritus	Comments
Diphenhydramine, cimetidine (H1 and H2 antagonists)	Urticaria, allergic drug reactions, palliative patients with advanced disease	May cause drowsiness
Corticosteroids	Inflammatory pruritus, local skin reactions	Can be given orally or topically as a cream rubbed onto the pruritic skin
Naloxone and methylnaltrexone (opioid antagonists), butorphanol (kappa opioid receptor agonist)	Opioid-induced pruritus related to mu-receptor agonists	Pruritus in up to 50% of patients receiving opioids; if pruritus is caused by an opioid and symptom management has failed, consider switching to another opioid May reverse analgesic effect so use with caution
Capsaicin	Postherpetic neuralgia, psoriasis	Helpful for treating chronic and localized pruritus
Aprepitant (substance P neurokinin receptors)	Sezary syndrome, cutaneous T-cell lymphoma, metastatic cancer, erlotinib-induced itch	Clinical trials needed to verify efficacy
Mirtazapine	Cancer-related itch, nocturnal itch	Other antidepressants may potentially help with itch

Adapted from Tey, H. L., & Yosipovitch, G. (2011). Targeted treatment of pruritus: A look into the future. *British Journal of Dermatology, 165*(1), 5–17.

V. Interventions to facilitate patient and family coping
   A. Teaching about behavioral interventions that may distract from the pruritus: imagery, television, reading, crafts
   B. Encouraging relaxation, stress reduction; referral to psychosocial services, if needed.

EVALUATION

The oncology nurse systematically and regularly evaluates the patient's and family's responses to interventions to prevent or manage pruritus toward the goal of comfort. Data about the risks and characteristics of pruritus are assessed on an ongoing basis to achieve optimal comfort. Nursing diagnoses, outcomes, and plans of care are reviewed and revised, as necessary.

Fatigue

OVERVIEW

I. Definition—Cancer-related fatigue is defined as "a distressing, persistent, subjective sense of physical, emotional, and/or cognitive tiredness or exhaustion related to cancer or cancer treatment that is not proportional to recent activity and interferes with usual functioning" (NCCN, 2013)
II. Physiology
   A. The physiology of cancer-related fatigue is not well understood.
   B. New theories suggest many reasons for fatigue (Wang, 2008).
      1. Release of inflammatory cytokines, interleukins (ILs), and tumor necrosis factor (TNF) may affect muscle function and metabolism, leading to fatigue.
      2. Vascular endothelial growth factor (VEGF) levels have been associated with fatigue, causing impaired thyroid blood flow and leading to hypothyroidism.
      3. Prolonged fatigue following treatment may be the result of elevated proinflammatory cytokine release factors (Barsevick et al., 2010).
   C. Fatigue is often seen with other symptoms related to cancer and its treatment.
      1. Pain, distress, and sleep disturbances have been found to cluster with fatigue (Brant et al., 2011; Kwekkeboom, Cherwin, Lee, & Wanta, 2010).
   D. Anemia-related fatigue is caused by a decrease in the hemoglobin and hematocrit levels, which causes fatigue and shortness of breath.
      1. Red blood cell (RBC) production has been shown to be suppressed by the presence of IL-1, IL-6, and TNF (Barsevick et al., 2010).
III. Risk factors (Campos, Hassan, Riechelmann, & Del Giglio, 2011)
   A. Disease-related factors

1. 70% to 80% of patients with cancer report fatigue at some point (Liu et al., 2012).
   a. Fatigue has been identified not only as an acute finding during treatment but also as a persistent, chronic condition seen up to 10 years after treatment (Harrington, Hansen, Moskowitz, Todd, & Feuerstein, 2010).
2. Fatigue precedes and accompanies most malignancies and is dependent on the stage and duration of illness.
3. Comorbidities and underlying diseases may increase fatigue.
   B. Treatment-related factors (Campos et al., 2011)
      1. Chemotherapy
         a. Drugs crossing the blood-brain barrier may cause neurotoxic effects, leading to fatigue.
         b. Nausea, vomiting, diarrhea, and anemia and end products from tumor death are thought to contribute to fatigue.
      2. Immunotherapy or biotherapy
         a. Fatigue is a common dose-limiting side effect in up to 70% of patients undergoing treatment with these agents.
         b. Interferon may also cause hypothyroidism, potentiating fatigue even more in these individuals.
      3. Hormone therapy
         a. Treatments aimed at suppressing hormone-dependent cancers may cause fatigue, as seen in breast and prostate cancers.
      4. Fatigue has been reported in up to 80% of those undergoing radiation therapy (Barbarino et al., 2013).
      5. Surgery
         a. Immobilization, anxiety, pain control, anesthesia, and infection
         b. Preoperative fatigue may affect postoperative fatigue.
      6. Medications—opioids, hypnotics, anxiolytics, antihistamines, antiemetics
   C. Lifestyle-related factors (Horneber, Fischer, Dimeo, Ruffer, & Weis, 2012; Kwekkeboom et al., 2010)
      1. Symptom clusters of fatigue, pain, and sleep disturbance common
      2. Decreased physical performance
      3. Emotional distress

ASSESSMENT

I. NCCN guidelines for fatigue assessment (NCCN, 2013)
   A. Assessment of each patient for the presence of fatigue and use a method for evaluating the extent and distress of the fatigue perceived by the patient
      1. Patient self-report—the gold standard
      2. Numeric scales or mild, moderate, or severe descriptors

3. Family and caregiver insight of the effect that fatigue has on the patient
   B. Focused history and physical examination
   1. Disease status, length and types of treatments, current comorbidities, or other health issues that may contribute to or potentiate fatigue
   2. Assessment of the degree of fatigue by evaluating onset, patterns, alleviating factors, duration, and the impact it has on overall functioning
   3. Impact of fatigue on quality of life (QOL)—patients may report fatigue to be more of a distressing symptom than pain
   C. Other contributing factors that may play into the fatigue (e.g., pain, nutritional issues, sleep disturbances, medications)
   D. Potential laboratory findings (Campos et al., 2011)
   1. Signs of anemia, such as low hemoglobin level
   2. Electrolyte disturbances
   3. Low levels of iron, vitamin B_{12}, folate
   4. Hypothyroidism and low hormone levels
   5. Low vitamin D levels (Dev et al., 2011)

PROBLEM STATEMENTS AND OUTCOME IDENTIFICATION

I. Ineffective Coping (NANDA-I), related to fatigue
   A. Expected outcome—patient copes with fatigue using individual and community support resources.
II. Activity Intolerance (NANDA-I)
   A. Expected outcome—patient performs ADLs and participates in desired activities at his or her level of ability or adapts to decreased energy levels.
III. Deficient Knowledge (NANDA-I), related to effective fatigue management strategies
   A. Expected outcome—patient recognizes fatigue as a manifestation of cancer and its treatment.
   B. Expected outcome—patient describes self-care measures for the management of fatigue.

PLANNING AND IMPLEMENTATION

I. Treatment of the malignancy or the underlying cause
II. Interventions to manage fatigue (NCCN, 2013)
   A. Erythropoiesis-stimulating agents (ESAs) (Mitchell, Beck, & Eaton, 2009)
   1. Patients with hemoglobin less than 10 g/dL most likely to benefit; evidence inconsistent when hemogloblin level is 11 to 12 g/dL.
   2. Potential for adverse events associated with ESAs, including thromboembolic events and hypertension
   3. Concerns that ESAs may support or extend tumor growth in some patients

B. Effectiveness of using psychostimulants or antidepressants not yet established
   C. Promise shown by vitamins and herbals, but trials have been small and limited.
   D. Blood transfusions—offer some relief of fatigue related to anemia (Preston, Hurlow, Brine, & Bennett, 2012)
   E. Nonpharmacologic management
   1. Exercise (Mitchell et al., 2009)
      a. Exercise is recommended several times per week during and following treatment for functionally able patients (Mishra et al., 2012).
      b. Recent studies report benefit from yoga (Bower et al., 2012).
   2. Energy conservation and activity management may improve fatigue.
   3. Relation, massage, and measures to improve sleep are likely to improve fatigue.
III. Interventions to increase knowledge of patient and family
   A. Discussing the potential for fatigue at the time of diagnosis and at treatment initiation
   B. Providing information to the patient and family about therapies known to cause fatigue
   C. Providing information about interventions used to treat fatigue
   D. Educating the patient and family about the management of fatigue
   1. Energy conservation—assisting the patient in prioritizing needs, planning, pacing the daily schedule, and modifying plans, if needed
   2. Exercise—having the patient maintain adequate activity to increase energy stores
   3. Nutrition—having the patient maintain adequate nutrition to promote ideal weight and energy
   4. Restoration of attention—reducing environmental demands (information, stimuli, distractions) to conserve attention for priority needs
   5. Sleep and rest—having the patient maintain adequate sleep and rest
IV. Interventions to facilitate patient and family coping
   A. Encouraging the patient and family to discuss fatigue and its impact on ADLs
   B. Consulting with psychosocial services when fatigue may be related to psychological and social factors such as depression, stress, or difficulty coping with the disease
   C. Administration of medical interventions in a timely and appropriate manner
   D. Acknowledging the potential for fatigue to interfere with sexuality

EVALUATION

The oncology nurse identifies individuals experiencing fatigue and generates an appropriate care plan to help patients increase activity and decrease fatigue by using evidence-based interventions. Periodic evaluation is imperative to ensure that the goals of the plan are met, thus improving patient satisfaction and quality of life.

Sleep Disorders

OVERVIEW

I. Definition (Irwin, Olmstead, Ganz, & Haque, 2013; Oncology Nursing Society [ONS], 2013)
   A. Sleep—natural process that is vital for brain function and restoration of the body and thought to be important for thermoregulation and immune function
II. Sleep disturbances—range from insomnia, being sleepy during daytime hours, abnormal movements and/or behaviors during rest
   A. Insomnia—defined as difficulty falling asleep staying asleep, non restorative sleep, resulting in daytime dysfunction, or a combination of all of these (Ancoli-Israel, 2009)
   B. Experienced by 30% to 75% of patients with cancer; has a significant negative impact on quality of life (ONS, 2013)
   C. Sleep problems not mentioned by many patients with cancer (Ancoli-Israel, 2009)
      1. 80% surveyed assumed sleep problems were caused by treatment.
      2. 60% wrongly assumed that the symptoms would be short-lived.
      3. Almost 50% thought that physicians cannot do anything to help.
III. Physiology (Page, Berger, & Johnson, 2006)
   A. Normal sleep-wake cycle
      1. Stages 1 through 4, cycles throughout the night or sleep time; stage 1 is the lightest level, progressing to stage 4, which is the deepest part of the sleep cycle
      2. Made of two different types of sleep, rapid eye movement (REM) and non–rapid eye movement (NREM)
      3. Typical sleep pattern in adults—4 to 6 cycles
   B. Other regulatory processes (Hansen et al., 2012; Miaskowski et al., 2011)
      1. Circadian rhythm and melatonin
         a. Hormone released by the pineal gland of the hypothalamus
         b. Low levels frequently associated with depression, insomnia
         c. Decreased levels of melatonin correlated with an increased risk of breast cancer, especially in those who work at night
      2. Clock genes—help regulate circadian rhythm
IV. Environmental factors—production of melatonin suppressed by exposure to light, either natural or artificial (Gooley et al., 2011)
V. Risk factors
   A. Disease-related factors
      1. Sleep disturbance related to the cancer in an estimated 52% to 58% of patients; one third complained of sleep problems prior to diagnosis (Ancoli-Israel, 2009)
      2. Presence of concurrent symptoms such as pain, nausea, fatigue, and depression
   B. Treatment-related factors (Page et al., 2006)
      1. Chemotherapy
      2. Hormones (e.g., tamoxifen)—may lead to imbalances that cause sweating and hot flashes, especially at night
      3. Cytokines or biotherapy—IL-2 and TNF-alpha associated with sleep disturbances
      4. Medications—analgesics, antidepressants, antiemetics, benzodiazepines, steroids, hypnotics
   C. Lifestyle-related and personal factors
      1. Psychological factors—sleep affected by diagnosis of cancer, depression, anxiety, life stressors, and other underlying psychiatric disorders
      2. Older age and female gender
      3. Exposure to light or having lights on before bed, which reduces melatonin excretion, delaying sleep or not allowing persons to rest
      4. Incidence higher in patients with lung or breast cancer (Irwin et al., 2013)

ASSESSMENT

I. History and physical information (National Cancer Institute [NCI], 2013)
   A. Paraneoplastic syndromes or presence of symptoms associated with tumor invasion (e.g., obstructions, pain, shortness of breath, pruritus, fatigue)
   B. Current or recent treatments for disease, including surgery (e.g., pain, unable to sleep in normal positions related to surgical site), chemotherapy, radiation
   C. Medications—opioids, sedatives or hypnotics, steroids, some antidepressants
   D. Herbal and nonpharmacologic use—caffeine or nicotine and dietary supplements, including some vitamins
   E. Environmental factors—hot, cold, too many lights on at night or during rest

F. Physical and psychological stressors (e.g., financial concerns, fear of job loss, death, depression, anxiety)

II. Characterization of sleep
   A. Usual patterns of sleep
   B. Routine before bed (e.g., food, bathing or self-care activities, medications)
   C. How long it takes to fall asleep
   D. Duration of sleep (frequency of awaking during night, ability to return to sleep, and usual time of getting up in the morning)
   E. Characteristics of disturbed sleep (changes following diagnosis, treatment, and hospitalization)
   F. Caregivers' observations of quantity and quality of patient's sleep
   G. Family or personal history of sleep disorders

III. Physical examination
   A. Observation of patient—dark circles under eyes, expressionless face, nystagmus, ptosis of the eyelids, frequent yawning, slurred speech, incorrect word usage
   B. Sleep studies—polysomnography

PROBLEM STATEMENTS AND EXPECTED OUTCOMES

I. Insomnia (NANDA-I)
   A. Expected outcome—patient is able to fall asleep and stay asleep.
   B. Expected outcome—patient identifies pharmacologic strategies to facilitate sleep.
   C. Expected outcome—patient describes specific behavioral and cognitive interventions to promote sleep.

II. Disturbed Sleep Pattern (NANDA-I)
   A. Expected outcome—patient states the risk factors of disease and treatment that may alter sleep patterns.
   B. Expected outcome—patient reports adequate sleep patterns.

PLANNING AND IMPLEMENTATION

I. Assessment and treatment of other underlying issues (e.g., supplemental oxygen for shortness breath, transfusions for anemia to counteract fatigue, medications for depression, financial counselors for issues related to job loss)

II. Interventions to promote sleep (Table 34-5)

Table 34-5

Nonpharmacologic Interventions to Promote Sleep

Intervention	Goal	Procedure
Stimulus control therapy	• Reassociate temporal (bedtime) and environmental (bed and bedroom) stimuli with rapid sleep onsets. • Establish a regular circadian sleep-wake rhythm.	Relax at least 1 hr before going to bed; develop a ritual prior to bed; go to bed only when sleepy; when unable to fall asleep or go back to sleep within 15 to 20 min, get out of bed, leave the bedroom, and return to bed only when sleepy; maintain a regular arising time in the morning; use the bed or bedroom for sleep and sex only (do not watch television, listen to the radio, eat, or read in bed); avoid naps during the day.
Sleep restriction procedures	• Curtail time in bed to the actual sleep time, thereby creating mild sleep deprivation, which results in more consolidated and more efficient sleep.	Restrict the amount of time spent in bed to the actual amount of time asleep; time in bed is progressively increased as sleep efficiency improves.
Relaxation training	• Reduce somatic and cognitive arousal interfering with sleep.	Attempt progressive muscle relaxation, autogenic training, biofeedback, imagery training, hypnosis, thought stopping.
Cognitive therapy	• Change dysfunctional beliefs and attitudes about sleep and insomnia that exacerbate emotional arousal, performance anxiety, and learned helplessness related to sleep (e.g., unrealistic sleep requirement expectations, faulty appraisals of sleep difficulties, misattributions of daytime impairments, misconceptions about the causes of insomnia).	Identify sleep cognitive distortions (mainly by self-monitoring); reframe dysfunctional thoughts about sleep into more adaptive thoughts by using cognitive restructuring techniques (e.g., decatastrophizing loss of sleep, reattribution, reappraisal, attention shifting).
Sleep hygiene education	• Change health practices and environmental factors that interfere with sleep.	Avoid stimulants (e.g., caffeine, nicotine) and alcohol around bedtime; do not eat heavy or spicy meals too close to bedtime; exercise regularly but not too late in the evening; maintain a dark, quiet, comfortable sleep environment.

Adapted from Ancoli-Israel, S. (2009). Recognition and treatment of sleep disturbances in cancer. *Journal of Clinical Oncology, 27*(35), 5864–5866; Page, M. S., Berger, A. M., & Johnson, L. B. (2006). Putting evidence into practice: Evidence-based interventions for sleep-wake disturbances. *Clinical Journal of Oncologic Nursing, 10*(6), 753–767; Oncology Nursing Society. (2013). *Putting evidence into practice: Sleep-wake disturbances.* https://www.ons.org/practice-resources/pep/sleep-wake-disturbances.

A. Cognitive behavioral therapy—includes behavioral strategies that promote sleep
B. Education regarding sleep hygiene and relaxation techniques to promote sleep; limiting time spent in bed that is not sleep-related
C. Encouraging patient to go to bed and wake up at regular times
D. Creating a dark, comfortable sleep environment to promote melatonin release
E. Having the patient avoid watching television in bed
F. Ensuring that the patient gets ample daylight while awake to keep circadian rhythm in balance
G. Having the patient avoiding naps, if possible, or limiting duration of naps
H. Having the patient limit or avoid caffeine
I. Restricting regular exercise to 3 hours before bedtime

III. Interventions to manage sleep pharmacologically
A. Lack of large trials or research studies to support the use of medications to induce and promote sleep in patients with cancer (Page et al., 2006)
B. Drug classes to treat insomnia (NCI, 2013)
  1. Nonbenzodiazepine benzodiazepine receptor agonists—extended-release medications may lead to excessive morning drowsiness
  2. Benzodiazepines
    a. Carry a much higher risk of tolerance, dependence, and withdrawal associated with the risk of seizures and death
    b. Extreme caution required with use in patients with a history of substance abuse
    c. Caution necessary in those with underlying respiratory issues because they cause respiratory depression
  3. Antihistamines—not widely used; caution necessary with use in older adults because these agents may cause confusion, delirium, or both
  4. Antidepressants and antipsychotics—used for their sedative properties but have narrow window for dosing; side effects may not outweigh the benefits
  5. Melatonin—natural hormone that promotes sleep with minimal side effects

IV. Interventions to increase patient and family knowledge
A. Informing the patient about the need to report sleep disturbance
B. Informing the patient about strategies for stimulus control and improved sleep

V. Interventions to maximize patient comfort
A. Synchronizing nursing interventions to prevent unnecessary interruption of sleep
B. Implementing pain and symptom management interventions in a timely and appropriate manner to control pain and concurrent symptoms

C. Administering sleeping medications in a timely and appropriate manner
D. Providing a restful environment
  1. Decreasing light and noise factors
  2. Maintaining the patient's room temperature
  3. Providing clean bed linens and straightening them
  4. Encouraging the practice of a normal bedtime routine

EVALUATION

The oncology nurse identifies those who are experiencing sleep disturbances and formulates an appropriate care plan, which includes appropriate, evidence-based interventions. Frequent reassessment ensures that interventions are successful in promoting adequate rest to improve the patient's quality of life.

References

American Pain Society. (2008). *Principles of analgesic use in the treatment of acute pain and cancer pain* (6th ed.). Glenview, IL: APS Press.

Ancoli-Israel, S. (2009). Recognition and treatment of sleep disturbances in cancer. *Journal of Clinical Oncology, 27*(35), 5864–5866. http://dx.doi.org/10.1200/jco.2009.24.5993.

Barbarino, R., Janniello, D., Morelli, P., Falco, M. D., Cicchetti, S., Di Murro, L., et al. (2013). Fatigue in patients undergoing radiation therapy: An observational study. *Minerva Medica, 104*(2), 185–191.

Barsevick, A., Beck, S. L., Dudley, W. N., Wong, B., Berger, A. M., Whitmer, K., et al. (2010). Efficacy of an intervention for fatigue and sleep disturbance during cancer chemotherapy. *Journal of Pain and Symptom Management, 40*(2), 200–216. http://dx.doi.org/10.1016/j.jpainsymman.2009.12.020.

Beijers, A. J., Jongen, J. L., & Vreugdenhil, G. (2012). Chemotherapy-induced neurotoxicity: The value of neuroprotective strategies. *Netherlands Journal of Medicine, 70*(1), 18–25.

Bennett, M. I., Rayment, C., Hjermstad, M., Aass, N., Caraceni, A., & Kaasa, S. (2012). Prevalence and aetiology of neuropathic pain in cancer patients: A systematic review. *Pain, 153*(2), 359–365. http://dx.doi.org/10.1016/j.pain.2011.10.028.

Bower, J. E., Garet, D., Sternlieb, B., Ganz, P. A., Irwin, M. R., Olmstead, R., et al. (2012). Yoga for persistent fatigue in breast cancer survivors: A randomized controlled trial. *Cancer, 118*(15), 3766–3775. http://dx.doi.org/10.1002/cncr.26702.

Brant, J. M. (2010). Practical approaches to pharmacologic management of pain in older adults with cancer. *Oncology Nursing Forum, 37*(Suppl.), 17–26. http://dx.doi.org/10.1188/10.onf.s1.17-26.

Brant, J. M. (2011). Pain and discomfort in cancer survivors. In J. L. Lester & P. Schmitt (Eds.), *Cancer rehabilitation and survivorship* (pp. 37–48). Pittsburgh: Oncology Nursing Society.

Brant, J. M. (2012). Strategies to manage pain in palliative care. In M. O'Connor, S. Lee, & S. Aranda (Eds.), *Palliative care nursing: A guide to practice.* (3rd ed., pp. 93–113). Victoria, Australia: Ausmed.

Brant, J. M. (2014). Pain. In B. G. C. H. Yarbro & D. Wujcik (Eds.), *Cancer symptom management* (pp. 69–91). Burlington, VT: Jones and Bartlett.

Brant, J. M., Beck, S. L., Dudley, W. N., Cobb, P., Pepper, G., & Miaskowski, C. (2011). Symptom trajectories during chemotherapy in outpatients with lung cancer colorectal cancer, or lymphoma. *European Journal of Oncology Nursing, 15*(5), 470–477. http://dx.doi.org/10.1016/j.ejon.2010.12.002 S1462-3889(10)00172-9.

Burris, H. A., 3rd., & Hurtig, J. (2010). Radiation recall with anticancer agents. *The Oncologist, 15*(11), 1227–1237. http://dx.doi.org/10.1634/theoncologist.2009-0090.

Campos, M. P., Hassan, B. J., Riechelmann, R., & Del Giglio, A. (2011). Cancer-related fatigue: A review. *Revista Da Associacao Medica Brasileira, 57*(2), 211–219.

Chauhan, A., Weiss, J., & Warrier, R. (2010). Effective management of pain in pediatric hematology and oncology. *Asian Pacific Journal of Cancer Prevention, 11*(2), 577–579.

Cunha, P. R., & Delfini Filho, O. (2012). Pruritus: Still a challenge. *Anais Brasileiros de Dermatologia, 87*(5), 735–741. http://dx.doi.org/S0365-05962012000500011.

Curtiss, C. P. (2010). Challenges in pain assessment in cognitively intact and cognitively impaired older adults with cancer. *Oncology Nursing Forum, 37*(Suppl.), 7–16. http://dx.doi.org/10.1188/10.ONF.S1.7-16 Y811R2M486485616.

Deer, T. R., Smith, H. S., Burton, A. W., Pope, J. E., Doleys, D. M., Levy, R. M., et al. (2011). Comprehensive consensus-based guidelines on intrathecal drug delivery systems in the treatment of pain caused by cancer pain. *Pain Physician, 14*(3), E283–E312.

Dev, R., Del Fabbro, E., Schwartz, G. G., Hui, D., Palla, S. L., Gutierrez, N., et al. (2011). Preliminary report: Vitamin D deficiency in advanced cancer patients with symptoms of fatigue or anorexia. *The Oncologist, 16*(11), 1637–1641. http://dx.doi.org/10.1634/theoncologist.2011-0151.

Epstein, J. B., Thariat, J., Bensadoun, R. J., Barasch, A., Murphy, B. A., Kolnick, L., et al. (2012). Oral complications of cancer and cancer therapy: From cancer treatment to survivorship. *CA Cancer Journal for Clinicians, 62*(6), 400–422. http://dx.doi.org/10.3322/caac.21157.

Gooley, J. J., Chamberlain, K., Smith, K. A., Khalsa, S. B., Rajaratnam, S. M., Van Reen, E., et al. (2011). Exposure to room light before bedtime suppresses melatonin onset and shortens melatonin duration in humans. *Journal of Clinical Endocrinology and Metabolism, 96*(3), E463–E472. http://dx.doi.org/10.1210/jc.2010-2098.

Hansen, M. V., Madsen, M. T., Hageman, I., Rasmussen, L. S., Bokmand, S., Rosenberg, J., et al. (2012). The effect of MELatOnin on Depression, anxietY, cognitive function and sleep disturbances in patients with breast cancer. The MELODY trial: Protocol for a randomised, placebo-controlled, double-blinded trial. *BMJ Open, 2*(1), e000647. http://dx.doi.org/10.1136/bmjopen-2011-000647.

Harrington, C. B., Hansen, J. A., Moskowitz, M., Todd, B. L., & Feuerstein, M. (2010). It's not over when it's over: Long-term symptoms in cancer survivors—a systematic review. *International Journal of Psychiatry in Medicine, 40*(2), 163–181.

Hayek, S. M., Deer, T. R., Pope, J. E., Panchal, S. J., & Patel, V. B. (2011). Intrathecal therapy for cancer and non-cancer pain. *Pain Physician, 14*(3), 219–248.

Horneber, M., Fischer, I., Dimeo, F., Ruffer, J. U., & Weis, J. (2012). Cancer-related fatigue: Epidemiology, pathogenesis, diagnosis, and treatment. *Deutsches Ärzteblatt International, 109*(9), 161–171. http://dx.doi.org/10.3238/arztebl.2012.0161 quiz 172.

International Association for the Study of Pain (IASP). (2012). *Definition of pain. IASP taxonomy.* www.iasp-pain.org/Content/NavigationMenu/GeneralResource Links/PainDefinitions/default.htm.

Irwin, M. R., Brant, J. M., & Eaton, L. H. (2011). *Putting evidence into practice: Improving oncology patient outcomes.* Pittsburgh: ONS Press.

Irwin, M. R., Olmstead, R. E., Ganz, P. A., & Haque, R. (2013). Sleep disturbance, inflammation and depression risk in cancer survivors. *Brain, Behavior, and Immunity, 30*(Suppl.), S58–S67. http://dx.doi.org/10.1016/j.bbi.2012.05.002.

Kwekkeboom, K. L., Cherwin, C. H., Lee, J. W., & Wanta, B. (2010). Mind-body treatments for the pain-fatigue-sleep disturbance symptom cluster in persons with cancer. *Journal of Pain and Symptom Management, 39*(1), 126–138. http://dx.doi.org/10.1016/j.jpainsymman.2009.05.022.

Lawson, E. F., & Wallace, M. S. (2010). Current developments in intraspinal agents for cancer and noncancer pain. *Current Pain and Headache Reports, 14*(1), 8–16. http://dx.doi.org/10.1007/s11916-009-0092-z.

Lema, M. J., Foley, K. M., & Hausheer, F. H. (2010). Types and epidemiology of cancer-related neuropathic pain: The intersection of cancer pain and neuropathic pain. *The Oncologist, 15*(Suppl. 2), 3–8. http://dx.doi.org/10.1634/theoncologist.2009-S505.

Liu, L., Rissling, M., Natarajan, L., Fiorentino, L., Mills, P. J., Dimsdale, J. E., et al. (2012). The longitudinal relationship between fatigue and sleep in breast cancer patients undergoing chemotherapy. *Sleep, 35*(2), 237–245. http://dx.doi.org/10.5665/sleep.1630.

Loftus, L. S., Edwards-Bennett, S., & Sokol, G. H. (2012). Systemic therapy for bone metastases. *Cancer Control, 19*(2), 145–153.

Roqué I Figuls, M., Martinez-Zapata, M. J., Scott Brown, M., & Alonso-Coello, P. (2011). Radioisotopes for metastatic bone pain. *Cochrane Database of Systematic Reviews,* (7), 1–68. http://dx.doi.org/10.1002/14651858.CD003347.pub2.

Maccauro, G., Spinelli, M. S., Mauro, S., Perisano, C., Graci, C., & Rosa, M. A. (2011). Physiopathology of spine metastasis. *International Journal of Surgical Oncology, 2011,* 107969. http://dx.doi.org/10.1155/2011/107969.

McCaffery, M., & Pasero, C. (1999). Assessment. In M. McCaffery & C. Pasero (Eds.), *Pain: Clinical manual.* (2nd ed., pp. 35–102). St. Louis: Mosby.

Mercadante, S. (2011). Managing breakthrough pain. *Current Pain and Headache Reports, 15*(4), 244–249. http://dx.doi.org/10.1007/s11916-011-0191-5.

Merkel, S., Voepel-Lewis, T., Shayevitz, J., & Malviya, S. (1997). The FLACC: A behavioral scale for scoring postoperative pain in young children. *Pediatric Nursing, 23*(3), 293–297.

Miaskowski, C., Lee, K., Dunn, L., Dodd, M., Aouizerat, B. E., West, C., et al. (2011). Sleep-wake circadian activity rhythm parameters and fatigue in oncology patients before the initiation of radiation therapy. *Cancer Nursing, 34*(4), 255–268. http://dx.doi.org/10.1097/NCC.0b013e3181f65d9b.

Mishra, S. I., Scherer, R. W., Geigle, P. M., Berlanstein, D. R., Topaloglu, O., Gotay, C. C., et al. (2012). Exercise interventions on health-related quality of life for cancer survivors. *Cochrane Database of Systematic Reviews, 8*, CD007566. http://dx.doi.org/10.1002/14651858.CD007566.pub2.

Mitchell, S. A., Beck, S. L., & Eaton, L. H. (2009). *Fatigue.* Pittsburgh: Oncology Nursing Society.

National Cancer Institute (NCI). (2013). *Sleep disorders.* cancer.gov/cancertopics/pdq/supportivecare/sleepdisorders/healthprofessional.

National Comprehensive Cancer Network (NCCN). (2010). *Clinical practice guidelines.* www.nccn.org/professionals/physician_gls/pdf/pain.pdfed.

Oncology Nursing Society (ONS). (2013). *Putting evidence into practice: Sleep-wake disturbances.* https://www.ons.org/practice-resources/pep/sleep-wake-disturbances.

Page, M. S., Berger, A. M., & Johnson, L. B. (2006). Putting evidence into practice: Evidence-based interventions for sleep-wake disturbances. *Clinical Journal of Oncology Nursing, 10*(6), 753–767.

Preston, N. J., Hurlow, A., Brine, J., & Bennett, M. I. (2012). Blood transfusions for anaemia in patients with advanced cancer. *Cochrane Database of Systematic Reviews, 2*, CD009007. http://dx.doi.org/10.1002/14651858.CD009007.pub2.

Ryan, J. L. (2012). Ionizing radiation: The good, the bad, and the ugly. *Journal of Investigative Dermatology, 132*(3 Pt 2), 985–993. http://dx.doi.org/10.1038/jid.2011.411.

Seccareccia, D., & Gebara, N. (2011). Pruritus in palliative care: Getting up to scratch. *Canadian Family Physician, 57*(9), 1010–1013, e1316-1019. http://dx.doi.org/57/9/1010.

Squiers, L. B., Holden, D. J., Dolina, S. E., Kim, A. E., Bann, C. M., & Renaud, J. M. (2011). The public's response to the U.S. Preventive Services Task Force's 2009 recommendations on mammography screening. *American Journal of Preventative Medicine, 40*(5), 497–504. http://dx.doi.org/S0749-3797(11)00045-6.

Tey, H. L., & Yosipovitch, G. (2011). Targeted treatment of pruritus: A look into the future. *British Journal of Dermatology, 165*(1), 5–17. http://dx.doi.org/10.1111/j.1365-2133.2011.10217.x.

Wang, X. S. (2008). Pathophysiology of cancer-related fatigue. *Clinical Journal of Oncology Nursing, 12*(Suppl.), 11–20. http://dx.doi.org/10.1188/08.cjon.s2.11-20.

Weisshaar, E., Szepietowski, J. C., Darsow, U., Misery, L., Wallengren, J., Mettang, T., et al. (2012). European guideline on chronic pruritus. *Acta Dermato-Venereologica, 92*(5), 563–581. http://dx.doi.org/10.2340/00015555-1400.

World Health Organization (WHO). (2012). *WHO's pain ladder.* www.who.int/cancer/palliative/painladder/en/.

Yu, H. H., Tsai, Y. Y., & Hoffe, S. E. (2012). Overview of diagnosis and management of metastatic disease to bone. *Cancer Control, 19*(2), 84–91.

CHAPTER 35

Cultural, Spiritual, and Religious Diversity

Lori Johnson

OVERVIEW

I. All human beings are unique individuals, yet each of us interacts with the world around us according to values, beliefs, and social norms that are influenced by our spiritual, religious, and cultural perspective.

II. Oncology nurses at all levels and in all settings recognize the importance of spiritual, religious, and cultural diversity and apply the nursing process to meet the unique needs of patients and caregivers with sensitivity and an understanding of interventions that support optimal outcomes.

III. Definitions—understanding diversity in health care begins with establishing a common language to ensure clear communication among different people. *Culture* can be defined as a world view of set traditions, attitudes, and practices, which are transmitted from generation to generation by a particular society, group of people, institution or organization (Merriam-Webster, 2013). *Religion* is an organized system of worship. Definitions for culture and religion are fairly uniform throughout current literature. However, defining *spirituality* proves somewhat more elusive; available peer-reviewed literature is consistent in reporting that *spirituality* is defined in different ways, depending on the group or person defining it. The following definitions will be used throughout this chapter as a means of focusing information in a way that is meaningful for oncology nurses providing patient and family-centered care.

A. Diversity
1. Condition of being composed of differing elements, especially the inclusion of people of different races or cultures in a group (Merriam-Webster, 2013)

B. Culture
1. Beliefs, values, and customs of a particular society or group; a way of thinking, behaving, or working that exists in a place or organization (Merriam-Webster, 2013)

2. Learned and passed from one generation to the next and, as such, changes over time in response to environmental or societal influences
3. Encompasses a group's world view, religion, economy, language, environment, use of technology, and social structure
   a. As an example, nursing culture varies from one practice area to another.

C. Race
1. Refers to populations identified based on phenotype (physical attributes), rather than genetics
2. "Race is socially defined, based on appearance" (Heurtin-Roberts, 2004).
3. One racial group may include more than one ethnic subgroup; for example, Asian American and Pacific Islanders include 57 different ethnic groups, speaking more than 100 languages (U.S. Census Bureau, 2012).
4. Skin color is most often used to define racial groups; however, definitions are fluid, and often disputed by the population being defined (Heurtin-Roberts, 2004).

D. Ethnicity
1. A subcultural group within a multicultural society
2. Largely based on a common national heritage and determined by a shared culture or cultural heritage
3. Ethnic groups comprising more than one racial group—for example, Cubans as an ethnic group including multiple racial groups (Heurtin-Roberts, 2004)

E. Spirituality
1. Refers to how a person perceives their place in the world and determines how a person relates to, and interacts with, other people, animals, nature, and the world around them
2. According to the North American Nursing Diagnosis Association (NANDA), refers to

the principles that guide an individual's sense of self and place in the world, and it "transcends one's biological and psychological nature" (Carroll-Johnson, Gorman, & Bush, 2006; Herdman, 2012)

F. Religion
1. An organized system of beliefs, ceremonies, and rules used to worship a god, a group of gods, or other higher being (Merriam-Webster, 2013)

G. Sacred
1. "A divine being or Ultimate Reality or Ultimate Truth as perceived by the individual" (Larson, Swyers, & McCullough, 1998)

H. Caregiver
1. In this chapter, the term *caregiver* refers to members of the patient's personal support system, whether the caregiver is the significant other, family member, a friend, or member of the patient's congregation or spiritual group.

I. Socioeconomic status (SES)
1. Includes annual income, level of education, type of employment, and other social factors (Elk & Landrine, 2012)

J. Poverty
1. In the United States (U.S.), poverty refers to a single person earning $11,490 or less per year.
2. For each additional person in a household, an amount of $4020 is added; for example, a family of four living in poverty would thus have an annual income of $23,550 per year or less.
3. In Alaska, the guidelines for determining poverty have set $14,350 as annual income for a single person, with $5030 added for each additional family member.
4. In Hawaii, the base amount is $13,230 annual income for a single person, with $4,620 for each additional household member (U.S. Department of Health & Human Services [DHHS], 2013).
5. The culture of poverty crosses racial and ethnic groups and has a major impact on health status (World Health Organization [WHO], 2013).

IV. Ethnic diversity in cancer
A. It was estimated that over 1.6 million Americans would be diagnosed with cancer and over 580,000 people would die from the disease in 2013 (American Cancer Society [ACS], 2013).
1. People living in poverty have a disproportionately high rate of cancer morbidity and mortality.

2. The most frequently reported cancer diagnoses and deaths by race and ethnicity are as follows (National Cancer Institute [NCI], 2013):
a. For men in all racial and ethnic groups, lung and bronchial, prostate, and colorectal cancer are among the top five diagnosed cancers.
b. Prostate cancer is the most frequently diagnosed cancer in Native American, African American, Filipino, Japanese, non-Hispanic white, and Hispanic men.
c. Lung and bronchial cancer account for the majority of newly diagnosed cancer among men in all other racial and ethnic groups, except for Native Americans.
   (1) For Native American men, the majority of cancer-related deaths are caused by prostate, stomach, and liver cancers.
d. Prostate and colorectal cancers rank second in mortality for men in most other racial and ethnic groups.
   (1) The exception to this is that liver cancer is the second leading cause of cancer-related death among Chinese men.
e. With the exception of African American, Filipino, and non-Hispanic white males, stomach cancer is in the top five diagnoses resulting in death.
f. Pancreatic cancer ranks in the top five for cancer-related mortality for all groups except Alaska Natives, Native Americans, and Filipinos.
g. For women, lung cancer is the number one cause of cancer-related death in most racial and ethnic groups.
h. For most groups, breast cancer is the second leading cause of cancer-related deaths, except for Filipina and Hispanic women, for whom breast cancer ranks first in cancer-related mortality.
i. Alaska Native women experience the highest cancer mortality from colorectal cancer. Colorectal cancer ranks among the top five in mortality for all groups except for Native Americans, for whom pancreatic cancer is in the top five causes of cancer-related deaths.

V. Cultural diversity
A. Health care consumers in the U.S. include increasingly diverse populations.
1. In 2010, the U.S. Census Bureau defined the Hispanic or Latino population as "a person of Cuban, Mexican, Puerto Rican, South or Central American, or other Spanish culture or

origin regardless of race" (U.S. Census Bureau, 2011).
  a. In 2010, the Hispanic population increased by 43%, accounting for over half of the total population growth since 2000.
  b. Hispanics account for 16.3% of the U.S. population.
  2. Asians account for 4.6% of the total population, totaling 14.67 million people.
  3. Native Hawaiian and other Pacific Islanders represent 0.2% of the total population.
  4. Over 9 million people in the U.S. identify themselves as being of combined or mixed race.
    a. More than 7% identify themselves as being of three races, and 91.7% identify themselves as being of two races.
  5. Between one third and one half of the total U.S. population identify themselves as other than non-Hispanic white alone.
    a. These groups, representing the minority population, increased from 86.9 million in 2000 to 111.9 million in 2010 (U.S. Census Bureau, 2011).
B. Cultural norms influence relationships between health care practitioners and patients or caregivers.
  1. Cultural factors include multiple aspects, from race and ethnicity to gender, sexual orientation, age, geographic region, and socioeconomic status.
  2. Although traditions and trends emerge in various groups, it is impossible to make sweeping generalities across populations.
  3. Learned values and beliefs give meaning to life events and to relationships.
    a. Some cultures place a high value on commitment to long-term relationships.
      (1) A strong bond exists within the community, and the relationships are more important than tasks.
      (2) Shifts or loss of interest in relationships may signal depression (Reinschmidt, Chong, & Nichter, 2013).
C. Culture affects time orientation to past, present, or future.
  1. In some cultures, time is fluid and flexible, and the process takes priority over the task at hand.
D. Cultural norms vary. Below are some examples (Management Sciences for Health, 2008; Vermont Department of Health, 2013).
  1. Cultures hold wide-ranging beliefs about personal space and eye contact.
    a. In some cultures, closeness, touching, and eye contact are a source of comfort and support.

  b. Other cultures are not demonstrative, and direct eye contact or touching is considered intrusive.
  2. Facial expressions have a wide range of meanings.
    a. Some cultures view smiling as an expression of happiness, but other cultures may smile during uncomfortable experiences as a nervous reaction or to divert attention from sadness.
    b. Winking means different things in different cultures.
      (1) As a sexual invitation
      (2) To convey a shared joke
      (3) May be viewed as a rude gesture
  3. Hand gestures hold meanings unique to a culture.
    a. The hand signal that people in the U.S. use to mean "OK" is the symbol for money in some cultures, and in other cultures, it is used as an offensive gesture to indicate a bodily orifice.
    b. "Thumbs up" gesture widely recognized in the U.S. as a congratulatory gesture has vulgar connotations in other cultures.
    c. Many cultures view pointing with a single finger as rude and prefer using the entire hand to point to something or indicate direction.
  4. Touch has specific meaning in cultures, and what is acceptable varies widely.
    a. In some cultures, touching, including kissing, is appropriate between people who have just met, whereas other cultures disapprove of touching between acquaintances.
  5. Posture and physical position have varying significance in different cultures.
    a. Showing the bottom of the feet to others may be seen as rude in some cultures.
    b. In some cultures, it is important to be facing the person to whom you are speaking.
    c. Hand position may also represent specific meaning.
    d. In some cultures, placing hands on the hips while speaking to someone is indicative of anger or confrontation.
VI. Poverty as a culture and cancer
  A. Poverty is considered a culture that affects the health status of people.
    1. Access to health care services is a major determinant of health status.
      a. Cancer prevention through early screening is not available to people without access to

primary health care (Freeman, 2004; World Health Organization, 2013).

(1) The poor lack access to quality health care.

(2) Poor people often do not seek health care if they are not able to pay for it.

(3) Pursuing health care services is often not a priority for poor people who are occupied with obtaining food and shelter.

(4) The poor have a higher risk for illness, including cancer, because of personal and environmental factors, including poor nutrition, being more likely to being exposed to carcinogens in the workplace, and having poor health habits such as smoking.

(5) People living in poverty are more often diagnosed with cancer in advanced stages.

2. Cancer prevention, defined as health-seeking behaviors and early screening, is a major determinant of risk for cancer (Elk & Landrine, 2012).

VII. Responses to the cancer experience

A. The meaning of a life-threatening diagnosis such as cancer is largely influenced by culture.

B. Cultural norms and behaviors have a major impact on all aspects of the cancer experience, including screening, seeking diagnosis, treatment options, symptom management, response to advanced cancer, hospice use, and end-of-life care (Carroll-Johnson et al., 2006; Kagawa-Singer, 2000).

C. Cancer prevention behaviors

1. Cultures that do not trust the conventional medicine system in the U.S. may not participate in screening.

2. Some cultures rely heavily on traditional (unlicensed) healers and may choose not to pursue traditional models of health and wellness.

3. Individuals or groups who are recent immigrants to the U.S. may lack knowledge about cancer screening.

4. Some cultures may hold a fatalistic view of cancer.

a. They may view cancer as being synonymous with certain death, and they may not believe that anything can be done to change their fate. This belief may keep them from participating in screening.

D. Response to diagnosis of cancer

1. Diagnosis of cancer is most often considered devastating news.

a. Depending on an individual's culture, the response may range from one of stoic acceptance to one that is highly demonstrative.

(1) Studies showed that Euro-American women responded very differently from how Chinese-American and Japanese-American women did when diagnosed with cancer.

(a) Both groups coped in a positive way, even though each response was very different.

(i) Euro-American women accessed an extensive personal support system and verbalized their intent to fight the disease, viewing it as the enemy.

(ii) Chinese-American and Japanese-American women proceeded with similar treatment decisions in a quietly stoic manner, without garnering a wide circle of support, and they did not talk about their disease or suffering.

E. Participation in clinical trials

1. Clinical trials are the foundation on which evidence-based practice is built.

2. Cultural influences determine the response to clinical trials as a health care option, and cultural factors present barriers to patient participation in clinical trials.

a. Participation in a clinical trial is considered an altruistic service to future patients.

b. Some patients will pursue all possible clinical trials in the hopes of benefiting from a treatment to achieve a cure.

c. Some patients enroll in a clinical trial to gain access to treatment that they are not otherwise able to pay for.

F. Coping with advanced cancer and end of life

1. Cultural and religious beliefs and norms lead to varied responses to advanced cancer and end of life.

2. These responses range on a continuum from fighting (as in combat) to passively waiting for death (Chiu, Donoghue, & Chenoweth, 2005).

VIII. Spiritual and religious diversity

A. Definitions

1. *Spirituality* and *religion* are often used interchangeably.

a. Although the two concepts are not mutually exclusive, one cannot be substituted for the other.

b. *Religion* describes organized systems of faith and worship that follow regulated practices intended to enhance spirituality.
   (1) For this reason, religiosity is rarely discussed without spirituality being at the core of the discussion.
   (2) A person may consider himself or herself a spiritual being without belonging to an organized religion.
   (3) As defined in this chapter, spirituality applies to all persons, whether they consider themselves spiritual or not.
2. Spirituality is "the personal quest for understanding answers to ultimate questions about life, about meaning, and about relationships to the sacred or transcendent, which may or may not lead to or arise from the development of religious rituals and the formation of community" (Koenig, McCullough, & Larson, 2001).
3. Spirituality "may be experienced with or without conceptual philosophy and named deity or deities. Spiritual values include honesty, trust, kindness, generosity, tolerance, patience, humility, perseverance, hope, courage, nonviolence, gratitude, compassion, moderation, connection, service, joy, love, and faith" (Williams-Orlando, 2012).

B. Spirituality and religiosity may influence a person's health-seeking behaviors with regard to cancer prevention.
1. Spirituality and religiosity have been identified as strong influences in health-related decision making (Gullatte, Brawley, Kinney, Powe, & Mooney, 2010; Peteet & Balboni, 2013).
2. A fatalistic view associated with spiritual or religious beliefs may result in a delay in seeking medical care.

C. Spirituality and religiosity influence the patient's adjustment to cancer.
1. Ability to cope with the initial diagnosis of cancer and to make decisions regarding cancer treatment independent of other cultural factors
2. May have a positive impact on the patient's response to cancer and its treatment (Carroll-Johnson et al., 2006; Harandy et al., 2010)
3. May experience spiritual distress associated with a cancer diagnosis for a variety of reasons
   a. A sense of abandonment by the greater power they believe in
   b. Inability to find meaning in their cancer diagnosis

c. Feel that they are being punished, justly or unjustly

D. The patient with cancer may experience a heightened sense of spirituality associated with a cancer diagnosis. Patients may:
1. Find joy in discovering that they are loved and cared for by family and friends, and by their community.
2. Experience a new or amplified connection with nature or the world around them.
3. Discover an intensified sense of spirituality or faith.
4. Feel a greater sense of appreciation for simple pleasures of life.

E. People who view cancer as "the will of God" may respond with either enhanced participation in their cancer treatment or by taking a passive, nonparticipative role in cancer screening, diagnosis, and subsequent treatment, depending on religious and other cultural influences (Harandy et al., 2010).
1. Patients and caregivers may view cancer as a punishment for sins committed (Harandy et al., 2010).
2. Viewing cancer as a just punishment may lead patients to take a passive stance, believing that the greater power they believe in has a plan for them and may not be motivated to participate in treatment.
3. Viewing cancer as an unjust punishment may cause patients to feel betrayed. The result may be spiritual distress that prevents the patient from finding meaning in their illness.

F. Spirituality and religiosity also influence how caregivers perceive the cancer experience.
1. Spirituality and religion may be a source of strength for caregivers.
2. Caregivers may have negative responses to the cancer caregiving experience in the context of spirituality or religion.
   a. Caregivers may experience guilt that they are healthy when their loved one is suffering.
   b. Caregivers may experience spiritual distress related to a perception of an unjust greater power.
3. Caregivers may feel overwhelmed by the responsibility of giving love, coupled with the perception that their loved one is no longer able to return their love.
4. Caregivers may feel that they are being punished.

G. Spirituality and religiosity may have a beneficial or harmful impact on the patient's and caregiver's adjustment to cancer and their participation in treatment (Maliski, Connor, Williams, & Litwin, 2010; Thuné-Boyle, Stygall, Keshtgar, Davidson, & Newman, 2013).

1. Relying on faith as a coping mechanism may help patients to overcome the initial shock and distress related to a new diagnosis of cancer.
2. Acceptance of the cancer diagnosis related to a belief in a higher power as being in control of life and death has been shown to correlate with better adjustment to illness.
3. Patients whose faith include the belief that they have an obligation to self-care to be worthy of divine intervention are more likely to be active participants in their cancer treatment.
4. Patients may transfer their faith in a higher power to faith in their physician to be able to cure their disease (Maliski et al., 2010).
5. Feeling punished, abandoned, or both has been shown to contribute to higher levels of distress for patients and may function as a barrier to active participation in treatment.

H. Spirituality and religiosity may have a beneficial or harmful influence on responses to end-of-life issues.

1. Patients who believe in existence after death may find joy in the prospect of the afterlife.
2. Patients whose belief system does not include an afterlife may feel despondent about the finality of death.

ASSESSMENT

I. Assessment includes the cultural, spiritual and religious beliefs of patients and caregivers and incorporates assessment findings into their nursing diagnoses and nursing plan of care (Dossey & Keegan, 2012).

A. The oncology nurse first recognizes his or her own culture, spirituality, and religiosity and how this may affect his or her perception of others.
B. The oncology nurse recognizes that culture, spirituality, and religiosity are part of the whole person and, as such, are assessed in the context of the human experience.
C. Assessment of the patient and caregivers includes, but is not limited to, the patient's support system, cultural beliefs and practices, philosophical or religious belief system, sense of belonging, and love for self and others.
D. The oncology nurse's spiritual assessment is performed without judgment and includes the following (Carroll-Johnson et al., 2006; Dossey & Keegan, 2012; NCI, 2012):

1. Identification of patient's and caregivers' spiritual support system; may include family, friends, congregation, or other group that patient and caregivers identify
2. Religious denomination, if any; also religious or spiritual practices or daily rituals, along with any related needs to support such practices
3. Beliefs of philosophy of life as pertaining to meaning and purpose
4. Exploration of the meaning of the cancer diagnosis for the patient and caregivers
5. Presence of spiritual distress, or loss of faith, experienced by the patient and caregivers
6. Presence of deepening of spirituality or religious faith as a result of the cancer diagnosis
7. Conflicts between spiritual or religious beliefs and cancer treatments
8. Spiritually related coping strategies used by the patient and caregivers; expression of inner strength(s) or ability to manifest joy or peace
9. Concerns about death or afterlife
10. Ways that the oncology nurse may support the patient and caregivers' spiritual needs

PROBLEM STATEMENTS AND OUTCOME IDENTIFICATION

I. Risk for Spiritual Distress and Impaired Religiosity (NANDA-I)

A. Expected outcomes

1. The patient states conflicts or disturbances related to practice of her or his belief system.
2. The patient discusses beliefs about spiritual issues.
3. The patient states feelings of trust in self, God, or other beliefs.
4. The patient continues spiritual practices not detrimental to health, treatment, or both.
5. The patient discusses feelings about death.
6. The patient displays a mood appropriate for the situation.

PLANNING AND IMPLEMENTATION

I. Interventions to enhance spirituality or religiosity and hopefulness.

A. Respecting patient's spiritual and religious beliefs and planning care that honors these beliefs

1. Creating time, space, and privacy, as needed, for spiritual or religious rituals
2. When appropriate (per patient request), praying with patient, caregivers, or both as a sincere, genuine gesture
3. Encouraging patient and caregivers to speak with their spiritual or religious leader

B. Avoiding proselytizing—the nurse does not impose his or her own spiritual or religious beliefs on patients and caregivers

Part 5

C. Supporting the patient's use of spiritual coping
   1. Referring the patient and caregivers to a hospital chaplain or support group that can support coping with spiritual issues
D. Assisting the patient in exploring modalities to enhance spiritual well-being
   1. Meditation (e.g., mindfulness meditation)
   2. Yoga
   3. Prayer
   4. Expressive therapies
      a. Art therapy
      b. Music therapy
      c. Journaling
         (1) Gratitude journaling
         (2) Expressive journaling

EVALUATION

The oncology nurse systematically and regularly evaluates the patient's and family's responses to interventions to determine progress toward the achieving a sense of hope, locus of control, and spiritual peace. Relevant data are collected, and actual findings are compared with expected findings. Nursing diagnoses, outcomes, and plans of care are reviewed and revised, as necessary.

References

American Cancer Society (ACS). (2013). *Cancer facts & figures 2013.* http://www.cancer.org/acs/groups/content/@epidemiologysurveilance/documents/document/acspc-036845.pdf.

Carroll-Johnson, R. M., Gorman, L. M., & Bush, N. J. (2006). *Psychosocial nursing care along the cancer continuum.* Pittsburgh: Oncology Nursing Society.

Chiu, Y. Y., Donoghue, J., & Chenoweth, L. (2005). Responses to advanced cancer: Chinese-Australians. *Journal of Advanced Nursing, 52*(5), 498–507.

Dossey, B. M., & Keegan, L. (2012). *Holistic nursing: A handbook for practice* (6th ed.). Sudbury, MA: Jones and Bartlett.

Elk, R., & Landrine, H. (2012). *Cancer disparities: Causes and evidence-based solutions.* New York: Springer.

Freeman, H. P. (2004). Poverty, culture, and social injustice: determinants of cancer disparities. *CA: A Cancer Journal for Clinicians, 54*(2), 72–77.

Gullatte, M. M., Brawley, O., Kinney, A., Powe, B., & Mooney, K. (2010). Religiosity, spirituality, and cancer fatalism beliefs on delay in breast cancer diagnosis in African American women. *Journal of Religion and Health, 49*, 62–72.

Harandy, T. F., Ghofranipour, F., Montazeri, A., Anoosheh, M., Bazargan, M., Mohammadi, E., et al. (2010). Muslim breast cancer survivor spirituality: Coping strategy or health-seeking behavior hindrance? *Health Care for Women International, 31*, 88–98.

Herdman, T. H. (2012). *NANDA international nursing diagnoses: Definitions and classification, 2012-2014.* Oxford: Wiley-Blackwell.

Heurtin-Roberts, S. (2004). *Race and ethnicity in health and vital statistics.* http://www.ncvhs.hhs.gov/040902p1.pdf.

Kagawa-Singer, M. (2000). *A socio-cultural perspective on cancer control issues for Asian Americans.* http://www.ncbi.nlm.nig.gov/pmc/articles/PMC1618773/.

Koenig, H. G., McCullough, M. E., & Larson, D. B. (2001). *Handbook of religion and health.* New York: Oxford University Press.

Larson, D. B., Swyers, J. P., & McCllough, M. E. (1998). *Scientific research on spirituality and health: A consensus report (pp. 68-82).* Rockville, MD: National Institute on Healthcare Research.

Maliski, S. L., Connor, S. E., Williams, L., & Litwin, M. S. (2010). Faith among low-income, African American/black men treated for prostate cancer. *Cancer Nursing, 33*(6), 470–478.

Management Sciences for Health. (2008). The provider's guide to quality and culture. http://erc.msh.org/mainpage.cfm?file=4.6.0.htm&module=provider&language=English.

Merriam-Webster. (2013). *Merriam-Webster online: Dictionary and thesaurus.* http://www.merriam-webster.com/.

National Cancer Institute (NCI). (2013). *Health disparities defined.* http://crchd.cancer.gov/disparities/defined.html.

National Cancer Institute (NCI). (2012). *Spirituality in cancer care.* http://www.cancer.gov/cancertopics/pdq/supportivecare/spirituality/HealthProfessional/page1/AllPages/Print.

Peteet, J. R., & Balboni, M. J. (2013). Spirituality and religion in oncology. *CA: a Cancer Journal for Clinicians, 63*(4), 280–289.

Reinschmidt, K. M., Chong, J., & Nichter, M. (2013). Monitoring shifts in social relations among chronically ill Mexican-Americans as a culturally sensitive indicator of depression. *Practicing Anthropology, 35*(3), 33–37.

Thuné-Boyle, I. C. V., Stygall, J., Keshtgar, M. R. S., Davidson, T. I., & Newman, S. P. (2013). Religious/spiritual coping resources and their relationship with adjustment in patients newly diagnosed with breast cancer in the UK. *Psycho-Oncology, 22*, 646–658.

U.S. Census Bureau. (2011). *Overview of race and Hispanic origin: 2010.* http://www.census.gov/prod/cen2010/briefs/c2010br-02.pdf.

U.S. Census Bureau. (2012). *The Asian population 2010.* www.census.gov/prod/cen2010/briefs/c2010br-11.pdf.

U.S. Department of Health and Human Services (DHHS). (2013). *2012 HHS poverty guidelines.* http://aspe.hhs.gov/poverty/12poverty.shtm.

Vermont Department of Health. (2013). *Health screening recommendations for children and adolescents: Cultural differences in non-verbal communication.* http://healthvermont.gov/family/toolkit/tools%5CF-6%20Cultural%20Differences%20in%20Nonverbal%20Communic.pdf.

Williams-Orlando, C. (2012). Spirituality in integrative medicine. *Integrative Medicine, 11*(4), 34–41.

World Health Organization. (2013). *Health topics: Poverty.* http://www.who.int/topics/poverty/en/.

CHAPTER 36

Altered Body Image

Elizabeth A. Freitas

Neoplastic Alopecia

OVERVIEW

I. Definition—treatment related hair loss, temporary or permanent, on any location on the body
II. Risk factors
  A. Undergoing treatments that affect rapidly dividing cells, damage hair follicles, or shift hair into shedding phase
    1. Radiation therapy (RT)
      a. Dosage greater than 30 to 35 Gy may cause temporary hair loss.
      b. Dosage greater than 40 Gy usually causes permanent hair loss in treated area from scarring of scalp.
      c. Craniospinal irradiation increases risk of permanent alopecia.
    2. Chemotherapy
      a. Agent or dose dependent
      b. Normally occurs 1 to 3 weeks after chemotherapy starts
      c. Typically has a sudden onset
      d. Increases with administration of multiple chemotherapy agents
      e. Classes of chemotherapeutic agents that often cause alopecia—alkylating agents, anthracyclines, antibiotics, antimetabolites, vinca alkaloids, and taxanes

ASSESSMENT

I. History—current hair growth, style, and color
II. Physical examination—location of thinning hair or complete hair loss
  A. Use of chemotherapy-induced alopecia grading scale
  B. Psychosocial assessment—perceptions of client before and after hair loss regarding self-concept, body image, perceived sexuality, and responses of others to hair loss (Atay, Conk, & Bahar, 2012)

PROBLEM STATEMENTS AND OUTCOME IDENTIFICATION

I. Interruption of Integumentary Function
  A. Expected outcome—hair loss is minimized.
II. Ineffective Coping (NANDA-I)
  A. Expected outcome—patient identifies measures to adapt to or cope with alopecia.
  B. Expected outcome—patient accesses community resources, insurance benefits, others who also have dealt with hair loss issues.
  C. Expected outcome—patient demonstrates acceptance of change or loss and an ability to adjust to lifestyle change.

PLANNING AND IMPLEMENTATION

I. Interventions to prevent hair loss
  A. Scalp cooling—for patients undergoing chemotherapy, moderately effective in minimizing hair loss (van den Hurk et al., 2012), although not approved by the U.S. Food and Drug Administration (FDA)
    1. Success dependent on chemotherapy agent, doses and duration of infusion, and the patient's liver function (Kargar, Sarvestani, Khojasteh, & Heidari, 2011)
    2. Risk of scalp metastases limited (Lemieux, Desbiens, & Hogue, 2011)
    3. Not recommended for hematologic malignancies
  B. RT—if feasible, maximum dose of less than 16 Gy at less than 5 mm under the surface of skin to minimize damage to the hair follicle (Rogers, 2011)
II. Interventions to protect the bare head
  A. Sunscreen (at least sun protection factor [SPF] 15) that offers both ultraviolet A (UVA) and UVB protection
  B. Head coverings
III. Interventions to improve coping
  A. Before chemotherapy—anticipating hair loss (computer imaging) and evaluating for likely

reactions; providing a list of local resources, for example, "Look Good/Feel Better" and Internet sites; recommending research of wigs before hair loss; and considering potential need for additional psychological support (McGarvey et al., 2010)

   B. During and after chemotherapy—having the patient acknowledge hair loss; inquiring about coping; considering dermatologic evaluation; and continuing to offer support and resources

IV. Interventions to camouflage—wigs: human or animal hair or synthetic (synthetic are not heat resistant); turbans: polyester, nylon or cotton (cotton slips less) and hats (Yeager & Olsen, 2011)

EVALUATION

The oncology nurse assesses the client's initial risk for alopecia and regularly evaluates the client's responses to interventions to determine progress toward the achievement of expected outcomes, keeping in mind that clients may have a more significant response to hair loss than anticipated. After assessment, actual findings are compared with expected findings, nursing diagnoses, and outcomes and the plans of care are reviewed and revised, as necessary.

Altered Body Image

OVERVIEW

  I. Definition
    A. Response to actual or perceived change in body structure or function, such as weight gain or loss, amputation, infertility, or cognitive dysfunction, which may manifest as dysfunctional perceptions, cognitions, emotions, or behaviors that affect one's daily functioning and quality of life (Ridolfi, & Crowther, 2012)
    B. Impact of the changes—may last for years and change over time (Molassiotis, Wengström, & Kearney, 2010)
  II. Risk factors—loss of organ or scarring, a change that is visible such as mastectomy, amputation, head and neck cancer, colostomy/ileostomy, or lymphedema (Flynn et al., 2011; Ridner, Bonner, Deng, & Sinclair, 2012)
  III. Potential impact on treatment decisions
    A. Breast cancer patients—need to know pros and cons of nipple-sparing mastectomy (and whether this is an appropriate clinical option) (Long, 2013)
    B. Testicular prosthesis—goal is to look normal and whole (Harrington, 2011)
  IV. Cancer treatments' impact on body image
    A. Aggressiveness of surgery
      1. Mastectomy distress greater compared with breast-conserving treatments; response regarding impact on body image mixed—not significant for some racial groups but significant for others

      2. Total abdominal hysterectomy body image worse compared with total laparoscopic hysterectomy (Janda et al., 2010)
      3. Ileo-conduit for bladder cancer and stoma for colon cancer more distressing (Fitch, Miller, Sharir, & McAndrew, 2010; Sharpe, Patel, & Clark, 2011)
    B. Hormone therapy—negative body image because of weight gain (Flynn et al., 2011; Harrington, 2011; Ervik, & Asplund, 2012).
    C. Different perceptions of patients and health care professionals—concerns of patients with head and neck cancer related to function (speech and exercise tolerance) and health care professionals' concerns for patients related to anatomic defects and patients' body image (Tschiesner, Becker, & Cieza, 2010)

ASSESSMENT

  I. Use of a standardized scale
    A. Body image scale (Hopwood et al., 2010)
    B. Site-specific scales—breast, head and neck
    C. Population-specific scales—Portuguese, Korean, and population-specific side effects
    D. Side effect specific scales—hair loss
    E. Patients' expectation that providers ask about body image issues (Cohen et al., 2012)
  II. Patients' baseline functional status and initial distress—may affect body image (Härt et al., 2010); low quality of life linked to problems with body image (Grant et al., 2011); self-compassion—may lessen a patients' body image disturbance (Przezdziecki et al., 2012)

PROBLEM STATEMENTS AND OUTCOME IDENTIFICATION

  I. Disturbed Body Image (NANDA-I)
    A. Expected outcome—patient demonstrates acceptance of change of appearance, loss of function, or both, and an ability to adjust to lifestyle change.
    B. Expected outcome—patient returns to prior level of social involvement.

PLANNING AND IMPLEMENTATION

  I. Interventions related to acceptance of change of appearance, loss of function, or both
    A. Assessment of patient's perception of the change and its impact on activities of daily living (ADLs), social behavior, personal relationships, and work
    B. Encouraging verbalization of positive and negative feelings about the actual or perceived changes (Konradsen, Kirkevold, McCallin, Cayé-Thomasen, & Zoffmann, 2012)
    C. Teaching adaptive behaviors
      1. Use of adaptive equipment
      2. Use of wigs, head coverings, cosmetics

3. Care of prosthesis or other adaptive devices—well-fitting prosthesis improves psychological coping: confidence, normalcy, and self-esteem (Hsu, Wang, Chu, & Yen, 2010; Fitch et al., 2012)

D. Introduction of adjuvant therapies

   1. Counseling—intracouple communication, information needs about intimacy and how to manage treatment-related sexual challenges and with partners (Cochrane, Lewis, & Griffith, 2011; Galbraith, Fink, & Wilkins, 2011; Kaplan & Pacelli, 2011)

   2. Support from family and friends (Haisfield-Wolfe, Mcguire, & Krumm, 2012)

   3. Complementary health approaches

      a. Art therapy—assists patient to integrate body image and create insights regarding recovery and survival (Thibeault, & Sabob, 2012)

      b. Strength training and physical exercise—help maintain function, socialization, and a sense of normalcy (Duijts, Faber, Oldenburg, van Beurden, & Aaronson, 2011)

      c. Mindfulness—decreases perceived stress and anxiety (Matchim, Armer, & Stewart, 2011)

E. Referring patients to resources and support groups, as appropriate

EVALUATION

The oncology nurse systematically and regularly evaluates the patient's and family's responses to cognitive and physical interventions to determine progress toward the achievement of a healthy body image, maintains social activity, and adjusts plans to meet expected outcomes. After relevant body image data are collected, actual findings are compared with expected findings, nursing diagnoses, and outcomes, the plans of care are reviewed and revised, as necessary.

References

Atay, S., Conk, Z., & Bahar, Z. (2012). Identifying symptom clusters in paediatric cancer patients using the Memorial Symptom Assessment Scale. *European Journal of Cancer Care, 21*, 460–468. http://dx.doi.org/10.1111/j.1365-2354.2012.01324.x46.

Cochrane, B., Lewis, F., & Griffith, K. (2011). Exploring a diffusion of benefit: Does a woman with breast cancer derive benefit from an intervention delivered to her partner? *Oncology Nursing Forum, 38*(2), 207–214. http://dx.doi.org/10.1188/11.ONF.207-214.

Cohen, M., Anderson, R., Jensik, K., Xiang, Q., Pruszynski, J., & Walker, A. (2012). Communication between breast cancer patients and their physicians about breast-related body image issues. *Plastic Surgical Nursing, 32*(1), 101–105. http://dx.doi.org/10.1097/PSN 0b013e3182650994.

Duijts, S., Faber, M., Oldenburg, H., van Beurden, M., & Aaronson, N. (2011). Effectiveness of behavioral techniques

and physical exercise on psychosocial functioning and health-related quality of life in breast cancer patients and survivors: A meta-analysis. *Psycho-Oncology, 20*, 115–126. http://dx.doi.org/10.1002/pon.1728.

Ervik, B., & Asplund, K. (2012). Dealing with a troublesome body: A qualitative interview of men's experiences living with prostate cancer treated with endocrine therapy. *European Journal of Oncology Nursing, 16*(2), 103–108. http://dx.doi.org/10.1016/j.ejon.2011.04.005.

Fitch, M., McAndrew, A., Harris, A., Anderson, J., Kubon, T., & McCleenen, J. (2012). Perspectives of women about external breast prostheses. *Canadian Oncology Nursing Journal, 22*(3), 162–174.

Fitch, M., Miller, D., Sharir, S., & McAndrew, A. (2010). Radical cystectomy for bladder cancer: A qualitative study of patient experiences and implications for practice. *Canadian Oncology Nursing Journal, 20*(4), 177–181. http://dx.doi.org/10.5737/1181912x204177181.

Flynn, K., Jeffery, D., Keefe, F., Porter, L., Shelby, R., Fawzy, M., et al. (2011). Sexual functioning along the cancer continuum: Focus group results from the Patient Reported Outcomes Measurement Information System (PROMISTM). *Psycho-Oncology, 20*(4), 378–386. http://dx.doi.org/10.1002/pon.173.

Galbraith, M., Fink, R., & Wilkins, G. (2011). Couples surviving prostate cancer: Challenges in their lives and relationships. *Seminars in Oncology Nursing, 27*(4), 300–308. http://dx.doi.org/10.1016/j.soncn.2011.07.008.

Grant, M., McMullen, C., Altschuler, A., Mohler, M., Hornborook, M., Herrinton, L., et al. (2011). Gender differences in quality of life among long-term colorectal cancer survivors with ostomies. *Oncology Nursing Forum, 38*(5), 587–596. http://dx.doi.org/10.1188/11. ONF.587-596.

Haisfield-Wolfe, M., Mcguire, D., & Krumm, S. (2012). Perspectives on coping among patients with head and neck cancer receiving radiation. *Oncology Nursing Forum, 39*(3), E249–E257. http://dx.doi.org/10.1188/12.ONF.E249-E257.

Harrington, J. (2011). Implications of treatment on body image and quality of life. *Seminars in Oncology Nursing, 4*, 290–299. http://dx.doi.org/10.1016/j.soncn.2011.07.007.

Härt, K., Engel, J., Herschbach, P., Reinecker, H., Sommer, H., & Friese, K. (2010). Personality traits and psychosocial stress: Quality of life over 2 years following breast cancer diagnosis and psychological impact factors. *Psycho-Oncology, 19*, 160–169. http://dx.doi.org/10.1002/pon.1536.

Hopwood, P., Haviland, J., Sumo, G., Mills, J., Bliss, J., & Yarnold, J. (2010). Comparison of patient-reported breast, arm, and shoulder symptoms and body image after radiotherapy for early breast cancer: 5-year follow-up in the randomized Standardization of Breast Radiotherapy (START) trials. *Lancet Oncology, 11*, 231–240. http://dx.doi.org/10.1016/S1470- 2045(09)70382-1.

Hsu, S., Wang, H., Chu, S., & Yen, H. (2010). Effectiveness of informational and emotional consultation on the psychological impact on women with breast cancer who underwent modified radical mastectomy. *Journal of Nursing Research, 18*(3), 215–225. http://dx.doi.org/10.1097/JNR.0b013e3181ed57d0.

Janda, M., Gebski, V., Brand, A., Hogg, R., Jobling, T., Land, R., et al. (2010). Quality of life after total laparoscopic hysterectomy versus total abdominal hysterectomy for stage I endometrial cancer: A randomized trial. *The Lancet Oncology, 11*(8), 772–780. http://dx.doi.org/10.1016/S1470-2045(10)70145-5.

Kaplan, M., & Pacelli, R. (2011). The sexuality discussion: Tools for the oncology nurse. *Clinical Journal of Oncology Nursing, 15*(1), 15–17. http://dx.doi.org/10.1188/11.CJON.15-17.

Kargar, M., Sarvestani, R., Khojasteh, H., & Heidari, M. (2011). Efficacy of penguin cap as scalp cooling system for prevention of alopecia in patients undergoing chemotherapy. *Journal of Advanced Nursing, 67*(11), 2473–2477. http://dx.doi.org/10.1111/j.1365 2648.2011.05668.x.

Konradsen, H., Kirkevold, M., McCallin, A., Cayé-Thomasen, P., & Zoffmann, V. (2012). Breaking the silence: Integration of facial disfigurement after surgical treatment for cancer. *Qualitative Health Research, 22*(8), 1037–1046. http://dx.doi.org/10.1177/1049732312 448545.

Lemieux, J., Desbiens, C., & Hogue, J. (2011). Breast cancer scalp metastasis as first metastatic site after scalp cooling: Two cases of occurrence after 7- and 9-year follow-up. *Breast Cancer Research and Treatment, 128*, 563–566. http://dx.doi.org/10.1007/s10549-011-1453-y.

Long, L. (2013). The use of nipple-sparing mastectomy in patients with breast cancer. *Clinical Journal of Oncology, 17*(1), 68–73. http://dx.doi.org/10.1188/13.CJON.68-72.

Matchim, Y., Armer, J., & Stewart, R. (2011). Mindfulness-based stress reduction among breast cancer survivors: A literature review and discussion. *Oncology Nursing Forum, 38*(2), E61–E71. http://dx.doi.org/10.1188/11.ONF.E61-E71.

McGarvey, E., Leon-Verdin, M., Baum, L., Bloomfield, K., Brenin, D., Koopman, C., et al. (2010). An evaluation of a computer-imaging program to prepare women for chemotherapy-related alopecia. *Psycho-Oncology, 19*, 756–766. http://dx.doi.org/10.1002/pon.1637.

Molassiotis, A., Wengström, Y., & Kearney, N. (2010). Symptom cluster patterns during the first year after diagnosis with cancer. *Journal of Pain and Symptom Management, 39*(5), 847–858. http://dx.doi.org/10.1016/j.jpainsymman.2009.09.012.

Przezdziecki, A., Sherman, K., Baillie, A., Taylor, A., Foley, E., & Stalgis-Bilinsk, K. (2012). *My changed body: Breast cancer, body image, distress and self-compassion.* http://dx.doi.org/10.1002/pon.3230.

Ridner, S., Bonner, C., Deng, J., & Sinclair, V. (2012). Voices from the shadows: Living with lymphedema. *Cancer Nursing, 35*(1), E18–E26. http://dx.doi.org/10.1098/NCC. 06013c31821404c0.

Ridolfi, D., & Crowther, J. (2012). The link between women's body image disturbances and body-focused cancer screening behaviors: A critical review of the literature and a new integrated model for women. *Body Image, 10*(2), 149–162. http://dx.doi.org/10.1016/j.bodyim. 2012.11.003.

Rogers, S. (2011). Comparison of permanent hair loss in children with standard risk PNETS of the posterior fossa following radiotherapy after surgical resection. *Pediatric Blood & Cancer, 57*(6), 1074–1076. http://dx.doi.org/10.1002/pbc.22992.

Sharpe, L., Patel, D., & Clark, S. (2011). The relationship between body image disturbance and distress in colorectal cancer patients with and without stomas. *Journal of Psychosomatic Research, 70*(5), 395–402. http://dx.doi.org/10.1016/j.jpsychores.2010.11.003.

Thibeault, C., & Sabob, B. (2012). Art, archetypes and alchemy: Images of self following treatment for breast cancer. *European Journal of Oncology Nursing, 16*, 153–157. http://dx.doi.org/10.1016/j.ejon.2011.04.009.

Tschiesner, U., Becker, S., & Cieza, A. (2010). Health professional perspective on disability in head and neck cancer. *Archives of Otolaryngology—Head & Neck Surgery, 136*(6), 576–583. http://dx.doi.org/10.1001/archoto.2010.78.

van den Hurk, C., Peerbooms, M., van de Poll-Franse, L., Nortier, J., Coebergh, & Breed, W. (2012). Scalp cooling for hair preservation and associated characteristics in 1411 chemotherapy patients. Results of the Dutch Cooling Registry. *Acta Oncologica, 51*, 497–504. http://dx.doi.org/10.3109/0284186X.2012.658966.

Yeager, C., & Olsen, E. (2011). Treatment of chemotherapy-induced alopecia. *Dermatologic Therapy, 24*, 432–442. http://dx.doi.org/10.1111/j.1529-8019.2011.01430.x.

CHAPTER 37

Coping Mechanisms and Skills

Geline Joy Tamayo and Ellen Carr

OVERVIEW

I. Prevalence and frequency
   A. All patients, no matter what stage of disease, experience some form or level of distress related to their diagnosis or treatment and so are faced with coping challenges (Cohen & Bankston, 2011; National Comprehensive Cancer Network [NCCN], 2013).
   B. Unidentified and untreated psychosocial distress can increase morbidity, mortality, and the duration and cost of treatment or compromise quality of life (QOL) and compliance (Pedersen, Olesen, Hanson, Zachariae, & Vedsted, 2013).

II. Definitions (related to oncology clinical care)
   A. Distress
      1. Multifactorial unpleasant emotional experiences of a psychological (cognitive, behavioral, emotional), social, and spiritual nature may interfere with the ability to cope effectively with cancer, its physical symptoms, and its treatment.
      2. Distress extends along a continuum, ranging from common normal feelings of vulnerability, sadness, and fears to problems that may become disabilities such as depression, anxiety, panic, social isolation, and existential and spiritual crises (NCCN, 2013; Rokach, Findler, Chin, Lev, & Kollender, 2013).
   B. Coping
      1. Types (Cohen & Bankston, 2011; Tucci, 2012)
         a. Problem-focused—directed toward reducing or eliminating a stressor
         b. Emotion-focused—directed toward changing one's own emotional reaction
         c. Meaning-focused—deriving meaning from the stressful experience
      2. Situational coping—a dynamic process that constantly changes as an individual confronts different stressful demands (McSorley et al., 2014)
   C. Post-traumatic stress disorder

1. Traumatic event or experience prompting specific clinical response
   a. Cognitive (e.g., forgetful, distracted, cannot concentrate)
   b. Behavioral (e.g., fight-or-flight response, avoidance, isolation)
   c. Emotional (e.g., numbing feeling, irritable, angry outbursts)
   d. Physiologic (e.g., insomnia, nightmares, agitated)
2. Response manifested by intense fear, helplessness, horror, reliving the event or experience, or all of these responses (Lelorain, Tessier, Florin, & Bonnaud-Antignac, 2012; Schmidt, Blank, Bellizi, & Park, 2012)

   D. Adaptation
      1. Ability to minimize disruptions to social roles, regulate experience of emotional distress, and maintain active engagement in meaningful life activities (Cohen & Bankston, 2011)

III. Factors influencing coping in oncology patients and their family members (Cohen & Bankston, 2011; National Cancer Institute [NCI], 2011a)
   A. Cancer diagnosis–related (Andreu et al., 2012; Cheng et al., 2013)
      1. Prevailing perception that diagnosis of cancer is a death sentence
      2. Lack of knowledge of the disease process
      3. Physiologic effects of the disease
      4. Unknown prognosis or expected outcome (Llewelyn et al., 2013; Van Laarhoven et al., 2011)
   B. Treatment-related—oncology (Boinon et al., 2014)
      1. Fear of the effects of treatment (Cheung et al., 2012)
         a. Chemotherapy and biotherapy (Andreu et al., 2012)
         b. Radiation therapy (McSorley et al., 2014)
         c. Surgery (Sterba et al., 2013)
         d. Post-treatment (survivorship) (Parelkar, Thompson, Kaw, Miner, & Stein, 2013)

C. Psychological
1. Comorbidities—psychological adjustment disorders (Singer et al., 2013)
2. Various adjustment disorders—criteria or symptoms based on American Psychiatric Association's *Diagnostic and Statistical Manual of Mental Disorders* (DSM-5) (American Psychiatric Association [APA], 2013)
   a. Development of emotional or behavioral symptoms in response to an identifiable stressor(s) occurring within 3 months of the onset of the stressor(s)
      (1) Symptoms or behaviors clinically significant; marked distress in response to stressor
      (2) Significant impairment in social or occupational functioning
      (3) In general, acute disturbance <6 months—chronic disturbance >6 months—with predominant symptoms such as anxiety and depressed mood (alone or combined), conduct, emotion disturbance, or all of these (APA, 2013)
3. Ineffective coping—may occur in crisis situation and may lead to suicidal ideation (Cohen & Bankston, 2011; NCI, 2011c)

D. Social factors (Boinon et al., 2014; Lelorain et al., 2012; Schmidt et al., 2012)
1. Roles—maintaining or changing
2. Health routine tasks, family issues, financial management, and living conditions that affect the individual's ability to cope
3. Family influences

E. Cultural factors (Davis, Rust, & Darby, 2013; Itano, 2011; Lee & Jin, 2013; Rosario & de la Rosa, 2014; Wenzel et al., 2012; see Chapter 35)
1. Issues of social organization, communication, healing practices, and beliefs

F. Factors influenced by gender (Cheng et al., 2013; Hoyt, Stanton, Irwin, & Thomas, 2013)

INEFFECTIVE COPING

I. Anxiety—fear (Cohen & Bankston, 2011; NCI, 2011a; Phelps, Bennett, Hood, Brian, & Murray, 2013)
A. Signs of anxiety
1. Agitation or restlessness
2. Sleep disturbances
3. Excessive autonomic activity
   a. Sweating
   b. Shortness of breath
   c. Lightheadedness; palpitations
4. Weight gain or loss
5. Mood changes
B. Patient's perception of disease and treatment (Pedersen et al., 2013)

1. The conscious or unconscious attempt to deny the knowledge or meaning of an event to reduce anxiety or fear, but leading to the detriment of health
   a. Delays seeking health care attention
   b. Displaced fears of the impact of the disease
   c. Limited perception of relevance of symptoms

II. Depression (Boyajian, 2010; Hamilton et al., 2013; Holslander & McMillan, 2011; NCI, 2011c; Rokach et al., 2013; Van Laarhoven et al., 2011)
A. Symptoms (patients may feel at least one of the following symptoms, lasting for a week or more)
1. Worthlessness
2. Low spirits
3. Inability to sleep, early awakening
4. Decreased or increased appetite
5. Irritability
6. Loss of pleasure in life
7. Withdrawal from others
8. Feelings of sadness, tendency to cry easily
9. Oversleeping
10. Negative viewing of events
11. Self-blame or self-criticism
12. Death thoughts
B. Causes of depression at time of cancer diagnosis
1. Poorly controlled pain
2. Advanced stage of cancer
3. Additional concurrent life stressors
4. Increased physical impairment or discomfort
5. Pancreatic cancer
6. Being unmarried
7. Having head and neck cancer
8. Treatment with certain medications
9. Treatment with certain chemotherapeutic agents
10. Metabolic changes
11. Endocrine abnormalities (Cohen & Bankston, 2011; NCI, 2011c)
C. Risk assessment and interventions (Rodriguez et al., 2012)
1. Indicators of depression that require more focused or involved interventions (Box 37-1)
2. Possible medical causes of cancer-related depression (Box 37-2)
3. Use of common antidepressants (Box 37-3)
D. Suicidal ideation
1. Screen for risk factors—gender (more often men), age, diagnosis, social supports, stressful life events (Cole, Bowling, Paletta, & Balzer, 2014) ⚠

III. Denial (Pedersen et al., 2013)
A. Conscious or unconscious attempt to deny the knowledge or meaning of an event to reduce anxiety or fear, but leading to the detriment of health
1. Delays seeking health care attention
2. Displaces fears of the impact of the disease

Box 37-1

Depression Indicators

Indicators of Depression, Requiring More Focused or Involved Interventions

- History of depression
- Weak social support system (e.g., not married, few friends, solitary work environment)
- Evidence of persistent irrational beliefs or negativistic thinking regarding the diagnosis
- More serious prognosis
- Greater dysfunction related to cancer
- Depressed mood for most of the day on most days

General Symptoms for More Than 2 Weeks

- Diminished pleasure or interest in most activities
- Significant change in appetite and sleep patterns
- Psychomotor agitation or slowing
- Fatigue

- Feelings of worthlessness or excessive, inappropriate guilt
- Poor concentration
- Recurrent thoughts of death or suicide

Because the risk of suicide is elevated in individuals with cancer, patients whose screens suggest suicide risk should be asked about suicidal ideation as part of their clinical evaluation.

Adapted from Cohen, M. & Bankston, S. (2011). Cancer-related distress. In C. H. Yarbro, D. Wujcik & B. H. Gobel. (Eds.). *Cancer nursing: Principles and practice* (7th ed., pp. 667–684) Sudbury, MA: Jones and Bartlett; National Cancer Institute. (2011c). *Depression (PDQ)*. www.cancer.gov/cancertopics/pdq/supportivecare/depression/Patient; Oncology Nursing Society. (2013). Implementing screening for distress: The joint position statement from the american psychosocial oncology society, Association of Oncology Social Work, and Oncology Nursing Society. *Oncology Nursing Forum*, 40(5), 423–424.

Box 37-2

Possible Medical Causes of Cancer-Related Depression

Treatment with Certain Medications

- Corticosteroids
- Interferon-alpha and aldesleukin (interleukin-2 [IL-2])
- Methyldopa
- Reserpine
- Barbiturates
- Propranolol
- Some antibiotics (e.g., amphotericin B)

Treatment with Certain Chemotherapeutic Agents

- Procarbazine
- L-asparaginase
- Interferon-alpha
- IL-2

Metabolic Changes

- Hypercalcemia

- Sodium or potassium imbalance
- Anemia
- Vitamin B_{12} or folate deficiency
- Fever

Endocrine abnormalities

- Hyperthyroidism or hypothyroidism
- Adrenal insufficiency

Adapted from National Cancer Institute. (2011c). *Depression (PDQ)*. www.cancer.gov/cancertopics/pdq/supportivecare/depression/Patient; Zhang, A., Gary, F. & Zhu, H. (2012). What precipitates depression in African-American cancer patients? Triggers and stressors. *Palliative & Supportive Care*, 10(4), 279–286; Lee, H. Y. and S. W. Jin. (2013). Older Korean Cancer survivors' depression and coping: Directions toward culturally competent interventions. *Journal of Psychosocial Oncology*, 31(4), 357–376; Boyajian, R. (2010). Depression's impact on survival in patients with cancer. *Clinical Journal of Oncology Nursing*, 14(5), 649–652.

---

    3. Does not perceive personal relevance of symptoms
    4. Uses self-treatment
  B. Denial not necessarily considered dysfunctional coping (Faller et al., 2013; Tallman, 2013; Tucci, 2012)

ASSESSMENT

I. Assessment and screening
  A. Standards of care established (Brown, 2014; Fischbeck et al., 2013, Holland, 2013; Knobf, Major-Campos, Chaqpar, Seigerman, & McCorkle, 2014; Lazenby, 2014; Muehlbauer, 2013)
  B. Assessment tools

    1. Interview, questionnaire, checklists, psychological tests, observation, metrics (biofeedback, psychoneuroimmunology)
  C. Commonly used assessment tools
    1. NCCN Distress Thermometer (DT) (NCCN, 2013; Tavernier, 2014)
      a. 0 (no distress) to 10 (severe distress) measurement, with accompanying simple questions identifying source of distress
      b. Recommendation that score of 4 or more triggers further physician or nurse evaluation, referral to psychosocial services, or both

---

Box 37-3

Selected Antidepressants

Tricyclic Antidepressants
- Amitriptyline (Elavil)
- Clomipramine (Anafranil)
- Desipramine (Norpramin)
- Doxepin (Sinequan)
- Imipramine (Tofranil)
- Nortriptyline (Pamelor)

Selective Serotonin Reuptake Inhibitors
- Citalopram (Celexa)
- Fluoxetine (Prozac)
- Fluvoxamine (Luvox)
- Paroxetine (Paxil)
- Sertraline (Zoloft)

Monoamine Oxidase Inhibitors
- Tranylcypromine (Parnate)
- Phenelzine (Nardil)

Atypical Antidepressants
- Bupropion (Wellbutrin)
- Trazodone (Desyrel)
- Nefazodone (Serzone)
- Mirtazapine (Remeron)
- Maprotiline (Ludiomil)
- Venlafaxine (Effexor)

Adapted from National Cancer Institute. (2011c). *Depression (PDQ)*. www.cancer.gov/cancertopics/pdq/supportivecare/depression/Patient; Van Laarhoven, H.., Schilderman, J., Bleijenberg, G, Donders, R. Vissers, K.., Verhagen, C. & Prins, J. (2011). Coping, quality of life, depression, and hopelessness in cancer patients in a curative and palliative, end-of-life care setting. *Cancer Nursing, 34*(4), 302–314; Cohen, M. & Bankston, S. (2011). Cancer-related distress. In C. H. Yarbro, D. Wujcik & B. H. Gobel. Cancer nursing: principles and practice (7th ed., pp. 667–684) Sudbury, MA: Jones and Bartlett.

---

2. Hospital Anxiety and Depression Scale (HADS) (Carlson, Waller, & Mitchell, 2012)
  a. 14-item scale (7 questions: anxiety; 7 questions: depression)
  b. Score from 0 to 21 (0 to 3 per question) to evaluate anxiety or depression levels

II. Components of assessment (Brown, 2014; Holland, 2013; Fischbeck et al., 2013; Lazenby, 2014; Muehlbauer, 2013)
  A. Assessment of psychosocial distress
    1. Identification of psychosocial needs that affect QOL and activities of daily living (ADLs)
  B. Identification of patterns of coping
  C. Observing for contributing factors to ineffective coping (see Ineffective Coping section above)
    1. Anxiety, depression, insomnia
    2. Previous stressors and the coping mechanisms used
    3. Diagnosis of mental disorders
  D. Providing opportunities for patient to discuss the meaning of the situation for him or her
    1. Self-described definitions of well-being and QOL
  E. Identifying contributors to distress
    1. Social factors contributing to distress
    2. Presence of family and community support (Zabalegui, Cabrera, Navarro, & Cebria, 2013)

PROBLEM STATEMENT AND OUTCOME IDENTIFICATION

I. Infective Coping (NANDA)
  A. Expected outcome—patient develops coping skills to process information and make appropriate decisions.
  B. Expected outcome—patient will be independent with ADLs and new skills.
  C. Expected outcome—patient socializes with family and friends.
  D. Expected outcome—patient returns to previous work or activities or occupational training for alternative work and leisure activities.
  E. Expected outcome—patient participates in support groups and informational systems to assist in problem solving, lifestyle changes, and adjustment.
  F. Expected outcome—family or caregivers demonstrate improved emotional health and well-being by expressing that they have better mood and outlook.
  G. Expected outcome—patient describes plan for follow-up care

II. Ineffective Self-Health Management (NANDA)
  A. Expected outcome—client describes integration of therapeutic regimen into daily living.
  B. Expected outcome—client demonstrates continued commitment to integration of therapeutic regimen into daily living routines.

III. Social Isolation (NANDA)
  A. Expected outcome—patient expresses enhanced personal well-being.
  B. Expected outcome—patient exhibits enhanced social interaction skills and involvement.

IV. Caregiver Role Strain (NANDA)
  A. Expected outcome—caregiver expresses increased feelings of support, reports low feelings or no feelings of burden, maintains own physical and psychological health, identifies resources available to help giving care, and verbalizes mastery of the

care situation, feeling confident and competent to provide care.

PLANNING AND IMPLEMENTATION

I. Providing effective communication and emotional support (Fischbeck et al., 2013; Given & Northouse, 2011; Holslander & McMillan, 2011; NCI, 2011b; Parelkar et al., 2013; Semple et al., 2013; Tallman, 2013)

    A. Use of verbal and nonverbal therapeutic communication approaches, including empathy, active listening, and confrontation to encourage patient and family to express emotions and solve problems

        1. Encouraging the patient to express feelings and thoughts

        2. Exploring the meaning of the person's illness experience and identifying uncertainties and needs (Butt, 2011)

        3. Providing information on possible disease trajectories to allow planning for future management

        4. Providing honest perception of reality and feedback about symptoms and behavior

        5. Encouraging the patient to explore adaptive behaviors to optimize functioning and accomplish ADLs

    B. Collaborating with the patient to identify strengths (Chen & Chang, 2012)

        1. Ability to relate the facts of the contributing stress factors

        2. Ability to recognize the source of the stressors

        3. Assisting the patient to expand personal skills and knowledge (Schmidt et al., 2012; Tallman, 2013)

    C. Being supportive of coping behaviors (Chen & Chang, 2012; Lelorain et al., 2012)

        1. Methods to self-manage distress (Garssen et al., 2013)

        2. Assisting the patient to set realistic goals related to cancer diagnosis and treatment

        3. Participating in planning care and scheduled activities

            a. Supporting decisions regarding patient's method of integrating therapeutic regimens

        4. Encouraging opportunities for social support (Zabalegui et al., 2013)

    D. Supporting spiritual needs, faith, and inquiry (Candy et al., 2012; Maliski, Connor, Williams, & Litwin, 2010; Puchalski, 2012)

    E. Initiating and coordinating referrals to counseling, psychotherapy, and support

    F. Providing and encouraging the use of available resources (Sterba et al., 2013; Wenzel et al., 2012)

        1. Providing the patient and family with a list of appropriate community-based resources (e.g., housing, home health care)

II. Patient and family education (Epiphaniou et al., 2012; Northouse et al., 2013; Rydahl-Hansen, 2013)

    A. Providing verbal and written information to the client and family about the disease, process, therapy, and effects of therapy

    B. Providing verbal and written information to the client and family about treatment, medications, side effects, and management

    C. Offering instructions regarding standard and alternative coping strategies

III. Referrals or counseling (Harvey, Rogak, Ford, & Holland, 2013; Holland, 2013; Tucci, 2012)

    A. Coordinating referral appointments

    B. Providing documentation or assessment to support counseling or therapy referral

IV. Support groups (Emilsson, Svensk, Tavelin, & Lindh, 2012; Rosario & de la Rosa, 2014; Sautier, Mehnert, Hocker, & Schilling, 2014)

    A. Psychosocial support groups and resources are available to patients across the continuum of cancer care, including spiritual, well-being, cultural, age-specific, exercise, movement, emotional, and sexual preference groups, caregivers, and disease-specific care.

    B. Support groups provide patients and caregivers a place to share experiences and obtain knowledge from those with similar situations.

    C. Support groups have a positive effect on an individual's coping while receiving chemotherapy (Schou et al., 2013; Breitbart et al., 2010).

    D. Support groups offer inspiration through witnessing the motivation to fight, experiencing the courage of others, and exposure to role modeling of others with cancer.

    E. Participation in a support group promotes a community feeling and a safe place to expose feelings and affirm each other.

        1. Online and social media connections provide additional venues for support (Seçkin, 2013).

V. Self-care

    A. Self-care skill building (Parelkar et al., 2013; Phelps et al., 2013)

        1. Multifocused education programs show merit in building coping skills (preparatory education, cognitive restructuring, building on current coping skills, guided imagery) (Garssen et al., 2013; Gatson-Johansson et al., 2013).

        2. Identifying strengths and recognizing and managing the source of stressors (Chen & Chang, 2012; Garsen et al., 2013; Parelkar et al., 2013; Phelps et al., 2013)

Part 5

B. Complementary and alternative medicine (CAM) and treatment (Decker & Lee, 2011; see Chapter 26)
   1. Various strategies effective; individual preference (Arthur et al., 2012; Kligler et al., 2011; Rausch et al., 2011)
   2. CAM use common, especially documented among women with breast cancer (Wanchai, Armer, & Stewert, 2010)
   3. Cognitive behavioral interventions or biofeedback shown to be effective (Cohen, 2010)

VI. Nursing research—interventions (Phelps et al., 2013; Rottmann et al., 2012; Rydahl-Hansen, 2013; Schou et al., 2013; Semple et al., 2013)
   A. Studies needed to show the effectiveness of psychosocial interventions, especially with specific client populations
   B. Difficult to draw conclusions about effectiveness, so more research on effective coping strategies needed

VII. Distress management standards or guidelines
   A. Established guidelines support evidence-based practice (Clark et al., 2012; Hammelef, Friese, Breslin, Riba, & Schneider, 2014; Holland, 2013; Lazenby, 2014).
   B. American College of Surgeons (ACS) Cancer Program Standards
      1. As of 2015, standards require that all cancer patients be routinely screened with validated tools during pivotal medical visits for psychological distress (ACS, 2012; Brown, 2014; Wagner, Spiegel, & Pearman, 2013).
         a. Patients have access to psychosocial services.
         b. Services are essential and are provided throughout the continuum of care.
         c. Services are provided either on site or via referral.
         d. Screening, referrals, provision for care documented in the patient's medical record
   C. Statement standards from the International Psycho-Oncology Society (IPOS, 2013)
      1. Distress considered the sixth vital sign to be assessed and measured
   D. NCCN Distress Management Guidelines (Hammelef et al., 2014; NCCN, 2013)
      1. It is important to recognize, monitor, document, and promptly treat at all stages of disease and in all settings.
      2. Screening should be done at the initial visit, with appropriate intervals, and as clinically indicated, especially with changes in disease status (remission, recurrence, progression).
      3. Standards should be implemented toward individual treatment plans for patients, with interdisciplinary guidance.
   4. Referrals should be readily available—licensed and/or certified psychologists or spiritual professionals
   E. Joint Position Statement, Implementing Screening for Distress: American Psychosocial Oncology Society, Association of Oncology Social Work, and Oncology Nursing Society (ONS, 2013)
      1. It is important to provide support for universal definition of distress.
      2. Validated tools should be used to screen for distress, covering a broad variety of symptoms over the continuum of cancer diagnosis and care.
      3. Response to screening data should be prompt, with licensed mental health professionals available to intervene.
      4. Suicide ideation is part of all clinical evaluations

EVALUATION

The oncology nurse systematically assesses the patient's coping patterns. The nurse can be instrumental in directing the patient and family and thus provide coping strategies. The patient can identify risks, adjust to changes, and perform ADLs within his or her physical capacity and has improved social interaction. In addition, nurses play a vital role in educating the patient and family about support groups. The nurse identifies and refers the patient to the appropriate support group. In addition, the nurse is qualified to participate directly in support groups as a facilitator, educator, consultant, social network, or resource.

References

American College of Surgeons (ACS). (2012). *Cancer Program Standards 2012: Ensuring patient-centered care, v. 1.2.1. Standard 3.2: Psychosocial distress screening.* (pp. 76–77). www.facs.org/cancer/coc/programstandards2012.pdf.

American Psychiatric Association (APA). (2013). *Diagnostic and statistical manual of mental disorders* (DSM-5); (5th ed.). Washington, DC: American Psychiatric Association.

Andreu, Y., Galdón, M., Dura, E., Martinez, P., Perez, P., & Murgui, S. (2012). A longitudinal study of psychosocial distress in breast cancer: Prevalence and risk factors. *Psychology & Health, 27*(1), 72–87.

Arthur, K., Belliard, C., Hardin, S., Khecht, K., Chen, C., & Montgomery, S. (2012). Practices, attitudes, and beliefs associated with complementary and alternative medicine (CAM) use among cancer patients. *Integrative Cancer Therapies, 11*(3), 232–242.

Boinon, D., Sultan, S., Charles, C., Stulz, A., Guillemeau, C., Delaloge, S., et al. (2014). Changes in psychological adjustment over the course of treatment for breast cancer: The predictive role of social sharing and social support. *Psycho-Oncology, 3* (23), 291–298.

Boyajian, R. (2010). Depression's impact on survival in patients with cancer. *Clinical Journal of Oncology Nursing, 14*(5), 649–652.

Breitbart, W., Rosenfeld, B., Gibson, C., Pessin, H., Poppito, S., Nelson, C., et al. (2010). Meaning-centered group psychotherapy for patients with advanced cancer: A pilot randomized controlled trial. *Psycho-Oncology, 19*(1), 21–28.

Brown, C. (2014). Screening and evidence-based interventions for distress in patients with cancer: Nurses must lead the way. *Clinical Journal of Oncology Nursing, 18*(1, Suppl.), 23–25.

Butt, C. M. (2011). Hope in adults with cancer. *Oncology Nursing Forum, 38*(5), E341–E350.

Candy, B., Jones, L., Varagunam, M., Speck, P., Tookman, A., & King, M. (2012). Spiritual and religious interventions for well-being of adults in the terminal phase of disease. *Cochrane Database of Systematic Reviews*, (5), CD007544.

Carlson, L., Waller, A., & Mitchell, A. (2012). Screening for distress and unmet needs in patients with cancer; Review and recommendations. *Journal of Clinical Oncology, 30*, 1160–1177.

Chen, P. Y., & Chang, H. C. (2012). The coping process of patients with cancer. *European Journal of Oncology Nursing, 16*(1), 10–16.

Cheng, C., Wang, T., Link, Y., Lin, H., Wung, S., & Liang, S. (2013). The illness experience of middle-aged men with oral cancer. *Journal of Clinical Nursing, 22*(23/24), 3549–3556.

Cheung, Y. T., Shwe, M., Chui, W. K., Chay, W. Y., Ang, S. F., Dent, R. A., et al. (2012). Effects of chemotherapy and psychosocial distress on perceived cognitive disturbances in Asian breast cancer patients. *Annals of Pharmacotherapy, 46*(12), 1645–1655.

Clark, P., Bolte, S., Buzablo, J., Golant, M., Daratosos, L., & Loscalzo, M. (2012). From distress guidelines to developing models of psychosocial care: Current best practices. *Journal of Psychosocial Oncology, 30*(6), 694–714.

Cohen, M. (2010). A model of group cognitive behavioral intervention combined with bio-feedback in oncology settings. *Social Work in Health Care, 49*(2), 149–164.

Cohen, M., & Bankston, S. (2011). Cancer-related distress. In C. H. Yarbro, D. Wujcik, & B. H. Gobel (Eds.), *Cancer nursing: Principles and practice* (7th ed., pp. 667–684). Sudbury, MA: Jones and Bartlett.

Cole, T., Bowling, J., Paletta, M., & Balzer, D. (2014). Risk factors for suicide among older adults with cancer. *Aging & Mental Health*, March 7: E.

Davis, C., Rust, C., & Darby, K. (2013). Coping skills among African-American breast cancer survivors. *Social Work in Health Care, 52*(5), 434–448.

Decker, G., & Lee, C. (2011). Complementary and alternative medicine (CAM) therapies in integrative oncology. In C. H. Yarbro, D. Wujcik, & B. H. Gobel (Eds.), *Cancer nursing: Principles and practice* (7th ed., pp. 626–654). Sudbury, MA: Jones and Bartlett.

Emilsson, S., Svensk, A., Tavelin, B., & Lindh, J. (2012). Support group participation during the post-operative radiotherapy period increases levels of coping resources among women with breast cancer. *European Journal of Cancer Care, 21*(5), 591–598.

Epiphaniou, E., Hamilton, D., Bridger, S., Robinson, V., Rob, G., Beynon, T., et al. (2012). Adjusting to the caregiving role: The importance of coping and support. *International Journal of Palliative Nursing, 18*(11), 541–545.

Faller, H., Schuler, M., Richard, M., Heckl, U., Weis, J., & Kuffner, R. (2013). Effects of psycho-oncologic interventions on emotional distress and quality of life in adult patients with cancer: Systematic review and meta-analysis. *Journal of Clinical Oncology, 31*(6), 782–792.

Fischbeck, S., Maier, B., Reinholz, U., Nehring, C., Schwab, R., Beutel, M., et al. (2013). Assessing somatic, psychosocial, and spiritual distress of patients with advanced cancer: Development of the Advanced Cancer Patients' Distress Scale. *American Journal of Hospice and Palliative Medicine, 30*(4), 339–346.

Garssen, B., Boomsma, M., Meezenbroek, E., Porsild, T., Berkhof, J., Berbee, M., et al. (2013). Stress management training for breast cancer surgery patients. *Psycho-Oncology, 22*(3), 572–580.

Gatson-Johansson, F., Fall-Dickson, J., Nanda, J., Sarenmalm, E., Maria Browall, M., & Goldstein, N. (2013). Long-term effect of the self-management comprehensive coping strategy program on quality of life in patients with breast cancer treated with high-dose chemotherapy. *Psycho-Oncology, 22*, 530–539.

Given, B., & Northouse, L. (2011). Who cares for family caregivers of cancer patients? *Clinical Journal of Oncology Nursing, 15*(5), 451–452.

Hamilton, J., Deal, A., Moore, A., Best, N. C., Galbraith, K. V., & Muss, H. (2013). Psychosocial predictors of depression among older African American patients with cancer. *Oncology Nursing Forum, 40*(4), 394–402.

Hammelef, K., Friese, C., Breslin, T., Riba, M., & Schneider, S. (2014). Implementing distress management guidelines in ambulatory oncology. *Clinical Journal of Oncology Nursing, 18*(1, Suppl.), 31–36.

Harvey, E., Rogak, L., Ford, R., & Holland, J. (2013). Rapid access to mental health professionals with experience in treating cancer-related distress: The American Psychosocial Oncology Referral Helpline. *Journal of the National Comprehensive Cancer Network, 11*(11), 1358–1361.

Holland, J. C. (2013). Distress screening and the integration of psychosocial care into routine oncologic care. *Journal of the National Comprehensive Cancer Network, 11*(5), 687–689.

Holslander, L., & McMillan, S. (2011). Depressive symptoms, grief and complicated grief among family caregivers of cancer patients three months into bereavement. *Oncology Nursing Forum, 38*(1), 60–65.

Hoyt, M., Stanton, A., Irwin, M., & Thomas, K. (2013). Cancer-related masculine threat, emotional approach coping, and physical functioning following treatment for prostate cancer. *Health Psychology, 32*(1), 66–74.

International Psycho-Oncology Society (IPOS). (2013). *Statement on standards and clinical practice guidelines in cancer care.* wpanet.org/detail.php?section_id=7&content_id=1087.

Itano, J. (2011). Cultural diversity among individuals with cancer. In C. H. Yarbro, D. Wujcik, & B. H. Gobel (Eds.), *Cancer nursing: Principles and practice* (7th ed., pp. 71–94). Sudbury, MA: Jones and Bartlett.

Kligler, B., Homel, P., Harrison, L., Sackett, E., Levenson, H., Kenney, J., et al. (2011). Impact of the Urban Zen Initiative on patients' experience of admission to an inpatient oncology floor: A mixed-methods analysis. *Journal of Alternative and Complementary Medicine, 17*(8), 729–734.

Knobf, T., Major-Campos, M., Chaqpar, A., Seigerman, A., & McCorkle, R. (2014). Promoting quality breast cancer care: Psychosocial distress screening. *Palliative & Supportive Care, 12*(1), 75–80.

Part 5

Lazenby, M. (2014). The international endorsement of US distress screening and psychosocial guidelines in oncology: A model for dissemination. *Journal of the National Comprehensive Cancer Network, 12*(2), 221–227.

Lee, H. Y., & Jin, S. W. (2013). Older Korean cancer survivors' depression and coping: Directions toward culturally competent interventions. *Journal of Psychosocial Oncology, 31*(4), 357–376.

Lelorain, S., Tessier, P., Florin, A., & Bonnaud-Antignac, A. (2012). Posttraumatic growth in long-term breast cancer survivors: Relation to coping, social support and cognitive processing. *Journal of Health Psychology, 17*(5), 627–639.

Llewelyn, C. D., Horney, D. J., McGurk, M., Weinman, J., Herold, J., Altman, K., et al. (2013). Assessing the psychological predictors of benefit finding in patients with head and neck cancer. *Psycho-Oncology, 22*(1), 97–105.

Maliski, S., Connor, S., Williams, L., & Litwin, M. (2010). Faith among low-income, African American/black men treated for prostate cancer. *Cancer Nursing, 33*(6), 470–478.

McSorley, O., McCaughan, E., Prue, G., Parahoo, K., Bunting, B., & O'Sullivan, J. (2014). A longitudinal study of coping strategies in men receiving radiotherapy and neo-adjuvant androgen deprivation for prostate cancer: A quantitative and qualitative study. *Journal of Advanced Nursing, 70*(3), 625–638.

Muehlbauer, P. (2013). Screen for psychosocial distress in patients with cancer. *ONS Connect, 28*(1), 34.

National Cancer Institute. (2011a). *Adjustment to cancer: Anxiety and distress (PDQ)*. www.cancer.gov/cancertopics/pdq/supportivecare/adjustment/HealthProfessional.

National Cancer Institute. (2011b). *Communication in cancer care (PDQ)*. www.cancer.gov/cancertopics/pdq/supportivecare/communication/healthprofessional.

National Cancer Institute. (2011c). *Depression (PDQ)*. www.cancer.gov/cancertopics/pdq/supportivecare/depression/Patient.

National Comprehensive Cancer Network (NCCN). (2013). *Distress management. Ver 2.2013*. www.nccn.org.

Northouse, L., Mood, W., Schafenacker, A., Kalemkerian, G., Zalupski, M., LoRusso, P., et al. (2013). Randomized clinical trial of a brief and extensive dyadic intervention for advanced cancer patients and their family caregivers. *Psycho-Oncology, 22*(3), 555–563.

Oncology Nursing Society (ONS). (2013). Implementing screening for distress: The joint position statement from the American Psychosocial Oncology Society, Association of Oncology Social Work, and Oncology Nursing Society. *Oncology Nursing Forum, 40*(5), 423–424.

Parelkar, P., Thompson, N., Kaw, C. K., Miner, K., & Stein, K. (2013). Stress coping and changes in health behavior among cancer survivors: A report from the American Cancer Society's Study of Cancer Survivors-II (SCS-II). *Journal of Psychosocial Oncology, 31*(2), 136–152.

Pederson, A., Olesen, F., Hanson, R., Zachariae, R., & Vedsted, P. (2013). Coping strategies and patient delay in patients with cancer. *Journal of Psychosocial Oncology, 31*(2), 204–218.

Phelps, C., Bennett, P., Hood, K., Brian, K., & Murray, A. (2013). A self-help coping intervention can reduce anxiety and avoidant health behaviours whilst waiting for cancer genetic risk information: Results of a phase III randomised trial. *Psycho-Oncology, 22*(4), 837–844.

Puchalski, C. M. (2012). Spirituality in the cancer trajectory. *Annals of Oncology, 23*(3), 49–55.

Rausch, S., Winegardner, F., Kruk, K., Phatak, V., Wahner-Roedler, D., Bauer, B., et al. (2011). Complementary and alternative medicine: Use and disclosure in radiation oncology community practice. *Supportive Care in Cancer, 19*(4), 521–529.

Rodriguez Vega, B., Orgaz Barnier, P., Bayon, C., Palao, A., Torres, G., Hospital, A., et al. (2012). Differences in depressed oncologic patients' narratives after receiving two different therapeutic interventions for depression: A qualitative study. *Psycho-Oncology, 21*(12), 1292–1298.

Rokach, A., Findler, L., Chin, J., Lev, S., & Kollender, Y. (2013). Cancer patients, their caregivers and coping with loneliness. *Psychology, Health & Medicine, 18*(2), 135–144.

Rosario, A. M., & de la Rosa, M. (2014). Santería as informal mental health support among U.S. Latinos with cancer. *Journal of Religion and Spirituality in Social Work, 33*(1), 4–18.

Rottmann, N., Dalton, S. O., Bidstrup, P. E., Würtzen, H., Høybye, M. T., Ross, L., et al. (2012). No improvement in distress and quality of life following psychosocial cancer rehabilitation. A randomised trial. *Psycho-Oncology, 21*(5), 505–514.

Rydahl-Hansen, S. (2013). Conditions that are significant for advanced cancer patients' coping with their suffering—as experienced by relatives. *Journal of Psychosocial Oncology, 31*(3), 334–355.

Sautier, L., Mehnert, A., Hocker, A., & Schilling, G. (2014). Participation in patient support groups among cancer survivors: Do psychosocial and medical factors have an impact? *European Journal of Cancer Care, 23*(1), 140–148.

Schmidt, S., Blank, T., Bellizzi, K., & Park, C. (2012). The relationship of coping strategies, social support, and attachment style with posttraumatic growth in cancer survivors. *Journal of Health Psychology, 17*(7), 1033–1040.

Schou, B., Karesen, R., Smeby, N. A., Espe, R., Sørensen, E. M., Amundsen, M., et al. (2014). Effects of psychoeducational versus a support group intervention in patients with early-stage breast cancer: Results of a randomized controlled trial. *Cancer Nursing, 37*(3), 198–207.

Seçkin, G. (2013). Satisfaction with health status among cyber patients: Testing a mediation model of electronic coping support. *Behaviour & Information Technology, 32*(1), 91–101.

Semple, C., Parahoo, K., Norman, A., McCaughan, E., Humphris, G., & Mills, M. (2013). Psychosocial interventions for patients with head and neck cancer. *Cochrane Database of Systematic Reviews, (7)*, CD009441.

Singer, S., Szalai, C., Briest, S., Brown, A., Dietz, A., Einenkel, et al. (2013). Co-morbid mental health conditions in cancer patients at working age—prevalence, risk profiles, and care uptake. *Psycho-Oncology, 22*(10), 2291–2297.

Sterba, K., Zapka, J., Gore, E., Ford, M., Ford, D., Thomas, M., et al. (2013). Exploring dimensions of coping in advanced colorectal cancer: Implications for patient-centered care. *Journal of Psychosocial Oncology, 31*(5), 517–539.

Tallman, B. A. (2013). Anticipated posttraumatic growth from cancer: The roles of adaptive and maladaptive coping strategies. *Counselling Psychology Quarterly, 26*(1), 72–88.

Tavernier, S. (2014). Translating research on the distress thermometer into practice. *Clinical Journal of Oncology Nursing, 18*(1, Suppl.), 26–30.

Tucci, R. (2012). Distress: Assessing the effects of coping with cancer. *Oncology Nurse Advisor, 26–28*, Jan/Feb. 2012.

Van Laarhoven, H., Schilderman, J., Bleijenberg, G., Donders, R., Vissers, K., Verhagen, C., et al. (2011). Coping, quality of life, depression, and hopelessness in cancer patients in a curative and palliative, end-of-life care setting. *Cancer Nursing, 34*(4), 302–314.

Wagner, L. I., Spiegel, D., & Pearman, T. (2013). Using the science of psychosocial care to implement the new American College of Surgeons Commission on Cancer Distress Screening Standards. *Journal of the National Comprehensive Cancer Network, 11*(2), 214–221.

Wanchai, A., Armer, J., & Stewert, B. (2010). Complementary and alternative medicine use among women with breast cancer: A systematic review. *Clinical Journal of Oncology Nursing, 14*(4), E45–E55.

Wenzel, J., Jones, R., Klimmek, R., Krumm, S., Darrell, L., Song, D., et al. (2012). Cancer support and resource needs among African American older adults. *Clinical Journal of Oncology Nursing, 16*(4), 372–377.

Zabalegui, A., Cabrera, E., Navarro, M., & Cebria, M. I. (2013). Perceived social support and coping strategies in advanced cancer patients. *Journal of Research in Nursing, 18*(5), 409–420.

Zhang, A., Gary, F., & Zhu, H. (2012). What precipitates depression in African-American cancer patients? Triggers and stressors. *Palliative & Supportive Care, 10*(4), 279–286.

CHAPTER 38

Psychosocial Disturbances and Alterations

Kathleen Murphy-Ende

Emotional Distress

OVERVIEW

I. Distress
   A. Psychological distress and existential concerns common in patients with cancer
   B. A combination of psychological, social, spiritual, physical, and financial stressors that strain the individual and family's coping abilities
   C. Defined as "severe pressure of trouble, pain, sickness or sorrow" (Oxford University Press, 2013)
   D. Used to describe the unpleasant emotional experience associated with the stressors that patients face when living with cancer
   E. Reflects a normative response different from psychological or psychiatric diagnoses such as clinical depression, adjustment disorder, post-traumatic stress disorder (PTSD), delirium, and anxiety disorder

II. Risk factors
   A. Disease and stage (Cohen & Bankston, 2011)
      1. Highest level of distress reported in patients with lung cancer
      2. Higher level of distress in patients in advanced stage of disease
      3. Impact of physical symptoms such as poor pain control
   B. Situational
      1. Personal meaning of the diagnosis
      2. Resources—emotional and practical support, spiritual guidance, and financial security
      3. Changes in roles—occupation, within family, between friends, altered physical capacity and cognitive functioning
   C. Developmental
      1. Age-specific developmental life tasks disrupted by diagnosis and treatment
      2. Personality and coping style

III. General treatment approaches
   A. Psychotherapeutic interventions that have been effective in the cancer population—individual supportive psychotherapy, cognitive-behavioral therapy, and group therapy (Osborn, Demoncada & Feuerstein 2006)
   B. Family psychotherapy
   C. Psychoeducational approaches
   D. Spiritual counseling
   E. Support groups
   F. Relaxation exercises, including meditation and guided imagery

IV. Potential sequelae of emotional distress
   A. Chronic emotional distress
   B. Development of major psychiatric disorders—anxiety, depression, adjustment disorder, and suicidal ideation or suicide
   C. PTSD—may occur in cancer survivors with similar experiences of those in military combat or natural disasters
   D. Somatic symptoms such as sleep disturbance, fatigue, loss of appetite, and gastrointestinal (GI) disturbances
   E. Declined performance at home, school, or work
   F. Nonadherence or misunderstanding of health information

ASSESSMENT

I. Screening
   A. National Comprehensive Cancer Network (2013) Guideline
      1. All patients should be routinely screened to identify the level and source of their distress so that further evaluation can be completed.
      2. Identifying and treating psychological issues is a complex process; appropriate referrals should be made to mental health specialists such as licensed clinical psychologists or psychiatrists.

3. Psychological needs vary, depending on the individual, developmental stage, phase of disease trajectory, past coping skills, and available emotional and practical resources.

B. Screening tools for distress
   1. Information obtained from screening checklists useful for identifying specific concerns and needs, rather than identifying a clinical diagnosis
   2. Distress Thermometer (Roth et al., 1998)—a unidimensional screening tool in which the patient is asked to indicate the severity of distress in the domains of emotional, spiritual, physical, practical, and family matters
      a. Designed for rapid assessment of patient distress; well-validated in patients with cancer
      b. Can be used as a one-item scale assessing the level of distress
      c. Contains a problem list in which the source of distress can be identified
      d. Sensitive to changes over time and only takes a few minutes to complete
      e. Not useful for identifying specific psychiatric disorders such as major depression
      f. Clinical pathways for the Distress Thermometer available to guide the follow-up assessment and management of distress (Holland, 1999); can be downloaded as part of the Distress Guidelines through the website for the NCCN (NCCN, 2013)

II. History
   A. Age, diagnosis, stage of disease, and treatment regimen
   B. Presence of risk factors
   C. Distressing thoughts, feelings, and behaviors such as nervousness, worry, jitteriness, tearfulness, hopelessness, difficulty concentrating, irritability, social withdrawal, ruminating, thoughts of death, suicidal ideation, self-harm, or harm to others

III. Pattern of emotional distress
   A. Distress occurs across the disease continuum, accompanied by the following feelings: vulnerability, sadness, fear of disability, worry of becoming a burden to others, depression, anxiety, panic, social isolation, and existential and spiritual crises.
   B. For each specific distressing symptom, the following should be assessed: frequency and intensity of specific distress, associated symptoms, and precipitating and alleviating factors.
   C. Duration of symptoms is assessed to determine if the symptoms are episodic or prolonged.
      1. Episodic symptoms often occur during disease transitions such as diagnosis or relapse.

2. Persistent symptoms may represent a psychiatric disorder, and the patient should be referred to a psychologist or psychiatrist.

IV. Impact on functional status—physical, interpersonal, occupational, academic performance, and spiritual practices

PROBLEM STATEMENTS AND OUTCOME IDENTIFICATION

I. Hopelessness (NANDA-I)
   A. Expected outcome—patient will maintain or develop a sense of hope.
   B. Expected outcome—patient will adjust or adapt to stressful events.
II. Risk for Post-Trauma Syndrome (NANDA-I), also known as PTSD
   A. Expected outcome—patient will verbalize improvement or resolution of their symptoms of post-traumatic syndrome.
III. Ineffective Role Performance (NANDA-I)
   A. Expected outcome—patient will verbalize realistic role expectations for current situation.
   B. Expected outcome—patient will identify the specific transitions that are likely to take place in his or her role.

PLANNING AND IMPLEMENTATION

I. Interventions to address hopelessness
   A. Identifying which dimension (affective, cognitive, behavioral, affiliative, temporal, or contextual) applies to the patient and then supporting and facilitating the individual's hope; professionals may increase cancer patients' sense of hope by being present, giving accurate information, and showing that they care.
   B. Assisting the patient to explore his or her value system, purpose, and meaning in life
   C. Promoting goal setting
   D. Offering psychological support programs that are grounded on the construct of hope and have successfully helped cancer patients to gain hope
II. Interventions to address PTSD
   A. Assisting the patient in identifying perceived threats and providing accurate information on actual risks
   B. Providing an opportunity for patients to give a narrative of their experience with support in the form of family and friends, nursing staff, support groups, and individual psychotherapy
   C. Offering supportive and expressive group therapy
III. Interventions to address ineffective role performance
   A. Assisting the patient in identifying realistic goals based on what he or she wants to accomplish in the current role

B. Asking the patient to list the priorities within his or her personal, professional, and social roles

C. Referring the patient to his or her employer's human resource department to assist with job schedule and duty changes

D. Referral to occupational rehabilitation psychologist, if indicated

EVALUATION

The oncology nurse systematically and regularly evaluates the client's and family's responses to interventions for distress to determine progress toward overcoming hopelessness and resolving PTSD. Relevant data are collected, and actual findings are compared with expected findings. Outcomes and plans of care are reviewed and revised, as necessary.

Anxiety

OVERVIEW

I. Definition—Anxiety is a "a mood state characterized by apprehension and somatic symptoms of tension in which an individual anticipates impending danger, catastrophe, or misfortune. The future threat may be real or imagined, internal or external. It may be an identifiable situation or a more vague fear of the unknown." (American Psychiatric Association [APA], 2007)

A. Commonly associated with cancer

B. Characterized by a high negative affect in which the patient may experience feeling distressed, fearful, hostile, jittery, nervous, and scornful

C. Anxiety frequently occurs with depression.

II. Risk factors

A. Disease related

1. Disease trajectory points—new diagnosis, initiation of treatment, completion of treatment, recurrent disease, advanced phase, and end of life

2. Physical symptoms—pain, insomnia and dyspnea, urinary retention, and pruritus

3. Abnormal metabolic states—hyperthyroidism, hormone-secreting tumors, paraneoplastic syndromes, electrolyte imbalance, hypoxia, sepsis, delirium, and hypoglycemia

4. Psychiatric disorders such as depression, delirium, paranoia, and persecution delusions, which may predispose the patient to anxiety

5. Preexisting anxiety disorders, genetics, age, and gender influence the expression and manifestation of anxiety (Murphy-Ende, 2012).

B. Treatment related

1. Patients undergoing palliative chemotherapy, radiation, or phase I or II clinical trials (Roth & Massie, 2009)

2. Prolonged treatment and hospitalization, blood and marrow transplantation, major surgery, or prolonged phase of recovery

3. Medications—corticosteroids, neuroleptics causing akathisia, thyroxine, bronchodilators, antihistamines, decongestants, beta-adrenergic stimulants, opioids that induced hallucinations

4. Opioid, alcohol, or benzodiazepine withdrawal

5. Body image changes from mastectomy, orchiectomy, colostomy, alopecia, skin changes, amputation, and weight loss or gain

6. Failure of therapy, progression of disease, or relapse

C. Intrapersonal related

1. Concern about future health, relationships, finances, and social or occupational roles and responsibilities

2. Loss of independence and perceived loss of sense of control

3. Limited coping skills

4. Cumulative losses that contribute to social isolation

5. Limited social resources

III. General treatment approaches

A. Treatment should be aimed at the exact cause, whenever possible.

B. Physical symptoms such as pain, insomnia, pruritus, urinary retention, dyspnea, and infection should be treated.

C. Psychoeducational interventions, including a focus on providing information about the medical system and treatment process and anticipatory guidance are likely to reduce anxiety. (Murphy-Ende, 2012).

1. Orientation to the health care setting and oncology team

2. Providing information about support groups may reduce anxiety.

D. Written or Internet education materials about specific types of cancer, treatment, and side effects should be provided.

E. Self-care and relaxation techniques need to be taught to the patient.

F. The patient and family should be instructed about managing and treating the side effects of chemotherapy and radiation therapy.

G. Referral to a licensed psychologist is facilitated for individual cognitive-behavioral therapy (Moorey & Greer, 2012), cognitive-existential group psychotherapy, or family psychotherapy and counseling.

H. Referral is made to cancer support groups to provide anxiety management techniques and coping skills.

I. Pharmacologic management is accomplished with anxiolytics, azapirones, antihistamines, antidepressants or atypical neuroleptics.

J. Complementary therapies such as exercise, art therapy, massage, music therapy, meditation, and progressive muscle relaxation may promote relaxation.

IV. Potential sequelae of anxiety (APA, 2013)

A. Somatic symptoms—nausea, vomiting, headaches, change in bowel habits

B. Behavioral issues—substance use, altered eating habits, self-harm, and social dysfunction

C. Cognitive effects—difficulty concentrating and making decisions, poor attention span, and impaired memory

D. Anxiety disorders—may occur as a maladaptive response; include adjustment disorder with anxious mood, generalized anxiety disorder, panic attacks, phobias, obsessive-compulsive disorder, PTSD, and depression

E. Interference with performance at home, school, or work

ASSESSMENT

I. Presence of risk factors

II. Subjective symptoms

A. Persistently tense, unable to relax, worried, easily excitable, having poor concentration or poor attention, indecisive, easily overwhelmed, and irritable; experiencing panic attacks, loss of control, insomnia, eating disturbances, palpitations, feelings of suffocation, dizziness, fatigue or exhaustion, difficulty swallowing, and a sense of impending doom; crying easily

III. Objective symptoms.

A. Facial tension or flushing, pallor, tremors, twitches, pacing, restlessness, nail biting, wringing of hands, voice quivering, rapid heart rate, increased respirations, increased blood pressure, constricted pupils, and cold hands

PROBLEM STATEMENTS AND OUTCOME IDENTIFICATION

I. Anxiety (NANDA-I)

A. Expected outcome—patient is able to express his or her emotions and identify the source of anxiety and coping responses that are likely to reduce anxiety.

B. Expected outcome—patient and family verbalize an understanding of therapeutic plans, options, goals, and expectations.

II. Death Anxiety (NANDA-I)

A. Expected outcome—patient will communicate fears about dying and identify specific issues that can be solved.

B. Expected outcome—patient will verbalize less anxiety and an overall reduction in psychological distress.

PLANNING AND IMPLEMENTATION

I. Interventions to address anxiety

A. Providing a safe environment ⚠

1. Assessment of the potential for self-harm

2. Providing a subdued space with reduced stimuli or providing gentle diversion

B. Use of active and empathic listening skills

C. Use of positive interpersonal skills—calm demeanor, speaking slowly with an even voice, listening, encouragement to identify the cause of anxiety, normalizing or affirming fears, assisting the patient to identify past effective coping skills

D. Assisting the patient to identify overwhelming feelings such as vulnerability, hopelessness, helplessness, fear, loss of control, and fear of the unknown

E. Administering medications, as ordered, monitoring for side effects, and evaluating effectiveness

1. Explaining the rationale for medications provided, including psychopharmacology information to patient and family

F. Providing information about psychological resources

G. Addressing iatrogenic causes of anxiety (medications or physical symptoms)

H. Addressing spiritual needs

II. Interventions to address death anxiety

A. Considering the developmental differences in conceptualizing death

B. Establishing a nurturing and supportive relationship

1. Providing continuity of care by assigning the same staff and avoiding the introduction of new staff members

C. Assisting the patient to contain the anxiety associated with impending death by listening to the concerns and being present

1. Allowing the patient to have frank discussions about his or her fears concerning dying

2. Facilitating open communication with family

D. Encouraging family and friends to visit if the patient obtains comfort from visitors

1. Facilitating open communication

2. Providing privacy

E. Assisting the patient to identify and address practical concerns around the issue of death

F. Assisting the patient to identify finding pleasure in short-term goals

1. Providing information about predictable physical symptoms

2. Reassuring the patient that pain and other symptoms will be assessed and addressed

G. Explaining common emotional phases that patients may face
  1. Acknowledging defense mechanisms as denial, which is a possible adaptive response to impending death
H. Encouraging the patient to identify his or her spiritual belief system that helps face the transition of death
  1. Offering to arrange for clergy services, as needed.
  2. Asking patient how faith-based interventions can be incorporated into care
I. Referral to palliative care or a psychologist to provide short-term psychological interventions

EVALUATION

The oncology nurse systematically and regularly evaluates the client's and family's responses to interventions for anxiety to determine progress toward the achievement of reducing anxiety and positive coping. Relevant data are collected, and actual findings are compared with expected findings. Problem statements and outcome identification, outcomes, and plans of care are reviewed and revised, as necessary.

Depression

OVERVIEW

I. Depression
  A. A mood state of feeling sad, discouraged, hopeless, and worthless
    1. May vary from mild and transient emotional distress to a major psychiatric illness
    2. Several types of depressive disorders that may affect one's physical, affective, cognitive and social well-being
    3. Reactive depression—a normal response to a precipitating event or situation, and can be a response to the cancer diagnosis, prognosis, treatment, fear of the unknown, cumulative losses, or fear of death
    4. Depression characterized by low positive affect, with symptoms of anhedonia and cognitive and motor slowing
  B. Evaluation of patient by a qualified mental health practitioner such as a psychologist or psychiatrist critical for accurate diagnosis and treatment
    1. Clinicians and patients may mistakenly believe that depression is normal in those who have cancer, which may be one barrier to accurate evaluation and effective treatment.
    2. Nurses may underestimate the level of depressive symptoms in patients with moderate or severe depression; however, nurses are in a key position to identify patients who are at risk and make referrals for further evaluation.

3. The *Diagnostic and Statistical Manual of Mental Disorders* (DSM-V) criteria for a diagnosis of a major depressive disorder are as follows:
    a. Have a depressed mood or loss of interest in or pleasure in nearly all activities for at least 2 weeks
    b. Have five or more of the following symptoms—change in appetite or weight change (5% or more in a month), insomnia or hypersomnia nearly every day, psychomotor agitation or retardation nearly every day (observable by others), decreased energy, feelings of worthlessness or guilt, difficulty concentrating or making decisions; and recurrent thoughts of death, suicidal ideation, or plans or attempts (APA, 2013)
  4. The symptoms listed above do not meet the diagnostic criteria if they are caused by the direct physiologic effects of a substance or a general medical condition or if the symptoms are accounted for by bereavement.
  5. It is often difficult to determine if physical symptoms are caused by the cancer and its treatment or by a mood disorder such as major depression.
    a. Many patients with cancer have physical symptoms and anxiety; psychologists should use clinical judgment and other diagnostic criteria besides the DSM-V.
II. Mood disorder
  A. Caused by a medical condition with depressive features
  B. Defined as depression that has a cause in a medical illness or is caused by a direct biologic condition, and the full criteria for a major depressive episode are not met (APA, 2013)
III. Adjustment disorder with depressed mood
  A. Considered acute if lasts less than 6 months
  B. Considered chronic when the symptoms last for 6 months or longer (APA, 2013)
IV. Demoralization
  A. Defined as the loss of meaning, which is a different construct from depression and should be considered a separate syndrome
  B. Characterized by loss of meaning, purpose, and hope
  C. Patient may still be able to experience pleasure in the present (Kissane, Treece, Breitbart, McKeen, & Chochinov, 2009)
V. Risk factors (Murphy-Ende, 2012)
  A. History and situational
    1. Personal history of major depression
    2. Previous suicide attempt
    3. Family history of depression
    4. Comorbid medical conditions (e.g., major medical illness, substance abuse)

5. Sleep deprivation
6. Social isolation
7. Other unexpected life events (e.g., changes in role, relationships, occupation, or living arrangement)
8. Spouse with an illness
9. Numerous cumulative losses of friends and family members
   B. Disease- and treatment-related
      1. Severe active disease—may lead to feelings of uncertainty about the future
      2. Pancreatic, lung, and central nervous system tumors and head and neck cancer
      3. Younger adult patients with cancer (Wilson, Chochinv, & Skirko, 2007)
      4. Poorly controlled pain, nausea, or dyspnea
      5. Physical limitations or restrictions
      6. Prolonged treatment or treatment failure
      7. Medications—use of biologic agents, chemotherapy, hormone therapy (antiestrogens), corticosteroids, benzodiazepines, and opioids
VI. General treatment approaches
   A. Referral of patients who express thoughts of suicide or desire to hasten death for immediate psychological evaluation ⚠
   B. Treatment for underlying medical conditions and physical symptoms
   C. Providing patient and family with education about depression, treatment, and reason for referral for further evaluation and treatment
   D. Coordinating psychological or psychiatric care
   E. Providing education about prescribed medications and their expected effects, time for response, importance of regular dosing, and possible side effects
      1. Explaining the rationale for not stopping the medication without first discussing this with the prescriber
   F. Monitoring the patient for side effects and assessing for positive response to medication, such as improved mood, appetite, and sleep
   G. Facilitating individual cognitive behavioral therapy, behavioral therapy, or psychotherapy, as well as family therapy, by a highly trained mental health specialist
   H. Providing pharmacologic management of depression with selective serotonin reuptake inhibitors, tricyclic antidepressants, serotonin-norepinephrine reuptake inhibitors, atypical antipsychotics, central nervous system stimulants
VII. Potential sequelae of depression
   A. Suicide or self-harm
   B. Altered sleep patterns
   C. Inability to maintain current role—functional disability

D. Poor quality of life
E. Social withdrawal
F. Adherence issues
G. Increased morbidity and mortality (Rosenstein, 2011)

ASSESSMENT

I. History
   A. Presence of risk factors for depression
   B. Presence of either a depressed mood or loss of interest or pleasure and at least five of the defining symptoms of depression for a period of 2 consecutive weeks or more (see above, Overview of Depression)
   C. Variation in cultural groups in their interpretations with regard to the meaning of depressive symptoms and use of different terms to describe symptoms
   D. Suicidal ideation, suicide attempt, suicide plan, means and motive to commit suicide ⚠
   E. Past use of effective or noneffective treatment for depression
   F. Concept and meaning of depression
   G. Impact of depressive symptoms on individual role and interpersonal communications or relationships
II. Symptoms and signs (APA, 2013)
   A. Subjective symptoms—report of depressed mood or anhedonia, insomnia, social withdrawal, fatigue, sense of worthlessness or guilt, difficulty concentrating, thoughts of death, suicide ideation, irritability, and somatic complaints without cause
   B. Objective symptoms—depressed or flat affect, crying, weight loss or gain, slow speech, and psychomotor excitation or retardation
III. Laboratory or measurement findings
   A. Medical laboratory testing—cortisol level, thyroid-stimulating hormone, complete blood cell count, or chemistry panel
   B. Mental status examination—changes may be indicative of depression or early delirium
   C. Depression screening instruments—Geriatric Depression Scale, Zung Self-Rating Depression Scale, Beck Depression Inventory, and Hospital Anxiety and Depression Scale
   D. Functional rating scales—Eastern Cooperative Oncology Group (ECOG0 Scale) Karnofsky Rating Scale and Palliative Performance Scale (PPS)

PROBLEM STATEMENTS AND OUTCOME IDENTIFICATION

I. Risk for Suicide (NANDA-I) ⚠
   A. Expected outcome—patient is protected from self-harm.

B. Expected outcome—patient identifies the complications of depression and verbalizes a plan for what to do if he or she becomes suicidal.

C. Expected outcome—patient or family is able to identify situations that require professional interventions.

D. Expected outcome—patient agrees to adhere to the follow-up treatment plans.

E. Expected outcome—patient has a stable and supportive living situation and available psychiatric care.

II. Risk for Situational Low Self-Esteem (NANDA-I)

A. Expected outcome—patient will maintain and increase self-efficacy and self-esteem.

PLANNING AND IMPLEMENTATION

I. Interventions to address risk of suicide ⚠

A. Staying with the patient and keep him or her safe from self-harm

B. Obtaining immediate psychological or psychiatric referral

C. Providing the patient and family with information on suicide prevention and a contact number for a clinician who is available 24 hours a day

D. Identifying and modifying the patient's psychological pain by assisting in altering the stressful environment and obtaining aid from significant other, family, or friends

E. Building a trusting relationship and offering realistic support by recognizing or validating the patient's concerns and struggles

F. Coordinating care with mental health providers

II. Interventions to address situational low self-esteem

A. Facilitating expression of feelings by acknowledging the patient's pain and despair and engaging in active listening

B. Reinforcing that depression may be self-limiting and that effective treatment exists

C. Assisting the patient to identify his or her strengths and accomplishments

D. Collaborating with the patient to identify factors that cause low self-esteem—for example, interpersonal deficits, role transitions, role disputes, marital conflict, and grief

E. Assisting the patient to identify personal growth goals and strategies for problem solving

EVALUATION

The oncology nurse systematically and regularly evaluates the client's and family's responses to depression interventions to determine progress toward the achievement of expected outcomes of safety from self-harm and improved mood. Relevant data are collected, and actual findings are compared with expected findings. Problem statements and outcome identification, outcomes, and plans of care are reviewed and revised, as necessary.

Loss of Personal Control

OVERVIEW

I. Loss of personal control

A. People facing cancer often feel a loss of control over their situation, a loss of ability to cope with current and future events, or both.

1. Loss of personal control is the perception that one's own actions will not significantly affect an event or an outcome.

2. Having a perceived lack of control may influence one's level of optimism, motivation level, and goals.

3. The concept of internal-external locus of control, which is a personality trait conceptualized by Rotter (1966), considers how much an individual believes that outcomes depend on his or her own actions or on circumstances outside the individual's control.

4. Self-efficacy is the perceived ability to cope with specific situations.

5. Concept of powerlessness is generally situationally determined.

B. People tend to be strongly motivated to gain control over their circumstances.

C. The perception of lack of control has negative effects on the well-being of individuals.

D. The belief that an event or one's reaction to it can be controlled may facilitate adjustment.

E. Personal control is correlated with better emotional well-being and health outcomes, enhanced ability to cope with stress, and improved motor and intellectual tasks in those living with a serious illness.

F. Some patients may have a perceived sense of control to inappropriately blame themselves for negative outcomes, which may result in guilt, remorse, and emotional distress.

G. The response to the situation and level of perceived control is influenced by the meaning of the event, comparison of similar events, patterns of coping, personality, support system, and available resources.

II. Risk factors

A. Disease related

1. Unexpected diagnosis and lack of understanding of the disease and treatment

2. Uncertainty of the prognosis

3. Inability to perform usual activities or a change in routine

4. Physical disability or cognitive impairment

5. Frequent hospitalizations or placement in an intensive care unit

6. Terminal phase of illness

B. Treatment related

1. Insufficient understanding about the treatment, side effects, and expected outcomes

2. Lengthy treatment course, travel to treatment site, and need for assistance with occupation and domestic responsibilities during treatment phase
3. Unexpected or poorly controlled side effects of treatment
4. Treatment failure
5. Body image issues such as weight loss or gain, alopecia, loss of limb

C. Situation related
   1. Dependency on others and loss of independence
   2. Loss of decision-making capacity
   3. Lack of privacy

D. Developmental, personality, and culture related
   1. Age-specific considerations
      a. Young children tend to be externally controlled.
      b. Adolescents tend to depend on peers for approval, and they test their independence.
      c. Young adults concerned about launching often conceptualize illness as a disruption of roles.
      d. Adults may be responsible for family members (children and aging parents) and conceptualize illness as a disruption of productivity in family and work.
      e. Older adults are often facing retirement and comorbid illnesses and conceptualize illness and possible death as separation from family and friends.
   2. Personality—degree of internal-external locus of control and other traits such as neuroticism, extraversion, openness, agreeableness, and conscientiousness
   3. Cultural differences from the health care providers or health care system that may affect communication and choices—dominant language, gender roles, high-risk behaviors, spiritual concerns, and basic value or belief system

III. General treatment approaches
   A. Patient and family education
      1. Encouraging questions and providing time for it
      2. Explaining that education is an ongoing process
   B. Assisting patient and family in decision making by explaining options, risks, and benefits
   C. Offering to arrange for individual counseling with a mental health specialist
   D. For the pediatric population, providing opportunities to make choices and express concerns through play and expressive arts (e.g., art therapy)
   E. Encouraging verbalization of feelings, providing emotional support, and assisting in basic problem solving

IV. Potential sequelae of prolonged loss of personal control
   A. Lowered self-esteem
   B. Helplessness and hopelessness
   C. Nonadherence or delay in treatment
   D. Depression, anxiety, or both
   E. Cancer fatalism with avoidance of health-promoting behaviors and cancer screening practices

ASSESSMENT

I. History (Loney & Murphy-Ende 2009)
   A. Presence of risk factors

II. Symptoms and signs
   A. Subjective characteristics of loss of personal control
      1. Overt or covert statements that suggest a loss of control
      2. Expressed frustration or dissatisfaction with care
      3. Anger or criticism toward staff
   B. Presence of objective characteristics of loss of personal control
      1. Refusal or reluctance to participate in decision making
      2. Refusal or reluctance to participate in activities of daily living (ADLs)
      3. Reluctance to express emotions
      4. Behavioral responses may include apathy, resignation, withdrawal, uneasiness, anxiety, and aggression.
      5. Responses to limitations on personal control may include attempts to circumvent limits, increased attempts to exercise control, and ignoring of limits.
      6. Nonadherence with the medical treatment regimen

III. Patient's problem-solving abilities
   A. Ability to identify the sense of powerlessness and insight into the contributing factors
   B. Past coping behaviors during other uncontrollable events
   C. Ability to identify aspects of care that the individual is able to make choices about
   D. Identification of other people or events that will reduce feelings of powerlessness

PROBLEM STATEMENTS AND OUTCOME IDENTIFICATION

I. Powerlessness (NANDA-I)
   A. Expected outcome—patient expresses a sense of control and participates in decision making.
   B. Expected outcome—patient identifies specific factors that are within his or her control.
   C. Expected outcome—patient or activated power of attorney of health care (POAHC) makes timely decisions.

Part 5

II. Impaired Resilience (NANDA-I)
 A. Expected outcome—patient participates in measures to minimize his or her sense of loss of control.
 B. Expected outcome—patient verbalizes his or her capabilities.
 C. Expected outcome—patient describes and initiates alternative coping strategies.

PLANNING AND IMPLEMENTATION

I. Interventions to address powerlessness
 A. Providing patient and family with orientation to the health care system and health education on the diagnosis, treatment, and expected outcomes
 B. Providing updated information on the current plan of care
 C. Providing opportunities for the patient to control decisions
 D. Assisting patient to identify the factors that can be controlled
 E. Reassuring patient or POAHC that he or she has the right to make decisions regarding medical care and will be assisted in the decision-making process
II. Interventions to address impaired individual resilience
 A. Assisting the patient in identifying past successful coping techniques
 B. Asking the patient to list his or her coping strengths
 C. Providing positive reinforcement when the patient demonstrates resilient behavior

EVALUATION

The oncology nurse systematically and regularly evaluates the client's and family's responses to interventions that address loss of self-control to determine progress toward the achievement of an increased sense of self control. Relevant data are collected, and actual findings are compared with expected findings. Problem statements, outcomes, and plans of care are reviewed and revised, as necessary.

Loss and Grief

OVERVIEW

I. Loss, grief, bereavement, and anticipatory grief
 A. Loss involves any perceived or experienced change in function, role, relationship, or lifestyle and implies separation from the people and things that are meaningful (Kubler-Ross, 1969).
  1. Although loss is a part of normal growth and development as attachments are given up, the sudden or cumulative losses associated with cancer are often distressing.
 B. Grief is the active, adaptive process of recognizing, coping with, and reconciling to loss (Kubler-Ross, 1969).

  1. The individual's reaction to the loss is often based on his or her perception of the loss.
  2. Grief response may be affected by personality, coping skills, and available supportive resources.
 C. Bereavement is deprivation of something or someone, such as a relation or friend, especially by death (Oxford University Press, 2013).
  1. A bereft person is deprived of nonmaterial assets and may feel robbed of someone, something important, and future plans.
 D. Anticipatory grief begins in response to the awareness of the impending loss of a loved one and acknowledgment of future losses.
II. Risk factors
 A. Disease-related and treatment-related
  1. Unexpected diagnosis, high risk of recurrence, and advanced disease or poor prognosis
  2. Changes in body structure, function, or image (e.g., amputation, mastectomy, colostomy, alopecia, cachexia, or cognition)
  3. Poor pain control or chronic pain
  4. History of psychiatric illness
 B. Situational and social
  1. Loss of a person through death, divorce, or separation
  2. Loss of something considered valuable, such as pet, home, or possessions
  3. Nature of the relationship with lost person
  4. Cumulative losses
  5. Limited social support
  6. Occupational or employment restrictions
 C. Developmental (Loney & Murphy-Ende, 2009)
  1. Younger than 2 years—self-centered and sees loss as deprivation of needs or separation
  2. 2 to 5 years—concept is temporary and concrete; and may express little distress of not being loved
  3. 5 to 9 years—concept is concrete and logical may see loss as fear of punishment or bodily harm
  4. 9 to 12 years—concept is realistic; may perceive loss as separation
  5. 12 to 18 years—concept is abstract and realistic; may perceive loss as a threat to independence
  6. 18 to 25 years—impact of loss is complex, with disruption in lifestyle
  7. 25 to 45 years—impact of loss may represent a threat to future
  8. 45 to 65 years—loss or death represents disruption of productivity in family or work
  9. 65 to death—concept of loss may be philosophical, with death perceived as separation
 D. Risk for complicated grief
  1. Perception of death as preventable

2. Ambivalent relationship to the deceased
3. Coexisting medical conditions
4. Coexisting financial or legal problems
III. General treatment approaches
  A. Providing basic information (verbal and written) on the grief process
  B. Exploring spiritual beliefs that may offer a sense of comfort, and referral to spiritual care
  C. Referral to grief counselor or psychologist for individual or family counseling
  D. Referral to support groups in the community
  E. Offering music or art therapy
  F. Providing pharmacologic management of severe symptoms
IV. Potential sequelae of loss and grief
  A. Complicated grief
  B. Depression or anxiety
  C. Denial
  D. Self-neglect or inability to take care of others
  E. Social isolation
  F. Physical symptoms
  G. Cognitive symptoms
  H. Substance abuse
  I. Suicidal ideation or attempt

ASSESSMENT

I. History
  A. Presence of risk factors, including previous losses
  B. Nature and meaning of the loss
  C. Personality and past coping responses
  D. Family characteristics and communication style
II. Symptoms and signs (Loney & Murphy-Ende, 2009)
  A. Cognitive—lack of concentration, distractibility, preoccupation with loss, searching for meaning, intrusive thoughts, or psychiatric symptoms
  B. Physical—fatigue, headache, shortness of breath, gastrointestinal complaints, sleep disturbance, cardiac symptoms, and fatigue or exhaustion
  C. Psychological—shock, denial, guilt, anger, hostility, ambivalence, sadness, shame, depression, preoccupation, ruminating, anxiety, or dulled senses
  D. Social—dependency on or avoidance of others and occupational lapses
  E. Spiritual distress—searching for meaning or change in views or beliefs
III. Stage of grief (Parkes, 1987)
  A. Alarm—a physiologic response
  B. Searching—episodes of psychological pain, with obtrusive wish for the person who was lost
  C. Mitigation—feeling comfort in sensing the presence of the deceased
  D. Anger and guilt—may be angry at others or self
  E. Gaining a new identity—recovery of lost functions and adaptation to new roles

IV. Patient and family level of understanding of their grief
V. Meaning of the loss
VI. Impact of losses and grief on routine, roles, relationships, occupation, and school

PROBLEM STATEMENTS AND OUTCOME IDENTIFICATION

I. Grieving (NANDA-I)
  A. Expected outcome—patient and family will identify the loss and its significance and express feeling validated in their loss.
  B. Expected outcome—patient and family will move through the stages of grief without developing complicated grief.
  C. Expected outcome—patient will be able to use his or her emotions to develop new coping strategies and manage the threats associated with the loss.
  D. Expected outcome—patient and family will identify personal strengths and effective coping mechanisms.
  E. Expected outcome—patient and family will adapt to the new living situation.
II. Interrupted Family Processes (NANDA-I)
  A. Expected outcome—family maintains its ability to function as a family system and be supportive to each other.
  B. Expected outcome—family expresses grief to each other and the professional staff.
  C. Expected outcome—family identifies the impact of the loss on the family structure and function.
  D. Expected outcome—family identifies the strengths and weakness of their family function.
  E. Expected outcome—family is knowledgeable of community resources and self-help methods (e.g., books, health care media) and support groups.

PLANNING AND IMPLEMENTATION

I. Interventions to address grieving
  A. Establishing a trusting relationship and encouraging the patient and family to share their grief without imposing own values or judgment
  B. Validating the grief and encouraging ways to express it
  C. Being prepared for negative affect such as anger, increased demands, irritability, sarcasm, and blaming
  D. Remaining calm during patient's behavioral outbursts and setting limits on inappropriate or dangerous behavior
  E. Conveying acceptance and empathetic concern
  F. Assisting patient and family in exploring coping methods
  G. Providing anticipatory guidance prior to loss—discussion of impending loss, review of significance of past losses and responses to those losses, providing information on mourning process, and assisting in formulating coping strategies

II. Interventions to address interrupted family processes
   A. Providing privacy for expression of feelings
   B. Encouraging family members to share their perceptions with each other and reminding them that everyone grieves in unique ways
   C. Validating each member's grief
   D. Considering cultural, religious, and social customs of mourning
   E. Referring the family to professional family or individual bereavement counseling

EVALUATION

The oncology nurse systematically and regularly evaluates the client's and family's responses to interventions that address loss and grief to determine progress toward the achievement of optimal functioning and grief resolution. Relevant data are collected, and actual findings are compared with expected findings. Problem statements, outcomes, and plans of care are reviewed and revised, as necessary.

References

American Psychiatric Association. (2007). *APA dictionary of psychology* (p. 63). Washington, DC: American Psychological Association, Author.

American Psychiatric Association (APA). (2013). *Diagnostic and statistical manual of mental disorders* (5th ed.; DSM-V). Washington, DC: American Psychiatric Association.

Cohen, M. Z., & Bankston, S. (2011). Cancer-related distress. In C. Yarbro, D. Wujcki, & B. Gobel (Eds.), *Cancer nursing: Principles and practice* (pp. 667–684). Boston: Jones and Bartlett.

Holland, J. (1999). Update: National Comprehensive Network guidelines for the management of psychosocial distress. *Oncology*, *13*(11A), 495–507.

Kissane, D. W., Treece, C., Breitbart, W., McKeen, N. A., & Chochinov, H. M. (2009). Dignity, meaning and demoralization: Emerging paradigms in end-of-life care. In H. M. Chochinov, & W. Breitbart (Eds.), *Handbook of psychiatry in palliative medicine* (pp. 324–340). New York: Oxford University Press.

Kubler-Ross, E. (1969). *On death and dying.* New York: Macmillan.

Loney, M., & Murphy-Ende, K. (2009). Death, dying, and grief in the face of cancer. In C. Burke (Ed.), *Psychosocial dimensions of oncology nursing care* (pp. 159–185). Pittsburgh: Oncology Nursing Society.

Moorey, S., & Greer, D. (2012). *Cognitive behavioral therapy for people with cancer.* Oxford, England: Oxford University Press.

Murphy-Ende, K. (2012). Mental health issues in cancer. In J. Payne (Ed.), *Contemporary issues in oncology* (pp. 165–190). Pittsburgh: Oncology Nursing Press.

National Comprehensive Cancer Network (NCCN). (2013). *Distress management (version 1.2013).* www.nccn.org/professionals/physician_gls/pdf/distress.pdf.

Osborn, R. L., Demoncada, A. C., & Feuerstein, M. (2006). Psychological interventions for depression, anxiety, and quality of life in cancer survivors: Meta-analysis. *International Journal Psychiatry Medicine*, *36*, 13–34.

Oxford University Press (2013). *Oxford English Dictionary.* dictionary.oed.com.

Parkes, C. (1987). *Bereavement: Studies of Grief in Adult Life.* Madison, CT: International University Press.

Rosenstein, D. (2011). Depression and end-of-life care for patients with cancer. *Dialogues in Clinical Neuroscience*, *13*(1), 101–108.

Roth, A. J., Kornblith, A. B., Batel-Copel, L., Peabody, E., Scher, H., & Holland, J. (1998). Rapid screening for psychological distress in men with prostate carcinoma: A pilot study. *Cancer*, *82*(10), 1904–1908.

Roth, A., & Massie, M. J. (2009). Anxiety in palliative care. In Chochinov, & W. Breitbert (Eds.), *Handbook of Psychiatry in Palliative Medicine.* (2nd ed., pp. 69–80). Oxford: University Press.

Rotter, J. (1966). Generalized expectations for internal versus external control of reinforcement. *Psychological Monographs*, *80*(1), 1–28.

Wilson, K., Chochinov, H., & Skirko, M. (2007). Depression and anxiety disorders in palliative care. *Journal of Pain and Symptom Management*, *33*, 118–129.

CHAPTER 39
Sexuality

Patricia W. Nishimoto, HaNa Kim, and Francisco A. Conde

OVERVIEW

I. Projected 18 million cancer survivors in the United States (U.S.) in 2022 (American Cancer Society [ACS], 2012)
   A. With improved survival, it is important for nurses to be aware of the long-term effects of cancer and its treatment on sexuality (Van de Poll-Franse et al., 2011).
      1. Cancer advocacy has resulted in more patients asking questions about how treatment might affect the sexual aspects of their lives (Hautamaki-Lamminen, Lipiainen, Beaver, Lehto, & Kellokumpu-Lehtinen, 2013).
      2. Across all cancer types, 66% of patients reported that patient-oncology provider conversations on sexual issues were important (Flynn et al., 2012).
      3. With interventions provided by health care providers, 70% of patients with cancer can have their sexual function return to baseline. Without interventions, functioning decreases over time (Cleary, Hegarty, & McCarthy, 2013).
      4. Patients' decreasing sexual functioning may increase the risk of emotional morbidity.
   B. Sexuality is an important component of quality of life (QOL) (Julien, Thom, & Kline, 2010; Zebrack, Foley, Wittmann, & Leonard, 2010).
   C. Not informing patients about possible adverse effects of cancer treatment on sexual function and fertility may result in legal liability (Crockin, 2005).
II. Sexuality as an important aspect of health care
   A. The World Health Organization (WHO) defines sexual health as integration of the somatic, emotional, intellectual, and social aspects of a sexual being (Olsson, Berglund, Larsson, & Athlin, 2012).
   B. The Oncology Nursing Society (ONS) has developed standards of care for sexuality (Brant & Wickham, 2013).

III. Nurses' difficulty discussing and addressing patients' sexual concerns (Saunamäki, Andersson, & Engström, 2010)
   A. Staff beliefs may prevent them from addressing patient's sexual concerns (Box 39-1) (Cavello, 2013; Julien et al., 2010; Olsson et al., 2012; White, Faithfull, & Allan, 2013; Zeng, Li, & Loke, 2011).
   B. When nurses do not initiate the conversation, it can lead to patient believing in the following:
      1. Sexuality is not a legitimate topic to discuss.
      2. Loss of sexual functioning is a "cost" of treatment.
      3. No effective treatment for sexual dysfunction exists, so it is not necessary to discuss it (Bober & Varela, 2012).
IV. Physiologic effects of cancer treatment on sexuality
   A. Hormone therapy
      1. Effects of endocrine therapy in men—gynecomastia, feminization, erectile dysfunction, decreased fertility, penile or testicular atrophy, decrease or loss of libido (Kumar, 2005)
      2. Effects of endocrine therapy in women—decreased vaginal lubrication, vaginal atrophy, change in libido, masculinization, amenorrhea, temporary or permanent menopause that may include menopausal symptoms of mood swings, hot flashes, sleep disturbance, and dyspareunia (Bowles et al., 2012)
   B. Radiation therapy
      1. Radiation therapy to the pelvis may cause temporary or permanent erectile dysfunction or decreased vaginal lubrication from vascular or nerve damage to pelvic structures.
      2. Amount of radiation therapy to the bulb of penis correlates to risk of erectile dysfunction resulting from destruction of nitric oxide–producing cells by radiation (Roach et al., 2004; Wernicke, Valicenti, DiEva, Houser, & Pequignot, 2004).

Box 39-1

Nursing Beliefs that Inhibit Addressing Patients' Sexual Concerns

1. Someone else will do it
2. Patients never bring up the subject
3. Patients are not worried about it
4. Nurses' personal biases regarding age, partner status, or discomfort discussing sexuality
5. Patients should be grateful to be alive. Belief priority should be on treatment and not "frivolous" matters
6. Patients may feel offended if asked and may even sue the nurse
7. Lack of knowledge or expertise, time, privacy, and administrative support

   a. Erection of penis during sexual stimulation is mediated by nitric oxide released from nerve endings close to the blood vessels of the penis.
3. Changes in sexual functioning have been shown to significantly decline in the first 2 years after external beam radiation therapy for prostate cancer (Siglin, Kubicek, Leiby, & Valicenti, 2010).
4. Prostate brachytherapy causes erectile dysfunction in 6% to 61% of men.
   a. It may also cause absence of or weak orgasm, painful ejaculation, decreased ejaculate volume, and decreased orgasmic quality.
   b. Age 70 years and older was a significant predictor of progressive erectile dysfunction following prostate brachytherapy (Matsushima et al., 2013).
5. Radiation-induced sexual dysfunction in cervical cancer ranges from 30% to 90%.
6. Brachytherapy for cancers of the cervix and uterus may cause dyspareunia and vaginal stenosis (Cleary et al., 2013).
7. Pelvic radiation in women may cause decreased vaginal lubrication (Bober & Varela, 2012), hardened clitoris (White et al., 2013), dyspareunia, change in vaginal sensation, risk of infection because of decreased vaginal lubrication, change in usual sexual expression, shortening of vaginal vault, decreased elasticity of vagina or vaginal stenosis, increased vaginal irritation, urinary incontinence, and/or bowel changes (Howlett et al., 2010).

C. Chemotherapy
1. In men, chemotherapy may cause decrease or loss of libido, retarded ejaculation or inhibition of ejaculation, and erectile dysfunction.
2. In women, chemotherapy may cause premature menopause, decreased libido, changes in body image, decreased vaginal distensibility and capacity, lubrication, and dyspareunia (Metzger et al., 2013).
3. Antimetabolites and antitumor antibiotics as single agents do not directly cause sexual dysfunction but may potentiate dysfunction when given with alkylating agents.
4. Chemotherapy side effects of oral stomatitis, dry mouth, nausea, fluid retention, fatigue, pain, and others may affect sexual functioning, libido, or both.

D. Surgery
1. When surgery disrupts the vascular system, the sympathetic nervous system, or the parasympathetic nervous system, it may affect the sexual response cycle (Davis, Meneses, & Messias, 2010).
2. Prostatectomy may cause retrograde ejaculation, erectile dysfunction if there is damage to autonomic nerve plexus, and diminished orgasm intensity.
   a. Prostatectomy may cause urinary incontinence, which could affect self-esteem, and the odor of urine on clothes may affect the libido of the patient and the partner.
3. Orchiectomy
   a. Unilateral orchiectomy for testicular cancer may not result in infertility or sexual dysfunction if the contralateral testis is normal and the patient is fertile at diagnosis (Krebs, 2011).
   b. Bilateral orchiectomy may decrease libido and cause atrophy of the penis.
4. Cystectomy
   a. Loss of vaginal lubrication in women (Bhatt et al., 2006; Zippe et al., 2004b) or erectile dysfunction in men (Zippe et al., 2004a) because of damage to nerves
   b. Change in vaginal diameter and length
   c. Retrograde ejaculation
5. Head and neck surgery (Low et al., 2009; O'Brien, Roe, Low, Deyn, & Rogers, 2012)
   a. Appearance affects body image and the way in which others view the patient
   b. Change in speech and ability to whisper during lovemaking
   c. Removal of spinal accessory nerve, which affects ability to turn the head
   d. Change in smell and taste sensations
   e. Drooling or the sensation of respirations on the neck of partner may affect partner's sexual desire
   f. Decreased saliva, halitosis, or both, which may affect kissing

6. Ostomy surgery (Den Oudsten et al., 2012)
   a. If woman has a colostomy, vaginal scarring may change the angle and distensibility of the vagina as well as body image.
   b. In women, decreased blood flow to the vagina may affect lubrication and cause dyspareunia.
   c. In men, decreased blood flow to the penis may affect erection.
   d. The appliance may "stick" to the body of the patient or the partner because of sweat.
7. Lumpectomy or mastectomy
   a. Numbness in previously sensitive breast, which may affect sexual pleasure
   b. In case of mastectomy, phantom nipple sensations
   c. May have "rubbery" sensation or occasional "electric shock–like" sensations

E. Other physiologic factors that affect sexuality—fatigue, pain, nerve damage, sleep deprivation, stenosis, scarring, organ loss, constipation, diarrhea, respiratory compromise, alopecia, fistulas or draining wounds, neuropathy, lymphedema, dyspareunia, muscle atrophy, hormone levels, menopausal symptoms, decreased blood cell counts, severity of cancer, comorbidities (Bober & Varela, 2012; Sandhu, Melman, & Mikhail, 2011; Tang, Lai, & Chung, 2010; Vitrano, Catania, & Mercadante, 2013)

V. Psychological effects of cancer treatment on sexuality
   A. Multiple factors that negatively affect body image
      1. Psychological and emotional response of the partner to the treatment-related physical changes (e.g., mastectomy, colostomy) experienced by the patient
      2. Physical changes resulting from cancer treatment
         a. Alopecia—whether partial or complete, may affect not only the patient but also the partner
            (1) Loss of eyelashes may cause constant blinking, which may affect attractiveness.
            (2) Loss of pubic hair may make the patient feel childlike and affect sexual desire; may affect partner's perception of adult versus child and affect relationship.
         b. Having an ostomy—may change body image such as the change in how clothes fit on the patient because of appliance
            (1) Patient may feel embarrassed and ashamed because of the presence of the ostomy.

c. Hysterectomy, prostatectomy, sterility from radiation therapy or chemotherapy
   (1) Inability to have children may influence how both men and women view their sexuality and sense of self.

B. Other psychological factors that affect sexuality — anxiety, fear of pain, fear of premature death, post-traumatic stress disorder (PTSD), depression, change in affect or personality, grief, shame, low self-esteem, feelings of isolation, cultural or religious beliefs, relationship discord, change in body image, fear of transmitting cancer, heightened sense of vulnerability, withdrawal (Bober & Varela, 2012; Cleary et al., 2013; Fallbjork, Salander, & Rasmussen, 2012; Jeffries & Clifford, 2011; Street et al., 2010; Zebrack et al., 2010)

VI. Reproductive and fertility issues
   A. Infertility is defined as the inability to conceive after 1 year of intercourse without contraception (Lee et al., 2006).
   B. It is estimated that 1,660,290 new cancer cases will be diagnosed in 2013 (ACS, 2013a).
      1. Of those diagnosed, 4% (approximately 66,000) are younger than 39 years.
      2. Most common cancers of people diagnosed who are younger than 40 years are breast cancer, melanoma, cervical cancer, non-Hodgkin lymphoma, and leukemia (Lee et al., 2006).
   C. Risk factors for cancer-related and cancer treatment–related infertility (Krebs, 2011; Lee et al., 2006; Metzger et al., 2013) include the following:
      1. Cancers of the genitourinary system such as bladder cancer, testicular cancer, and prostate cancer
      2. Gynecologic malignancies such as cancers of the uterine, ovaries, and cervix
      3. Exposure to radiation from diagnostic workups, radiation therapy, or both
         a. Depends on the location and dose of radiation
         b. Radiation therapy
            (1) In males receiving pelvic radiation
               (a) Age of male does not affect risk of sterility.
               (b) Less than 4 Gy results in temporary sterility.
               (c) More than 5 Gy results in permanent sterility (Krebs, 2011).
            (2) In females
               (a) Age and total amount of radiation dosage affect risk of sterility.
               (b) Of women younger than 40 years receiving 20 Gy fractionated over 5 to 6 weeks, 95% will have sterility.

(c) In those older than 40 years, a dose of 6 Gy affects sterility (Krebs, 2011).
(3) Field of radiation therapy (e.g., abdomen or pelvis)
(a) Of men and women receiving radiation below the diaphragm, 25% risk sterility.
4. Chemotherapy
a. Depends on type and dose of chemotherapy
(1) Lomustine, doxorubicin, and melphalan can suppress gonadal function.
(2) Cyclophosphamide, cytarabine, and fluorouracil usually have reversible germ cell toxicity.
(3) Childhood treatment of sarcoma with high-dose cyclophosphamide has high risk of gonadal dysfunction for males because of depletion of germinal epithelium and for females because of fall in estradiol and progesterone levels and elevation in follicle-stimulating hormone (FSH) and luteinizing hormone (LH) (Krebs, 2011) levels.
(4) Of men and women who receive mechlorethamine, oncovin (vincristine), procarbazine, prednisone (MOPP) combination therapy, 80% have fertility affected.
(5) Fertility is affected in 35% of men treated with doxorubicin (Adriamycin), bleomycin, vinblastine, dacarbazine (ABVD) combination therapy; fertility is usually recovered after cessation of treatment.
(6) Severity of pretreatment of oligospermia and cumulative dose affect spermatogenesis.
(7) Fertility may return as late as 4 years after treatment, so serial measurements of serum FSH levels and sperm counts need to be done.
5. Hormone or endocrine therapy
6. Stem cell and marrow transplantation
7. Biologic response modifiers and targeted therapies
8. Surgery to pelvis, reproductive organs (e.g., orchiectomy, hysterectomy), and those that affect the prostatic nerve plexus or presacral sympathetic nerves
D. Over 50% of cancer patients do not recall having a discussion about fertility risk when diagnosed (Campo-Engelstein, 2010).

E. The American Society of Clinical Oncology (ASCO) has made recommendations regarding fertility preservation in cancer patients.
1. Prior to start of cancer therapy, oncologists should discuss with patients the possibility of infertility and fertility preservation options and should make appropriate referrals to reproductive specialists (Lee et al., 2006).
F. Cancer and cancer treatment during pregnancy involves the following:
1. Risk factors depend on trimester of pregnancy.
a. Diagnostic tests
(1) The tests may present a risk to the fetus.
(2) Radioactive iodine is contraindicated for staging in pregnant woman.
(3) Diagnosis of cancer itself may be more difficult because of pregnancy changes.
(a) At the time of diagnosis, 1% to 4% of women with breast cancer are pregnant.
(b) Diagnosis of breast cancer may be delayed because of vascular, lymphatic, and density changes in the breast associated with pregnancy.
(c) Diagnostic tests may be delayed because of pregnancy, which may affect the survival of the patient.
b. Chemotherapy agents
(1) The type of agent used influences the risk to the fetus.
(a) Antimetabolites (especially methotrexate), alkylating agents, and folic acid antagonists should be avoided in the first trimester.
(b) Radiolabeled monoclonal antibodies should be avoided.
(c) The teratogenic potential of the agents is affected by drug dosage, ability of drug to enter fetal circulation, and route of administration.
(2) The first trimester is the time of greatest risk for negative health effects on the developing fetus.
(a) Patients with high-grade lymphoma during the first trimester should not delay therapy.
(b) Slower growing tumors may allow treatment to be delayed until the second trimester or after delivery.
c. Radiation therapy
(1) Usually delayed until after delivery
(2) Risk depends on field and dose of radiation
VII. Risk of human immunodeficiency virus (HIV) and sexually transmitted diseases (see Chapter 18)

ASSESSMENT

I. History and physical examination
- A. Assessment for factors that may affect sexuality and fertility—age, past medical and surgical history, cancer type and treatments, side effects, social history (including relationship status and quality of the relationship), cultural and religious beliefs
- B. In men, assessment for desire for children, erectile dysfunction
- C. In women, assessment for desire for children, pregnancy status, menopause or menopausal symptoms

II. Models for sexual assessment (Krebs, 2011)
- A. Three commonly used models for sexual assessment—ALARM, BETTER, and PLEASURE (Box 39-2)
  1. Each model assesses current sexual activities and practices, sexual attitudes and desire, and current medical issues.

PROBLEM STATEMENT AND OUTCOME IDENTIFICATION

I. Nursing diagnoses
- A. Ineffective Sexuality Pattern (NANDA-I)
- B. Disturbed Body Image (NANDA-I)
- C. Alterations in Sensation or Perception
- D. Risk for Ineffective Childbearing Pattern

II. Expected outcomes
- A. Patient identifies potential or actual alterations (changes in sexual function and desire, body image, sensation, perception, fertility) caused by disease or treatment. (*Note:* These outcomes are specific to Western culture and may not be appropriate for all patients.)

Box 39-2

Models for Sexual Assessment

ALARM	**A**ctivity, **L**ibido, **A**rousal and orgasm, **R**esolution, and **M**edical history relevant to sexuality
BETTER	**B**ringing up the topic, **E**xplaining that sexuality is part of quality of life (QOL) and nursing care, **T**elling the patient about resources, **T**iming the discussion to the patient's preference, **E**ducating the patient about the side effects of treatment that have impact on sexuality, and **R**ecording, which should be made in the patient notes that the topic has been discussed
PLEASURE	**P**artner, **L**ovemaking, **E**motions, **A**ttitudes, **S**ymptoms, **U**nderstanding, **R**eproduction, **E**nergy

---

- B. Patient expresses feelings about alterations in sexuality, body image, sensation, and fertility.
- C. Patient describes strategies and resources that he or she can use in response to actual or potential alterations.
- D. Patient identifies satisfactory alternative methods for expressing sexuality.
- E. Patient engages in open communication with partner about these matters.

PLANNING AND IMPLEMENTATION

I. Use of the PLISSIT (P = permission, LI = limited information, SS = specific suggestions, IT = intensive therapy) model for sexuality counseling (Annon, 1976; Oskay, Beji, Bal, & Yilmaz, 2011)
- A. Useful model for levels of nursing intervention based on the nurse's comfort and expertise with subject of sexuality
- B. Referral to another provider at any level of intervention after verifying the skill of the provider.
  1. P = Permission
     - a. First level of intervention
       (1) All nurses are able to provide this level of intervention of normalizing concerns (Davis et al., 2010).
       (2) It is permission to discuss the topic, not blanket permission for all behaviors.
       (3) Nurses initiate discussion to convey acceptability that discussing sexual changes caused by diagnosis or treatment is appropriate.
       (4) Permission includes giving patients permission to not engage in sexual activity.
     - b. To effectively intervene, nurses need to know basic knowledge about sexuality.
       (1) Anatomy and physiology
       (2) How disease, treatments, and age affect sexual functioning
       (3) Sexual response cycle
     - c. Example—"We've talked together about how chemotherapy can affect your body, but another important aspect is how it can affect how you feel about yourself as a man and how it may impact on your role as a husband."
  2. LI = Limited Information
     - a. Second level of intervention
       (1) Most nurses are able to intervene at this level.
       (2) Providing limited information may positively affect self-image, relationship, and ability to enjoy sex; decrease fear; increase communication; and increase knowledge (Cleary, Hegarty, & McCarthy, 2011).

Part 5

(3) This level of intervention addresses concerns, questions, myths, and misconceptions.
    b. Need for nurses to know how diagnosis and treatment can affect sexuality
    c. Example—"You asked a very good question about what type of birth control to use to prevent pregnancy while on chemotherapy. You have Hodgkin disease, which means you could use birth control pills or other hormonal methods. It may put you at increased risk of infection to use an intrauterine device or even a diaphragm, so perhaps it is better not to use one of those. And if you gain or lose weight, it could cause the diaphragm to not fit and so not be effective." (LI level)
3. SS = Specific Suggestions
    a. Third level of intervention
        (1) Many experienced or advanced practice nurses are able to intervene at this level. Otherwise, patients are referred to gynecologists for health interventions such as oral contraceptive pills.
        (2) Suggestions need to be appropriate for the following:
            (a) Cultural and religious beliefs
            (b) Patient and partner's value system, preferences, and priorities
    b. Opportunity to consider different options, but nurse does not impose them
    c. Example—suggestions to decrease pain during coitus include use of pillows to cushion joints and taking pain medication prior to sexual activity.
4. IT = Intensive Therapy
    a. Requires in-depth knowledge level about sexuality and counseling
    b. Usually needed for long-standing or severe concerns
    c. Example—if treatment brings up issues of childhood abuse, intensive therapy is needed.
5. Approximately 80% to 90% of sexual problems identified by patients may be solved with use of the first three levels (Cleary et al., 2013).
II. Interventions related to Ineffective Sexuality Pattern
    A. Prevention
        1. Education and anticipatory guidance—may decrease fear and distress while facilitating open communication with the partner (Cleary et al., 2013)
            a. Patients report that they are more receptive to discussing sexuality with nurses (Cleary et al., 2011).
            b. The physiology of sexual functioning and ways in which diagnosis and treatment may

affect functioning in both positive and negative ways should be explained to the patient. Including this as part of pretreatment counseling potentiates the ability of the patient to give fully informed consent (Cavello, 2013).
            c. It should not be assumed that the patient already has basic information on sexuality.
                (1) Models or drawings may be used.
                (2) Handouts or website information should be made available.
            d. Myths or misconceptions (e.g., fear that anal stimulation may cause rectal cancer) should be dispelled.
        2. Encouraging communication between the couple (Davis et al., 2010)
            a. The nurse could serve as a role model for the couple by speaking openly when discussing sexual functioning.
            b. A nonjudgmental approach should be used by the nurse as the couple discusses fears or feelings. The nurse should build a rapport to build trust.
            c. The couple should be allowed to conduct role playing in a safe environment; the nurse may demonstrate how they may begin the conversation about changes in sexual functioning.
            d. Attendance at classes or support groups where sexuality is openly discussed should be encouraged.
        3. Being a patient advocate
            a. Being aware of medications that affect sexual functioning (e.g., narcotics, hormones, sedatives, antidepressants)
            b. Suggesting alternative medications that may have fewer side effects
            c. Being aware of studies that are being done on equipment or devices that improve sexual function and lessen treatment-related impact on sexuality (e.g., Eros is an FDA-approved device that mechanically increases blood flow to the clitoris and external genitalia)
            d. Encouraging the couple to speak with the surgeon before surgery about the benefits and risks of procedures that can preserve sexual function
    B. Interventions related to sexual dysfunction
        1. Conducting a sexual history
        2. Intervention using the PLISSIT model
            a. Incorporating the patient's value system and cultural beliefs into intervention
            b. Supporting the patient in considering options to meet her or his sexual needs and that accommodate to changes in sexual function

(1) Massage, fantasy, change in positions, use of sexy lingerie to cover incision site or stoma

(2) For vaginal dryness in women—use of water-based lubricants, vaginal dilators, relaxation techniques, topical estrogen if not contraindicated

(3) Referrals for medical intervention for pelvic floor muscle exercises and manometric biofeedback, penile implants, penile injections, vacuum devices, and vaginal reconstruction

c. Strategies to expand patient's knowledge base

(1) Encouraging attendance at support groups; psychoeducational support plays a role in improving alterations in sexual functioning, especially for female patients (Incrocci & Jensen, 2013).

(2) Providing written or Internet resources on sexuality and cancer; verbal counseling combined with written information is more effective (Bober & Varela, 2012; Cleary et al., 2011).

(3) Providing a list of resources (Bober & Varela, 2012)

(4) Including sexual health as part of the survivorship plan of care (Cavello, 2013)

II. Interventions related to Disturbed Body Image

A. Referral to the ACS's Look Good Feel Better Program

B. Helping patient obtain information about reconstructive surgical options, as appropriate (e.g., penile graft, breast reconstruction)

C. Providing considerations or suggestions to address concerns about the impact of ostomy on sexual health

1. Ensuring tight seal of appliance to decrease odor
2. Emptying appliance before sexual activity
3. Avoiding certain foods that cause flatulence or increased odor

D. If patient has a scar, providing information about ways of using makeup or clothing in a manner that enhances self-image and alleviates feelings of shame or embarrassment

III. Interventions related to Alterations in Sensation or Perception

A. Use of the ALARM, BETTER, or PLEASURE model to assess for any changes in taste, hearing, smell, or touch that could affect patient's sexual functioning

1. For example, metallic after-taste or dry mouth resulting from chemotherapy may affect romantic interactions—for example, decreased ability to enjoy a food with a partner or difficulty kissing for an extended period

2. Nerves severed after surgery may cause hyperalgesia, numbing, and peripheral neuropathy, which may decrease sexual pleasure.

B. Discussing the importance of bringing up concerns related to sexuality as they arise

1. Providing educational materials and resources on sensory changes that may occur as a result of cancer treatment interventions

2. For patients who have had laryngectomy—suggesting wearing a scarf around the neck to hide the stoma during sex to help decrease self-consciousness and embarrassment (ACS, 2013b)

3. If patient unable to whisper or speak during sex, suggesting use of touch and other nonverbal behaviors as part of foreplay and intimacy

4. Suggesting use of cologne or perfume to mask any stoma odors and avoidance of odorous foods prior to initiating sex

5. Suggesting that during foreplay, partner could be asked to use soft materials such as rabbit fur or silk on areas of hyperalgesia or neuropathy that could be exacerbated with pressure or touch

6. Recommending novel ways of engaging in lovemaking to prevent sexual pain associated with a certain position or tender area

7. Suggesting use of a vaginal moisturizer on a daily basis to help lubricate the vaginal lining and prevent vaginal dryness and dyspareunia

a. Vaginal moisturizers can be used in conjunction with a water- or silicone-based lubricant during sexual intercourse.

8. Informing patient that worsening of vaginal atrophy after radiation therapy can be prevented by estrogen cream (if not contraindicated) and vaginal dilation (Katz, 2009)

a. A dilator should be used twice a day if penile intercourse is not an option.

9. Recommending that patient set aside blocks of "date time" to help enhance low desire or libido without the pressure of engaging in sexual intercourse

IV. Interventions related to Risk for Ineffective Childbearing Pattern

A. Discussing the importance of not becoming pregnant during and after treatment (specific time based on type of treatment given and follow-up needed, such as scans that have radiation risk)

1. Providing counseling regarding use of birth control strategies

a. Referral to primary care providers or gynecologist for pharmacologic interventions
2. Use of the PLISSIT model for intervention management
B. Prevention of complications in pregnant women with cancer
   1. Diagnostic test considerations
      a. Discussing or asking provider (physician, nurse practitioner, physician assistant) if diagnostic workup can be modified to reduce risk to fetus
         (1) Requesting ultrasonography instead of radiography, if possible
         (2) Use of magnetic resonance imaging (MRI) instead of computed tomography (CT) to prevent radiation exposure to fetus
         (3) If early-stage disease, omitting late-stage workup (e.g., bone scan)
      b. May be able to modify diagnostic test procedure (e.g., shield fetus)
      c. Unreliability of serum tumor markers when patient is pregnant
      d. Consultation with the obstetrician when making diagnostic decisions and in management of pregnant patient receiving cancer therapy
   2. Chemotherapy and molecular-targeted therapy agents
      a. Usually safer to give chemotherapy and molecular-targeted therapy during the second or third trimester (McGrath & Ring, 2011)
      b. May increase risk of the following to fetus:
         (1) Low birth weight—increases risk of admission to neonatal intensive care unit with attendant risks of preterm delivery
         (2) Mutagenesis
         (3) Teratogenic effects
      c. Risks and benefits of various regimens
      d. Delay of treatment initiation, if possible
      e. Addressing issue of pregnancy termination, keeping in mind cultural and religious beliefs
      f. Being aware of risk to fetus from antiemetics, growth factors, analgesics
   3. Radiation therapy
      a. Shielding of fetus, if possible
      b. Delaying therapy until after delivery, if possible
      c. Use of machine with low leakage; considering target dose, size of radiation therapy field, and distance of the field edges from fetus
   4. Surgery
      a. Timing of surgery (trimester of pregnancy)
      b. Type of surgery

c. Anesthetic agent used
   (1) Need to adjust for pregnancy-induced physiologic and anatomic changes
d. Length of surgery
5. Ostomy patients may have trouble "pushing" for a vaginal delivery because of removal of muscles.
C. Management of pregnant patient during cancer treatment
   1. Pregnant patient with cancer optimally managed by a multidisciplinary team that includes oncologists, hematologists, perinatologists, family physicians, psychologists, social workers, and nurses
      a. Nurses play an important role as patient advocate within the team.
   2. High-risk prenatal care if the patient remains pregnant
      a. Risk of thrombocytopenia
      b. Risk of disseminated intravascular coagulation
      c. Risk of premature delivery because of physical stress of illness, treatment, or side effects
   3. Evaluation of treatment options with patient and describing the one with lowest risk to fetus
   4. Initiating discussion about whose life is a priority if an emergency occurs
   5. Careful evaluation of each drug with regard to safety
      a. Assessing if drug crosses placental barrier
         (1) Example—lorazepam, which increases risk of floppy baby syndrome
      b. After delivery, need to counsel mother about risk to baby if she breastfeeds while receiving chemotherapy
         (1) Potential for immunosuppression or neutropenia
         (2) Unknown effect on growth and development
         (3) Possible risk of carcinogenesis
   6. Counseling mother that breast irradiation may result in little or no breast milk production
D. Interventions to prevent cancer treatment–related infertility
   1. Choosing the treatment with least risk to fertility, when possible, and discussing whether fertility preservation is the highest priority for the patient
      a. Assessing and discussing insurance coverage (Campo-Engelstein, 2010) and risks for infertility such as age and type of treatment (Quinn et al., 2011)
         (1) Fertile Hope—a national LIVESTRONG program that may provide financial assistance for fertility preservation to

citizens or permanent residents of the U.S. with cancer

   b. Referral to reproductive specialist (Quinn et al., 2011)

2. Use of oophoropexy to protect the ovaries from radiation injury (Lee et al., 2006; Tulandi, Huang, & Tan, 2008)

   a. Referral to gynecologic oncologist, if required

3. Shielding to prevent or reduce radiation exposure to testes, if possible

4. Methods to preserve fertility

   a. Strategies to preserve male fertility

      (1) Sperm banking—most successful and only established fertility preservation (Fertile Hope, 2013a)

      (2) Obtaining sperm through testicular extraction or electroejaculation under sedation an option, especially in men with neurologic impairment

      (3) Testicular tissue freezing—still experimental

   b. Strategies to preserve female fertility

      (1) Standard options—egg harvesting, in vitro fertilization (IVF), and embryo freezing for later implantation (Fertile Hope, 2013b)

      (2) Eggs donated by another woman

      (3) Gestational surrogacy—another woman carrying the pregnancy

      (4) GnRH (gonadotropin-releasing hormone) agonist or cyclic oral contraceptives—may be used to protect ovaries during chemotherapy (Chen, Li, Cui, & Hu, 2011; Yang et al., 2013)

5. Referral to organizations such as Fertile Hope for resources on cancer treatment-related infertility and preservation strategies

E. Management of cancer treatment–related infertility

1. Grief counseling for loss of fertility

2. Treatment for retrograde ejaculation to restore fertility

   a. Certain drugs (e.g., sympathomimetic phenylpropanolamine) that can temporarily close the sphincter to enable sperm ejaculation

EVALUATION

The oncology nurse systematically and regularly evaluates the patient's and the family's responses to interventions to determine progress toward the achievement of expected outcomes. Relevant data are collected, and actual findings are compared with expected findings. Nursing diagnoses, outcomes, and plans of care are reviewed and revised, as necessary.

Internet Resources

American Association of Sexuality Educators, Counselors and Therapists
www.aasect.org
American Cancer Society
www.cancer.org
American Society of Clinical Oncology
www.cancer.net
Fertile Hope
www.fertilehope.org
Fertility concerns
www.Fertilehope.com
Gay and Lesbian Ostomates
www.glo-uoaa.org/
National Sexuality Resource Center
www.nsrc.sfsu.edu
Oncolink
www.oncolink.com
Out With Cancer
www.outwithcancer.com
Pregnant Women with Cancer
www.pregnantwithcancer.org
Women's Cancer Network
www.wcn.org

References

American Cancer Society. (2012). *Cancer treatment and survivorship facts & figures 2012–2013.* Atlanta: Author.

American Cancer Society. (2013a). *Cancer facts & figures, 2013.* Atlanta: Author.

American Cancer Society. (2013b). *Moving on after treatment for laryngeal or hypopharyngeal cancers.* http://www.cancer.org/cancer/laryngealandhypopharyngealcancer/overviewguide/laryngeal-and-hypopharyngeal-cancer-overview-after-follow-up.

Annon, J. (1976). The PLISSIT model: A proposed conceptual scheme for the behavioral treatment of sexual problems. *Journal of Sex Education and Therapy, 2*(2), 1–15.

Bhatt, A., Nandipati, K., Dhar, N., Ulchaker, J., Jones, S., Rackley, R., et al. (2006). Neurovascular preservation in orthotopic cystectomy: Impact on female sexual function. *Urology, 67*(4), 742–745.

Bober, S. L., & Varela, V. S. (2012). Sexuality in adult cancer survivors: Challenges and intervention. *Journal of Clinical Oncology, 30*(30), 3712–3719.

Bowles, E. J. A., Boudreau, D. M., Chubak, J., Yu, O., Fujii, M., Chestnut, J., et al. (2012). Patient-reported discontinuation of endocrine therapy and related adverse effects among women with early-stage breast cancer. *Journal of Oncology Practice, 8*(6), e149–e157.

Brant, J. M., & Wickham, R. (Eds.). (2013). *Statement on the scope and standards of oncology nursing practice: Generalist and advanced practice.* Pittsburgh: Oncology Nursing Society.

Campo-Engelstein, L. (2010). Consistency in insurance coverage for iatrogenic conditions resulting from cancer treatment including fertility preservation. *Journal of Clinical Oncology, 28* (8), 1284–1286.

Cavello, J. (2013). Sexual health after cancer: Communicating with your patients. *The ASCO Post, 4*(6), 1; 26.

Chen, H., Li, J., Cui, T., & Hu, L. (2011). Adjuvant gonadotropin-releasing hormone analogues for the prevention of chemotherapy induced premature ovarian failure in premenopausal women. *Cochrane Database of Systematic Reviews,* (11), CD008018.

Cleary, V., Hegarty, J., & McCarthy, G. (2011). Sexuality in Irish women with gynecologic cancer. *Oncology Nursing Forum, 38* (2), E87–E96.

Cleary, V., Hegarty, J., & McCarthy, G. (2013). How a diagnosis of gynaecological cancer affects women's sexuality. *Cancer Nursing Practice, 12*(1), 32–37.

Crockin, S. L. (2005). Legal issues related to parenthood after cancer. *Journal of the National Cancer Institute Monographs, 2005* (34), 111–113.

Davis, S. C., Meneses, K., & Messias, H. (2010). Exploring sexuality & quality of life in women after breast cancer surgery. *The Nurse Practitioner, 35*(9), 25–31.

Den Oudsten, B. L., Traa, M. J., Thong, M. S. Y., Martijn, H., De Hingh, I. H. S. T., Bosseha, K., et al. (2012). Higher prevalence of sexual dysfunction in colon and rectal cancer survivors compared with the normative population: A population-based study. *European Journal of Cancer, 48,* 3161–3170.

Fallbjork, U., Salander, P., & Rasmussen, B. H. (2012). From "no big deal" to "losing oneself": Different meanings of mastectomy. *Cancer Nursing, 35*(5), E41–E48.

Fertile Hope. (2013a). *Male reproductive options.* http://www.fertilehope.org/healthcare-professionals/clinical-tools/male_options_v3.pdf.

Fertile Hope. (2013b). *Female reproductive options.* http://www.fertilehope.org/healthcare-professionals/clinical-tools/male_options_v3.pdf.

Flynn, K. E., Reese, J. B., Jeffery, D. D., Abernethy, A. P., Lin, L., Shelby, R. A., et al. (2012). Patient experiences with communication about sex during and after treatment for cancer. *Psycho-Oncology, 21,* 594–601.

Hautamaki-Lamminen, K., Lipiainen, L., Beaver, K., Lehto, J., & Kellokumpu-Lehtinen, P. (2013). Identifying cancer patients with greater need for information about sexual issues. *European Journal of Oncology Nursing, 17,* 9–15.

Howlett, K., Koetters, T., Edrington, J., West, C., Paul, S., Lee, K., et al. (2010). Changes in sexual function on mood and quality of life in patients undergoing radiation therapy for prostate cancer. *Oncology Nursing Forum, 37*(1), E58–E66.

Incrocci, L., & Jensen, P. T. (2013). Pelvic radiotherapy and sexual function in men and women. *The Journal of Sexual Medicine, 10*(S1), 53–64.

Jeffries, H., & Clifford, C. (2011). A literature review of the impact of a diagnosis of cancer of the vulva and surgical treatment. *Journal of Clinical Nursing, 20,* 31–3142.

Julien, J. O., Thom, B., & Kline, N. E. (2010). Identification of barriers to sexual health assessment in oncology nursing practice. *Oncology Nursing Forum, 37*(3), E186–E190.

Katz, A. (2009). Interventions for sexuality after pelvic radiation therapy and gynecological cancer. *The Cancer Journal, 15,* 45–47.

Krebs, L. (2011). Sexual and reproductive dysfunction. In C. H. Yarbro, D. Wujcik, & B. H. Gobel (Eds.), *Cancer nursing: Principles and practice* (pp. 879–911). Sudbury, MA: Jones and Bartlett.

Kumar, R. J. (2005). Adverse events associated with hormonal therapy for prostate cancer. *Reviews in Urology, 7*(Suppl. 5), S37–S43.

Lee, S. J., Schover, L. R., Partridge, A. H., Patrizio, P., Wallace, W. H., Hagerty, K., et al. (2006). American Society of Clinical Oncology recommendations on fertility preservation in cancer patients. *Journal of Clinical Oncology, 24*(18), 2917–2931.

Low, C., Fullarton, M., Parkinson, E., O'Brien, K., Jackson, S. R., Lowe, D., et al. (2009). Issues of intimacy and sexual dysfunction following major head and neck cancer treatment. *Oral Oncology, 45*(10), 898–903.

Matsushima, M., Kikuchi, E., Maeda, T., Nakashima, J., Sugawara, A., Ando, T., et al. (2013). A prospective longitudinal survey of erectile dysfunction in patients with localized prostate cancer treated with permanent prostate brachytherapy. *The Journal of Urology, 189,* 1014–1018.

McGrath, S. E., & Ring, A. (2011). Chemotherapy for breast cancer in pregnancy: Evidence and guidance for oncologists. *Therapeutic Advances in Medical Oncology, 3*(2), 73–83.

Metzger, M. L., Meacham, L. R., Patterson, B., Casillao, J. C., Constine, L. S., Hijya, N., et al. (2013). Female reproductive health after childhood, adolescent and young adult cancers: Guidelines for the assessment and management of female reproductive complications. *Journal of Clinical Oncology, 31,* 1–9.

O'Brien, K., Roe, B., Low, C., Deyn, L., & Rogers, S. N. (2012). An exploration of the perceived changes in intimacy of patients' relationships following head and neck cancer. *Journal of Clinical Nursing, 21*(17–18), 2499–2508.

Olsson, C., Berglund, A., Larsson, M., & Athlin, E. (2012). Patient's sexuality—a neglected area of cancer nursing? *European Journal of Oncology Nursing, 16,* 426–431.

Oskay, U. Y., Beji, N. K., Bal, M. D., & Yilmaz, S. D. (2011). Evaluation of sexual function in patients with gynecologic cancer and evidence-based nursing interventions. *Sexuality and Disability, 29,* 33–41.

Quinn, G. P., Vadaparampil, S. T., Gwede, C. K., Reinecke, J. D., Mason, T. M., & Silvo, C. (2011). Developing a referral system for fertility preservation among patients with newly diagnosed cancer. *Journal of the National Comprehensive Cancer Network, 9*(11), 1219–1225.

Roach, M., Winter, K., Michalski, J. M., Cox, J. D., Purdy, J. A., Bosch, W., et al. (2004). Penile bulb dose and impotence after three-dimensional conformal radiotherapy for prostate cancer on RTOG 9406: Findings from a prospective, multi-institutional, phase I/II dose-escalation study. *International Journal of Radiation Oncology, Biology, Physics, 60*(5), 1351–1356.

Sandhu, K. S., Melman, A., & Mikhail, M. S. (2011). Impact of hormones on female sexual function and dysfunction. *Female Pelvic Medicine & Reconstructive Surgery, 17*(1), 8–16.

Saunamäki, N., Andersson, M., & Engström, M. (2010). Discussing sexuality with patients: Nurses' attitudes and beliefs. *Journal of Advanced Nursing, 66*(6), 1308–1316.

Siglin, J., Kubicek, G. J., Leiby, B., & Valicenti, R. K. (2010). Time of decline in sexual function after external beam radiotherapy for prostate cancer. *International Journal of Radiation Oncology, Biology, Physics, 76*(1), 31–35.

Street, A. F., Couper, J. W., Love, A. W., Bloch, S., Kissane, D. W., & Street, B. C. (2010). Psychosocial adaptation in female partners of men with prostate cancer. *European Journal of Cancer Care, 19,* 234–242.

Tang, C. S., Lai, B. P. Y., & Chung, T. K. H. (2010). Influences of mastery, spousal support, and adaptive coping on sexual drive and satisfaction among Chinese gynecologic cancer survivors. *Archives of Sexual Behavior, 39,* 1191–1200.

Tulandi, T., Huang, J. Y., & Tan, S. L. (2008). Preservation of female fertility: An essential progress. *Obstetrics and Gynecology, 112*(5), 1160–1172.

Van de Poll-Franse, L. V., Mols, F., Gundy, C. M., Creutzberg, C. L., Nout, R. A., Verdonck-de Leeuw, I. M., et al. (2011). Normative data for the EORTC QLC-C30 and EROTC-sexuality items in the general Dutch population. *European Journal of Cancer, 47,* 667–675.

Vitrano, V., Catania, V., & Mercadante, S. (2013). Sexuality in patients with advanced cancer: A prospective study in a population admitted to an acute pain relief and palliative care unit. *American Journal of Hospice & Palliative Care, 28*(3), 198–202.

Wernicke, A. G., Valicenti, R., DiEva, K., Houser, C., & Pequignot, E. (2004). Radiation dose delivered to the proximal penis as a predictor of the risk of erectile dysfunction after three-dimensional conformal radiotherapy for localized prostate cancer. *International Journal of Radiation Oncology, Biology, Physics, 60*(5), 1357–1363.

White, I. D., Faithfull, S., & Allan, H. (2013). The re-construction of women's sexual lives after pelvic radiotherapy: A critique of social constructionist & biomedical perspectives on the study of female sexuality after cancer treatment. *Social Science & Medicine, 76,* 188–196.

Yang, B., Shi, W., Yang, J., Liu, H., Zhao, H., Li, X., et al. (2013). Concurrent treatment with gonadotropin-releasing hormone agonists for chemotherapy-induced ovarian damage in premenopausal women with breast cancer: A meta-analysis of randomized controlled trials. *The Breast, 22*(2), 150–157.

Zebrack, B. J., Foley, S., Wittmann, D., & Leonard, M. (2010). Sexual functioning in young adult survivors of childhood cancer. *Psycho-Oncology, 19,* 814–822.

Zeng, Y. C., Li, D., & Loke, A. Y. (2011). Life after cervical cancer: Quality of life among Chinese women. *Nursing & Health Sciences, 13,* 296–302.

Zippe, C. D., Raina, R., Massanyi, E. Z., Agarwal, A., Jones, J. S., Ulchaker, J., et al. (2004). Sexual function after male radical cystectomy in a sexually active population. *Urology, 64*(4), 682–685.

Zippe, C. D., Raina, R., Shah, A. D., Massanyi, E. Z., Agarwal, A., Ulchaker, J., et al. (2004). Female sexual dysfunction after radical cystectomy: A new outcome measure. *Urology, 63*(6), 1153–1157.

Part 5

CHAPTER 40

Metabolic Emergencies

Kristen W. Maloney

Disseminated Intravascular Coagulation

OVERVIEW

I. Definition—disseminated intravascular coagulation (DIC) marked by intravascular activation of coagulation; consumes coagulation factors and platelets within the body, which leads to potential bleeding and hemorrhage; process may be more gradual in the patient with cancer (Levi, 2009)

II. Pathophysiology of DIC
   A. Multiple underlying causes of DIC, risk may increase as cancer treatment continues (Levi, 2009)
   B. Activation of coagulation pathways
      1. Extrinsic pathway (factor VII) activated with damage to endothelial lining of blood vessels
      2. Intrinsic pathway (factor XII) activated with damage to subendothelial tissue
      3. Extrinsic and intrinsic pathways comprise the common pathway.
      4. Results in clot formation and activation of coagulation cascade
         a. Fibrin clots are formed, accumulate in body's circulatory system
         b. Clots consume available platelets and coagulation proteins.
         c. Normal coagulation is disrupted; abnormal bleeding occurs.

III. Causes of DIC
   A. DIC is always secondary to an underlying disorder that causes an activation of coagulation (Levi & van der Poll, 2013).
   B. Common causes include sepsis, severe infection, vascular abnormalities, severe allergic reactions, severe immunologic reactions, and malignancy, both solid tumors and leukemia (Levi & van der Poll, 2013).

IV. Diagnostic strategies
   A. Laboratory studies (Table 40-1)
      1. Intravascular clotting—platelet count, fibrinogen level, thrombin time, protein C level, protein S level
      2. Depletion of clotting factors—prothrombin time (PT), activated partial thromboplastin time (aPTT), international normalized ratio (INR)
      3. Accelerated fibrinolysis—fibrin degradation products (FDPs), D-dimer assay, antithrombin III level.
      4. Looking at clinical effects of cell destruction—schistocytes on peripheral smear, bilirubin level, blood urea nitrogen level

V. Management and treatment strategies
   A. Key to treatment of DIC is to treat the underlying cause; once the underlying cause is managed, DIC will likely correct itself (Levi, Toh, Thachil, & Watson, 2009).
   B. Laboratory data, patient condition and underlying cause should be used to determine effective treatment strategies.
      1. Transfusions of platelets, fresh frozen plasma (FFP), cryoprecipitate
      2. Use of anticoagulants (e.g., heparin, low-molecular-weight heparin)—controversial because studies show effects on laboratory data but lack a clinically significant patient outcome (Levi et al., 2009)
      3. Use of fibrinolytic agents (e.g., epsilon-aminocaproic acid, tranexamic acid)—can be used in severe cases, in which bleeding does not respond to other therapies (Levi & van der Poll, 2013)
      4. Anticoagulant factor concentrates (e.g., recombinant human-activated protein C)—have potential to improve DIC but not proven to reduce mortality (Levi & van der Poll, 2013).

Table 40-1

Normal Laboratory Values Related to Coagulation

Laboratory Test	Results
Platelet count	150,000-400,000/mm^3
Fibrinogen	200-400/100 mL
Thrombin time	7-12 sec
Protein C level	4 µg/mL
Protein S level	23 µg/mL
Prothrombin time	11-15 sec
Activated partial thromboplastin time	30-40 sec
International normalized ratio	1-1.2 times normal
Fibrin degradation products	<10 mg/mL
D-dimer assay	<50 µg/dL
Bilirubin level	0.1-0.2 mg/dL
Blood urea nitrogen	8-20 mg/dL

Adapted from Morton, P. G., Fontaine, D. K., Hudak, C. M., & Gallo, B. M. (Eds.). (2005). *Critical care nursing: A holistic approach* (8th ed.). Philadelphia: Lippincott, Williams and Wilkins.

Table 40-2

Laboratory Results with Disseminated Intravascular Coagulation

Increased Values	Decreased Values	Other
Thrombin time	Platelet count	Schistocytes present on peripheral smear
Prothrombin time	Fibrinogen level	
Activated partial thromboplastin time	Protein C level	
International normalized ratio	Protein S level	
Fibrin degradation products	Antithrombin III level	
D-dimer assay		
Bilirubin level		
Blood urea nitrogen		

ASSESSMENT

I. Physical examination
   A. Skin symptoms—pallor, petechiae, jaundice, ecchymosis, hematomas, acral cyanosis (irregularly shaped blue or gray discolored areas on extremities), bleeding from any site of invasive procedures
   B. Eyes, ears, mouth, nose, and throat symptoms—visual disturbances, scleral injection, periorbital edema, subconjunctival hemorrhage, eye or ear pain, petechiae on nasal or oral mucosa, epistaxis, tenderness or bleeding from gums
   C. Cardiac symptoms—tachycardia, hypotension, diminished peripheral pulses, changes in color and temperature of extremities
   D. Respiratory symptoms—dyspnea, tachypnea, hypoxia, hemoptysis, cyanosis, shortness of breath
   E. Gastrointestinal (GI) symptoms—tarry stools, hematemesis, abdominal pain, abdominal distention, positive results of guaiac stool test
   F. Genitourinary symptoms—hematuria (burning, dysuria and frequency associated with hematuria), decreased urinary output
   G. Musculoskeletal symptoms—joint pain and stiffness
   H. Neurologic symptoms—headache, restlessness, confusion, lethargy, altered level of consciousness, obtundation, seizures, coma
II. Laboratory data—indicative of DIC occurring in patient (Table 40-2)

PROBLEM STATEMENTS AND OUTCOME IDENTIFICATION

I. Risk for Bleeding (NANDA-I)
   A. Expected outcome—patient will identify risk factors for bleeding.
   B. Expected outcome—patient will remain hemodynamically stable.
II. Risk for Ineffective Peripheral Tissue Perfusion (NANDA-I)
   A. Expected outcome—patient will show signs of appropriate perfusion through stabilization of organ systems.
III. Anxiety (NANDA-I)
   A. Expected outcome—patient will verbalize awareness of his or her own coping abilities.
   B. Expected outcome—patient will demonstrate effective coping skills.

PLANNING AND IMPLEMENTATION

I. Interventions to manage sites of active bleeding
   A. Application of pressure to sites of bleeding via pressure dressing or sandbag
   B. Intravenous (IV) fluids, as needed, for volume repletion
   C. Oxygen therapy, as needed
   D. Blood products, as needed
   E. Anticoagulant, as ordered
II. Interventions for patient safety ⚠
   A. Assistance with activities of daily living (ADLs)
   B. If hospitalized, bed in low locked position, two side rails up, call bell within reach

Part 6

C. Educating patient and caregiver on risk for injury
D. Providing close supervision for mobilization with appropriate device and footwear needed for ambulation
E. Scheduling a home assessment with home nursing care and physical therapy

III. Interventions to assist in coping
A. Assessment of available resources for patient and caregivers
B. Providing education specific to DIC and its signs and symptoms
C. Providing emotional support for patient and caregivers

EVALUATION

The oncology nurse systematically and regularly evaluates patient and family responses to interventions related to DIC to determine progress toward the achievement of hemodynamic stability. Relevant data are collected, and actual findings are compared with expected findings. Nursing diagnoses, outcomes, and plans of care are reviewed and revised, as necessary.

Thrombotic Thrombocytopenic Purpura (TTP)

OVERVIEW

I. Definition—a disorder of platelet aggregation, in which thrombosis of the microvasculature may occur (Kessler, Khan, & Lai-Miller, 2012)
II. Pathophysiology of TTP
A. Rare disease, difficult to understand; theories exist regarding pathophysiology
1. ADAMTS13 regulates the length and binding accessibility of both von Willebrand factor (VWF) and ultralarge multimers of von Willebrand factor (ULVWFs) (Rizzo et al., 2012).
2. With lack of ADAMTS13 in TTP, ULVWFs are not broken down and, instead, continue to stick to the endothelium, collecting platelets that pass by, which results in formation of thrombi (Rizzo et al., 2012).
B. VWF was first described in 1924; it is divided into two categories, hereditary and acquired TTP.
III. Causes of TTP
A. Hereditary
1. Hereditary TTP is an autosomal recessive disorder, accounting for only 1% of cases (Kessler et al., 2012).
a. Hereditary TTP is caused by a deficiency of ADAMTS13, a regulator of von Willebrand factor secreted by endothelial cells, and manifests in childhood or young adulthood, typically after an event (i.e., surgery or infectious process).

b. ADAMTS13 has been studied closely; multiple mutations have been linked to TTP.
B. Acquired
1. Acquired TTP is consistent with severe VWF cleaving protease deficiency.
a. Autoimmune diseases
b. Drug-induced
c. Cancer
d. Pregnancy
e. Infection
C. Hemolytic uremic syndrome (HUS)
1. May be typical or atypical
2. Both associated with lower ADAMTS13 activity and have very similar symptoms to acquired TTP; differential diagnosis may be challenging (Shah and Sarode, 2013).
IV. Diagnostic strategies
A. ADAMTS13 assays important in diagnosis; however, multiple versions of the assay exist, and testing takes time.
1. Improved reliability and timeliness of ADAMTS13 testing
2. ADAMTS13 deficiency alone not necessarily enough to determine TTP, but is a valuable test (Shah and Sarode, 2013)
B. Laboratory studies
1. Complete blood cell count (CBC)
2. Peripheral smear
3. Hemolysis laboratory tests (e.g., lactate dehydrogenase [LDH], bilirubin, reticulocyte count)
4. Basic metabolic panel
5. Urinalysis
6. Coagulation studies
7. Direct Coombs test
V. Management and treatment strategies
A. Goal of TTP management is to normalize the platelet count (Kessler et al., 2012)
B. Plasma exchange the first method to use in management of TTP
C. FFP used to replace the plasma removed in plasma exchange (plasmapheresis)
D. High-dose steroids shown to be effective in treatment
E. Platelet transfusions only used in life-threatening emergencies in which the patient has severe bleeding or hemorrhage
F. Rituximab—used in patients with autoimmune TTP (Kessler et al., 2012)
G. Cyclosporine is a potential prophylactic treatment; can be used in conjunction with plasma exchange

ASSESSMENT

I. Physical examination
A. Skin symptoms—jaundice, pallor, and ecchymosis

B. Neurologic symptoms—headache, confusion, seizures, paresthesia, fever, altered level of consciousness

C. Musculoskeletal symptoms—weakness

D. Gastrointestinal symptoms—nausea, vomiting, diarrhea, abdominal pain

II. Laboratory data

A. Decreased hemoglobin or hematocrit

B. Decreased platelet count (<50,000, or 50% decrease from previous count) (Kessler et al., 2012)

C. Elevated LDH

D. Elevated bilirubin

E. Elevated reticulocyte count

F. Elevated blood urea nitrogen (BUN) and creatinine

G. Presence of red blood cells (RBCs), proteinuria in urinalysis

H. Normal to slightly elevated FDPs

I. Negative direct Coombs test

J. Schistocytes on peripheral smear (Munoz & Hughes, 2012)

PROBLEM STATEMENTS AND OUTCOME IDENTIFICATION

I. Risk for Ineffective Gastrointestinal, Renal, Peripheral Tissue, or Cerebral Tissue Perfusion or Risk for Decreased Cardiac Tissue Perfusion (NANDA-I)

A. Expected outcome—patient will show signs of appropriate perfusion through stabilization of organ systems.

II. Risk for Bleeding (NANDA-I) ⚠

A. Expected outcome—patient will identify risk factors for bleeding.

B. Expected outcome—patient will demonstrate appropriate behaviors to prevent or minimize bleeding.

III. Risk for Injury (NANDA-I)

A. Expected outcome—patient will demonstrate appropriate personal safety.

PLANNING AND IMPLEMENTATION

I. Interventions to monitor for bleeding

A. Monitoring laboratory values, specifically platelet count

B. Inspection of skin, wounds, insertion sites for bleeding

II. Interventions to promote patient safety ⚠

A. Safety intervention (see list under DIC)

III. Interventions to assist in coping

A. Assessment of available resources for patient and caregivers

B. Education specific to TTP and its signs and symptoms

C. Positive feedback to patients and caregivers through coaching and listening

D. Suggesting resources such as psychological counseling and pastoral care services

IV. Monitoring sites of active bleeding

A. Application of pressure to sites of bleeding via pressure dressing or sandbag

B. IV fluids, as needed, for volume repletion

C. Oxygen therapy, as needed

D. Blood products (i.e., fresh frozen plasma), as needed

EVALUATION

The oncology nurse systematically and regularly evaluates patient and family responses to interventions for TTP to determine progress toward the achievement of hemodynamic stability. Relevant data are collected, and actual findings are compared with expected findings. Nursing diagnoses, outcomes, and plans of care are reviewed and revised, as necessary.

Syndrome of Inappropriate Antidiuretic Hormone (SIADH)

OVERVIEW

I. Definition—an endocrine paraneoplastic syndrome that results from inappropriate secretion of antidiuretic hormone (ADH) from either the posterior pituitary gland or from an ectopic source, leading to hyponatremia.

II. Pathophysiology of SIADH

A. ADH is also known as arginine vasopression (AVP) in its active form.

B. ADH completes synthesis in the hypothalamus and is stored and released for the posterior pituitary gland; ADH is released in its activated form (AVP) when stimulated, causing renal tubules to absorb more sodium and water.

1. AVP is released in response to:
   a. Changes in plasma osmolality
   b. Changes in plasma volume

C. In SIADH, ADH is secreted even though the osmolality is normal; in addition, aldosterone secretion is decreased, and atrial natriuretic peptide (ANP) increases (Esposito, Piotti, Bianzina, Malul, & Dal Canton, 2011), which combine to worsen hyponatremia.

D. Cancerous cells have the ability to release AVP.

1. Results in an increase in free water in extracellular fluid
2. Causes plasma hypo-osmolality and serum hyponatremia
3. Sodium excreted from the kidneys
4. Intracellular edema—as fluid shifts from extracellular to intracellular spaces, cerebral edema occurs.

III. Causes of SIADH

A. Cancerous causes of SIADH (Castillo, Vincent, & Justice, 2012)

1. Lung cancer, both small cell and non–small cell (most common type of cancer to cause SIADH)
2. Also seen in various solid tumor cancers and some hematologic malignancies
3. Chemotherapeutic agents—vinca alkaloids (vincristine, vinblastine), platinum compounds (cisplatin, carboplatin), alkylating agents (cyclophosphamide, ifosfamide, melphalan), methotrexate

B. Noncancerous causes of SIADH
1. Drugs—antidepressant agents (selective serotonin reuptake inhibitors [SSRIs], tricyclic antidepressants), carbamazepine, hydrochlorothiazide, nonsteroidal anti-inflammatory drugs (NSAIDs), neuroleptic agents, desmopressin, oxytocin (Gross, 2012)
2. Central nervous system—trauma, infection, Guillain-Barré syndrome, vasculitis
3. Other—human immunodeficiency virus (HIV), acquired immunodeficiency syndrome (AIDS), chronic obstructive pulmonary disease (COPD)

IV. Diagnostic strategies
A. Laboratory studies
1. Basic metabolic panel
2. CBC
3. Urinalysis—urine osmolality, urine specific gravity, urine sodium

V. Management and treatment strategies
A. Treatment of underlying cause of SIADH
B. Treatment dependent on severity (mild, moderate, severe) of hyponatremia
1. Mild SIADH (sodium level = 125-134 mEq/L)
   a. Fluid restriction to 1000 mL/day; water intake should not exceed the urine output (Gross, 2012).
   b. Review of current medications for underlying cause
   c. Neurologic assessment
   d. Monitoring of sodium levels
2. Moderate SIADH (sodium level = 115-124 mEq/L)
   a. Fluid restriction to 1000 mL/day; water intake should not exceed the urine output (Gross, 2012).
   b. Review of current medications for underlying cause
   c. Neurologic assessment.
   d. Demeclocycline, 300 to 600 mg twice daily (Esposito et al., 2011)
      (1) May cause nephrogenic diabetes insipidus, resulting in the treatment of hyponatremia; not used frequently because of side effects
   e. Monitoring of sodium levels
3. Severe SIADH (sodium level < 110-115 mEq/L)

   a. Fluid restriction to 1000 mL/day; water intake should not exceed the urine output (Gross, 2012).
   b. Review of current medications for underlying cause
   c. Frequent neurologic assessments
   d. 3% hypertonic saline infusion—dosing recommendations 0.5 to 1 mL/kg body weight/hr (Gross, 2012); infused this way to prevent increase of serum sodium too rapidly and to prevent pulmonary edema, both potential side effects of hypertonic saline infusion
   e. Loop diuretics (e.g., furosemide)—ability to increase free water excretion through hypertonic diuresis (Esposito et al., 2011)
   f. Monitoring of sodium levels

ASSESSMENT

I. Physical examination
A. Signs and symptoms of SIADH—primarily neurologic and gastrointestinal (GI) systems
B. Neurologic—personality changes, headache, decreased mentation, lethargy, disorientation, confusion
C. Severe neurologic symptoms—seizures and coma
D. GI—abdominal cramps, nausea, vomiting, diarrhea, anorexia

II. Laboratory data
A. Serum osmolality (<275 mOsm/kg)
B. Serum sodium (<130 mEq/L)
C. Urine osmolality greater than serum osmolality
D. Decreased BUN
E. Decreased creatinine
F. Decreased uric acid
G. Decreased albumin

PROBLEM STATEMENTS AND OUTCOME IDENTIFICATION

I. Risk for Electrolyte Imbalance (NANDA-I)
A. Expected outcome—patient will verbalize signs and symptoms related to electrolyte imbalance.
B. Expected outcome—patient will regain appropriate laboratory values through treatment.

II. Risk for Imbalanced Fluid Volume (NANDA-I)
A. Expected outcome—patient will maintain adequate hydration based on laboratory values.
B. Expected outcome—patient will identify risk factors related to fluid intake.

III. Risk for Acute Confusion (NANDA-I)
A. Expected outcome—patient will identify resources available to assist during potential period of confusion.
B. Expected outcome—patient will remain safe during periods of confusion. ⚠

PLANNING AND IMPLEMENTATION

I. Interventions to monitor for electrolyte abnormalities
   A. Monitoring laboratory values
   B. Observing for signs and symptoms of hyponatremia
      1. Nausea or vomiting
      2. Headache
      3. Confusion
      4. Fatigue
      5. Restlessness
      6. Seizures
II. Interventions to monitor and manage fluid retention
   A. Restriction of fluid intake
   B. Daily weighing
   C. Auscultating for lung sounds
   D. Maintaining accurate intake and output records
III. Interventions to manage neurologic problems
   A. Frequent neurologic assessment
   B. Placing patient on seizure precautions when SIADH is severe ⚠

EVALUATION

The oncology nurse systematically and regularly evaluates patient and family responses to SIADH interventions to determine progress toward electrolyte balance. Relevant data are collected, and actual findings are compared with expected findings. Nursing diagnoses, outcomes, and plans of care are reviewed and revised, as necessary.

Systemic Inflammatory Response Syndrome (SIRS): Sepsis and Septic Shock

OVERVIEW

I. Definitions
   A. Criteria to assist in recognizing progression to sepsis (Table 40-3)
   B. Sepsis—a response to infection, evidenced by elevated temperature, heart rate, and respiratory rate, which can progress to severe sepsis
   C. Severe sepsis—defined as sepsis with organ dysfunction, hypotension, or hypoperfusion (Zhao et al., 2012)

Table 40-3

Systemic Inflammatory Response Syndrome (SIRS) Criteria

Temperature	>38° C or <36° C
Heart rate	>90 beats/min
Respiratory rate	>20 breaths/min
White blood cell count	>12,000 cells/mm^3

   D. Septic shock—defined as hypotension that is refractory to adequate fluid resuscitation, requiring vasopressor therapy, or both (Mann-Salinas, Engebretson, & Batchinsky, 2013)
II. Pathophysiology
   A. Bacterial, viral, or fungal invasion, leading to release of endotoxin and other cell components into the bloodstream (e.g., plasma cells, neutrophils, macrophages, monocytes); release of components causes multiple actions to take place within the body (Lam, Bauer, & Guzman, 2013).
      1. Vasodilation
      2. Increased vascular permeability
      3. Decreased arterial or venous tone
      4. Clot formation
      5. End-organ damage
      6. Cell death
   B. Process begins with an infection and escalates to various levels.
      1. Early recognition of SIRS is important for patient outcome (Ibrahim & Claxton, 2009).
      2. SIRS is recognized when the following criteria are met:
         a. Temperature greater than 38° C or less than 36° C
         b. Heart rate greater than 90 beats per minute
         c. Respiratory rate greater than 20 breaths per minute
         d. White blood cell (WBC) count greater than 12,000 cells/mm^3
      3. SIRS progresses to sepsis when at least two of the above criteria are assessed in a particular patient.
      4. Sepsis develops into severe sepsis when one or more organ systems experience dysfunction.
      5. Severe sepsis becomes septic shock when acute circulatory failure is present, characterized by hypotension that is unresponsive to fluid hydration.
      6. Septic shock may result in multiple organ dysfunction syndrome, which may lead to death.
   C. Infection type
      1. Gram-negative organism
      2. Gram-positive organism (increase in prevalence because of increased use of access devices)
      3. Fungus
      4. Virus
III. Risk factors for SIRS, sepsis, or septic shock
   A. Recent antineoplastic treatment resulting in neutropenia
   B. Medical devices—central venous catheter, urinary catheter, drains
   C. Respiratory infection
   D. Urinary tract infection
   E. Mucositis

F. Age older than 65 years

G. Poor nutritional status

H. Hospitalization

I. Concurrent immunosuppressive diseases

IV. Diagnostic studies

  A. Basic metabolic panel

  B. CBC

  C. Coagulation studies

  D. Lactic acid

  E. Arterial blood gases

  F. Tests used to determine potential areas of infection:

    1. Blood cultures

    2. Urinalysis or urine culture

    3. Wound culture (if applicable)

    4. Computed tomography (CT)

    5. Chest radiography

    6. Sputum analysis

    7. Stool analysis

V. Management and treatment strategies

  A. Fluid resuscitation, as part of early goal-directed therapy, for hypotension or lactic acid > 4 mmol/L (Smith, 2013)

    1. Crystalloid solution as first-line therapy (e.g., normal saline)

  B. Establishing vascular access (if not already in place)

  C. Broad-spectrum antimicrobial therapy within first 45 minutes of recognition

  D. Move to an intensive care setting if vasopressor, arterial catheters, mechanical ventilation needed for treatment

  E. Vasopressor therapy to maintain a mean arterial pressure (MAP) of 65 mm Hg

    1. Norepinephrine as first-line therapy (Dellinger et al., 2013)

    2. Arterial catheter placed if administering vasopressors

  F. Inotropic therapy (e.g., dobutamine) added on the basis of ongoing signs of hypoperfusion (Dellinger et al., 2013)

  G. Oxygen therapy (e.g., nasal cannula, nonrebreather mask, or mechanical ventilation, if needed)

  H. Supportive therapy

    1. Blood product administration

      a. RBC transfusion, for hemoglobin less than 7 g/dL (Dellinger et al., 2013)

      b. Fresh frozen plasma to correct coagulopathies

      c. Platelet transfusion used when less than 10,000/mm^3; if active bleeding, platelet goal should be less than 50,000/mm^3

    2. Glucose control; important in patients with or without diabetes

3. Renal replacement therapy or intermittent hemodialysis

4. Deep vein thrombosis prophylaxis

5. Nutrition

ASSESSMENT

I. Physical examination (Aitken et al., 2011)

  A. In addition to the SIRS criteria, the following are signs and symptoms of sepsis:

    1. Central nervous system—confusion, agitation, chills

    2. Cardiovascular—sinus tachycardia, hypotension

    3. Respiratory—tachypnea, hypoxia on room air, decreased breath sounds

    4. Renal—decreased urine output

    5. Skin—dry, warm, flushed

    6. GI—nausea, vomiting

  B. The following are signs and symptoms of septic shock:

    1. Central nervous system—obtundation, coma

    2. Cardiovascular—tachycardia, arrhythmias, hypotension

    3. Respiratory—shortness of breath, decreased breath sounds, crackles or wheezes, pulmonary edema, acute respiratory distress syndrome (ARDS)

    4. Renal—oliguria or anuria, acute renal failure

    5. Skin—cold, pale, decreased perfusion, mottling

    6. GI—decreased GI motility, jaundice

II. Laboratory data

  A. Indicative of sepsis

    1. Prolonged PT or aPTT

    2. Decreased platelets

    3. Decreased fibrinogen

    4. Hyperglycemia

    5. Increased lactic acid

    6. Positive blood cultures

    7. Increase in WBC in urinalysis

    8. Increased WBC in CBC

  B. In addition to the above, the following are indicative of septic shock:

    1. Elevated liver function test results

    2. Increased levels of BUN or creatinine

    3. Decreased hemoglobin or hematocrit

    4. Late stages showing decrease in blood glucose

PROBLEM STATEMENTS AND OUTCOME IDENTIFICATION

I. Impaired Gas Exchange (NANDA-I)

  A. Expected outcome—patient will verbalize signs and symptoms of potential respiratory distress.

  B. Expected outcome—patient will demonstrate appropriate oxygenation through laboratory values and symptomatology.

II. Decreased Cardiac Output (NANDA-I)

A. Expected outcome—patient will demonstrate increased activity tolerance.

B. Expected outcome—patient will remain hemodynamically stable, as evidenced by laboratory values and vital signs.

III. Risk for Ineffective Peripheral Tissue Perfusion (NANDA-I)

A. Expected outcome—patient will show signs of appropriate perfusion through stabilization of organ systems.

IV. Impaired Spontaneous Ventilation (NANDA-I)

A. Expected outcome—patient will maintain adequate gas exchange while on mechanical ventilation.

B. Expected outcome—patient will not develop complications while on mechanical ventilation.

V. Anxiety, Fear (NANDA-I)

A. Expected outcome—patient will verbalize awareness of his or her own coping abilities.

B. Expected outcome—patient will demonstrate effective coping skills

VI. Risk for Infection (NANDA-I)

A. Expected outcome—patient will verbalize signs and symptoms of infection.

B. Expected outcome—patient will demonstrate behaviors to decrease risk for infection.

VII. Risk for Imbalanced Body Temperature (NANDA-I)

A. Expected outcome—patient will report elevated temperature to appropriate health care provider. ⚠

B. Expected outcome—patient will verbalize signs and symptoms of a fever.

PLANNING AND IMPLEMENTATION

I. Interventions to monitor for SIRS and early signs and symptoms of sepsis

A. Monitoring laboratory values

B. Monitoring vital signs, more frequently in patients at risk for infection

C. Assessing potential sites of infections; cultures, as ordered

II. Prevention of infection in patients with neutropenia, per institution protocol (see Chapter 4)

III. Interventions to education patients and caregivers on infection control

A. Hand hygiene

B. If patient is at home, instructing patient to monitor temperature

C. Promoting hygiene care, specifically perineal care

IV. Interventions to manage sepsis or septic shock

A. Administering antibiotics, as ordered

B. Monitoring for organ system failure

C. Monitoring for signs and symptoms of fluid overload
  1. Daily weight
  2. Strict monitoring of intake and output

D. Monitoring for oxygen saturation; administering oxygen therapy, as needed

V. Interventions to provide emotional support to patients and caregivers

A. Assessment for current coping strategies and encourage use

B. Providing supportive resources, as needed

EVALUATION

The oncology nurse systematically and regularly evaluates patient and family responses to interventions to prevent and manage SIRS and sepsis and to determine progress toward hemodynamic stability. Relevant data are collected, and actual findings are compared with expected findings. Nursing diagnoses, outcomes, and plans of care are reviewed and revised, as necessary.

Tumor Lysis Syndrome (TLS)

OVERVIEW

I. Definition—an oncologic emergency resulting from cancer treatment, in which large amounts of tumor cells are destroyed, resulting in electrolyte abnormalities

II. Pathophysiology of TLS

A. Antineoplastic agents are given for cancer treatment, causing rapid cell kill.

B. After cells are lysed, cellular contents are released into the bloodstream.

C. Contents include deoxyribonucleic acid (DNA), potassium, phosphate, and cytokines (Howard, Jones, & Pui, 2011)
  1. DNA is metabolized into adenosine and guanosine; both converted to xanthine
  2. Xanthine is oxidized by xanthine oxidase; leads to uric acid production
  3. Uric acid is then excreted by the kidneys.

D. When accumulation of cellular contents is more rapid than excretion, TLS develops (Howard et al., 2011) and causes the following:
  1. Hyperkalemia
  2. Hyperphosphatemia
  3. Hyperuricemia
  4. Hypocalcemia

III. Risk factors for TLS

A. Severity of TLS dependent on type of cancer mass with the potential for the tumor cell to lyse; patient comorbidities may contribute (Howard et al., 2011).

B. Types of cancer with high potential for tumor lysis
  1. High-grade lymphomas (e.g., Burkitt lymphoma)
  2. Acute leukemia
  3. Any cancer with large, bulky tumor mass

C. Pre-existing conditions that place patients at higher risk
  1. Chronic renal insufficiency (Howard et al., 2011)

2. Oliguria
3. Dehydration
4. Hypotension
5. Acidic urine
6. Exposure to nephrotoxins (e.g., vancomycin, aminoglycosides, contrast agents for diagnostic purposes)
7. Splenomegaly
8. Extensive lymphadenopathy
9. Ascites

D. Treatments, used in combination or alone, with high risk for development of TLS
1. Chemotherapy (e.g., cisplatin, etoposide, (Mackiewicz, 2012), cytarabine for treatment of acute myelogenous leukemia (Montesinos et al., 2008)
2. Immunotherapy
3. Monoclonal antibodies (e.g., rituximab) (Yang et al., 2012)
4. Radiation therapy
5. Hormone therapy

IV. Diagnostic strategies
A. Laboratory studies
1. Basic metabolic panel
2. Liver function tests
3. Urinalysis

V. Management and treatment strategies
A. Monitoring of laboratory values vital in management and treatment of TLS
1. Depending on severity of TLS, laboratory values may be monitored every 6 to 12 hours (Howard et al., 2011).
B. Preventative strategies key to TLS treatment
1. Hydration via IV fluids
   a. IV fluids are administered 24 to 48 hours before therapy begins and may continue for up to 72 hours after therapy is completed; dosage of 3 L/m^2 daily is recommended (Lewis, Hendrickson, & Moynihan, 2011; Maloney & Denno, 2011).
   b. Monitoring of intake and output, along with daily weighing, is important for potential impact of fluid overload.
   c. Loop diuretics are used to decrease fluid retention and aid in excretion of cellular contents.
2. Allopurinol
   a. Administered in 600- to 800-mg daily doses, beginning 24 to 48 hours prior to treatment (Kennedy & Ajiboye, 2010)
   b. Inhibits the enzyme xanthine oxidase, which in turn blocks conversion of particular enzymes to uric acid, assisting in the decrease of uric acid in the body (Maloney & Denno, 2011)
3. Urate oxidase (Rasburicase)

a. Used as an alternative to allopurinol
b. Works by converting uric acid to allantoin, which is then easily excreted in urine; unlike allopurinol, has ability to lower existing uric acid level and prevent further accumulation
c. Administered intravenously (0.2 mg/kg) over 30 minutes (McCurdy & Shanholtz, 2012)
d. Not used in patients with a glucose-6-phosphate dehydrogenase (G6PD) deficiency

C. Further treatment withheld until resolution of TLS
D. Management of hyperkalemia
1. Review of medications contributing to elevated potassium levels
2. Restriction of dietary intake of potassium-rich foods
3. Monitoring electrocardiography (ECG) changes
4. Dialysis—may be initiated if potassium level greater than 7 mEq/L, serum uric acid level greater than 10 mg/dL, or serum phosphorus level greater than 10 mg/dL (Maloney & Denno, 2011)
5. Pharmacologic treatment
   a. Polystyrene sulfonate
   b. Calcium gluconate
   c. Sodium bicarbonate
   d. Loop diuretic (e.g., furosemide)
   e. Regular insulin

E. Management of hyperphosphatemia
1. Restriction of dietary intake of food high in phosphorus
2. Pharmacologic treatment
   a. Phosphate-binding antacids (e.g., oral aluminum hydroxide) (Colen, 2008)

F. Management of hyperuricemia
1. Continuation of hydration via IV fluids
2. Pharmacologic treatment
   a. Increased allopurinol dosing
   b. Urate oxidase

G. Management of hypocalcemia
1. Monitoring of ECG changes
2. Pharmacologic treatments—calcium gluconate

ASSESSMENT

I. Physical examination
A. Signs and symptoms of electrolyte imbalance key in identification of TLS, in addition to laboratory values (Table 40-4)
1. Signs and symptoms of hyperkalemia
   a. ECG changes
   b. Muscle weakness, cramping, or both
   c. Twitching, tingling, paresthesias
   d. Nausea, vomiting, diarrhea
   e. Lethargy
   f. Syncope

Table 40-4

Signs and Symptoms of Electrolyte Imbalance in Tumor Lysis Syndrome (TLS)

Electrolyte Imbalance	Signs and Symptoms
Hyperkalemia	Electrocardiography (ECG) changes, muscle weakness and/or cramping, twitching, tingling, paresthesia, nausea, vomiting, diarrhea, lethargy, syncope
Hyperphosphatemia	Oliguria or anuria, hypertension, edema
Hyperuricemia	Nausea, vomiting, diarrhea, anorexia, edema, flank pain, hematuria, lethargy, malaise, fatigue, weakness, pruritus
Hypocalcemia	Tetany, positive Chvostek and Trousseau signs, twitching, paresthesia, muscle cramps, seizure, syncope, hypotension, anorexia, ECG changes, irritability, anxiety, confusion, hallucinations, diarrhea

2. Signs and symptoms of hyperphosphatemia
   a. Oliguria or anuria
   b. Hypertension
   c. Edema
3. Signs and symptoms of hyperuricemia
   a. Nausea, vomiting, diarrhea
   b. Anorexia
   c. Edema
   d. Flank pain
   e. Hematuria
   f. Lethargy, malaise
   g. Fatigue, weakness
   h. Pruritus
4. Signs and symptoms of hypocalcemia
   a. Tetany
   b. Positive Chvostek and Trousseau signs
   c. Twitching
   d. Paresthesia
   e. Muscle cramps
   f. Seizure
   g. Syncope
   h. Hypotension
   i. Anorexia
   j. ECG changes
   k. Irritability, anxiety, confusion, hallucinations
   l. Diarrhea
II. Laboratory data.
   A. Hyperkalemia
   B. Hyperphosphatemia
   C. Hyperuricemia
   D. Hypocalcemia
   E. Elevated LDH
   F. Decrease in creatinine clearance
   G. Uric acid crystals in urinalysis

PROBLEM STATEMENTS AND OUTCOME IDENTIFICATION

I. Risk for Electrolyte Imbalance (NANDA-I)
   A. Expected outcome—patient will verbalize signs and symptoms related to electrolyte imbalance.
   B. Expected outcome—patient will regain appropriate laboratory values.
II. Risk for Imbalanced Fluid Volume (NANDA-I)
   A. Expected outcome—patient will maintain adequate hydration based on laboratory values.
   B. Expected outcome—patient will identify risk factors related to dehydration.
III. Fatigue (NANDA-I)
   A. Expected outcome—patient will identify risk factors associated with fatigue.
   B. Expected outcome—patient will verbalize methods to conserve energy to participate in daily activities.
IV. Risk for Activity Intolerance (NANDA-I)
   A. Expected outcome—patient will have an increase in activity.
   B. Expected outcome—patient's body will respond to treatments, reflected in laboratory data.
V. Nausea (NANDA-I)
   A. Expected outcome—patient will report decrease in nausea and/or vomiting.
   B. Expected outcome—patient will maintain balanced diet for nutritional needs.

PLANNING AND IMPLEMENTATION

I. Interventions to monitor for TLS
   A. Monitoring laboratory values for electrolyte imbalance
   B. Assessment for signs and symptoms indicative of electrolyte imbalances
      1. Cardiac monitoring, as needed
      2. Neurologic assessment
      3. Monitoring renal function
      4. Monitoring for weight gain
      5. Monitoring for decreased urine output
II. Interventions to manage fluid balance
   A. Adequate hydration to prevent TLS
   B. Strict monitoring of intake and output
   C. Daily weighing
   D. Treatment for nausea and vomiting
III. Interventions for patient and family education
   A. Reporting signs and symptoms of electrolyte imbalance to the health care team
   B. Providing instructions on adequate fluid intake during cancer treatment
   C. Diet modifications to reduce intake of potassium and phosphorus, if indicated

EVALUATION

The oncology nurse systematically and regularly evaluates patient and family responses to TLS interventions to determine progress toward electrolyte balance. Relevant data are collected, and actual findings are compared with expected findings. Nursing diagnoses, outcomes, and plans of care are reviewed and revised, as necessary.

Hypersensitivity

OVERVIEW

I. Definition—an undesirable reaction produced by normal immune system in response to exposure to an antigen or allergen; may refer to allergic reactions or infusion-related reactions; linked to certain types of antineoplastic therapy

II. Pathophysiology
  A. Reactions divided into four categories:
    1. Type I—immediate immunoglobulin E (IgE)—mediated
      a. Most common type associated with antineoplastic agents
      b. Results from exposure to an antigen with formation of IgE antibodies, attached to receptors on mast cells and basophils (Van Gerpen, 2009)
      c. Further exposure to the same antigen—creates a reaction with release of histamines, leukotrienes, prostaglandins, and other inflammatory mediators
    2. Type II—IgG or IgM antibody–mediated
    3. Type III—immune complex–mediated
    4. Type IV—cell-mediated or delayed
  B. Categorized as uniphasic (occurring while treatment is being delivered, resolving within hours) or biphasic (reoccurrence of symptoms hours 1 to 72 hours after resolution of original symptoms) (Viale & Yamamoto, 2010)
  C. Reactions to antineoplastic agents considered anaphylactoid, not anaphylactic; *anaphylactoid* indicates that the patient has had no prior exposure to the drug that he or she is receiving.
    1. Anaphylactoid and anaphylactic reactions have similar signs and symptoms and are treated in the same way (Van Gerpen, 2009).
  D. Severe symptoms of hypersensitivity indicate anaphylaxis (see next section).
  E. Cytokine release syndrome also important in management of oncology patients
    1. Release of cytokines from targeted cells cause this syndrome.
    2. Symptoms such as fever, nausea, chills, hypotension, dyspnea, and scratchy throat may result (Breslin, 2007).
    3. Management similar to a hypersensitivity reaction; however, severe cases may require management similar to anaphylaxis.

III. Risk factors
  A. Hypersensitivity reaction caused by a variety of antineoplastic agents (Lee, Gianos, & Klaustermeyer, 2009; Lenz, 2007; Van Gerpen, 2009)
    1. Platinums (e.g., carboplatin, oxaliplatin)
      a. Consistent with type I reactions because most typically occur after multiple cycles of therapy
      b. Most reactions to oxaliplatin occur within the first minutes of infusion
      c. Studies on desensitization protocols for platinum agents completed
    2. Taxanes (e.g., paclitaxel, docetaxel)
      a. Paclitaxel treatment—should include premedication to prevent reactions as well as a longer infusion time
      b. Unclear if reaction is to drug or diluent
      c. Desensitization protocols used for paclitaxel administration
      d. Most severe reactions—occur with the first or second dose within the first minutes of infusion
    3. L-Asparaginase
      a. Higher risk when given intermittently rather than daily; IV administration poses higher risk than intramuscular or subcutaneous route.
      b. Intradermal skin testing performed prior to administration
    4. Procarbazine
      a. Corticosteroid recommended before infusion
    5. Epipodophyllotoxins (e.g., etoposide)
      a. Reactions within first few minutes or hours after infusion; more commonly occur after multiple doses
    6. Monoclonal antibodies (e.g., rituximab, cetuximab)
      a. Type of biotherapy—murine (mouse protein), chimeric (7%-9% mouse protein), humanized or fully humanized; makeup of the monoclonal antibodies may lead to hypersensitivity reaction; higher content of murine protein correlates with a higher risk of reaction.
      b. Most reactions within 30 to 120 minutes of the first infusion of rituximab
      c. Most reactions related to cytokine release rather than murine exposure; reaction is greater during first treatment.
  B. Other factors that indicate a greater risk
    1. History of hypersensitivity reactions
    2. Repeated exposure to a particular agent

3. IV administration
4. Short interval between exposures (Van Gerpen, 2009)
5. Medical products (e.g., latex)
6. Blood products
7. Certain foods

IV. Diagnostic studies
   A. Test doses via skin testing

V. Management and treatment
   A. Pharmacologic management used for pretherapy delivery to assist in prevention of a reaction
      1. Corticosteroids
      2. Histamine 1 (H_1) antagonists (e.g., diphenhydramine)
      3. H_2 antagonists (e.g., ranitidine, famotidine)
      4. Antipyretics (e.g., acetaminophen)
   B. Nonpharmacologic management
      1. Cessation of current infusion and initiation of normal IV saline.
      2. Emergency equipment at bedside
      3. Maintaining airway; oxygen, if needed
   C. Pharmacologic interventions in the event of a hypersensitivity reaction
      1. Epinephrine
      2. H_1 antagonists
      3. H_2 antagonists
      4. Corticosteroids
      5. Albuterol (for inhalation)

ASSESSMENT

I. Physical examination
   A. Signs and symptoms of hypersensitivity may be very similar to, yet not as severe as, those of anaphylaxis.
   B. Symptoms of hypersensitivity reaction (allergic reaction) may include transient flushing or rash, fever less than 100.4°F, urticaria, bronchospasm, hypotension, edema, or angioedema (Lenz, 2007).
   C. Symptoms of an acute infusion reaction may include itching, rash, urticaria, rigors, chills, headache, fatigue, dizziness, sweating, nausea, vomiting, cough, dyspnea, bronchospasm, hypotension, hypertension, tachycardia, flushing, and back pain (Lenz, 2007).

II. Laboratory data
   A. Positive or negative skin test

PROBLEM STATEMENTS AND OUTCOME IDENTIFICATION

I. Risk for Allergy Response (NANDA-I)
   A. Expected outcome—patient will identify risk factors for allergy response.
   B. Expected outcome—patient will verbalize signs and symptoms of allergic and/or hypersensitivity reaction.

II. Impaired Gas Exchange (NANDA-I)
   A. Expected outcome—patient will verbalize signs and symptoms of potential respiratory distress.
   B. Expected outcome—patient will demonstrate appropriate oxygenation through laboratory values and symptomatology.

III. Ineffective Breathing Pattern (NANDA-I)
   A. Expected outcome—patient will verbalize signs and symptoms of respiratory distress.

IV. Anxiety, Fear (NANDA-I)
   A. Expected outcome—patient will verbalize awareness of coping abilities.
   B. Expected outcome—patient will demonstrate effective coping skills.

PLANNING AND IMPLEMENTATION

I. Interventions to prevent a hypersensitivity reaction
   A. Having baseline knowledge of hypersensitivity risk associated with medications to be administered
   B. Being aware of the patient's current allergies
   C. Obtaining baseline vital signs and additional vital signs per infusion protocol for specific medication

II. Interventions to manage a hypersensitivity reaction
   A. Stopping medication administration
   B. Taking vital signs
   C. Administering additional medications for treatment of reaction
   D. Monitoring airway for potential compromise
   E. Maintaining patent airway
   F. Administering IV fluids, as needed
   G. Notifying primary care provider about signs and symptoms observed
   H. Restarting infusion, potentially at a slower rate, based on orders

III. Interventions to manage potential anxiety or fear
   A. Assisting patient in identifying appropriate coping strategies
   B. Providing relaxation methods, as appropriate
   C. Acknowledging the patient's feelings as they are expressed

EVALUATION

The oncology nurse systematically and regularly evaluates patient and family responses to interventions for hypersensitivity reactions to minimize complications and keep the patient safe. Relevant data are collected, and actual findings are compared with expected findings. Nursing diagnoses, outcomes, and plans of care are reviewed and revised, as necessary.

Anaphylaxis

OVERVIEW

I. Definition—an allergic reaction that potentiates a life-threatening emergency; may be a generalized or

systemic hypersensitivity reaction (Younker &
Soar, 2010)
II. Pathophysiology
  A. IgE antibody is developed after first exposure to an
  antigen.
  B. At next exposure, the IgE antibody binds to mast
  cells and basophils.
  C. This triggers release of inflammatory mediators,
  including histamine, tryptase, leukotrienes,
  prostaglandins, and platelet activating factor
  (Simons & Sheikh, 2013).
  D. The release of substances causes systemic
  vasodilation, increased capillary permeability,
  bronchoconstriction, and coronary
  vasoconstriction.
III. Risk factors
  A. Various antigens may provoke an anaphylactic
  response, and route of administration may vary
  (Arnold and Williams, 2011; Younker & Soar, 2010).
    1. Allergy testing
    2. Antibiotics (most common are beta-lactams
    [e.g., penicillins, cephalosporins])
    3. Anesthetics or anesthetic adjuncts
    4. Antineoplastic agents (e.g., chemotherapy,
    biotherapy)
    5. Blood products
    6. Contrast media used for radiographic testing
    7. Foods (e.g., egg, fish, food additives, peanuts,
    shellfish, milk)
    8. Insect venom
    9. Latex
IV. Diagnostic studies
  A. Test doses performed for particular medications
V. Management and treatment strategies
  A. Epinephrine—first-line pharmacologic therapy
  (Sheikh, 2013; Simons & Sheikh, 2013)
    1. Works through alpha- and beta-adrenergic
    properties; increases peripheral
    vasoconstriction and bronchodilation,
    reduction of mast cells
    2. Begins working within seconds to minutes of
    administration
    3. Can be administered intravenously by health
    care provider trained in management of
    vasopressors; also given intramuscularly in the
    anterolateral aspect of the thigh
    4. Injection may be repeated after 5 minutes and
    up to 15 minutes
  B. Nonpharmacologic therapy
    1. Emergency equipment at bedside to monitor
    patient
    2. Oxygen to be given via 100% nonrebreather
    mask (or highest concentration possible)
    3. Stopping of current infusion that potentially
    caused anaphylaxis
    4. IV normal saline given as fast as possible

  C. Other pharmacologic treatments
    1. H1 receptor antagonist—to improve cutaneous
    erythema and decrease itching (Arnold &
    Williams, 2011)
    2. Corticosteroids—to prevent biphasic reactions

ASSESSMENT
I. Physical examination
  A. Signs and symptoms (Simons & Sheikh, 2013,
  Arnold & Williams, 2011).
    1. Dermatologic symptoms—flushing, itching,
    urticaria, morbilliform rash, angioedema
    2. Ophthalmologic symptoms—periorbital
    edema, infected conjunctiva, tears
    3. Respiratory symptoms—bronchospasm,
    chest tightness, tachypnea, throat or nasal
    itching, congestion, sneezing, dysphonia,
    hoarseness, dry cough, stridor, cyanosis,
    respiratory arrest
    4. Cardiovascular symptoms—chest pain,
    tachycardia, diaphoresis, hypotension, cyanosis,
    dysrhythmias, palpitations, shock
    5. GI symptoms—nausea, vomiting, diarrhea,
    abdominal pain
    6. Neurologic symptoms—headache, dizziness,
    uneasiness, lightheadedness, confusion, tunnel
    vision, loss of consciousness
    7. Other symptoms—metallic taste, feeling of
    impending doom
II. Laboratory data.
  A. Result of test dose studies

PROBLEM STATEMENTS AND OUTCOME IDENTIFICATION
I. Impaired Gas Exchange (NANDA-I)
  A. Expected outcome—patient will verbalize signs
  and symptoms of respiratory distress.
  B. Expected outcome—patient will demonstrate
  appropriate oxygenation through laboratory values
  and symptomatology.
II. Ineffective Breathing Pattern (NANDA-I)
  A. Expected outcome—patient will verbalize signs
  and symptoms of respiratory distress.
III. Impaired Spontaneous Ventilation (NANDA-I)
  A. Expected outcome—patient will maintain airway
  with appropriate breath sounds.
IV. Anxiety, Fear (NANDA-I)
  A. Expected outcome—patient will verbalize
  awareness of coping abilities.
  B. Expected outcome—patient will demonstrate
  effective coping skills.

PLANNING AND IMPLEMENTATION
I. Interventions to prevent anaphylaxis
  A. Having knowledge of reaction potential for
  specific medication being administered

B. Obtaining baseline vital signs and additional vital signs per infusion protocol for specific medication

II. Interventions to manage anaphylaxis
   A. Emergency equipment placed at bedside or available
   B. Institutional protocol for anaphylactic emergencies
   C. Stopping current infusion
   D. Maintaining patent airway
   E. Taking vital signs
   F. Notifying primary care provider of signs and symptoms observed
   G. Initiating a rapid response or code call, if needed
   H. Administering emergency medications, as ordered
   I. Administering IV fluids
   J. Monitoring oxygen saturation; administering supplemental oxygen, as needed
   K. Performing cardiopulmonary resuscitation (CPR), when needed

III. Interventions for potential anaphylaxis occurring in the community
   A. Patient should have emergency numbers available.
   B. Patient should have emergency medications available if high risk (e.g., EpiPen).

IV. Interventions to provide emotional support to patients and caregivers
   A. Assessment of coping mechanisms
   B. Educating patient and caregivers on support available
   C. Providing therapeutic relaxation, as needed
   D. Assisting patient and caregivers in identifying appropriate coping strategies

EVALUATION

The oncology nurse systematically and regularly evaluates patient and family responses to prevent anaphylaxis and safely manage anaphylactic reactions when they occur. Relevant data are collected, and actual findings are compared with expected findings. Nursing diagnoses, outcomes, and plans of care are reviewed and revised, as necessary.

Hypercalcemia

OVERVIEW

I. Definition—abnormally high level of calcium (>10.5 mg/dL); most common oncologic emergency occurring in 10% to 20% of all cancer patients (Foulkes, 2010)

II. Pathophysiology
   A. Calcium and bone metabolism regulated by parathyroid hormone (PTH), 1,25-dihydroxyvitamin D, and calcitonin (LeGrand, 2011)
      1. PTH stimulates calcium reabsorption from bones and kidneys.

2. When the body detects low calcium levels, 1,25-dihydroxyvitamin D works on the gut and stimulates absorption of dietary calcium intake for body needs.
   3. Calcitonin works to decrease serum calcium levels by suppressing bone and renal reabsorption of calcium.
   4. PTH, 1,25-dihydroxyvitamin D, and calcitonin work to maintain calcium homeostasis within the body.
   B. Two different mechanisms that cause hypercalcemia of malignancy
      1. Humoral hypercalcemia of malignancy (HHM)—accounts for approximately 80% of hypercalcemia of malignancy cases
         a. Most often the cause in patients with little to no bone metastases
         b. Parathyroid hormone–related protein (PTHrP)—produced by many solid tumors; acts very similarly to PTH, resulting in increased renal and bone reabsorption of calcium
      2. Local osteolytic hypercalcemia (LOH)—accounts for approximately 20% of hypercalcemia of malignancy cases
         a. In LOH, bone provides a place for tumor growth; tumor cells produce various cytokines that lead to calcium reabsorption from the bones (Khoury, Chang, Gru, & White, 2012).
         b. Osteoclasts are active at the site of tumor cells, resulting in breakdown of bone and increase in calcium levels.

III. Risk factors
   A. Solid tumors—those that commonly metastasize to the bone
      1. Breast
      2. Lung
      3. Prostate
   B. Hematologic malignancies
      1. Multiple myeloma
      2. Lymphoma
   C. Nononcologic diagnoses
      1. Hyperparathyroidism (most common)

IV. Diagnostic strategies
   A. Basic metabolic panel (to include serum calcium)
   B. Serum albumin and prealbumin
      1. Important to adjust serum calcium for low serum albumin, as is experienced by many patients with cancer
      2. Formula—(base albumin concentration [4 mg/dL] − measured serum albumin concentration [g/dL]) × 0.8 mg/dL + reported serum calcium
   C. PTH level

V. Management and treatment strategies

A. Hydration with IV fluids—0.9% normal saline
 1. This will begin rehydration and diuresis (LeGrand, 2011).
 2. Rate of infusion of fluid is dependent on level of serum calcium, severity of dehydration, and patient's ability to tolerate high rates of infusion.
 3. Loop diuretic (e.g., furosemide) is added, if necessary, to reduce volume overload after rehydration.
B. Bisphosphonates
 1. Inhibit bone reabsorption through osteoclast activity
 2. Administered intravenously
 3. Zoledronic acid proven to be more effective than pamidronate
  a. Dosing of zoledronic acid—4 mg over 15 minutes (LeGrand, 2011)
  b. Normal calcium levels maintained for at least 4 to 6 weeks
C. Denosumab
 1. A fully humanized monoclonal antibody that inhibits osteoclast production and survival (Boikos & Hammers, 2012)
 2. Potential to cause severe hypocalcemia
 3. Dosing—120 mg subcutaneous injection every 4 weeks (Clemons, Gelmon, Pritchard, & Paterson, 2012)
D. Calcitonin
 1. Rapid onset of action; decreases serum calcium levels by inhibiting osteoclasts in bone and increasing urinary excretion of calcium (Clines, 2011);.
 2. Corticosteroid—may be given in conjunction to allow for a longer effect of calcitonin (LeGrand, 2011)
 3. Tachyphylaxis occurs quickly (Behl, Hendrickson, & Moynihan, 2010).
E. Gallium nitrate
 1. Used in quick relapse of hypercalcemia after initial use of bisphosphonate
 2. Has prolonged infusion time (LeGrand, 2011)
 3. Nephrotoxicity major complication in the use of this medication

ASSESSMENT

I. Physical examination
 A. Signs and symptoms of hypercalcemia (Foulkes, 2010)
  1. Mild (10.5-11.5 mg/dL)
   a. GI symptoms—anorexia, nausea, vomiting, abdominal cramping, loss of appetite
   b. Neurologic symptoms—restlessness, difficulty concentrating, lethargy, confusion
   c. Muscular symptoms—fatigue and generalized weakness
   d. Renal symptoms—frequent urination, nocturia, polydipsia
   e. Cardiovascular symptoms—orthostatic hypotension
  2. Moderate (11.5-13.5 mg/dL), in addition to symptoms listed for mild
   a. GI symptoms—constipation, bloating, increasing abdominal pain
   b. Neurologic symptoms—psychosis, drowsiness, mental status changes
   c. Muscular symptoms—increased weakness
   d. Renal symptoms—dehydration
   e. Cardiovascular symptoms—ECG abnormalities (i.e., prolonged P-R interval, widened QRS, shortened Q-T, S-T intervals), hypertension, cardiac arrhythmias
  3. Severe (>13.5 mg/dL), in addition to mild and moderate symptoms
   a. GI symptoms—ileus
   b. Neurologic symptoms—seizures and coma
   c. Muscular symptoms—ataxia and pathologic fractures
   d. Renal symptoms—oliguric renal failure and renal insufficiency
   e. Cardiovascular symptoms—ECG abnormalities (e.g., widened T waves, heart block, ventricular arrhythmias) and cardiac arrest
II. Laboratory data
 A. Increased serum calcium level
 B. Low levels of PTH, except in rare cases of PTH-secreting tumor (LeGrand, 2011)

PROBLEM STATEMENTS AND OUTCOME IDENTIFICATION

I. Risk for Electrolyte Imbalance (NANDA-I)
 A. Expected outcome—patient will verbalize signs and symptoms related to electrolyte imbalance.
 B. Expected outcome—patient will regain appropriate laboratory values.
II. Fatigue (NANDA-I)
 A. Expected outcome—patient will identify risk factors associated with fatigue.
 B. Expected outcome—patient will verbalize methods to conserve energy to participate in daily activities.
III. Risk for Acute Confusion (NANDA-I)
 A. Expected outcome—patient will identify resources available for assistance during potential periods of confusion.
 B. Expected outcome—patient will remain safe during episodes of confusion. ▲
IV. Risk for Falls (NANDA-I) ▲
 A. Expected outcome—patient will verbalize risk factors for falling.
 B. Expected outcome—patient will demonstrate appropriate personal safety measures.

V. Nausea (NANDA-I)
   A. Expected outcome—patient will report decrease in nausea and/or vomiting.
   B. Expected outcome—patient will maintain balanced diet for nutritional needs.

PLANNING AND IMPLEMENTATION

I. Interventions to maintain patient personal safety if confusion arises ⚠
   A. If hospitalized, bed in low locked position with two side rails up, call bell within reach
   B. Close monitoring for safety
II. Interventions to maintain activity level, as tolerated by patient
   A. Partnering with physical therapy, occupational therapy, or both, as needed
   B. Monitoring for fall risk ⚠
      1. Assessment of current medications that place patient at higher risk of fall
      2. Assessment of current gait and activity ability
      3. Assessment of current mental status and orientation
      4. If risk identified, placing patient on fall precautions to alert staff of risk for fall
      5. Educating patient and caregiver on fall precautions and importance of safety
III. Interventions to manage fluid and electrolyte balance
   A. Monitoring intake and output closely
   B. Daily weighing
   C. Administering IV fluids for hydration, as ordered
   D. Administering loop diuretic, as needed, if volume overload exists

EVALUATION

The oncology nurse systematically and regularly evaluates patient and family responses to interventions for hypercalcemia to determine progress toward electrolyte balance and safety. Relevant data are collected, and actual findings are compared with expected findings. Nursing diagnoses, outcomes, and plans of care are reviewed and revised, as necessary.

References

Aitken, L. M., Williams, G., Harvey, M., Blot, S., Kleinpell, R., Labeau, S., et al. (2011). Nursing considerations to complement the surviving sepsis campaign guidelines. *Critical Care Medicine, 39*(7), 1800–1818.

Arnold, J. J., & Williams, P. M. (2011). Anaphylaxis: Recognition and management. *American Family Physician, 84*(10), 1111–1118.

Behl, D., Hendrickson, A. W., & Moynihan, T. J. (2010). Oncologic emergencies. *Critical Care Clinics, 26*(1), 181–205.

Boikos, S. A., & Hammers, H. J. (2012). Denosumab for the treatment of bisphosphonate-refractory hypercalcemia. *Journal of Clinical Oncology: Official Journal of the American Society of Clinical Oncology, 30*(29), e299.

Breslin, S. (2007). Cytokine-release syndrome: Overview and nursing implications. *Clinical Journal of Oncology Nursing, 11*(1 Suppl), 37–42.

Castillo, J. J., Vincent, M., & Justice, E. (2012). Diagnosis and management of hyponatremia in cancer patients. *The Oncologist, 17*(6), 756–765.

Clemons, M., Gelmon, K. A., Pritchard, K. I., & Paterson, A. H. (2012). Bone-targeted agents and skeletal-related events in breast cancer patients with bone metastases: The state of the art. *Current Oncology (Toronto, Ont.), 19*(5), 259–268.

Clines, G. A. (2011). Mechanisms and treatment of hypercalcemia of malignancy. *Current Opinion in Endocrinology, Diabetes, and Obesity, 18*(6), 339–346.

Colen, F. N. (2008). Oncologic emergencies: Superior vena cava syndrome, tumor lysis syndrome, and spinal cord compression. *Journal of Emergency Nursing: JEN: Official Publication of the Emergency Department Nurses Association, 34*(6), 535–537.

Dellinger, R. P., Levy, M. M., Rhodes, A., Annane, D., Gerlach, H., & Opal, S. M. (2013). Surviving sepsis campaign: International guidelines for management of severe sepsis and septic shock: 2012. *Critical Care Medicine, 41*(2), 580–637.

Esposito, P., Piotti, G., Bianzina, S., Malul, Y., & Dal Canton, A. (2011). The syndrome of inappropriate antidiuresis: Pathophysiology, clinical management and new therapeutic options. *Nephron Clinical Practice, 119*(1), c62–c73, discussion c73.

Foulkes, M. (2010). Nursing management of common oncological emergencies. *Nursing Standard (Royal College of Nursing (Great Britain): 1987), 24*(41), 49–56.

Gross, P. (2012). Clinical management of SIADH. *Therapeutic Advances in Endocrinology and Metabolism, 3*(2), 61–73.

Howard, S. C., Jones, D. P., & Pui, C. H. (2011). The tumor lysis syndrome. *The New England Journal of Medicine, 364*(19), 1844–1854.

Ibrahim, S., & Claxton, D. F. (2009). SIRS criteria in prediction of septic shock in hospitalized patients with hematologic malignancies. *Cancer Biology & Therapy, 8*(12), 1101.

Kennedy, L. D., & Ajiboye, V. O. (2010). Rasburicase for the prevention and treatment of hyperuricemia in tumor lysis syndrome. *Journal of Oncology Pharmacy Practice: Official Publication of the International Society of Oncology Pharmacy Practitioners, 16*(3), 205–213.

Kessler, C. S., Khan, B. A., & Lai-Miller, K. (2012). Thrombotic thrombocytopenic purpura: A hematological emergency. *The Journal of Emergency Medicine, 43*(3), 538–544.

Khoury, N., Chang, J., Gru, A. A., & Whyte, M. P. (2012). Resorptive hypercalcemia in post-essential thrombocythemia myelofibrosis: Treatment with denosumab. *The Journal of Clinical Endocrinology and Metabolism, 97*(9), 3051–3055.

Lam, S. W., Bauer, S. R., & Guzman, J. A. (2013). Septic shock: The initial moments and beyond. *Cleveland Clinic Journal of Medicine, 80*(3), 175–184.

Lee, C., Gianos, M., & Klaustermeyer, W. B. (2009). Diagnosis and management of hypersensitivity reactions related to common cancer chemotherapy agents. *Annals of Allergy, Asthma & Immunology: Official Publication of the American College of Allergy, Asthma, & Immunology, 102*(3), 179–187.

Legrand, S. B. (2011). Modern management of malignant hypercalcemia. *The American Journal of Hospice & Palliative Care*, *28*(7), 515–517.

Lenz, H. J. (2007). Management and preparedness for infusion and hypersensitivity reactions. *The Oncologist*, *12*(5), 601–609.

Levi, M. (2009). Disseminated intravascular coagulation in cancer patients. *Best Practice & Research. Clinical Haematology*, *22*(1), 129–136.

Levi, M., Toh, C. H., Thachil, J., & Watson, H. G. (2009). Guidelines for the diagnosis and management of disseminated intravascular coagulation. British Committee for Standards in Haematology. *British Journal of Haematology*, *145*(1), 24–33.

Levi, M., & van der Poll, T. (2013). Disseminated intravascular coagulation: A review for the internist. *Internal and Emergency Medicine*, *8*(1), 23–32.

Lewis, M. A., Hendrickson, A. W., & Moynihan, T. J. (2011). Oncologic emergencies: Pathophysiology, presentation, diagnosis, and treatment. *CA: A Cancer Journal for Clinicians*, *61*(5), 287–314.

Mackiewicz, T. (2012). Prevention of tumor lysis syndrome in an outpatient setting. *Clinical Journal of Oncology Nursing*, *16*(2), 189–193.

Maloney, K., & Denno, M. (2011). Tumor lysis syndrome: Prevention and detection to enhance patient safety. *Clinical Journal of Oncology Nursing*, *15*(6), 601–603.

Mann-Salinas, L. E., Engebretson, J., & Batchinsky, A. I. (2013). A complex systems view of sepsis: Implications for nursing. *Dimensions of Critical Care Nursing: DCCN*, *32*(1), 12–17.

McCurdy, M. T., & Shanholtz, C. B. (2012). Oncologic emergencies. *Critical Care Medicine*, *40*(7), 2212–2222.

Montesinos, P., Lorenzo, I., Martin, G., Sanz, J., Perez-Sirvent, M. L., Martinez, D., et al. (2008). Tumor lysis syndrome in patients with acute myeloid leukemia: Identification of risk factors and development of a predictive model. *Haematologica*, *93*(1), 67–74.

Morton, P. G., Fontaine, D. K., Hudak, C. M., & Gallo, B. M. (2005). *Critical care nursing: A holistic approach* (8th ed.). Philadelphia: Lippincott, Williams and Wilkins.

Munoz, J., & Hughes, A. (2012). Thrombotic thrombocytopenic purpura after autologous peripheral stem cell transplantation. *Blood*, *119*(24), 5620.

Rizzo, C., Rizzo, S., Scire, E., Di Bona, D., Ingrassia, C., Franco, G., et al. (2012). Thrombotic thrombocytopenic purpura: A review of the literature in the light of our experience with plasma exchange. *Blood Transfusion = Trasfusione del Sangue*, *10*(4), 521–532.

Shah, N., & Sarode, R. (2013). Thrombotic thrombocytopenic purpura—what is new? *Journal of Clinical Apheresis*, *28*(1), 30–35.

Sheikh, A. (2013). Emergency management of anaphylaxis: Current pharmacotherapy and future directions. *Expert Opinion on Pharmacotherapy*, *14*(7), 827–830.

Simons, F. E., & Sheikh, A. (2013). Anaphylaxis: The acute episode and beyond. *BMJ (Clinical Research Ed.)*, *346*, f602.

Smith, J. S. (2013). Current recommendations for diagnosis and management of sepsis and septic shock. *JAAPA: Official Journal of the American Academy of Physician Assistants*, *26*(10), 42–45.

Van Gerpen, R. (2009). Chemotherapy and biotherapy-induced hypersensitivity reactions. *Journal of Infusion Nursing: The Official Publication of the Infusion Nurses Society*, *32*(3), 157–165.

Viale, P. H., & Yamamoto, D. S. (2010). Biphasic and delayed hypersensitivity reactions. *Clinical Journal of Oncology Nursing*, *14*(3), 347–356.

Yang, B., Lu, X. C., Yu, R. L., Chi, X. H., Zhang, W. Y., Zhu, H. L., et al. (2012). Diagnosis and treatment of rituximab-induced acute tumor lysis syndrome in patients with diffuse large B-cell lymphoma. *The American Journal of the Medical Sciences*, *343*(4), 337–341.

Younker, J., & Soar, J. (2010). Recognition and treatment of anaphylaxis. *Nursing in Critical Care*, *15*(2), 94–98.

Zhao, H., Heard, S. O., Mullen, M. T., Crawford, S., Goldberg, R. J., Frendl, G., et al. (2012). An evaluation of the diagnostic accuracy of the 1991 American College of Chest Physicians/Society of Critical Care Medicine and the 2001 Society of Critical Care Medicine/European Society of Intensive Care Medicine/American College of Chest Physicians/American Thoracic Society/Surgical Infection Society sepsis definition. *Critical Care Medicine*, *40*(6), 1700–1706.

CHAPTER 41
Structural Emergencies

Wendy H. Vogel

Increased Intracranial Pressure (ICP)

OVERVIEW

I. Definition—a potentially life-threatening neurologic event that occurs with an increase in brain tissue, blood, cerebrospinal fluid (CSF), or all of these in the intracranial cavity, resulting in nerve cell damage, permanent neurologic deficits, and death

II. Pathophysiology
   A. The intracranial cavity is a nonexpandable chamber that contains brain tissue, blood, and CSF (Smith & Amin-Hanjani, 2013).
   B. An increase in ICP (with or without displacement of intracranial structures) occurs with an increase in the volume of any of the three components.
   C. Causes of ICP in the oncology setting include primary or metastatic tumors within the intracranial cavity, leptomeningeal metastases, blood clots, posterior reversible encephalopathy syndrome, infection, or a metabolic disorder (Giglio & Gilbert, 2010; Li, Jenny, & Castaldo, 2012; Schimpf, 2012; Smith & Amin-Hanjani, 2013). ICP occurs once compensatory mechanisms are exhausted because of the following:
      1. Displacement or edema of brain tissue
      2. Obstruction of CSF outflow
      3. Increased vascularity associated with tumor growth
   D. Brain injury results from brainstem compression, reduction in cerebral blood flow, or both, which leads to tissue necrosis (Smith & Amin-Hanjani, 2013).

III. Principles of diagnosis and medical management
   A. Diagnostic tests
      1. Diagnostic scanning—may include contrast-enhanced magnetic resonance imaging (MRI) (often preferred), computed tomography (CT), cerebral angiography, or positron emission tomography (PET) with CT (Giglio & Gilbert, 2010); a negative finding does not rule out ICP (Smith & Amin-Hanjani, 2013). ⚠
      2. ICP monitoring—per intraventricular, intraparenchymal, subarachnoid, or epidural site (Schimpf, 2012; Smith & Amin-Hanjani, 2013); goal is to keep ICP at less than 20 mm Hg and cerebral perfusion pressure (CPP) between 60 and 75 mm Hg (Schimpf, 2012)
      3. CT- or MRI-guided stereotactic biopsy for tissue diagnosis if malignancy is suspected cause
      4. CSF examination if leptomeningeal metastasis or meningitis is suspected (Giglio & Gilbert, 2010; Shelton, Ferrigno, & Skinner, 2013)
   B. Nonpharmacologic interventions
      1. Therapy directed at cause of ICP
      2. Surgery (Giglio & Gilbert, 2010)
         a. Emergent surgery to resect or debulk the tumor, if necessary, if life-threatening increased ICP present; could include removal of tumor or clot
         b. Shunt placement—provides an alternate pathway for CSF
         c. Ommaya reservoir placement for intrathecal chemotherapy administration
      3. Hyperventilation—the most rapid, short-term method to decrease ICP by causing vasoconstriction, which decreases cerebral blood volume and ICP; requires patient to be sedated, intubated, and ventilated to a partial pressure of carbon dioxide (P_{CO_2}) between 26 and 30 mm Hg (Smith & Amin-Hanjani, 2013)
      4. Radiation therapy (RT)—may be used if tumor is radiosensitive
         a. Primary treatment or palliative treatment for metastatic disease, depending on radiosensitivity of tumor; RT should never be started if elevation of ICP is uncontrolled,

because this may cause acute herniation and death (Giglio & Gilbert, 2010). ⚠

  b. Adjuvant treatment with either surgery or chemotherapy

  c. Specialized RT approaches for brain metastases

    (1) Stereotactic radiosurgery, including CyberKnife (Giglio & Gilbert, 2010)

    (2) Brachytherapy (Khan, Khan, Almasan, Singh, & Macklis, 2011)

  5. Removal of offending agent (as with posterior reversible encephalopathy syndrome) (Li et al., 2012; Tlemsani et al., 2011)

C. Pharmacologic interventions

  1. Chemotherapy or targeted therapy

    a. Most antineoplastic agents do not cross the blood-brain barrier; nitrosoureas and procarbazine are exceptions (Lee, 2012).

    b. Targeted therapies such as epidermal growth factor receptor (EGFR) inhibitors and the *HER2neu* and *BRAF* inhibitors are showing promise for brain metastasis.

    c. Regional drug delivery such as through the intrathecal or intraventricular (via CSF) routes, circumvents the blood-brain barrier (Clarke, 2012; Giglio & Gilbert, 2010).

  2. Corticosteroids (Giglio & Gilbert, 2010)

    a. Used to decrease inflammation, with resultant decrease in symptoms

    b. Emergent treatment often started prior to other modalities and may be tapered.

    c. May require maintenance doses for residual tumor; dependence may develop from long-term use.

  3. Osmotherapy (Smith & Amin-Hanjani, 2013; Torre-Healy, Marko, & Weil, 2012)

    a. Reduces intracellular water of brain, thus reducing brain volume

    b. Mannitol most frequently used hyperosmotic agent; caution needed in patients with renal insufficiency because it may cause acute renal failure and electrolyte disturbances ⚠

    c. Loop diuretics (e.g., furosemide)—may exacerbate dehydration and hypokalemia ⚠

    d. Bolus doses or infusion of hypertonic saline—may be used in combination, before or after mannitol; may cause renal failure, electrolyte disturbances, acute red blood cell (RBC) lysis, or phlebitis ⚠

    e. Maintenance of euvolemia—all free water (e.g., D5W, 0.45% saline, and enteral free water) to be avoided; only isotonic fluids (e.g., 0.9% normal saline) to be used

  4. Anticonvulsant therapy as prophylaxis in high-risk cases or treatment

  5. Antipyretic therapy to reduce fever

  6. Sedative agents

ASSESSMENT

I. Identification of patients at risk (Giglio & Gilbert, 2010; Shelton et al., 2013)

  A. Patients with cancers of the lung, breast, and kidney, and melanoma who have increased risk for metastases to the brain

  B. Patients with primary tumors of brain or spinal cord

  C. Patients with a diagnosis of leukemia, lymphoma, or neuroblastoma

  D. Oncology patients with thrombocytopenia, platelet dysfunction, or disseminated intravascular coagulation (DIC) may have bleeding that may cause increased ICP.

  E. Patients with infections such as encephalitis, meningitis, or systemic candidiasis, especially immunocompromised patients

  F. Patients with syndrome of inappropriate antidiuretic hormone secretion (see Chapter 40)

  G. Patients with history of RT

  H. Patients with occluded Ommaya reservoir

II. Physical examination—signs and symptoms depend on volume, location, and rate of ICP (see Table 41-1)

  A. Early signs and symptoms (Li et al., 2012; Shelton et al., 2013; Smith & Amin-Hanjani, 2013); if ICP suspected, minimization of further elevations through careful positioning and sedation (see Interventions) ⚠

    1. Headaches

      a. Often worse in early morning; moderate to severe in intensity; global or localized

      b. May be initiated or aggravated by Valsalva maneuver, coughing, vomiting, exercise, or bending over

      c. Pain may be described as dull, sharp, or throbbing

      d. May increase in severity, frequency, and duration over time

    2. Neurologic

      a. Blurred vision (diplopia), photophobia, contralateral pupillary dilation, decreased visual fields

      b. Extremity drifts, ipsilateral weakness

      c. Lethargy, apathy, confusion, restlessness

      d. Speech alterations such as slowed or delayed responses, word confusion

      e. Level of consciousness—sensitive index of the patient's neurologic status

    3. Gastrointestinal (GI)

      a. Loss of appetite

      b. Nausea and vomiting; vomiting may be projectile, sudden, and unexpected, not related to food intake.

Table 41-1

Key Physical Assessment Data in Suspected Structural Oncologic Emergencies

Body System	Assessment Data
Skin	Temperature, turgor, wounds, sites of central or intravenous lines, rash, cyanosis, flushing, diaphoresis
Head	Trauma, facial edema, dysphagia, hoarseness
Eyes	Pupil size, shape, reactivity; extraocular movements, papilledema, vision changes, diplopia, periorbital or orbital edema, ptosis
Ears and nose	Cerebrospinal fluid or blood
Neck	Jugular venous distention, masses, bruits, nuchal rigidity
Chest	Heart rate, rhythm, murmurs, gallops or rubs; respiratory rate, ease, use of accessory muscles, adventitious sounds, cough, pain
Abdomen	Masses, distention, bowel sounds, hepatomegaly, splenomegaly, incontinence, nausea, vomiting
Renal	Incontinence, decreased urinary output, retention
Musculoskeletal	General weakness, asymmetric weakness or deficits, tremor, edema, paralysis, handwriting change, gait changes, pain
Vascular	Edema, decreased or absent pulses, vital signs, dilated veins
Neurologic	Cranial nerves, reflexes, sensation, strength, Glasgow Coma Scale, mental status, level of consciousness, seizures, syncope
Psychiatric	Anxiety, depression, behavioral changes, aphasia

From Grecu, L. (2012). Cardiac tamponade. *International Anesthesiology Clinics*; Kaplan, M. (2013). Spinal cord compression. In M. Kaplan (editor). *Understanding and Managing Oncologic Emergencies*. Pittsburgh: Oncology Nursing Society; Schimpf, M. (2012). Diagnosing increased intracranial pressure. *Journal of Trauma Nursing*; Shelton, B. (2013). Superior vena cava syndrome. In M. Kaplan (editor). *Understanding and Managing Oncologic Emergencies*. Pittsburgh: Oncology Nursing Society; Story, K. (2013). In M. Kaplan (editor). *Understanding and Managing Oncologic Emergencies*. Pittsburgh: Oncology Nursing Society.

B. Late signs and symptoms (Li et al., 2012; Shelton et al., 2013; Smith & Amin-Hanjani, 2013)
   1. Cardiovascular—bradycardia, widening pulse pressure; as ICP increases, blood pressure rises.
   2. Respiratory—slow shallow respirations; tachypnea; Cheyne-Stokes respirations
   3. Neurologic—decreased ability to concentrate; decreased level of consciousness; personality changes; hemiplegia; hemiparesis; seizures; pupillary changes; papilledema (considered cardinal sign of increased ICP); papilledema, which is a swelling of the optic nerve where it meets the eye (the optic disc) and usually noted bilaterally
   4. Glasgow Coma Scale score less than 8 (Table 41-2)
   5. Abnormal posturing
   6. Temperature elevations
   7. Cushing triad (bradycardia, respiratory depression and hypertension)—a poor prognostic sign requiring emergent intervention ⚠

PROBLEM STATEMENTS AND OUTCOME IDENTIFICATION

See Shelton et al., 2013.

I. Risk for Ineffective Cerebral Tissue Perfusion (NANDA-I)
   A. Expected outcome—tissue perfusion will be adequate to prevent permanent neurologic damage.
   B. Expected outcome—progressive perfusion deficit will be recognized early and managed promptly.

Table 41-2

Glasgow Coma Scale

	Score
Eye Opening	
Spontaneous	4
Response to verbal command	3
Response to pain	2
No eye opening	1
Best Verbal Response	
Oriented	5
Confused	4
Inappropriate words	3
Incomprehensible sounds	2
No verbal response	1
Best Motor Response	
Obeys commands	6
Localizing response to pain	5
Withdrawal response to pain	4
Flexion to pain	3
Extension to pain	2
No motor response	1

Glasgow Coma Scale score—lowest score is 3 (worst) and highest is 15 (best). Record by the three parameters: eye opening (E); verbal response (V) and motor response (M). (Example E4V4M4 is a score of 12.) A score of 13 or higher correlates with mild brain injury, scores of 9 to 12 correlate with moderate brain injury, and a score of 8 or less correlates with severe brain injury.

II. Disturbed Thought Processes
   A. Expected outcome—patient and family identify appointed designee for decision making regarding treatment and subsequent care needs.

B. Expected outcome—patient will maintain reality orientation and communication with others.

C. Expected outcome—patient will communicate needs to participate in care.

III. Impaired Physical Mobility and Risk for Injury (NANDA-I) ⚠

    A. Expected outcome—risk of falls is minimized.

    B. Expected outcome—skin integrity is maintained.

    C. Expected outcome—patient participates in strategies to maximize safety and comfort in the acute care setting and at home.

IV. Deficient Knowledge (NANDA-I) of disease process and interventions

    A. Expected outcome—client or family identifies signs and symptoms of increased ICP to report to health care team.

    B. Expected outcome—patient participates in decision making about care, discharge planning, and life activities.

PLANNING AND IMPLEMENTATION

I. Interventions to monitor and manage inadequate cerebral tissue perfusion

    A. Monitoring for mental status changes

    B. Monitoring for changes of decreasing cardiac output (changes in vital signs, decreased urinary output, changes in mentation)

    C. Instructing the patient to avoid Valsalva maneuver

    D. Administering stool softeners, as ordered, to prevent constipation and straining; avoiding taking rectal temperatures

    E. Administering antiemetics, as ordered, to relieve nausea and vomiting

    F. Monitoring activities and positioning to minimize increased ICP

        1. Use of log roll technique when turning patients, keeping patient passive

        2. Avoiding head and neck flexion or extension, rotating the head, or both

        3. Elevating head of bed (HOB) 30 degrees to promote venous drainage

        4. Having patient avoid prone position or activities that exert pressure on the abdomen

        5. Implementing measures to decrease stress

            a. Maintaining a calm environment

            b. Minimizing external stimulation—light, noise, touch, temperature extremes

            c. Encouraging calm interactions between the patient and others

            d. Teaching about stress reduction strategies to patient and family

        6. Monitoring for sensory or motor changes—changes in visual acuity, pupil reactions, verbal expression; decrease in muscle strength, coordination, movement

        7. Assessment for associated symptoms such as nausea, vomiting, and headache

        8. Monitoring for seizure activity

II. Interventions to prevent injury

    A. Maintaining bed rest with increasing ICP and progressive symptoms; elevation of HOB

    B. Keeping bed in lowest position with side rails elevated

    C. Developing a daily schedule of activities with appropriate rest periods

    D. Use of assistive devices, as needed

    E. Use of bed alarms to monitor patient activity

III. Interventions for disturbed thought processes

    A. Monitoring of progressive mental status changes

    B. Explaining care procedures in clear, simple terms

    C. Reassuring patient that close monitoring will occur

    D. Assessment of patient's ability for self-care and safety in current environment

IV. Interventions to facilitate physical mobility and prevent injury

    A. Assessment of skin integrity regularly; inspecting pressure points and immobile extremities

    B. Use of pressure-distributing devices or padding, as needed

    C. Change of position every 2 hours

    D. Instructing patient about proper use of assistive devices

    E. Assisting patient and family to set realistic goals to maintain optimal activity and self-care levels within limitations imposed by the disease

    F. Assisting patient and family to assess physical environment in acute care setting and home and make appropriate changes to promote safety

        1. Encouraging situating major living area on ground level in the home

        2. Removal of scatter rugs from floors

        3. Encouraging use of rubber-soled, tie shoes and assistive devices

        4. Orienting patient to person, time, and place, as needed

        5. Reinforcing safe environment needs should seizures occur

        6. Referral to appropriate supportive services

            a. Physical therapy for activity program and use of assistive devices

            b. Services for community and social support, financial evaluation

            c. Palliative care consultation, as appropriate

V. Interventions to manage acute pain

    A. Assessment of pain with the use of an appropriate pain scale

    B. Implementation of measures to control discomfort caused by headaches

C. Measurement of efficacy of interventions with the use of a pain scale

D. Assessment, reduction, and elimination of common side effects of narcotics

E. Implementation of noninvasive pain relief measures such as relaxation or distraction

F. Administration of analgesics, as ordered

VI. Interventions to address knowledge deficit

A. Instructing patient in critical signs and symptoms that might indicate progressive disease

B. Including family or significant other in educational process

C. Assessment of readiness to learn and preferred learning method

D. Instructing patient in self-care measures, community resources, and contacts for emergencies

E. Providing information about disease process, interventions, and expectations of outcome

EVALUATION

The oncology nurse systematically and regularly evaluates patient and family responses to interventions related to increased ICP to determine progress toward the achievement of expected outcomes. Relevant data are collected, and actual findings are compared with expected findings. Nursing diagnoses, outcomes, and plans of care are reviewed and revised, as necessary.

Spinal Cord Compression

OVERVIEW

I. Definition—a neurologic emergency that occurs when the spinal cord or cauda equina is compromised by direct pressure, vertebral collapse, or both caused by metastatic spread or direct extension of a malignancy; compression results in compromised neurologic function if not treated promptly (Kilbride, Cox, Kennedy, Lee, & Grant, 2010; National Institute for Health and Clinical Excellence [NICE], 2010).

II. Pathophysiology (Hammack, 2012; Killbride et al., 2010; McCurdy & Shanholtz, 2012)

A. The spinal cord is a cylindric body of nervous tissue that occupies the upper two thirds of the vertebral canal.

B. The spinal cord has motor, sensory, and autonomic functions.

C. Compression of the spinal cord may occur as a result of tumor invasion of the vertebrae and results from subsequent collapse of the spinal cord that causes increased pressure or as a result of primary tumors of the spinal cord.

D. Compression of the spinal cord may result in minor changes in motor, sensory, and autonomic

function or complete paralysis. Spinal cord compression is the second most frequent neurologic complication of metastatic cancer.

E. Ambulatory status at diagnosis is directly related to prognosis and quality of life.

III. Principles of medical management

A. Emergent treatment required within 24 hours of signs of neurologic compromise; negative outcomes and deterioration in motor and autonomic function associated with delays in initiating treatment (NICE, 2010)

B. Diagnostic tests (Dimopoulous, et al., 2009; Hammack, 2012; Killbride, et al., 2010; McCurdy & Shanholtz, 2012; NICE, 2010)

1. High level of clinical suspicion key to successful outcomes because prognosis is dependent on prompt diagnosis

2. MRI—diagnostic procedure of choice for evaluating spinal cord compression; entire spine should be assessed

3. CT—may be an alternative when MRI is unavailable or contraindicated; less sensitive

4. Myelography—used with or without CT when MRI and other imaging modalities are nondiagnostic

5. Spinal radiography—shows bone abnormalities or soft tissue masses; should not be used to diagnose or rule out spinal metastasis

6. PET—both sensitive and specific but less available than MRI; should not be used alone for diagnosis or treatment guidance

C. Nonpharmacologic interventions

1. RT (McCurdy & Shanholtz, 2012)

a. For radiosensitive tumors such as lymphoma, myeloma, breast and prostate cancers, and small cell lung carcinoma (SCLC)

b. Treatment of choice for most epidural metastases and cord compressions (Shiue et al., 2010)

c. Used alone when no evidence of spinal instability or radical spinal compression.

d. Most common dose is 30 Gy given in 10 fractions (Hammack, 2012)

2. Surgery (Akram & Allibone, 2010; NICE, 2010)

a. Laminectomy—used to decompress a vertebral body; urgency of surgery dependent on neurologic compromise

b. Used if tumor is not responsive to RT

c. Used if recurrent tumor is in an area previously treated with RT (maximal safe RT dose has already been received by spinal cord)

3. Surgery followed by RT

D. Pharmacologic interventions (Hammack, 2012; McCurdy & Shanholtz, 2012)

1. Corticosteroids
   a. Almost always the initial treatment to relieve or stabilize neurologic deficits; reduce spinal cord edema and pain
   b. High initial dose; intravenous (IV) bolus dose given as soon as SCC is suspected; patients may experience a sudden, intense burning or tingling perineal discomfort; slow IV administration may lesson or eliminate this sensation. ⚠
   c. Subsequent regular dosing until treatment concludes, followed by tapering of dose; monitoring of blood glucose levels; assessment for other adverse events such as mania and insomnia ⚠
   e. GI prophylaxis with proton pump inhibitors
2. Chemotherapeutic agents (Hammack, 2012; Kaplan, 2013)
   a. Limited role because of slower and unpredictable results; could be considered in highly chemosensitive tumors and if patient has minimal neurologic deficits
   b. May be used as an adjuvant treatment to radiation and surgery for tumors such as lymphomas, germ cell tumors, and neuroblastoma responsive to anti neoplastics
   c. May be used if recurrence of tumor is at a site of previous surgery or RT
3. Analgesics—more than 95% of patients with spinal cord compression have pain.
   (see Chapter 34)
   a. Management guided by type of pain as described in the World Health Organization (WHO) pain relief ladder; opioids often required (NICE, 2010; Taylor & Schiff, 2010)
   b. Observation for adverse events such as constipation, nausea, somnolence, and pruritus ⚠
   c. Adjuncts to opioids help with neuropathic pain
      (1) Anticonvulsants
      (2) Antidepressants
4. Anticoagulants—patients with SCLC are at high risk for deep venous thrombosis (DVT) or pulmonary embolus; prophylactic treatment with low-molecular-weight heparin (Hammack, 2012; NICE, 2010; Taylor & Schiff, 2010)
5. Bone remodeling agents—for patients with metastatic bone lesions (Taylor and Schiff, 2010)

ASSESSMENT

I. Factors for identification of patients at risk (Kaplan, 2013; McCurdy & Shanholtz, 2012)
   A. Cancers that have a natural history for metastasizing to the bone—breast, lung, prostate, renal, melanoma, non-Hodgkin lymphoma, myeloma
   B. Cancers that metastasize to the brain and spinal cord—lymphoma, seminoma, neuroblastoma
   C. Primary cancers of the spinal cord—ependymoma, astrocytoma, glioma
   D. History of vertebral compression fractures
II. Pertinent history (Kaplan, 2013)
   A. Histology of primary tumor, date of diagnosis, stage at diagnosis, treatment history, history of metastatic disease; responses to treatment and survival following treatment vary among types of cancer.
   B. Time since onset of symptoms; level and degree of compression
   C. Comprehensive pain assessment, including onset, duration, location, intensity, description, and exacerbating and relieving factors
   D. Pre-existing medical problems and current medications
III. Physical examination—presenting signs and symptoms vary, depending on the location and severity of the compression (Kaplan, 2013; Kilbride et al., 2010) (see Table 41-1).
   A. Early signs and symptoms
      1. Neck or back pain—always requires prompt evaluation in a patient with cancer; back pain the first symptom in 96% of patients and may be local, radicular, or both; pain may precede other symptoms by up to 2 months (Hammack, 2012; Kaplan, 2013; McCurdy & Shanholtz, 2012)
         a. Gentle percussion and palpation of the vertebral column, neck flexion, and straight leg raises—may indicate the level of cord compression
         b. Localized pain—constant, dull, aching; usually progressive
         c. Radicular pain—may be constant or initiated with movement; may be shooting in nature; radiates along the dermatome of the affected nerve root
         d. Pain usually worse in supine position; may awaken patient at night
         e. Pain exacerbated by straining, coughing, or flexion of neck; pain only with movement may indicate spinal instability that needs surgical intervention.
      2. Motor weakness or dysfunction—may present as heaviness, stiffness, or weakness of extremities and lead to loss of coordination and ataxia (Table 41-3)
      3. Sensory loss—with regard to light touch, pain, or temperature
   B. Late signs and symptoms (Hammack, 2012; Kaplan, 2013)—ominous; treatment must be instituted on an emergent basis. ⚠

Table 41-3

Assessment of Motor and Sensory Function

Function	Assessment Techniques
Muscle strength	Upper extremities—ask patient to grip your finger as firmly as possible. Lower extremities—ask patient to resist plantar flexion of his or her feet.
Coordination of hands and feet	Ask patient to touch each finger to his or her thumb in rapid sequence. Ask patient to turn hand over and back as quickly as possible. Ask patient to tap your hand as quickly as possible with the ball of each foot.
Sensory perception	Touch patient along length of extremities and trunk with the blunt and sharp ends of a safety pin, and ask patient to identify as either sharp or dull. Ask patient to report the sensation of touch when touched with a wisp of cotton. Move one of the patient's fingers, and ask if the finger is being moved up or down. Touch skin of patient with test tube of hot water and then cold water; ask the patient to describe the temperature.

1. Loss of sensation for deep pressure, vibrations, position
2. Incontinence or retention of urine or stool
3. Sexual impotence
4. Paralysis
5. Muscle atrophy
6. Loss of sweating below lesion

PROBLEM STATEMENTS AND OUTCOME IDENTIFICATION

I. Acute Pain (NANDA-I)
   A. Expected outcome—pain is regularly assessed; treatment is prompt; pain is then reassessed for intervention efficacy.
   B. Expected outcome—patient achieves acceptable pain control.
   C. Expected outcome—patient and family identify complementary or integrative health programs or approaches to care (e.g., pain management, relaxation).
II. Impaired Physical Mobility (NANDA-I)
   A. Expected outcome—patient maintains optimal level of physical mobility.
   B. Expected outcome—patient and family participate in rehabilitation program designed to promote adaptation to residual limitations associated with spinal cord compression.
III. Impaired Neurologic Function
   A. Expected outcome—patient carries out acceptable bowel and urinary elimination.

IV. Deficient Knowledge (NANDA-I), related to early signs and symptoms of spinal cord compression and care after spinal cord compression
   A. Expected outcome—patient lists signs and symptoms that should be reported to the health care team.
   B. Expected outcome—patient describes strategies to minimize sequelae of spinal cord compression.

PLANNING AND IMPLEMENTATION

I. Interventions to manage pain and increase comfort (see Chapter 34)
II. Interventions to promote physical mobility
   A. Mobilizing the patient on the basis of findings of stable or unstable spine
   B. Maintaining neutral spine alignment by using log roll technique until neurologically stable (NICE, 2010) (Table 41-4)
   C. Ongoing assessment of motor functions (Kaplan, 2013)
   D. Initiating a consultation with physical and occupational therapy as soon as the spine is stabilized (Shiue et al, 2010); immobility increases the risk for thromboembolic events, pneumonia, and sepsis (Taylor & Schiff, 2010). ⚠
   E. Assisting patient to maintain a safe level of independence within the limitations imposed by the cord compression
   F. Encouraging patient and family to express concerns about the effect of residual limitations on activities of daily living (ADLs) and lifestyle

Table 41-4

Mobility Interventions

Unstable Spine	Stable Spine
Place sandbags on either side of the head to limit movement.	Initiate range of motion exercises after physical therapy evaluation and with a physician's order.
Use cervical collar to support cervical spine.	Instruct patient and family in isometric exercises.
Support head and neck during all movement.	Provide personal assistance with ambulation.
Use no pillows.	Instruct patient and family in use of assistive devices with ambulation.
Maintain alignment when turning or positioning.	Maintain proper alignment while in bed, turning, or positioning.
Use a log roll, pull sheet, or transfer board when turning or positioning.	
Place patient on special bed, as indicated—Stryker frame or CircOlectric bed.	

III. Interventions to improve or maintain neurologic function (Kaplan, 2013)
  A. Monitoring for progression of motor or sensory deficits every 8 hours
    1. Decrease in muscle strength and coordination
    2. Decrease in perception of temperature, touch, position
    3. Change in level of consciousness
  B. Monitoring bowel and urinary elimination patterns and effectiveness
    1. Recording intake and output every 8 hours; monitoring nutrition and fluid status
    2. Palpation for bladder distention if interval between voiding increases
    3. Recording frequency and characteristics of stool with each bowel movement
    4. Conducting gentle digital rectal examination to check for impaction if no bowel movement within 3 days, unless neutropenic or thrombocytopenic
    5. Instituting a bowel and urinary elimination program
IV. Interventions to improve or maintain skin integrity
  A. Regularly assessing skin integrity and evaluating intervention
  B. Instituting a skin care regimen
  C. Providing instructions to the patient and family about assessing the pressure and temperature of objects coming in contact with the patient's areas of compromised feeling or sensation
V. Interventions to increase knowledge of disease process and therapeutic interventions
  A. Providing education about reporting any changes in bowel and urinary elimination patterns, pain, sensory and motor function, skin integrity, or sexual dysfunction
  B. Providing education about treatment modalities, potential adverse events, and self-care
VI. Interventions to preserve self-image and role performance
  A. Supporting patient and caregiver in acceptance of functional limitations
  B. Facilitating patient and caregivers end-of-life discussions

EVALUATION

The oncology nurse systematically and regularly evaluates the patient's responses to spinal cord compression interventions to determine progress toward the achievement of individual patient goals. Relevant data are collected, and actual findings are compared with expected findings. Nursing diagnoses, outcomes, and plans of care are reviewed and revised, as necessary.

Superior Vena Cava Syndrome (SVCS)

OVERVIEW

I. Definition—occurs as a result of compromised venous drainage of the head, neck, upper extremities, and thorax through the superior vena cava (SVC) because of compression or obstruction of the vessel by, for example, tumor or thrombus
II. Pathophysiology
  A. The SVC is a thin-walled major vessel that carries venous drainage from the head, neck, upper extremities, and upper thorax to the heart (McCurdy & Shanholtz, 2012; Shelton, 2013).
  B. The SVC is located in the mediastinum and is surrounded by the rigid structures of the sternum, trachea, and vertebrae and the aorta, right bronchus, lymph nodes, and pulmonary artery (Lepper et al., 2011).
  C. The SVC is a low-pressure vessel that is easily compressed; compression (acute or gradual) can occur from direct tumor invasion, enlarged lymph nodes, or a thrombus within the vessel (Brumbaugh, 2011). Right-sided lung cancers are responsible for most cases of SVCS (Drews & Rabkin, 2013).
  D. When obstruction of the SVC occurs, venous return to the heart from the head, neck, thorax, and upper extremities is impaired (Lepper et al., 2011; Shelton, 2013).
    1. Venous pressure and congestion in head, neck, upper extremities, and upper thorax increase.
    2. Decreased cardiac filling and output may ensue.
    3. Blood flow diverts to multiple smaller collaterals to the azygos vein or the inferior vena cava.
III. Principles of medical management
  A. Goals of treatment include relief of the obstruction and treatment of the underlying cause and presenting symptoms (Shelton, 2013).
  B. Treatment and prognosis are determined by rapidity of onset and cause of obstruction (McCurdy & Shanholtz, 2012). Histologic diagnosis is necessary for treatment of the causes of the primary tumor (Shelton, 2013).
  C. Diagnostic tests (Brumbaugh, 2011; Drews & Rabkin, 2013; Shelton, 2013) include the following:
    1. CT of the thorax (contrast or helical)—the preferred diagnostic test; often identifies cause of SVCS and may define anatomy of a mediastinal mass
    2. MRI—sensitive for SVCS and beneficial in those who cannot tolerate contrast, but may be complicated by inability to tolerate supine position, longer scanning time and higher cost (Bockorny, Kourelis, & Bockorny, 2012)

3. PET is useful when planning the radiation field and to determine if the cause is malignant or benign.
4. Contrast venography is more invasive but useful to determine the extent of thrombus formation and if stent placement or surgery is planned.
5. Chest radiography results are usually abnormal, showing mediastinal widening and pleural effusion.
6. Additional tests to determine the histologic diagnosis of the primary condition include bronchoscopy, bone marrow biopsy, mediastinoscopy, thoracentesis, sputum analysis, and needle biopsy of palpable lymph nodes (Lepper et al., 2011; Shelton, 2013).

D. Nonpharmacologic interventions (Brumbaugh, 2011; Shelton, 2013; Venturini, Becuzzi, & Magni, 2012, Drews & Rabkin, 2013)
1. RT is considered the primary treatment for SVCS if the patient has non–small cell lung cancer and is often used in other types of malignancies as well. RT may also be used as initial treatment if a histologic diagnosis cannot be made or the clinical status of the patient is deteriorating.
2. To avoid embolization, along with anticoagulation therapy, the central venous catheter should be removed in catheter-induced SVCS. Thrombolytic therapy or tissue plasminogen activators may be used to treat a thrombosis that is catheter-induced.
3. Percutaneous intravascular stent placement is useful when urgent intervention needed. Percutaneous balloon angioplasty may be necessary to enlarge the vascular lumen prior to stent placement.
4. Surgical reconstruction of SVC is rarely required because of effectiveness of stent placement. Surgical resection of the tumor is rare because of the poor prognosis in many patients with SVCS.
5. Oxygen therapy is provided to relieve dyspnea.

E. Pharmacologic interventions (Bockorny et al., 2012; Drews & Rabkin, 2013; Lepper et al., 2011; Shelton, 2013)
1. Anti neoplastic therapy alone in patients who have had previous maximum mediastinal RT or as initial therapy for those who have chemosensitive disease such as SCLC, non-Hodgkin lymphoma, or germ cell cancer
2. Anti neoplastic therapy in conjunction with RT
3. Corticosteroids—may reduce edema or inflammation (e.g., to prevent postradiation edema); useful in steroid-responsive malignancies
4. Diuretics—may reduce edema and intravascular volume
5. Thrombolytic therapy when the cause is a thrombus

ASSESSMENT

I. Identification of patients at risk (Drews & Rabkin, 2013; Shelton, 2013)
A. Presence of non–small cell lung cancer (NSCLC) and SCLC, breast cancer, lymphoma involving the mediastinum, germ cell tumors, thyroid and GI cancers, melanoma, and Kaposi sarcoma
B. Presence of central venous catheters and pacemakers
C. Previous RT to the mediastinum
D. Associated conditions such as histoplasmosis, mediastinal fibrosis, fungal infection, benign tumors, and aortic aneurysm

II. Physical examination—progression of physical signs can be slow or acute; slow progression allows collateral blood flow to develop; when this occurs, symptoms regress.
A. Early signs and symptoms of SVCS (Shelton, 2013)
1. Symptoms more pronounced in the morning or when bending over and improve after being upright for several hours
2. Redness and edema in conjunctivae and around the eyes and face
3. Swelling of the neck, arms, hands; men may have problems buttoning shirt collars (Stoke sign)
4. Neck and thoracic vein distention—visible collateral veins on the chest, breast, or both
5. Dyspnea—most common symptom
6. Nonproductive cough
7. Hoarseness, occasionally dysphagia
8. Cyanosis of upper torso
9. Nasal stuffiness, fullness in head
10. Women may experience swelling of their breasts

B. Late signs and symptoms of SVCS (Brumbaugh, 2011; Shelton, 2013)
1. Symptoms of increased ICP—severe headache, visual disturbances, blurred vision, dizziness, syncope
2. Irritability, changes in mental status, or both
3. Stridor, signs of congestive heart failure
4. Tachycardia, tachypnea, orthopnea
5. Hypotension, absence of peripheral pulses
6. Dysphagia, hoarseness, hemoptysis
7. Progressive cyanosis, facial edema
8. Horner syndrome (Kinnard, 2012)—the combination of drooping of the eyelid (ptosis) and constriction of the pupil (miosis), sometimes accompanied by decreased sweating (anhidrosis) of the face on the same side

III. Evaluation of laboratory data—comparison of available laboratory data against previous and normal values
  A. Arterial blood gases
  B. Electrolytes, kidney function
  C. Complete blood cell count (CBC)
  D. Coagulation studies

PROBLEM STATEMENTS AND OUTCOME IDENTIFICATION

I. Impaired Gas Exchange (NANDA-I)
  A. Expected outcome—respiratory rate is within normal limits (WNL).
  B. Expected outcome—patient reports relief from dyspneic symptoms.
II. Decreased Cardiac Output (NANDA-I)
  A. Expected outcome—cardiac rate, rhythm, and blood pressure are WNL.
III. Anxiety (NANDA-I)
  A. Expected outcome—patient relates increased psychological comfort.
IV. Deficient Knowledge (NANDA-I), related to disease process and therapeutic interventions
  A. Expected outcome—patient verbalizes critical signs and symptoms to report to health care team.
  B. Expected outcome—patient describes plans for continued follow-up care.
  C. Expected outcome—patient participates in decision making about care, discharge planning, and life activities.

PLANNING AND IMPLEMENTATION

I. Interventions to maintain adequate gas exchange (Lepper et al., 2011)
  A. Maintenance of airway
  B. Fowler or semi-Fowler position to decrease edema, dyspnea, hydrostatic pressure
  C. Instructions to the patient to avoid Valsalva maneuver or other straining activities
  D. Assistance with ADLs to conserve breathing and energy
  E. Assessment for progressive respiratory distress
  F. Administration of oxygen, as ordered
II. Interventions to maintain adequate cardiac output
  A. Monitoring for changes in tissue perfusion (decreased peripheral pulses, decrease in blood pressure, cyanosis)
  B. Monitoring for changes of decreasing cardiac output (changes in vital signs, decreased urinary output, changes in mentation)
  C. Monitoring intake, output, and weight
III. Interventions to decrease anxiety
  A. Explaining care procedures in clear, simple terms
  B. Encouraging patient to ask questions about care and changes in condition
  C. Providing a quiet, nonstimulating environment

IV. Interventions to increase knowledge of disease process and therapeutic interventions (Shelton, 2013)
  A. Providing information about critical signs and symptoms that might indicate progressive disease
  B. Inclusion of family or significant other in educational process
  C. Assessment of readiness to learn and preferred learning method
  D. Instructing patient in self-care measures, community resources, and emergent contacts
  E. Educating patient about disease process, interventions, expectations of outcome
V. Interventions to prevent injury (Lepper et al., 2011; Shelton, 2013)
  A. Avoiding venipunctures, IV fluid administration, or measurement of blood pressure in the upper extremities
  B. Removing jewelry (e.g., rings) and restrictive clothing
  C. Assessment for changes in neurologic or mental status
  D. Monitoring for signs and symptoms of adverse effects of anticoagulant therapy—petechiae; ecchymosis; bleeding of gums, nose, urinary tract, or GI system
  E. Monitoring for signs and symptoms of adverse effects of steroid therapy—muscle weakness, mood swings, steroid-induced glycosuria, dyspepsia, insomnia

EVALUATION

The oncology nurse systematically and regularly evaluates the patient's responses to interventions for SVCS to determine progress toward the achievement of adequate perfusion. Relevant data are collected, and actual findings are compared with expected findings. Nursing diagnoses, outcomes, and plans of care are reviewed and revised, as necessary.

Cardiac Tamponade

OVERVIEW

I. Definition—a life-threatening situation of excessive accumulation of fluid in the pericardial sac exerting extrinsic pressure on the cardiac chambers, resulting in decreased cardiac output and compromised cardiac function
II. Pathophysiology
  A. The pericardium is a two-layered sac (parietal and visceral layers) surrounding the heart (Grecu, 2012; Schairer, Biswas, Keteyian, & Ananthasubramaniam, 2011; Story, 2013).
    1. The space between the two layers is the pericardial cavity.

2. The cavity normally is filled with 10 to 50 mL of fluid produced by the mesothelial cells of the visceral pericardium. This fluid between opposing layers of the heart allows the heart to move without friction.
3. Recesses and sinuses may accommodate a limited increase of pericardial fluid.

B. An increase in the intrapericardial pressure may occur because of the following (Grecu, 2012; Story, 2013):
1. Fluid accumulation in the pericardial sac secondary to the following:
   a. Increased capillary permeability from chemotherapy or biotherapy
   b. Direct trauma to the chest
   c. Improper insertion of central line or pacemaker
2. Direct or metastatic tumor invasion to the pericardial sac
3. Fibrosis of the pericardial sac related to RT
4. Infections causing pericardial effusions
5. Obstruction of mediastinal lymph nodes

C. As intrapericardial pressure increases, the following occur:
1. Cardiac chambers are compressed, and left ventricular filling decreases.
2. The ability of the heart to pump decreases.
3. Cardiac output decreases, and blood pressure falls.
4. Impaired systemic perfusion occurs, and cardiogenic shock may follow.
5. Rate of pericardial fluid increase is more important than volume accrued because the slow accumulation allows time for the pericardium to expand. Acute increases may cause severe symptoms, even with a small amount of fluid (Bodson, Bouferrache, & Vieillard-Baron, 2011; Grecu, 2012).

III. Principles of medical management
A. Diagnostic tests (Bodson et al., 2011; Grecu, 2012; Khandaker et al., 2010; Schairer et al., 2011)
1. Chest radiography shows enlarged pericardial silhouette after more than 200 mL of fluid has accumulated; however, it is not a definitive diagnostic tool.
2. CT is very useful because it can also reveal pleural effusion, masses, or pericardial thickening; however, it may overestimate the volume of effusion. It can reveal whether effusion is hemorrhagic and estimate pericardial thickness.
3. Echocardiography is the initial and most precise diagnostic test and should be repeated frequently to monitor for progression. Effusion, collapse of right or left atrium, respiratory variation in flow velocities, and dilation of inferior vena cava may be seen.

4. Electrocardiography (ECG) results vary, depending on the extent of the tamponade; signs similar to pericarditis (ST elevation and PR depression) may be seen. Typically, sinus tachycardia, low QRS voltage, and electrical alternans are present.
5. MRI is very sensitive in the detection of effusions as small as 30 mL; however, it requires more time and involves increased cost.
6. Pericardiocentesis and cytology testing of fluid are also performed.
   a. Bloody fluid is associated with a positive cytology test result.
   b. Cytology testing has a significant false-negative rate.

B. Nonpharmacologic interventions (Grecu, 2012; Story, 2013)
1. Pericardiocentesis is the temporary removal of excess pericardial fluid.
   a. It is important to be aware of possible delay in scheduling the procedure and to ensure patient stability. Local anesthesia is preferred because anesthesia may cause life-threatening hypotension and cardiac arrest. Pericardiocentesis may be contraindicated in thrombocytopenia and anticoagulation therapy (Loukas et al., 2012). ⚠
2. The pericardial window is a surgical opening of the pericardium to allow fluid drainage.
3. Total pericardectomy is the removal of the pericardial sac for patients with constrictive or chronic pericarditis.
4. Percutaneous balloon pericardiotomy (an alternative to surgical pericardial window) involves a balloon being used to create a pericardial window by stretching the pericardium.
5. RT may be performed to treat radiosensitive tumors of the pericardium. RT is contraindicated in radiation pericarditis and when area involved has previously received radiation. ⚠
6. Volume resuscitation is done to correct hypovolemia (Bodson et al., 2011). Any changes in vital signs might indicate hemodynamic impairment. ⚠

C. Pharmacologic interventions (Lewis, Hendrickson, & Moynihan, 2011; Story, 2013)
1. Pericardial sclerosis (to prevent recurrence of pericardial effusion) is an instillation through a pericardial catheter of agent (e.g., doxycycline [Doxy 100], thiotepa [Thioplex], bleomycin [Blenoxane], mitomycin C [Mitomycin], sterile talc) that cause inflammation and subsequent fibrosis.

2. Systemic anti neoplastic therapy may be used for treating chemotherapy-sensitive malignancies such as lymphoma, breast cancer, or SCLC.
3. Corticosteroids may be used after drainage of the effusion but are not used in urgent treatment (Bodson et al. 2011).

ASSESSMENT

I. Identification of patients at risk (Story, 2013)
  A. Patients with primary tumors of the heart, including mesothelioma and sarcomas (including Kaposi sarcoma)
  B. Patients with metastatic tumors to the pericardium—lung, breast, GI tract, leukemia, Hodgkin or non-Hodgkin lymphoma, sarcoma, melanoma
  C. Patients who have received more than 4000 cGy of radiation to a field in which the heart is included
  D. Patients receiving chemotherapy or biotherapy associated with increased capillary permeability (e.g., anthracyclines, interferon, interleukin, granulocyte-macrophage colony-stimulating factor)
  E. Those with comorbidities such as heart disease, connective tissue disorders, myxedema (dry, waxy, nonpitting edema with abnormal deposits of mucin in the skin often associated with hypothyroidism), tuberculosis, aneurysms, renal failure, and history of cardiac surgery (e.g., valve surgery)
II. Physical examination
  A. Early signs and symptoms (Khandaker et al., 2010; Story, 2013)
    1. Retrosternal chest pain relieved by leaning forward and intensified when lying supine or by inspiration; may radiate to neck and jaw; chest pain may be difficult to differentiate from a myocardial infarction. ⚠
    2. Dyspnea with exertion
    3. Muffled heart sounds, pericardial friction rub
    4. Tachycardia, with weak or absent apical and peripheral pulses, heart palpitations
    5. Fatigue, malaise
    6. Vague, right upper quadrant pain resulting from hepatic venous congestion
    7. Mild jugular venous distention
    8. May be asymptomatic
  B. Late signs and symptoms (Khandaker et al., 2010; Story, 2013)
    1. Tachycardia—more than 100 beats/min; a protective mechanism; any intervention that lowers the heart rate (e.g., beta blocker or anesthesia) could cause dangerous decrease in cardiac output. ⚠

2. Tachypnea, orthopnea
3. Decreased systolic pressure and rising diastolic pressure (narrow pulse pressure)
4. Pulsus paradoxus greater than 10 mm Hg—classic for cardiac tamponade; pulsus paradoxus is an ominous finding. ⚠
5. Increased central venous pressure (CVP)
6. Altered levels of consciousness
7. Oliguria
8. Peripheral edema
9. Diaphoresis
10. Cyanosis
11. Anxiety and agitation, mental status changes
12. Hiccups
13. Hoarseness, dysphagia
14. Beck triad forms the classic signs of cardiac tamponade—elevated CVP, hypotension, and distant heart sounds; all three of these signs occur only in advanced cardiac tamponade.
15. Chest pain—may disappear
16. Increased jugular venous distention
III. Evaluation of laboratory data—review of laboratory data and comparison of results with previous values and normal parameters (Kaplow, 2011; Story, 2013)
  A. Arterial blood gas values if patient has respiratory distress
  B. Electrolyte values

PROBLEM STATEMENTS AND OUTCOME IDENTIFICATION

I. Decreased Cardiac Output (NANDA-I)
  A. Expected outcome—patient will maintain optimal cardiac output.
II. Ineffective Breathing Pattern (NANDA-I)
  A. Expected outcome—patient will maintain optimal respiratory status.
III. Anxiety (NANDA-I)
  A. Expected outcome—patient relates increased psychological comfort.
IV. Deficient Knowledge (NANDA-I), related to cardiac tamponade and its management
  A. Expected outcome—patient identifies signs and symptoms to be reported to the health care team.
  B. Expected outcome—patient describes the effects of cardiac tamponade or treatment on ADLs and lifestyle.

PLANNING AND IMPLEMENTATION

I. Interventions to maintain cardiac output
  A. Frequent, regular assessment of cardiovascular, status, evaluating for instability (e.g., sinus tachycardia, drop in blood pressure) (Schairer et al., 2011; Story, 2013)
  B. Following pericardiocentesis, observation for complications such as bleeding, change in vital

signs, cardiac arrhythmias, infection, and abdominal or shoulder pain (Loukas et al., 2012)
  C. Assessment of character and amount of drainage from pericardial catheter, if present
  D. Assessment of catheter site for signs and symptoms of infection
II. Interventions to maintain optimal respiratory function (Story, 2013)
  A. Frequent, regular assessment of respiratory status, evaluating for changes
  B. Administration of oxygen therapy, as ordered
  C. Positioning with HOB elevated
  D. Instructing patient in energy conservation, relaxation techniques; ensuring adequate rest
III. Interventions to increase comfort
  A. Instituting nonpharmacologic methods of pain control (see Chapter 34)
  B. Assisting patient to positions of comfort; maintenance of proper body alignment
  C. Administering analgesics, as ordered
  D. Evaluation of effectiveness of interventions
IV. Interventions to decrease anxiety
  A. Explaining care procedures in clear, simple terms to decrease anxiety
  B. Reassuring patient that close monitoring will occur
  C. Encouraging patient to ask questions about care measures, changes in condition, or both
  D. Providing a quiet, nonstimulating environment
V. Interventions to increase knowledge of disease process and therapeutic interventions
  A. Educating patient and caregiver about disease process, treatment, and self-care
  B. Educating patient and caregiver about signs and symptoms that require emergent health care
  C. Assessment of readiness to learn and preferred learning method
  D. Providing information about community resources and emergency contacts
VI. Interventions to reduce risk for injury
  A. Assisting patient with ADLs and ambulation, as needed
  B. Keeping bed in low position, with side rails up
  C. Encouraging patient and family to communicate concerns about the condition and the treatment with a member of the health care team

EVALUATION

The oncology nurse systematically and regularly evaluates the patient's responses to interventions for cardiac tamponade to determine progress toward the achievement of adequate perfusion and comfort. Relevant data are collected, and actual findings are compared with expected findings. Nursing diagnoses, outcomes, and plans of care are reviewed and revised, as necessary.

References

Akram, H., & Allibone, J. (2010). Spinal surgery for palliation in malignant spinal cord compression. *Clinical Oncology, 22,* 792–800. http://dx.doi.org/10.1016/j.clon.2010.07.007.

Bockorny, M., Kourelis, T., & Bockorny, B. (2012). Superior vena cava syndrome caused by colon adenocarcinomas metastasis: A case report and review of literature. *Connecticut Medicine, 76*(2), 77–80.

Bodson, L., Bouferrache, K., & Vieillard-Baron, A. (2011). *Current Opinion in Critical Care, 17,* 416–424. http://dx.doi.org/10.1097/MCC.0b013e3283491f27.

Brumbaugh, H. (2011). Superior vena cava syndrome. In C. H. Yarbor, D. Wujcik, & B. H. Goel (Eds.), *Cancer nursing: principles and practice* (7th ed., pp. 995–1004). Burlington, MA: Jones and Bartlett.

Clarke, J. (2012). Leptomeningeal metastasis from systemic cancer. *Continuum, 18*(2), 328–342. http://dx.doi.org/10.1212/01.CON.0000413661.58045.e7.

Dimopoulos, M., Terpos, E., Comenzo, R., Tosi, P., Beksac, M., Sezer, O., et al. (2009). International myeloma working group consensus statement and guidelines regarding the current role of imaging techniques in the diagnosis and monitoring of multiple myeloma. *Leukemia, 23*(9), 1545–1556. http://dx.doi.org/10.1038/leu.2009.89.

Drews, R., & Rabkin, D. (2013). *Malignancy-related superior vena cava syndrome.* www.uptodate.com.

Giglio, P., & Gilbert, M. (2010). Neurologic complications of cancer and its treatment. *Current Oncology Reports, 12,* 50–59. http://dx.doi.org/10.1007/s11912-009-0071-x.

Grecu, L. (2012). Cardiac tamponade. *International Anesthesiology Clinics, 50*(2), 59–77. http://dx.doi.org/10.1097/AIA.0b013e318254053e.

Hammack, J. (2012). Spinal cord disease in patients with cancer. *Continuum, 18*(2), 312–327. http://dx.doi.org/10.1212/01.CON.0000413660.58045.ae.

Kaplan, M. (2013). Spinal cord compression. In M. Kaplan (Ed.), *Understanding and managing oncologic emergencies,* (2nd ed., pp. 337–383). Pittsburgh: Oncology Nursing Society.

Kaplow, R. (2011). Cardiac tamponade. In C. H. Yarbor, D. Wujcik, & B. H. Goel (Eds.), *Cancer nursing: Principles and practice* (7th ed., pp. 915–927). Burlington, MA: Jones and Bartlett.

Khan, N., Khan, M., Almasan, A., Singh, A., & Macklis, R. (2011). The evolving role of radiation therapy in the management of malignant melanoma. *International Journal of Radiation Oncology, 80*(3), 645–654. http://dx.doi.org/10.1016/j.ijrobp.2010.12.071.

Khandaker, M., Espinosa, R., Nishimura, R., Sinak, L., Hayes, S., Melduni, R., et al. (2010). Pericardial disease; diagnosis and management. *Mayo Clinic Procedures, 85*(6), 572–593. http://dx.doi.org/10.4065/mcp.2010.0046.

Kilbride, L., Cox, M., Kennedy, C., Lee, S., & Grant, R. (2010). Metastatic spinal cord compression: A review of practice and care. *Journal of Clinical Nursing, 19,* 1767–1783. http://dx.doi.org/10.1111/j.1365-2702.2010.03236.x.

Kinnard, E. (2012). Superior vena cava syndrome in the cancer patient: A case study. *Journal for the Advanced Practitioner in Oncology, 3*(6), 385–387.

Part 6

Lee, S. (2012). Role of chemotherapy on brain metastasis. *Progress in Neurological Surgery*, *25*, 110–114. http://dx.doi.org/10.1159/000331183.

Lepper, P., Ott, S., Hoppe, H., Schumann, C., Stammberger, U., Bugalho, A., et al. (2011). Superior vena cava syndrome in thoracic malignancies. *Respiratory Care*, *56*(5), 653–666. http://dx.doi.org/10.4187/respcare.00947.

Lewis, M., Hendrickson, A., & Moynihan, T. (2011). Oncologic emergencies: Pathophysiology, presentation, diagnosis and treatment. *CA: A Cancer Journal for Clinicians*, *61*, 287–314. http://dx.doi.org/10.3322/caac.20124.

Li, Y., Jenny, D., & Castaldo, J. (2012). Posterior reversible encephalopathy syndrome: Clinicoradiological spectrum and therapeutic strategies. *Hospital Practice*, *40*(1), 202–213. http://dx.doi.org/10.3810/hp.2012.02.961.

Loukas, M., Walters, A., Boon, J., Welch, T., Meiring, J., & Abrahams, P. (2012). Pericardiocentesis: A clinical anatomy review. *Clinical Anatomy*, *25*, 872–881. http://dx.doi.org/10.1002/ca.22032.

McCurdy, M., & Shanholtz, C. (2012). Oncologic emergencies. *Critical Care Medicine*, *40*(7), 2212–2222.

National Institute for Health and Clinical Excellence (NICE). (2010). *Metastatic spinal cord compression: Diagnosis and management of adults at risk of and with metastatic spinal cord compression.* http://guidance.nice. org.uk/CG75/Guidance/pdf/English.

Schairer, J., Biswas, S., Keteyian, S., & Ananthasubramaniam, K. (2011). A systematic approach to evaluation of pericardial effusion and cardiac tamponade. *Cardiology in Review*, *19*(5), 233–238. http://dx.doi.org/10.1097/CRD.0b013e31821 e202c.

Schimpf, M. (2012). Diagnosing increased intracranial pressure. *Journal of Trauma Nursing*, *19*(3), 160–167. http://dx.doi.org/10.1097/JTN.0b013e318261cfb4.

Shelton, B. (2013). Superior vena cava syndrome. In M. Kaplan (Ed.), *Understanding and managing oncologic emergencies* (2nd ed., pp. 385–410). Pittsburgh: Oncology Nursing Society.

Shelton, B., Ferrigno, C., & Skinner, J. (2013). Increased intracranial pressure. In M. Kaplan (Ed.), *Understanding and managing oncologic emergencies* (2nd ed., pp. 157–197). Pittsburgh: Oncology Nursing Society.

Shiue, K., Sahgal, A., Chow, E., Lutz, S., Chang, E., Mayr, N., et al. (2010). Management of metastatic spinal cord compression. *Expert Reviews*, *10*(5), 697–708. http://dx.doi.org/10.1586/era.10.47.

Smith, E., & Amin-Hanjani, S. (2013). *Evaluation and management of elevated intracranial pressure in adults.* www.uptodate.com.

Story, K. (2013). Cardiac tamponade. In M. Kaplan (Ed.), *Understanding and managing oncologic emergencies* (2nd ed., pp. 43–68). Pittsburgh: Oncology Nursing Society.

Taylor, J., & Schiff, D. (2010). Metastatic epidural spinal cord compression. *Seminars in Neurology*, *30*(3), 245–253. http://dx.doi.org/10.1055/s-0030-1255221.

Tlemsani, C., Mir, O., Boudou-Rouquette, P., Huillard, O., Maley, K., Ropert, S., et al. (2011). Posterior reversible encephalopathy syndrome induced by anti-VEGF agents. *Targeted Oncology*, *6*, 253–258. http://dx.doi.org/10.1007/s11523-011-0201-x.

Torre-Healy, A., Marko, N., & Weil, R. (2012). Hyperosmolar therapy for intracranial hypertension. *Neurocritical Care*, *17*, 117–130. http://dx.doi.org/10.1007/s12028-011-9649-x.

Venturini, E., Becuzzi, L., & Magni, L. (2012). Catheter-induced thrombosis of the superior vena cava. *Case Reports in Vascular Medicine*, *2012*, 469619. http://dx.doi.org/10.1155/2012/469619.

CHAPTER 42
Survivorship

Denice Economou and Stacie Corcoran

OVERVIEW

I. Definition of cancer survivor
   A. A cancer patient is considered a survivor from the time of diagnosis through the rest of his or her life. Significant others, family, and caregivers are also affected by the cancer diagnosis and are included in this definition (Hewitt, Greenfield, & Stoval, 2006; National Coalition for Cancer Survivorship [NCCS], 2013; National Comprehensive Cancer Network [NCCN], 2013a).

II. Statistics on cancer survivors (Siegel et al., 2012)
   A. In 2012, cancer survivors in the United States (U.S.) numbered over 13 million.
      1. Number of cancer survivors in the U.S. will rise to 18 million by 2022.
   B. 59% of cancer survivors are 65 years of age or older.
   C. 64% of cancer survivors have survived 5 years or more.
   D. Most common cancer sites in the survivor population are breast (22%), prostate (20%), colorectal (9%), and gynecologic (8%).

III. Long-term and late effects of cancer treatment
   A. Definitions (Aziz & Rowland, 2003; Carver, Szalda, & Ky, 2013; Hewitt et al., 2006; Jacobs et al., 2009; Landier & Smith, 2011)
      1. Long-term side effects begin as a complication of treatment, persist throughout treatment, and may continue after treatment is completed.
      2. Late effects are those that begin after treatment is completed, may be absent or subclinical at the end of treatment, and may manifest years later.
   B. Cancer survivors are at risk for long-term and late effects related to their cancer and its treatment (McCabe, Faithfull, Makin, & Wengstrom, 2013b; Palos & Zandstra, 2013).
   C. Long-term and late effects associated with cancer—vary according to disease, treatment, comorbid conditions, and age of patient (Campo et al., 2011; Carver et al., 2013; Economou, Hurria, & Grant, 2012; Miller & Triano, 2008; Stein, Syrjala, & Andrykowski, 2008)

   D. Lasting effects of cancer and its treatment(s) on patient's quality of life (Figure 42-1)
   E. Long-term and late effects of cancer treatment
      1. Physical consequences (Landier & Smith, 2011; Miller & Triano, 2008; Stein et al., 2008)
         a. Cardiovascular—congestive heart failure, cardiomyopathy, carotid artery disease, valvular heart disease, electrical or conductive system disease
         b. Pulmonary—pulmonary fibrosis, restrictive lung disease, dyspnea
         c. Gastrointestinal (GI)—malabsorption, dysphagia, gastroesophageal reflux disease (GERD), hepatitis, constipation, diarrhea, weight gain, cachexia
         d. Bone—osteopenia or osteoporosis, avascular necrosis
         e. Endocrine—hypothyroidism, adrenal insufficiency, diabetes mellitus
         f. Genitourinary—chronic kidney disease, proteinuria or albuminuria, incontinence
         g. Oral—xerostomia, dental caries, osteonecrosis of the jaw
         h. Sensory, neurologic, or other—fatigue, hearing loss, visual changes, taste changes or loss, neuropathy, lymphedema, insomnia
         i. Reproductive, fertility, and sexuality—hormonal deficits, sexual dysfunction, loss of libido, changes in body image (see Chapter 39)
      2. Psychological concerns (Stein et al., 2008)
         a. Anxiety
         b. Depression
         c. Worry
         d. Fear of recurrence
      3. Social concerns
         a. Changes in roles and relationships
         b. Workplace discrimination
         c. Financial burden of treatment, job loss, or both
      4. Cognitive impairment (Asher, 2011)
         a. Forgetfulness or problems with memory

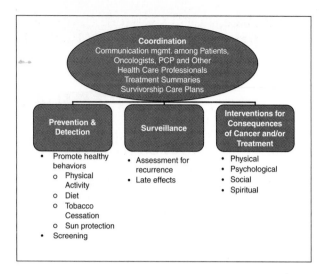

Figure 42-1 Quality of life model applied to cancer survivors.

b. Inability to concentrate

c. Difficulty finding words or expressing thoughts

5. Financial issues (Leigh, 2005)

  a. Change in employment status

  b. Reduced schedule; lack of employment

  c. Inability to obtain and retain insurance coverage

  d. Prescription and device costs

  e. Impact on family and lifestyle

6. Spiritual concerns (Ferrell, Dow, & Grant, 1995; Frost et al., 2012)

  a. Meaning of illness

  b. Transcendence

  c. Finding inner strength

  d. Religious faith

F. Risk of recurrence and secondary malignancy ⚠

1. Adult survivors of childhood cancers have the greatest risk of developing one or more secondary malignancies, and this accounts for 20% of deaths (Mertens et al., 2008).

  a. Patients with Hodgkin lymphoma have an increased risk for recurrence and secondary malignancies related to chemotherapy and radiation.

  b. Women who received chest radiation as children or adolescents have a significantly increased risk for developing breast cancer.

    (1) The risk is comparable to that in women who are *BRCA1*- and *BRCA2*-positive (Campo et al., 2011).

2. Secondary malignancies associated with radiation therapy within the treatment field include skin cancers, sarcomas, thyroid cancer, breast cancer, and lung cancer (McCabe et al., 2013b; Miller & Triano, 2008; Stein et al., 2008).

  a. Surveillance recommendations for young women who have received chest radiation

    (1) In women who received a radiation dose of 20 Gy or higher to the chest, mammography, with or without magnetic resonance imaging (MRI), should be performed, starting at age 25 years or 8 years after initial cancer therapy (Campo et al., 2011).

  b. Surveillance recommendations for patients who have received radiation dose of 30 Gy or more to their colon or rectum

    (1) These women should be screened with colonoscopy every 5 years starting at age 35 years or 10 years after radiation (Campo et al., 2011).

IV. Survivorship care

A. Survivorship is recognized as a distinct phase of the cancer trajectory, providing multiple opportunities to promote a healthy lifestyle, monitor for recurrence, and identify and manage long-term and late effects (Figure 42-2) (American Cancer Society [ACS], 2011; Hewitt et al., 2006).

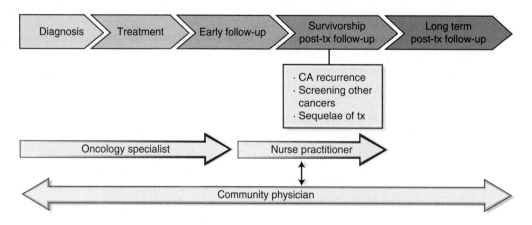

Figure 42-2 Survivorship as a distinct phase of the cancer trajectory.

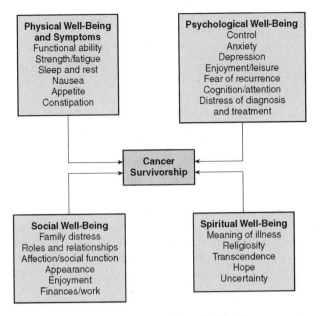

Figure 42-3 Institute of Medicine (IOM): Components of survivorship care. *From Grant, M., Sun, V. (2010). Advances in quality of life at the end of life.* Seminars in Oncology Nursing, *26(1), 26–35.*

1. Many settings institute survivorship care at treatment completion or transition to maintenance therapy (e.g., androgen-blocking treatment for prostate cancer) (McCabe, Bhatia, Oeffinger et al., 2013a).
B. Essential components of survivorship care (Figure 42-3) (Hewitt et al., 2006)
   1. Assessment to detect recurrence of cancer
   2. Identification and management of long-term and late effects
   3. Screening recommendations for other cancers
   4. Health promotion recommendations related to nutrition, exercise, and smoking cessation
   5. Treatment summary and follow-up care plan
   6. Communication with primary care physician and other providers
C. Major barriers to the provision of survivorship care for the future
   1. Oncology care needed for aging Americans but deficits in the workforce anticipated by 2020 (Hortobagyi, 2007).
   2. Number of oncologists available to care for these survivors expected to be inadequate.
   3. Fewer geriatricians in light of the increasing number of cancer survivors who are older than 60 years, with additional comorbidities of normal aging (Hortobagyi, 2007)

ASSESSMENT

I. Data collection
   A. Clinical data
      1. Demographic information

2. Providers' names, specialty area (e.g., primary care provider, gynecologist, cardiologist), and contact information
3. Past medical history
   a. Comorbidities
   b. Family history, including cancer diagnoses or other major illnesses
   c. Genetic history, if available
   d. Cancer diagnosis, including multiple primaries or relapses
   e. Type and duration of treatment—chemotherapy, surgery, radiation therapy, hormone therapy
4. Health behaviors (e.g., smoking, alcohol intake, diet, physical activity)
5. Receipt of preventive health services (e.g., colonoscopy, mammography, immunizations)
6. Genetic testing, as appropriate, for patients with breast, ovarian, or colon cancer (NCCN, 2013b)
7. Medication reconciliation (including complementary and alternative medicine [CAM])
8. Allergies
   B. Focused review of symptoms
II. Psychosocial assessment
   A. Social history—occupation, living situation, financial concerns
   B. Past coping skills
   C. Risk for anxiety, depression, fear of recurrence
      1. Use of patient self-assessment tool (e.g., NCCN distress thermometer, Hospital Anxiety and Depression Scale [HADS]), per institutional practices
   C. Support systems—identification of available support from family members, friends, peers, church
III. Physical assessment
   A. Assessment for long-term and late effects of cancer and its treatment
IV. Imaging and laboratory tests
   A. Assessment for recurrent disease based on established guidelines (e.g., NCCN or the American Society of Clinical Oncology [ASCO]), or as developed or adapted by individual institutions or practices

PROBLEM STATEMENTS AND OUTCOMES IDENTIFICATION

I. Risk of Injury (NANDA-I), related to cancer, cancer treatment, or both
   A. Expected outcome(s)—patient will have decreased severity and/or relief of any adverse effects of cancer and/or cancer treatment.
II. Deficient Knowledge (NANDA-I), related to follow-up surveillance, potential late effects of cancer and its treatment, health promotion, health maintenance activities, and available resources

A. Expected outcomes
1. Patient verbalizes an understanding of late and long-term effects of the cancer treatment.
2. Patient adheres to recommended follow-up surveillance.
3. Patient exhibits promotion of healthy lifestyle changes in his or her life.
4. Patient demonstrates compliance with cancer screening recommendations.
5. Patient uses appropriate services, as directed, such as physical therapy, social work, smoking cessation specialist (Rock et al., 2012).
III. Communication and Coordination of Care among Health Care Providers
A. Expected outcomes—patient identifies the appropriate health care provider to consult for health prevention, promotion, and monitoring and for new acute concerns.
IV. Nursing diagnosis based on treatment modalities (Table 42-1)

PLANNING AND IMPLEMENTATION

I. Interventions to decrease severity and relieve any ongoing adverse effects of cancer and its treatment
A. Assessment for any ongoing physiologic, psychological, emotional, social, spiritual, and financial issues

B. Nonpharmacologic and pharmacologic interventions, as necessary
C. Referral to appropriate specialists (e.g., physical or occupational therapist, mental health provider, chaplain, pain and palliative care specialist, speech and swallow therapist), as appropriate
D. Encouraging all patients to be physically activity and return to daily activities as soon as possible
1. Physical activity recommendations for cancer survivors (NCCN, 2013a)
a. Overall volume of weekly activity of at least 150 minutes of moderate-intensity activity or 75 minutes of vigorous-intensity activity or equivalent combination
b. Two to three weekly sessions of strength training that involves major muscle groups
c. Stretch major muscle groups and tendons
d. For physically inactive survivors, beginning with one to three light to moderate-intensity exercises, 20-minute sessions per week, with progression based on tolerance, as outlined in the above guidelines
II. Interventions related to knowledge deficit
A. Assessment of motivation and willingness of patient and caregivers to learn
B. Determination of cultural influences on health teaching
1. Providing interpreter services, as needed
2. Providing culturally appropriate educational materials to reinforce education
C. Providing and discussing the cancer survivorship care plan (CSCP) (Hewitt et al., 2006; McCabe et al., 2013a; McCabe et al., 2013b; Oeffinger & McCabe, 2006; Stricker, Jacobs, & Palmer, 2012)
1. The CSCP should include the following:
a. Treatment summary—cancer site, type and stage of cancer, date of diagnosis, and any treatment(s) received
b. Written information about long-term and late effects of treatment
c. Recommended follow-up surveillance and intervals for disease recurrence or progression
d. Based on established national guidelines
e. Recommended health promotion behaviors (e.g., smoking cessation, nutrition, physical activity, and safe use of CAM) and health maintenance activities (e.g., cancer screening, bone health screening, and being current with immunizations)
f. List of health care team providers with their contact information
g. Institutional and community resources and referral to support groups, as needed

Table 42-1

Nursing Diagnoses Based on Cancer Treatment Modalities

Treatment Modality	Potential Nursing Diagnoses
Chemotherapy	• Fatigue • Impaired Memory • Risk for Injury • Risk for Infection • Risk for Peripheral Neurovascular Dysfunction • Decreased Cardiac Output
Radiation therapy	• Impaired Skin Integrity • Impaired Mobility
Surgery	• Acute or Chronic Pain • Disturbed Body Image • Sexual Dysfunction
Endocrine therapy	• Increased Risk for Osteoporosis • Disturbed Sleep Pattern
Stem cell transplantation	• Risk for Infection • Risk for Injury • Risk for Bleeding • Impaired Gas Exchange • Risk for Impaired Liver Function • Electrolyte Imbalance • Activity Intolerance
Molecular targeted therapy	• Decreased Cardiac Output • Risk for Impaired Skin Integrity

III. Interventions to improve communication and coordination among providers
  A. Providing a copy of the survivorship care plan to the patient, primary care provider, and any specialists involved in patient's care via fax, mail, or electronic communication

EVALUATION

The oncology nurse plays an active and critical role in the evaluation of a patient's physical, psychological, emotional, spiritual, and social well-being. Continuous assessment of the patient's status is performed, and relevant data are collected. An individualized cancer survivorship care plan of care is developed on the basis of the cancer site and treatment(s) received. Evidence-based interventions are performed to address the specific physical and psychosocial needs of the patient, family members, or both. The oncology nurse evaluates the interventions on the basis of achievement of expected outcomes and makes revisions to the plan of care, as necessary (see table below for additional resources):

ADDITIONAL RESOURCES

Organization	Website
American Cancer Society	www.cancer.org
American Society of Clinical Oncology (ASCO)	http://www.asco.org/advocacy-practice/cancer-survivorship
Cancer Care	http://www.cancercare.org/
Cancer Legal Resource Center	http://www.disabilityrightslegalcenter.org/cancer-legal-resource-center
Cancer Control Planet	www.cancercontrolplanet.cancer.gov
Centers for Disease Control and Prevention (CDC) Survivorship Area	www.cdc.gov/cancer/survivorship
Children's Oncology Group	http://www.childrensoncologygroup.org/index.php/survivorshipguidelines
City of Hope Pain and Palliative Care Resource Center	http://prc.coh.org/
Fertile Hope	http://www.fertilehope.org/healthcare-professionals/index.cfm
Memorial Sloan-Kettering Cancer Center	www.mskcc.org/livingbeyondcancer
National Cancer Institute Office of Cancer Survivorship	http://dccps.nci.nih.gov/ocs
National Coalition for Cancer Survivorship	www.canceradvocacy.org
National Comprehensive Cancer Network (NCCN) Survivorship Guidelines	http://www.nccn.org/professionals/physician_gls/f_guidelines_nojava.asp#supportive
ONS Putting Evidence into Practice (PEP)	http://www2.ons.org/Research/PEP
Young Survival Coalition	http://www.youngsurvival.org/

Survivorship Care Plan Resources

ASCO Care Plan	http://www.asco.org/advocacy-practice/cancer-survivorship
Journey Forward	www.journeyforward.org
LIVESTRONG Care Plan	www.livestrongcareplan.org

References

American Cancer Society (ACS). (2011). *Cancer screening guidelines.* www.cancer.org.

Asher, A. (2011). Cognitive dysfunction among cancer survivors. *American Journal of Physical Medicine & Rehabilitation*, 90(5), S16–S26.

Aziz, N. M., & Rowland, J. H. (2003). Trends and advances in cancer survivorship research: Challenge and opportunity. *Seminars in Radiation Oncology*, 13(3), 248–266.

Campo, R. A., Rowland, J. H., Irwin, M. L., Nathan, P. C., Gritz, E. R., & Kinney, A. Y. (2011). Cancer prevention after cancer: Changing the paradigm–a report from the American Society of Preventive Oncology. *Cancer Epidemiology, Biomarkers and Prevention*, 20(10), 2317–2324. http://dx.doi.org/10.1158/1055-9965.EPI-11-0728.

Carver, J. R., Szalda, D., & Ky, B. (2013). Asymptomatic cardiac toxicity in long-term cancer survivors: Defining the population and recommendations for surveillance. *Seminars in Oncology*, 40(2), 229–238. http://dx.doi.org/10.1053/j.seminoncol.2013.01.005.

Economou, D., Hurria, A., & Grant, M. (2012). Integrating a cancer-specific geriatric assessment into survivorship care. *Clinical Journal of Oncology Nursing*, 16(3), E78–E85. http://dx.doi.org/3739XN0221005818.

Ferrell, B. R., Dow, K. H., & Grant, M. (1995). Measurement of the quality of life in cancer survivors. *Quality of Life Research*, 4(6), 523–531.

Frost, M. H., Johnson, M. E., Atherton, P. J., Petersen, W. O., Dose, A. M., Kasner, M. J., et al. (2012). Spiritual well-being and quality of life of women with ovarian cancer and their spouses. *The Journal of Supportive Oncology*, 10(2), 72–80.

Hewitt, M., Greenfield, S., & Stoval, E. (2006). *From cancer patient to cancer survivor: Lost in transition.* Washington, D.C.: National Academies Press.

Hortobagyi, G. N. (2007). A shortage of oncologists? The American Society of Clinical Oncology workforce study. *Journal of Clinical Oncology*, 25(12), 1468–1469. http://dx.doi.org/10.1200/JCO.2007.10.9397.

Part 7

Jacobs, L. A., Palmer, S. C., Schwartz, L. A., DeMichele, A., Mao, J. J., Carver, J., et al. (2009). Adult cancer survivorship: Evolution, research, and planning care. *CA: A Cancer Journal for Clinicians, 59*(6), 391–410. http://dx.doi.org/59/6/391, [pii]10.3322/caac.20040.

Landier, W., & Smith, S. (2011). Late effects of cancer treatment. In C. H. Yarbro, D. Wujcik, & B. H. Gobel (Eds.), *Cancer Nursing: Principles and Practice* (7th ed.). Sudbury, MA: Jones and Bartlett.

Leigh, S. (2005). Coping: Survivorship issues and financial concerns. In J. Itano & K. Taoka (Eds.), *Core curriculum for oncology nursing* (4th ed., pp. 80–88). Philadelphia: Elsevier Saunders.

McCabe, M. S., Bhatia, S., Oeffinger, K. C., Reaman, G. H., Tyne, C., Wollins, D. S., et al. (2013a). American Society of Clinical Oncology statement: Achieving high-quality cancer survivorship care. *Journal of Clinical Oncology, 31*(5), 631–640. http://dx.doi.org/JCO.2012.46.6854, [pii]10.1200/JCO.2012.46.6854.

McCabe, M. S., Faithfull, S., Makin, W., & Wengstrom, Y. (2013b). Survivorship programs and care planning. *Cancer, 119*(Suppl. 11), 2179–2186. http://dx.doi.org/10.1002/cncr.28068.

Mertens, A. C., Liu, Q., Neglia, J. P., Wasilewski, K., Leisenring, W., Armstrong, G. T., et al. (2008). Cause-specific late mortality among 5-year survivors of childhood cancer: The Childhood Cancer Survivor Study. *Journal of the National Cancer Institute, 100*(19), 1368–1379. http://dx.doi.org/djn310, [pii]10.1093/jnci/djn310.

Miller, K. D., & Triano, L. R. (2008). Medical issues in cancer survivors—a review. *Cancer Journal, 14*(6), 375–387. http://dx.doi.org/10.1097/PPO.0b013e31818ee3dc.

National Coalition for Cancer Survivorship (NCCS). (2013). *Survivorship.* http://www.canceradvocacy.org/.

National Comprehensive Cancer Network (NCCN). (2013a). *Survivorship version 1.2013.* http://www.nccn.org/professionals/physician_gls/pdf/survivorship.pdf.

National Comprehensive Cancer Network (NCCN). (2013b). *Genetic/familial high-risk breast and ovarian version 4.2013.* http://www.nccn.org/professionals/physician_gls/pdf/genetics_screening.pdf.

Oeffinger, K. C., & McCabe, M. S. (2006). Models for delivering survivorship care. *Journal of Clinical Oncology, 24*(32), 5117–5124.

Palos, G. R., & Zandstra, F. (2013). Call for action: Caring for the United States' aging cancer survivors. *Clinical Journal of Oncology Nursing, 17*(1), 88–90. http://dx.doi.org/10.1188/13.CJON.88-90.

Rock, C. L., Doyle, C., Demark-Wahnefried, W., Meyerhardt, J., Courneya, K. S., Schwartz, A. L., et al. (2012). Nutrition and physical activity guidelines for cancer survivors. *CA: A Cancer Journal for Clinicians, 62*(4), 243–274. http://dx.doi.org/10.3322/caac.21142.

Siegel, R., DeSantis, C., Virgo, K., Stein, K., Mariotto, A., Smith, T., et al. (2012). Cancer treatment and survivorship statistics, 2012. *CA: A Cancer Journal for Clinicians, 62*(4), 220–241. http://dx.doi.org/10.3322/caac.21149.

Stein, K. D., Syrjala, K. L., & Andrykowski, M. A. (2008). Physical and psychological long-term and late effects of cancer. *Cancer, 112*(11 Suppl.), 2577–2592. http://dx.doi.org/10.1002/cncr. 23448 [doi].

Stricker, C. T., Jacobs, L. A., & Palmer, S. C. (2012). Survivorship care plans: An argument for evidence over common sense. author reply 1393-1395. *Journal of Clinical Oncology, 30*(12), 1392–1393. http://dx.doi.org/JCO.2011.40.7940

CHAPTER 43

Palliative and End-of-Life Care

Debra E. Heidrich

OVERVIEW

I. Palliative care
   A. An essential component of quality care for persons with advanced cancer and for their family members
   B. Defined by the Center for Medicare and Medicaid Services (CMS) and the National Quality Forum (as cited in National Consensus Project for Quality Palliative Care [NCP], 2013), means patient and family-centered care that optimizes quality of life by anticipating, preventing, and treating suffering; throughout the continuum of illness involves addressing physical, intellectual, emotional, social, and spiritual needs and facilitating patient autonomy, access to information, and choice
   C. Summary of key features (NCP, 2013; National Comprehensive Cancer Network [NCCN], 2013; World Health Organization [WHO], n.d.)
      1. Patient and family are the focus of care.
      2. Symptoms are anticipated, prevented, and treated skillfully.
      3. Psychosocial, emotional, and spiritual symptoms are as important as physical symptoms.
      4. Patient autonomy is respected, requiring access to information to assist with decision-making.
      5. Care is provided by an interdisciplinary team of providers.
      6. Life is affirmed and death is accepted as a normal process.
      7. Bereavement counseling for both the patient and the family are included as part of the plan of care.
   D. Palliative care—a continuum of care that includes hospice care and bereavement counseling, as illustrated in Figure 43-1
      1. Palliative care begins at the time of diagnosis of a life-threatening illness, along with disease-directed, life-prolonging therapies.
      2. Palliative care may be initiated by the primary oncology team and is augmented by palliative care experts, based on the patient's and family's needs.
      3. Palliative care expert consultation should be considered in these key areas in patients with a cancer diagnosis (Ramchandran & von Roenn, 2013):
         a. Advanced disease with a prognosis of less than 1 year
         b. Significant symptom burden from disease or from treatment
         c. Significant social or psychosocial distress
         d. Impaired performance status (Eastern Cooperative Oncology Group Performance Status score of 3 or higher or a Karnofsky Performance Scale score of less than 50%) (Tables 43-1 and 43-2)
      4. Palliative care becomes the main focus of care when disease-directed, life-prolonging therapies are no longer effective, appropriate, or desired. At this time, referral may be made to hospice care programs.
      5. Palliative care is a growing specialty.
         a. Certification in hospice and palliative care is available for physicians, nurses at all levels (nursing assistants, licensed practical nurses, registered nurses, and advanced practice nurses), social workers, and chaplains (Center to Advance Palliative Care [CAPC], n.d.a).
         b. Palliative care programs are found in multiple settings (CAPC, n.d.b).
            (1) Consultative teams in acute care settings, including intensive care units and emergency departments
            (2) Ambulatory care clinics, as a separate entity or integrated within other specialty practices or clinics (e.g., oncology, heart failure, chronic lung disease)
            (3) Home-based primary care programs
            (4) Long-term care or nursing home programs

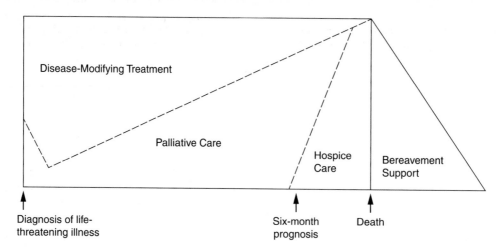

Figure 43-1 The Palliative Care Continuum. *Adapted from National Consensus Project for Quality Palliative Care (NCP). (2009). Clinical practice guidelines for quality palliative care (2nd ed.). Pittsburgh: Authors; and Ferris, F. D., Bruera, E., Cherny, N., Cummings, C., Currow, D., Dudgeon, D., & Von Roenn, J. H. (2009). Palliative care a decade later: Accomplishments, the need, next steps—from the American Society of Clinical Oncology.* Journal of Clinical Oncology, 27, 3052–3058.

Table 43-1

Eastern Cooperative Oncology Group (ECOG) Performance Status

Grade	Performance Status
0	Fully active, able to carry on all predisease performance without restriction
1	Restricted in physically strenuous activity but ambulatory and able to carry out work of a light or sedentary nature (e.g., light housework, office work)
2	Ambulatory and capable of all self-care but unable to carry out any work activities; up and about more than 50% of waking hours
3	Capable of only limited self-care, confined to bed or chair more than 50% of waking hours
4	Completely disabled; cannot carry on any self-care; totally confined to bed or chair
5	Dead

From Oken, M.M., Creech, R.H., Tormey, D.C., Horton, J., Davis, T.E., McFadden, E.T., & Carbone, P.P. (1982). Toxicity and response criteria of the Eastern Cooperative Oncology Group. *American Journal of Clinical Oncology, 5,* 649–655.

Table 43-2

Karnofsky Performance Scale

Percentage of Normal Performance Status	Definitions
100	Normal; no complaints; no evidence of disease
90	Able to carry on normal activity; minor signs or symptoms of disease
80	Normal activity with effort; some signs or symptoms of disease
70	Cares for self; unable to carry on normal activity or do active work
60	Requires occasional assistance but is able to care for most of needs
50	Requires considerable assistance and frequent medical care
40	Disabled; requires special care and assistance
30	Severely disabled; hospitalization is indicated, although death is not imminent
10	Moribund; fatal process progressing rapidly
0	Dead

Adapted from Lehne, R. (2013). *Pharmacology for nursing care* (8th ed.). Philadelphia: Saunders.

E. Positive impact of palliative care on cancer patient outcomes supported by research (Bakitas et al., 2009; Bischoff, Weinberg, & Rabow, 2013; Bukki, et al., 2013; Follwell et al., 2009; Temel, et al., 2010)
   1. Lower symptom intensity
   2. Improved quality of life
   3. Longer survival
   4. Less aggressive end-of-life care
   5. Improved patient and family satisfaction with care

F. Standards for palliative care in oncology (NCCN, 2013)
   1. Institutions should develop processes for integrating palliative care into cancer care as part of usual oncology care and for patients with specialty palliative care needs.
   2. All patients with cancer should be screened for palliative care needs at the initial visit, at appropriate intervals, and as clinically indicated.
   3. Patients and families should be informed that palliative care is an integral part of their comprehensive cancer care.
   4. Educational programs should be provided to all health care professionals and trainees so that they can develop effective palliative care knowledge, skills, and attitudes.
   5. Palliative care specialists and interdisciplinary palliative care teams, including board-certified palliative care physicians, advanced practice nurses, and physician assistants, should be readily available to provide consultative or direct care to patients and families who request or require their expertise.
   6. Quality of palliative care should be monitored by institutional quality improvement programs.

II. Hospice care
A. Hospice is both a philosophy of care and a regulated insurance benefit. As a philosophy of care, it is the model of high-quality, compassionate care, which helps patients and families live as fully as possible when cure is not possible (National Hospice and Palliative Care Organization [NHPCO], n.d.a).
   1. Hospice care started as a grassroots movement to improve the quality of the dying experience as an alternative to the traditional curative model of care.
   2. Hospice care is based on the understanding that dying is part of the life cycle and that meticulous management of physical, psychosocial, and spiritual symptoms will promote quality of living for the patient-family system.

3. As an organized model of care, the hospice movement is about 50 years old. Following is a brief history of hospice care; more detailed information is available on the NHPCO website (NHPCO, n.d.b).
   a. The modern hospice movement started in the 1960s through the work of Dame Cicely Saunders and the establishment of St. Christopher Hospice in London, England.
   b. Dr. Florence Wald, Dean of the Yale School of Nursing, pioneered the hospice movement in the United States (U.S.). The Connecticut Hospice opened in 1974 and was the first U.S. hospice program.
   c. The Medicare hospice benefit was approved by Congress in 1982 after demonstration projects showed that interdisciplinary care focused on quality of living and addressing the multiple symptoms of terminal illness improved outcomes and cost less than usual care.
   d. The Medicare benefit became permanent in 1986, providing a stable source of payment for hospice care. This supported a steady growth of hospice programs throughout the U.S.

B. Hospice care is part of the palliative care continuum of care (see Figure 43-1).
   1. The same key features of palliative care apply to hospice care.
   2. Hospice care is focused on the last phase of life.
      a. The Medicare Hospice Benefit stipulates that the patient must have a prognosis of 6 months or less of remaining life to be eligible for this benefit.
      b. Eligibility criteria should not be confused with length of service; patients can receive hospice care for as long as they meet eligibility criteria (NHPCO, n.d.a).
      c. Late referrals to hospice are very common. The median length of stay in 2012 was only 18.7 days, with 35.5% of patients dying or discharged within 7 days of admission (NHPCO, 2013).
      d. Physicians are often overly optimistic when estimating prognosis. Stiel et al. (2010) showed that on average, physicians overestimate survival time by a factor of 4.
      e. Asking the "surprise question" (i.e., "Would I be surprised if this patient died in the next year?") helps identify patients who might be appropriate for a hospice referral (Moss et al., 2010).

3. The focus of interventions in hospice care is relief of distressing symptoms and enhancement of quality of life for both the patient and the family.

   a. Advanced cancer and its treatment are associated with multiple distressing physical, psychosocial, emotional, and spiritual symptoms, requiring a multidimensional interdisciplinary approach to care.

   b. Persons experience these symptoms during the living-dying interval in their own unique ways within their own family, social, and cultural structure. Respect for the individual includes honoring these unique experiences.

   c. No therapies are specifically excluded in hospice; disease-modifying or life-prolonging therapies may be part of the plan of care if these therapies are the best approach for relief of distressing symptoms or enhancement of the quality of life (Egan City & Labyak, 2010).

4. Medicare Hospice Benefit

   a. Eligibility criteria (CMS, 2013)

      (1) The patient must be eligible for Medicare Part A.

      (2) The referring physician and hospice medical director certify, to the best of their knowledge, that the patient has a prognosis of 6 months or less of remaining life if the disease runs its natural course.

      (3) The patient chooses hospice care for the treatment of the terminal illness (i.e., waives right to traditional Medicare for the treatment of the terminal illness and its symptoms).

   b. Services include (CMS, 2013) the following:

      (1) Nursing care

      (2) Physician services

      (3) Social services

      (4) Counseling services including, but not limited to, bereavement counseling, dietary counseling, and spiritual counseling

      (5) Medical equipment and supplies

      (6) Medications for symptom control

      (7) Home health and homemaker services

      (8) Physical, occupational, and speech therapy

      (9) Dietary or nutrition counseling

      (10) Grief and loss counseling

      (11) Volunteer service

      (12) Short-term inpatient care for pain and symptom control

      (13) Short-term respite care

   c. Four different levels of care—reflecting the variations in care intensity required to meet patient's and family's needs (City Egan & Labyak, 2010)

      (1) Routine home care—care provided in the patient's place of residence, including private home, nursing home, and residential care setting

      (2) Continuous home care—care provided in the patient's place of residence during a time of crisis requiring predominantly continuous nursing care

      (3) General inpatient care—care provided in an inpatient facility for pain or symptom control when the symptom(s) cannot be managed at home

      (4) Inpatient respite care—care provided in an approved facility on a short-term basis to give respite to the family caregiver

III. Grief and bereavement

   A. Definitions (Corless, 2010; Buglass, 2010)

      1. Loss—the absence of an object, position, ability, or attribute

      2. Grief—the psychological, social, and somatic responses to loss

      3. Anticipatory grief—the psychological, social, and somatic responses to an anticipated loss

      4. Mourning—the outward and active expression of grief through participation in various death and bereavement rituals, which vary by culture

      5. Bereavement—the state of having suffered a loss; the period during which grief and mourning occur, the first year after a loss generally being the most difficult

      6. Complicated grief—a disturbance in the normal process of grief

         a. Prolonged grief—persistent and severe yearning for the deceased beyond 6 to 12 months after the loss (Bryant, 2013); recognized as a mental disorder causing significant distress and disability and included in the *Diagnostic and Statistical Manual*, 5th edition (Bryant, 2013; Waldrop & Kutner, 2013a)

         b. Disenfranchised grief—grief that occurs when the loss cannot be openly acknowledged; examples include death of a person in a nonsanctioned relationship such as an extramarital affair or homosexual relationship, loss resulting from miscarriage or abortion, and loss of the essence of the individual before actual death, as in severe dementia

B. Manifestations of acute grief
  1. Social
    a. Restlessness and inability to sit still
    b. Uncomfortable around other people or social withdrawal
    c. Feeling of not wanting to be alone
    d. Lack of ability to initiate and maintain organized patterns of activity
  2. Physical
    a. Anorexia and weight loss or the opposite, overeating and weight gain
    b. Heart palpitations; nervousness, tension, panic
    c. Shortness of breath
    d. Tightness in throat
    e. Inability to sleep
    f. Lack of energy and feelings of physical exhaustion
    g. Headaches, muscular aches, gastrointestinal distress
  3. Cognitive-emotional
    a. Sadness and crying
    b. Forgetfulness or difficulty concentrating
    c. Feelings of anger or guilt
    d. Mood swings
    e. Sense of helplessness
    f. Yearning for the deceased
    g. Dreams of the deceased
C. Theories of the grief process—help explain the reactions and responses to grief
  1. Kubler-Ross (1969) described phases or stages of grief. This theory assists in understanding the kinds of reactions observed in persons experiencing loss. These stages are not linear and often overlap, and they do not necessarily occur sequentially.
    a. Denial—"No, it can't be true."
    b. Anger—"Why me?"
    c. Bargaining—"Please, God."
    d. Depression—"I just don't care anymore."
    e. Acceptance—"I can't change it, but here's what I can do."
  2. Worden (2002) described grief work in terms of tasks to accomplish for grief to be resolved.
    a. Accepting the reality of the loss
    b. Experiencing the pain of grief
    c. Adjusting to the environment without the deceased person
    d. Withdrawing emotionally from the deceased by forming an ongoing relationship with the memories of the deceased in a way that allows the bereaved person to continue with life; referred to as *relocation* by Worden
  3. The dual process model of coping with bereavement shows the dynamic nature of grief. The bereaved person oscillates between loss-oriented coping and restoration-oriented coping. Both loss- and restoration-oriented processes are necessary for adjustment to the loss.
    a. Loss-oriented coping—concentrating on and working through some aspect of the loss experience itself (e.g., crying, yearning, relocation)
    b. Restoration-oriented coping—mastering new tasks, reorganizing life, and developing a new identity
D. Support interventions for the person experiencing grief
  1. Counseling of patients and families to express feelings and heal relationships while the patient has the physical and mental capacity to participate in these conversations—"five things" of relationship completion introduced by Byock (1997) and used by many hospice professionals; encouraging patients and families to address these five things may assist with finding meaning and assuaging guilt.
    a. I forgive you.
    b. Forgive me.
    c. Thank you.
    d. I love you.
    e. Good-bye.
  2. Support of individuals to participate in mourning practices (i.e., the cultural practices and rituals associated with death, dying, and burial) that are meaningful to the individual(s)
  3. Encouraging expression of thoughts and feelings in an accepting environment; grieving person usually benefits from the opportunity to "tell his or her story."
    a. Referrals to layperson or professionally led support groups
    b. Assessment of desire for clergy visit or referral
    c. When appropriate for the setting and the relationship, planning a bereavement visit or telephone call from nurse case manager
    d. Encouraging the individual to identify one or more family members, neighbors, friends, or faith community members with whom they can express their feelings
  4. Counseling interventions that may be helpful
    a. Interventions to encourage expression of thoughts, feelings, or anger to the deceased that may or may not have been expressed previously (Corless, 2010)
      (1) Letter writing
      (2) Talking to an empty chair or to a picture

Part 8

(3) Journal writing

(4) Venting anger—banging a pillow on the mattress, screaming at home or in a parked car, crying loudly at home

b. Interventions to assist in finding meaning in past or current events

(1) Guided imagery

(2) Journal writing

(3) Analysis of role changes

(4) Drawing pictures

IV. Community resources for palliative and hospice care

A. Medicare-certified hospice programs

1. Patients who meet the eligibility criteria for hospice and are accepting of the hospice philosophy of care should be referred to a certified hospice care program.

2. Certification ensures that the program meets the standards, as defined by the CMS.

3. Hospice organizations range from small, independent organizations, to organizations affiliated with larger health care systems, to very large corporations with multiple offices throughout a region or across the U.S.

4. Hospices that are members of NHPCO may be found by searching a zip code on the NHPCO website.

B. Palliative care programs

1. Acute care hospital-based programs

a. According to CAPC (2012), 66% of hospitals with more than 50 beds have a palliative care program.

b. These programs range from single-professional (usually nurse or physician) consultations, to interdisciplinary consultation teams, to programs that include specialty palliative care units.

c. The Joint Commission launched a certification process for hospice inpatient palliative care programs in 2011. This certification sets standards for information management, access to services, communication, patient-directed care using an interdisciplinary team, coordination of services, and performance improvement (CAPC, 2011). Although certification ensures that programs meet these standards, many palliative care programs are not yet certified.

C. Ambulatory palliative care (Rabow, 2013)

1. Outpatient provision of palliative care in practices and clinics is in early development, and the prevalence of ambulatory palliative care programs is unknown.

2. Most of the best-evaluated practices are part of a cancer center.

3. The structure and function vary, depending on such factors as affiliation with an established inpatient palliative care program, number of disciplines involved in the care, referral sources, and model of care (consultative versus co-management of patients).

4. There is no certification process for ambulatory palliative care.

D. Community-based, non-hospice palliative care

1. Home-based and nursing home–based palliative care programs exist (Sefcik, Rao, & Ersek, 2013; Zhang et al., 2013).

2. These models of care have the potential to increase quality of care for persons with chronic progressive illnesses, especially for patients who do not meet hospice eligibility criteria but who have significant symptom burden.

3. No certification process exists for non-hospice, community-based palliative care.

E. Nurses caring for patients with advanced, progressive illnesses—those not in hospice or palliative care programs must be aware of other potential resources for patient-family needs; resources that may be available in the community include the following:

1. Home care services for those with a home need for skilled nursing care or therapies

2. Home health aide, homemaker services, or a combination of both, which may or may not be covered by insurance, depending on identified needs and insurance plan

3. Social services agencies

4. Area Agency on Aging, which may provide a wide array of services, including meals, home health care or homemaker service, caregiver support, legal advice, and transportation services

5. Agencies that provide support specifically to persons with a cancer diagnosis—for example, American Cancer Society or the Cancer Support Community

6. Layperson-led and professional-led grief support programs—hospices often accept families into their grief support programs, even if the patient was not enrolled in a hospice.

V. Reimbursement

A. Hospice services

1. The Medicare Hospice Benefit pays the hospice a daily rate based on the level of care the patient is receiving—that is, routine home care, continuous home care, general inpatient care, or inpatient respite care. This capitated rate must cover all hospice services, as listed under section II.B.4 above.

2. The model of reimbursement accepts that some patients' care will cost more than the hospice will be paid and some patients' care will cost less than the hospice will be paid, so that the hospice can cover the overall costs of providing care to all patients.
3. Most private insurance hospice policies are modeled after the Medicare Hospice Benefit.
4. The Medicare Hospice Benefit does not pay for room and board, treatment or medications aimed at curing the terminal illness, or any care for the terminal illness that is not arranged by the hospice and part of the hospice plan of care (CMS, 2013).

B. Palliative care services
1. Payment for palliative care services varies across settings.
2. Physicians and advanced practice nurses may be able to bill for consultations under insurance plans such as Medicare Part A for inpatient care or Part B for ambulatory or home-based care.
3. The revenue that palliative care programs generate via billing is usually not sufficient to sustain a program of care. The most significant financial benefit for hospital-based palliative care services comes from cost savings while improving the quality of care (CAPC, n.d.c).

VI. Caregiver support
A. Family members and friends (informal caregivers) often assume caregiving roles for persons with advanced progressive illnesses. This caregiving is associated with significant physical, psychosocial, and financial burden, as well as some positive benefits (Waldrop & Kutner, 2013b).
1. Informal caregivers are at risk for increased cardiovascular disease, psychosocial stress, fatigue, and depression.
2. Some caregivers showed decreased mortality, positive affect, and pride in accomplishments, suggesting that in some circumstances, providing direct care can provide positive benefits.
3. Factors that may influence the impact of caregiving include the following:
   a. General caregiver resilience
   b. Relationship with the patient
   c. Presence of difficult-to-manage symptoms
   d. Degree of challenge in everyday caregiving (e.g., amount of physical assistance required or the presence of dementia)
   e. Financial impact of loss of patient and caregiver income, as well as costs of medical care

f. Degree to which caregivers think that they have access to needed information and professional support
   g. Degree to which caregivers think that they are carrying out patients' wishes
   h. Social support available to the caregiver
B. Supportive interventions for caregivers (Waldrop & Kutner, 2013b; Waldrop & Kutner, 2013c).
1. Evaluation of the patient-family unit, including the caregiver's physical and mental health, family functioning and presence of any conflict within the family, nature of the relationship between the patient and caregiver, financial situation, and difficulty of caregiving requirements
2. Assisting the caregiver to feel competent in providing care
   a. Demonstrating physical caregiving (e.g., changing sheets on occupied bed, catheter care, dressing change) and having the caregiver do a return demonstration with professional caregiver available for coaching and support
   b. Providing written instructions for reinforcement
   c. Reinforcing teaching with each interaction
   d. Providing positive feedback
   e. Ensuring that caregiver knows who to call with questions
3. Addressing the physical burden of caregiving
   a. Promoting the use of assistive devices that make caregiving less strenuous
   b. Physical or occupational therapy referral to teach caregiver safe transfer techniques and to encourage as much self-care by the patient within the limits of the disease
   c. Augmentation of caregiving with home health aides, personal care assistants, or homemaker services
   d. Encouraging the caregiver to call on extended family members, friends, and faith community networks for assistance with direct caregiving or household tasks
4. Anticipating and treating symptoms
   a. Providing clear instruction on when and how to use medications and nonpharmacologic interventions for symptom control
   b. Demonstrating and requesting return demonstration to ensure that caregiver feels competent to give the medication or treatment
   c. Ensuring that caregiver knows who to call if plan of care for symptom control is not working or a new symptom develops, whatever the time of day

d. Increasing the level of care if symptoms are not responding to usual treatment (e.g., palliative care or hospice referral, transfer to an inpatient facility, initiation of continuous hospice care at home)

5. Providing psychosocial and emotional support for the caregiver
   a. Actively listening to fears, concerns, expression of grief
   b. Clarifying patient and family goals, including advance care planning, to ensure plan of care is congruent with patient and family goals
   c. Providing information to clarify any misperceptions or misunderstandings
   d. Augmentation of support services by making referrals to social worker, chaplain, counselors, and community resources
   e. Encouraging caregivers to accept assistance so that they have time for self-care, including sleeping, eating, and other restorative activities
   f. Use of hospice inpatient respite level of care, when indicated
   g. Communicating changes in patient condition, especially signs and symptoms of imminent death, so that caregivers feel as prepared as possible

VII. Interdisciplinary team
   A. Interdisciplinary care is an essential component of comprehensive palliative care programs and is required for certification of hospice and palliative care services (CAPC, 2011; CMS, 2013; NCCN, 2013; NCP, 2013).
   B. The expertise of several disciplines is required to meet the varied physical, psychological, emotional, and spiritual needs of the patient-family system (Egan City & Labyak, 2010).
   C. In contrast to multidisciplinary care, where each discipline assesses the patient and formulates a plan in a specific area of expertise, the interdisciplinary approach requires that the various disciplines collaborate with all disciplines involved to create a patient and family-directed plan of care. The patient and family are part of the palliative care interdisciplinary team (Egan City & Labyak, 2010).
   D. Interdisciplinary care requires that each discipline expand and blend their traditional roles in care with those of other disciplines (Egan City & Labyak, 2010) (Table 43-3).

VIII. Comfort measures
   A. Palliative care is based on the effective management of pain and other distressing symptoms throughout the continuum of care. Management of many of these symptoms is addressed elsewhere in this text. In this section, symptoms commonly seen in the final stages of life are addressed.
   B. The emphasis of symptom management is quality of life.
      1. Interventions are ideally aimed at addressing the underlying cause rather than treating the outward symptom. For example, restlessness related to the discomfort from urinary retention is best treated with catheterization rather than administering a benzodiazepine. When the underlying cause is not identifiable or the underlying cause is cancer that has proven to be unresponsive to treatment, the focus will shift to the outward symptom.
      2. Interventions that carry a significant burden are avoided. For example, although radiation therapy may be effective for treating bone pain, the discomfort and disruptions associated with being transported to daily radiation therapy may be burdensome for some individuals, especially at the end of life; an adjustment in analgesics may be a better option in such cases.
      3. Interventions that may have been helpful earlier in the disease process may no longer improve quality of life. For example, individuals with a low hematocrit may no longer get effective symptom relief from transfusions, and they may even feel worse if the transfusion leads to fluid overload caused by poor kidney function.

Table 43-3

Interdisciplinary Team Collaboration in Palliative Care

Dimension of Care	Team Members Involved
Physical or symptom	Physician, nurse, pharmacist, therapist, nutritionist, volunteers
Functional	Nurse, nursing assistants or aides, therapists, homemakers, volunteers
Interpersonal	Counselors, social workers, psychologist, chaplains, volunteers
Well-being	Counselors, social workers, psychologist, chaplains, volunteers
Transcendent	Chaplain, counselors, social worker, psychologist, volunteers

Adapted from Egan City, K. & Labyak, M. J. (2010). Hospice palliative care for the 21st century: A model for quality end-of-life care. In B. R. Ferrell & N. Coyle (Eds.). *Oxford textbook of palliative nursing* (3rd ed. pp. 13–52). New York: Oxford University Press.

Nutrition and Hydration Issues in Advanced Cancer

OVERVIEW AND ASSESSMENT

See Chapter 28.

PROBLEM STATEMENTS AND OUTCOME IDENTIFICATION

I. Imbalanced Nutrition: Less than Body Requirements (NANDA-I), related to pain, nausea, constipation, anorexia, weakness, dysphagia, cancer cachexia, or the dying process
   A. Expected outcome—patient will maintain intake that promotes physical and emotional comfort.
   B. Expected outcome—patient will be able to safely eat those foods that provide pleasure.
   C. Expected outcome—physical discomforts interfering with eating or caused by eating are treated when possible.
   D. Expected outcome—patient and family express understanding of the irreversible nature of refractory cachexia in advanced cancer.

II. Impaired Swallowing (NANDA-I), related to obstruction, pain caused by infection, xerostomia, or generalized weakness
   A. Expected outcome—patient will be able to swallow safely and comfortably for as long as possible.
   B. Expected outcome—if chemotherapy or radiation therapy is used, the benefits of the treatment outweigh the burdens and side effects are managed.
   C. Expected outcome—patient does not experience significant aspiration.
   D. Expected outcome—the oral mucosa is moist and free from infection and lesions.
   E. Expected outcome—no delay occurs in switching essential medications from the oral route to an alternative route when patient is too weak to swallow.

III. Risk for Deficient Fluid Volume (NANDA-I), related to excessive fluid loss from nausea and vomiting, diarrhea, diaphoresis, diuresis, or diminished fluid intake
   A. Expected outcome—patient will not experience any uncomfortable symptoms associate with dehydration or overhydration.
   B. Expected outcome—patient does not report a dry mouth or thirst.
   C. Expected outcome—patient does not exhibit any uncomfortable signs and symptoms of dehydration.
   D. Expected outcome—patient does not exhibit any signs of opioid toxicity that can be associated with dehydration.
   E. Expected outcome—patient does not exhibit any signs and symptoms of fluid overload if artificial fluids are administered.

PLANNING AND IMPLEMENTATION

I. Interventions to address nutritional issues at the end of life
   A. Treatment for any uncomfortable symptoms interfering with adequate intake (e.g., pain, nausea, constipation)
   B. Consultation with a registered dietician with experience in caring for persons with advanced progressive diseases for appropriate suggestions on food choices to maximize nutritional intake, being cognizant that nutritional intake does not reverse cancer cachexia (Isenring & Teleni, 2013)
   C. Discontinuation of interventions that no longer provide comfort
   D. Implementation of aspiration precautions in persons with weakness or dysphagia
   E. Allowing as much, or as little, intake as the patient desires for comfort; encouraging family to provide favorite foods, recognizing that cancer cachexia may cause taste changes
   F. Good oral care
   G. Maintaining a pleasant environment (sights, smells, sounds)
   H. Evaluation of the effectiveness of any appetite stimulants (e.g., corticosteroids or progestational agents); effects of these agents are short-lived and show no clear improvement in quality of life or prolongation of survival (Barcos, 2013).
   I. Providing education to the patient and family about cancer cachexia, emphasizing that the weight loss and poor appetite are caused by the disease
      1. Avoiding using, and correcting the family when they use, the term *starvation*; cancer cachexia is a different process and is not reversible in advanced stages (Barcos, 2013).
      2. Assisting the family in understanding the nature of refractory cancer cachexia to avoid conflicts between the patient and family with regard to food intake
      3. Avoiding use of enteral feeding tubes in persons with limited prognoses and poor functional status because these measures do not improve survival or quality of life (Bozzetti et al., 2009)

II. Interventions to address difficulty swallowing at the end of life
   A. Obtaining appropriate medical orders to treat any treatable causes
      1. If dysphagia is caused by obstruction by tumor, the patient may or may not be a candidate for additional antitumor treatments. Patients whose tumors have progressed on treatment are less likely to get benefits for additional treatment. Corticosteroids may be helpful to decrease inflammation around the tumor and provide some relief.
      2. Orders for antifungal medication to be obtained if signs and symptoms of candidiasis are present

B. Obtaining order for viscous lidocaine for oral pain

C. Treatment for xerostomia (see Chapter 28)

D. Evaluation and recommendations by speech therapist for measures that make swallowing more effective and prevent aspiration, as well as recommendations on food choices and consistencies

E. Keeping oral mucosa clean

F. Encouraging patient to take frequent sips of water or suck on ice if the patient is not at high risk for aspiration

G. Obtaining order for administration of artificial saliva

H. Implementation of aspiration precautions

I. Anticipating that patient will lose the ability to swallow as death approaches and work with prescriber to obtain orders for alternative routes of essential medication that are currently administered via the oral route; alternative routes may include sublingual, buccal, rectal, transdermal, subcutaneous, or intravenous; less invasive routes preferred for home administration

III. Interventions to address fluid loss at the end of life

A. Assessment of the underlying cause of excessive fluid loss and obtaining appropriate medical orders to treat the underlying cause or the symptom itself

1. Numerous potential causes of nausea and vomiting—medication side effect, paraneoplastic syndromes such as hypercalcemia and syndrome of inappropriate antidiuretic hormone, constipation, bowel obstruction, and increased intracranial pressure; thorough assessment essential to differentiate among these causes; when the underlying cause cannot be treated, antiemetics are essential.

2. Assessment of the amount, frequency, consistency, and odor of diarrhea to assist in determining the cause; administration of anti-infectives and antidiarrheal medications, as ordered

3. Assessment for amounts and patterns of diaphoresis

   a. Obtaining orders for antipyretics when fever is present and causing discomfort—for persistent fever, antipyretics around the clock to avoid the discomfort of repeat sweating and chilling during defervescence; alternatively, if patient asymptomatic, discontinuation of the antipyretic, which may actually improve overall comfort (Pittelkow & Loprinzi, 2010)

   b. Discussing the potential of using an anticholinergic medication such as scopolamine, atropine, or hyoscyamine to dry secretions; use of anticholinergics in the palliative setting based on anecdotal reports only

4. Assessment for underlying cause of diuresis

   a. If the underlying cause is the syndrome of inappropriate antidiuretic hormone, obtaining an order for demeclocycline or urea (Bower & Cox, 2010)

   b. If the underlying cause is overuse of diuretics, obtaining an order to discontinue the diuretics

5. Encouraging fluid intake, depending on the patient's ability to tolerate oral fluids

   a. Reinforcing to patient and family that a decrease in oral intake is part of the natural dying process

   b. Explaining that this "natural dehydration" has some benefits such as less pulmonary congestion, edema, ascites, and nausea or vomiting, as well as less need to urinate

   c. Providing thorough oral care to keep lips and oral mucosa moist

   d. Providing education and emotional support to the family because issues related to hydration may be a source of worry or concern

6. Monitoring for any discomfort associated with dehydration—for example, dizziness, confusion, agitated delirium, headache, and somnolence

   a. In the absence of adequate fluids, patients may not be able to clear the active metabolites of medications.

   b. Opioid toxicity is recognized as a potential problem in this population. Accumulation of the active metabolites of morphine and other opioids may lead to myoclonus, hyperalgesia and allodynia, profound sedation, and respiratory depression (Gelfman & Chai, 2013; Juba, Wahler, & Daron, 2013).

   c. Reduction of the opioid dose or rotation to a different opioid with the prescriber should be discussed with opioid toxicity; benzodiazepine administration is another option. Hydration to help eliminate these active metabolites should also be considered (Teuteberg, 2005).

7. Providing artificial fluids via the intravenous or subcutaneous route if patient exhibits any of the discomforts associated with dehydration

   a. Monitoring to ensure that fluids are contributing to comfort and not causing discomfort

   b. Discontinuing artificial fluids if patients develop signs of overhydration such as increases in pulmonary secretions, edema, ascites, or nausea and vomiting

   c. Educating patients and family members about the pros and cons of artificial fluids at initiation of this therapy and indicators used to determine when fluids are no longer providing comfort

EVALUATION

The oncology nurse systematically and regularly evaluates the patient's and family's responses to nutritional interventions to achieve the patient's individual comfort goal. Nutritional needs are assessed, data are collected, and the nutritional plan is continuously modified to meet the goal for the patient.

Cardiopulmonary Symptoms at End of Life

OVERVIEW AND ASSESSMENT

See Chapter 32.

PROBLEM STATEMENTS AND OUTCOME IDENTIFICATION

I. Ineffective Breathing Pattern (NANDA-I), related to underlying disease process, anemia, generalize weakness, or the dying process
   A. Expected outcome—patient reports relief from dyspnea.
   B. Expected outcome—patient exhibits regular, unlabored respirations, without excessive use of accessory muscles. There is an absence of increased work of breathing.
   C. Expected outcome—patient has minimal noisy breathing at end of life; when noisy breathing occurs, family understands that it is not distressing to the patient.
   D. Expected outcome—patient (as able) and family understand the purpose of any medications used to treat dyspnea or lessen secretions.
II. Decreased Cardiac Output and Ineffective Peripheral Tissue Perfusion (NANDA-I), caused by organ failure and the dying process
   A. Expected outcome—patient will not experience discomfort during the dying process.
   B. Expected outcome—family will be aware of the signs and symptoms of imminent death and be prepared for the patient's death.

PLANNING AND IMPLEMENTATION

I. Interventions to address pulmonary symptoms
   A. Monitoring respiratory rate and the work of breathing.
   B. Repositioning patient to lessen work of breathing (e.g., head of bed elevated, leaning forward over bedside table, supporting with pillows)
   C. Collaborating with medical team to treat any treatable causes of dyspnea
      1. The appropriateness of therapies is determined by the patient's prognosis, always balancing benefits and burdens.
         a. When the cause of dyspnea is progression of the cancer, additional antineoplastic agents may not provide any benefit. The focus will be on symptomatic relief of dyspnea (see below) (Smith & Jackson, 2013).
         b. The potential use of corticosteroids should be discussed with the medical team because this class of medications is reported to be helpful in some circumstances (Lin, Adelman, & Mehta, 2012).
      2. If dyspnea is caused by pneumonia, the benefits and burdens of treating with anti-infectives, based on the patient's life expectancy, should be discussed with team.
         a. If the goal of care is quality of life and treatment of the pneumonia will not achieve this goal, it may be considered futile care. Identifying patient and family goals of care is an ongoing process that evolves over time as the disease progresses. With each sign of progressive disease, it is important to evaluate the patient's perceived quality of life and to provide information to the patient and the family about the patient's current condition and anticipated outcomes, with and without treatment of acute events. An ethics consultation may be helpful if any disagreements exist about the appropriateness of medical interventions among the health care team or the family.
         b. With or without treatment with anti-infectives, measures should be taken to relieve dyspnea symptomatically (see below) and antipyretics administered, as needed, for fever.
      3. If dyspnea is caused by pleural effusions or ascites, it is necessary to assess if draining the effusion is appropriate at this time, recognizing that malignant effusions tend to recur.
         a. If death is imminent, drainage of the effusion may not be appropriate.
         b. When life expectancy is relatively short, a one-time removal of accumulated fluid may be sufficient for symptom relief.
         c. If the patient has a longer life expectancy, the benefits and burdens of chemosclerosis or an indwelling drainage catheter should be evaluated (Thai & Damant, 2006).
      4. If the dyspnea is caused by low hemoglobin, it is necessary to evaluate if the patient is a good candidate for a transfusion.
         a. As mentioned above, the goal of a transfusion is to improve quality of living. If a transfusion increases hemoglobin but has little effect on overall quality of life, additional transfusions may be inappropriate.
         b. Fluid overload with transfusions should be monitored for.

5. If the patient is hypoxic, it is necessary to maintain, or obtain an order for, oxygen therapy, as appropriate.
   a. Patients who have required oxygen therapy throughout the course of their disease usually require continuation of oxygen therapy throughout dying process.
   b. Patients who have not required oxygen therapy throughout the course of their disease may benefit as much from air blowing in the face or air via nasal cannula, as from oxygen (Brennan & Mazanec, 2011; Philip et al., 2006).
   c. Masks should be avoided because they may be uncomfortable for the patient and may contribute to agitation and restlessness.

6. If signs of fluid overload are present, diuretics should be administered, as ordered; this is especially important in patients with heart failure. Artificial fluids are discontinued if they are contributing to fluid overload.

D. Symptomatic treatment for dyspnea
   1. Providing a cool sensation to the face—for example, with the use of a fan blowing air toward the face or cool compresses on the cheeks (Galbraith, Fagan, Perkins, Lynch, & Booth, 2010)
   2. Administering oral or parenteral opioids, as ordered, for dyspnea, and titrating, as needed, for comfort (Brennan & Mazanec, 2011; Chan, Tse, Sham, & Thorsen, 2010); most studies have been conducted using morphine, but other opioids may be used.
      a. In the opioid-naïve patient, the starting dose is equivalent to morphine 5 to 10 mg orally or 1 to 2 mg intravenously given on an as-needed basis.
      b. Patients receiving opioids for pain will require 25% to 50% higher doses than their baseline requirements for pain control.
      c. Orders should be obtained to increase dose, as needed, for comfort.
      d. Short-acting opioids are recommended when initiating treatment. Patients requiring routine, stable doses for dyspnea may be converted to a long-acting formulation.
      e. Evidence has shown that nebulized morphine is not effective. Nebulized fentanyl is reported to be helpful, but more studies are needed (Brennan & Mazanec, 2011).
   3. Administering benzodiazepines only if a significant anxiety component to dyspnea is present; little evidence exists to support the use of benzodiazepines for dyspnea (Brennan & Mazanec, 2011).
   4. Providing reassurance, presence, and support to lessen the anxiety associated with dyspnea

E. Treatment for noisy breathing caused by secretions that collect at the back of the throat when swallowing is impaired.
   1. Elevating head of bed or placing patient in the side-lying position to promote drainage
   2. Providing emotional support to family
      a. Acknowledging the difficulty in listening to this noisy breathing; reassuring family that the noisy breathing is believed not to cause discomfort to the patient
      b. Avoiding using the term *death rattle*, because this can be perceived as distressing to patient
   3. Requesting an order for an anticholinergic medication to dry secretions (Smith & Jackson, 2013).
      a. Little evidence has shown that use of anticholinergic agents for noisy breathing actually improves comfort (Campbell & Yarandi, 2013). The lack of evidence and potential for side effects has led some practitioners to avoid using them.
      b. Home hospice settings frequently use atropine eye drops given sublingually. Other medications include hyoscyamine, scopolamine, and glycopyrrolate.
      c. The side effects of anticholinergics, especially agitation, should be monitored; the medicine is discontinued if side effects outweigh benefits.
      d. Good mouth care should be provided because anticholinergics may make the mouth uncomfortably dry.
   4. Deep suctioning is avoided because it causes discomfort and stimulates the mucosa to produce additional secretions.

II. Interventions to address decreased cardiac output and poor tissue perfusion
   A. Explaining that changes in skin temperature and color are part of the dying process
      1. The skin may be cold, clammy, and become slightly cyanotic or mottled, starting at the periphery and moving inward (Smith & Jackson, 2013).
      2. The core body temperature usually does not drop below normal during the dying process, and it is believed the patient does not experience a sensation of being cold.
      3. Heating devices and extra blankets are not helpful at this time. Generally, whatever layers of bed covers were comfortable for the patient throughout the care should be maintained during the dying process. Heavy layers of covers should be avoided because they can actually make the work of breathing harder.
   B. Monitoring for progression of mottling and reinforcing that this is an indication of imminent death

C. Providing good skin care to minimize risk of skin breakdown, especially when the dying process appears to be prolonged

D. Explaining that the Cheyne-Stokes breathing pattern is an additional sign that circulation is slowing

   1. The periods of apnea in the dying person may be very difficult for family members to deal with, especially when these periods are prolonged.

   2. Each breath may appear to be the last one. If this pattern continues for hours, the family needs extra support.

E. Discontinuation of routine monitoring of vital signs because this may be disruptive to the patient and family and does not change the plan of care; explaining this change in plan to family members so that they do not perceive this as cessation of adequate care

EVALUATION

The oncology nurse systematically and regularly evaluates the patient's and family's responses to decreased cardiopulmonary functioning. Breathing, cardiac output, and tissue perfusion are assessed, data are collected, and the cardiopulmonary plan is continuously modified to ensure patient comfort.

Perception and Cognition Issues at End of Life

OVERVIEW AND ASSESSMENT

See Chapters 37 and 38.

PROBLEM STATEMENTS AND OUTCOME IDENTIFICATION

I. Risk for Acute Confusion (NANDA-I), related to presence of multiple predisposing and precipitating factors for delirium

A. Expected outcome—patient will not experience delirium when it is avoidable.

B. Expected outcome—distress associated with delirium is minimized by prompt recognition of delirium and prompt treatment.

C. Expected outcome—patient remains oriented to person and surroundings for as long as possible.

PLANNING AND IMPLEMENTATION

I. Interventions to address acute confusion or delirium

A. Monitoring for signs and symptoms of delirium routinely

   1. Recognizing the diagnostic criteria for delirium (American Psychiatric Association, 2013)

      a. Disturbance in attention (reduced ability to direct, focus, sustain, and shift attention) and awareness (reduced orientation to environment)

      b. Develops in a short period, represents a change from baseline, and tends to fluctuate during the course of the day

      c. Additional disturbance in cognition (e.g., memory deficit, disorientation, language, visuospatial ability or perception)

      d. Disturbances in criteria *a* and *c* not explained by another pre-existing, established, or evolving neurocognitive disorder and not occurring in the context of a severely reduced level of arousal, such as coma

      e. Evidence from the history, physical examination, or laboratory findings that the disturbance is a direct physiologic consequence of another medical condition, substance intoxication or withdrawal (i.e., because of drug or related to a medication), or exposure to a toxin or has multiple causes

   2. Conducting ongoing assessment, including review the patient's history, physical examination data, and laboratory findings to search for a cause of the delirium

      a. Delirium can be a physiologic consequence of a general condition (e.g., urinary tract infection), may be caused by organ failure, intoxication, or medications, or may have more than one cause.

      b. Screening tools based on the above diagnostic criteria for delirium such as the Confusion Assessment Method (CAM) and Delirium Observation Scale (and others) are incorporated into daily or shift assessments.

      c. A single question such as "Do you feel that (the patient's name) has been more confused today?" may be a good quick screen to determine if a more formal evaluation is appropriate (Sands, Dantoc, Hartshom, Ryan, & Lujic, 2010; Weckmann & Morrison, 2013a). The family may notice subtle changes before they are recognized by health care professionals (Szarpa et al., 2013).

   3. Considering the three subtypes of delirium—hyperactive, hypoactive, and mixed—in ongoing assessment

      a. *Hyperactive delirium* is often associated with medication side effects and drug withdrawal (Blazer & van Nieuwenhuizen, 2012).

      b. *Hypoactive delirium* occurs more frequently in older adults and is associated with metabolic abnormalities and dehydration. Because these patients appear lethargic and confused, they are often misdiagnosed as having dementia or depression (Blazer & van Nieuwenhuizen, 2012; Heidrich & English, 2010).

      c. The mixed subtype exhibits features of both hyperactive and hypoactive delirium.

Part 8

B. Eliminating as many factors that contribute to delirium as possible (Heidrich & English, 2010)
1. Multiple factors such as age, cognitive status, functional status, malnutrition, and organ system failure may not be controlled.
2. Many of the medications used for symptom control, such as opioids, benzodiazepines, and anticholinergic agents, contribute to delirium.
   a. Each medication should be evaluated for its effectiveness and side effects.
   b. Orders should be obtained to discontinue medications that are no longer helpful or when burdens outweigh benefits.
C. Treating constipation, pain, infections, hypoxia, fever, dehydration, and metabolic abnormalities, as appropriate, depending on the patient's life expectancy; for example, bisphosphonate to treat hypercalcemia is not appropriate if the patient has a prognosis of less than 2 to 3 weeks of life remaining.
D. Avoiding overstimulation caused by noise, obnoxious lighting, and constant interruptions; facilitating adequate sleep
1. For mild delirium, elimination of contributing factors and providing a calm, safe environment may be sufficient (Weckmann & Morrison, 2013b).
E. Avoiding use of bladder catheters, when possible
F. Avoiding use of physical restraints
G. Orientation cues (ideally provided by familiar persons), frequent reassurances about safety; touch
H. Obtaining an order for an antipsychotic medication to treat delirium, when needed, for patient comfort and safety
1. When patient shows signs of distress, a trial with an antipsychotic is indicated; usually patients with hyperactive delirium may be extremely distressed as well (Weckmann & Morrison, 2013b).
2. Haloperidol is the most frequently used antipsychotic for delirium, but others in this class may be used.
   a. Exception—quetiapine (Seroquel) is the drug of choice if the patient has Parkinson disease.
   b. Frequent doses may be required.
   c. Patients should have at least two normal assessments before an attempt is made to wean them off antipsychotics.
3. Although benzodiazepines contribute to delirium, they are sometimes added to antipsychotics to treat extreme agitation and to reduce the extrapyramidal side effects of haloperidol (Weckmann & Morrison, 2013b).
4. Sedation may be required to treat refractory delirium when antipsychotics and benzodiazepines are not effective. Medications for deep sedation include phenobarbital and propofol.

EVALUATION

The oncology nurse systematically and regularly evaluates the patient's and family's responses to acute confusion. Cognition and delirium are assessed, data are collected, and the plan is continuously modified to maintain patient orientation as long as possible.

References

American Psychiatric Association. (2013). *Diagnostic and statistical manual of mental disorders* (5th ed.; DSM-5). Washington DC: American Psychiatric Association.

Bakitas, M., Lyons, K. D., Hegel, M. T., Balan, S., Barnett, K. N., Brokaw, F. C., et al. (2009). The project ENABLE II randomized controlled trial to improve palliative care for rural patients with advanced cancer: Baseline finding, methodological challenges, and solutions. *Palliative & Supportive Care, 7*, 75–86. http://dx.doi.org/10.1017/S1478951509000108.

Barcos, V. E. (2013). What medications are effective in improving anorexia and weight loss in cancer? In N. E. Goldstein & R. S. Morrison (Eds.), *Evidence-based practice of palliative medicine* (pp. 153–157). Philadelphia: Elsevier.

Bischoff, K., Weinberg, V., & Rabow, M. W. (2013). Palliative and oncologic co-management: Symptom management for outpatients with cancer. *Supportive Care in Cancer, 21*(11): 3031–3037. http://dx.doi.org/10.1007/s00520-013-1838-z.

Blazer, D. G., & van Nieuwenhuizen, A. O. (2012). Evidence for the diagnostic criteria of delirium: An update. *Current Opinion in Psychiatry, 25*, 239–243.

Bower, M., & Cox, S. (2010). Endocrine and metabolic complications of advanced cancer. In G. Hanks, N. I. Cherny, N. A. Christakis, M. Fallon, S. Kaasa, & R. K. Portenoy (Eds.) *Oxford textbook of palliative medicine* (4th ed., pp. 1013–1033). New York: Oxford University Press.

Bozzetti, F., Arends, J., Lundholm, K., Micklewright, A., Zurcher, G., Muscaritoli, M., et al. (2009). ESPEN guidelines on parenteral nutrition: Non-surgical oncology. *Clinical Nutrition, 28*, 445–454. http://dx.doi.org/10.1016/j.clnu.2009.04.011.

Brennan, C. W., & Mazanec, P. (2011). Dyspnea management across the palliative care continuum. *Journal of Hospice and Palliative Nursing, 13*, 130–139.

Bryant, R. A. (2013). Is pathological grief lasting more than 12 months grief or depression? *Current Opinion in Psychiatry, 26*, 41–46. http://dx.doi.org/10.1097/YCO.0b013e32835b2ca2.

Buglass, E. (2010). Grief and bereavement theories. *Nursing Standard, 24*(41), 44–47.

Bukki, J., Scherbel, J., Stiel, S., Klein, C., Meidenbauer, N., & Ostgathe, C. (2013). Palliative care needs, symptoms, and treatment intensity along the disease trajectory in medical oncology outpatients: a retrospective chart review. *Supportive Care in Cancer, 21*, 1743–1750. http://dx.doi.org/10.1007/s00520-013-1721-y.

Byock, I. (1997). *Dying well.* New York: Riverhead Books.

Campbell, M. L., & Yarandi, H. N. (2013). Death rattle is not associated with patient respiratory distress: Is pharmacologic treatment indicated? *Journal of Palliative Medicine, 16*, 1255–1259. http://dx.doi.org/10.1089/jpm.2011.0394.

Center for Medicare and Medicaid Services. (2013). *Hospice medicare services.* www.medicare.gov/Pubs/pdf/02154.pdf.

Center to Advance Palliative Care. (2011). *A guide to help palliative care programs successfully complete The Joint Commission certification process.* www.capc.org/palliative-care-professional-development/Licensing/joint-commission/tjc-guide-2011.pdf.

Center to Advance Palliative Care (CAPC). (2012). *Growth of palliative care in U.S. hospitals 2012 snapshot.* www.capc.org/capc-growth-analysis-snapshot-2011.pdf.

Center to Advance Palliative Care (CAPC). (n.d.a). *Certification and licensing.* www.capc.org/palliative-care-professional-development/Licensing.

Center to Advance Palliative Care (CAPC). (n.d.b). *Palliative care across the continuum.* www.capc.org/palliative-care-across-the-continuum.

Center to Advance Palliative Care (CAPC). (n.d.c). *Benefits to hospitals.* www.capc.org/building-a-hospital-based-palliative-care-program/case/hospitalbenefits.

Chan, K., Tse, D. M. W., Sham, M. M. K., & Thorsen, A. B. (2010). Palliative medicine in malignant respiratory diseases. In G. Hanks, N. I. Cherny, N. A. Christakis, M. Fallon, S. Kaasa, & R. K. Portenoy (Eds.), *Oxford textbook of palliative medicine* (4th ed., pp. 1107–1144). New York: Oxford University Press.

Corless, I. G. (2010). Bereavement. In B. R. Ferrell, & N. Coyle (Eds.), *Oxford textbook of palliative nursing* (3rd ed., pp. 597–611). New York: Oxford University Press.

Egan City, K., & Labyak, M. J. (2010). Hospice palliative care for the 21st century: A model for quality end-of-life care. In B. R. Ferrell & N. Coyle (Eds.), *Oxford textbook of palliative nursing* (3rd ed., pp. 13–52). New York: Oxford University Press.

Ferris, F. D., Bruera, E., Cherny, N., Cummings, C., Currow, D., Dudgeon, D., et al. (2009). Palliative care a decade later: Accomplishments, the need, next steps—from the American Society of Clinical Oncology. *Journal of Clinical Oncology, 27,* 3052–3058. http://dx.doi.org/10.1200/JCO.2008.20.1558.

Follwell, M., Burman, D., Le, L. W., Wakimoto, K., Seccareccia, D., Bryson, J., et al. (2009). Phase II study of an outpatient palliative care intervention in patients with metastatic cancer. *Journal of Clinical Oncology, 27,* 206–213.

Galbraith, S., Fagan, P., Perkins, P., Lynch, A., & Booth, S. (2010). Does the use of a handheld fan improve chronic dyspnea? A randomized, controlled, crossover trial. *Journal of Pain and Symptom Management, 39,* 831–838. http://dx.doi.org/10.1016/j.jpainsymman.2009.09.024.

Gelfman, L. P., & Chai, E. J. (2013). Which opioids are safest and most effective in renal failure? In N. E. Goldstein & R. S. Morrison (Eds.), *Evidence-based practice of palliative medicine* (pp. 28–33). Philadelphia: Elsevier.

Heidrich, D. E., & English, N. (2010). Delirium, confusion, agitation, and restlessness. In B. R. Ferrell & N. Coyle (Eds.), *Oxford textbook of palliative nursing* (3rd ed., pp. 449–467). New York: Oxford University Press.

Isenring, E. A., & Teleni, L. (2013). Nutritional counseling and nutritional supplements: A cornerstone of multidisciplinary cancer care for cachectic patients. *Current Opinion in Supportive & Palliative Care, 7,* 390–395. http://dx.doi.org/10.1097.SPC.0000000000000016.

Juba, K. M., Wahler, R. G., & Daron, S. M. (2013). Morphine and hydromorphone-induced hyperalgesia in a hospice patient. *Journal of Palliative Medicine, 17,* 809–812.

Kuebler-Ross, E. (1969). *On death and dying.* New York: Macmillan.

Lin, R. J., Adelman, R. D., & Mehta, S. S. (2012). Dyspnea in palliative care: Expanding the role of corticosteroids. *Journal of Palliative Medicine, 15,* 834–837.

Moss, A. H., Lunney, J. R., Culp, S., Auber, M., Kurian, S., Rogers, J., et al. (2010). Prognostic significance of the "surprise" question in cancer patients. *Journal of Palliative Medicine, 13,* 837–840. http://dx.doi.org/10.1089/jpm.2010.0018.

National Comprehensive Cancer Network (NCCN). (2013). *NCCN guidelines version 2.2013: Palliative care.* www.nccn.org/professionals/physician_gls/pdf/palliative.pdf.

National Consensus Project for Quality Palliative Care (NCP). (2009). *Clinical practice guidelines for quality palliative care* (2nd ed.). Pittsburgh: Authors.

National Consensus Project for Quality Palliative Care. (2013). *Clinical practice guidelines for quality palliative care* (3rd ed.). Pittsburgh: Authors.

National Hospice and Palliative Care Organization. (2013). *NHPCO facts and figures on hospice care.* www.nhpco.org/sites/default/files/public/Statistics_Research/2013_Facts_Figures.pdf.

National Hospice and Palliative Care Organization (n.d.a). *Key hospice messages.* www.nhpco.org/press-room/key-hospice-messages.

National Hospice and Palliative Care Organization (n.d.b). *History of hospice care.* www.nhpco.org/history-hospice-care.

Oken, M.M., Creech, R.H., Tormey, D.C., Horton, J., Davis, T.E., McFadden, E.T., & Carbone, P.P.: Toxicity And response criteria of the Eastern Cooperative Oncology Group. *American Journal of Clinical Oncology, 5,* 649–655.

Philip, J., Gold, M., Milner, A., DiIulio, J., Miller, B., & Spruyt, O. (2006). A randomized, double-blind, crossover trial of the effect of oxygen on dyspnea in patients with advanced cancer. *Journal of Pain and Symptom Management, 32,* 541–550.

Pittelkow, M. R., & Loprinzi, C. L. (2010). Pruritus and sweating in palliative medicine. In G. Hanks, N. I. Cherny, N. A. Christakis, M. Fallon, S. Kaasa, & R. K. Portenoy (Eds.), *Oxford textbook of palliative medicine* (4th ed., pp. 934–951). New York: Oxford University Press.

Rabow, M. W. (2013). What new models exist for ambulatory palliative care? In N. E. Goldstein & R. S. Morrison (Eds.), *Evidence-based practice of palliative medicine* (pp. 468–473). Philadelphia: Elsevier.

Ramchandran, K. J., & von Roenn, J. H. (2013). What is the role for palliative care in patients with advanced cancer? In N. E. Goldstein & R. S. Morrison (Eds.), *Evidence-based practice of palliative medicine* (pp. 276–280). Philadelphia: Elsevier.

Sands, M. B., Dantoc, B. P., Hartshorn, A., Ryan, C. J., & Lujic, S. (2010). Single question in delirium (SQiD): Testing its efficacy against psychiatrist interview, the Confusion Assessment Method and the Memorial Delirium Assessment Scale. *Palliative Medicine, 24,* 561–565. http://dx.doi.org/10.1177/0269216310371556.

Sefcik, J. S., Rao, A., & Ersek, M. (2013). What models exist for delivering palliative care and hospice in nursing homes? In N. E. Goldstein & R. S. Morrison (Eds.), *Evidence-based practice of palliative medicine* (pp. 450–457). Philadelphia: Elsevier.

Smith, L. N., & Jackson, V. A. (2013). How do symptoms change for patients in the last days and hours of life? In N. E. Goldstein & R. S. Morrison (Eds.), *Evidence-based practice of palliative medicine* (pp. 218–226). Philadelphia: Elsevier.

Stiel, S., Bertram, L., Neuhaus, S., Nauck, F., Ostgathe, C., Elsner, F., & Radbruch, L. (2010). Evaluation and comparison of two prognostic scores and the physicians' estimate of survival in terminally ill patients. *Supportive Care in Cancer, 18*, 43–49. http://dx.doi.org/10.1007/s00520-009-0628-0.

Szarpa, K. L., Kerr, C. W., Wright, S. T., Luczkiewicz, D. L., Hand, P. C., & Ball, L. S. (2013). The prodrome to delirium: A grounded theory study. *Journal of Hospice and Palliative Nursing, 6*, 332–337. http://dx.doi.org/10.1097/NJH.0b013e31828fdf56.

Temel, J. S., Greer, J. A., Muzikansky, A., Gallagher, E. R., Admane, S., Jackson, V. A., et al. (2010). Early palliative care for patients with metastatic non-small-cell lung cancer. *New England Journal of Medicine, 363*, 733–742. http://dx.doi.org/10.1056/NEJMoa1000678.

Teuteberg, W. G. (2005). *Opioid-induced hyperalgesia. Fast facts and concepts.* www.eperc.mcw.edu/EPERC/FastFactsIndex/ff_142.htm.

Thai, V., & Damant, R. (2006). *Malignant pleural effusions. Fast facts and concepts.* www.eperc.mcw.edu/EPERC/FastFactsIndex/ff_157.htm.

Waldrop, D., & Kutner, J. S. (2013a). What is prolonged grief disorder and how can its likelihood be reduced? In N. E. Goldstein & R. S. Morrison (Eds.), *Evidence-based practice of palliative medicine* (pp. 436–442). Philadelphia: Elsevier.

Waldrop, D., & Kutner, J. S. (2013b). What is the effect of serious illness on caregivers? In N. E. Goldstein & R. S. Morrison (Eds.), *Evidence-based practice of palliative medicine* (pp. 421–428). Philadelphia: Elsevier.

Waldrop, D., & Kutner, J. S. (2013c). What can be done to improve outcomes for caregivers of patients with serious illness? In N. E. Goldstein & R. S. Morrison (Eds.), *Evidence-based practice of palliative medicine* (pp. 429–435). Philadelphia: Elsevier.

Weckmann, M. T., & Morrison, R. S. (2013a). What is delirium? In N. E. Goldstein & R. S. Morrison (Eds.), *Evidence-based practice of palliative medicine* (pp. 198–204). Philadelphia: Elsevier.

Weckmann, M. T., & Morrison, R. S. (2013b). What pharmacological treatments are effective for delirium? In N. E. Goldstein & R. S. Morrison (Eds.), *Evidence-based practice of palliative medicine* (pp. 205–210). Philadelphia: Elsevier.

Worden, J. W. (2002). *Grief counseling and grief therapy: A handbook for the mental health practitioner* (3rd Ed.). New York: Springer.

World Health Organization (WHO) (n.d.). *WHO definition of palliative care.* www.who.int/cancer/palliative/definition/en.

Zhang, M., Smith, K. L., Cook-Mack, J., Wajnberg, A., DeCherrie, L. B., & Soriano, T. A. (2013). How can palliative care be integrated into home-based primary care programs? In N. E. Goldstein & R. S. Morrison (Eds.), *Evidence-based practice of palliative medicine* (pp. 458–467). Philadelphia: Elsevier.

CHAPTER 44

Evidence-Based Practice and Standards of Oncology Nursing

Rita Wickham

I. Synopsis
   A. Standards—developed by the Oncology Nursing Society (ONS), in collaboration with the American Nurses Association, in 1979; revised in 1987, 1996, 2004, and 2013; the newest version includes the oncology nurse generalist and advanced practice oncology nurses (APNs)—nurse practitioner (NP) and clinical nurse specialist (CNS)
   B. Applicable to all roles and in all settings where oncology nurses care for patients
   C. Emphasize the importance of the following:
      1. Intraprofessional and interprofessional collaboration and collegiality
      2. Ethical practice
      3. Recognition of racial and ethnic diversity and the need for diversity awareness
      4. Ensuring quality cancer care
      5. Appropriate resource use (Brant & Wickham, 2013)
   D. Serve as a powerful guide for ensuring evidence-based quality cancer nursing care
   E. Indicate to society at large that oncology nursing is able to define and govern the quality of oncology nursing practice (Schultz, 2012)
II. Definitions
   A. *Standards*—authoritative statements that delineate duties that all registered nurses (RNs) are expected to perform competently; in this case, oncology nursing standards, which are articulated and disseminated by ONS, offer a mechanism by which to judge the quality of practice (Brant & Wickham, 2013).
   B. *Patient*—the individual, family, group, or community for whom the nurse provides specifically planned services (Brant & Wickham, 2013)

III. Components of each standard
   A. Standard statement
   B. Rationale—explanation of the underlying reason for the standard
   C. Measurement criteria—relevant, measurable indicators that demonstrate adherence to the standard
IV. Standards of care (Box 44-1)
   A. Encompass the professional nursing actions and activities as carried out by the oncology nurse and include the following:
      1. Assessment
      2. Diagnosis
      3. Outcome identification
      4. Planning
      5. Implementation
      6. Evaluation (Brant & Wickham, 2013)
   B. Address each of the 14 high-incidence problem areas common to patients cared for by oncology nurses and include the following:
      1. Health promotion
      2. Patient and family education
      3. Coping
      4. Comfort
      5. Nutrition
      6. Complementary and alternative medicine
      7. Protective mechanisms
      8. Mobility
      9. Gastrointestinal (GI) and urinary function
      10. Sexuality
      11. Cardiopulmonary function
      12. Oncologic emergencies
      13. Palliative and end-of-life care
      14. Survivorship (Brant & Wickham, 2013)
   C. Purpose
      1. Oncology nursing (generalist and APN) Standards of Care
         a. Serve as a guide for providing quality cancer care within the framework of

Box 44-1

Standards of Care

Standard I: Assessment

The oncology nurse systematically and continually collects data regarding the physical, psychological, social, spiritual, and cultural health status of the patient, including in-depth data specific to the disease and treatment experience of the patient with cancer.

Standard II: Diagnosis

The oncology nurse analyzes assessment data to determine nursing diagnoses.

Standard III: Outcome Identification

The oncology nurse identifies expected outcomes individualized to the patient, family, or both.

Standard IV: Planning

The oncology nurse develops an individualized and holistic plan of care that prescribes interventions to attain expected outcomes, focusing on the 14 high-incidence areas.

Standard V: Implementation

The oncology nurse implements the plan of care to achieve the identified expected outcomes for the patient.

Standard VI: Evaluation

The oncology nurse systematically and regularly evaluates the patient's response to interventions to determine progress toward achievement of expected outcomes.

From Brant, J.M. & Wickham, R.S. (Eds.). (2013). *Statement on the scope and standards of oncology nursing practice* (pp. 21–43). Pittsburgh: Oncology Nursing Society.

the nursing process by ensuring the following:
  (1) Data collection is systematic, characterized by diversity awareness, continuous, collected from multiple sources, documented, and communicated with members of the multidisciplinary cancer care team.
  (2) Nursing and collaborative diagnoses are derived from interpretation of presenting data and reflect the patient's actual or potential health problems.
  (3) Identified outcomes, which flow from nursing and collaborative diagnoses, are individualized to the patient's needs.
  (4) The plan of care results from current knowledge of the nursing, biologic, social, behavioral, cultural, and physical sciences.
  (5) The plan of care reflects the patient's priorities and prescribed nursing strategies to achieve health promotion, maintenance, and restoration across the cancer continuum.
  (6) The plan of care is implemented in concordance with the patient's needs.
  (7) The patient actively participates in all aspects of plan development, implementation, and evaluation.
  (8) Patient progress is evaluated jointly by the nurse and patient.
  (9) Evaluation of patient outcomes directs reassessment and revision of the plan of care.
  b. Facilitates professional development by doing the following:
   (1) Identifying gaps in the nurse's knowledge base
   (2) Determining range of practice for which the individual oncology nurse is prepared
 2. Oncology nursing Standards of Care
  a. Provide a basis for the development of job descriptions, performance appraisals, evaluation instruments, and peer review
  b. Present a basis for quality assessment and quality improvement
  c. Generate research questions
  d. Stimulate research to validate practice and provide the foundation of evidence-based practice
  e. Provide a basis for program evaluation
  f. Promote intra- and interprofessional collaboration
  g. Provide a basis for organizational policies, procedures, and protocols
 3. For the patient, standards ensure the following:
  a. Participation in health promotion; health protection; cancer prevention; cancer treatment; symptom management; and survivor care, palliative care, or both
  b. Quality of care consistent with existing standards
V. Standards of Professional Performance (Box 44-2)
 A. Provide the framework for the oncology nurse to develop ethically sound practice, confront ethical challenges, use resources wisely, and assume a leadership role in the evolving future health care; describe competent behaviors of the oncology nurse's role as a professional nurse and include the following:
  1. Ethics
  2. Education

Box 44-2

Standards of Professional Performance

Standard VII: Ethics

The oncology nurse uses ethical principles as a basis for decision making and patient advocacy.

Standard VIII: Education

The oncology nurse acquires and expands a personal knowledge base that reflects the current evidence-based state of cancer care and oncology nursing and that incorporates enhanced competence and critical-thinking skills. The oncology nurse contributes to the professional development of licensed peers, assistive personnel, and interprofessional colleagues.

Standard IX: Evidence-Based Practice and Research

The oncology nurse contributes to the scientific base of cancer nursing practice, education, management, quality improvement, and research through multiple avenues: identifying clinical dilemmas and problems appropriate for rigorous study, collecting data, critiquing existing research, and integrating relevant research into clinical practice to improve patient outcomes.

Standard X: Quality of Practice

The oncology nurse systematically evaluates the quality, safety, and effectiveness of oncology nursing practice within all practice settings and across the continuum of cancer care.

Standard XI: Communication

The oncology nurse interacts and communicates effectively with the interprofessional health care team and with the patient and family and uses a variety of strategies to foster mutual respect and shared decision making that enhance clinical outcomes and patient satisfaction in all practice settings.

Standard XII: Leadership

The oncology nurse demonstrates leadership in the practice setting and in the nursing profession by actively acknowledging the dynamic nature of cancer care and the necessity to prepare for evolving technologies, modalities of treatment, and supportive care.

Standard XIII: Collaboration

The oncology nurse partners with the patient and family, the interprofessional team, and community resources to optimize cancer care.

Standard XIV: Professional Practice Evaluation

The oncology nurse consistently evaluates his or her own nursing practice in relation to national oncology nursing professional standards and guidelines, the state nurse practice act, relevant statewide regulatory requirements, and job-specific performance expectations.

Standard XV: Resource Utilization

The oncology nurse considers factors related to safety, efficiency, effectiveness, and cost in planning and delivering care to patients.

Standard XVI: Environmental Health

The oncology nurse practices in an environmentally safe and healthy manner.

From Brant, J.M. & Wickham, R.S. (Eds.). (2013). *Statement on the scope and standards of oncology nursing practice* (pp. 45–63). Pittsburgh: Oncology Nursing Society.

---

   3. Evidence-based practice and research
   4. Quality of practice
   5. Communication
   6. Leadership
   7. Collaboration
   8. Professional practice evaluation
   9. Resource utilization
   10. Environmental health (Brant & Wickham, 2013)

VI. Examples of application of the Standards of Care and Standards of Professional Performance in oncology nursing practice

   A. Application of Standard of Care III (Outcome Identification) to guide development of practice setting–specific plans of care for various aspects of the 14 high-incidence problem areas.

      1. To affect a high-incidence problem area (e.g., protective mechanisms), nurses can use the Centers for Disease Control (CDC) guideline for preventing intravascular catheter-related infection—an interprofessionally developed, evidence-based publication—to develop teaching materials for patients with central venous catheters (CVCs) and practice procedures or guidelines (O'Grady et al., 2011) (Box 44-3).

   B. Application of Standard of Professional Performance V (Quality of Practice) as a framework for a practice setting quality improvement program

      1. Use of the measurement criteria of each standard of care as a statement of acceptable practice

      2. Use of the 14 high-incidence problem areas to identify potential indicators (well-defined, measurable dimensions of quality and appropriate patient care; can be measurable

Box 44-3

Application of Evidence-Based Practice Resources

A national interprofessionally diverse panel, in collaboration with several other agencies, met to develop a guideline for prevention of infections related to intravascular catheters for health care personnel who insert intravascular catheters (IVCs) and individuals responsible for surveillance and infection control in hospital, outpatient, and home health care settings (O'Grady et al., 2011). They performed an extensive systematic review of the research and clinical reports related to IVCs. The trustworthiness of the group and the process are demonstrated by the committee members' reports of potential conflicts of interest.

The working group categorized their recommendations in a manner similar to other efforts to rate evidence in the literature:

Category IA recommendations are strongly supported by well-designed experimental, clinical, or epidemiologic studies and recommended for implementation.

Category IB statements are also strongly recommended for implementation based on some experimental data, clinical or epidemiologic studies, and a strong theoretical rationale. In other cases, category IB recommendations are accepted practice (e.g., aseptic technique) with limited evidence for their support.

Category IC recommendations are requirements mandated by state or federal regulations, rules, or standards.

Category II recommendations are "suggested" for implementation and supported by suggestive clinical or epidemiologic studies or have a theoretical rationale.

Unresolved Issues, where evidence is insufficient or there is no consensus about efficacy.

The summary recommendations focus on education and training, catheter type (only recommendations that are applicable to cancer patients with long-term CVCs are included here), hygiene, skin preparation, and dressings. Note that many of the recommendations are not 1A.

Education, Training, and Staffing

1. Health care personnel should be educated about indications for IVC use, appropriate insertion and maintenance procedures, and infection control measures to prevent catheter-related infections. (Category IA recommendation)
2. Knowledge and guideline adherence should be periodically assessed in all personnel who insert and/or maintain IVCs. (Category IA recommendation)
3. Only trained personnel who demonstrate competence for insertion and/or maintenance of peripheral and central IVCs should be designated to provide this care. (Category IA recommendation)

Peripheral and Midline Catheters

1. Catheters should be selected based on intended purpose and duration of use, recognized infectious and noninfectious complications (e.g., phlebitis and infiltration), and experience of individual catheter users. (Category IB recommendation)
2. Steel needles should be avoided when vesicants are being administered. (Category IA recommendation)

Central Venous Catheters (CVCs)

1. The risks and benefits of a central venous catheter (CVC) should be weighed to reduce infectious complications versus mechanical complications (e.g., pneumothorax, thrombosis, air embolism, and catheter misplacement). (Category IA recommendation)
2. No recommendation exists regarding a preferred site of insertion to minimize infection risk for a tunneled CVC. (Unresolved Issue)
3. A CVC should be used with the minimum number of ports or lumens essential to management of the patient. (Category IB recommendation)

Hand Hygiene and Aseptic Technique

1. Hand hygiene, either washing hands with soap and water or alcohol-based hand rubs (ABHRs), should be done before and after inserting, replacing, accessing, repairing, or dressing an intravascular catheter. The insertion site should not be palpated after antiseptic is applied unless aseptic technique is maintained. (Category IB recommendation)
2. Aseptic technique should be maintained during insertion and care of intravascular catheters. (Category IB recommendation)
3. Clean or sterile gloves should be worn when changing an intravascular catheter dressing. (Category IC recommendation)

Skin Preparation

1. Clean skin should be prepped with an antiseptic (70% alcohol, tincture of iodine, or alcoholic chlorhexidine solution) before peripheral venous catheter insertion. (Category IB recommendation)
2. Clean skin should be prepped with a >0.5% chlorhexidine preparation with alcohol before CVC insertion and dressing changes. If chlorhexidine is contraindicated, tincture of iodine, iodophor, or 70% alcohol can be used. (Category IA recommendation)
3. No comparisons of chlorhexidine preparations and alcohol-povidone-iodine to prepare clean skin exist. (Unresolved Issue)
4. Antiseptics should be allowed to dry (according to the manufacturer's recommendation) prior to placement of a catheter. (Category IB recommendation)

Box 44-3

Application of Evidence-Based Practice Resources—cont'd

Catheter Site Dressing Regimens

1. Catheter sites should be covered with sterile gauze or sterile, transparent, semipermeable dressing. (Category IA recommendation)
2. If a patient is diaphoretic or the catheter site is bleeding or oozing, a gauze dressing should be used. (Category II recommendation)
3. Damp, loosened, or visibly soiled catheter site dressings should be replaced. (Category IB recommendation)
4. Topical antibiotic ointments or creams should not be used on insertion sites because they may promote fungal infections and antimicrobial resistance. (Category IB recommendation)
5. The catheter or catheter site should not be submerged in water, but showering should be permitted if precautions to reduce the likelihood of introducing organisms into the catheter are taken (e.g., catheter and connecting device are protected with an impermeable cover during the shower). (Category IB recommendation)
6. Transparent dressings on tunneled or implanted CVC sites should not be changed more than once per week (unless the dressing is soiled or loose) until the insertion site has healed. (Category II recommendation)
7. No recommendation exists about the need for any dressing on well-healed exit sites of long-term cuffed and tunneled CVCs. (Unresolved Issue)
8. Catheter site care must be compatible with the catheter material. (Category IB recommendation)
9. The catheter site should be visually monitored when changing the dressing or by palpation through an intact dressing on a regular basis, depending on the clinical situation of the individual patient. If a patient has insertion site tenderness, fever without obvious source, or other manifestations suggesting local or bloodstream infection, the dressing should be removed to allow thorough examination of the site. (Category IB recommendation)
10. Patients should be instructed to report any changes in catheter site or new discomfort. (Category II recommendation)

Antibiotic Lock Prophylaxis, Antimicrobial Catheter Flush, and Catheter Lock Prophylaxis

1. Prophylactic antimicrobial lock solution should be used in patients with long-term catheters and a history of multiple catheter-related bloodstream infections (CRBSIs) despite optimal maximal adherence to aseptic technique. (Category II recommendations)

Needleless Intravascular Catheter Systems

1. Needleless components should be changed at least as often as the administration set; changes more frequently than every 72 hours are not beneficial. (Category II recommendation)
2. Needleless connectors should be changed no more frequently than every 72 hours or per manufacturer's recommendations to reduce infection rates. (Category II recommendation)
3. It must be ensured that all system components are compatible to minimize leaks and breaks. (Category II recommendation)
4. To minimize contamination risk, access ports should be scrubbed with an appropriate antiseptic (see above) and accessed using sterile technique. (Category IA recommendation).

care processes, clinical events, complications, or outcomes) that can be used to monitor oncology nursing care
3. Determining a threshold (a pre-established aggregate level of performance that should be achieved) for action
4. Collection of data that monitor the quality and effectiveness of oncology nursing care
5. Analysis of data to identify areas to improve care
6. Formulating recommendations to improve client outcomes and satisfaction with care
7. Implementation of recommendations and evaluate effectiveness

C. Application of Standards of Care and Standards of Professional Performance to education

1. Use of the Standards of Care and Standards of Professional Performance to develop curricular content outlines for generalist oncology nursing education, staff development, and continuing education programs.
2. Use of the measurement criteria as learner objectives for nurse and client education

D. Application of Standards of Care and Standards of Professional Performance to nursing management and leadership

1. Use of the Standards of Care and Standards of Professional Performance as a framework to develop staff performance evaluation instruments
2. Use of Standards of Professional Performance Evaluation and Resource Utilization (XV) to

justify resources required to provide oncology nursing care

E. Application of Standard of Professional Performance IX (Evidence-Based Practice and Research) to facilitate application of evidence-based practice as well as the conduct of oncology nursing research
1. Evidence-based practice (EBP) has its basis in evidence-based medicine, first developed as a method for clinical learning in the 1980s at McMaster University in Hamilton, Ontario, Canada.
2. The primary goal of EBP in oncology nursing is to guide nursing interventions that are demonstrated to enhance the quality and outcomes of cancer care (Mallory, 2010).
3. Definition and components of EBP include the following:
   a. Integration of the best possible research evidence with clinical expertise and patient needs (Porter-O'Grady, 2010)
   b. A problem-solving approach for clinical practice, which answers a pertinent question related to a nurse's personal clinical expertise as well as the patient's preference and values and that incorporates relevant evidence gathered by a systematic search and critical appraisal (Melnyk, Fineout-Overholt, 2005)
   c. A systematic approach to practice, which emphasizes using best evidence in combination with clinical experience and patient preferences and values to make decisions about care and treatment (Leufer & Cleary-Holdforth, 2009)
   d. Essential components—a systematic review and synthesis of research that results in a systematic process for change, including systematic and rigorous assessment, implementation, and evaluation of outcomes (Boucher, Underhill, Roper, & Berry, 2013)
4. The oncology nursing profession has mandated the inclusion of EBP in its standards. For the oncology nurse generalist, these mandates are a component of each of the six Standards of Care.

F. Application of Standard of Professional Performance IX (Evidence-Based Practice and Research)—"The oncology nurse contributes to the scientific base of cancer nursing practice, education, management, quality improvement, and research through multiple avenues: identifying clinical dilemmas and problems appropriate for rigorous study, collecting data, critiquing existing research, and integrating relevant research into clinical practice to improve patient outcomes" (Brant & Wickham, 2013).

G. Application of ONS Standards of Oncology Nursing Education: Oncology Generalist Level Education
1. Standard II (Resources)—the Standards of Oncology Nursing Education state: "Educational materials specific to oncology nursing are peer-reviewed, evidence-based, current, available, and accessible to the faculty and students" (Jacobs, 2002).
2. Standard V (student, the oncology nurse generalist)—the Standards of Oncology Nursing Education also state that graduates of generic nursing programs should be able to assume nursing care responsibilities that include the following:
   a. Use of research evidence to collect and analyze client-related data
   b. Development and evaluation of an evidence-based plan of care
   c. Participation in oncology nursing research through identification of research questions, implementing research findings, and evaluating outcomes of interventions (Jacobs, 2002)

VII. Need for EBP based on changing health care practices, economic considerations, quality outcomes, and information, including the following:
A. The Institute of Medicine has mandated that 90% of all health care decisions in the United States will be evidence-based by 2020 (Olsen, Aisner, & McGinnis, 2007).
B. EBP fosters comprehensive, outcomes-driven health care.
C. Health outcomes may be seriously jeopardized and health care costs may soar without EBP.
D. Pay for performance programs, incentives for clinicians to follow evidence-based guidelines, and nonpayment for preventable nosocomial events are increasing (Melnyk Fineout-Overholt, Stillwell, & Williamson, 2009).

VIII. Use of evidence to inform clinical practice—a multistep process that includes the following:
A. Precise description of the client or clinical problem
B. Identification of information needed to solve the problem
C. Efficient search of the literature for relevant studies
1. Data sources for EBP include, but are not limited to the following:
   a. Research-based evidence
      (1) Prospective, randomized controlled trials
      (2) Observational studies

      (3) Descriptive studies

      (4) Correlational studies

    b. Theoretic evidence

      (1) Propositions based on empiric knowledge

      (2) Propositions based on nonempiric knowledge

    c. Nonresearch evidence

      (1) Retrospective or concurrent chart review

      (2) Quality improvement and risk data

      (3) Cost-effective analysis

      (4) Benchmarking data

      (5) International, national, and local standards of care

      (6) Case reports or clinical expertise

      (7) Principles of pathophysiology

      (8) Infection control data

      (9) Regulatory and legal data

  D. Evaluation of the validity of these studies

    1. Studies may range from meta-analyses and integrative reviews to case reports and may include both qualitative and quantitative research (Fawcett & Garity, 2009).

  E. Identification of the clinical relevance or "message"

  F. Development of a clinical protocol to guide client care

  G. Implementation of the protocol

  H. Evaluation or audit of processes and outcomes

IX. Need for nurses to cultivate a spirit of inquiry and make a commitment to ask appropriate questions that lay the groundwork for EBP within an individual health care setting; steps for developing EBP include the following:

  A. Step 1—asking clinical question(s) of interest in the PICOT format:

    P—Patient population of interest

    I—Intervention or area of interest

    C—Comparison intervention or group

    O—Outcome

    T—Time

  B. Step 2—searching for the best evidence

    1. Identifying key words and phrases in electronic databases to conduct a focused literature search

    2. Use of both filtered (e.g., Cochrane reviews) and unfiltered (e.g., PubMed articles) sources

  C. Step 3—critically appraising publications or evidence to determine which are most reliable and valid, relevant, and applicable to the question

  D. Step 4—integrating the evidence with clinical expertise and patient preferences and values

  E. Step 5—evaluating the outcomes of practice changes or decisions based on ongoing monitoring of positive and negative effects of the change

  F. Step 6—sharing information gained from change with colleagues (disseminating findings) (Melnyk Fineout-Overholt, Stillwell, & Williamson, 2010)

X. Potential research roles of the oncology nurse generalist that can facilitate EBP:

  A. Identification of practice problems by observation of patient populations and quality improvement activities; examples of practice problems include the following:

    1. Developing and testing an intervention to improve patient adherence to oral chemotherapy that includes a model for symptom management (Spoelstra et al., 2013)

    2. Developing, implementing, and evaluating an in-hospital, standardized antibiotic order set to reduce time to administration of initial doses for adult patients admitted with febrile neutropenia (Best et al., 2011)

  B. Participation in evaluation of existing research or clinical evidence

    1. Use of identified measurement criteria to outline staff nurse roles and responsibilities in oncology nursing research

    2. Assisting in studies related to high-incidence problem areas or oncology nursing priorities (Berger, Cochrane, & Mitchell, 2009)

      a. Considering which nursing interventions promote optimal client outcomes

      b. Determining the need for any additional high-incidence problem areas beyond the 14 identified

    3. Use of standards to identify possible oncology nursing–related research questions:

      a. Defining oncology nurses' roles and actions in facilitating discussions about palliative care, advance directives, or end-of-life care with patients when they are decisional

      b. Determining how to develop a survivorship care plan that addresses not only being cancer-free, but potential long-term effects of cancer therapies and psychological responses to cancer and cancer treatment

  C. Collaboration with other health care providers or nurse researchers to identify and implement a potential solution to a specific clinical problem

  D. Participation in research activities under the guidance of a qualified researcher that may lead to practice changes and add to EBP

    1. Conceptualization and design of a research study

      a. Establishing that the problem is clinically significant and that a gap exists in the current literature

b. Assessing the feasibility of the methods and procedures for the proposed study

2. Implementation of a nursing research study
   a. Identifying and enrolling patients
   b. Implementing protocol-specific orders
   c. Collecting study data
   d. Educating patients, caregivers, and other health care team members about the study

E. Role of oncology nurses in medical clinical trials that focus on the following:

1. Cancer prevention and screening for early detection, cancer diagnosis, cancer treatment, supportive care, or survivorship

2. Medical clinical trials of drugs, which occur in four consecutive phases of investigation, three of them before U.S. Food and Drug Administration (FDA) approval
   a. Phase I trials—assess and document drug toxicities and determine maximally tolerated dose (MTD) of a *new compound* (term used before drug is named)
   b. Phase II trials—new compound given to patients with specific tumor types (some patients may have had some response in phase I studies) and continuing to monitor toxicities
   c. Phase III trials—random assignment to one of two or more treatment arms to determine the following:
      (1) The effects of treatment in comparison to another treatment arm
      (2) Whether a new treatment has less toxicity (morbidity) than a "standard" therapy
      (3) Pivotal phase III trials that may lead to FDA approval of a new drug
   d. Phase IV trials—implemented after FDA approval, evaluate new indications for a drug or device and also collect additional data related to use in a greater number of patients (Green, Benedetti, Smith, & Crowley, 2012)

XI. Critiquing research reports for applicability to EBP
A. Research reports critiqued to carry out the following:

1. Evaluate the believability of the results
2. Decide if the study is applicable to this practice setting and patient group
3. Determine if the study could be replicated in this practice, if appropriate
4. Decide if the findings are consistent with other research findings on the topic
5. Decide what, if any, new knowledge can be gained from the research

6. Identify whether the findings are sufficiently mature or complete for practice implementation (Greenhalgh, 2010)

B. Steps for evaluating a research report
1. Reviewing and critiquing the entire report, not just individual components
2. Closely reviewing how the report is laid out (e.g., contains all the necessary components and are logically ordered) and the information presented
3. Identifying whether the information is of value to clinical practice
4. Objectively identifying the study's strengths and weaknesses (Fawcett & Garity, 2009)

C. Guidelines and exact questions for completing a critique—these vary, depending on the study methodology, and include evaluation of the following:

1. Research problem or purpose
   a. Is the purpose explicit and include study variables and the population to be studied?
   b. Does the problem have significance for nursing?
   c. Are there formally stated hypotheses or research questions that directly relate to the research problem? (Burns & Grove, 2011; Oman, 2003)

2. Theoretic framework (most common in nursing research; medical studies do not typically include it)
   a. Is a theoretic framework identified?
   b. Does the framework support the hypothesis, research statement, or question?

3. Design or method
   a. Is the study design well-suited to the research problem?
      (1) Qualitative research is done to describe or explore phenomena and to gain understanding.
         (a) Characteristics—process-focused, subjective, and not generalizable
         (b) Types—descriptive, survey, phenomenology, content analysis
      (2) Quantitative research is done to describe relationships between variables, examine cause and effect, and identify facts.
         (a) Characteristics—outcome-focused, objective, may be generalizable
         (b) Types—quasiexperimental, experimental, correlational

b. Is the method adequate to answer the research question or phenomenon being studied?

4. Sampling
   a. Are criteria for participant selection clearly identified? For a qualitative study, was purposive sampling done?
   b. Is participant selection appropriate for the research purpose and method?
   c. Is the sample representative of a larger population?

5. Data collection
   a. Are data collection criteria and procedures clearly identified?
   b. Do data collection tools seem appropriate for research question and methodology?
   c. Are the tools valid and reliable, and is information about this clear?
   d. Is protection of human subjects (e.g., informed consent, protected health information) clearly addressed?
   e. For qualitative research, is data saturation described?

6. Data analysis—will differ depending on whether a qualitative or quantitative method is used
   a. Qualitative
      (1) Is the data analysis strategy compatible with the study purpose?
      (2) Are the findings presented in a manner that allows the reader to verify the researcher's theoretic conclusions?
      (3) Do the conclusions, implications, and recommendations reflect the findings of the study?
      (4) Would a quantitative approach be more appropriate?
   b. Quantitative
      (1) Does the report include the appropriate statistics?
      (2) Were the results of any statistical tests significant, and was this information adequately reported?
      (3) Could the study have been strengthened by including qualitative data?

7. Findings, implications, and recommendations
   a. Are important results presented, and is their interpretation consistent with the results?

b. Are specific limitations of the study presented?
c. Are identified implications appropriate, particularly as related to specified study limitations?
d. Are implications for nursing practice discussed?
e. Are specific recommendations for future research discussed?

XII. Questions to ask before implementing research findings into nursing practice:
   A. Are the results clinically significant and can they be generalized?
   B. Are the implementation strategies discussed by the researcher desirable and feasible in practice?
   C. Are institutional support and resources adequate to implement the study findings?
   D. Can the outcome of implementing study findings be measured?

XIII. Need for nurses to recognize barriers to implementation of EBP, which can be institutional or individual (Morgan, 2012)
   A. Lack of time during their work shift
   B. Insufficient knowledge or skills to do research
   C. Lack of support
   D. Limited access to information

XIV. Many resources available to nurses to gain knowledge and aid in implementing EBP, including the following:
   A. Information regarding nursing research priorities may provide potential sources of evidence identified by ONS and the National Institute of Nursing Research (NINR) (Table 44-1) (Berger et al., 2009; NINR, 2011)
   B. Cochrane Collaboration—http://www.cochrane.org
   C. Agency for Healthcare Research and Quality (AHRQ)—http://www.ahcpr.gov/
   D. National Guidelines Clearing House—http://www.guideline.gov/
   E. Online Journal of Knowledge Synthesis for Nursing—www.stti.iupui.edu
   F. Evidence-Based Healthcare Information—www.mlanet.org
   G. ONS Putting Evidence into Practice (20 resources designed to offer evidence-based interventions; e.g., for patient care and teaching, staff development)—http://www.ons.org/Research/PEP

Table 44-1

Nursing Research Priorities

National Institute of Nursing Research 2004 Priorities (NINR, 2011)	2009–2013 Research Agenda for Oncology Nursing (Berger, Cochrane, & Mitchell, 2009)
• Advance the science of health—promotion of health and quality of life and, simultaneously, contain costs • Promote health and prevent disease • Improve quality of life through better management of the symptoms of acute and chronic illness • Advance palliative and end-of-life care • Role of innovation and technology and information needs of patients, families, communities, and caregivers	• Health promotion—develop or test interventions to adopt or maintain health behaviors, or increase first-time or interval cancer screening (especially in underserved and understudied populations). • Cancer symptoms and side effects—in children and adults across cultures and ethnicities • Late effects of cancer treatment, long-term survivorship issues—develop or test interventions to minimize adverse outcomes and risks associated with development of comorbid illnesses. • End-of-life issues—develop knowledge about the mechanisms and management of symptoms in patients near end of life. • Psychological and family issues—design or test interventions to reduce negative and improve positive outcomes. • Nursing-sensitive patient outcomes—evaluate the effect of nursing care on promoting and maintaining treatment adherence. • Translation science—develop implementation science methods and techniques to improve clinical capacity to screen, assess, deliver effective interventions, and optimize oncology nursing care quality and outcomes.

Adapted from Berger, A.M., Cochrane, B., & Mitchell, S.A. (2009). The 2009-2013 research agenda for oncology nursing. *Oncology Nursing Forum, 36,* E274–E282; National Institute of Nursing Research. (NINR) (2011). *Strategic plan.* http://www.ninr.nih.gov/researchandfunding/grant-development-and-management-resources.

References

Berger, A. M., Cochrane, B., & Mitchell, S. A. (2009). The 2009-2013 research agenda for oncology nursing. *Oncology Nursing Forum, 36,* E274–E282.

Best, J. T., Frith, K., Anderson, F., Rapp, C. G., Rioux, L., & Ciccarello, C. (2011). Implementation of an evidence-based order set to impact initial antibiotic time intervals in adult febrile neutropenia. *Oncology Nursing Forum, 38,* 661–668.

Boucher, J., Underhill, M., Roper, K., & Berry, D. (2013). Science and practice aligned within nursing. Structure and process for evidence-based practice. *Journal of Nursing Administration, 43,* 229–234.

Brant, J. M., & Wickham, R. S. (Eds.). (2013). *Statement on the scope and standards of oncology nursing practice* (2nd ed.). Pittsburgh: Oncology Nursing Society.

Burns, N., & Grove, S. K. (2011). *Understanding nursing research* (5th ed.). Philadelphia: Elsevier.

Fawcett, J., & Garity, J. (2009). *Evaluating research for evidence-based nursing practice.* Philadelphia: F.A. Davis.

Green, S., Benedetti, J., Smith, A., & Crowley, J. E. (2012). *Clinical trials in oncology* (3rd ed.). Boca Raton, FL: Chapman & Hall/C.R.C.

Greenhalgh, T. (2010). *How to read a paper. The basics of evidence-based medicine* (4th ed.). Hoboken, NJ: Wiley-Blackwell.

Jacobs, L. A. (Ed.). (2002). *Standards of oncology nursing education: Generalist and advanced practice levels* (3rd ed.). Pittsburgh: Oncology Nursing Society.

Leufer, T., & Cleary-Holdforth, J. (2009). Evidence-based practice: Improving patient outcomes. *Nursing Standard, 23*(32), 35–39.

Mallory, G. A. (2010). Professional nursing societies and evidence-based practice: Strategies to cross the quality chasm. *Nursing Outlook, 58,* 279–286.

Melnyk, B., & Fineout-Overholt, E. (2005). *Evidence-based practice in nursing and healthcare: A guide to best practice.* Philadelphia: Lippincott: Williams and Wilkins.

Melnyk, B. M., Fineout-Overholt, E., Stillwell, S. B., & Williamson, K. M. (2009). Igniting a spirit of inquiry: An essential foundation for evidence-based practice. *American Journal of Nursing, 109*(11), 49–52.

Melnyk, B. M., Fineout-Overholt, E., Stillwell, S. B., & Williamson, K. M. (2010). The seven steps of evidence-based practice. *American Journal of Nursing, 110*(1), 51–53.

Morgan, L. A. (2012). A mentoring model for evidence-based practice in a community hospital. *Journal of Nurses Staff Development, 28*(5), 233–237.

National Institute of Nursing Research (NINR) (2011). *Strategic plan.* http://www.ninr.nih.gov/researchandfunding/grant-development-and-management-resources.

O'Grady, N. P., Alexander, M., Burns, L. A., Dellinger, P., Garland, J., & Saint, S. (2011). *Guidelines for the prevention of intravascular catheter-related infections, 2011.* http://stacks.cdc.gov/view/cdc/5916/.

Olsen, L., Aisner, D., & McGinnis, J. M. (2007). *IOM roundtable on evidence-based medicine. The learning healthcare system.* Retrieved June 21, 2013 from, http://www.nap.edu/catalog/11903.html.

Oman, K. S. (2003). Reading, understanding, and critiquing research reports. In K. S. Oman, M. E. Krugman, & R. M. Fink (Eds.), *Nursing research secrets* (pp. 37–45). Philadelphia: Hanley & Belfus.

Porter-O'Grady, T. (2010). Introduction to evidence-based practice in nursing and health care. In K. Malloch, & T. Porter-O'Grady (Eds.). *Quantum leadership: A resource for health care innovation.* (3rd ed., pp. 1–30). Sudbury, MA: Jones and Bartlett.

Schultz, M. (2012). Image of nursing: Influences of the present. In J. Zerwekh, & J. C. Claborn (Eds.), *Nursing today: Transitions and trends* (7th ed., pp. 173–189). St. Louis: Elsevier Saunders.

Spoelstra, S. L., Given, B. A., Given, C. W., Grant, M., Sikorskii, A., & Decker, V. (2013). An intervention to improve adherence and management of symptoms for patients prescribed oral chemotherapy agents. *Cancer Nursing, 36,* 18–28.

CHAPTER 45

Education Process

Diane G. Cope

OVERVIEW

I. Educational theory should provide the foundation for any formal (and many informal) educational interventions, whether they are aimed at an individual patient, staff, nurse, or community. Learning theories that can be useful for formulating teaching strategies in clinical practice are listed below. For others, see Olson & Hergenhahn (2009), Santrock (2008), Slavin (2009), and Syx (2008).

A. Behavioral learning theory (operant conditioning, classical conditioning) posits that learning is based on observable behaviors that are reinforced to increase the strength of the behavior (Braungart & Braungart, 2008; Miller & Stoeckel, 2011; Omrod, 2008). Examples of behavioral interventions are relaxation techniques, biofeedback, and visual imagery. Behavioral interventions are often used to help pediatric patients with cancer to cope with painful procedures; adult patients with cancer can use them to reduce stress, pain, and anxiety and to increase coping ability.

B. Cognitive learning theory describes the internal process that leads to learning (Braungart & Braungart, 2008; Miller & Stoeckel, 2011; Omrod, 2008; Watson & McKinstry, 2009). It requires attention, thought, and reasoning for information to be retrieved and applied. An example of cognitive learning is the creation of a mnemonic for symptoms that should trigger a phone call to the physician or other health care provider. A patient's ability to differentiate systemic from local treatment demonstrates cognitive learning.

C. Social learning theory describes learning that takes place based on watching and imitating others (Bandura, 1977). Three core concepts of social learning theory exist and include the following:
   1. Individuals can learn through observation.
   2. This process involves internal mental states and processing.
   3. Something that is learned does not always result in a change in behavior.

D. Motivational learning theory is concerned with the processes that describe why and how human behavior is activated and directed. Motivation can result from internal cues or drive (e.g., "I want to be here for my children, so I've got to stop smoking") or environmental (external) cues (e.g., "I have to stop smoking because my workplace has a nonsmoking policy and I hate sneaking out for a cigarette") that activate behavior (Pinto & Floyd, 2008).

E. Humanistic learning theory posits that that each individual is unique and all individuals have a desire to learn and grow in a positive manner. It is a learner-directed approach and is based on spontaneity, the importance of emotions and feelings, the right of individuals to make their own choices, and human creativity (Rogers, 1994). A patient expressing fear of dying and needing better coping mechanisms is an example of humanistic learning theory.

F. Adult learning theory (andragogy) describes the adult learner as someone who is self-directed, independent, and problem-centered (Knowles, 1970). Learning is based on past experience. An example of an adult learning experience would be an independent Internet search for information related to a new cancer diagnosis.

II. Patient education

A. Needs assessment (Kitchie, 2008; Miller & Stoeckel, 2011; Muma, 2012)
   1. Questions to be answered include the following:
      a. What does the patient know? The patient needs to be asked what he or she understands about the diagnosis, tests, treatment, needed self-care, and follow-up.
      b. What does the patient want to know? This may be different from what the nurse thinks the patient wants to know.
      c. Will any cultural or religious beliefs or practices affect the teaching or learning process (Bastable, 2008; Knoerl, Esper, & Hasenau, 2011; Kulwicki, 2009)? For example, alternative supplements may be a traditional

and important part of the patient's belief system, but these supplements may interfere with chemotherapy drugs.

   d. What language does the patient speak? If the nurse does not speak the same language, what is the alternative teaching plan (Miller & Stoeckel, 2011)? The availability of translators on site should be explored.

   e. Does the patient have a physical (e.g., hearing, vision, mobility, dexterity) or cognitive (e.g., stroke, confusion, somnolence) impairment that might impede learning?

   f. Does the patient have a preferred learning style (e.g., visual, aural, or kinesthetic—seeing, hearing, doing; global or analytic—big picture, component parts) (Inott & Kennedy, 2011)?

   g. What is the educational background of the patient?

2. Methods (Kitchie, 2008)

   a. Individual assessment involves specific questions such as the following: What is the most important thing you want to learn now? Will you be able to carry on your normal activities during chemotherapy treatments?

   b. Family or caregiver assessment. Are you able to assist the patient? What information do you want to learn to assist in your care?

   c. Community assessment before development of targeted patient education program or materials (Keller, Strohschein, & Briske, 2008; Miller & Stoeckel, 2011)

     (1) Survey or checklist

     (2) Interested party analysis

     (3) Interview and key informant

     (4) Focus group

3. Nursing diagnosis—based on the needs assessment; leads to the goals and objectives of teaching plan (Herdman, 2012).

B. Goals and objectives (also called *outcome criteria* or *outcome objectives*) (Heinrich, Molenda, Russell, & Smaldino, 2001; Miller & Stoeckel, 2011)

1. Goals

   a. SMART

     S—specific

     M—measureable

     A—attainable

     R—realistic

     T—timely

   b. Providing a global view of intended outcomes—for example, ability for self-care after discharge

2. Objectives (Bastable & Doody, 2014; Heinrich et al., 2001; Miller & Stoeckel, 2011)

   a. "Who" will do "what" by "when" and "to what extent" (effective objectives follow the ABCD rule):

     A—audience (who the learner is)

     B—behavior (what the learner is to do)

     C—condition (under what circumstances)

     D—degree (how much; to what extent the learner is to perform)

   b. Specific assessment criteria; for example, ability to state four foods with high iron content after reading information regarding foods with high iron content

C. Teaching plan—decisions involve the following:

1. Who will do the teaching (e.g., staff nurse, patient educator, patient-to-patient volunteer)?

2. How it will be taught, based on patient's preference, health literacy, and availability of alternative methods (e.g., one-on-one, group, demonstration and return demonstration, self-instruction activities, video, computer, print, combination)?

3. Preparing for teaching by reviewing evidence-based teaching practices in the literature (professional journal articles or recent textbooks), standards of care, and hospital procedure manuals and consulting experts (e.g., advanced practice nurses, physicians)

4. Organizing and practicing all teaching sessions before the actual teaching

5. Planning the teaching to coincide with a teachable moment when the learner might be most likely to be receptive to the message (e.g., smoking cessation in family members when a patient is diagnosed with lung cancer; self-care skills before discharge; cancer screening to coincide with a public awareness campaign)

D. Evaluation

1. Determination of ways to measure learning (e.g., learner explains in own words, return demonstration, quiz, behavior change)

2. Documentation of learning outcomes (e.g., patient can state the side effects of the medication; patient can demonstrate correct catheter care technique) on care plan, documentation form, or nursing notes

3. Reassessment and reinforcement of teaching and learning at next available opportunity

III. Family education—family members or significant others may have the same or different learning needs; addressing these learning needs especially important if the family member or significant other has a role in caring for the patient at home

A. Needs assessment with, or independent of, the patient

B. Identification of overlapping and separate needs

C. Obtaining patient's permission to include family in teaching (Health Insurance Portability and Accountability Act [HIPAA])

D. Scheduling teaching sessions when family can be available

E. Assessment of learning; reinforcement, as necessary

F. Documentation as indicated by needs and relationship with patient (e.g., caregiver)

IV. Staff education (Avillion, 2009)

A. Categories of staff learning needs assessment
   1. Orientation for new staff nurses
   2. Needs assessment, including individual needs, for all staff nurses
   3. Targeted needs assessment for learning objectives such as those related to critical events, new or revised policies or procedures, and new treatment

B. Methods for assessing staff learning needs
   1. Intuition (e.g., new staff nurses must understand hospital policies; staff nurses must be informed when nursing policies or procedures change)
   2. Self-assessment (e.g., nurses evaluate their own learning needs based on the type of patient for whom they will provide care; nurses identify learning needs based on interest)
   3. Diagnostic methods (e.g., nurses are tested for competence in specific areas; nurses are observed in practice)
   4. Performance analysis (e.g., information is obtained from quality improvement and incident reports; infection control data are analyzed)

C. Teaching plan
   1. Use of principles of adult learning (Knowles, 1970)
      a. Adults should understand why they must learn something.
      b. Adults should be self-directed.
      c. Teaching plan should consider prior learning and experience.
      d. Educators should create a learning environment and culture.
   2. Determination of objectives of teaching (e.g., nurse will demonstrate venipuncture technique; nurse will identify components of a patient's admission assessment)
   3. Determination of teaching method (e.g., class, one on one, print or computer, self-directed or teacher-directed, games and simulations, grand rounds, panels and seminars, case studies, webinars)
   4. Establishment of evaluation criteria (e.g., test, observation, dialogue, learner satisfaction, performance improvement, patient satisfaction)

V. Community education

A. Community health nursing
   1. Community can be defined geographically (e.g., New York City, state of Missouri), by ethnic or religious group (e.g., African Americans, evangelical Christians), and by interest or characteristics (e.g., sexual orientation, occupation), among many others.
   2. The role of the nurse in community health is defined by many organizations, including the American Nurses Association (http://www.ana.org), the American Public Health Association (http://www.apha.org), and state and local departments of health. Many definitions include the word "populations" as the target of nursing interventions.

B. Healthy People 2020—national priorities established by the U.S. Department of Health and Human Services (DHHS, 2010) to improve health and reduce health disparity

C. Models for health education and promotion (Millar & Warner, 2014)
   1. Models of individual health behavior
      a. Health belief model—states that people change behavior based on perceived susceptibility to a condition, its perceived severity, the perceived benefits to reducing risk behaviors, and the perceived barriers to reducing the risk (Miller & Stoeckel, 2011)
      b. Theory of reasoned action—proposes that variables such as demographics, attitudes, and personality traits affect health beliefs and motivations (Miller & Stoeckel, 2011)
      c. Social cognitive theory (Bandura, 1977) (see I.C. above)
   2. Models of community health behavior change
      a. PRECEDE-PROCEED—PRECEDE: Predisposing, Reinforcing, and Enabling Constructs in Educational Diagnosis and Evaluation, outlines a diagnostic planning process to assist in the development of targeted and focused public health programs; PROCEED: Policy, Regulatory, and Organizational Constructs in Educational and Environmental Development, guides the implementation and evaluation of the programs designed using PRECEDE (Green & Kreuter, 2005; Tramm, McCarthy, & Yates, 2012; Weir, McLeskey, Brunker, Brooks, & Supiano, 2011)
      b. Diffusion of innovations—identifies stages of change (awareness, interest, trial, decision, adoption) and places people on a continuum (innovators, early adopters, early majority, late majority, laggers) (Dearing, 2009); the

stages through which a technologic innovation passes are as follows:

(1) Knowledge (exposure to its existence, and understanding of its functions)
(2) Persuasion (the forming of a favorable attitude to it)
(3) Decision (commitment to its adoption)
(4) Implementation (putting it to use)
(5) Confirmation (reinforcement based on positive outcomes)

D. Community assessment
   1. Identification of pertinent information
      a. Descriptive data (e.g., demographics, history, ethnicity, values and beliefs, physical environment, health and social services)
      b. Illness prevalence data
      c. Health learning needs (e.g., human immunodeficiency virus [HIV] and acquired immunodeficiency syndrome [AIDS] prevention, smoking prevention in teens)
   2. Analysis of data
      a. Identification of common health problems (e.g., high incidence of heart disease, tuberculosis)
      b. Development of a community health diagnosis; for example, senior citizens at risk for social isolation because of lack of public transportation

E. Intervention
   1. Generally aimed at primary, secondary, or tertiary prevention
   2. Working with community (e.g., key informants, leaders, health care community, schools) to prioritize and develop interventions to meet health needs identified in assessment
   3. Plan implemented using community resources, advocates, and agencies

F. Evaluation
   1. Intervention is evaluated for impact on identified health need.
   2. Intervention may be modified for ongoing health needs. Is it cost-effective? Were objectives met? What are the long-term implications of continuing or not continuing the intervention?

References

Avillion, A. E. (2009). *Learning styles in nursing education: Integrating teaching strategies into staff development.* Marblehead, MA: HCPro.

Bandura, A. (1977). Self-efficacy: Toward a unifying theory of behavioral change. *Psychological Review, 84*(2), 191–215.

Bastable, S. B. (2008). Gender, socioeconomic, and cultural attributes of the learner. In S. Bastable (Ed.), *Nurse as educator: Principles of teaching and learning for nursing practice* (pp. 285–338). Sudbury, MA: Jones and Bartlett.

Bastable, S. B., & Doody, J. A. (2008). Behavioral objectives. In S. Bastable (Ed.), *Nurse as educator: Principles of teaching and learning for nursing practice* (pp. 384–427). Sudbury, MA: Jones and Bartlett.

Braungart, M. M., & Braungart, R. G. (2008). Applying learning theories to healthcare practice. In S. Bastable (Ed.), *Nurse as educator: Principles of teaching and learning for nursing practice* (pp. 51–89). Sudbury, MA: Jones and Bartlett.

Dearing, J. W. (2009). Applying diffusion of innovation theory to intervention development. *Research on Social Work Practice, 19*(5), 503–518. http://dx.doi.org/10.1177/1049731509335569.

Green, L. W., & Kreuter, M. W. (2005). *Health promotion planning: An educational and ecological approach* (4th ed.). New York: McGraw-Hill.

Heinrich, R., Molenda, M., Russell, J., & Smaldino, S. (2001). *Instructional methods and technologies for learning* (7th ed.). Englewood Cliffs, NJ: Prentice Hall.

Herdman, T. H. (Ed.). (2012). *International nursing diagnoses: Definitions and classification, 2012-2014.* Oxford, England: Wiley-Blackwell.

Inott, T., & Kennedy, B. B. (2011). Assessing learning styles: Practical tips for patient education. *Nursing Clinics of North America, 3*(46), 313–320.

Keller, L. O., Strohschein, S., & Briske, L. (2008). Population-based public health nursing practice: The intervention wheel. In M. Stanhope, & J. Lancaster (Eds.), *Public health nursing: Population-centered health care in the community.* (7th ed., pp. 187–214). St. Louis: Mosby Elsevier.

Kitchie, S. (2008). Determinants of learning. In S. Bastable (Ed.), *Nurse as educator: Principles of teaching and learning for nursing practice* (pp. 93–146). Sudbury, MA: Jones and Bartlett.

Knoerl, A. M., Esper, K. W., & Hasenau, S. M. (2011). Cultural sensitivity in patient health education. *Nursing Clinics of North America, 3*(46), 335–340.

Knowles, M. S. (1970). *The modern practice of adult education: From pedagogy to andragogy* (2nd ed.). New York: Adult Education Company.

Kulwicki, A. (2009). Culture and ethnicity. In P. A. Potter, & A. Perry (Eds.), *Fundamentals of nursing.* (7th ed., pp. 106–120). St. Louis: Mosby Elsevier.

Millar, D. J., & Warner, K. D. (2014). Health promotion: Achieving change through education. In J. A. Mender, C. Rector, & K. D. Warner (Eds.), *Community and public health nursing: Promoting the public's health* (8th ed., pp. 349–383). Philadelphia: Lippincott Williams and Wilkins.

Miller, M. A., & Stoeckel, P. A. (2011). *Patient education: Theory and practice.* Sudbury, MA: Jones and Bartlett.

Muma, R. D. (2012). An approach to patient education. In R. D. Muma, & B. A. Lyons (Eds.), *Patient education: A practical approach* (pp. 3–9). Sudbury, MA: Jones and Bartlett.

Olson, M. H., & Hergenhahn, B. R. (2009). *An introduction to theories of learning* (8th ed.). Englewood Cliffs, NJ: Pearson Education.

Omrod, J. E. (2008). *Human learning* (5th ed.). Englewood Cliffs, NJ: Pearson Education.

Pinto, B. M., & Floyd, A. (2008). Theories underlying health promotion interventions among cancer survivors. *Seminars in Oncology Nursing, 24*(3), 153–163. http://dx.doi.org/10.1016/j.soncn.2008.05.003.

Rogers, C. (1994). *Freedom to learn.* New York: Merrill.

Santrock, J. W. (2008). *A topical approach to life-span development* (4th ed.). Boston: McGraw-Hill.

Slavin, R. E. (2009). *Educational psychology theory and practice* (9th ed.). Upper Saddle River, NJ: Pearson Education.

Syx, R. L. (2008). The practice of patient education: The theoretical perspective. *Orthopaedic Nursing, 27*(1), 50–54.

Tramm, R., McCarthy, A., & Yates, P. (2012). Using the PRECEDE-PROCEED model of health program planning in breast cancer nursing research. *Journal of Advanced Nursing, 68*(8), 870–1880. http://dx.doi.org/10.111/j.1365-2648.2011.05888.

U.S. Department of Health and Human Services (DHHS). (2010). *Healthy people 2020.* http://www.healthypeople.gov/2020/default.aspx.

Watson, P. W. B., & McKinstry, B. (2009). A systematic review of interventions to improve recall of medical advice in healthcare consultations. *Journal of the Royal Society of Medicine, 102*(6), 235–243. http://dx.doi.org/10.1258/jrsm.2009.090013.

Weir, C., McLeskey, N., Brunker, C., Brooks, D., & Supiano, M. A. (2011). The role of information technology in translating educational interventions into practice: An analysis using the PRECEDE/PROCEED model. *Journal of the American Medical Information Association, 18*, 827–834. http://dx.doi.org/10.1136/amiajnl-2010-000076.

CHAPTER 46
Legal Issues

Julie Ponto

OVERVIEW

I. "Nursing requires specialized knowledge, skill, and independent decision making... because health care poses a risk of harm to the public if practiced by professionals who are unprepared or incompetent, professionals are governed by laws and rules designed to minimize the risk." (Russell, 2012)

II. Regulation of nursing practice
   A. State Boards of Nursing (BoN)—provide oversight of nursing practice by enforcing the State Nurse Practice Act to protect the health, welfare, and safety of the public
      1. State BoN typically have employed staff (e.g., executive officer, attorney, administrative staff) and appointed or elected representatives of various nursing groups (e.g., registered nurses, licensed practical or vocational nurses, advanced practice registered nurses)
      2. Membership, selection, and length of term of appointed or elected members are determined by the state and vary by state.
      3. Nurses can influence practice and policy by being active in the State BoN (e.g., appointed or elected member; attending public meetings of the BoN; communicating with BoN regarding issues important to cancer care and cancer nursing).
   B. Nurse Practice Acts—define nursing roles, titles, and scopes of practice; define educational program standards, requirements for licensure, and grounds for disciplinary action
   C. National Council of State Boards of Nursing (NCSBN)—develops the National Council Licensure for Registered Nurses (NCLEX-RN) examination, encourages consistency among state BoNs (e.g., provides model language for Nurse Practice Acts) (NCSBN, 2011)
   D. Definitions of regulatory terms
      1. Sources of law—laws governing practice come from a variety of sources, including statute
         a. Statute—"written law passed by Congress or state legislature and signed into law by the president or state governor" (NOLO, 2013)
         b. Common law—law based on court decisions and custom compared with legislative actions; often serves as the basis for malpractice litigation
      2. Administrative rule or regulation—a statement adopted by a government sanctioned agency (e.g., BoN) intended to make the law (e.g., Nurse Practice Act) more specific, or to explain the agency's organization or procedures
         a. Administrative rules relate to specific statutes and undergo a process allowing for public comment (Russell, 2012).
         b. Administrative rules have the force and effect of law once they are enacted.
   E. Categories of common BoN disciplinary cases in nursing practice (Russell, 2012)
      1. Practice related
      2. Drug related
      3. Boundary violations
      4. Sexual misconduct
      5. Abuse
      6. Fraud
      7. Positive criminal background checks
   F. Potential disciplinary actions by BoNs (Russell, 2012)
      1. Fine or civil penalty
      2. Referral to alternative-to-discipline program
      3. Public reprimand or censure
      4. Requirements for monitoring, remediation, education
      5. Limitation or restriction of practice
      6. Separation from practice (e.g., suspension, loss of license)

III. Patient's Bill of Rights in Health Care
   A. A variety of documents from national organizations and health care institutions outline

what consumers can expect from the healthcare environment.

B. The Affordable Care Act legislated a new set of patient's rights in the health care environment (Department of Health and Human Services [DHHS], 2012).

1. Provides coverage to Americans with pre-existing conditions
2. Protects consumers choice of doctors
3. Keeps young adults covered
4. Ends lifetime limits on coverage
5. Ends pre-existing condition exclusions for children.
6. Ends arbitrary withdrawals of insurance coverage.
7. Reviews premium increases.
8. Helps consumers get the most from their premium dollars.
9. Restricts annual dollar limits on coverage.
10. Removes insurance company barriers to emergency services.

C. Individuals who are hospitalized have the right to the following (American Hospital Association, 2003):

1. High quality hospital care
2. A clean and safe environment
3. Involvement in their care
4. Protection of their privacy
5. Help when leaving the hospital
6. Help with billing claims

IV. Standards of practice—outline nationally determined practice expectations for individuals or organizations; provide guidance for nurses, employers, and educators, and often used in legal situations to determine whether an individual or organization met what is regarded as the standard of care

A. Nursing professional practice standards

1. Nursing—scope and standards of practice (American Nurses Association [ANA], 2010a)
2. Guide to the code of ethics for nurses—interpretation and application (ANA, 2008)
3. Nursing's social policy statement—the essence of the profession (ANA, 2010b)

B. Oncology nursing standards of practice or position statements (Table 46-1)

1. Cancer pain management (Oncology Nursing Society [ONS], 2013a).

Table 46-1

Oncology Nursing Society Position Statements

Position Statement Title	Position Statement Description
Cancer pain management (ONS, 2013a).	This position statement addresses the essential nature of pain management in oncology nursing and includes the educational, ethical, legal, and socioeconomic components of pain management
Education of the RN who administers and cares for the individual receiving chemotherapy and biotherapy (ONS, 2012).	This position statement supports specialized education for nurses who administer chemotherapy and biotherapy and includes introductory and annual competence assessment and outlines the recommended components of oncology nursing chemotherapy or biotherapy education and competence assessment.
Lifelong learning for professional oncology nurses (ONS, 2013b).	This statement describes the importance of ongoing formal and informal education for oncology nurses to remain current in oncology knowledge and outlines a variety of methods for ongoing knowledge development and dissemination, including obtaining and maintaining oncology nursing certification, using novel education methods, and participating in a range of scholarly activities.
Oncology certification for nurses (ONS, 2013c).	This position statement describes the contribution of specialized oncology nursing certification to safe and effective cancer care. The statement describes the establishment of the Oncology Nursing Certification Corporation (ONCC) and the rigorous processes used by ONCC to demonstrate legally defensible and psychometrically sound examinations. The statement encourages nurses in oncology to be certified and employers to encourage oncology certification.
Palliative and end-of-life care (ONS, 2010).	This position statement describes the contribution of specialized oncology nursing certification to safe and effective cancer care. The statement describes the establishment of the ONCC and the rigorous processes used by ONCC to demonstrate legally defensible and psychometrically sound examinations. The statement encourages nurses in oncology to be certified and employers to encourage oncology certification.
2013 Updated American Society of Clinical Oncology/Oncology Nursing Society chemotherapy administration safety standards including standards for the safe administration and management of oral chemotherapy (Neuss et al., 2013).	This paper describes the recommended components of safe administration of enteral and parenteral chemotherapy including policies and procedures outlining staff training and continuing education, chemotherapy preparation, chemotherapy administration, and patient management guidelines.

2. Education of the RN who administers and cares for the individual receiving chemotherapy and biotherapy (ONS, 2012).
3. Lifelong learning for professional oncology nurses (ONS, 2013b).
4. Oncology certification for nurses (ONS, 2013c).
5. Palliative and end-of-life care (ONS, 2010).
6. 2013 Updated American Society of Clinical Oncology/Oncology Nursing Society chemotherapy administration safety standards, including standards for the safe administration and management of oral chemotherapy (Neuss et al., 2013)

C. Accreditation and certification agencies or programs for healthcare institutions
1. The Joint Commission (www.jointcommission.org)
2. National Patient Safety Goals (NPSG) (www.jointcommission.org)
3. Magnet Recognition Program (www.nursecredentialing.org/Magnet)
4. Occupational Safety and Health Administration (OSHA) (www.osha.gov)
5. Centers for Disease Control and Prevention (CDC) (www.cdc.gov)
6. Department of Health and Human Services (DHHS) (www.hhs.gov)
7. National Institutes of Health (NIH) (www.nih.gov)
8. Centers for Medicare and Medicaid (CMS) (www.cms.gov)
9. National Institute for Occupational Safety and Health (NIOSH) (www.cdc.gov/niosh)

D. Oncology-specific accreditation and certification agencies and programs
1. Oncology Nursing Certification Corporation (ONCC) (www.oncc.org)
2. American College of Surgeon – Commission on Cancer (ACS-COC) (www.facs.org/cancer/)
3. Quality Oncology Practice Initiative (QOPI) (www.qopi.asco.org)

V. Legal issues for individuals with cancer (Cancer Legal Resource Center [CLRC], 2010; Prince, 2011; Retkin, Antoniadis, Pepitone, & Duval, 2010; Sandel et al., 2010)
A. Advance directives
B. Bankruptcy—cancer survivors two times more likely to experience bankruptcy than the general public (Ramsey et al., 2013)
C. Competence for decision making
D. Disability insurance
E. Employment discrimination
F. Genetic discrimination
G. Hospital-acquired conditions (HACs) (Fife et al., 2010)
H. Human subjects research
I. Informed consent for chemotherapy (oral and parenteral)
J. Living wills
K. Organ and tissue donation
L. Privacy and confidentiality
M. Survivorship care planning
N. Time off from work (Family & Medical Leave Act [FMLA])
O. Withdrawing treatment—courts have consistently confirmed the right of both competent and incompetent individuals to receive or discontinue treatment (McGowan, 2011)

VI. Professional practice issues in oncology nursing with legal implications (Polovich, Whitford, & Olsen, 2009; Schulmeister, 2011)
A. Adverse drug events
B. Chemotherapy medication errors
C. Drug (substance) diversion
D. Electronic health record—ANA condones the involvement of RNs in the "product selection, design, development, implementation, evaluation and improvement of information systems and electronic patient care devices used in patient care settings" (ANA, 2009; Madison & Staggers, 2011)
E. Malpractice
F. Mandatory reporting (State regulations requiring nurses and other healthcare providers to report certain conditions or events [e.g. suspected child, sexual, domestic, or elder abuse, communicable diseases, death) (Black & Hawks, 2008)
G. Occupational and environmental hazards
H. Off-label drug or device use (Stafford, 2012)
I. Risk evaluation and mitigation strategies (REMS)
J. Scope of practice
K. Social media (Lambert, Barry, & Stokes, 2012; National Council of State Boards of Nursing [NCSBN], 2011)
L. Staff competence (e.g., chemotherapy administration, patient safety, preventing iatrogenic conditions)
M. Vesicant extravasation
N. Withholding and withdrawing life support
O. Workplace behavior and performance issues—lateral violence, bullying, verbal intimidation
1. Can range in severity from disruptive behaviors to assault
2. Currently no national workplace laws governing workplace bullying, but some state laws have established penalties for workplace bullying (Matt, 2012)

3. Occupational Safety and Health Administration (OSHA)—requires employers to provide a workplace free from hazards and recommends policies and procedures that reflect "zero-tolerance for all forms of violence from all sources" (OSHA, 2004)

4. Need for all staff to receive education and training to ensure a clear understanding of their role in situations involving lateral violence, bullying, and intimidation (Matt, 2012)

VII. Legislative policy issues affecting oncology care (ONS, n.d.; Robert Wood Johnson Foundation [RWJF], 2013)

A. Access to cancer care

B. Cancer and cancer care disparities

C. Cancer prevention and early detection

D. Costs of cancer care

E. Oncology drug shortages

F. Pain management

G. Risk evaluation and mitigation strategies (REMS)

H. Tobacco products

I. Workforce issues (e.g., aging workforce; diversity; practicing at the full scope of education and training; increasing number of baccalaureate-prepared nurses in the workforce to 80% by 2020 [National Academies of Science, 2010])

VIII. Legal liability terms and definitions (www.law.com)

A. Negligence—deviation from the acceptable standard of care that a reasonable person would use in a specific situation

B. Malpractice—deviation from a professional standard of care

C. Duty—care relationship between patient and provider

D. Breach of duty—failure to meet an acceptable standard of care

E. Defamation—the act of harming the reputation of another by making false statements to a third person

F. False imprisonment—a restraint of a person in a bounded area without justification or consent

G. Slander—a defamatory statement expressed in a transitory form, especially speech

H. Proximate cause—the cause that directly produces an event and without which the event would not have occurred

I. Civil—of or pertaining to private rights and remedies that are sought by action or suit, but distinct from criminal proceedings

J. Assault—the threat of, or use of, force on another that causes that person to have a reasonable apprehension of imminent harmful or offensive contact

IX. Common causes of litigation against nurses (Austin, 2010; Canadian Nurses Association [can] Healthpro & Nurses Service Organization, 2011)

A. Scope of practice issues

B. Inadequate or inappropriate patient assessment or monitoring

C. Inadequate or inappropriate treatment or care

D. Medication administration—errors of omission or commission

E. Failure to rescue

F. Inappropriate delegation—lack of consideration for delegating the right task, to the right person, at the right time, under the right circumstances, and providing the right supervision

G. Documentation deficiencies—contribute to many liability claims

X. Strategies for minimizing risk of malpractice or disciplinary action (Austin, 2010; Brous, 2012; Palatnik, 2012)

A. Development of skills in interpersonal communication—positive relationships with patients and families reduce the likelihood of a patient-family complaint.

1. Communicating clearly when educating patients and families

2. Listening carefully to family member questions and concerns

B. Maintaining knowledge and skills

1. Attending relevant continuing education programs

2. Obtaining specialty certification

3. Obtaining an advanced or graduate degree

4. Joining relevant professional associations (e.g., Oncology Nursing Society, Hospice and Palliative Nurses Association, American Society for Pain Management Nursing)

5. Becoming involved in advocacy initiatives with nursing professional organizations

C. Verifying that job description fits within state-defined scope of practice

D. Maintaining individual professional liability insurance—can protect a nurse beyond what employer policies may cover

E. Maintaining a "job well done" file—keeping letters of commendation, thank-you notes or cards from patients and family members, colleagues, and supervisors

F. Keeping list of community service activities which demonstrate civic mindedness (e.g., participation in cancer screening activities; teaching community basic life support classes; leading cancer support groups)

G. Maintaining positive relationship with supervisor—demonstrating willingness to contribute to the professional environment (e.g., serving on unit or institutional committees; leading journal club)

    1. Demonstrating effective follower behaviors (e.g., offering constructive feedback; participating in workplace decision-making; offering creative solutions to problems in the workplace)

  H. Keeping abreast of current regulatory and practice issues through state BoN

   I. Maintaining professional boundaries with patients

   J. Respecting physical limitations (e.g., fatigue related to rotating shifts, overtime)

XI. Role of documentation in reducing legal risks

  A. Written documentation—a "powerful communication tool" and also "provides evidence of the work of the nurse" (Jefferies, Johnson, & Griffiths, 2010)

  B. Can be used in legal disputes to determine whether a standard of care was met

  C. Seven essentials of quality nursing documentation revealed by a meta-analysis (Jefferies et al., 2010):

    1. Patient centered
    2. Contained the actual work of nurses including education and psychosocial support
    3. Written to reflect the objective clinical judgment of the nurse
    4. Presented in logical and sequential manner
    5. Written as events occur
    6. Reflected variances in the patient's condition (e.g., changes in patient response or nursing interventions)
    7. Fulfilled legal requirements

XII. Resources

  A. American Association of Legal Nurse Consultants—www.aalnc.org

  B. American Hospital Association—www.aha.org

  C. American Nurses Association—www.ana.org

  D. Cancer Legal Resource Center—www.disabilityrightslegalcenter.org/cancer-legal-resource-center

  E. National Cancer Legal Services Network—www.nclsn.org

  F. National Council of State Board of Nursing—www.ncsbn.org

  G. Oncology Nursing Society—www.ons.org

  H. Oncology Nursing Certification Corporation—www.oncc.org

   I. Quality Oncology Practice Initiative—www.qopi.asco.org

References

American Hospital Association. (2003). *The patient care partnership: Understanding expectations, rights and responsibilities.* Retrieved from the AHA website: http://www.aha.org/content/00-10/pcp_english_030730.pdf.

American Nurses Association. (2008). *Guide to the code of ethics for nurses: Interpretation and application.* Silver Spring, MD: ANA.

American Nurses Association. (2010a). *Nursing: Scope and standards of practice* (2nd ed.). Silver Spring, MD: ANA.

American Nurses Association. (2010b). *Nursing's social policy statement: The essence of the profession.* Silver Spring, MD: ANA.

Austin, S. (2010). Seven legal tips for safe nursing practice. *Nursing Critical Care, 5,* 15–20.

Black, J., & Hawks, J. H. (2008). *Medical-surgical nursing: Clinical management for positive outcomes* (8th ed.). St. Louis, MO: Elsevier Saunders.

Brous, E. (2012). Professional licensure protection strategies. *American Journal of Nursing, 112,* 43–47.

Canadian Nurses Association Healthpro and Nurses Service Organization. (2011). *Understanding Nurse Liability, 2006-2010: A Three-Part Approach.* Retrieved from NSO website: http://www.nso.com/nurseclaimreport2011.

Cancer Legal Resource Center (CLRC). (2010). *The HCP manual: A legal resource guide for oncology health care professionals.* Los Angeles: Cancer Legal Resource Center.

Department of Health and Human Services (DHHS). (2012). *Patient's bill of rights.* Retrieved from U.S. DHHS Healthcare.gov website: http://www.healthcare.gov/law/features/rights/bill-of-rights/.

Fife, C. E., Yankowsky, K. W., Ayello, E. A., Capitulo, K. L., Fowler, E., Krasner, D. L., et al. (2010). Legal issues in the care of pressure ulcer patients: Key concepts for healthcare providers – a paper from the International Expert Wound Care Advisory Panel. *Advances in Skin & Wound Care, 23,* 493–507.

Jefferies, D., Johnson, M., & Griffiths, R. (2010). A meta-study of the essentials of quality nursing documentation. *International Journal of Nursing Practice, 16,* 112–124. http://dx.doi.org/10.1111/j.1440-172X.2009.01815.x.

Lambert, K. M., Barry, P., & Stokes, G. (2012). Risk management and legal issues with the use of social media in the healthcare setting. *Journal of Healthcare Risk Management, 31,* 41–47.

Madison, M. P., & Staggers, N. (2011). Electronic health records and the implications for nursing practice (2011). *Journal of Nursing Regulation, 1,* 54–60.

Matt, S. B. (2012). Ethical and legal issues associated with bullying in the nursing profession. *Journal of Nursing Law, 15*(1), 9–13.

McGowan, C. M. (2011). Legal aspects of end-of-life care. *Critical Care Nurse, 31*(5), 64–69. http://dx.doi.org/10.4037/ccn2011550.

National Academies of Science. (2010). *The future of nursing: Leading change, advancing health. Committee on the Robert Wood Johnson Foundation Initiative on the Future of Nursing, at the Institute of Medicine.* Retrieved from National Academies Press: http://www.nap.edu/catalog.php?record_id=12956.

National Council of State Boards of Nursing (NCSBN). (2011). *White paper: A nurse's guide to the use of social media.* Retrieved from NCSBN website: https://www.ncsbn.org/Social_Media.pdf.

Neuss, M. N., Polovich, M., McNiff, K., Esper, P., Gilmore, T., LeFebvre, K. B., et al. (2013). 2013 Updated American Society of Clinical Oncology/Oncology Nursing Society chemotherapy administration safety standards including standards for the safe administration and management of oral chemotherapy. *Oncology Nursing Forum, 40,* 225–233.

NOLO. (2013). *Nolo's plain-English law dictionary.* Retrieved from NOLO website: http://www.nolo.com/dictionary/statute-term.html.

American Nurses Association. (2009). *Electronic health record: ANA position statement.* Retrieved from ANA website: http://nursingworld.org/MainMenuCategories/Policy-Advocacy/Positions-and-Resolutions/ANAPositionStatements/Position-Statements-Alphabetically/Electronic-Health-Record.html.

Oncology Nursing Society. (2010). *Palliative and end-of-life care.* Retrieved from ONS website: http://www.ons.org/Publications/Positions/EndOfLife.

Oncology Nursing Society. (2013a). *Cancer pain management.* Retrieved from ONS website: http://www.ons.org/Publications/Positions/Pain.

Oncology Nursing Society. (2013b). *Lifelong learning for professional oncology nurses.* Retrieved from ONS website: http://www.ons.org/Publications/positions/LifelongLearning.

Oncology Nursing Society. (2013c). *Oncology certification for nurses.* Retrieved from ONS website: http://www.ons.org/Publications/Positions/Certification.

Occupational Safety and Health Administration (OSHA). (2004). *Guidelines for preventing workplace violence for health care & social service workers.* http://www.osha.gov/Publications/OSHA3148/osha3148.html.

Oncology Nursing Society (n.d.). Legislative action center. Retrieved from Oncology Nursing Society website: http://www.ons.org/LAC.

Oncology Nursing Society. (2012). *Education of the RN who administers and cares for the individual receiving chemotherapy and biotherapy.* Retrieved from ONS website: http://www.ons.org/Publications/Positions/RNed.

Palatnik, A. M. (2012). Reducing your liability risk. *Nursing Critical Care, 7,* 4.

Polovich, M., Whitford, J. M., & Olsen, M. (Eds.), (2009). *Chemotherapy and biotherapy guidelines and recommendations for practice.* (3rd ed.). Pittsburgh, PA: Oncology Nursing Society.

Prince, A. (2011). The cancer legal resource center: A tool for oncology professionals. *Journal of the Advanced Practitioner in Oncology, 2,* 282–284.

Ramsey, S., Blough, D., Kirchhoff, A., Kreizenbeck, K., Fedorenko, C., Snell, K., et al. (2013). Washington State cancer patients found to be at greater risk for bankruptcy than people without a cancer diagnosis. *Health Affairs.* http://dx.doi.org/10.1377/hlthaff.2012.1263. Advance online publication.

Retkin, R., Antoniadis, D., Pepitone, D. F., & Duval, D. (2010). Legal services: A necessary component of patient navigation. *Seminars in Oncology Nursing, 29,* 149–155.

Robert Wood Johnson Foundation (RWJF). (2013). *Health policy.* Retrieved from Robert Wood Johnson Foundation website: http://www.rwjf.org/en/topics/rwjf-topic-areas/health-policy.html.

Russell, K. A. (2012). Nurse practice acts guide and govern nursing practice. *Journal of Nursing Regulation, 3,* 36–42.

Sandel, M., Hansen, M., Kahn, R., Lawton, E., Paul, E., Parker, V., et al. (2010). Medical-legal partnerships: Transforming primary care by addressing the legal needs of vulnerable populations. *Health Affairs, 29,* 697–1705.

Schulmeister, L. C. (2011). Legal issues. In C. H. Yarbro, D. Wujcik, & B. H. Gobel (Eds.), *Cancer nursing: principles and practice.* (7th ed.). Burlington, MA: Jones and Bartlett.

Stafford, R. S. (2012). Off-label use of drugs and medical devices: A review of policy implications. *Clinical Pharmacology & Therapeutics.* http://dx.doi.org/10.1038/clpt.2012.22. Advance online publication.

CHAPTER 47
Ethical Issues

Paula Nelson-Marten and Jacqueline J. Glover

I. Clinical ethics (Nelson-Marten & Braaten, 2008; Nelson-Marten & Glover, 2005)
   A. Ethical issues occur frequently in oncology nursing practice and will only increase as scientific and technologic advances are made and resources become more restricted
   B. An understanding of clinical ethics is important for the oncology nurse so that he or she can apply this knowledge in daily nursing practice and advocate for clients and families to enhance care and quality of life.
   C. The terms *morals* and *ethics* are often used interchangeably, but historically each term has a distinct meaning.
      1. Morals—taken from the Latin word *mores*, which means customs
         a. Personal values or rules that are based on an individual's upbringing, conscience, and cultural and religious beliefs
         b. Serves as a guide to individual moral choice and behavior
      2. Ethics—derived from the Greek term *ethos*, which means conduct, customs, and character
         a. The study or practice of intentionally and critically analyzing moral choices
         b. A process for deciding the best course of action when faced with conflicting choices; involves principles to guide rational deliberation and facilitate dialogue
   D. The American Nurses Association (ANA) Code of Ethics for Nurses with Interpretive Statements provides a framework for ethical nursing practice. The newest version (ANA, 2001) is available online at www.nursingworld.org.
      1. The ANA Code of Ethics makes the values of nursing explicit and describes the purpose of the code and the history of the development of the code.
      2. A guide to the Code of Ethics for Nurses, which includes cases to guide in the interpretation and application of the code, is also available. It is available at www.nursingworld.org.

   3. The nine provisions in the code with interpretative statements for each are as follows:
      a. Practices with compassion and respect
      b. Primary commitment is to the client
      c. Promotes health and safety
      d. Responsible for individual nursing practice
      e. Owes same duties to self as to others
      f. Establishes and maintains health care environments
      g. Advances the profession through practice, education, administration, and knowledge development
      h. Collaborates to meet health needs
      i. Responsible for maintaining the profession
II. Ethical knowledge base
   A. Ethical theories
      1. Ethical theories provide a vocabulary and an organizational framework to help assess moral behavior in particular circumstances.
      2. Ethical theories are not mutually exclusive claims to moral truths; rather, they are important but partial contributions to a comprehensive, although necessarily fragmented, moral vision (Steinbock, London & Arras, 2012).
   B. Two major types of ethical theories
      1. Utilitarianism—Jeremy Bentham (1748-1832) and John Stuart Mills (1806-1873) credited with this theory
         a. Holds that actions are right in proportion because they tend to promote happiness; actions are wrong if they tend to produce the reverse of happiness.
         b. Is a consequentialist theory in that it judges the appropriateness of an action by the consequence of what will happen if the action is or is not performed
      2. Deontologic theories (formalism)—based on a calculation of duties (the Greek word for duty is *deon*), rather than on consequences

a. Begins with the assumption that what makes an action better or worse is some intrinsic property of the action itself

b. Famous deontologic moral theorist Immanuel Kant (1724–1804)—the end never justifies the means; if you want to know if a proposed action is morally permissible, the right question to ask is not "What are the likely consequences?" but "Can I, as a rational agent, consistently will that everyone in a similar situation should act this way?" (similar to a universal golden rule); alternatively, "Is this action in accord with the requirement to treat other people as ends in themselves and not merely as means?"

C. Many approaches to health care ethics

1. Principle-based—exemplified in Beauchamp and Childress's *Principles of Biomedical Ethics* (Beauchamp & Childress, 2012)

a. Approach involves analyzing how the various principles apply to a given situation and determining how they should be balanced

b. Five core ethical principles identified:

(1) Respect for persons or respect for autonomy (self-rule)—honoring client confidences, practicing shared decision making, communicating honestly

(2) Nonmaleficence (not harming)—ensuring that anticipated treatment benefits outweigh any anticipated harms, offering only potentially therapeutic interventions

(3) Beneficence (promoting good)—acting in the best interests of others

(4) Justice (fairness)—allocating scarce resources fairly, abiding by institutional and insurance allocation policies

(5) Veracity—following the obligation to tell the truth

2. Casuistry—case-based approach to ethical decision making; exemplified in *Bioethics: An Introduction to the History, Methods and Practice,* 3rd edition (Jecker, Jonsen, & Pearlman, 2011)

3. Focuses on practical decision making in particular cases and uses paradigm cases for comparison and analysis

4. Ethics of care—exemplified in the works of Carol Gilligan and Nel Noddings (Gilligan, 1993; Noddings, 2003).

a. Emphasizes importance of focusing on the client in the context of his or her relationships; focuses on emotional commitment and a willingness to act unselfishly for the benefit of others; emphasizes sympathy, compassion, fidelity, discernment, and love; has its roots in a theologic ethic of love and, more recently, in some feminine or feminist writings (Tong, 1993)

5. Virtue-based ethics—exemplified in the ethics of Aristotle and Alistair MacIntyre (2007)

a. Emphasizes the goal of living a good life by the development of good character; emphasizes the agents who perform actions and make choices; presumes that morally appropriate decisions occur as a result of being decided by morally sensitive and skilled people; virtue theorists focus on education and development of the character of the agent making the decision

6. Narrative-based ethics—exemplified in the work of Sally Gadow (1999)

a. Puts emphasis on learning the client's story; client's illness is the telling of a story that requires empathy and compassion; narrative ethics can increase sensitivity to details of a "case" and help the nurse understand the ethical values involved

D. Framework for ethical decision making (Scanlon & Glover, 1995) (Box 47-1)

E. Ethics committees

1. Most hospitals and many nursing homes, long-term care organizations, and hospices have a designated committee to help professionals, patients, and families address ethical issues.

a. The Joint Commission (TJC) now includes standards that require a "mechanism" to address ethical issues (TJC, n.d.).

2. Three functions of an ethics committee (Hester & Schonfeld, 2012)

a. Case consultation

b. Policy development

c. Education

3. Core competencies for health care ethics consultation (American Society for Bioethics and Humanities [ASBH], n.d.)

III. Oncology nursing clinical practice issues requiring an ethical perspective

A. Communication

1. Communication is a two-way process. Nurses need to be effective listeners as well as effective communicators of information.

2. Nurses should pay close attention to indirect communication (body language). Approximately 80% of communication is of a nonverbal nature.

Box 47-1

Framework for Ethical Decision Making

Step 1—Ethical question(s), "should" questions such as "Who should decide?" "What should they do?"

Step 2—Gut check; what is your first reaction to this case? What is your gut telling you to do on an "emotive" level?

Step 3—What are the known clinically relevant facts? What facts do you need to gather?

Step 4—What are the values at stake for all the relevant parties?

What are values? Many people use the terms *values* and *principles* interchangeably. We use values in this framework to broaden the scope of ethical "content" to include other actions or traits of character that promote the good, are good, or are otherwise meant to describe actions that are right. In addition to the four principles (Respect for Autonomy, Beneficence, Nonmaleficence, and Justice), examples of other values include veracity (truth telling), fidelity (keeping promises), respect for life, privacy, confidentiality, integrity, family relationships, compassion, kindness, health care relationships, trust, courage, and generosity.

Step 5—What could you do? List all options.

Step 6—What should you do? Make a choice among the options listed in step 5, and include a description of how you would actually do it (the process).

Step 7—Justify your choice; give reasons to support your choice. Refer back to the values in step 4. Anticipate objections and respond to them.

Step 8—How could this ethical issue have been prevented? Would any policies, guidelines, or practices be useful in changing any systemic problems?

Adapted from Scanlon, C., & Glover, J. J. (1995). A professional code of ethics: Providing a moral compass in turbulent times. *Oncology Nursing Forum, 22*(10), 1515–1521.

3. Shared decision making between health care professionals and clients requires open and ongoing communication about all aspects of client health care.

4. Nurses have an obligation to communicate honestly with clients (principle of veracity in the ANA Code of Nursing Ethics (ANA, 2001).

5. Communicating bad news (Buckman, 1992)
   a. Definition—any news that will potentially, drastically, and negatively alter a client's view of his or her future
   b. Buckman's six-step protocol
      (1) Step 1—getting started, getting the physical context right, where the meeting is held, and having the right people there
      (2) Step 2—finding out how much the client knows
      (3) Step 3—finding out how much the client wishes to know
      (4) Step 4—sharing the information; aligning and educating
      (5) Step 5—responding to the client's feelings
      (6) Step 6—Planning and follow-through

6. Nurse's role in communication
   a. Being an advocate for the client in discussions or decisions that may affect the client's health and well-being; showing sensitivity and support for the client who is receiving "bad" news
   b. Concurrently, being supportive of the work of the interdisciplinary team caring for the client and work to facilitate "open," honest communication (unless the client wishes "not to know" or a cultural imperative exists)

B. Confidentiality and privacy issues
   1. Confidentiality and privacy are values related to the ethical principle of autonomy. They both play important roles in providing respect and autonomy for persons.
   2. Confidentiality includes protecting a client's information that is critical in the health care context but should not be revealed outside this context.
   3. Privacy refers to protection of the client from having to reveal personal information that is not needed in the health care context. Privacy also includes protection of a client from viewing by others.
   4. Confidentiality and privacy requirements were emphasized in the 1996 federal law—Health Insurance Portability and Accountability Act (HIPAA, 1996). HIPAA requires the protection and confidential handling of protected health information (PHI).
   5. What does this law mean for nursing? It means that a client's health information is to be kept confidential and protected (PHI); only the minimum information necessary to provide appropriate care for the patient is to be shared. PHI relates to the sharing of a person's information in all forms— electronic, by phone, written, and verbally (HIPAA, 1996).

C. Cultural assessment—the nurse's role
   1. Everyone has a personal culture. A health care professional culture also exists.
   2. Culture plays an important role in the values, beliefs, and behaviors of individuals. These values, beliefs, and behaviors are often demonstrated when one is ill.

3. Knowing how and when to do a cultural assessment is important for the nurse.

4. Arthur Kleinman, a physician and medical anthropologist at Harvard University, developed an "explanatory model of illness" to elicit a client's perspective of his or her illness. The model includes eight questions to ask a client with the goal of learning beliefs about illness from a cultural perspective (Kleinman, 1988; Kleinman & Benson, 2006).

5. Another term may need to be substituted for *sickness*. The eight questions are as follows:
   a. What do you call the problem?
   b. What do you think has caused the problem?
   c. Why do you think it started when it did?
   d. What do you think that the sickness does?
   e. How severe is the sickness? Will it have a short or long course?
   f. What kind of treatment do you think you (or the patient, if asking a family member) should receive? What are the most important results you hope to receive from this treatment?
   g. What are the chief problems that the sickness has caused?
   h. What do you fear most about the sickness?

6. What should the nurse do with the cultural knowledge that is learned? The nurse should use the knowledge in being an advocate for the client through inclusion of the client's cultural assessment or knowledge by way of the following:
   a. Communication with the health care team
   b. Documentation in the client's medical records
   c. Including the family, significant others, as appropriate, in client's care or goals for care
   d. Obtaining an interpreter
   e. Providing education materials in the client's language

7. Increasing one's own cultural competence should be a continuous process (National Center for Cultural Competence, http://nccc.georgetown.edu, n.d.)

D. Informed consent—both an ethical and a legal consideration; all major ethical principles, autonomy, beneficence, nonmaleficence, justice, and veracity play an important role.

1. Definition—an ethical and legal concept that requires the health care professional to provide sufficient information regarding the client's condition and recommended treatments or interventions, including benefits, risks, and alternatives, that enable the client to make an informed decision to accept or reject proposed recommendations

2. What constitutes an informed decision—open to interpretation by all parties to the situation; what constitutes informed varies by individual values, beliefs, and culture
   a. Reasonable person standard—disclosure of what an ordinary person in the client's position would consider significant in deciding whether or not to consent to the procedure or treatment
   b. Subjective standard—what a particular client may need or want to know to make a decision

3. Purpose of informed consent
   a. To enable autonomous choice
   b. To promote good client care as defined by the client
   c. To protect client from harm
   d. To ensure responsible health care professional actions
   e. To avoid exploitation
   f. To encourage self-scrutiny by health care professionals

4. Elements of informed consent
   a. Decision-making capacity
      (1) Decision maker must possess a set of values and goals and the ability to do the following:
         (a) Understand information and communicate.
         (b) Reason and deliberate concerning one's choices.
      (2) Decision-making capacity may be determined by a member of the health care team familiar with the process, including the nurse.
      (3) Decision-making capacity is not absolute or permanent. Decision-making capacity is often task-specific.
      (4) Loss of decision-making capacity may be situational and may be related to medication use, anesthesia, or numerous types of medical procedures and may be caused by the current health state.
      (5) Clients experiencing depression, other mental illness, dementia, or chronic illnesses or disabilities may have decision-making capacity; assessment of capacity needs determination on an individual basis.
   b. Competency differs from capacity to make decisions. Decision-making capacity is a clinical judgment. Determining competency or incompetency is done by a court.

5. Barriers to obtaining informed consent
   a. Inadequate time allowed for discussion and decision making
   b. Failure to access the client's understanding and to improve knowledge as needed
   c. Failure to acknowledge uncertainty
   d. Framing information so that biases are present or the client is pressured to decide
   e. Language or cultural barriers
   f. Client's altered level of consciousness— confusion, disorientation, experiencing side effects of medications, and effects of illness or disease process
   g. Failure to address vulnerability—for example, feelings of loss of control, loss of power, and fear of situation, or helplessness
6. Exceptions to the requirement to obtain informed consent
   a. In an emergency—consent implied in an emergency if immediate threat to the client's life or permanent functioning exists
   b. Waiver of consent—client waives his or her right to disclosure and authorizes someone else to receive the information
   c. Legal requirements—for example, police orders for alcohol levels or statutory requirements for screening
   d. Therapeutic privilege (rarely, if ever, justified)—withholding of information based on possible harm that may occur by giving information to the client
7. Role of the oncology nurse in informed consent
   a. Disclosure—physicians, advanced practice nurses (APNs), or both responsible for explaining medical treatments and procedures
      (1) Knowing what was said— reinforcing and clarifying information presented
      (2) Notifying physician or APN if not able to validate the client's understanding
      (3) Informing physician or APN of possible medication administration that may interfere with the client's comprehension
      (4) Confirming documentation of informed consent in the medical record
   b. Advocacy—be an advocate for the client and family in relation to informed consent; soliciting client's value system; respecting client's right to choose; assessing anxiety or ambivalence related to the procedure or treatment; and ensuring client confidentiality; actively addressing any intervention, act, or policy that has the potential to violate the client's rights
   c. Presence—nurse must be aware of his or her own value system, beliefs, and biases and consider these when working with client decision making, informed consent, or both; may need to ask to be relieved of care for the client if his or her values, beliefs, and biases would impede the provision of quality care

IV. Issues in clinical research for the oncology nurse (Nelson-Marten & Glover, 2005; National Cancer Institute [NCI], 2012)
   A. Oncology nurses may find themselves caring for clients who are involved in either research studies or clinical trials. Good nursing care requires knowledge of the ethical issues inherent in these studies. The nurse's first obligation is to care for the client but he or she may also have obligations to the research study or clinical trial. These obligations can result in a balancing act (NCI, 2012).
   B. Clinical trials are research studies that are conducted to gain new knowledge for the benefit of future clients; the client involved in the trial may or may not receive benefit.
      1. Considerations for the oncology nurse
         a. Do you understand the purpose(s) of the study, potential side effects, and outcomes for your client or patient?
         b. Will you be comfortable answering questions that the patient or family may have?
         c. Has the patient met with the research or clinical trials' physician or nurse? Does the patient understand his or her role in the trial and potential side effects and outcomes?
         d. Has the patient signed an informed consent document?
      2. Potential risks of a clinical trial
         a. Side effects that were not expected or that are worse than standard care
         b. New drugs or therapies may not be superior to standard care.
         c. The trial being randomized and the participant not being able to choose a study arm
         d. Insurer and drug company not covering all of the involved costs
         e. Involvement requiring more health care visits than standard care
         f. The trial being the "last treatment option"—if the study or trial does not offer a potential benefit, the participant may be faced with the need to decide on palliative and end-of-life care.
      3. Potential benefits of a clinical trial
         a. Access to a new drug or therapy may be only available in the research study or clinical trial.

b. The new drug or therapy may be more effective than standard care.

c. The participant may benefit from the drug or therapy under study.

d. The participant may receive more health care attention than standard care provides.

C. Role of the oncology nurse in assisting with a research study or clinical trial

1. Advocating for the client and family for issues related to the study or trial and participation

2. Ensuring that informed consent is obtained and documented

3. Maintaining current knowledge of the treatment and interventions

4. Assessing and documenting the client's response to the treatment or intervention

5. Assisting the client in managing symptoms

6. Providing physical, psychological, and spiritual care, as needed

7. Ensuring confidentiality and anonymity

8. Being present or offering support for client and family needs to communicate thoughts or feelings regarding the study or trial and/or personal responses to the study or trial

D. Ethical considerations in research studies or clinical trials

1. Belmont Report (n.d.)—outlined ethical principles and guidelines for the protection of human subjects in research. The report described the principles and how they are meant to protect the research participant. This report led to the federal government's mandate that meeting Institutional Review Board (IRB) and informed consent guidelines be a prerequisite before conducting either research studies or clinical trials (http://www.hhs.gov/ohrp/archive/irb/irb_introduction.htm).

2. Three ethical principles involved—respect for persons, beneficence, and justice

3. Need for oncology nurse to be familiar with the Belmont Report—how the three ethical principles relate to his or her role in client protection and use of the principles

V. Ethical issues in palliative care and end-of-life care

A. Distinction among curative care, palliative care, and end-of-life care is important; confusion of terms may lead to potential ethical issues for clients and families (Beltran & Coluzzi, 1997; Center to Advance Palliative Care [CAPC], 2013).

1. Curative care—type of care typically given by the U.S. health care system

a. Primary goal—reversal of the disease process and to prolong life; cure, if possible

b. Secondary goal—symptom management

2. Palliative care—"specialized medical care for people with serious illnesses"; "focused on providing patients with relief from the symptoms, pain, and stress of a serious illness—whatever the diagnosis. The goal is to improve quality of life for both the patient and the family" (CAPC, 2013).

a. Good symptom management is the cornerstone of palliative care.

b. Active palliative care may include curative goals with the goal of restoration rather than cure (Beltran & Coluzzi, 1997).

3. End-of-life care—the type of care given at the end of life is "comfort care," sometimes referred to as *palliative care*; the term *palliative care* used in this way refers to comfort care.

a. Comfort care is best delivered through a hospice setting.

b. Primary goal is symptom control or comfort and psychosocial and spiritual support.

c. Secondary goal is providing a "good death" for the client and support for the family.

B. Advance directives—since the passage of the federal Patient Self-Determination Act (PSDA), effective December 1, 1991, all health care institutions receiving federal funds are required to give clients written information about their right to participate in their own health care decisions and to complete advance directives (PSDA, 1994).

1. Role of the nurse

a. Educating the client and family regarding the use of advance directives

b. Referring the client to an appropriate resource for initiating an advance directive

c. Ensuring that the health care team is aware of the existence and content of advance directives

2. Living will

a. Written document that directs a person's physician to withhold or withdraw life-prolonging interventions (e.g., cardiopulmonary resuscitation [CPR], kidney dialysis, feeding tubes, breathing machines) if he or she is terminally ill or (in some states) permanently unconscious

b. Instructs person's physician to provide only those treatments that will relieve pain and provide comfort

c. Differing state laws regarding when a living will is valid and what provisions are acceptable; some states require special documentation of desires related to the medical provision of hydration and nutrition; information and forms from all 50 states available from the National Hospice and Palliative Care Organization (http://www.caringinfo.org)

Part 9

3. Medical power of attorney
   a. Written document that allows a person to name another individual to make health care decisions for him or her if he or she is unable to make them
   b. Special state provisions about what kinds of decisions a medical power of attorney representative can make and under what circumstances; information and forms from all 50 states available from the National Hospice and Palliative Care Organization (http://www.caringinfo.org)
C. Do not attempt resuscitation (DNAR) orders
   1. A physician's order not to perform cardiopulmonary resuscitation (CPR) in the event that a client's pulse, respirations, or both cease
   2. DNARs considered by some to be a kind of advance directive because clients must indicate their wishes before CPR is necessary; however, DNARs are different in that they are physicians' orders and must be written by a physician, based on the values and preferences of the client as expressed by a client with capacity or his or her legal representative.
   3. Many states laws allow for out of hospital DNARs, which are respected by emergency medical professionals.
   4. Critical to discuss goals of treatment with clients with potentially life-limiting illnesses; CPR an important, but not the only, part of this discussion; provision of all therapies to be guided by the client's values, goals, and preferences
D. Physician Orders for Life-Sustaining Treatment (POLST) paradigm—more extensive physician order sets to direct treatment in some states (http://polst.org, n.d.)
   1. These forms useful for some clients to have their actual wishes documented in the form of physicians' orders that are transportable among health care settings; not for everyone, but only for clients who have a need for standing medical orders
   2. Role of the nurse with regard to DNARs and POLST forms
      a. Ensuring that a clear understanding exists among physicians, clients, and family members regarding CPR and other scope of treatment orders
      b. Promoting values—driving decision making throughout treatment by encouraging clients and family members to communicate openly with the health care team
      c. Ensuring proper documentation and appropriate renewal procedures of DNARs

and POLST orders according to institutional policies
      d. Respecting cultural values regarding death and dying
      e. Validating emotional responses of clients and family members to resuscitation and other scope of treatment orders
      f. Referring the client and family to other appropriate resources (spiritual care, social work, other support services)
      g. Being an advocate for the client and the family
VI. Ethics and the oncology nurse in palliative and end-of-life care (ANA, 2001; Nelson-Marten & Glover, 2005)
A. The oncology nurse needs to be aware of potential ethical issues in end-of-life care, be able to weigh benefits and burdens of particular treatments, and take into consideration the client's beliefs, values, and preferences. The nurse needs to separate out his or her beliefs and not allow them to influence the nursing care he or she provides
B. Potential ethical issues may arise with the following:
   1. Extraordinary versus ordinary care—distinguishing between treatments morally required and treatments that are extraordinary or optional based on burden to the client and family
   2. Withholding versus withdrawing—no ethical or legal distinction between these two terms and corresponding categories of therapies
   3. Requests for palliative sedation—appropriate for cases of extreme suffering—that is, having pain and other types of suffering
   4. Requests to relieve extreme suffering and the principle of double effect
C. The ANA has published several position statements related to ethics and end-of-life care. The oncology nurse should refer to and use the position statements for guidance when ethical issues arise in caring for clients.
   1. Euthanasia, assisted suicide, and aid in dying—approved in April 2013
   2. Foregoing nutrition and hydration—revised in March 2011
   3. Nursing care and do not resuscitate (DNR) orders and allowing natural death decisions—revised in March 2012
   4. Registered nurses' roles and responsibilities in providing expert care and counseling at the end of life—approved in June 2010
VII. Ethical issues in pediatric oncology
A. Parents are usually regarded as the appropriate decision makers for their infants and children with cancer (Committee on Bioethics of the American Academy of Pediatrics, 1995).

1. The appropriate framework for decision making is the best interest standard.
   a. *Best interest* refers to the balancing of potential benefits with potential harms in a decision to promote the well-being of infants and children with cancer.
   b. It is a calculus of what can be done (and the likelihood that it can happen) with what the infant or child has to go through in terms of risks (and their likelihood).
2. The presumption is that older children and adolescents should be involved in decisions to the extent that they would want to be involved.
   a. Families differ in the extent that they involve their older children and adolescents in decisions of all kinds, and health care decision making is particularly difficult.
   b. Health care professionals should work with families who are reluctant to share information and involve older children and adolescents who want to be informed and involved.
   c. Health care professionals should work with families who want to involve them in deceiving older children and adolescents. Truth telling and trust are central values and should be respected.
3. The literature in pediatric advance care planning is emerging (Hammes, Klevan, Kempf, & Williams, 2005).
4. Sometimes health care professionals may believe that family decisions are harming their infants, children, and adolescents.
   a. Conflicts among members of the team or between the team and the family can be emotionally charged. Collaboration among all team members is critical. Resolving conflict with the family regarding their decisions may involve intensive work on the part of one or more members of the health care team (e.g., with the nurse, social worker, and chaplain).
   b. Children not only belong to their families, they are also members of the broader community. Health care professionals have independent obligations to promote the welfare of the infants, children, and adolescents in their care. A classic example is when a child requires a blood transfusion to survive or prevent further health decline. The health care team believes that the transfusion should be given and the parents of the child refuse for whatever reason, such as religious beliefs. In this situation, the health care team has an ethical obligation to promote what is best for the child's welfare.

   c. When efforts to negotiate with families about treatment choices fail, it may be appropriate to seek state intervention through a court order for treatment. This is a last resort and should only be attempted in the following circumstances (Diekema, 2004):
      (1) Significant risk for serious harm
      (2) Imminent harm
      (3) Intervention that the parents have refused as being necessary to prevent serious harm
      (4) Intervention that the parents have refused as being of proven efficacy
      (5) Benefits and likely burdens of providing the intervention significantly more favorable than the option chosen by the parents
      (6) No other options that would prevent serious harm and are less intrusive and more acceptable to the family
      (7) State intervention in this case can be generalized to other similar situations.
      (8) Agreement of most parents that state intervention is reasonable in this particular situation
B. Pediatric oncology research
   1. Separate regulations exist for research with children, who are defined as a vulnerable population.
      a. Risks must be minimal or a moderate increase over minimal risk.
      b. *Minimal risk* means that the probability and magnitude of harm or discomfort anticipated in the research is not greater in and of themselves than those ordinarily encountered in daily life or during the performance of routine physical or psychological examinations or tests.
      c. Parents or guardians provide consent (Eder, Yamokoski, Wittmann, & Kodish, 2007).
      d. Children who are capable must provide consent.
   2. Children are a vulnerable population, the benefits of the research should outweigh the risks, and risk should be minimized. However, research is necessary as a matter of justice, because children are not little adults and have unique treatment needs.

References

American Nurses Association. (2001). *Code of Ethics for nurses with interpretative statements.* http://www.nursingworld.org.

American Society for Bioethics and Humanities (ASBH). (n.d.). *Core competencies for health care ethics consultation.* http://www.asbh.org.

Beauchamp, T. L., & Childress, J. F. (2012). *Principles of biomedical ethics* (7th ed.). New York: Oxford University Press.

Belmont Report. Retrieved from http://www.hhs.gov/ohrp/archive/irb/irb_introduction.htm.

Beltran, J. E., & Coluzzi, P. H. (1997). Medical ethics: A model for comprehensive palliative care. *The Talbert Journal of Health Care, Spring/Summer,* 47–57.

Buckman, R. (1992). *How to break bad news: A guide for healthcare professionals.* Baltimore: John Hopkins University Press.

Center to Advance Palliative Care (CAPC). (2013). *Building a hospital-based palliative care program.* http://www.capc.org/building-a-hospital-based-palliative-care-program/.

Committee on Bioethics, American Academy of Pediatrics. (1995). Informed consent, parental permission, and assent in pediatric practice. *Pediatrics, 95,* 314–317.

Diekema, D. S. (2004). Parental refusals of medical treatment: The harm principle as threshold for state intervention. *Theoretical Medicine and Bioethics, 25*(4), 243–264.

Eder, M. L., Yamokoski, A. D., Wittmann, P. W., & Kodish, E. D. (2007). Improving informed consent: Suggestions from parents of children with leukemia. *Pediatrics, 19,* e849–e859.

Gadow, S. (1999). Relational narrative: The postmodern turn in nursing ethics. *Scholarly Inquiry for Nursing Practice, 13*(1), 57–70.

Gilligan, C. (1993). *In a different voice: Psychological theory and women's development.* Boston: Harvard University Press.

Hammes, B. J., Klevan, J., Kempf, M., & Williams, M. S. (2005). Pediatric advance care planning. *Journal of Palliative Medicine, 8,* 766–773.

Health Insurance Portability and Accountability Act (HIPAA). (1996). Public Law No. 104-191.

Hester, D. M., & Schonfeld, T. (2012). *Guidance for healthcare ethics committees.* Cambridge: Cambridge University Press.

Jecker, N. S., Jonsen, A. R., & Pearlman, R. A. (2011). *Bioethics: An introduction to the history, methods and practice* (3rd ed.). Boston: Jones and Bartlett.

Kleinman, A. (1988). *The illness narratives: Suffering, healing, and the human condition.* New York: Basic Books.

Kleinman, A., & Benson, P. (2006). Anthropology in the clinic: The problem of cultural competency and how to fix it. *PLoS Medicine, 3*(10), 1673–1676.

MacIntyre, A. C. (2007). *After virtue: A study in moral theory* (3rd ed.). Notre Dame, Indiana: University of Notre Dame Press.

National Cancer Institute. (2012). *A balancing act: Nursing and ethics in clinical trials.* http://www.cancer.gov/ncicancerbulletin/072412/page6.

National Center for Cultural Competence. (n.d.). http://nccc.georgetown.edu.

Nelson-Marten, P., & Braaten, J. S. (2008). Advance directives, end-of-life decisions, and ethical dilemmas. In R. A. Gates, & R. M. Fink (Eds.), *Oncology nursing secrets* (3rd ed., pp. 619–630). St. Louis: Mosby/Elsevier.

Nelson-Marten, P., & Glover, J. (2005). Ethical considerations. In M. E. Langhorne, J. S. Fulton, & S. E. Otto (Eds.), *Oncology nursing* (5th ed., pp. 648–658). St. Louis: Mosby/Elsevier.

Noddings, N. (2003). *Caring: A feminine approach to ethics and moral education* (2nd ed.). Berkeley, CA: University of California Press.

Patient Self-Determination Act (PSDA). (1994). Public Law No. 101–508, '4206, 4751 (hereinafter OBRA) 104 Stat. 1388–115 to 117, 1388–204 to 206 (codified at 42 U.S.C.A. '1395 cc(f) (l) & id'.1396a(a) (West Supp. 1994).

Physician orders for life-sustaining treatment (POLST). (n.d.) *More extensive physician order sets to direct treatment in some states.* http://polst.org.

Scanlon, C., & Glover, J. J. (1995). A professional code of ethics: Providing a moral compass in turbulent times. *Oncology Nursing Forum, 22*(10), 1515–1521.

Steinbock, B., London, A. J., & Arras, J. D. (2012). *Ethical issues in modern medicine: Contemporary readings in bioethics* (8th ed.). New York: McGraw-Hill.

The Joint Commission (TJC). (n.d.). http://www.jointcommission.org.

Tong, R. (1993). *Feminine and feminist ethics.* Belmont, CA: Wadsworth.

CHAPTER 48

Professional Issues

Darlena D. Chadwick and Lani Kai Clinton

QUALITY IMPROVEMENT

I. Impact of medical errors
   A. Approximately 200,000 people die in hospitals each year as a result of medical errors that could have been prevented (Andel, Davidow, Hollander, & Moreno, 2012).
   B. Financial cost of medical errors is estimated to be $19.5 billion annually from expenses of additional care, lost income, and disability.
   C. Nonfinancial costs of medical errors include loss of trust in the health care system, low morale in hospital employees, and lower levels of health in the general population.

II. Types of errors
   A. Diagnostic
      1. Error or delay in diagnosis
      2. Failure to use indicated tests
      3. Use of outmoded tests or therapy
      4. Failure to act on results of monitoring or testing
   B. Treatment
      1. Error in the performance of an operation, procedure, or test
      2. Error in administering the treatment
      3. Error in the dose or method of using a drug
      4. Avoidable delay in treatment or in responding to an abnormal test
      5. Inappropriate (not indicated) care
   C. Preventive
      1. Failure to provide prophylactic treatment
      2. Inadequate monitoring or follow-up of treatment
      3. Inadequate risk assessment, such as risk for falls, suicide, nutritional deficiency, and infection
   D. Other types of errors
      1. Failure of communication
      2. Equipment failure or malfunction

III. Several strategies for improvement provided by the Institute of Medicine (IOM) report, *To Err is Human: Building a Safer Health System* (IOM, 1999)
   A. National focus to increase the knowledge about safety
      1. Creation of Center for Patient Safety tasked with setting national safety goals and tracking their progress
   B. Improved identification of errors
      1. Mandated reporting system
      2. Voluntary reporting system with confidentiality to improve participation
   C. Raising performance standards and expectations
   D. Implementing safety systems
      1. Developing a "culture of safety" where safety is an explicit organizational goal

IV. IOM report, *Delivering High-Quality Cancer Care: Charting a New Course for a System in Crisis* (IOM, 2013)
   A. Conceptual framework for high-quality cancer care delivery system (Figure 48-1)
      1. Applies to all health care professions across all cancer care settings
      2. Quality improvement efforts by oncology nurses important to meet the recommended changes in the health care delivery system
   B. Six key elements of the model (IOM, 2013)
      1. Engaged patients
         a. Patients and families should receive understandable information about the cancer, prognosis, treatment, risks and benefits of treatment, palliative care, psychosocial support, and estimated costs of treatment (Ferrell, McCabe, & Levit, 2013).
      2. Adequately staffed, trained, and coordinated workforce
         a. Coordinated team-based cancer care to implement patient care plans and deliver patient-centered care
         b. All individuals caring for patients with cancer should have appropriate core competencies.
      3. Evidence-based cancer care
         a. Research should include patient-reported outcomes.
         b. Older adult patients with cancer and those with multiple comorbidities should be included in cancer clinical trials.

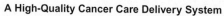

A High-Quality Cancer Care Delivery System

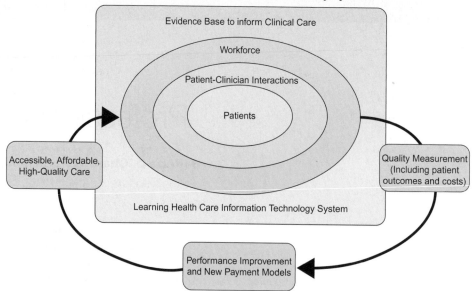

Figure 48-1 Conceptual framework: High-quality cancer care delivery system. *From Institute of Medicine (2013).* Delivering high-quality cancer care: Charting a new course for a system in crisis. *Washington, DC: National Academies Press.*

4. A learning health care information technology (IT) system for cancer care
   a. Need to develop health care IT system that meets "meaningful use" criteria and provides the following:
      (1) Real-time analysis of data from patients
      (2) Patient outcome data rapidly available to clinicians
5. Translation of evidence into clinical practice, quality measurement, and performance improvement
   a. Development of a national quality reporting program for cancer care
      (1) Reporting of quality measures
      (2) Clinicians to use patient outcome data to provide future care to patients with cancer
6. Accessible, affordable cancer care
   a. Reduction in disparities in access to cancer care for vulnerable and underserved populations
   b. Improvement in the affordability of cancer care by reforming traditional fee-for-service payment reimbursements to new payment models and eliminate waste
C. Key elements for oncology nurses (Ferrell et al., 2013)
   1. Oncology nurses play a key role in providing education and supporting patients and their families during the decision-making process with regard to treatment and costs of care.

2. Oncology nurses provide psychosocial support to patients and their families during the entire cancer trajectory, including end-of-life and timely referral to hospice for end-of-life care.
   a. Patients should receive end-of-life care that is consistent with their needs, values, and preferences.
3. Comprehensive and formal training in end-of-life communication for physicians and nurses is needed.
4. Oncology nurses play a vital role in multidisciplinary collaboration and coordination of care among cancer care team, primary care physicians, and other specialists.
5. The need for oncology nurses to obtain certification in oncology nursing is growing.
6. Patient-centered outcomes, older adults with cancer, and those with multiple comorbidities are areas that need to be included in nursing research studies.
V. Model for quality improvement
   A. Plan-Do-Study-Act (PDSA) model (Langley, Nolan, Nolan, Norman, & Provost, 2009)
      1. Developed by Associates in Process Improvement
      2. Consists of two main parts (Figure 48-2)
         a. Three fundamental questions
            (1) What is our goal?
               (a) Setting aims that are time-specific and measurable

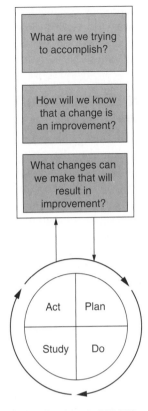

Figure 48-2 Plan-Do-Study-Act (PDSA) model for quality improvement. *From Sorensen, R., & Iedema, R., (2008).* Managing clinical processes in health services. *London: Churchill Livingstone Elsevier.*

(2) How will we know that a change is an improvement? How will we measure our outcome?
   (a) Use of quantitative tools to determine whether change has led to an improvement
(3) What changes can we make that will result in improvement?
   (a) Obtaining ideas for change from staff who work in the system, from colleagues who have successfully improved their system, or from change models or techniques
b. PDSA cycle
   (1) Planning
      (a) Identifying what needs to be improved
      (b) Planning who, what, where, when
      (c) Planning what data to collect and how to collect the data
   (2) Doing
      (a) Implementing the plan
   (3) Studying
      (a) Analyzing the data
      (b) Comparing data with baseline information or predictions

(4) Acting
   (a) Based on the results, determine what changes will be made, and carry out the changes.
   (b) Continuation of data collection to monitor sustainability of the change

MULTIDISCIPLINARY COLLABORATION

I. Related professional standards
   A. Oncology Nursing Society (ONS) *Statement on the Scope and Standards of Oncology Nursing Practice: Generalist and Advanced Practice* (Brant & Wickham, 2013). Collaboration involves the following:
      1. The oncology nurse partners with patients, families, interdisciplinary team, and community resources to provide optimal care.
         a. Rationale—the complexity of oncology care requires coordinated, ongoing interaction among patients, families, interdisciplinary cancer care team, and community; through the collaborative process, health care providers use their diverse abilities to assess, plan, implement, and evaluate oncology care.
      2. The oncology nurse collaborates with patients, families, and interdisciplinary team to formulate desired outcomes of care, the treatment plan, an evaluation of the quality of care, and other decisions related to patient care.
      3. The oncology nurse consults with other health care providers and makes appropriate referrals, including provisions for continuity of care, such as home care, hospice, rehabilitation, palliative care, and community-based support groups to enhance patient care.
      4. The oncology nurse collaborates with other health care providers in educational programs, consultation, management, and research endeavors.
II. Barriers to the development of collaborative relationships
   A. Lack of identification with one's own profession
   B. Tendency to regard professional expertise as bias
   C. Discomfort with responsibility
   D. Felt discrimination in relationships
   E. Failure of others to value one's profession
   F. Competency inconsistencies within one's profession with lack of uniform preparation
   G. Lack of clearly defined, distinct domain of influence
   H. Lack of understanding regarding scope of practice (Schadewaldt, McInnes, Hiller, & Gardner, 2013)
   I. Overlapping and changing domains of practice that produce competition
   J. Perceived threats of autonomy

K. Lack of administrative support for collaborative relationships
L. Lack of recognition for knowledge and expertise
M. Role confusion (role extension versus role expansion) within or among professions
N. Legal responsibility (Schadewaldt et al., 2013)

III. Opportunities for collaboration
A. Potential for collaboration among health care providers and agencies exists whenever and with whomever the patient and family have contact.
   1. Although emphasis is often placed on physician-nurse collaboration, nurses have the opportunity for collaborative relationships with any member of the multidisciplinary health care team.
B. Nurse-to-nurse collaboration may be influenced by the following roles:
   1. Clinician, educator, researcher, administrator—examples include the following:
      a. Clinician-researcher collaboration in the identification of a clinical problem and evaluation of applicable research findings to address the problem
      b. Educator-administrator-clinician collaboration in the development, implementation, and evaluation of staff graduate orientation
      c. Clinician-administrator-researcher collaboration in the development and testing of a patient acuity classification system
   2. Domain of responsibility, such as shift and performance standards—examples include the following:
      a. Day, evening, and night shift nurses collaborate to develop change-of-shift report guidelines.
      b. Primary nurse and associate nurse collaborate on the nursing process.
   3. Specialization such as collaboration among nurses with different specialties
   4. Subspecialization such as collaboration among nurses within a subspecialty (e.g., medical oncology, surgical oncology, radiation oncology, biotherapy) in the development of educational cancer care materials for patients and families
   5. Practice settings, including acute care, outpatient, home care, hospice, ambulatory cancer treatment center, community hospital, and rural community
      a. For example, collaboration among nurses from a variety of practice settings to develop a chronic pain protocol
      b. Collaborative relationships may extend beyond health care providers to members of advocacy agencies and organizations, including collaborating with patients in the development and implementation of patient and family support groups.

C. Future of oncology nursing depends on critical collaborative partnerships being formed within the clinical practice arenas, as well as partnerships with other organizations.

NAVIGATION THROUGHOUT THE CANCER CONTINUUM

I. History of patient navigation programs
A. In 1990, patient navigation was initiated by Harold P. Freeman at the Harlem Hospital Center in New York for patients with breast cancer (Freeman, 2004).
   1. Patient navigation program was developed to address barriers faced by cancer patients—for example, lack of health insurance, fear and distrust of the medical system, and cultural and communication barriers.
   2. Lay navigators were used to reduce health care access barriers, which resulted in increased screening rates among underserved populations, reduced treatment delay following cancer diagnosis, and an improvement in overall 5-year survival (Freeman, 2004).
B. In 2005, the Patient Navigator Outreach and Chronic Disease Prevention Act was passed.
   1. Legislation provided funding for patient navigation demonstration projects.
C. In 2012, the American College of Surgeons Commission on Cancer (ACoSCoC) developed a new standard, to be phased in 2015, requiring cancer programs to implement a patient navigation process to address health care disparities and barriers to cancer care in order to obtain or maintain accreditation (ACoSCoC, 2012).
D. In 2013, the American College of Surgeons National Accreditation Program for Breast Centers (ACoS NAPBC) included patient navigation as one of the essential components of its accredited breast centers.

II. Cancer care continuum
A. Cancer care continuum model (Figure 48-3)
   1. Prevention and risk reduction—includes tobacco control, nutrition, physical activity
   2. Screening—includes age, gender-specific screening, and genetic testing
   3. Diagnosis—biopsy and staging process
   4. Treatment
   5. Survivorship—surveillance for recurrences and secondary malignancies, management of long-term effects
   6. End-of-life care—implementation of advance care planning (e.g., completion of advance health care directive and will) and hospice care
B. Patient navigators—play an important role in assisting patients and their families or caregivers

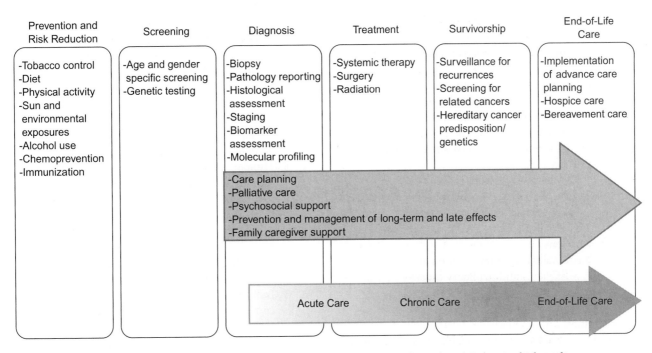

Figure 48-3 Cancer care continuum model. *From Institute of Medicine. (2013).* Delivering high-quality cancer care: Charting a new course for a system in crisis. *Washington, DC: National Academies Press.*

access to quality cancer care across the cancer care continuum (from prevention and risk reduction to end-of-life care)

III. Types of navigators

A. Oncology nurse navigator—professional registered nurse (RN) with specialty training in oncology who offers individualized assistance to patients, families, and caregivers to overcome health care system barriers

   1. Able to provide education and resources to facilitate patient decision making and access to quality health and psychosocial care throughout the cancer continuum

B. Lay navigator—trained nonprofessional or volunteer who offers individualized assistance to patients, families, and caregivers to overcome health care system barriers facilitate patient access to quality health and psychosocial care throughout the cancer continuum

IV. Core competencies of oncology nurse navigator (ONS, 2013)

A. Four competency categories

   1. Professional role—demonstrates professionalism within the workplace and community; examples include the following:

     a. Promotes lifelong learning and evidence-based practice

     b. Contributes to oncology nurse navigation program development, implementation, and evaluation within the health care system and community

     c. Participates in the tracking of metrics and patient outcomes to evaluate outcomes of the navigation program

     d. Obtains or develops oncology-related educational materials

     e. Builds partnerships with local agencies and groups that support patient care and educational needs

   2. Education—provides education to patients, families, and caregivers to facilitate informed decision making; examples include the following:

     a. Assesses educational needs of patients while considering barriers to care—for example, literacy, language, socioeconomic status, cultural influences

     b. Provides education about diagnosis, treatment options, side effect management, follow-up care, and survivorship

     c. Promotes healthy lifestyle choices and self-care strategies and makes appropriate referrals to ancillary services

     d. Promotes awareness of clinical trials

   3. Coordination of care—facilitates efficient delivery of health care services; examples include the following:

     a. Identifies potential and actual barriers to care and provides appropriate services and referrals to meet the needs of the patient

     b. Facilitates timely scheduling of appointments, diagnostic testing, procedures, and treatments

     c. Participates in coordination of the plan of care with the multidisciplinary team

d. Uses clinical guidelines
e. Ensures smooth transition from active treatment into survivorship or end-of-life care

4. Communication—demonstrates interpersonal communication skills with patients, families, and colleagues; examples include the following:
   a. Builds therapeutic and trusting relationships through effective communication and listening skills
   b. Advocates for patients
   c. Provides psychosocial support and makes appropriate referrals
   d. Ensures communication is culturally sensitive
   e. Facilitates communication among members of the multidisciplinary cancer care team

PATIENT ADVOCACY

I. Definition
   A. In the broadest terms, advocacy is support for a particular cause.
   B. Advocacy involves use of ethical principles, which include the following:
      1. Beneficence—the principle of doing good
      2. Nonmaleficence—the principle of doing no harm
      3. Utilitarianism—an ethical doctrine in which actions are focused on accomplishing the greatest good for the greatest number of people
   C. In patient care, advocacy carries a connotation of social responsibility, of helping people, especially when they are unable to speak for themselves.
   D. Being on the front lines of patient care, oncology nurses fulfill a key role in patient advocacy.
   E. Advocacy is a core value of many professional organizations such as the ONS.
      1. ONS promotes advocating for patients.
         a. Maximizing quality of life
         b. Optimizing patient access to excellent care
         c. Advocating for public policy, especially with respect to health issues
      2. ONS promotes advocating for nurses.
         a. Supporting and respecting oncology nurses
         b. Promoting access to continuing education
         c. Emphasizing a safe work environment and fair compensation

II. Types of advocacy
   A. Simplistic advocacy—one person pleading the cause of another
   B. Paternalistic advocacy—doing something for or to another without that person's consent on the premise that it serves the person's own good
   C. Consumer advocacy—ensuring that patients have adequate information to make their decisions
   D. Consumer centric advocacy—providing information and then supporting the patient in his or her decision
   E. Existential advocacy—acknowledging that various experiences in health care such as the definition of health versus illness, pain versus suffering, and the experience of dying are highly personal; ensuring that the patient's beliefs are accepted and supported
   F. Human advocacy—as a personal extension of self, disclosing one's own views on health issues and life as a means to connect more deeply with the patient

III. Risks of advocacy
   A. Nurses may lack autonomy to take moral actions.
   B. Conflicting demands of different patients may create ethical conflicts.
   C. Independent action may be restricted by conflicting accountability to public, employer, and patients.
   D. Supporting the ideas or well-being of another person may lead to personal difficulty and sacrifice.
   E. Oncology nurses often must deal with very difficult and controversial issues such as pain management, end-of-life care, and ethical decision making.

IV. Avenues to be advocates
   A. Within one's own work setting
      1. By listening and speaking out for the needs expressed by patients and their families, thereby empowering patients and their families
      2. By keeping abreast of current knowledge and sources of information on clinical trials, newly available evidence-based treatments, health legislation that affects practice and health care delivery, hospice and other resources that can benefit patients and families under their care
   B. Within one's own community
      1. By volunteering or practicing in minority, underserved, medically disadvantaged, or vulnerable populations to decrease health disparities in cancer and other areas that affect health and well-being
      2. By becoming active politically to ensure that legislation protects the health of his or her community, state, and nation
   C. Within professional organizations
      1. By becoming actively involved in organizational legislative committees advocating for nurses, cancer care, and patients
      2. By using avenues available to ONS, American Nurses Association (ANA), and other professional organizations to provide testimony or letters to state legislators, congressional representatives, or both groups to support health care and health care initiatives and reform

EDUCATIONAL AND PROFESSIONAL DEVELOPMENT

I. Synopsis
   A. As the U.S. health care system evolves, the role of nurses must simultaneously evolve.
   B. The way nurses are trained is changing to keep pace with changing patient needs and expectations, technologic advances, and increasing specialization.
   C. Key recommendations of the IOM report, *The Future of Nursing: Leading Change, Advancing Health* (IOM, 2011), are as follows:
      1. Nurses practice to the full potential of their education and training.
      2. Nurses achieve higher levels of education and training through improved education systems.
      3. Nurses engage as full partners with physicians and health care professionals in redesigning health care.
      4. Nurses develop effective workforce planning and policy making through better data collection and information infrastructure.
   D. Barriers to practice
      1. Variability in educational pathways leading to entry-level RN licensure
      2. Variability in licensure requirements of advanced practice RNs (APRNs) among states
      3. Variability in advanced certification requirements across specialties

II. Educational development
   A. Need for the proportion of nurses with a bachelor of science degree in nursing (BSN) to increase to 80% by 2020 (IOM, 2011)
      1. Strategies include the following:
         a. RN to BSN or master of science in nursing (MSN) degree programs—some nursing schools offer these programs to provide an efficient bridge for nurses with an associate degree (AD) to obtain their BSN or MSN degree.
         b. BSN at community colleges—some community colleges offer AD students a streamlined, automatic transition to universities to obtain BSN degrees.
   B. Participation in organizational, local, and national educational and professional seminars, webinars, workshops, and conferences to expand knowledge base in oncology and to obtain continuing education credits for relicensure
   C. Graduate education
      1. Formalized university or college education to increase depth of professional knowledge and skills
      2. Formalized university or college education to redirect career path or fulfill career development plan

III. Professional development
   A. Obtaining certification in oncology nursing
      1. Certification—assures public that the certified nurse has the knowledge and qualifications needed to practice in his or her clinical area of nursing (Summers, 2013)
      2. Provided by the Oncology Nursing Certification Corporation (ONCC)
      3. Six certifications available in oncology nursing (ONCC, 2013a)—Oncology Certified Nurse (OCN, Advanced Oncology Certified Nurse Practitioner (AOCNP), Advanced Oncology Certified Clinical Nurse Specialist (AOCNS), Certified Pediatric Hematology Oncology Nurse (CPHON), Certified Breast Care Nurse (CBCN), and the Blood and Marrow Transplant Certified Nurse (BMTCN)
      4. Initial certifications in Certified Pediatric Oncology Nurse (CPON) and Advanced Oncology Certified Nurse (AOCN) no longer available, but renewals are available for nurses who currently hold these credentials
      5. Requirements for OCN, CPON, CPHON, CBCN, and BMTCN certifications (ONCC, 2013b)
         a. Current, active, unrestricted RN license at the time of application and examination
         b. Minimum of 1 year of experience as an RN within the 3 years prior to application
         c. Minimum of 1000 hours of practice in the area of certification applying for within the 2½ years (30 months) prior to application
         d. Completion of a minimum of 10 contact hours in the area of certification applying for within the 3 years (36 months) prior to application
      6. Requirements for AOCNS and AOCNP certifications (ONCC, 2013b)
         a. Current, active, unrestricted RN license at the time of application and examination
         b. Graduate degree from an accredited APRN program
         c. Practice hours
            (1) If graduated from an accredited NP or CNS program with concentration in adult oncology, 500 hours supervised clinical practice as adult CNS or NP obtained within the graduate program, following the graduate program, or both
            (2) If graduated from an accredited NP or CNS program with non-oncology concentration, 1000 hours supervised clinical practice as adult CNS or NP obtained within and/or following the graduate program
         a. One graduate level oncology course of at least 2 credits or 30 hours oncology continuing education units

B. Membership and participation in local, state, national, and international professional organizations such as the Oncology Nursing Society (ONS), American Nurses Association (ANA), American Society of Clinical Oncology (ASCO), and American Society of Hematology (ASH)

Internet Resources

Agency for Healthcare Research and Policy (AHRQ)
www.ahrq.gov
American Academy of Nursing
www.aannet.org
American College of Surgeons Commission on Cancer
www.facs.org/cancer
American Nurses Credentialing Center (ANCC)
www.nursecredentialing.org
American Organization of Nurse Executives
www.aone.org
American Society of Clinical Oncology
www.asco.org
National Council of State Board of Nurses
www.ncsbn.org
National Institutes of Health
www.nih.gov
Oncology Nursing Certification Corporation
www.oncc.org
Oncology Nursing Society
www.ons.org

References

American College of Surgeons Commission on Cancer. (2012). *Cancer program standards 2012: Ensuring patient-centered care.* Chicago: Author.

American College of Surgeons National Accreditation Program for Breast Centers. (2013). *2013 breast center standards manual.* Chicago: Author.

Andel, C., Davidow, S. L., Hollander, M., & Moreno, D. A. (2012). The economics of health care quality and medical errors. *Journal of Health Care Finance, 39*(1), 38–50.

Brant, J. M., & Wickham, R. (Eds.), (2013). *Statement on the scope and standards of oncology nursing practice: Generalist and advanced practice.* Pittsburgh: Oncology Nursing Society.

Ferrell, B., McCabe, M. S., & Levit, L. (2013). The Institute of Medicine report on high-quality cancer care: Implications for oncology nursing. *Oncology Nursing Forum, 40*(6), 603–609.

Freeman, H. P. (2004). A model patient navigation program. *Oncology Issues,* 44–46.

Institute of Medicine. (1999). *To err is human: Building a safer health system.* Washington, DC: National Academies Press.

Institute of Medicine. (2011). *The future of nursing: Leading change, advancing health.* Washington, DC: National Academies Press.

Institute of Medicine. (2013). *Delivering high-quality cancer care: Charting a new course for a system in crisis.* Washington, DC: National Academies Press.

Langley, G. L., Nolan, K. M., Nolan, T. W., Norman, C. L., & Provost, L. P. (2009). *The improvement guide: A practical approach to enhancing organizational performance.* San Francisco: Jossey-Bass.

Oncology Nursing Certification Corporation. (2013a). *General information.* www.oncc.org/TakeTest.

Oncology Nursing Certification Corporation. (2013b). *Eligibility.* www.oncc.org/Eligibility.

Oncology Nursing Society. (2013). *Oncology nurse navigator core competencies.* Pittsburgh: Oncology Nursing Society.

Schadewaldt, V., McInnes, E., Hiller, J. E., & Gardner, A. (2013). Views and experiences of nurse practitioners and medical practitioners with collaborative practice in primary health care—an integrative review. *BMC Family Practice, 14*(1), 132.

Summers, B. L. (2013). Scope of practice. In J. M. Brant & R. Wickham (Eds.), *Statement on the scope and standards of oncology nursing practice: Generalist and advanced practice.* Pittsburgh: Oncology Nursing Society.

Index

Note: Page numbers followed by *b* indicate boxes, *f* indicate figures and *t* indicate tables.